Tumor Board
Case Management

Tumor Board
Case Management

Editors

David P. Winchester, M.D., F.A.C.S.
Professor and Chairman
Department of Surgery
Evanston Hospital
Evanston, Illinois

Murray F. Brennan, M.D., F.A.C.S.
Chairman, Department of Surgery
Memorial Sloan-Kettering Cancer Center
New York, New York

Gerald D. Dodd, Jr., M.D.
Emeritus Professor and Head
Department of Diagnostic Imaging
University of Texas M.D. Anderson Cancer Center
Singleton Professor of Radiology
St. Luke's Episcopal Hospital
Houston, Texas

Donald E. Henson, M.D.
Early Detection Branch
Division of Cancer Prevention and Control
National Cancer Institute
Bethesda, Maryland

B. J. Kennedy, M.D.
Emeritus Regent's Professor of Medicine
Department of Medicine
University of Minnesota School of Medicine
Minneapolis, Minnesota

Glenn D. Steele, Jr., M.D., F.A.C.S.
President of Medical Affairs
Dean and Richard T. Crane Professor
Biological Sciences Division
University of Chicago
Chicago, Illinois

J. Frank Wilson, M.D., F.A.C.R.
Professor and Chairman
Department of Radiation Oncology
Director, Cancer Center
Medical College of Wisconsin
Milwaukee, Wisconsin

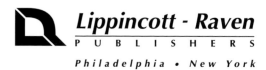

Lippincott - Raven
P U B L I S H E R S
Philadelphia • New York

Acquisitions Editor: J. Stuart Freeman, Jr.
Developmental Editor: Eileen Wolfberg Jackson
Manufacturing Manager: Dennis Teston
Production Manager: Lawrence Bernstein
Production Editor: Lawrence Bernstein
Cover Designer: Emily Adler
Indexer: Jayne Percy
Compositor: Lippincott-Raven Electronic Production
Printer: Quebecor-Kingsport

Library of Congress Cataloging-in-Publication Data

Tumor board case management / editors, David Winchester . . . [et al.].
      p. cm.
   Includes bibliographical references and index.
   ISBN 0-397-51340-2
   1. Cancer—Case studies.   I. Winchester, David, 1937–
   [DNLM: 1. Neoplasms—case studies.   QZ 200 T9305 1996]
RC262.T79   1996
616.99′209—dc20
DNLM/DLC
For Library of Congress   96-23252
                                                       CIP

Contents

Head and Neck

Esophagus

Stomach

Pancreas

Rectum

Anal Canal

Lung

Mediastinum

Bone (Adult)

Soft Tissue Sarcoma (Adult)

Melanoma

Cervix

Uterus

Ovary

Prostate

Testis

Bladder

Kidney

Spinal Cord

Brain

Complex Cancer Management

Adrenal Gland

Contributors

Herand Abcarian, M.D.
Turi Josefsen Professor and Head
Department of Surgery
University of Illinois College of Medicine
840 South Wood Street, M/C 958
Chicago, Illinois 60612

Martin D. Abeloff, M.D.
Department of Medical Oncology
Johns Hopkins University Hospital
600 North Wolfe Street
Baltimore, Maryland 21205

Andre A. Abitbol, M.D.
Associate Director
Regional Cancer Treatment Center
Baptist Hospital of Miami
8900 North Kendall Drive
Miami, Florida 33176

Yousif A. Abubakr, M.D.
Assistant Professor of Medicine
Department of Internal Medicine
Wayne State University
401 Brush South
3990 John R 4-Brush South
Detroit, Michigan 48201

Pasha Agarwal, M.D.
Associate Pathologist
St. Joseph Hospital
215 North 12th Street
Reading, Pennsylvania 19603

Muhyi Al-Sarraf, M.D. , F.R.C.P.S., F.A.C.P.
Medical Director
Providence Cancer Center
Clinical Professor
Division of Hematology and Oncology
Department of Medicine
Wayne State University School of Medicine
Detroit, Michigan 48201

Willie A. Andersen, M.D., F.A.C.S.
Associate Professor
Division of Gynecologic Oncology
University of Virginia Health Sciences Center
Charlottesville, Virginia 22908

Deborah K. Armstrong, M.D.
Assistant Professor
Department of Medical Oncology
Johns Hopkins Medical Institute
600 North Wolfe Street, Room 2-127
Baltimore, Maryland 21287

Illias Athanasiadis, M.D.
Department of Medicine
Northwestern University Medical School
Veterans Affairs Lakeside Medical Center
Chicago, Illinois 60611

Hervy E. Averette, M.D., F.A.C.S.
Division of Gynecologic Oncology
Department of Obstetrics and Gynecology
University of Miami/Jackson Memorial Medical
  Center
1475 NW 12th Avenue (D-52)
Miami, Florida 33136

Charles M. Balch, M.D.
Executive Vice President
University of Texas M. D. Anderson Cancer
  Center
1515 Holcombe Boulevard
Houston, Texas 77030

Robert M. Barone, M.D., F.A.C.S.
Director, Surgical Oncology Services
Sharp Healthcare
8008 Frost Street, Suite 300
San Diego, California 92123

John G. Batsakis, M.D.
Professor and Chairman
Department of Pathology
University of Texas M. D. Anderson Cancer
   Center
1515 Holcombe Boulevard
Houston, Texas 77030

Oliver H. Beahrs, M.D.
Professor of Surgery, Emeritus
Department of Surgery
Mayo Medical School
200 First Street Southwest
Rochester, Minnesota 55905

Robert W. Beart, Jr., M.D.
Department of Surgery
University of Southern California
Kenneth Norris Jr. Cancer Hospital
1441 Eastlake Avenue
Los Angeles, California 90033

Edwin Beckman, M.D.
Pathology Department
Ochsner Clinic
1514 Jefferson Highway
New Orleans, Louisiana 70121

John R. Benfield, M.D.
Professor and Chief
Department of Surgery
Division of Cardiothoracic Surgery
University of California, Davis
4301 X Street, Suite 2250
Sacramento, California 95817

Al B. Benson III, M.D.
Director of Clinical Investigations
   Program
Department of Medicine
Robert H. Lurie Cancer Center
Associate Professor
Division of Hematology and Oncology
Northwestern University
233 East Erie Street
Chicago, Illinois 60611

Jordan D. Berlin, M.D.
Assistant Professor
Oncology Section
Department of Medicine
University of Wisconsin
600 Highland Avenue
Madison, Wisconsin 53792

Kirby I. Bland, M.D.
J. Murray Beardsley Professor and Chairman
Department of Surgery
Brown University School of Medicine
Executive Surgeon-in-Chief
Memorial Hospital of Rhode Island
The Miriam Hospital
Roger Williams Medical Center
VA Medical Center
Surgeon-in-Chief
Rhode Island Hospital
593 Eddy Street
Providence, Rhode Island 02903

George E. Block, M.D., F.A.C.S.
(Deceased)
Department of Surgery
University of Chicago Medical Center
5841 South Maryland
Chicago, Illinois 60637

Michael D. Blum, M.D., F.A.C.S.
Clinical Associate
Department of Urology
Northwestern University Medical School
250 East Superior Street
Chicago, Illinois 60611

Leslie H. Blumgart, M.D.
Chief of Hepatobiliary Service
Department of Surgery
Memorial Sloan-Kettering Cancer Center
1275 York Avenue
New York, New York 10021

John S. Bolton, M.D.
Clinical Assistant Professor of Surgery
Department of Surgery
Alton Oschner Medical Foundation
Louisiana State University Medical School
1516 Jefferson Highway
New Orleans, Louisiana 70121

John W. Braasch, M.D. Ph.D.
Assistant Clinical Professor
Department of General Surgery
Harvard Medical School
Lahey Hitchcock Clinic
41 Mall Road
Burlington, Massachusetts 01805

David G. Bragg, M.D.
Professor and Chairman
Department of Radiology
University of Utah Health Sciences Center
50 North Medical Drive
Salt Lake City, Utah 84132

Richard F. Branda, M.D.
Professor of Medicine and Pharmacology
Department of Medicine
University of Vermont
Genetics Laboratory
32 North Prospect Street
Burlington, Vermont 05401

Murray F. Brennan, M.D., F.A.C.S.
Professor and Chairman
Department of Surgery
Memorial Sloan-Kettering Cancer Center
1275 York Avenue
New York, New York 10021

J. Ralph Broadwater, M.D.
Associate Professor
Vice-Chairman for Clinical Affairs
Department of Surgery
University of Arkansas for Medical Sciences
4301 West Markham, Slot 725
Little Rock, Arkansas 72205

William E. Burak, Jr., M.D.
Assistant Professor
Division of Surgical Oncology
Department of Surgery
Arthur G. James Cancer Hospital and Research
  Institute
The Ohio State University
410 West 10th Avenue
Columbus, Ohio 43210

Dennis K. Burns, M.D.
Associate Professor of Pathology
Department of Pathology
University of Texas Southwestern Medical
  Center
5323 Harry Hines Boulevard
Dallas, Texas 75235

Linda J. Burns, M.D.
Assistant Professor of Medicine
Department of Medicine
Division of Medical Oncology
University of Minnesota Hospital and Clinic
Harvard Street at East River Road
Minneapolis, Minnesota 55455

Michael Burt, M.D., Ph.D.
Attending Surgeon
Department of Surgery, Thoracic Service
Memorial Sloan-Kettering Cancer Center
1275 York Avenue
New York, New York 10021

Robert M. Byers, M.D.
Professor
Department of Head and Neck Surgery
University of Texas M. D. Anderson Cancer
  Center
1515 Holcombe Boulevard
Houston, Texas 77030

Roger W. Byhardt, M.D.
Professor
Department of Radiation Oncology
Medical College of Wisconsin
8700 West Wisconsin Avenue
Milwaukee, Wisconsin 53226

Blake Cady, M.D.
Professor
Department of Surgery
Harvard Medical School
New England Deaconess Hospital
110 Francis Street, Suite 2H
Boston, Massachusetts 02215

Richard G. Caldwell, A.B.. M.D., M.S.
Clinical Associate Professor
Department of Surgery
University of Chicago
Lutheran General Hospital
1775 Dempster Street
Park Ridge, Illinois 60068

John L. Cameron, M.D.
Professor and Chairman
Department of Surgery
Johns Hopkins University Hospital
Richard Ross Research Building
720 Rutland Avenue, Room 759
Baltimore, Maryland 21205

George Canellos, M.D.
Medical Oncologist
Dana-Farber Cancer Institute
44 Binney Street
Boston, Massachusetts 02115

Joseph A. Caprini, M.D.
Professor of Clinical Surgery
Department of Surgery
Glenbrook Hospital
Northwestern University
2100 Pfingsten Road
Glenview, Illinois 60025

Paul P. Carbone, M.D.
Department of Medical Oncology
University of Wisconsin Hospital
600 Highland Avenue
Madison, Wisconsin 53792

Robert W. Carey, M.D.
Associate Clinical Professor of Medicine
Department of Medicine
Massachusetts General Hospital
100 Blossom Street
Boston, Massachusetts 02114

C. H. Carrasco, M.D.
Department of Diagnostic Imaging
University of Texas M. D. Anderson Cancer
  Center
1515 Holcombe Boulevard
Houston, Texas 77030

John M. Cassel, M.D., F.A.C.S.
Clinical Associate of Plastic Surgery
University of Miami School of Medicine
8950 North Kendall Drive, #106
Miami, Florida 33176

William J. Catalona, M.D.
Division of Urologic Surgery
Washington University School of
  Medicine
4960 Children s Place
Saint Louis, Missouri 63110

Gunnar J. Cederbom, M.D.
Head, Breast Imaging Section
Department of Radiology
Ochsner Clinic and Ochsner Foundation
  Hospital
1514 Jefferson Highway
New Orleans, Louisiana 70121

Lawrence M. Cher, M.D.
Department of Neurology
Neuro-Oncology Service
Massachusetts General Hospital
Harvard Medical School
Boston, Massachusetts 02114

Gene Chiao, M.D.
Department of Medicine
Evanston Hospital
2650 Ridge Avenue
Evanston, Illinois 60201

Vincent P. Chuang, M.D.
Professor of Radiology
Department of Diagnostic Radiology
University of Texas M. D. Anderson Cancer
  Center
1515 Holcombe Boulevard, Box 57
Houston, Texas 77030

Ivan Ciric, M.D.
Bennett-Tarkington Professor of
  Neurosurgery
Northwestern University Medical School
Chief, Division of Neurosurgery
Evanston Hospital
2650 Ridge Avenue
Evanston, Illinois 60201

Orlo H. Clark, M.D., F.A.C.S.
Department of Surgery
University of San Francisco
Mt. Zion Medical Center
P.O. Box 7921
San Francisco, California 94120

Alfred M. Cohen, M.D.
Professor
Department of Surgery
Cornell University Medical College
Chief, Colorectal Service
Memorial Sloan-Kettering Cancer Center
1275 York Avenue
New York, New York 10021

Lawrence R. Coia, M.D.
Senior Member and Vice-Chairman
Department of Radiation Oncology
Fox Chase Cancer Center
7701 Burholme Avenue
Philadelphia, Pennsylvania 19111

Daniel G. Coit, M.D.
Professor
Department of Surgery
Memorial Sloan-Kettering Cancer Center
1275 York Avenue
New York, New York 10021

Jay S. Cooper, M.D.
Professor and Director
Division of Radiation Oncology
New York University-Tisch Hospital
560 First Avenue
New York, New York 10016

Edward M. Copeland III, M.D.
The Edward R. Woodward Professor and
  Chairman
Department of Surgery
University of Florida College of Medicine
P.O. Box 100286
Gainesville, Florida 32610

A. Benedict Cosimi, M.D.
Claude E. Welch Professor of Surgery
Department of Surgery
Harvard Medical School
Massachusetts General Hospital
32 Fruit Street
Boston, Massachusetts 02114

James D. Cox, M.D., F.A.C.R.
Professor and Chairman
Department of Radiation Oncology
University of Texas M. D. Anderson Cancer
  Center
1515 Holcombe Boulevard
Houston, Texas 77030

William T. Creasman, M.D.
Sims-Hester Professor and Chair
Department of Obstetrics and Gynecology
Medical University of South Carolina
171 Ashley Avenue
Charleston, South Carolina 29425

Mary K. Cullen, M.D.
Clinical Instructor of Dermatology
Barnes Jewish Hospital
Research Associate
Department of Cell Biology and Physiology
Washington University School of Medicine
660 South Euclid Avenue
St. Louis, Missouri 63110

Francis J. Cummings, M.D.
Associate Professor of Medicine
Roger Williams Medical Center
Brown University
825 Chalkstone Avenue
Providence, Rhode Island 02908

John P. Curtin, M.D.
Assistant Professor of Obstetrics and Gynecology
Cornell University Medical Center
Associate Attending Surgeon
Gynecology Service, Department of Surgery
Memorial Sloan-Kettering Cancer Center
1275 York Avenue
New York, New York 10021

John M. Daly, M.D., F.A.C.S.
Chairman
Department of Surgery
Cornell Medical Center
Surgeon-in-Chief
New York Hospital
525 East 68th Street
New York, New York 10021

Michael A. Warso, M.D.
Department of Surgical Oncology
University of Illinois at Chicago
840 South Wood Street (M/C 820)
Chicago, Illinois 60612

Lawrence W. Davis, M.D.
Professor
Department of Radiation Oncology
Emory University
1365 Clifton Road
Atlanta, Georgia 30322

Michele D. Davis, M.D.
The Genesee Hospital
224 Alexander Street
Rochester, New York 14607

Ronald C. DeConti, M.D.
Professor of Medicine
Division of Medical Oncology
H. Lee Moffitt Cancer Center and Research
  Institute
University of South Florida
12902 Magnolia Drive
Tampa, Florida 33612

Jerome J. DeCosse, M.D., Ph.D.
Professor
Department of Surgery
New York Hospital-Cornell Medical
  Center
525 East 68th Street
New York, New York 10021

Michael J. Demeure, M.D., F.A.C.S.
Assistant Professor
Departments of Surgery and Cellular
  Biology/Anatomy
Medical College of Wisconsin
9200 West Wisconsin Avenue
Milwaukee, Wisconsin 53226

Louis F. Diehl, M.D.
Associate Professor of Clinical Medicine
Uniformed Services University of the Health
  Sciences
Chief, Hematology-Oncology Service
Walter Reed Army Medical Center
Washington, DC 20307

Philip J. DiSaia, M.D.
The Dorothy Marsh Chair in Reproductive
  Biology
Professor
Department of Obstetrics and Gynecology
University of California
Irvine Medical Center
101 The City Drive
Orange, California 92668

Gerald D. Dodd, Jr., M.D.
Emeritus Professor
Department of Diagnostic Radiology
University of Texas M. D. Anderson Cancer
  Center
1515 Holcombe Boulevard
Houston, Texas 77030
Singleton Professor of Radiology 2-256
St. Luke's Episcopal Hospital
6720 Bertner Street
Houston, Texas 77225

Dechen Dolkar
Medical Student
University of Southern California
Los Angeles, California

William L. Donegan, M.D.
Professor of Surgery
Medical College of Wisconsin
Sinai Samaritan Medical Center
945 North 12th
Milwaukee, Wisconsin 53233

John H. Donohue, M.D.
Consultant
Division of Gastroenterologic and General
  Surgery
Mayo Clinic and Mayo Foundation
Asssociate Professor of Surgery
Mayo Medical School
Department of Surgery
Mayo Clinic/Rochester Methodist
  Hospital
200 First Street Southwest
Rochester, Minnesota 55905

Douglas Dorsay, M.D.
Department of Surgery
University of South Carolina School of Medicine
2 Richland Medical Park, Suite 402
Columbia, South Carolina 29203

Harold O. Douglass, Jr., M.D.
Professor of Surgery
State University of New York at Buffalo
Associate Chief, Surgical Oncology
Chief, Upper Gastrointestinal Oncology
Department of Surgical Oncology
Roswell Park Cancer Institute
Elm and Carlton Streets
Buffalo, New York 14263

Robert Dreicer, M.D., FACP
Associate Professor of Medicine and Urology
Department of Internal Medicine
University of Iowa
200 Hawkins Drive
Iowa City, Iowa 52242

Francis G. Duhaylongsod, M.D.
Assistant Professor of Surgery
Duke University Medical Center
Durham, North Carolina 27710

John R. Durant, M.D.
Executive Vice President
American Society of Clinical Oncology
225 Reinekers Lane, Suite 650
Alexandria, Virginia 22314

James T. Eastman III, M.D.
Chairman
Department of Pathology
Lancaster General Hospital
555 North Duke Street
Lancaster, Pennsylvania 17604

Michael J. Edwards, M.D.
Associate Professor
Division of Surgical Oncology
Department of Surgery
University of Louisville
529 South Jackson Street, Room 318
Louisville, Kentucky 40202

G. Philip Engeler, M.D.
Department of Radiation Oncology
Firelands Community Hospital
1101 Decatur Street, C.N. 5005
Sandusky, Ohio 44870

Charles A. Enke, M.D.
Bishop Clarkson Hospital
44th and Dewey Avenue
Omaha, Nebraska 68105

Warren E. Enker, M.D.
Professor and Vice Chairman
Department of Surgery
Beth Israel Medical Center
Chief, Colorectal Surgery
Albert Einstein College of Medicine
350 East 17th Street, Baird Hall 1622
New York, New York 10003

Beth Erickson, M.D.
Associate Professor
Department of Radiation Oncology
Medical College of Wisconsin
Froedtert Memorial Lutheran Hospital
9200 West Wisconsin Avenue
Milwaukee, Wisconsin 53226

Carmelita P. Escalante, M.D.
Assistant Professor of Medicine
Department of Medical Specialties
University of Texas M. D. Anderson Cancer
* Center*
1515 Holcombe Boulevard, Box 40
Houston, Texas 77030

Ramon M. Esclamado, M.D.
Associate Professor and Director
Division of Head and Neck Surgery
Department of Otolaryngology - Head and Neck
* Surgery*
University of Michigan
1904 Taubman Center, Box 0312
Ann Arbor, Michigan 48109

Richard Essner, M.D.
Assistant Medical Director, Surgical
* Oncology*
John Wayne Cancer Institute
2200 Santa Monica Boulevard
Santa Monica, California 90404

James F. Evans, M.D., F.A.C.S
Director, Section of Surgical Oncology
Department of General Surgery
Geisinger Clinic
Clinical Assistant Professor
Jefferson Medical College
100 North Academy Avenue
Danville, Pennsylvania 17822

Robert C. Eyre, M.D.
Assistant Clinical Professor of Surgery
* (Urology)*
Harvard Medical School
Chief, Division of Urology
New England Deaconess Hospital
110 Francis Street, Suite 6E
Boston, Massachusetts 02215

Robert C. Eyerly, M.D., F.A.C.S.
Surgeon (retired)
Geisinger Medical Center
100 North Academy Boulevard
Danville, Pennsylvania 17822

L. Penfield Faber, M.D.
Professor of Surgery
Department of Cardiovascular—Thoracic
* Surgery*
Rush Medical College
1653 West Congress
Chicago, Illinois 60612

William R. Fair, M.D.
Chief, Urologic Surgery
Memorial Sloan-Kettering Cancer Center
1275 York Avenue
New York, New York 10021

Gist Farr, M.D.
Pathologist
Alton Oschner Medical Institute
1514 Jefferson Highway
New Orleans, Louisiana 70121

William B. Farrar, M.D., F.A.C.S.
Associate Professor
Department of Surgery
Arthur G. James Cancer Hospital and Research
* Institute*
The Ohio State University
410 West 10th Avenue
Columbus, Ohio 43210

Victor W. Fazio, M.D.
Rupert B. Turnbull, Jr., Chairman
Department of Colon and Rectal Surgery
The Cleveland Clinic Foundation
Professor of Surgery
Cleveland Clinic Health Sciences Center
Ohio State University School of Medicine
9500 Euclid Avenue
Cleveland, Ohio 44195

Willard E. Fee, Jr, M.D.
Edward C. and Amy H. Sewell Professor
Chairman
Division of Otolaryngology
Department of Surgery
Stanford University Medical Center
300 Pasteur Drive, Room R-135
Stanford, California 94305

L. Peter Fielding, M.D.
Chief, Department of Surgery
Genesee Hospital
222 Alexander Street, Suite 1105
Rochester, New York 14607

David J. Fillmore, M.D.
Assistant Professor
Department of Radiology
University of Utah Health Sciences Center
50 North Medical Drive
Salt Lake City, Utah 84132

Robert C. Flanigan, M.D.
Professor and Chairman
Department of Urology
Loyola University Medical Center
Chief, Department of Urology
Hines Veterans Administration Hospital
2160 South First Avenue
Maywood, Illinois 60153

John F. Foley, M.D., Ph.D.
Professor of Medicine
Department of Internal Medicine
Section of Oncology/Hematology
University of Nebraska Medical Center
600 South 42 Street, Box 983330
Omaha, Nebraska 68198

Yuman Fong, M.D.
Surgeon
Department of Surgery
Memorial Sloan-Kettering Cancer Center
1275 York Avenue
New York, New York 10021

Arlene A. Forastiere, M.D.
Associate Professor of Oncology
Department of Medical Oncology
Johns Hopkins Medical Institute
600 North Wolfe Street, Room 128
Baltimore, Maryland 21287

James H. Foster, M.D.
Emeritus Professor
Department of Surgery
University of Connecticut School of Medicine
435 Waterville Road
Avon, Connecticut 06001

Barbara Fowble, M.D.
Senior Member
Department of Radiation Oncology
Fox Chase Cancer Center
7701 Burhelm Avenue
Philadelphia, Pennsylvania 19104

Willard A. Fry, M.D., F.A.C.S.
Professor of Clinical Surgery
Northwestern University Medical School
Chief, Section of Thoracic Surgery
Evanston Hospital
2650 Ridge Avenue
Evanston, Illinois 60201

Karen K. Fu, M.D.
Professor
Department of Radiation Oncology
University of California, San Francisco
School of Medicine
505 Parnassus Avenue, L-08
San Francisco, California 94143

Adam S. Garden, M.D.
Assistant Professor of Radiotherapy
Department of Radiotherapy
University of Texas, M. D. Anderson Cancer
*   Center*
1515 Holcombe Boulevard, Box 97
Houston, Texas 77030

David H. Garfield, M.D.
Associate Clinical Professor
Department of Medicine
University of Colorado Health Sciences
*   Center*
4200 East 9th Avenue
Denver, Colorado 80262

John E. Garnett, M.D.
Assistant Clinical Professor
Department of Urology
Northwestern University
251 East Chicago Avenue, Suite 1430
Chicago, Illinois 60611

Marc B. Garnick, M.D.
Associate Professor
Harvard Medical School
Department of Medicine
Beth Israel Hospital
330 Brookline Avenue
Boston, Massachusetts 02215

Thomas A. Gaskin, M.D., F.A.C.S.
Department of Surgery
Princeton Baptist Health System
701 Princeton Avenue SW
Birmingham, Alabama 35211

Robert J. Ginsberg, M.D.
Chief, Thoracic Service
Memorial Sloan-Kettering Cancer Center
Professor
Department of Cardiothoracic Surgery
Cornell University Medical College
1275 York Avenue
New York, New York 10021

Eli Glatstein, M.D.
Professor, Vice Chairman and
*   Clinical Director*
Department of Radiation Oncology
University of Pennsylvania
3400 Spruce Street
2 Donner Building
Philadelphia, Pennsylvania 19104-4283

James F. Glenn, M.D.
Lucille P. Markey Cancer Center
University of Kentucky Medical Center
800 Rose Street
Lexington, Kentucky 40536

Helmuth Goepfert, M.D.
Professor of Surgery
Department of Head and Neck Surgery
University of Texas M. D. Anderson Cancer
*   Center*
1515 Holcombe Boulevard, Box 69
Houston, Texas 77030

Don R. Goffinet, M.D.
Professor
Department of Radiation Oncology
Stanford University Hospital
300 Pasteur Drive
Stanford, California 94305

David A. Goldfarb, M.D.
Staff Urologist
Department of Urology
Cleveland Clinic Foundation
9500 Euclid Avenue (A110)
Cleveland, Ohio 44195

Elizabeth M. Gore, M.D.
Assistant Professor
Department of Radiation Oncology
Medical College of Wisconsin
9200 West Wisconsin Avenue
Milwaukee, Wisconsin 53226

David B. Gough, M.B., M.Ch., Ph.D.,
*   **F.R.C.S.(I)***
Senior Lecturer in Surgery
University of Aberdeen Medical School
Foresterhill
Aberdeen AB9 2ZD
United Kingdom

Frederick L. Greene, M.D.
Professor
Department of Surgery
University of South Carolina School of
*   Medicine*
2 Medical Park, Suite 402
Columbia, South Carolina 29203

Perry W. Grigsby, M.D., M.B.A., F.A.C.R.
Professor of Radiology
Radiation Oncology Center
Washington University School of Medicine
4939 Childrens Place, Suite 5500
St. Louis, Missouri 63110

Leonard L. Gunderson, M.D., M.S.
Professor of Oncology
Chair of Radiation Oncology
Mayo Clinic and Mayo Medical School
Charlton Building, Desk R
Rochester, Minnesota 55905

George B. Haasler, M.D.
Associate Professor
Department of Cardiothoracic Surgery
Medical College of Wisconsin
9200 West Wisconsin Avenue
Milwaukee, Wisconsin 53226

Bruce G. Haffty, M.D.
Associate Professor
Department of Therapeutic Radiology
Yale University School of Medicine
333 Cedar Street, Box 208040
New Haven, Connecticut 06520

Daniel J. Haraf, M.D.
Assistant Professor
Department of Radiation Oncology
The University of Chicago
5841 South Maryland, MC 0085
Chicago, Illinois 60637

Jay R. Harris, M.D.
Professor of Radiation Oncology
Joint Center for Radiation Therapy
Harvard Medical School
330 Brookline Avenue
Boston, Massachusetts 02215

Jules E. Harris, M.D.
Professor
Department of Medicine
Rush-Presbyterian-St. Luke's Medical Center
1725 West Harrison Street
Chicago, Illinois 60612

John H. Healey. M.D.
Associate Professor of Surgery
Cornell University
Chief, Orthopedic Surgery
Memorial Sloan-Kettering Cancer Center
1275 York Avenue
New York, New York 10021

I. Craig Henderson, M.D.
Adjunct Professor
Department of Medicine
University of California, San Francisco
505 Parnassus Avenue, Box 1270
San Francisco, California 94143

Donald Earl Henson, M.D.
Early Detection Branch
Executive Plaza North, Room 305
6130 Executive Boulevard
Rockville, Maryland 20852

Fred H. Hochberg, M.D.
Department of Neurology
Neuro-Oncology Service
Massachusetts General Hospital
Harvard Medical School
Boston, Massachusetts 02114

Jerome Hoeksema, M.D.
Assistant Professor
Department of Urology
Rush Presbyterian<\#150>St. Luke's Medical
  Center
1653 West Congress Parkway
Chicago, Illinois 60612

John P. Hoffman, M.D., F.A.C.S.
Professor of Surgery
Department of Surgical Oncology
Temple University School of Medicine
Fox Chase Cancer Center
7701 Burholme Avenue
Philadelphia, Pennsylvania 19111

David C. Hohn, M.D.
Surgeon
University of Texas M. D. Anderson Cancer
  Center
1515 Holcombe Boulevard
Houston, Texas 77030

James M. Holland, M.D.
1000 Central Street
Evanston, Illinois 60201

E. Carmack Holmes, M.D.
Professor
Department of Surgery
UCLA Medical Center
10833 Le Conte Boulevard
Los Angeles, California 90024

Herbert C. Hoover, Jr., M.D.
Pennsylvania State University College of
  Medicine
Hershey, Pennsylvania
Chairman
Department of Surgery
Lehigh Valley Hospital
Cedar Crest and I-78, Box 689
Allentown, Pennsylvania 18105

John Horton, M.B.Ch.B., F.A.C.P.
Professor of Medicine
Associate Dean, Education
Department of Medical Oncology/Hematology
H. Lee Moffitt Cancer Center and Research
  Institute
12902 Magnolia Drive, Suite 3157
Tampa, Florida 33612

William J. Hoskins, M.D.
Professor of Obstetrics and Gynecology
Cornell University Medical College
Deputy Physician in Chief, Disease
  Management Teams
Chief, Gynecology Service
Department of Surgery
Avon Chair in Gynecologic Oncology
  Research
Memorial Sloan-Kettering Cancer Center
1275 York Avenue
New York, New York 10021

Roger D. Hurst, M.D., F.R.C.S.(Ed),
  F.A.C.S.
Assistant Professor
Department of Surgery
University of Chicago Medical Center
5841 South Maryland
Chicago, Illinois 60637

Frank Hussey, M.D.
Radiation Oncologist
Lutheran General Hospital
1775 West Dempster
Park Ridge, Illinois 60068

Jerry Hussong, M.D., D.D.S.
Division of Hematology/Oncology
Department of Medicine
Northwestern University Medical School
Veterans Affairs Lakeside Medical Center
Chicago, Illinois 60611

Robert V. P. Hutter, M.D.
Clinical Professor of Pathology
University of Medicine and Dentistry
New Jersey Medical School
Professor of Pathology (Adjunct)
Columbia University College of Physicians
  and Surgeons
Department of Pathology
St. Barnabas Medical Center
94 Old Short Hills Road
Livingston, New Jersey 07039

Samuel Idarraga
(chapter 122)

Jeffrey M. Ignatoff, M.D., F.A.C.S.
Associate Professor of Clinical Urology
Northwestern University Medical School
1000 Central Street, Suite 720
Evanston, Illinois 60201

Joseph P. Imperato, M.D.
Assistant Professor of Clinical Radiology
Department of Radiology
Northwestern University Medical School
Lake Forest Hospital
660 North Westmoreland Road
Lake Forest, Illinois 60045

Valerie K. Israel, M.S., D.O.
Assistant Professor of Medicine
Division of Medical Oncology
Department of Medicine
University of Southern California
Norris Comprehensive Cancer Center
1441 Eastlake Avenue, Room 3445, MS 34
Los Angeles, California 90033

J. Milburn Jessup, M.D.
Associate Professor
Department of Surgery
Harvard Medical School
Deaconess Hospital
110 Francis Street, Suite 3A
Boston, Massachusetts 02215

Walter B. Jones, M.D.
Attending Surgeon
Gynecology Service, Department of Surgery
Memorial Sloan-Kettering Cancer Center
1275 York Avenue
New York, New York 10021

Larry R. Kaiser, M.D., FACS
Professor of Surgery
Chief, General Thoracic Surgery
University of Pennsylvania Medical Center
3400 Spruce Street
Philadelphia, Pennsylvania 19104

Angelos A. Kambouris, M.D., F.A.C.S.
Clinical Associate Professor of Surgery
University of Michigan
Head, Division of General Surgery
Henry Ford Hospital
2799 West Grand Boulevard
Detroit, Michigan 48202

Lynne S. Kaminer, M.D.
Division of Hematology
Northwestern University Medical School
250 East Superior Street
Chicago, Illinois 60611

Constantine Karakousis, M.D., Ph.D.
Chief, Surgical Oncology
State University of New York
Millard Fillmore Hospital
3 Gates Circle
Buffalo, New York 14209

Martin S. Karpeh, Jr., M.D.
Assistant Attending Surgeon
Assistant Professor
Department of Surgery
Memorial Sloan-Kettering Cancer Center
1275 York Avenue, Box 438
New York, New York 10021

James W. Keller, M.D
Professor
Department of Radiation Oncology
Emory University School of Medicine
1365 Clifton Road
Atlanta Georgia, 30322

Mary Margaret Kemeny, M.D., F.A.C.S.
Chief of Surgical Oncology
North Shore University Hospital
300 Community Drive
Manhasset, New York 11030

B. J. Kennedy, M.D., M.Sc, M.A.C.P.
Regent's Professor of Medicine, Emeritus
Masonic Professor of Oncology, Emeritus
Division of Medical Oncology
Department of Medicine
University of Minnesota Medical School
420 Delaware Street Southeast, Box 286
Minneapolis, Minnesota 55455

Henry M. Keys, M.D.
Department of Radiation Oncology
Albany Medical Center
43 New Scotland Avenue
Albany, New York 12208

Janardan Khandekar, M.D.
Professor
Department of Medicine
Evanston Hospital/ North Western
*   University*
2650 Ridge Avenue
Evanston, Illinois 60201

Lyndon J. Kim, M.D.
Clinical and Research Fellow
Department of Neurology
Neuro-Oncology Service
Massachusetts General Hospital
Harvard Medical School
Boston, Massachusetts   02114

David Klimstra, M.D.
Department of Pathology
Memorial Sloan-Kettering Cancer Center
1275 York Avenue
New York, New York 10021

Douglas W. Klotch, M.D. F.A.C.S.
Associate Professor
Division of Otolaryngology
Department of Surgery
University of South Florida College of Medicine
Harbourside Medical Towers
4 Columbia Drive, Suite 730
Tampa, Florida 33606

Ira J. Kodner, M.D.
Professor
Department of Surgery
Section of Colon and Rectal Surgery
Washington University School of Medicine
Barnes-Jewish Hospital
216 South Kingshighway
St. Louis, Missouri 63110

Ritsuko Komaki, M.D., F.A.C.S.
Professor
Department of Radiation Oncology
University of Texas M. D. Anderson Cancer
*   Center*
1515 Holcombe Boulevard, Box 97
Houston, Texas 77030

William G. Kraybill, M.D.
Chief, Melanoma/Soft Tissue Service
Roswell Park Cancer Institute
Elm and Carlton Streets
Buffalo, New York 14263

Robert R. Kuske, Jr., M.D.
Clinical Associate Professor
Department of Radiology
Tulane University Medical Center
Chairman
Ochsner Center for Radiation Oncology
Ochsner Clinic and Medical Foundation
1516 Jefferson Highway
New Orleans, Louisiana 70121

Hau C. Kwaan, M.D., Ph.D.
Professor of Medicine
Northwestern University Medical Center
333 East Huron Street
Chicago, Illinois 60611

Robert A. Kyle, M.D.
Professor
Departments of Medicine, Laboratory
   Medicine, and Pathology
Mayo Medical School
200 First Street, Southwest
Rochester, Minnesota 55905

Paul H. Lange, M.D.
Chairman, Department of Urology
University of Washington School of
   Medicine
1959 Northeast Pacific, MS RL10
Seattle, Washington 98195

Jonathan F. Lara, M.D.
Clinical Assistant Professor
University of Medicine and Dentistry
Department of Pathology
St. Barnabas Medical Center
94 Old Short Hills Road
Livingston, New Jersey 07039

Richard H. Larson, M.D., F.A.C.S.
Senior Attending Surgeon
Department of Surgery
Evanston Hospital Corporation
2650 Ridge Avenue, Burch 104
Evanston, Illinois 60201

Walter Lawrence, Jr., M.D.
Professor (Surgical Oncology)
Director Emeritus
Massey Cancer Center
Department of Surgery
Medical College of Virginia
P.O. Box 980011, MCV
Richmond, Virginia 23298

Edward R. Laws, Jr., M.D.
Professor of Neurosurgery and Medicine
Department of Neurosurgery
University of Virginia Health Science Center
Box 212 H.S.C.
Charlottesville, Virginia 22908

LaSalle D. Leffall, Jr., M.D.
Charles R. Drew Professor
Department of Surgery
Howard University Hospital
2041 Georgia Avenue Northwest
Washington, DC 20060

William T. Leslie, M.D.
Assistant Professor
Section of Medical Oncology
Rush Medical College
1725 West Harrison, Room 821
Chicago, Illinois 60612

Bernard Levin, M.D.
Vice President
Division of Cancer Prevention
University of Texas M. D. Anderson Cancer
   Center
1515 Holcombe Boulevard, Box 203
Houston, Texas 77030

Seymour H. Levitt, M.D.
Department of Therapeutic Radiology-
   Radiation Oncology
University of Minnesota Hospital and Clinic
Box 494, UMHC
Harvard Street at East River Road
Minneapolis, Minnesota 55455

Norman B. Levy, M.D.
Associate Professor
Department of Pathology
Dartmouth-Hitchcock Medical Center
One Medical Center Drive
Lebanon, New Hampshire 03756

Robin Levy, M.D.
Department of Medicine
Evanston Hospital
2650 Ridge Avenue
Evanston, Illinois 60201

Alan A. Lewin, M.D., F.A.C.P.
Department of Radiation Oncology
Baptist Hospital of Miami
8900 North Kendall Drive
Miami, Florida 33176

Frank R. Lewis, Jr., M.D.
Professor
Department of Surgery
Henry Ford Hospital
2799 West Grand Boulevard
Detroit, Michigan 48202

John L. Lewis, M.D.
Department of Surgery
Memorial Sloan-Kettering Cancer Center
1275 York Avenue
New York, New York 10021
Leslie A. Litzky, M.D.
Assistant Professor
Departments of Pathology and Laboratory
    Medicine
University of Pennsylvania Medical Center
6 Founders Pavilion
3400 Spruce Street
Philadelphia, Pennsylvania 19104

Robert B. Livingston, M.D.
Professor
Department of Medicine
Head, Division of Oncology
University of Washington
1959 Northeast Pacific Street
Seattle, Washington 98195

Joseph LoCicero III, M.D.
Associate Professor of Surgery
Harvard Medical School
Chief, General Thoracic Surgery
Deaconess Hospital
110 Francis Street, Suite 2C
Boston, Massachusetts 02215

Gershon Y. Locker, M.D.
Associate Professor of Medicine
Northwestern University Medical School
Evanston Hospital
2650 Ridge Avenue
Evanston, Illinois 60201

**Arthur S. Ludwig, Jr., M.D., C.A.P.,
    A.S.C.P.**
Chairman
Department of Pathology
Princeton Baptist Health System
701 Princeton Avenue Southwest
Birmingham, Alabama 35211

John R. Lurain, M.D.
John and Ruth Brewer Professor of Gynecology
    and Cancer Research
Section Head, Gynecologic Oncology
Northwestern University Medical School
Prentice Women s Hospital
333 East Superior Street
Chicago, Illinois 60611

Michael Lyster, M.D.
Fellow, Division of Hematology and Oncology
Department of Medicine
Northwestern University
250 East Superior Street
Chicago, Illinois 60611

Ann G. Martin, M.D.
Division of Dermatology
Box 8123
Washington University School of Medicine
660 South Euclid Avenue
St. Louis, Missouri 63110

Nael Martini, M.D.
Professor of Surgery
Cornell University Medical College
Attending Thoracic Surgeon
Memorial Sloan-Kettering Cancer Center
1275 York Avenue
New York, New York 10021

L. Stewart Massad, M.D.
Division of Gynecologic Oncology
Department of Obstetrics and Gynecology
Cook County Hospital
1835 West Harrison Street
Chicago, Illinois 60612

Robert J. Mayer, M.D.
Chief, Division of Clinical Oncology
Dana-Farber Cancer Institute
Professor of Medicine
Harvard Medical School
44 Binney Street
Boston, Massachusetts 02115

Ann McCunniff, M.D.
Department of Radiation Oncology
Bowman Gray School of Medicine
Medical Center Boulevard
Winston-Salem, North Carolina 27157

Minesh P. Mehta, M.B.Ch.B.
Associate Professor
Department of Human Oncology
University of Wisconsin
600 Highland Avenue K4/B100
Madison, Wisconsin 53792

Mick Meiselman, M.D.
Department of Medicine
Evanston Hospital
2650 Ridge Avenue
Evanston, Illinois 60201

Douglas E. Merkel, M.D.
Evanston Hospital
Department of Medical Oncology
2650 Ridge Avenue
Evanston, Illinois 60201

John S. Metcalf, M.D.
Associate Professor and Director
Department of Surgical Pathology
Medical University of South Carolina
171 Ashley Avenue
Charleston, South Carolina 29425

Michael M. Method, M.D.
Division of Gynecologic Oncology
Department of Obstetrics and Gynecology
University of Miami/Jackson Memorial Medical
* Center*
1475 Northwest 12th Avenue (D-52)
Miami, Florida 33136

Richard A. Michaelson, M.D.
Chief Medical Officer
Cancer Center, Department of Medicine
St. Barnabas Medical Center
94 Old Short Hills Road
Livingston, New Jersey 07039

Joseph Miller, M.D.
Surgeon
Emory University School of Medicine
1440 Clifton Road
Atlanta, Georgia 30322

Letha E. Mills, M.D.
Medical Oncologist
Mary Hitchcock Memorial Hospital
One Medical Center Drive
Lebanon, New Hampshire 03756

Bruce Minsky, M.D.
Department of Radiation Oncology
Memorial Sloan-Kettering Cancer Center
1275 York Avenue
New York, New York 10021

Bharat Mittal, M.D.
Chief, Division of Radiation Oncology
Northwestern University Medical School
303 East Chicago Avenue
Chicago, Illinois 60611

Frederick L. Moffat, Jr., M.D., F.A.C.S.,
** F.R.C.S.(C)**
Associate Professor of Surgery
University of Miami School of Medicine
Sylvester Comprehensive Cancer Center
Surgical Oncology (310T), Room 3550
1475 NW 12th Avenue
Miami, Florida 33136

Michael J. Moffett, M.D.
Division of Hematology
Albany Medical College
Albany, New York 12208

Jeffrey F. Moley, M.D.
Washington University School of Medicine
Barnes Hospital
One Barnes Hospital Plaza
St. Louis, Missouri 63110

Terence N. Moore, M.D., F.A.C.R.
Radiation Oncologist
Division of Radiation Oncology
Lancaster General Health Campus
2102 Harrisburg Pike
Lancaster, Pennsylvania 17601

A. R. Moossa, M.D.
Professor and Chairman
Department of Surgery
University of California
San Diego Medical Center
200 West Arbor Drive
San Diego, California 92103

Brian J. Moran, M.D.
Alexian Brothers Regional Cancer Care
* Center*
800 West Biesterfeld Road
Elk Grove Village, Illinois 60007

William Moran, M.D.
Department of Surgery
Section of Otolaryngology
University of Chicago Hospitals
5841 South Maryland
Chicago, Illinois 60637

Monica Morrow
Associate Professor
Department of Surgery
Northwestern University Medical School
250 East Superior Street
WESL 201
Chicago, Illinois 60611

Donald L. Morton, M.D.
Medical Director and Surgeon-in-Chief
John Wayne Cancer Institute
2200 Santa Monica Boulevard
Santa Monica, California 90404

Kevin J. Murray, M.D.
Associate Professor of Radiation Oncology
Medical College of Wisconsin
9200 West Wisconin Avenue
Milwaukee, Wisconsin 53226

Hyman B. Muss, M.D.
Comprehensive Cancer of Wake Forest
  University
Medical Center Boulevard.
Winston-Salem, North Carolina 27157

Rudolph M. Navari, M.D., Ph.D.
Director
Bone Marrow Transplant Center
Princeton Baptist Health System
701 Princeton Avenue Southwest
Birmingham, Alabama 35211

Scott M. Noel, M.D.
Pathology medical Services
1919 South 40th Street, Suite 333
lincoln, Nebraska 68506

William R. Noyes, M.D.
Department of Human Oncology
University of Wisconsin
Madison, Wisconsin 53792

Paul H. O'Brien, M.D.
Professor
Department of Surgery
Medical University of South Carolina
171 Ashley Avenue
Charleston, South Carolina   29425

Carl A. Olsson, M.D.
Professor and Chairman
Department of Urology
Columbia University College of Physicians and
  Surgeons
630 West 168th Street
New York, New York 10032

Mark B. Orringer, M.D.
Department of Surgery
University of Michigan Hospital
1500 East Medical Center Drive
Ann Arbor, Michigan 48109

Robert T. Osteen, M.D.
Department of Surgery
Brigham and Women s Hospital
75 Francis Street
Boston, Massachusetts 02115

William R. Panje, M.D.
Department of Otolaryngology
Rush-Presbyterian-St. Luke's Medical Center
1725 West Harrison, Suite 340
Chicago, Illinois 60612

Roy A. Patchell, M.D.
Neuro-Oncologist
University of Kentucky Hospital
800 Rose Street
Lexington, Kentucky 40536

G. Alex Patterson, M.D.
Surgeon
Washington University School of Medicine
660 South Euclid Avenue
St. Louis, Missouri 63110

Carlos A. Perez, M.D.
Director
Radiation Oncology Center
Washington University Medical Center
4511 Forest Park, Suite 200
St. Louis, Missouri 63108

Ryan S. Perkins, M.D.
Department of Radiation Oncology
St. Vincent s Medical Center
1800 Barrs Street
Jacksonville, Florida 32204

Lester J. Peters, M.D.
Department of Radiotherapy
University of Texas M. D. Anderson Cancer
  Center
1515 Holcombe Boulevard
Houston, Texas 77030

Bruce A. Peterson, M.D.
Division of Medical Oncology
University of Minnesota Hospitals
Box 348-UMHC
Harvard Street at East River Road
Minneapolis, Minnesota 55455

Carol Portlock, M.D.
Department of Medical Oncology
Memorial Sloan-Kettering Cancer Center
1275 York Avenue
New York, New York 10021

Julio Pow-Sang, M.D.
Associate Professor of Surgery
Division of Urology
H. Lee Moffitt Cancer Center and Research
  Institute
12902 Magnolia Drive
University of South Florida
Tampa, Florida 33612

Cary A. Presant, M.D.
President
California Cancer Medical Center
1250 South Sunset Avenue, Suite 303
West Covina, California 91790

Robert L. Quigley, M.D., Ph.D., F.A.C.S.
Department of Cardiothoracic Surgery
3 Yellow-Guthrie Clinic
Guthrie Square
Sayre, Pennsylvania 18840

Robert M. Quinlan, M.D., F.A.C.S.
Chief of Surgery
Medical Center of Central Massachusetts
67 Belmont Street
Worcester, Massachusetts 01605

Kanti R. Rai, M.D.
Medical Oncologist
Long Island Jewish Medical Center
270-05 76th Avenue
New Hyde Park, New York 11040

Wendy Recant, M.D.
Department of Pathology
University of Chicago Hospital
5841 South Maryland
Chicago, Illinois 60637

Carolyn E. Reed, M.D.
Division of Cardiothoracic Surgery
Medical University of South Carolina
171 Ashley Avenue
Charleston, South Carolina 29425

Laurel W. Rice, M.D.
Associate Professor
Department of Gynecologic Oncology
University of Virginia Health Sciences Center
Charlottesville, Virginia 22908

Jerome P. Ritchie, M.D.
Surgeon
Harvard Medical School
30 Binney Street
Boston, Massachusetts 02115

Kenneth B. Roberts, M.D.
Department of Therapeutic Radiology
Hunter Radiation Therapy
Yale-New Haven Hospital
Room HRT138
20 York Street
New Haven, Connecticut 06504

Michael Rodriguez, M.D.
Division of Gynecologic Oncology
Department of Obstetrics and Gynecology
University of Miami/Jackson Memorial Medical
  Center
1475 Northwest 12th Avenue (D-52)
Miami, Florida 33136

Marvin M. Romsdahl, M.D., Ph.D.
Department of Surgical Oncology
University of Texas M. D. Anderson Cancer
  Center
1515 Holcombe Boulevard, Box 106
Houston, Texas 77030

Stephen C. Rubin, M.D.
Professor and Director
Division of Gynecologic Oncology
University of Pennsylvania Medical Center
3400 Spruce Street
Philadelphia, Pennsylvania 19104

Benjamin F. Rush, Jr., M.D.
Distinguished Professor and Chair
Department of Surgery
University Hospital/University of Medicine and
  Dentistry of New Jersey
150 Bergen Street
Newark, New Jersey 07103

Homer H. Russ, M.D.
Radiation Therapy Department
St. Joseph s Hospital
611 St. Joseph Avenue
Marshfield, Wisconsin 54449

Christy A. Russell, M.D.
Assistant Professor
Division of Medical Oncology
Medical Oncology Fellowship Director
Department of Medicine
University of Southern California
Norris Comprehensive Cancer Center
1441 Eastlake Avenue, Room 3445, MS 34
Los Angeles, California 90033

Liisa Russell, M.D.
Division of Cardiothoracic Surgery
University of California at Davis School of
Medicine
Room 2250, Professional Building
4301 X Street
Sacramento, California 95817

William T. Sause, M.D., F.A.C.R.
Radiation Therapy Department
LDS Hospital
8th Avenue and C Street
Salt Lake City, Utah 84143

Raymond E. Sawaya, M.D.
Professor and Chairman
Department of Neurosurgery
University of Texas M.D. Anderson Cancer
Center
1515 Holcombe Boulevard
Houston, Texas 77030

Stephen I. Schabel, M.D.
Professor
Department of Radiology
Medical University of South Carolina
171 Ashley Avenue
Charleston, South Carolina 29425

Howard I. Scher, M.D.
Chief, Genitourinary Oncology Service
Department of Medicine
Memorial Sloan-Kettering Cancer Center
1275 York Avenue
New York, New York 10021

John E. Schiller, M.D.
Department of Radiation Oncology
The Penrose-St. Francis Healthcare System
P.O. Box 7021
Colorado Springs, Colorado 80933

Ken Schroer, M.D.
Department of Pathology
H. Lee Moffitt Cancer Center
University of South Florida
42902 Magnolia Drive
Tampa, Florida 33612

Christopher J. Schultz, M.D.
Assistant Professor of Radiation Oncology
Medical College of Wisconsin
8700 West Wisconsin Avenue
Milwaukee, Wisconsin 53226

James G. Schwade, M.D., F.A.C.R.
Chief, Radiation Oncologist
Miami Neuroscience Center
HealthSouth Doctors' Hospital
Coral Gables, Florida

Robert J. Schweitzer, M.D.
Professor of Surgery (Clinical)
University of California, Davis (East Bay)
Surgical Oncologist
Summit Medical Center
3232 Elm Street
Oakland, California 94609

Troy G. Scroggins, Jr., M.D.
Radiation Oncology
Ochsner Clinic
1514 Jefferson Highway
New Orleans, Louisiana 70121

Hilliard Seigler, M.D.
Department of Surgery
Duke University Medical Center
Box 3708
Durham, North Carolina 27710

Stephen F. Sener, M.D., F.A.C.S.
Associate Professor of Surgery
Northwestern University Medical School
Evanston Hospital
Burch #106
2650 Ridge
Evanston, Illinois 60201

Bernd-Uwe Sevin, M.D., Ph.D., F.A.C.S.
Division of Gynecologic Oncology
Department of Obstetrics and Gynecology
University of Miami/Jackson Memorial Medical
Center
1475 Northwest 12th Avenue (D-52)
Miami, Florida 33136

Jatin P. Shah, M.D.
E. W. Strong Chair in Head and Neck Oncology
Chief, Head and Neck Service
Memorial Sloan-Kettering Cancer Center
1275 York Avenue
New York, New York 10021

Ashok R. Shaha, MD. F.A.C.S.
Memorial Sloan-Kettering Cancer Center
Head and Neck Service
1275 York Avenue
New York, New York 10021

Charles Shapiro, M.D.
Dana Farber Cancer Institute
44 Binney Street
Boston, Massachusetts 02115

Daniel H. Shevrin, M.D.
Oncology Department
Evanston Hospital
2650 Ridge Avenue
Evanston, Illinois 60201

Rache Simmons, M.D.
Strang-Cornell Breast Center
428 East 72nd Street
New York, New York 10021

Scott Y. Sittler, MD
Assistant Professor of Clinical Pathology
Department of Pathology
University of Miami School of Medicine
1611 NW 12th Avenue
Miami, Florida 33136

Donald G. Skinner, M. D.
Professor and Chairman
Department of Urology
University of Southern California School of
* Medicine*
1441 Eastlake
Suite 7414
Los Angeles, California 90033

Lee E. Smith, M.D.
Professor of Surgery
George Washington University
2150 Pennsylvania Avenue NW
Washington, DC 20037

Steve Snyder, M.D.
Division of Medical Oncology
University of Minnesota Medical School
University Hospital
Minneapolis, MN 55455

Ronald H. Spiro, M.D.
Department of Surgery
Memorial Sloan-Kettering Cancer Center
1275 York Avenue
New York, New York 10021

Kasi Sridhar, M.D.
Professor of Medicine
University of Miami School of Medicine
Sylvester Comprehensive Cancer Center
Division of Hematology/Oncology (D8-4)
1475 NW 12th Avenue
Miami, Florida 33136

Glenn D. Steele, Jr., M.D., F.A.C.S.
Vice President of Medical Affairs
Dean, Biological Sciences Division
University of Chicago
5841 South Maryland. MC 1000
Chicago, Illinois 60637

F. Kristian Storm, M.D., F.A.C.S.
Department of Surgery, Section Oncology
University of Wisconsin School of Medicine
600 Highland Avenue
Madison, Wisconsin 53792

Oscar Streeter, M.D.
Assistant Professor of Clinical Oncology
Chief Physician
Department of Radiation Oncology
University of Southern California
Norris Comprehensive Cancer Center
1441 Eastlake Avenue, Room 3445, MS 34
Los Angeles, California 90033

Elliot W. Strong, M.D.
Department of Surgery
Memorial Sloan-Kettering Cancer Center
1275 York Avenue
New York, New York 10021

Steven J. Stryker, M.D.
Associate Professor of Clinical Surgery
676 North St. Clair
Suite 1525
Northwestern University Medical School
Chicago, Illinois 60611

Keith Stuart (chapter 33)

Paul H. Sugarbaker, M.D.
Chief, Surgical Oncology
Washington Hospital Center Cancer
* Institute*
110 Irving Street, NW
Washington, DC 20010

Carl M. Sutherland, M.D.
Department of Surgery
Tulane University Hospital
1415 Tulane Avenue
New Orleans, Louisiana 70112

Patrick J. Sweeney, M.D.
Instructor
Department of Radiation Oncology
The University of Chicago
5841 South Maryland MC0085
Chicago, Illinois 60637

Mark S. Talamonti, M.D.
Assistant Professor of Surgery
Department of Surgery
Northwestern University Medical School
Department of Surgery
250 East Superior Street, WESL 201
Chicago, Illinois 60611

John N. Tasiopoulos, D.O.
Department of Medicine
Evanston Hospital
2650 Ridge Avenue
Evanston, Illinois 60201

Marie E. Taylor, M.D.
Mallinckrodt Institute of Radiology
Washington University Medical Center
4939 Children's Place, Suite 5500
St. Louis, Missouri 63110

Peyton T. Taylor, Jr., M.D., F.A.C.S.
Richard N. and Louise R. Crockett Professor
  and Director
Division of Gynecologic Oncology
University of Virginia Health Sciences Center
Box 387
Charlottesville, Virginia 22908

John H. Texter, Jr., M.D.
Surgeon
Southern Illinois University Medical College
Division of Urology
P.O. Box 19230
Springfield, Illinois 62794

Maria Theodoulou, M.D.
Clinical Assistant Physician
Breast Oncology Service
Memorial Sloan-Kettering Cancer Center
1275 York Avenue
New York, New York 10021

Courtney M. Townsend, Jr., M.D.
Department of Surgery
University of Texas Medical Branch at
  Galveston
301 University Boulevard
Galveston, Texas 77555

Edward L. Trimble, M.D., M.P.H.
CIB, CTEP, DCTDC
National Cancer Institute
6130 Executive Boulevard
Executive Plaza North, Room 741, MSC 7436
Bethesda, Maryland 20892

Andrew M. Trotti, M.D.
Associate Professor
Division of Radiation Oncology
H. Lee Moffitt Cancer Center
University of South Florida
42902 Magnolia Drive
Tampa, Florida 33612

Donald Trump, M.D.
Professor of Medicine and Surgery
Deputy Director
University of Pittsburgh Cancer Institute
University of Pittsburgh
201 Kaufmann Building
Pittsburgh, Pennsylvania 15213

Roger Tutton, M.D.
Radiology Department
Ochsner Clinic
1514 Jefferson Highway
New Orleans, Louisiana 70121

Leo B. Twiggs, M.D.
Chief, Department of Gynecology
University of Minnesota Hospital
Box 604-UMHC
Harvard Street at East River Road
Minneapolis, Minnesota 55455

Jon A. van Heerden, M.B.,Ch.B., M.S.,
  F.R.C.S.(C),
F.A.C.S., Hon. F.C.M.(S.A.), Hon. F.R.C.S.
Fred C. Anderson Professor
Department of Surgery
Mayo Medical Center
200 First Street, Southwest
Rochester, Minnesota 55905

Anna L. Vaughn, R.N.
Department of Surgery
Duke University Medical Center
Durham, North Carolina 27710

Nicholas A. Vick, M.D.
Professor of Neurology
Northwestern University Medical School
Evanston Hospital
2650 Ridge Avenue
Evanston, Illinois 60201

Hugo V. Villar, M.D.
Department of Surgery
University Medical Center
1501 North Campbell Avenue
Tucson, Arizona 85724

Everett E. Vokes, M.D.
Professor
Department of Medicine
Section of Hematology/Oncology
University of Chicago
5841 South Maryland MC2115
Chicago, Illinois 60637

Charles F. von Gunten, M.D., Ph.D.
Hematology/Oncology
Northwestern University Medical School
233 East Erie Street, #700
Chicago, Illinois 60611

Reinhard W. von Roemeling, M.D.
Attending Physician
Department of Medical Oncology
Fox Chase Convention Center
7701 Burholme Avenue
Philadelphia, Pennsylvania 19111

Jamie H. Von Roenn, M.D.
Hematology/Oncology
Northwestern University Medical School
233 East Erie Street, #700
Chicago, Illinois 60611

Julie M. Vose, M.D.
Department of Medicine
University of Nebraska
600 South 42nd Street
Omaha, Nebraska 68198

Gaylord T. Walker, M.D.
Department of Surgery
University of South Alabama
159 Louiselle Street
Mobile, Alabama 36607

James R. Wallace, M.D., Ph.D
Associate Professor
Department of Surgery, Division of Trauma
Medical College of Wisconsin
9200 West Wisconsin Avenue
Milwaukee, Wisconsin 53226

Sidney Wallace, M.D.
Professor of Radiology
University of Texas M. D. Anderson Cancer Center
1515 Holcombe Boulevard
Houston, Texas 77030

Alexander J. Walt, M.D. (deceased)
Harper Hospital
3990 John R Street
Detroit, Michigan 48201

Harold J. Wanebo, M.D.
Director, Division of Surgical Oncology
Brown University
Roger Williams Medical Center
825 Chalkstone Avenue
Providence, Rhode Island 02908

Raymond P. Warrell, Jr., M.D.
Member and Professor of Medicine
Cornell University Medical College
Memorial Sloan-Kettering Cancer Center
1275 York Avenue
New York, New York 10021

Gregory Warren, M.D.
Indiana University School of Medicine and Cancer Center
550 North University Boulevard, Room 1640
Indianapolis, Indiana 46202

Robert S. Warren, M.D.
Associate Professor of Surgery
Chief of Surgical Oncology
Department of Surgery
University of California, San Francisco
533 Parnassus Avenue, Room U-372
San Francisco, California 94143

W. Bedford Waters, M.D.
Professor
Department of Urology
Foster G. McGaw Hospital
Loyola University of Chicago
2160 South First Avenue
Maywood, Illinois 60153

Irving J. Weigensberg, M.D.
Clinical Assistant Professor
University of Illinois College of Medicine
Medical Director
Department of Radiation Oncology
Methodist Medical Center of Illinois
221 Northeast Glen Oak Avenue<\#9>
Peoria, Illinois 61636

Ralph R. Weichselbaum, M.D.
Professor and Chairman
Department of Radiation Oncology
University of Chicago
5841 South Maryland MC0085
Chicago, Illinois 60637

Raymond B. Weiss, M.D.
Professor of Medicine
Hematology-Oncology Service
Uniformed Services
University of the Health Sciences
Walter Reed Army Medical Center
Washington, D.C.

Ilene Ceil Weitz, M.D.
Associate Clinical Professor of Medicine
Division of Hematology
University of Southern California School of
  Medicine
California Cancer Medical Center
1250 South Sunset Avenue
West Covina, California 91790

Samuel A. Wells, Jr., M.D.
Bixby Professor and Chairman
School of Medicine
Washington University
660 South Euclid Avenue, Box 8109
St. Louis Missouri 63110

Kent C. Westbrook, M.D.
Professor of Surgery
University of Arkansas for Medical Sciences
Chief, Division of Surgical Oncology
Director, Arkansas Cancer Research Center
4301 West Markham, Slot 623
Little Rock, Arkansas 72205

J. Taylor Wharton, M.D.
Professor and Chairman
Department of Gynecologic Oncology
University of Texas M.D. Anderson Cancer
  Center
1515 Holcombe Boulevard.
Houston, Texas 770300

Julia R. White, M.D.
Department of Radiation Oncology
John L. Doyne Hospital
8700 West Wisconsin Avenue
Milwaukee, Wisconsin 53226

Michael Whittaker, M.D.
Assistant Professor of Pathology
Medical College of Wisconsin
8700 West Wisconsin Avenue
Milwaukee, Wisconsin 53226

Morton C. Wilhelm, M.D.
Professor Emeritus
Department of Surgery
University of Virginia Medical Center
Health Science Center
Charlottesville, Virginia 22908

Christopher G. Willett, M.D.
Department of Radiation Oncology
Massachusetts General Hospital
323 Fruit Street
Boston, Massachusetts 02114

Richard D. Williams, M.D.
Professor and Head
Department of Urology
University of Iowa
200 Hawkins Drive
Iowa City, Iowa 52242

Stephen D. Williams, M.D.
Indiana University
School of Medicine and Cancer Center
550 North University Boulevard, Room 1640
Indianapolis, Indiana 46202

Charles B. Wilson, M.D.
Department of Neurosurgery
University of California, San Francisco
505 Parnassus Avenue
San Francisco, California 94143

J. Frank Wilson, M.D., F.A.C.R.
Professor and Chairman
Department of Radiation Oncology
Director, Cancer Center
Medical College of Wisconsin
8701 Watertown Plank Road
Milwaukee, Wisconsin 53226

David J. Winchester, M.D.
Assistant Professor of Surgery
Northwestern University Medical School
2650 Ridge Avenue
Evanston, Illinois 60201

Kenneth I. Wishnow, M.D.
Associate Professor
Harvard Medical School
110 Francis Street, Suite 3A
Boston, Massachusetts 02215

Walter G. Wolfe, M.D.
Professor of Surgery
Duke University Medical Center
Durham, North Carolina 27710

Stuart J. Wong, M.D.
Fellow
Department of Internal Medicine
Division of Hematology/Oncology
Medical College of Wisconsin
9200 West Wisconsin Avenue
Milwaukee, Wisconsin 53226

William C. Wood, M.D.
Surgeon
Emory University Hospital
1364 Clifton Road
Atlanta, Georgia 30322

Angela B. Wurster, R.N., M.S.N.
Departments of Surgery and Pathology and
 Laboratory Medicine
University of Pennsylvania School of Medicine
3400 Spruce Street
Philadelphia, Pennsylvania 19104

Robert C. Young, M.D.
Medical Oncologist and President
Fox Chase Cancer Center
7701 Burholme Avenue
Philadelphia, Pennsylvania 19111

Anthony L. Zietman, M.D.
Department of Radiation Oncology
Boston University Hospital
88 East Newton
Boston, Massachusetts 02118

Preface

Tumor Board Case Management follows the tumor conference format with its emphasis on case orientation and open exchange of views and recapitulates the conference's structure, philosophy, and purpose. The book, therefore, retains the reality of medical practice in which physicians treat patients one at a time. Most medical textbooks usually represent reviews of published reports and a summation of the author's experience, but they rarely deal with individual patients, the basis for medical decisions, or complications that confront physicians in treating the individual.

Tumor Board Case Management, a new approach to medical education, is designed to extend the management and educational benefits of the tumor board by presenting the most current information on pretreatment evaluation and multimodality therapy for a wide variety of cancers. Actual case histories of 152 patients that were presented at tumor boards were selected to emphasize specific and often difficult aspects of cancer patient management and to illustrate teaching examples, which give the most forceful educational information when supported by clinical trial data. Other more controversial cases required the selection, among several management options, of therapy based only on experience or on incomplete scientific data. The book thus contains standard cases in which there is agreement on treatment and problem cases for which precise treatment is not available.

Management problems for surgeons, oncologists, and radiotherapists are also included. The cases span a spectrum of clinical problems, covering cancer in nearly all anatomic sites and in different age groups and races, and in both sexes. The importance of the different histologic tumor types and the different tumor stages at presentation are taken into account. Patients with localized disease or with metastatic disease are discussed. Complications that can arise during treatment are also considered as well as specific approaches to complex situations, for example, the nonoperative management of obstruction or the treatment of cancer in the immunosuppressed patient.

Cases were selected based on disease prevalence (17 cases of breast cancer but only 4 of renal cancer were included) and to represent differing views, based from different institutions, including universities, small community hospitals, large urban hospitals, and cancer centers. Also included are cases of solid and nonsolid tumors to reflect the full range of malignant tumors, as well as cases of cancer patients with AIDS or other chronic debilitating diseases. Comments, designed to resolve controversies or to provide ancillary information such as the endocrine manifestations of the paraneoplastic syndromes, were obtained for each case from physicians representing different specialties of medicine, different treatment approaches, and different regions of the United States. In some cases, comments were from physicians not involved directly in cancer patient care, such as endocrinologists or cardiologists.

The cases are fully documented with roentgenograms and histologic slides that were actually shown at the tumor conference and presented in detail, including results of laboratory tests. The advantages and limitations of new technology are assessed. In many cases, a consensus on treatment and management does not exist. For example, how should early prostate cancer detected by minimally elevated levels of serum prostate-specific antigen (PSA) be treated—as in a case of a 60-year-old man who has a serum PSA level of 6.7 with a small focal defect in the prostate on ultrasound? For other cases, treatment course unfolds during the presentation. Therefore, depending on the case, the treatment and management decision will vary.

Deficiencies in patient workup or in the clinical-laboratory evaluation are noted as appropriate. Excessive or costly workup, inappropriate use of laboratory tests, and new treatment options are often considered. For example, should the timing of surgery for breast cancer depend on the menstrual cycle? Are premenopausal breast cancer patients with nodal involvement more likely to suffer recurrence if surgery is performed in the first half of the menstrual cycle? Ethical issues are also considered in some cases.

Much is to be learned from every case presentation—each contains an introduction and discussion. Although cases of individual cancer patients are discussed, the management principles may apply to similar cases encountered in a physician's practice, which is an advantage of this educational approach. *Tumor Board Case Management* also emphasizes the Physicians Data Query (PDQ), sponsored by the National Cancer Institute and now used in many hospitals, in disseminating new information on patient management and early detection.

The case presentations follow a standard format. There is a concise description of the history and physical findings, pertinent pretreatment evaluation and staging, multidisciplinary discussion of the management options, and final recommendations. When possible, references are included to support the recommendations.

David. P. Winchester, M.D., F.A.C.S.
Murray F. Brennan, M.D., F.A.C.S.
Gerald D. Dodd, Jr., F.A.C.S.
Donald E. Hensen, M.D.
B. J. Kennedy, M.D.
Glenn D. Steele, Jr., M.D., F.A.C.S.
J. Frank Wilson, M.D., F.A.C.R.

Introduction

No disease challenges the physician as much as cancer. Providing care for the cancer patient raises the most difficult questions about treatment, standards of care, consultation, cost, and follow-up. More than 60 years ago, to deal with this devastating disease, physicians instituted a system for interspecialty consultation known as the tumor conference or tumor board. With remarkable prescience, these physicians recognized that the care and management of cancer patients would transcend the expertise of the individual medical specialties.

Tumor conferences are forums for the interdisciplinary care of cancer patients, especially those with difficult management problems or unusual manifestations of cancer (1,2). They provide a mechanism for reaching a consensus on treatment through the empirical process of testing our opinions against one another and through facts. The mechanism follows democratic principles, that is, full and equal representation of all views. Although the size, structure, and method of operation may vary depending on the institution, tumor boards are conducted in a wide spectrum of hospitals and related institutions that vary in size and function. Of 1,330 selected hospitals surveyed by the National Cancer Institute (3), tumor conferences were regularly conducted in 1,267 (95%). Almost 400,000 patient cases, nearly one third of all cancer cases diagnosed in one year, are presented annually at tumor conferences.

PATIENT CARE

Tumor conferences provide a forum for pretreatment evaluation, for resolving controversial management problems, for estimating prognosis, for staging, for planning post-treatment follow-up, and for considering rehabilitation and other supportive care (4,5). Tumor conferences serve the needs of the oncologic specialists and primary care physicians who often serve as family physicians for cancer patients. Closely allied with the tumor conference is the tumor registry, which provides information on tumor incidence, patient follow-up, and statistical analyses.

Research indicates that physicians acquire information in one or more of the following ways: formal consultation, reading the literature, conversations with colleagues, and attendance at educational sessions (6,7,8). Tumor conferences have the potential to serve physicians in all these capacities.

Consultation

In many hospitals, outside consultants who provide additional expertise are often invited to participate in the tumor conference. Consultants are available from regional cancer centers, university hospitals, or through the American Cancer Society. As an established institution, tumor conferences promote consultation among surgeons, internists, radiologists, radiation oncologists, gynecologists, medical oncologists, and other specialists including social workers, nurses, and psychologists (9). Tumor conferences provide a setting for multispeciality consultation.

Literature Review

Besides considering new clinical protocols and reviewing diagnostic modalities, tumor conferences often present summaries of the recent published reports, especially with the aid of computer-generated data from Physicians Data Query (PDQ). Physicians are also apprised of new treatment protocols through newsletters, handouts, or announcements available at the conference. References or other sources of information are often cited by participants. Tumor conferences also provide a review of management practices and survival information condensed from published reports or analyzed from local or state tumor registries.

Interpersonnel Cooperation

Tumor conferences can enhance interdisciplinary and interpersonnel cooperation among the medical staff. Through open interaction, the tumor board fosters confidential exchange of views that focus on outcome, quality of care, referral patterns, and practice habits. In addition, tumor boards offer opportunities to review the process of decision making in medicine, evaluate various approaches to medical education, assess knowledge and improve leadership and communication skills (10,11).

By presenting follow-up data, tumor conferences provide not only a feedback on the results of therapy but also a mechanism for peer review and quality assurance. Tumor conferences are in a position to compare the expected outcomes for different management options.

Educational Benefits

Equally important are the educational benefits of the tumor conference. Through participation, physicians have the opportunity to learn about new diagnostic modalities, changing treatment patterns and new patient management principles. The natural history of various cancers and means to prevent the disease may be reviewed. Through didactic presentations, the tumor conference provides a setting for discussions on many issues in cancer patient management. These include the recent application of basic sciences to diagnosis or treatment, such as the identification of the *bcr* gene for the diagnosis of chronic myeloid leukemia or the role of suppressor gene mutations as potential prognostic markers for patients with breast cancer (12). The educational benefits may extend to other physicians, as the results of tumor conference case presentations are often published in clinical journals. According to theories on learning, adults acquire new information best when the relevance to their daily work can easily be seen.

The tumor conference with its inexhaustible variety of cases is an excellent problem-oriented learning resource for students, interns, residents and practicing physicians. By providing a forum for education, patterns of care and diffusion of new technology, tumor conferences also serve as a community-level focus for the local, regional and national network of information dissemination essential for reducing cancer morbidity and mortality (13). Tumor conferences are probably the largest source of continuing medical education in the United States Survey results indicate that 77% of hospital-wide conferences offer credits for continuing medical education (3)

Unlike many educational programs, tumor conferences extend our horizons beyond the bounds of patient care. They fortify knowledge, confirm experience, and deepen our sympathy for the human condition. In oncology education, personal computers, videocassettes, and videodisks are no substitute for the tumor conference.

UNIFYING INFLUENCE

Tumor boards serve as a unifying influence in medical practice because they bring together the different specialties in the search of optimal treatment for a difficult disease. With its multidisciplinary representation, no group other than the tumor conference is better prepared to treat the patient who may feel fragmented by the treatment approaches offered by the different medical specialties. Initial management decisions are often critical in determining ultimate outcome.

The professional medical societies have long recognized the importance of the tumor conference. The American College of Surgeons, as a requisite for approval for its hospital-based Cancer Program, requires an active tumor conference that meets at least monthly under the aegis of an interdisciplinary cancer committee (14). The College further requires a patient-oriented and consultative conference with didactic presentations not exceeding 25% of conference time. Ideally, the conference must be prospective with the focus on pretreatment evaluation and planning. Conferences must be documented and must include those cancer cases commonly seen at the institution during the year. To encompass all views on management, interdisciplinary participation is required. Without such participation, the tumor board cannot achieve its mission. Although opinions on optimal patient management are the object of the tumor conference, the College emphasizes that the final decisions on treatment are the responsibility of the primary treating physician and that the opinions are only recommendations made to the treating physician by the board or conference participants. In addition to the College of Surgeons, the College of American Pathologists encourages its members to participate actively in tumor conferences. Previously, the National Cancer Institute awarded grants to investigators to study and evaluate the methods most effective in allowing tumor boards to function as a key element in patient care decision making and in continuing professional education (15). Studies have shown that educational interventions can significantly impact on the clinical and educational effectivenes of hospital-based tumor conferences (16).

Tumor boards are held in many settings. The most common is the hospital-wide conference, which attracts many disciplines involved in cancer patient care. Joint tumor boards are similar but include two or more institutions as sponsors with cases selected from the institutions (17). Finally, the format of the tumor conference is used by many of the medical subspecialties for inter- and intradepartment conferences. Scientific interests and research areas are explored through site- or disease-oriented subspecialty departmental conferences that have evolved in larger institutions. Usually more focused on the disease process, these conferences often consider specific technical issues as well as problems in diagnosis and patient management (18). Interdisciplinary approaches to patient care are also found in hospital ethics (19) and in nursing (20).

CONTRIBUTIONS TO CARE

The resources devoted to the conduct of tumor conferences should not be underestimated. These resources represent a contribution from the medical profession to cancer patient care, a contribution not widely publicized nor recognized. Resources include the time and personal cost of physicians and other professionals in medicine who volunteer their services. Based on reported attendance, meeting frequency and meeting length, an estimated 1.25 million physician man-hours are allocated annually to the conference (3). Many nonphysician personnel, such as tumor registrars and oncology nurses, also contribute their time and effort. The tumor conference visibly reflects the interest and the dedication of physicians, nurses and others to the care and treatment of patients with cancer.

Based on survey results (3), an average of 20 physicians attend hospital-wide and joint tumor conferences, and 15 physicians attend departmental conferences. An average of 7.6 different medical disciplines are represented at a hospital-wide conference. The average number of nonphysician personnel attending each hospital-wide conference is 7.4. According to survey data, the average hospital-wide cancer conference involves the allocation of 50.8 hours of physician effort and 20.7 hours of nonphysician effort per month. In terms of figures available for 1990, the total contribution made by physicians and nonphysicians was nearly 600 million dollars annually to cancer patient management through tumor board participation. The overall cost of presenting each patient at the tumor conference is more than $12,000. The contributions made by the medical and allied professions participating in tumor conferences are substantial within the cancer care system (21).

Less than 1% of all hospitals charge the patient for consultation provided by his or her case presentation at the tumor board. Management recommendations made at the tumor conference may avoid unnecessary diagnostic evaluation, reducing the costs of care.

Tumor boards may have a greater impact on cancer patient management in smaller hospitals not affiliated with universities or cancer centers. These small hospitals utilize more outside consultants and present more cases at each tumor conference than larger institutions (13). They are also more likely sponsor joint conferences in conjunction with another hospital.

ESTABLISHED INSTITUTION

A tumor conference is an established institution for cancer patient care. The majority of hospitals in the United States conduct some type of tumor conference on a weekly or monthly basis. Many conferences have been in existence for more than 25 years. In many hospitals, tumor boards of variable size and purpose are the cornerstone for standard multidisciplinary management for patients with cancer (22). Tumor conferences benefit the patients, the physicians, the professional nonmedical staff, and the institution. Through the tumor board, physicians can offer the patient the most recent advances in all modalities of treatment, which is the only way to insure maximal response, highest quality of life and survival. It has been estimated that a minimum of 60% of cancer patients stand to benefit from multidisciplinary treatment planning. Perhaps just as important, patients appreciate the concern shown by physicians when their condition is discussed at the tumor conference.

In medicine, it is difficult to resist the pressure of experience as shared through the tumor board. When all the alternatives have been sifted, convergence of opinion becomes the accepted course of action. What matters is our loyalty to our patients, not our hope of curing all cancers. We converse at the tumor board to make further conversation unnecessary.

Donald E. Hensen, M.D.

REFERENCES

1. Fleming ID, Sumner S. The hospital cancer program: its benefits to patients. *Bull Am Coll Surg* 1980;65:10–3.
2. Gross EG. The role of the tumor board in a community hospital. *CA* 1987;37:88–92.
3. Henson DE, Frelick RW, Ford LG, et al. Results of a national survey of characteristics of hospital tumor conferences. *Surg Gynecol Obstet* 1990;170:1–6.
4. Berman HL. The tumor board; is it worth saving? *Milit Med* 1975; 140:529–31.
5. Fleming ID. Multidisciplinary treatment planning. Tumor boards. *Cancer* 1989;64(Suppl):279–81.
6. DaRosa DA, Mast TA, Dawson-Saunders B, et al. A study of the information-seeking skill of medical students and physician faculty. *J Med Educ* 1983;58:45–50.
7. McLaughlin CP, Ponshansky R. Diffusion of innovation in medicine. A problem of continuing education. *J Med Educ* 1965;40:437–47.
8. Stinson ER, Mueller DA. A survey of health professionals information habits and needs. *JAMA* 1980;243:140–3.
9. Muggia FM. Multidisciplinary considerations in cancer treatment: origin and scope. *Int J Radiat Oncol Biol Phys* 1984;1:31–3.
10. Kelsey JV, Beck JR. The effect of decision analysis on clinical uncertainty at tumor board. *J Cancer Educ* 1990;5:125–34.
11. Radecki SE, Nyquist JG, Gates JD. Educational characteristics of tumor conferences in teaching and non-teaching hospitals. *J Cancer Educ* 1995;9:204–216.
12. Thor AD, Moore DH II, Edgerton SM, et al. Accumulation of p53 tumor suppressor gene protein. An independent marker of prognosis in breast cancer. *JNCI* 1992;84:845–55.
13. Katterhagen JG, Wishart DL. The tumor board: how it works in a community hospital. *CA* 1977;27:201–4.
14. American College of Surgeons. *Cancer Program Manual*. Commission on Cancer, Chicago, 1991.
15. Nyquist JG, Gates JD, Radecki SE, Abrahamson S. Investigation into the education process of cancer case conferences. *Acad Med* 1990;65:535–6.
16. Nyquist JG, Radecki SE, Gates JD, Abrahamson S. An educational intervention to improve tumor conferences. *J Cancer Educ* 1995;10:71–77.
17. Rosenbaum EH, Rogers WL, Clever JA, et al. Experiment with a city wide tumor board (Meeting Abstract). *Proc Am Soc Clin Oncol* 1977;1:335.
18. Friedman E, Friedman C. Tumors of the head and neck: a 4-year study of a multidisciplinary approach. *Int J Oral Surg* 1978;7:291–5.
19. Cohen CB. Interdisciplinary consultation on the care of the critically ill and dying. The role of one hospital ethics committee. *Crit Care Med* 1982;10:776–84.
20. McCalla JL. A multidisciplinary approach to identification and remedial intervention for adverse late effects of cancer therapy. *Nurs Clin North Am* 1985;20:117–30.
21. Henson DE. Opportunities unexplored. The tumor conference. *Arch Pathol Lab Med* 1990;114:565.
22. Lambert JC, Abernathy C, Waddell WR. Cancer care in the small hospital. *Surg Clin North Am* 1979;59:441–7.

Acknowledgments

The educational value of the Tumor Board, a widely accepted, multidisciplinary format for the prospective discussion of the optimum treatment of the cancer patient, was conceived by Dr. Oliver H. Beahrs. Dr. Beahrs, a past President of the American College of Surgeons, recognized the collective clinical wisdom of Tumor Boards across the country. He challenged the staff of the Cancer Department of the American College of Surgeons to organize a textbook whose contributors were the principals of the Tumor Board.

Countless hours were contributed by busy cancer clinicians in the preparation of case presentations and commentaries. Especially noteworthy was the broad range of contributors, including attending physicians from community hospitals, faculty from community teaching hospitals, and academicians from major centers. Intellectually honest differences of opinions inevitably arise during Tumor Board deliberations. The willingness of case presenters to be critically analyzed by an "outside consultant" commentator enriched the educational message.

Cancer programs approved by the Commission on Cancer of the American College of Surgeons and one of the important, required components, The Tumor Board, rely heavily on the tumor registrar. These dedicated professionals contribute significantly to the quality care of the cancer patient through cancer registry operations and organization of the Tumor Board.

The staff of the Cancer Department, especially Deirdre McAllister, Lisa Richards and Carol H. Johnson, are to be commended for their diligence in the organization of this book. Also to be acknowledged is the staff of Lippincott-Raven under the leadership of Stuart Freeman.

To Dr. Beahrs, an educational innovator, and to the editors, case presenters, commentators, tumor registrars and staff, a sincere thank you.

David P. Winchester, M.D.
Editor

Tumor Board
Case Management

SECTION I

Head and Neck

1

Squamous Cell Carcinoma of the Lip

Frederick L. Moffat, Jr., Scott Y. Sittler, Kasi S. Sridhar, and John M. Cassel

Presenting the problem of neurotropism

CASE PRESENTATION

A 34-year-old Caucasian man presented in March 1991 with a 3-week history of a rapidly growing mass involving the left side of his lower jaw. The patient noted mild painless restriction in his ability to open his mouth. A Panorax film of the mandible performed by a dentist showed no evidence of bony destruction.

Past medical history was significant for a stage I (T1 N0 M0) squamous carcinoma of the left lower lip in January, 1990, treated by Mohs' surgery with clear surgical margins. The operator noted that the resultant defect measured 4.5 cm before primary repair. Perineural invasion was noted (Fig. 1–1A), but no further treatment had been given. In 1985, the patient had undergone radical orchiectomy, six cycles of cisplatin, bleomycin, and VP-16, and retroperitoneal lymphadenectomy for stage IV (T1 N2 M0) nonseminomatous (mixed type) carcinoma of the testis. He was free of testicular cancer at this time.

On examination, there was a 5-cm mass fixed to and protruding inferolaterally from the midhorizontal ramus of the left mandible, with fixation and violaceous discoloration of the overlying skin. The left lower lip scar was clinically tumor-free. Facial nerve function and the cervical nodes were normal. Examination of the oral cavity revealed advanced periodontal disease. The mass obliterated the left mandibular gingivobuccal sulcus and bulged into the left floor of mouth. No ulcerations or mucosal abnormalities were noted, and indirect laryngoscopy was unremarkable.

Needle aspiration cytology of the mass revealed squamous cell carcinoma, which with the clinical picture suggested metastatic lip cancer to facial artery lymph nodes (N2a). Chest roentgenogram and liver function tests were normal. Computed tomography (CT) of the head and neck demonstrated a 3.5 × 4.0 cm soft tissue mass wrapped around the inferior border of the left mandible. The bone was intact, but the overlying skin and the inferior pole of the parotid gland were invaded. Posteriorly, the mass impinged on the musculature of the base of tongue and oropharynx. There was no pterygoid involvement.

The patient was presented at the weekly Head and Neck Tumor Board conference. The treatment options favored by the discussants included radical surgery and postoperative radiotherapy versus neoadjuvant chemotherapy, radical surgery, and postoperative chemotherapy plus radiation. Because the explosive rate of tumor growth suggested high responsiveness to cytotoxic agents, the latter option was recommended by the Board and accepted by the patient.

The chemotherapy regimen included cisplatin, methotrexate, and 5-fluorouracil. Unfortunately, therapy was complicated by nausea, vomiting, and severe mucositis, and it became clear during the second cycle of chemotherapy that the tumor was again progressing rapidly. The patient noted increasing trismus due to tumor mass effect, the left mandibular teeth were becoming increasingly misaligned, and the skin overlying the tumor was starting to break down. Repeat CT scan (Fig. 1–2) showed the now 8.0 × 8.0 cm mass to extend from the lower vertical mandibular ramus down to the level of the hyoid bone. There was extensive skin involvement, mandibular destruction, and invasion of or encroachment on the deep musculature of the lateral oral and pharyngeal tongue. The cervical nodes remained within normal limits. The patient's course and status were presented to the Tumor Board, and radical surgical excision was recommended. The surgical approach was discussed in detail by the head

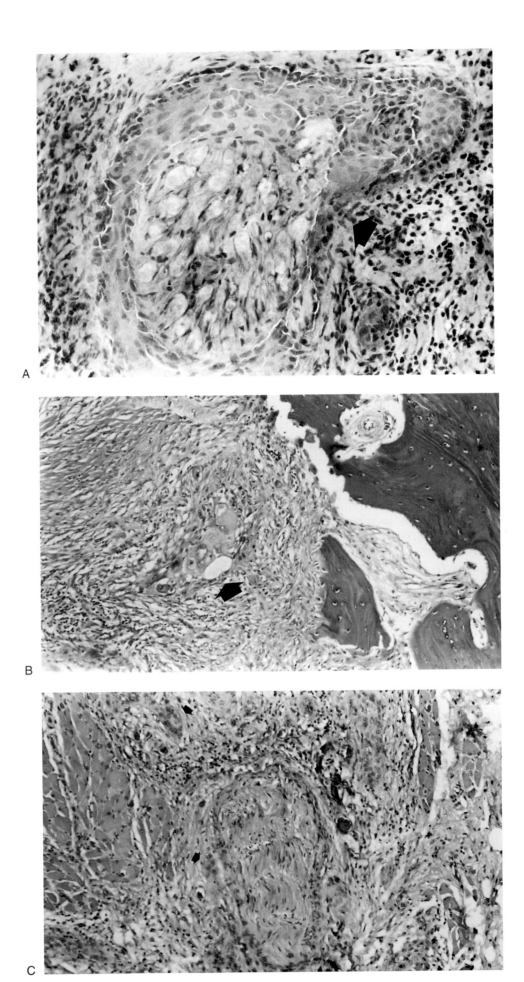

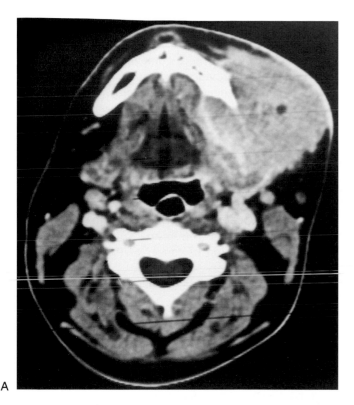
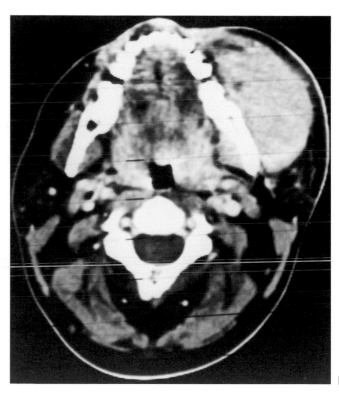

A

B

FIG. 1–2. Computed tomography scan of the tumor after two courses of chemotherapy, during which the lesion had progressed. The coronal view through the inferior border of the horizontal mandibular ramus (**A**) shows bony destruction, extensive skin involvement, invasion of the deep musculature of the floor of mouth and lateral anterior tongue, and possible encroachment on the oropharynx and base of tongue. Involvement of these latter structures is shown to better advantage on coronal section through the lower ascending mandibular ramus (**B**).

and neck surgeons, plastic surgeons, and oral surgeons in attendance. As the extent of soft tissue involvement would necessitate through-and-through resection of much of the cheek, a rectus abdominis myocutaneous free flap was recommended as the best of several reconstructive alternatives. Immediate mandibular reconstruction was deemed inadvisable because postoperative radiotherapy to high doses was planned, and the risk of microscopic margin involvement and early tumor relapse was high.

The operation consisted of tracheostomy and left radical neck dissection en bloc with resection of the tumor mass and left hemimandible from condylar neck to mentum, the inferior one half of the parotid, the cervicomandibular division of the facial nerve, cheek skin, left buccal mucosa, and floor of mouth, some deep musculature of the anterior and pharyngeal tongue, and the left hypoglossal nerve. The resulting defects in the oral mucosa and facial skin measured 6 × 9 cm and 12 × 24 cm, respectively. Frozen section histology confirmed that all surgical margins were free of tumor. All remaining teeth were extracted, and the oral cavity mucosal defect was closed primarily. In reconstructing the cheek, the rectus flap vessels were anastomosed to the spared left jugular vein and the transverse cervical artery.

The tumor mass, measuring 6 × 6 × 6 cm, had invaded and destroyed the mandible (see Fig. 1–1B). None of the 70 identified cervical lymph nodes was involved by tumor.

Recovery was uneventful with successful take of the flap. Postoperative radiotherapy consisted of 4 MeV photons through right and left lateral base of skull/upper neck ports to a dose of 30 Gy, and 18 MeV electrons to the left lateral base of skull and neck to a dose of 28.8 Gy.

FIG. 1–1. A: Photomicrograph of the original squamous cell lip cancer, demonstrating invasion of the perineural space (*arrow*) around a peripheral trunk of the mental nerve. **B:** Histopathology of the mandibular mass, showing infiltration and destruction of bone by poorly differentiated squamous cell carcinoma (*arrow*); note the extensive desmoplastic reaction in the marrow space around this nest of tumor cells. **C:** Photomicrograph of the resected lower lip recurrence showing tumor infiltration into the soft tissues and perineural spaces (*arrows*).

He remained clinically disease-free until December 1991 when he presented with a 1.0-cm nodule at the site of the previous lip surgery that had developed over the preceding week. There was no cervical adenopathy. Biopsy confirmed recurrent squamous cell carcinoma (rT1 N0 M0). Because of the rapidity of growth, immediate radical surgery was recommended; 75% of the lower lip was excised with preservation of the right oral commissure, suturing skin primarily to mucosa. Reconstruction was deferred pending histologic confirmation of complete excision of the recurrent tumor and a 6-month period of observation postoperatively.

Histopathology revealed a poorly differentiated squamous cell carcinoma with perineural invasion (see Fig. 1–1C). The surgical margins were free of disease, the closest margin being 1.3 cm from microscopic tumor.

He wore simple gauze dressings over the lip defect in the interim, and was able to control his oral incompetence using a variety of strategies. The lip was reconstructed in June, 1992, with a right fan flap (1) and a small left Estlander flap, providing good balance between upper and lower lips with moderate but acceptable microstomia. He recovered satisfactorily, with good oral competence due in part to the moderate degree of tautness in the reconstructed lower lip. He remains disease-free.

REFERENCES

1. Gillies Sir H, Millard DR Jr. *The Principles and Art of Plastic Surgery,* vol 1., Boston: Little, Brown & Co. 1957:507–8.

COMMENTARY by Jatin P. Shah

The first report of neoplastic invasion of nerves was made by Cruvhelhier in 1842 and, 20 years later, Newmann reported a case of carcinoma of the lower lip extending into both mental nerves (1,2). Spread of tumor along nerves was attributed to perineural lymphatic spread by Ernst (3). However, a more contemporary definition of neurotropism was provided by Jentzer, "Carcinoma cells have a particular tendency to grow along nerve trunks and their sheaths and to reproduce carcinomatous foci in nerves at a distance from the primary tumor" (4). The frequency of neurotropism varies tremendously and is reported to be as low as 2% for cancer of the lip and as high as 72% in patients with adenoid cystic carcinoma (5,6). Goepfert reported 14% of patients with skin carcinoma manifesting neurotropism and Soo reported 27% of patients with upper aerodigestive tract squamous cell carcinomas manifesting neurotropism (7,8). In a review of 80 patients with extension of cancer of the head and neck through peripheral nerves, Ballantyne reported a significant death rate and observed that perineural spread may be asymptomatic or patients may have minor complaints of burning, stinging, or shooting pain; however, numbness in the distribution of the nerve in question was reported as "almost pathognomic of nerve involvement" (9). In two different reports from the M.D. Anderson Hospital, it was noted that the head and neck is especially prone to perineural extension to the central nervous system and that in cancers of the lip and skin of the head and neck, nerve involvement is associated with a significant increase in lymph node metastasis (5,7). Neurotropism is also manifested in patients with malignant melanoma (10).

In the patient presented above, the potential for extension of squamous cell carcinoma of the lower lip along the mental nerve into the mandibular canal should have been suspected upon receipt of the histologic diagnosis of "squamous carcinoma of the lower lip with perineural invasion." In patients with such histologic diagnosis, it is imperative that adequate radiographic studies be performed to assess the potential invasion of the inferior alveolar nerve via the mental nerve. A simple panoramic X-

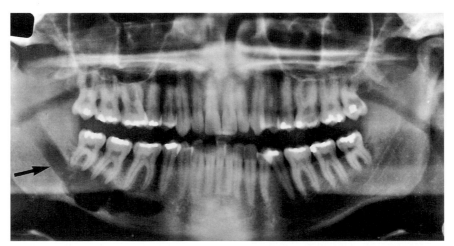

Fig. 1–3. Panoramic radiograph of the mandible showing expansion of the right inferior alveolar canal secondary to neural involvement from cancer of the lower lip.

ray of the mandible may reveal widening of the inferior alveolar canal secondary to nerve invasion long before the patient develops any symptoms (see Fig. 1–1). Once invasion of the inferior alveolar nerve is documented either by clinical findings, radiographic studies, or operative findings, the surgical procedure should encompass resection of the entire third division of the 5th cranial nerve up to the base of the skull. Often, skip areas of tumor invasion are observed in grossly normal looking nerve. Invasion of the mandibular canal and inferior alveolar nerve by cancer mandates a hemimandibulectomy to encompass all gross disease. The need for adjuvant radiation therapy is clear and should be considered in every instance in which soft tissue disease is documented along the mental foramen from recurrent cancer. The radiation portals in that situation should extend up to the base of the skull to include the gasserian ganglion, which may be the most proximal part of the central nervous system involved by recurrent cancer. Clearly, patients with tumor extension up to the base of the skull carry a significantly poor prognosis compared with those with limited neural invasion. Reconstruction of the resected mandible should be decided upon several factors, including the overall prognosis of the patient, the risk of local recurrence, general condition of the patient to withstand a microvascular composite free-flap reconstruction, and the suitability of the surgical defect in terms of the extent of bone loss, soft tissue loss, and mucosal or skin loss as a result of tumor resection.

Clearly, neurotropism by squamous carcinomas and melanomas of the skin, lip, and mucosa of the upper aerodigestive tract is an established phenomenon. Pathology reports of a primary tumor indicating "neural invasion" should alert the clinician regarding the possibility of cranial nerve involvement and the need for appropriate investigations to make an earlier diagnosis to implement aggressive treatment and potentially successful outcome.

REFERENCES

1. Cruvhelhier J. *Anatomic Pathologique du Corps Humain*. Paris, 1835.
2. Newmann E. *Arch Path Anat* 1862:24:201.
3. Ernst P. *Beitr Path Anat* 1905:Suppl. 7:29.
4. Jentzer A. *Schweiz Med Wchnschr* 1930:60:1050.
5. Byers RM, O'Brien J, Waxler J. The therapeutic and prognostic implications of nerve invasion in cancer of the lower lip. *Int J Rad Oncol Biol Phys* 1978:4:215–7.
6. Van der Waal JE, Snow GB, Van der Waal I. Intra-oral adenoid cystic carcinoma. *Cancer* 1920:66:2031–3.
7. Goepfert H, Dichtel WJ, Medina JE, et al. Perineural invasion in squamous cell carcinoma of the head and neck. *Am J Surg* 1984:148:542–7.
8. Soo KC, Carter RL, O'Brien CJ, et al. Prognostic implications of perineural spread in squamous carcinomas of the head and neck. *Laryngoscope* 1986:96:1145–8.
9. Ballantyne AJ, McCarten AB, Ibanez ML. The extension of cancer of the head and neck through peripheral nerves. *Am J Surg* 1963:106:651–67.
10. Reed RJ, Leonard DD. Neurotropic melanoma. *Am J Surg Pathol* 1979:3:301–11.

2

Stage II Squamous Cell Carcinoma of the Lateral Oral Tongue

Robert M. Byers

An ideal patient for surgical care

CASE PRESENTATION

A 21-year-old white man had a sore on the left side of his tongue for several months. The area persisted and slowly enlarged so that by 5 months later it was quite painful and made it difficult for him to articulate and swallow. He denies any associated ear pain, tongue numbness, paresthesia, weight loss, or bleeding. He has been in good general health with no associated medical problems and is taking no medications. A biopsy revealed poorly differentiated infiltrating squamous carcinoma grade III. The social history reveals that he has been smoking cigarettes since the age of 11, up to a pack per day. Intraoral exam shows a 2.5 × 2.5 × 1-cm lesion located in the middle third of the lateral border of the left side of his tongue with good mobility (Fig. 2–1). The lesion is ulcerative and does not extend down into the floor of the mouth. It does not cross the midline, is anterior to the circumvallate papillae, and infiltrates minimally into the substance of the tongue. The teeth are in good repair and examination with indirect laryngoscopy reveals no abnormalities. Examination of the neck reveals a 1-cm, very soft, subdigastric lymph node on the left side thought to be clinically negative (Fig. 2–2). The remainder of his complete physical examination is unremarkable. Thus, this patient has a T2 N0 biopsy-proven squamous cell carcinoma of the lateral oral tongue. His work-up included a chest roentgenogram, which was clear, and CBC, SMA, urinalysis, coagulation profile, all of which were within normal limits.

This patient was presented at the Planning Conference, which included surgeons, radiotherapists, and medical oncologists. The options concerning his treatment included radiotherapy alone, surgery alone, or combined treatment. The plan of treatment consisted of intraoral surgical resection of the primary and a supraomohyoid selective neck dissection (Fig. 2–3). Thirty-four lymph nodes were removed from the left side of his neck, none of which contained metastatic disease. The submandibular gland was unremarkable and the partial glossectomy revealed superficially invasive grade II–grade III squamous cell carcinoma, margins free (Fig. 2–4). His postoperative course was uneventful and he was discharged on the fourth postoperative day. Again, the patient was presented for discussion as to the follow-up treatment. Based on his pathologic findings, no postoperative radiation was suggested and he should be followed on a routine basis. I might add that because of his young age and the histologic appearance of the tumor, a neck dissection was suggested to be included with his primary resection. He has been followed on a routine basis since his surgery. Repeated chest roentgenograms were clear for 5 years. Two years postoperatively he developed some palpable lymphadenopathy in the submental triangle. They were removed under local anesthesia and revealed pathologically two lymph nodes, no tumor present. He has continued to be followed and was last seen 5 years postoperatively, at which time he was free of any disease, swallowing well, had good articulation, and was given a return for 1 year.

In summary, this is a young patient, under the age of 30 years, who developed squamous cell carcinoma of his oral tongue, was treated with surgery only, and is free of disease more than 5 years after completion of his treatment.

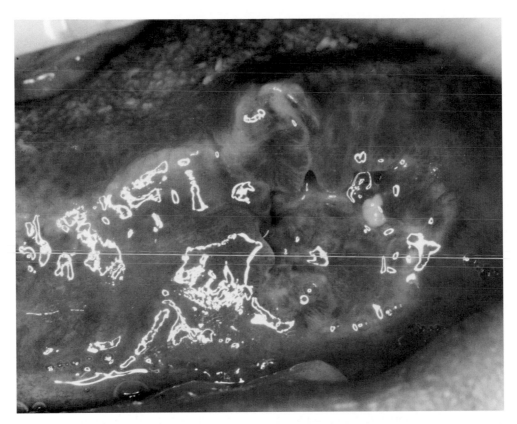

FIG. 2–1. Ulcerative squamous cell carcinoma of the lateral oral tongue in this young male patient.

COMMENTARY by William R. Panje

I concur with Dr. Byers' management of this case. The head and neck oncology literature likewise support this treatment. Transoral excisions of small (<4 cm) oral cavity cancers and a discontinuous supraomohyoid neck dissection performed properly are oncologically sound (1,2). The fact that radiation therapy was avoided, at least initially, is justifiable, based on the patient's young age and the presence of histopathologically negative upper cervical lymphatics.

Some points germane to this case include preoperative evaluation, transoral removal of oral cavity cancers,

Elective Neck Dissection
Percent Pathologically Positive Nodes

ORAL TONGUE

Type of Neck Dissection:

- Unilateral Supraomohyoid (regardless of T-stage)
- 4% Bilateral

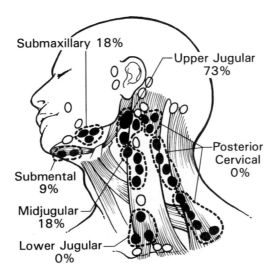

Submaxillary 18%

Upper Jugular 73%

Posterior Cervical 0%

Submental 9%

Midjugular 18%

Lower Jugular 0%

FIG. 2–2. Relative risk of each nodal group to contain occult disease if removed electively with a neck dissection.

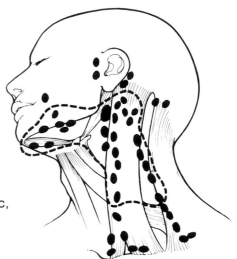

Supraomohyoid:

Lip, skin of face, oral cavity, oropharynx: submental, submandibular, subdigastric, midjugular, upper and middle posterior cervical.

FIG. 2–3. Nodal groups removed with a supraomohyoid neck dissection and the sites of the primary for which this selective neck dissection would be appropriate.

supraomohyoid neck dissection, and postoperative follow-up.

In the preoperative evaluation of this high-risk patient I would obtain a contrast-enhanced CT scan of the head and neck as well as perform endoscopy and tumor mapping under general anesthesia. An enhanced head and neck CT scan obtained before biopsy of the primary are useful in determining the tumor size and extension. Because tongue cancers have a high incidence of occult cervical metastasis (>55%) with contralateral spread, the infused CT scan is helpful in delineating potential pathological lymph nodes (3). Clinical detection of regional metastasis

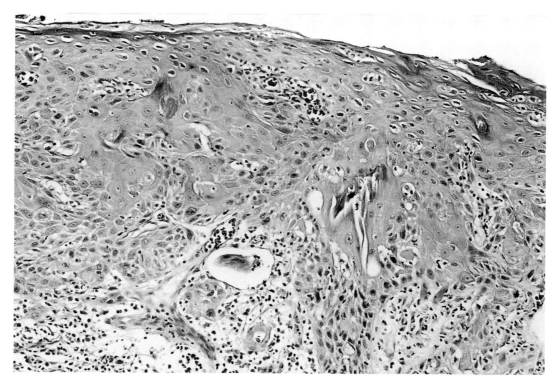

FIG. 2–4. Invasive grade II–III squamous carcinoma of tongue. Typical of oral mucosal squamous carcinoma, the lesion is heterogeneous and "zonated." The more superficial elements are relatively well differentiated. In contrast, tumor cells at the invasive interface between carcinoma and normal tissue are poorly differentiated. In addition, there is invasion of superficial lymphatics.

by palpation is highly unreliable. The importance of a complete preoperative evaluation, including endoscopy with tumor mapping, cannot be overemphasized. A 6% incidence of synchronous head and neck primaries with an exceptionally high incidence of secondary esophagus cancers with oral cavity cancer should encourage the head and neck surgeon to employ preoperative endoscopy. Tongue cancers are especially difficult to palpate in the awake patient. Pain and apprehension preclude any real meaningful digital or bimanual assessment of tumor infiltration or extension. General anesthesia allows for relaxation with a better overall assessment of tumor induration.

The transoral removal of small oral cavity neoplasms can offer a relatively less morbid and quicker approach to the primary cancer ablation (4). The high incidence of positive surgical margins and local-regional recurrences after excision of small oral cavity cancers suggest a technical rather than biologic basis (5,6). Exposure, immobility, and method of ablation are all important considerations in removing tongue cancers. Inadequate exposure, that is, the inability to see and palpate all sides of the lesion, are a contraindication to using a transoral approach for tumor ablation. The lesion is exposed and firmly held in position during the removal. General anesthesia with muscle paralysis helps to prevent tongue retraction and contraction, both primary reasons for a haphazard and incomplete removal. Instrumentation used in the transoral removal of cancers may also contribute to local regional recurrences. A clean cold knife excision of a tongue neoplasm is difficult because of bleeding. Diathermy or monopolar cautery ablation, although hemostatic, causes muscle contraction and retraction, potentiating unsure margins and possible cancer dissemination. Laser (CO_2, Nd-YAG, KTP) allows for microscopic hemostatic-controlled neoplasm removal without muscle contraction. Transgression of the cancer with a laser beam produces lymphatic "sealing" and prevents cancer seeding. The lesion can either be laser-removed as a specimen similar to a knife excision or vaporized and margins assessed intraoperatively. The head and neck laser surgeon should consult with the pathologist regarding specimen margin assessment after laser excision.

Because of limited space I will not expand on the rationale of supraomohyoid neck dissection other than to emphasize the works of Byers and Barton. The report of Byers et al. on histopathologic examination of neck dissection specimens as related to primary site of origin revealed no lower jugular or posterior triangle nodes in N0-electively dissected neck specimens for oral tongue primaries (7). A supraomohyoid neck dissection removes ipsilateral nodal stations associated with small oral tongue cancers. Schuller believes that a supraomohyoid neck dissection is adequate for treating T1 and T2 oral cavity cancers (8). Barton addressed the surgical management of small oral cavity cancer in continuity with a supraomohyoid neck dissection (Mono bloc dissection)

(9). Essentially, the technique is an oncologically valid method for managing T1 and T2 oral cavity cancers with histologically negative cervical adenopathy. Controversy surrounds the issue of supraomohyoid neck dissections (10).

Finally, the head and neck oncologic surgeon should perform surveillance and chemoprevention. The excellent work of Ki Hong substantiates that chemoprevention is useful in managing precancerous and second malignancies of the upper aerodigestive tract (11,12). Other oncologists are finding vitamin A derivatives as well as vitamins C and E and selenium, in addition to cruciferous vegetables, important nutritional sources in preventing upper aerodigestive tract cancer. Discontinuance of tobacco and excessive alcohol as well as avoidance of exposure to other carcinogens (i.e., asbestos) is important for any head and neck cancer patient. Surveillance should include close follow-up using oral cavity microscopic and cytologic examination. The use of vital dyes [e.g., toluidine blue and photo active dyes (HPD)] are helpful in identifying precancerous and cancerous lesions of the upper aerodigestive tract.

REFERENCES

1. Strong MS, Vaughn CW, Healey GB, Shapshay SM, Jako GJ. Transoral management of localized carcinoma of the oral cavity using the CO_2 laser. *Laryngoscope* 1979:89:897–905.
2. Strong EW. Carcinoma of the tongue. *Otolaryngol Clin North Am* 1979:12:107–14.
3. Freidman M, et al. The Role of Computed Tomographic Scanning in Evaluating the Clinically Negative Neck. In: *Proc Head and Neck Cancer, vol 2, 1988.* Fee, Jr, WE, Ed. B.C. Decker, Inc; 1990:138–44.
4. Panje WR, Scher N, Karnell M. Transoral carbon dioxide laser for cancer, tumors, and other diseases. *Arch Otolaryngol* 1989:115: 681–8.
5. Berkett PR, Miller GF. Mucosal tattooing in oral cavity carcinoma. *Otolaryngol Head Neck Surg* 1979:87:775.
6. Panje WR, Smith B, McCabe BF. Epidermoid carcinoma of the floor of mouth: surgical therapy versus combination therapy versus radiation therapy. *Otolaryngol Head Neck Surg* 1980:88:714.
7. Byers RM, Wolf PF, Ballantyne AJ. Rationale for elective modified neck dissection. *Head Neck Surg* 1988:10:160–7.
8. Schuller DE, Caputo ME. Surgical management of the N0 neck. In: *Proc Head and Neck Cancer, Vol 2, 1988,* Fee, Jr, WE, ed. B.C. Decker Inc; 1990:150–2.
9. Barton RT, UcMakli A. The treatment of squamous cell carcinoma of the floor of the mouth. *Surg Gynecol Obstet* 1977:145:2127.
10. Collins SL: Controversies in management of cancer of the neck. In: *Comprehensive Management of Head and Neck Tumors.* S Thawley S, Panje W, eds. Philadelphia: WB Saunders; 1987:1386–43.
11. Hong WK, Lippman SM, Itri L, et al. Prevention of second primary tumors with isotretinoin in squamous cell carcinoma of the head and neck. *N Engl J Med* 1990:323:795.
12. Heyne LKE, Lippman EM, Hong WK. Chemoprevention in head and neck cancer. *Hematol/Oncol Clin North Am* 1991:5:783–5.

EDITORIAL BOARD COMMENTARY

Patients with head and neck cancers should be routinely evaluated for the development of second primary cancers of the head and neck.

3 Stage IV Carcinoma of the Posterior Third of the Tongue

Benjamin F. Rush, Jr.

Preservation of function is a primary goal

CASE PRESENTATION

Dr. Tavarone: W.B. is a 52-year-old Caucasian man with a long history of ethanol and tobacco abuse who presented with a 2-month history of pain on the left jaw and neck with increasing severity. He also suffered from crescendo dysphagia tolerant to soft foods and liquids at the time of admission. He had previously been seen at another hospital where a biopsy of the posterior tongue was reported as a poorly differentiated squamous cell carcinoma. Review of systems revealed a productive cough and mild dyspnea on exertion. There was no dyspnea at rest. The patient admitted to a 76 pack-per-year tobacco history with a heavy ethanol intake. The patient had undergone hip arthroplasty 5 years earlier and a tonsillectomy as a child.

Physical examination revealed a Caucasian man who appeared somewhat older than his stated age. His vital signs were normal. Examination of the eyes and ears was not remarkable. On examination of the oral cavity, it was noted that the patient had difficulty protruding his tongue past his lips and that there was a pronounced elevation on the left tongue posteriorly at the level of the circumvallate papillae. Bimanual palpation at this point showed a mass occupying the posterior third of the tongue and descending near but not to the vallecula. The mass extended to the left side of the tongue and was deeply invading the tongue muscle. It also crossed the midline. It should be noted that the patient's voice had a "potato in the mouth quality." There was no palpable cervical adenopathy. The remainder of the patient's physical exam was unremarkable, and he was admitted with a diagnosis of squamous cell carcinoma of the posterior

tongue that was considered stage IV based on the size of the lesion and the deep invasion of the glossal musculature. Laboratory reports were unremarkable except for mildly elevated liver function tests. Chest film showed no evidence of metastatic lesions. Fiberoptic laryngoscopy confirmed the presence of the large mass in the posterior tongue as well as a shallow ulceration at the left center of the posterior tongue area. A computerized tomography (CT) scan of the oral cavity and neck was obtained.

Dr. Lee (radiologist): As is clearly seen on the CT, the left side of the tongue is occupied by an enhancing mass that crosses over to the right side (Fig. 3–1). There is some thickening of the lateral pharyngeal wall, which may be edema or tumor invasion. Inferior cuts show the tumor invading deeply within the muscle, as was the impression on physical examination. There is no evidence of nodal involvement on either side of the neck.

Dr. Rush (surgical oncology): This patient was sent to me for consideration for operation. In patients such as this, there are several options available. Surgery as the initial step would require the removal of the entire tongue because the removal of most of the posterior and mid-tongue would have led to loss of the blood supply to the anterior tongue. Total glossectomy would have required relining of the floor of the mouth, probably by a pectoralis major myocutaneous flap. This still leaves the problem of how the patient will swallow without aspirating. In the past, the solution to this problem was always to do a total laryngectomy with the total glossectomy. The argument for this was that without a tongue the patient couldn't talk anyway. Another solution to the problem is to suture the epiglottis almost entirely closed

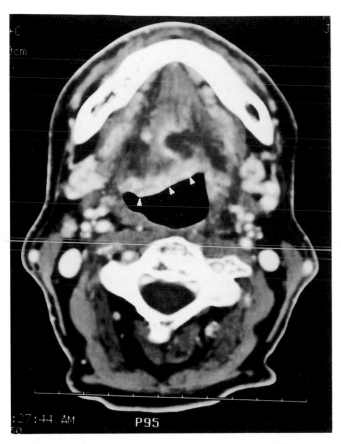

FIG. 3–1. Carcinoma of the posterior tongue. The tumor (*arrows*) shows an increased density because of the uptake of contrast material.

so it serves as a vent that rises above the fluids being swallowed. Patients can create sound through the vent but are unable to breathe through it, so a tracheostomy is required. Even without a tongue, patients can make themselves understood moderately well but usually only to people who know them and individuals who are used to dealing with severely impaired speech. The patient, of course, will have lost all taste and will be required to breathe through a tracheostomy. Another option would be to attempt organ preservation by primary treatment of the local lesion with radiation and/or chemotherapy, together with the treatment of cervical metastases through radical neck dissection. There is no evidence that survival by this technique is any better than with primary excision alone. However, control of primary lesions by combined radiochemotherapy has been excellent in recent trials, especially when radiation is boosted by brachytherapy because it offers the possibility of saving vital structures. After discussing all these options with the patient, he elected to attempt organ preservation and on September 3, 1992, the patient underwent a panendoscopy, repeat biopsy, and placement of mediport.

Dr. Pliner (medical oncology): The chemotherapy of choice for squamous cell carcinoma of the head and neck, currently, is cisplatin, 5-fluorouracil (5-FU), and leukovorin. The addition of leukovorin greatly enhances the effects of 5-FU and may result in an increased response rate. Previously untreated squamous cell cancers of the oral cavity and oral pharynx respond remarkably well to this regimen with total response rates as high as 90% reported by some. Complete response rates are between 50% and 60%. On the other hand, this is only a temporary response and even the complete responders can be expected to show an early recurrence after the termination of chemotherapy. The patient was begun on a week's course of cisplatin, 5-FU, and leukovorin while still in the hospital and was discharged after a week of treatment. He received a second course a month later and 3 weeks later had demonstrated an excellent regression of more than 50%, although tumor could still be palpated in the posterior tongue.

Dr. Cathcart (radiation oncologist): The patient was treated with opposed lateral portals of the oropharynx, which measured 12 × 12 cm. These fields included the primary tumor and upper lymphatics of the neck. The lower neck and supraclavicular lymphatics were treated with an adjoining AP field. After reaching a dose of 4,140 cGy, a cone-down of the lateral portals was done to exclude the spinal cord from photon irradiation. Radiation therapy to the primary tumor continued to a dose of 5,040 cGy with photon beam, and the posterior neck was treated with 8 MeV electrons to a dose of 5,040 cGy. A midline block was added to the supraclavicular field at 4500- cGy and the treatment continued to 5,040 cGy.

Dr. Rush (surgical oncology): On January 12, 1993, 1 month after his radiation was complete, he was readmitted to the surgical service to be evaluated for subsequent operation. At this time, he had lost 27% of his original body weight and was started on a course of enteral nutritional support for 2 weeks, which resulted in a weight gain of 15 pounds. On January 26, 1993, a radical neck dissection was performed together with a tracheostomy. After the neck dissection, a lateral pharyngoscopy was performed and a substantial biopsy taken from the midtongue. At this time, the tongue had regained partial mobility, although speech was still slurred. Biopsy was done in an area that appeared to be firm. Frozen section showed residual carcinoma. The radiotherapist placed several brachytherapy needles for subsequent implantation of iridium seeds. The incision in the hypopharynx was closed and the neck dissection flap was restored and sutured in place.

Dr. Cathcart (radiation oncology): Seventy-two hours after this surgery, iridium seeds were placed in the various catheters and a total additional dose of 3,000 cGy was delivered to the base of the tongue. Insertion of iridium seeds proceeded without incident and a distributed dose was delivered to the posterior third of the tongue (Fig. 3–2).

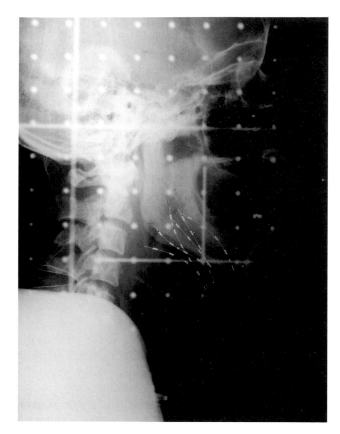

FIG. 3–2. Brachytherapy to the posterior tongue. The iridium seeds are distributed within the catheters embedded in the tumor.

Dr. Adesokan (pathologist): Examination of the biopsy specimen taken at surgery shows inflammation and scarring. There are still islands of squamous cell carcinoma scattered throughout the muscular bed of the tongue up to the edge of the biopsy specimen. Although the previous biopsy of the tongue had been read as an undifferentiated lesion, we concluded that this biopsy is moderately differentiated. There are not many keratin pearls, but there are numerous intracellular bridges (Fig. 3–3). There were 30 nodes removed at surgery, none of which contained cancer.

Rene Kaufman (speech pathologist): The patient is now more than a month since completion of therapy and at this time has regained a substantial amount of mobility in his tongue, although it is still somewhat tied down on the left. His speech has become much less slurred and his swallowing is normal. There is no evidence of aspiration or residual dysphasia. Much of the substantial weight loss observed during treatment resulted from this large tumor, which distorted his oral pharynx, and by the edema and inflammation produced by chemotherapy and radiation therapy.

Dr. Cathcart (radiation oncology): One of the hazards of radiation therapy in this area is the loss of nutrition provoked by the increasing inability to swallow. In the earlier days of radiation therapy up to a third of the patients would die during the course of treatment primarily from their depleted nutritional state, which led to pneumonia or other problems. The use of parenteral or enteral nutritional support either during or after radiation therapy has improved patient management.

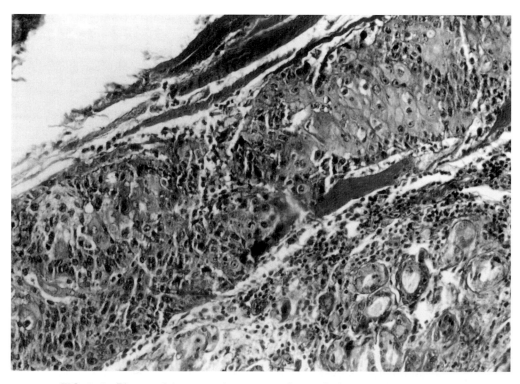

FIG. 3–3. Biopsy of the posterior tongue after radiation and chemotherapy.

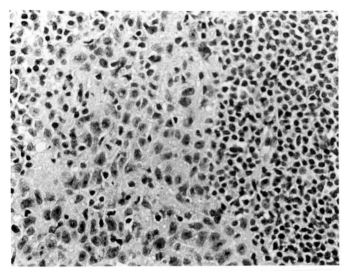

FIG. 4–1. Nonkeratinizing, poorly differentiated squamous cell carcinoma from a cervical lymph node (×200)

combination of chemotherapy and radiotherapy off protocol. The reverse sequence of the intergroup investigational arm was started.

Treatment

Induction chemotherapy with three cycles of cisplatin and 5-FU (cisplatin 100 mg/m^2 and 5-FU 1,000 mg/m^2 per day given by continuous infusion for 5 days) was given at 3-week intervals starting on April 27, 1992. This was followed by concomitant radiation therapy started 3 months later and cisplatin at the same dose given at 3-week intervals.

The patient underwent the prescribed course of therapy. The first cycle of induction chemotherapy was complicated by prolonged neutropenia and the cisplatin dose was decreased to 80 mg/m^2 in subsequent cycles. Other than mild, grade I mucositis, he had no problems during induction chemotherapy.

The cervical nodes disappeared completely after induction chemotherapy. Clinical otolaryngologic examination showed a small 1.0×0.5–cm lesion in the right fossa of Rosenmuller. CT scan (Fig. 4–3) showed regression of the primary tumor. No enlarged cervical lymph nodes were noted.

The combined radiation therapy and chemotherapy was complicated by mucositis and vomiting requiring intravenous fluids on one occasion. The patient also complained of loss of taste and developed thrush during the treatment. He lost 30 lbs (12% of body weight) by the end of treatment.

Radiation dose was 7,000 cGy to the primary site, 7,000 cGy to the left neck, 6,000 cGy to the right neck, and 5,000 cGy to the supraclavicular areas.

Nasopharyngoscopy after the completion of therapy showed a complete response with no evidence of tumor in the nasopharynx.

The patient is alive and free of disease 20 months post-treatment.

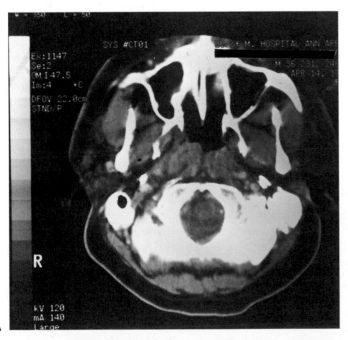
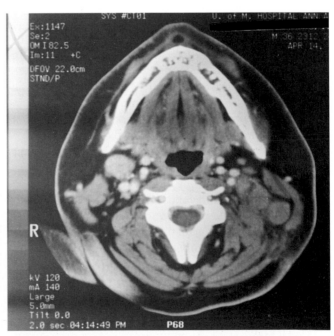

FIG. 4–2. CT of the head and neck. **A:** There is fullness of the posterior pharyngeal tissue. The mass is more prominent on the right in the region of the lateral pharyngeal recess. **B:** Extensive lymph node metastases, more prominent on the right than on the left.

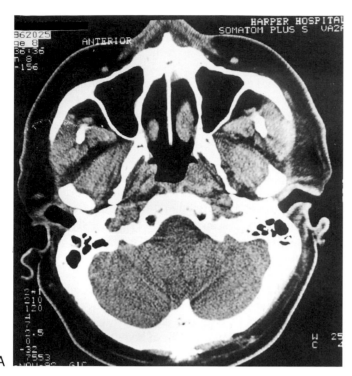
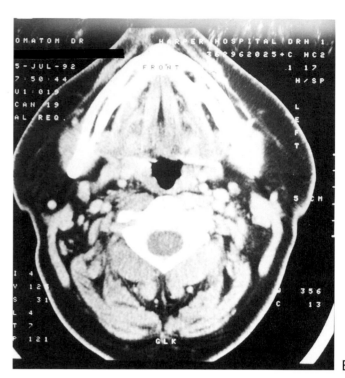

A

B

FIG. 4–3. Post-treatment CT. **A:** Regression of the nasopharyngeal mass. **B:** Post-treatment response of the enlarged cervical lymph nodes.

Discussion

Nasopharyngeal carcinoma (NPC) is a rare neoplasm of the head and neck region in the United States and Western Europe. It is more common among the Southern Chinese (Canton Province), Southeast Asian, Northern African, and Eskimo populations. It is a common tumor in the migrants of the countries to North America (i.e., Chinese in San Francisco and British Columbia) or Western Europe (i.e., Libyans in Italy; Algerians and Moroccans in France). With the increase of migration from Southeast Asia to Southern California and other coastal areas, there has been an increase in the incidence of NPC in these regions.

Nasopharyngeal cancer differs from other malignant tumors of the head and neck in many aspects. There is no clear association to smoking, the incidence of lymph node metastasis at presentation or overall nodal disease is much higher (80–90%), the incidence of systemic involvement is higher (>30%), and age of presentation, sex, and pathology differs. The most common pathologic types are:

1. Keratinizing squamous cell carcinoma (WHO I)
2. Nonkeratinizing squamous cell carcinoma or transitional cell carcinoma (WHO II)
3. Undifferentiated carcinoma or lympho-epithelioma (WHO III).

The last two pathologic types are the most common cancers reported from the high prevalence countries and in migrants of these countries to North America and Western Europe. Also, these two types may present in a much younger age group, with no differences in incidence between the sexes. Another difference is the high sensitivity of these lesions to radiotherapy.

Because of the location of these tumors, they are traditionally treated by radiotherapy (RT). The incidence of local control of NPC with radiation treatment is very high (75%). The incidence of locoregional control and 5-year survival for RT alone depend on the stage of the disease. Excellent results are observed for stage I (T1 N0 M0) and stage II (T2 N0 M0) cancers; however, the best 5-year survival reported for stage IV is less than 30%. Despite the high complete response of stages III and IV to RT, the rate of local failure is about 50% to 80%.

NPC is responsive to systemic chemotherapy, especially to platinol-based combinations. Because of the poor results obtained with RT in locally advanced stages, combined modality therapy with the addition of chemotherapy have produced good results. The most common sequence of treatments are induction chemotherapy followed by RT, or concurrent cisplatin and radiation treatment. The most common and effective induction chemotherapy given is cisplatin and 5-FU 120-hr infusion for two to three courses every 3 weeks. More recently, both induction and concurrent chemoradiotherapy have been piloted. The improved results of these phase II trials led to the initiation and activation of the

National Intergroup Nasopharyngeal Randomized Phase III Study.

SELECTED READINGS

1. Ho HC. Epidemiology of nasopharyngeal carcinoma. *J Roy Coll Surg* 1975:20:223.
2. Qin D, Hu Y, Yan J, et al. Analysis of 1379 patients with nasopharyngeal carcinoma treated by radiation. *Cancer* 1988:61:1117–24.
3. Decker D, Drelichman A, Al-Sarraf M, et al. Chemotherapy for nasopharyngeal carcinoma: a 10 year experience. *Cancer* 1983:52: 602–5.
4. Al-Kourainy K, Crissman J, Ensley J, et al. Excellent response to cis-platinum-based chemotherapy in patients with recurrent or previously untreated advanced nasopharyngeal carcinoma. *Am J Clin Oncol* 1988:11:553–7.
5. Al-Sarraf M, Pajak TF, Cooper JS, et al. Chemo-radiotherapy in patients with locally advanced nasopharyngeal carcinoma: a Radiation Therapy Oncology Group Study. *J Clin Oncol* 1990:8:1342–51.

COMMENTARY by Arlene Forastiere

This patient's presentation is typical for cancer of the nasopharynx (NPC). Cervical lymphadenopathy brings most patients to medical attention. Other common symptoms include nasal obstruction, serous otitis media, and conduction hearing loss (1). Anatomically, the nasopharynx has a dense plexus of lymphatic vessels that allow tumor to spread to the retropharyngeal, junctional, and jugulo-digastric nodes initially, and then to the internal jugular and spinal accessory chain. Bilateral nodal involvement is present at diagnosis in approximately 50% of patients with undifferentiated (WHO III) histology and unilateral involvement is seen in 90%. Data indicate that patients with low cervical (level 4) or supraclavicular nodes have a poor prognosis compared with those with high cervical nodes. Thus, location of adenopathy appears to have greater prognostic significance than unilaterality or bilaterality (1–3).

NPC should be thought of as two diseases. WHO I behaves similarly to squamous cell carcinomas from other sites in the head and neck whereas nonkeratinizing and undifferentiated, WHO II and III, are characteristically more radiosensitive, associated with positive Epstein-Barr virus serology, present with early and more advanced neck disease, and have a higher rate of distant metastases, but better 5-year survival. The most common site for distant metastasis is bone, followed by lung and liver (3,4). Systematic evaluations before treatment have shown that subclinical metastases are present in approximately 40% of patients with undifferentiated histology and N3 disease (5). Thus, routine staging procedures should include a CT scan or MRI of the head and neck, bone scan, chest and upper abdominal CT scans, complete blood count, and serum chemistries. Serologic markers, specifically immunoglobulin G (IgG) anti–Epstein-Barr nuclear antigen, IgG and IgA against viral capsid antigen, and early antigen constitute the anti–Epstein-Barr profile.

Titers are elevated in 85% of patients with type 2 and 3 histology and 35% with type 1 histology. When followed serially, these markers may have value in predicting early relapse after successful treatment (6).

Standard treatment for NPC is radiotherapy. Local control is excellent for T1 and T2 primary tumors (>80%); in contrast, local control for T3 and T4 disease ranges from 44% to 73% (7,8). Persistent or recurrent disease is related to initial stage with T3, T4, and N3 or bulky disease having the worst outcome. It is noteworthy that the patient in the case report had T2 N2c disease with the largest node measuring 2.0 cm on clinical exam. This disease volume may be effectively controlled with careful radiotherapy treatment planning using CT or MRI. Distant metastases, however, occur in approximately 35% of individuals so staged, with most failures observed within 3 years following treatment (3,4,9). Overall, the 5-year survival rate of patients with stage IV (M0) disease is approximately 30%. These factors account for the introduction of cisplatin-based chemotherapy into the management of newly diagnosed poor prognosis patients.

Three strategies have been employed in combined modality trials for NPC: (a) chemotherapy before radiotherapy (neoadjuvant); (b) chemotherapy simultaneous with radiotherapy (concomitant); and (c) chemotherapy after radiotherapy (adjuvant). WHO II and III NPC is highly sensitive to both chemotherapy and radiotherapy. Trials using the neoadjuvant approach have uniformly shown high response rates to chemotherapy (80–95%) and suggest survival benefit for patients with T3, T4, and advanced nodal disease when compared with historic controls (10). One large multicenter randomized trial comparing neoadjuvant bleomycin, epirubicin, and cisplatin followed by radiotherapy versus radiotherapy alone has shown a significant difference in disease-free survival at 3 years, 47.7% versus 30.5%, respectively (11). Further follow-up is needed to determine the impact of this neoadjuvant chemotherapy on survival.

The concomitant approach (simultaneous radiotherapy and chemotherapy) has been evaluated in uncontrolled trials, some compared with historic controls. Benefit for T3, T4 primaries, and advanced nodal disease is suggested by these analyses with better local control and perhaps survival as well (10,12). Adjuvant chemotherapy administered after completion of radiotherapy has been evaluated in one controlled trial that did not show benefit but the chemotherapy selected was not considered to be an optimal regimen (13). Other adjuvant trials employing historic controls have suggested improved survival (10,14).

The patient chose not to participate in a national random assignment trial of radiotherapy versus concomitant radiotherapy and chemotherapy followed by adjuvant chemotherapy. The physicians elected to treat the patient with neoadjuvant chemotherapy followed by concomitant radiotherapy and chemotherapy. Toxicity was typical—myelosuppression requiring dose reduction, mucositis, and weight loss. The patient had complete resolution of his cancer and was disease-free at 20 months.

Since the time this patient was treated, the randomized trial in which he was asked to participate has been closed and the results demonstrate a highly significant difference in survival. Patients with stages III and IV (M0) nasopharyngeal cancer were randomized to standard treatment with 70 Gy of radiation or to combined modality therapy consisting of cisplatin 100 mg/m^2 day 1, 22, and 43 during radiotherapy (70 Gy) followed by cisplatin 80 mg/m^2 day 1 and 5-fluorouracil 1,000 mg/m^2/day, days 1 to 4 every 3 weeks for 3 courses. The two treatment groups were well-balanced for T and N stage, performance status, and histology. At the first planned interim analysis of this study with a total of 150 patients and median follow-up of 4 years, median progression free survival was 13 months for RT versus 52 months for RT/ chemotherapy, p<0.0001; median survival was 30 months for RT and not reached for RT/chemotherapy, and 2-year survival was 55% versus 80%, respectively, p = 0.0007. Improved local–regional control and a decrease in distant metastatic rate was also observed in patients on the combined treatment arm. These results establish a new standard for treating patients with locally advanced nasopharyngeal cancer and should be adopted by the oncology community for treatment of this disease.

REFERENCES

1. Dickson RI. Nasopharyngeal carcinoma: an evaluation of 209 patients. *Laryngoscope* 1981:91:333.
2. Neel HB III, Taylor WF. New staging system for nasopharyngeal carcinoma: Long-term outcome. *Arch Otolaryngol Head Neck Surg* 1989:115:1293.
3. Sham JST, Choy D, Choi PHK. Nasopharyngeal carcinoma: the significance of neck node involvement in relation to the pattern of distant failure. *Br J Radiol* 1990:63:108–13.
4. Ahmad A, Stefani S. Distant metastases of nasopharyngeal carcinoma: a study of 256 male patients. *J Surg Oncol* 1986:33:194–7.
5. Micheau C, Boussen H, Klijanienko J, et al. Bone marrow biopsies in patients with undifferentiated carcinoma of nasopharyngeal type. *Cancer* 1987:60:2459–64.
6. Neel HB, Taylor WF. Epstein-Barr virus related antibody. Changes in titers after therapy for nasopharyngeal carcinoma. *Arch Orolaryngol Head Neck Surg* 1900:116:1287–90.
7. Lee AWM, Poon YF, Foo W, et al. Retrospective analysis of 5037 patients with nasopharyngeal carcinoma treated during 1976-1985: overall survival and patterns of failure. *Int J Radiat Oncol Biol Phys* 1992:23:261–70.
8. Hoppe RT, Goffinet DR, Bagshaw MA. Carcinoma of the nasopharynx. Eighteen years' experience with megavoltage radiation therapy. *Cancer* 1976:37:2605–12.
9. Teo P, Tsao SY, Shiu W, et al. A clinical study of 407 cases of nasopharyngeal carcinoma in Hong Kong. *Int J Radiat Oncol Biol Phys* 1989:17:515–30.
10. Dimery IW, Hong WK. Overview of combined modality therapies for head and neck cancer. *J Natl Cancer Inst* 1993:85:95–111.
11. Cvitkovic E. Neoadjuvant chemotherapy with epirubicin, cisplatin, bleomycin in undifferentiated nasopharyngeal cancer: preliminary results of an international phase III trial. *Proc Am Soc Clin Oncol* 1994:13:283.
12. Al-Sarraf M, Pajak TF, Cooper JS, et al. Chemoradiotherapy in patients with locally advanced nasopharyngeal carcinoma: a Radiation Therapy Oncology Group study. *J Clin Oncol* 1990:8:1342–51.
13. Rossi A, Molinari R, Boracchi P, et al. Adjuvant chemotherapy with vincristine, cyclophosphamide and doxorubicin after radiotherapy in local-regional nasopharyngeal cancer: result of a 4-year multicenter randomized study. *J Clin Oncol* 1988:10:1401–10.
14. Fandi A, Altun M, Azil N, et al. Nasopharyngeal cancer: Epidemiology, staging and treatment. *Semin Oncol* 1994:21:382–97.
15. Al-Sarraf M, Le Blanc M, Giri PGS, et al. Superiority of chemo-radiotherapy (CT-RT) vs radiotherapy (RT) in patients with locally advanced nasopharyngeal cancer (NPC). Preliminary results of intergroup (0099) (SWOG 8892, RTOG 8817, ECOG 2388) randomized study. *Proc Am Soc Clin Oncol* 1996:15:313.

5

T3 Lesion of the Larynx

Ryan S. Perkins and Roger W. Byhardt

Voice preservation via a clinical trial

CASE PRESENTATION

The patient, a 59-year-old black man with a long history of excessive smoking and drinking, presented to his physician with complaints of increasing hoarseness, sore throat, dysphagia, and right-sided otalgia over a 6-week period. He also noted a 20-lb weight loss.

His past medical history was remarkable for chronic schizophrenia, which was well controlled with Haldol. He denied any drug allergies. Family history was noncontributory. He had a greater than 50 pack-per-year smoking history and was smoking two packs of cigarettes per day. He had a prior history of alcohol dependence.

Physical examination at presentation revealed a thin man without any significant shortness of breath. Karnofsky performance score was 80. Dentition was poor. No oral cavity or oropharyngeal lesions were noted. Flexible nasopharyngoscopy revealed a large right-sided exophytic lesion involving the laryngeal surface of the epiglottis extending inferiorly over the aryepiglottic fold into the right arytenoid, false cord, and true cord. The right true vocal cord was immobile. A 2-cm mobile, firm, right inferior cervical lymph node was noted.

A computed tomography (CT) scan of the head and neck showed a large enhancing mass involving the right aryepiglottic fold, pre-epiglottic space, and false cord with extensive right spinal accessory lymphadenopathy (Fig. 5–1). Pharyngoesophagram revealed a 3.5 × 3.5 cm fungating mass that compressed the right pyriform sinus.

Direct laryngoscopy revealed a large exophytic tumor starting at the laryngeal surface of the epiglottis and extended inferiorly to involve the right false cord and true vocal cord. The medial wall of the pyriform sinus was also involved. Biopsy revealed a moderately differentiated squa-

mous cell carcinoma (Fig. 5–2). Because of the advanced periodontal disease and the extent of the primary cancer, and in anticipation of future radiotherapy treatments, he was edentulated at the time of the scoping procedure.

After reviewing the pertinent details of the patient's case at the multidisciplinary ENT Tumor Board Conference, the clinical stage was determined to be American Joint Committee on Cancer (AJCC) T3 N1 M0 (stage III). Treatment options were discussed, including total laryngectomy followed by postoperative radiation therapy or definitive radiation therapy. In view of the patient's desire for cure and to preserve his larynx the otolaryngologic surgeons, radiation oncologists, and medical oncologists collectively agreed to enroll the patient in the phase III RTOG trial (91-11), which is designed to investigate strategies to preserve the larynx. This study compares conventional irradiation, concomitant chemotherapy plus irradiation, and neoadjuvant chemotherapy followed by definitive irradiation. After signing an informed consent the patient was randomized to radiation therapy with cisplatin given on days 1, 22, and 43 of the radiotherapy schedule.

He was treated with two parallel-opposed lateral head and neck fields and an abutting anterior supraclavicular field. The primary tumor and draining lymphatics were treated to 40 Gy, after which off-cord lateral fields were used to 50 Gy. Reduced lateral boost fields directed at the primary tumor were continued for an additional 20 Gy, to give a total of 70 Gy to the primary lesion. The supraclavicular region received 50 Gy. The right and left posterior necks were boosted with electron fields; the right (the side of the adenopathy) received an additional 30 Gy with electrons to a total of 70 Gy; the left received an additional 10 Gy to a total of 60 Gy. Additionally, the tracheal stoma site was treated with electrons to a total of 60 Gy. A total dose

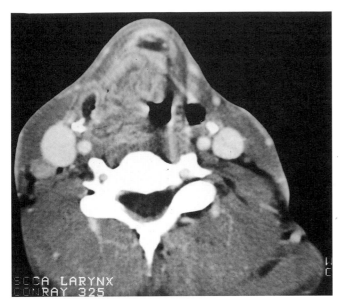

FIG. 5–1. Axial CT scan through the neck at the level of the epiglottis during the administration of intravenous contrast. There is a large enhancing mass involving the right aryepiglottic fold with extension anteriorly into the pre-epiglottic space and deformity and narrowing of the airway.

of 70 Gy in 35 fractions over 53 elapsed days was given to the area of the primary tumor and clinically involved nodes.

This therapy was tolerated well without any unusual or unexpected side effects. He was hospitalized during his cisplatin infusions. A G-tube was placed at the beginning of the treatment as acute reactions were anticipated using the combined approach. He gained 10 pounds during treatment. At completion of therapy his oral mucosa was erythematous and there were thick oral secretions. It was difficult to assess accurately the response of the tumor because of the pooled secretions. The right neck node was barely palpable.

At his first follow-up appointment 2 weeks after completing treatment, his voice quality was good and he denied any pain. The larynx was poorly visualized because of the persistent secretions. Direct laryngoscopy to biopsy any abnormal areas and to assess the response to therapy revealed an irregular area on the left laryngeal epiglottic surface with a small amount of white exudate. Biopsies were taken of this area. The arytenoids were markedly swollen but free of other abnormalities. The rest of the glottic and hypopharyngeal regions were normal appearing. A 1.5-cm firm, mobile neck mass in the right inferior neck was palpated and a fine needle aspiration was done for cytology.

The biopsies showed no residual tumor, but cytology demonstrated residual tumor of the neck node. After discussion at the ENT Tumor Board Conference, it was decided to do only a radical neck dissection to complete his treatment because the only persistent tumor was in the neck.

Thus, 7 weeks after completing his radiotherapy treatments, he had a functional right neck dissection. Sixteen lymph nodes were removed from the upper jugular, lower jugular, posterior triangle, and supraclavicular region. One lower jugular lymph node contained metastatic squamous cell carcinoma with extranodal extension into the surrounding soft tissue (Fig. 5–3).

After the neck dissection, the subcutaneous tissues became hard and edematous. His voice quality had become "gurgly." He had monthly follow-up visits in a combined ENT/radiation oncology head and neck clinic. He had increasing difficulty swallowing and, 6 months after therapy, his total nutritional input was through the G-tube. He denied any neck pain or odynophagia.

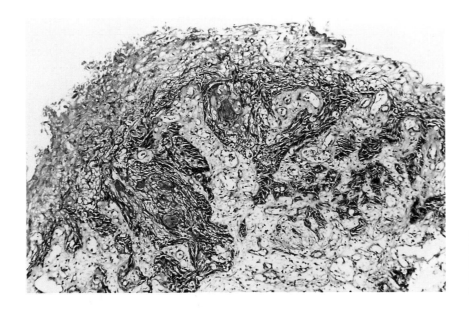

FIG. 5–2. Representative histology from the biopsied right supraglottic mucosa showing invasive moderately differentiated squamous cell carcinoma before radiation therapy. (H&E, × 60.)

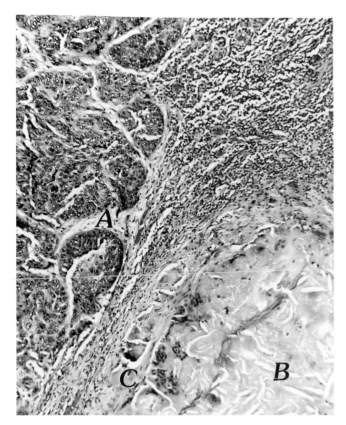

FIG. 5–3. Representative histology from the right neck lymph node after radiation therapy. There are nests of metastatic squamous cell carcinoma (**A**), and an area of tumor cell necrosis due to radiotherapy (**B**). The tumor cell necrosis is focally reacted with histiocytic foreign body giant cells (**C**). (H&E, × 60.)

A CT scan of the neck and soft tissues 16 months after treatment showed some soft tissue thickening in the pre-epiglottic and paralaryngeal tissue with thickening of the aryepiglottic folds and the vocal cords. There was no asymmetry to suggest possible malignancy. Chest roentgenograms were clear.

Eighteen months after completion of therapy, the patient is clinically and radiologically without evidence of recurrent disease. There is mild edema of the supraglottic larynx. His voice is clinically improving. He is eating pureed foods and relies less on his G-tube to maintain his weight. He continues to smoke one pack of cigarettes per day.

COMMENTARY by Ramon M. Esclamado

The patient examined is an excellent illustration of the current controversies in the management of advanced squamous cell carcinoma of the larynx. Several points in the case history are important and should be briefly reviewed. The patient has a prior history of alcohol dependence and chronic schizophrenia that was well controlled with Haldol. These factors may affect patient acceptance and compliance with any recommended treatment regimen and emphasizes the importance of identifying any patient treatment biases and wishes, coexisting medical problems, social history, and lack of support systems that may prevent successful completion of treatment.

Second, the patient's advanced periodontal disease was identified and tooth extraction was performed at the time of endoscopy; a G-tube was also placed in anticipation of significant treatment-related mucositis. These small but important points are essential for minimizing treatment-related complications of the recommended therapy in this case.

The tumor was clinically staged as T3 N1 M0 (stage III) and appears to be a supraglottic primary lesion. However, two important findings at direct laryngoscopy warrant special consideration. First, the tumor crosses the laryngeal ventricle to involve both the false and true vocal cords with vocal cord fixation. By definition, this is a deeply invasive transglottic tumor that has at least a 75% risk of cartilage invasion and extralaryngeal spread that, if present, would upstage the lesion to T4 N1 M0 (stage IV), and is associated with poorer outcome (1). The preoperative CT scan of the larynx is essential in assessing cartilage invasion or extralaryngeal spread. Second, this is a marginal zone supraglottic tumor that "spills over" to involve the medial wall of the pyriform sinus. It can escape the compartmentalization of the larynx and normal barriers to tumor spread, and behave as a more aggressive hypopharyngeal lesion (2). This finding is also important in salvage laryngectomy, as this surgical margin is often indistinct after previous chemotherapy and/or radiation. I have found it helpful to tattoo with India ink the extralaryngeal extent of tumor at the initial endoscopy to assist with defining the original extent of tumor should salvage surgery be necessary.

Standard therapy for this lesion is generally accepted as total laryngectomy, neck dissection, and postoperative radiation (3). This results in loss of normal laryngeal voice, decreased smell and taste, laryngectomy rhinitis, and creation of a tracheostoma with its attendant hygiene demands. To avoid the functional morbidity associated with total laryngectomy, the role of chemotherapy and radiation therapy as an alternative to surgery has been actively investigated.

The largest randomized prospective study available to date addressing this issue is the Veterans Affairs Laryngeal Cancer Study Group Trial (4). This was a prospective, randomized, multi-institutional study to determine if induction chemotherapy (CT) (cisplatin 100 mg/m^2 and 5-FU 1g/m^2 per day × 5 for three cycles) combined with definitive XRT (66–76 Gy) and surgery salvage was an effective organ preservation treatment strategy compared with conventional surgery and postoperative XRT in patients with stage III/IV laryngeal squamous carcinoma. Tumor response was assessed after two cycles of CT: responders received a third cycle followed by XRT; nonresponders underwent salvage laryngectomy. Final analysis of 332 patients (166 CT–XRT; 166 s–XRT) indicates similar 3-year survival rates of 53.3% for CT and 55.9% for S=XRT (π=7,967). Median follow-up is 60 months (range 24–75 months). Of the 166 CT patients, 63 (38%) required salvage laryngectomy. The larynx was preserved in 52 of 79 (66%) surviving patients (5). This study gave strong evidence that a carefully coordinated program of CT–XRT can preserve that larynx in most patients with advanced laryngeal cancer without compromising overall survival. The major unresolved issue raised in this study is whether the rate of laryngeal preservation with CT–XRT is superior to that of primary radiotherapy alone.

The best radiotherapy results report locoregional control rates of 40% for T3-T4 supraglottic cancers, and initial local control rates of approximately 50% in patients with T3 N0 and T4 N0 transglottic cancers (6). Despite these encouraging results, overall survival for patients with advanced laryngeal cancer treated with definitive XRT and surgical salvage is worse than patients treated with surgery and adjuvant XRT (2). Use of this treatment approach requires careful follow-up and patients must be willing to accept the tradeoff of potentially diminished survival and increased surgical morbidity.

Preliminary results have recently been reported in single arm phase I/II trials (7,8) evaluating the feasibility and efficacy of concomitant CT–XRT of advanced squamous cell cancer of the head and neck, including the larynx. In a limited number of patients, an approximate 2-year disease-free survival of 80% to 90% had been achieved with organ preservation.

The phase III TOG trial that this patient was entered into attempts to compare these three treatment strategies in a controlled, randomized fashion, and will hopefully answer some of the questions raised in this discussion. Other issues that require careful attention in evaluating the overall efficacy of any treatment regimen must consider overall cost and duration of treatment, speech and swallowing evaluation to determine that the organ preserved is actually functioning, and that the morbidity and complication rates associated with salvage surgery are acceptable. Future efforts should be focused toward developing strategies that will result not only in higher organ preservation rates, but also in improved overall survival.

REFERENCES

1. Kirchner JA, Cornog JL Jr, Holmes RE. Transglottic cancer: its growth and spread within the larynx. *Arch Otolaryngol* 1974:9:247.
2. Sasaki CT, Carlson RD. Malignant neoplasms of the larynx. In: *Otolaryngology Head and Neck Surgery,* 2nd ed. Cummings CW, et al., eds. St. Louis: Mosby Year Book; 1993:1925–54.
3. Wolf G, Lippman SM, Laramore G, Hong WK. Head and neck cancer. In: *Cancer Medicine,* 3rd ed. Holland JF, et al., eds. Philadelphia: Lea & Febiger; 1993:1211–75.
4. The Department of Veterans Affairs Laryngeal Cancer Study Group. Induction chemotherapy plus radiation compared with surgery plus radiation in patients with advanced laryngeal cancer. *N Engl J Med* 1991:324:1685–90.
5. Wolf G, Hong WK, Fisher S. et al., the VA Laryngeal Cancer Study Group. Larynx preservation with induction chemotherapy (CT) and radiation (XRT) in advanced laryngeal cancer: final results of the VA Laryngeal Study Group cooperative trial. *Proc Am Soc Clin Oncol* 1993:12:277.
6. Marks JE. Radiation therapy. In: *Otolaryngology Head and Neck Surgery,* 2nd ed. Cummings CW, et al., eds. St. Louis: Mosby Year Book; 1993:2122–47.
7. Forastiere AA, Koch W, Lee DJ, Cummings CW. Cisplatin and carboplatin with radiation to preserve organ function in patients with cancer of the oral cavity, oropharynx and hypopharynx. Fourth research workshop on the biology, prevention, and treatment of head and neck cancer abtracts. *Head Neck* 1994:16(5):490.
8. Adelstein DJ, Lavertu P, Saxton JP, et al. Concurrent combination chemotherapy (CT) and continuous course radiotherapy (RT) for treatment of squamous cell head and neck cancer (SCHNC): toxicity and results. Fourth research workshop on the biology, prevention, and treatment of head and neck cancer abtracts. *Head Neck* 1994:16(5):490.

6

T2 N1 M0 Laryngeal Carcinoma

Patrick J. Sweeney, Daniel J. Haraf, Everett E. Vokes, William Moran, and
Ralph R. Weichselbaum

Voice preservation treatment

CASE PRESENTATION

R.K. is a 55-year-old Caucasian man with a 60 pack-per-year smoking history who was admitted with a 2-month history of hoarseness. He was originally told by his family doctor that he had laryngitis but his symptoms persisted and he was referred to an otolaryngologist who diagnosed him as having vocal cord polyps. The patient then sought a second opinion by the ENT service at our institution. The patient denied hemoptysis, dysphagia, or otalgia. His past medical history was unremarkable except for an appendectomy and he takes no medications. He is employed as a policeman. In addition to the above described tobacco history, he reported consuming several vodka drinks daily for the past 4 years.

On examination, the patient was a healthy-appearing man. There was no palpable cervical or supraclavicular lymphadenopathy. The oral cavity was moist and the patient was edentulous. There were no visible lesions within the oropharynx or oral cavity. Palpation of the tongue and floor of mouth were unremarkable. Direct laryngoscopy demonstrated an exophytic mass involving the laryngeal surface of the epiglottis, left false cord, anterior commissure, and both true vocal cords. The vocal cords were mobile. The lungs, heart, and abdominal exams were normal. The neurologic exam, including cranial nerves, was normal.

The hematocrit value was 45%. The white cell count was 9,800. The liver function tests were normal. Chest roentgenograms revealed emphysematous changes but no evidence of neoplastic process. The barium swallow demonstrated asymmetry of the left aryepiglottic fold with mass effect and medial displacement of the left aryepiglottic fold (Fig. 6–1). A mass effect was also noted in the left arytenoid and left false cord with phonation. No abnormalities of the esophagus were noted. A computed tomography (CT) scan of the neck revealed a soft tissue prominence along the left anterior aspect of the vocal cord, with thickening of the anterior aspect of the right vocal cord (Fig. 6–2). There was no pre-epiglottic space invasion. There were bilateral jugulo-digastric nodes present, both measuring approximately 1 cm, that were not pathologic by size criterion. However, the left jugulo-digastric node demonstrated ring enhancement, suggestive of a necrotic center and infiltration (Fig. 6–3).

The patient subsequently underwent an examination under anesthesia with direct laryngoscopy and esophagoscopy. He was found to have an exophytic mass located on the left true vocal cord that extended to the anterior commissure as well as the right anterior true vocal cord. On the left, the mass extended superiorly to involve the ventricle, left false cord, and laryngeal surface of the epiglottis. Posterior extension to the vocal process of the left arytenoid was also noted. The esophagus was normal. Because of concern regarding the airway, a tracheostomy was placed. Biopsies were obtained revealing invasive, moderately differentiated squamous cell carcinoma involving the left false vocal cord and the left true vocal cord. The epicenter of the tumor was felt to be in the supraglottis with extension inferiorly to the glottis. The neck was negative for lymphadenopathy by physical exam but positive for a left jugulo-digastric node by CT scan. The clinical stage was therefore determined as T2,

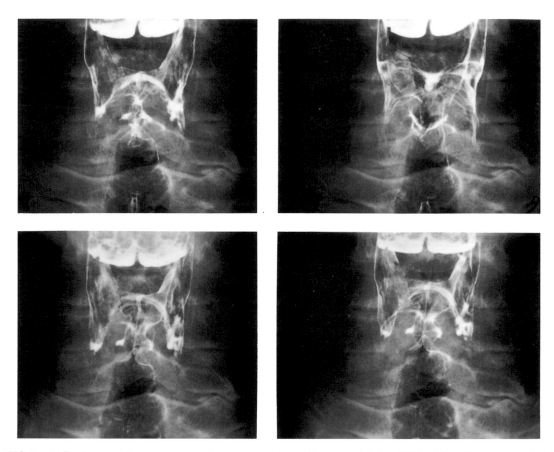

FIG. 6–1. Barium swallow demonstrating asymmetry of the aryepiglottic (AE) folds with a mass effect and medial displacement of the left AE fold. A mass effect is also seen in the subarytenoid region and at the level of the left false cord. Penetration of contrast into the larynx is probably secondary to incompetence of the AE fold closure.

N1, M0 stage III supraglottic carcinoma. The case was presented at the weekly head and neck tumor board for consideration of treatment options.

Surgical considerations for the primary tumor in this patient include a hemilaryngectomy or total laryngectomy. A modified neck dissection will be necessary as well because of the left-sided jugulo-digastric node with a necrotic center. The advantage of a hemilaryngectomy is that it allows for some preservation of voice. However, this patient is not a good candidate for this procedure: typically, hemilaryngectomies are reserved for lesions of a single vocal cord. This patient has extension to both vocal cords. Likewise, extension to the left true cord makes this patient inappropriate for a supraglottic laryngectomy. Thus, the best surgical procedure for this patient is a total laryngectomy and a left neck dissection. Although the procedure will sacrifice his voice, the ultimate local control is approximately 80% (1).

A total laryngectomy and neck dissection will result in the excellent local control stated above. However, depending on operative findings, postoperative radiotherapy may be required and this would expose the patient to the morbidity of both treatments. Definitive radiotherapy is also an

option. The advantages of radiation therapy over total laryngectomy as primary treatment are (a) voice preservation in most patients, (b) the potential to salvage irradiation failures with surgery, and (c) the ability to treat both sides of the neck. The disadvantages of radiotherapy are (a) a high incidence of xerostomia and (b) an increased risk of failure compared with surgery. Historically, local control with conventional radiotherapy is approximately 60% to 79% for T2 supraglottic lesions (2,3). However, many of the irradiation failures can be salvaged surgically with close follow-up and early detection of tumor recurrence.

To improve local control with radiotherapy, some have advocated altered fractionation schedules. Wang showed a 29% improvement in local control for T2 supraglottic cancers from 60% to 89% with twice-daily radiotherapy of 160 cGy per fraction compared with historical controls treated with conventional once-daily irradiation (2). Mendenhall et al. has also demonstrated slightly improved local control for T2 cancers with a nonconventional radiotherapy schedule compared with once-daily treatment (3).

The medical oncology service agrees with the desire for voice preservation but feels the patient should be consid-

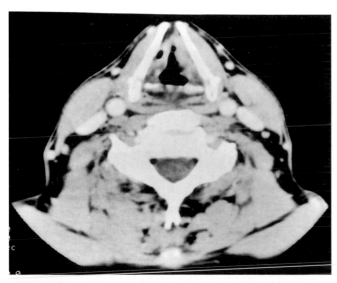

FIG. 6–2. Soft tissue prominence is seen along the left anterior aspect of the vocal cord, which crosses the midline and extends to the anterior right cord. The left cord is more extensively involved than the right.

ered for chemotherapy. Data supporting neoadjuvant chemotherapy is presented in the Veterans Affairs Study Group trial. Patients with stages III and IV larynx cancer had an equivalent survival when treated with laryngectomy and postoperative irradiation versus those receiving

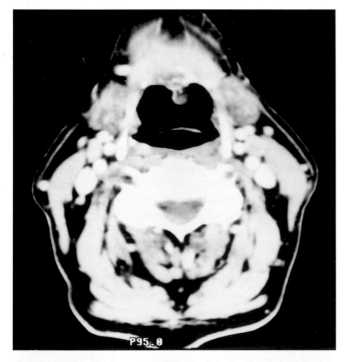

FIG. 6–3. Bilateral jugulo-digastric nodes are seen measuring approximately 1 cm in diameter. The left jugulo-digastric node is round and exhibits ring enhancement, suggestive of tumor infiltration.

induction chemotherapy followed by radiation therapy. An important finding was that the larynx was preserved in two thirds of the patients treated on the chemoradiotherapy arm (4). A second issue is whether this patient is at risk to develop distant metastases. Both radiotherapy and surgery are local treatments that do not address distant micrometastatic disease. A potential need to treat micrometastases is seen in the Head and Neck Contracts Study (5) and the study by Merlano et al. (6): (a) The Head and Neck Contracts study, although not showing a survival advantage between conventional treatment of advanced head and neck cancer (surgery or radiation) and either induction chemotherapy plus conventional treatment or induction and maintenance chemotherapy plus conventional treatment, did demonstrate a significant difference in the incidence of distant metastases favoring the induction and maintenance chemotherapy arm, and (b) the pilot study by Merlano et al. showed a survival benefit for alternating chemotherapy and radiotherapy over radiotherapy alone in advanced squamous cell cancer of the head and neck. A final issue to consider with regard to chemotherapy is the "radiation sensitizer" effect of a number of chemotherapeutic agents when given concomitantly with irradiation (7).

It was decided to treat the patient with an institutional protocol for previously untreated stages II to IV locally advanced head and neck cancer studying the efficacy of concomitant chemoradiotherapy with the goal of preserving organ function. The chemotherapy agents were hydroxyurea (1.0 gm PO q 12 h × 6 days) and 5-fluorouracil (800 mg/m^2/day × 5 days) given concurrent with irradiation. The radiotherapy consisted of 180 to 200 cGy fractions given for 5 consecutive days. Total dose received by the tumor was 70 Gy. Per protocol, the treatment was given in 14-day cycles: each cycle consisted of chemoradiotherapy for five consecutive days beginning on day 0. From day 6 through 14, no therapy was given to allow partial recovery from acute toxicities. Each cycle was then repeated until the end of the radiotherapy prescription for a total of 14 weeks or seven cycles.

The patient tolerated the therapy well. He developed the anticipated side effects of erythema in the neck over the irradiated area. He had no problems with dysphagia or weight loss and his blood counts remained stable. After four cycles of chemoradiotherapy he was noted to have a significant reduction in tumor mass on indirect laryngoscopy.

The patient is now 1 year postcompletion of chemoradiotherapy. He has been seen at regular intervals by his ENT physician. His voice quality is good and he is clinically without evidence of local or distant disease.

REFERENCES

1. DeSanto L. Cancer of the supraglottic larynx: a review of 260 patients. *Otolaryngol Head Neck Surg* 1985:93:705–11.

2. Wang CC. Carcinoma of the larynx. In: *Radiation Therapy for Head and Neck Neoplasms: Indications, Techniques, and Results*, 2nd ed. Chicago: Yearbook Medical Publishers; 1990:223–60.

3. Mendenhall WM, Parsons JT, Stringer SP, Cassisi NJ and Million RR: Carcinoma of the supraglottic larynx: a basis for comparing the results of radiotherapy and surgery. *Head Neck* 1990;12:204–9.

4. The Department of Veteran's Affairs Laryngeal Cancer Study Group: Induction chemotherapy plus radiation compared with surgery plus radiation in patients with advanced laryngeal cancer. *N Engl J Med* 1991;324:1685–90.

5. Head and Neck Contracts Program: Adjuvant chemotherapy for advanced head and squamous carcinoma. *Cancer* 1987;60:301–11.

6. Merlano M, Rosso R, Benasso M, et al. Alternating chemotherapy (CT) and radiotherapy (RT) vs RT in advanced inoperable SCC-HN: A cooperative randomized trial. *Proc Am Soc Clin Oncol* 1991;10:198(abstr).

7. Vokes E, Weichselbaum R. Concomitant chemoradiotherapy: concomitant chemoradiotherapy: rationale and clinical experience in patients with solid tumors. *J Clin Oncol* 1990;8:911–34.

COMMENTARY by Karen K. Fu

The clinical presentation of this patient was consistent with a primary arising from the glottic or supraglottic larynx. Although the epicenter of the tumor was felt to be in the supraglottis, symptoms of persistent hoarseness and the lack of symptoms of sore throat and odynophagia are more consistent with a primary in the glottic rather than the supraglottic larynx. In either case, this would be a T2 lesion. Although there was no palpable lymphadenopathy, CT scan showed changes consistent with metastasis in a left jugulo-digastric node. Thus, the tumor was T2 N1 M0 (clinical stage III).

The standard treatment for this patient would have been surgery and radiotherapy or radiotherapy alone. With involvement of both vocal cords, the patient was not eligible for laryngeal conservation surgery. Surgical treatment for this patient would have been a total laryngectomy and a modified left neck dissection. Postoperative radiotherapy would be indicated if there was tumor at or close (<5 mm) to surgical margins, cartilage invasion, involvement of the soft tissues of the neck, multiple (>1) lymph node metastases, extracapsular nodal extension, and perineural, lymphatic, or vascular invasion.

As pointed out by Dr. Sweeney and his colleagues, radiotherapy has the advantages of voice preservation and treatment of bilateral neck. For T2 carcinoma of the supraglottic larynx, recent results suggest similar local control rates with radiotherapy alone compared with surgery with or without adjuvant radiotherapy (1). Improved local control rates have also been reported with twice-daily hyperfractionated or accelerated fractionated radiotherapy compared with historical controls with once-daily conventional fractionated radiotherapy (2–4). Even if radiotherapy fails to control the local-regional disease, surgical salvage is usually successful with close follow-up and early detection of recurrent disease. The exophytic appearance of the tumor and the intact mobility of the vocal cords in this patient would suggest a favorable response to radiotherapy. Furthermore, with his profes-

sion as a policeman, voice preservation would be a significant factor in the selection of treatment modality.

The role of chemotherapy in the management of laryngeal cancer remains controversial. A randomized trial by the VA Laryngeal Cancer Study Group showed similar survival for patients with stage III/IV laryngeal squamous carcinoma treated with induction chemotherapy followed by definitive radiotherapy (CT–XRT) or surgery and postoperative radiotherapy (S–XRT) (5). Although the disease-free interval was significantly shorter in the CT–XRT group and 38% of the patients had required laryngectomy for salvage. The larynx was preserved in 66% of the patients who were alive at 4 years (6). However, it remains to be determined whether radiotherapy alone is as effective as induction chemotherapy and radiotherapy or concurrent chemotherapy and radiotherapy in laryngeal preservation. Such trial is currently in progress by the Head and Neck Intergroup.

One of the rationales for adding chemotherapy to standard therapy for head and neck cancer is to decrease distant metastasis. In the trial by the VA Laryngeal Cancer Study Group, although distant metastasis as the site of first tumor recurrence was more common after S–XRT than after CT–XRT, this difference in patterns of relapse disappeared over time (6). Four other randomized trials of induction or adjuvant chemotherapy in advanced head and neck cancer also suggest a decreased incidence of distant metastasis with chemotherapy (7–10). However, none of these trials showed a survival benefit.

Randomized trials thus far have shown no improvement of survival with neoadjuvant or adjuvant chemotherapy (11). However, several randomized trials of concomitant radiotherapy and single-agent chemotherapy demonstrated an improved local-regional control and/or disease-free survival (11,12). Improved overall survival has also been reported with 5-FU and bleomycin for carcinoma of the oral cavity and with methotrexate for carcinoma of the oropharynx. More recently, multidrug chemotherapy has been combined with concomitant radiotherapy in an attempt to further improve the results. However, when more than one chemotherapeutic agent is used during radiotherapy, increased toxicity necessitates the use of split-course radiotherapy with planned interruptions or an alternating chemotherapy and radiotherapy approach. Thus, the treatment is prolonged and this may adversely affect local control (13). Although the only randomized trial comparing alternating chemotherapy and radiotherapy to radiotherapy alone in advanced head and neck cancer showed an improved survival with the combined treatment, there was no significant difference in the incidence of distant metastases (7.5% vs. 6.5%) (14). The difference in survival was largely due to the poor local-regional control in the radiotherapy alone group. However, the delivery of radiotherapy in this trial was suboptimal. The median dose was only 62 Gy and treatment was delayed 1 week in 32%, for 2 weeks in 11%, and for more than 2 weeks in 14% of the patients in the radiotherapy alone group. At the present time, alternating chemotherapy and radiotherapy or split-course concomitant chemoradiotherapy should not be adapted for routine clinical practice except in the setting of a clinical trial, as was the case in this patient. Outside of a clinical trial setting, the preferred treatment for this patient would have been radiotherapy with laryngeal preservation, reserving surgery for salvage should radiotherapy fail to achieve local-regional control.

This patient is also at risk for the development of a second cancer. He should be advised to stop drinking and smoking. In addition, he should be considered for participation in a chemoprevention trial.

REFERENCES

1. Weems DH, Mendenhall WM, Parsons JT, et al. Squamous cell carcinoma of the supraglottic larynx treated with surgery and/or radiation therapy. *Int J Radiat Oncol Biol Phys* 1987:13:1483–7.
2. Wendt CD, Peters LJ, Ang KK, et al. Hyperfractionated radiotherapy in the treatment of squamous cell carcinomas of the supraglottic larynx. *Int J Radiat Oncol Biol Phys* 1989;17:1057–62.
3. Wang CC. Deciding on optimal management of supraglottic carcinoma. *Oncology* 1991:5:41–9.
4. Parsons JT, Mendenhall WM, Million RR, et al. Twice-a-day irradiation of squamous cell carcinoma of the head and neck. *Semin Radiat Oncol* 1992:2:29–30.
5. Wolf G, Hong W, Fisher S, et al. Larynx preservation with induction chemotherapy (CT) and radiation (XRT) in advanced laryngeal cancer: final results of the VA Laryngeal Cancer Study Group Cooperative Trial. *Proc ASCO* 1993:12:227.
6. Wolf GT, Hong WK. VA Laryngeal Cancer Study Group Cooperative Trial. Induction chemotherapy as part of a new treatment strategy to preserve the larynx in advanced laryngeal cancer. In: *Head and Neck Cancer,* Johnson JT, Didolkar MS, eds. The Netherlands: Elsevier Science; 1993;3:27–36.
7. Final Report of the Head and Neck Program. Adjuvant chemotherapy for advanced head and neck squamous carcinoma. *Cancer* 1987:60:301–11.
8. Schuller DE, Stein, DW, Metch B. Analysis of treatment failure patterns. *Arch Otolaryngol Head Neck Surg* 1989:15:834–6.
9. Laramore GE, Scott CB, Al-Sarraf M, et al. Adjuvant chemotherapy for resectable squamous cell carcinomas of the head and neck: report on intergroup study 0034. *Int J Radiat Oncol Biol Phys* 1992:23:705–13.
10. Jaulerry C, Rodriguez J, Brunin F, et al. Induction chemotherapy in advanced head and neck tumors: results of two randomized trials. *Int J Radiat Oncol Biol Phys* 1992:23:483–9.
11. Vokes EE, Weichselbaum RR, Lippman SM, et al. Head and neck cancer. *N Engl J Med* 1993;328:184–94.
12. Fu KK. Integration of chemotherapy and radiotherapy for organ preservation in head and neck cancer. In: *Head and Neck Cancer,* Johnson JT, Didolkar MS, eds. The Netherlands: Elsevier Science, 1993;3:27–36.
13. Fowler JF, Lindstrom MJ. Loss of local control with prolongation in radiotherapy. *Int J Radiat Oncol Biol Phys* 1992:23:457–67.
14. Merlano M, Vitale V, Rosso R, et al. Treatment of advanced squamous cell carcinoma of the head and neck with alternating chemotherapy and radiotherapy. *N Engl J Med* 1992;327:1115–21.

7

T3 Pyriform Sinus Carcinoma

Adam S. Garden and Lester J. Peters

Importance of clinical trials

CASE PRESENTATION

H.D. is a 64-year-old Caucasian man who was admitted in December, 1991, with a 6-month history of sore throat, 3 weeks of hoarseness, and a right upper neck mass. He had a slight decrease in appetite with a 5-pound weight loss over 3 months. Before his presentation in December, he underwent several courses of antibiotics, which did not alleviate his symptoms. He was found to have a lesion in the right pyriform sinus. He underwent a direct laryngoscopy under general anesthesia and a biopsy revealed poorly differentiated squamous cell carcinoma. Surgical resection involving total laryngectomy, partial pharyngectomy, and a right radical neck dissection was recommended. However, at the patient's request, he was referred to M.D. Anderson Cancer Center (MDACC) for a second opinion for possible nonsurgical management of his lesion.

The patient was born and raised in Louisiana and works as a general contractor. He had a 40 pack-per-year history of smoking, although he had discontinued this habit 10 years before to his presentation. He drinks one-half pint of alcohol a day. He has no significant past medical history nor family history.

On physical examination, a large mass was seen filling the pyriform sinus. The lesion appeared to arise from the medial wall of the right pyriform sinus, and extended onto and over the aryepiglottic fold involving the arytenoid on that side. The right hemilarynx was fixed. The left side was uninvolved. Examination of his neck revealed a 3-cm mobile upper jugular lymph node. The remainder of his physical examination was unremarkable.

Radiographic studies included computerized tomography (CT) of the head and neck, which revealed the tumor in the right pyriform sinus extending to the right aryepiglottic fold and involving the right paraglottic space with fixation of the right true cord (Fig. 7–1). Several lymph nodes were seen in the right upper and middle jugular chain with central necrosis. A chest roentgenogram was unremarkable. Screening blood work included a chemical survey and complete blood count, both of which were normal.

The patient was staged as T3 N1 M0, stage III squamous cell carcinoma of the right pyriform sinus. The patient was seen and examined by members of our multidisciplinary team, including head and neck surgeons, radiotherapists, and medical oncologists. The patient was offered participation in an institutional study for patients with locally advanced squamous cell carcinoma of the head and neck in whom standard treatment would require a laryngectomy. This was a Phase II study involving induction chemotherapy with cisplatin, 5-fluorouracil (5-FU), and high-dose l-leukovorin. Patients with a partial or complete response proceeded to radiotherapy delivered using twice-daily fractionation to a total dose of 76.6 Gy. Nonresponders proceeded to surgery. The patient agreed to participate in this study.

Before instituting chemotherapy, the patient had been seen by our dental oncology team, who recommended extraction of five teeth. This was done, and 10 days later, on December 31, 1991, the patient began his first cycle of chemotherapy, which consisted of cisplatin 25 mg/m^2 delivered for 5 days, 5-FU 800 mg/m^2 delivered over days 2 through 6, and l-leukovorin 250 mg^2 on days 1 through 6. On the sixth day, his hoarseness increased significantly, and on indirect laryngoscopy he was noted to have a great deal of supraglottic edema with marked narrowing of his airway. He was taken to the operating room

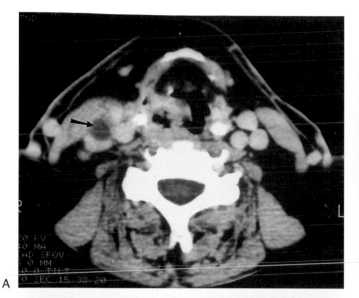

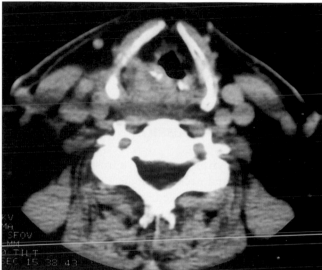

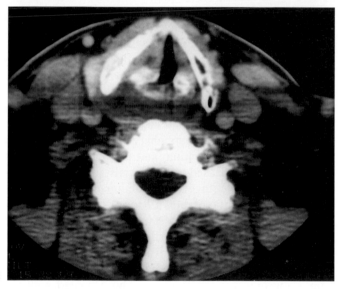

FIG. 7–1. CT scans of the right pyriform sinus lesion. **A:** Lesion in the vestibule of the right pyriform sinus and central necrosis of an adjacent upper jugular chain lymph node (*arrow*). **B:** Pyriform sinus lesion filling sinus and displacing the right arytenoid. **C:** Paraglottic involvement with right true vocal cord in a paramedian position due to fixation.

for an elective but urgent tracheostomy. Subsequently, the patient developed grade 4 neutropenia and grade 3 thrombocytopenia. Therefore, as per protocol, a planned dose reduction was made for the second and third cycles. This reduction was done by eliminating 1 day of treatment for each drug. The remainder of his chemotherapy was completed uneventfully.

On re-evaluation after his chemotherapy, the patient had a clinical complete response, and radiographically a near complete response was noted. The patient therefore proceeded to receive radiation therapy, which started on April 1, 1992, and was completed on May 18, 1992. Radiation was delivered using a pair of parallel opposed lateral fields that encompassed the primary lesion in the pyriform sinus and the draining lymph nodes of the neck, including the retropharyngeal nodes. These areas were treated to 55 Gy at 1.1 Gy per fraction twice daily. A reduction off the spinal cord was made after 44 Gy, and

the left neck posterior cervical strip was treated with 9 MeV electrons to 54 Gy. As there was concern that the off-cord fields' posterior border may be tight on the original gross nodal disease in the right neck, the right posterior cervical strip was supplemented to 70 Gy. This too was delivered with 9 MeV electrons. The original primary disease and right neck mass were then boosted through parallel opposed lateral fields at 1.2 Gy per fraction twice daily to the final dose of 76.6 Gy. The lower neck was treated to 50 Gy at 2 Gy per fraction. The initial fields were treated with cobalt 60 photons; the off-cord lateral fields and the boost fields were treated with 6 MV photons. The patient tolerated his radiation well, developing mucosal erythema and mild arytenoid edema as well as dry desquamation of the skin of his neck.

After resolution of his radiation reactions, the patient remained asymptomatic. Six months after his radiation, asymmetry of the larynx was noted. However, this was greater on the left side than on the right. The patient was observed closely over the next 3 months and these changes improved. Two years later the patient remains well, without evidence of recurrent disease or new primary cancers. There continues to be minimal asymmetry of the larynx, but this is asymptomatic.

TUMOR BOARD DISCUSSION

Cancers of the pyriform sinus are a frustrating group of cancers for head and neck oncologists to manage. They tend to present in advanced stages, and their local-regional management can entail considerable morbidity. In a series of more than 400 patients with pyriform sinus primaries who were admitted to the MDACC between 1949 and 1976, more than 80% had advanced local disease (stages III and IV) and more than 70% had clinical nodal involvement (1). In patients who do not have successful local-regional management, the distant failure rate is high.

Definitive radiotherapy produces good results in most patients who present with early stage disease (2). However, radiation therapy alone for T3 and T4 lesions and unfavorable large infiltrative T2 lesions achieves local control in only a minority of cases. Thus, standard treatment for patients who are medically operable is surgical resection.

Because of the location of these tumors, surgical treatment typically involves partial or total pharyngectomy with a laryngectomy. The improvements in microvascular grafting techniques that allow for replacement of the pharynx with either a free jejunal transfer or sometimes a soft tissue transfer have allowed cases that in previous decades might have been considered technically unresectable to become resectable. Many patients are thus able to learn to swallow and even with postoperative radiation therapy are able to return to relatively normal diets (3).

Most patients require postoperative radiotherapy as adverse features, such as close or positive margins, invasion into the soft tissues of the neck, invasion into the thyroid cartilage, multiple nodes involved, and/or extracapsular spread of nodal disease are found. These patients with advanced disease treated with surgery and postoperative radiotherapy will achieve local-regional control in 70% of the cases (4).

In recent years, there has been a considerable interest in using induction chemotherapy as a means of selecting patients with advanced cancers of the larynx and hypopharynx for larynx preservation even though multiple clinical trials have failed to show any overall survival benefit for this therapeutic approach (5). The large VA trial (6) demonstrated that induction chemotherapy with cisplatin and 5-FU followed by radiotherapy in complete responders resulted in larynx preservation in roughly 60% of the patients, with no detrimental effects on overall sur-

vival compared with standard surgery and postoperative radiotherapy. Based on the Phase III VA trials (6), the RTOG is now conducting a randomized Phase III larynx preservation trial investigating induction chemotherapy versus concurrent chemotherapy and radiation versus radiation only, with the latter as the control arm. The groups that they are studying, however, do not include patients with hypopharyngeal primaries.

At MDACC, several institutional trials have been undertaken evaluating the role of induction chemotherapy for larynx preservation in patients with advanced head and neck cancers of any site whose resection would require laryngectomy (7). Our initial trial used chemotherapy consisting of cisplatin, 5-FU, and bleomycin. However, when our results were compared with other published series, we concluded that bleomycin added only to toxicity, and this drug was dropped from the regimen for the second study. The third and most recent trial added high-dose l-leukovorin to cisplatin and 5-FU to help improve response rates. The results of this experience are still unreported. However, the former two trials confirmed the hypothesis that induction chemotherapy followed by radiation could spare some larynges without compromising survival in patients who were considered unsuitable for definitive radiotherapy and who otherwise would have undergone total laryngectomy. In particular, 28% of patients with hypopharyngeal cancer are alive with laryngeal preservation, and the overall 2-year survival rate is 46%. Based on these trials, we concluded that it was reasonable to offer induction chemotherapy to patients with unfavorable T2 or T3 hypopharyngeal lesions as an alternative to standard surgical resections, recognizing that many will still need surgery. However, for patients with very advanced lesions (T4), this approach is probably not valid because the outcome in this subgroup was worse than in those treated with primary surgery (8).

In our studies, hyperfractionated radiation was used after chemotherapy. There have been several reports using hyperfractionation as a sole modality of treatment for head and neck cancer, with most showing an advantage for hyperfractionation, both prospectively and retrospectively, compared with conventional once-a-day fractionation (9–11). However, the role of hyperfractionation in combination with either concurrent or sequential chemotherapy is undefined.

Conclusion

Primary surgery remains the standard treatment for advanced hypopharynx cancers but has considerable functional morbidity. Further studies investigating nonsurgical management are being performed, with a trend now toward using chemotherapy and radiation concurrently. However, this strategy can be recommended only for motivated patients who agree to participate in structured clinical trials.

REFERENCES

1. El Badawi SA, Goepfert H, Herson J, Fletcher GH, et al. Squamous cell carcinoma of the pyriform sinus. *Laryngoscope* 1982;92:357–64.
2. Garden AS, Morrison WH, Ang KK, Peters LJ. Hyperfractionated radiation in the treatment of squamous cell carcinomas of the head and neck: a comparison of two fractionation schedules. *Int J Radiat Oncol Biol Phys* 1995;31:493–502.
3. Cole CJ, Garden AS, Frankenthaler RA, Reece GP, et al. Postoperative radiation of free jejunal autografts in patients with advanced cancers of the head and neck. *Cancer* 1995;75:2356–60.
4. Peters LJ, Goepfert H, Ang KK, Byers RM, et al. Evaluation of the dose for postoperative radiation therapy of head and neck cancer: first report of a prospective randomized trial. *Int J Radiat Oncol Biol Phys* 1993;26:3–11.
5. Stell PM, Rawson NSB. Adjuvant chemotherapy in head and neck cancer. *Br J Cancer* 1990;61:779–87.
6. The Department of Veterans Affairs Laryngeal Study Group. Induction 000 chemotherapy plus radiation compared with surgery plus radiation in patients with advanced laryngeal cancer. *N Engl J Med* 1991;324:1685–90.
7. Shirinian MH, Weber RS, Lippman SM, Dimery IW, et al. Laryngeal preservation by induction chemotherapy plus radiotherapy in locally advanced head and neck cancer: the M.D. Anderson Cancer Center experience. *Head Neck* 1994;16:39–44.
8. Clayman GL, Weber RS, Guillamondegui O, Byers RM, et al. Laryngeal preservation for advanced laryngeal and hypopharyngeal cancers. *Arch Otolaryngol Head Neck Surg* 1995;121:219–23.
9. Horiot JC, LeFur R, N'Guyen T, Chenal C, et al. Hyperfractionation versus conventional fractionation in oropharyngeal carcinoma: final analysis of a randomized trial of the EORTC cooperative group of radiotherapy. *Radiother Oncol* 1992;25:231–41.
10. Parsons JT, Mendenhall WM, Stringer SP, Cassisi NJ, Million RR. Twice-a-day radiotherapy for squamous cell carcinoma of the head and neck: the University of Florida experience. *Head Neck* 1993;15:87–96.
11. Wendt CD, Peters LJ, Ang KK, Morrison WH, et al. Hyperfractionated radiotherapy in the treatment of sqamous cell carcinomas of the supraglottic larynx. *Int J Radiat Oncol Biol Phys* 1989;17:1057–62.

COMMENTARY by Karen K. Fu

Management of advanced carcinoma of the pyriform sinus remains a challenge to the head and neck oncologist. Although excellent local control with laryngeal voice preservation can be achieved with radiotherapy alone in most patients with T1 or T2 lesions (1), results of radiotherapy alone are inferior to those with combined surgery and postoperative radiotherapy for resectable T3 or T4 lesions (2–4). However, surgery for advanced carcinoma of the pyriform sinus usually requires total laryngectomy, partial pharyngectomy, and a radical neck dissection with loss of voice and impairment of swallowing function. Thus, there is a need for alternatives to surgery with the aim of preservation of organ function in patients with advanced carcinoma of the larynx and hypopharynx. In recent years, attempts to improve the results of radiotherapy for advanced head and neck cancer have usually involved the use of combined chemotherapy and radiotherapy or altered fractionation radiotherapy.

The VA Laryngeal Cancer Study Group conducted the first randomized trial comparing induction chemotherapy followed by definitive radiotherapy (CT–XRT) to surgery and postoperative radiotherapy (S–XRT) in patients with stage III or IV squamous cell carcinoma of the larynx (5,6). Although there was no significant difference in overall survival, the disease-free interval was significantly shorter in the CT–XRT group and 38% of the patients had required laryngectomy for salvage. At 4 years, the larynx was preserved in 66% of the patients who were still alive (6). Subsequently, a phase III trial was initiated by the Head and Neck Intergroup to determine the relative efficacy of induction chemotherapy and radiotherapy versus radiotherapy alone in laryngeal preservation for patients with T2-3 and N0-3 squamous cell carcinoma of the larynx. This trial is still in progress.

The use of induction chemotherapy followed by radiotherapy for laryngeal preservation in squamous cell carcinoma of the hypopharynx has also been evaluated in a randomized trial by the European Organization of Research on the Treatment of Cancer (EORTC 24891) (7). Preliminary results were presented at the 1994 Annual Meeting of the American Society of Clinical Oncology. Two hundred two patients with squamous cell carcinoma of the hypopharynx were randomized to receive total laryngectomy, partial pharyngectomy plus radical neck dissection (TLRND) and postoperative radiotherapy (XRT) (arm A), or induction chemotherapy followed by XRT in clinically complete responders or TLRND postoperative XRT in other cases. One hundred ninety seven patients (97 in arm A and 100 in arm B) were evaluable. Survival was the same for both arms: 54 patients in arm A and 53 patients in arm B were dead. Laryngeal preservation was achieved in 28% of the patients in arm B. Thus, it appears induction chemotherapy followed by definitive radiotherapy in patients who show complete response to chemotherapy may be an alternative to radical surgery and postoperative radiotherapy in patients with advanced squamous cell carcinoma of the hypopharynx. However, it remains to be proved whether similar results can be achieved with radiotherapy alone without the additional cost and toxicity of induction chemotherapy.

For patients with T3 carcinoma of the pyriform sinus, retrospective comparisons suggest an improved local control rate with hyperfractionated or accelerated fractionated radiotherapy compared with historical controls treated with conventional fractionated radiotherapy (4,8). However, this has not been established in prospectively randomized clinical trials. Thus far, phase III trials in head and neck cancer demonstrating an improved local-regional control with hyperfractionated radiotherapy have largely been limited to carcinoma of the oropharynx (9–11).

In this patient with clinically T3 N1 carcinoma of the pyriform sinus, both induction chemotherapy and hyperfractionated radiotherapy were used in the setting of an institutional phase II trial. The induction chemotherapy regimen differs from those used in the VA Laryngeal Cancer Study Group Trial and the EORTC Trial. Fortunately, the treatment appears to have been successful thus far and with preservation of organ function. Furthermore, he appears to have tolerated the induction chemotherapy and hyperfractionated radiotherapy well. In fact, there was no suggestion of increased acute radiation reactions commonly observed in patients receiving hyperfractionated radiotherapy. However, at the present time, the treatment this patient received remains experimental and should not be adapted for routine clinical practice. The efficacy of this experimental protocol treatment relative to other nonsurgical approaches such as conventional fractionated, hyperfractionated, or accelerated fractionated radiotherapy alone or combined with induction or concurrent chemotherapy in patients with advanced squamous cell carcinoma of the hypopharynx, remains to be established through prospectively randomized clinical trials.

REFERENCES

1. Mendenhall WM, Parsons JT, Stringer SP, et al. Radiotherapy alone or combined with neck dissection for T1-2 carcinoma of the pyriform sinus: an alternative to conservation surgery. *Int J Radiat Oncol Biol Phys* 1993;27(5):1017—27.
2. Garden AS, Morrison WH, Ang KK, Peters LJ. Hyperfractionated radiation in the treatment of squamous cell carcinomas of the head and neck: a comparison of two fractionation schedules. *Int J Radiat Oncol Biol Phys* 1995;31:493–502.
3. Cole CJ, Garden AS, Frankenthaler RA, Reece GP, et al. Postoperative radiation of free jejunal autografts in patients with advanced cancer of the head and neck. *Cancer* 1995;75:2356–60.
4. Wang CC. Carcinoma of the hypopharynx. In: *Radiation Therapy for Head and Neck Neoplasms: Indications, Techniques, and Results.* Chicago: Yearbook Medical Publishers; 1990:207–22.
5. The Department of Veterans Affairs Laryngeal Cancer Study Group. Induction chemotherapy plus radiation compared with surgery plus radiation in patients with advanced laryngeal cancer. *N Engl J Med* 1991;324:1685–90.
6. Wolf GT, Hong WK. VA Laryngeal Cancer Study Group Cooperative Trial. Induction chemotherapy as part of a new treatment strategy to preserve the larynx in advanced laryngeal cancer. In: *Induction Chemotherapy as Part of a New Treatment strategy to Preserve the Larynx in Advanced Laryngeal Cancer,* Johnson JT, Didolkar MS, eds. The Netherlands: Elsevier Science, 1993;3:27–36.
7. Lefebvre JL, Sahmoud T Larynx preservation in hypopharynx squamous cell carcinoma: preliminary results of a randomized study (EORTC 24891). *Proc ASCO* 1994;13:912.
8. Clayman GL, Weber RS, Guillamondegui O, Byers RM, et al. Laryngeal preservation for advanced laryngeal and hypopharyngeal cancers. *Arch Otolaryngol Head Neck Surg* 1995;121:219–23.
9. Horiot JC, Le-Fur R, Nguyen T, et al. Hyperfractionation versus conventional fractionation in oropharyngeal carcinoma: final analysis of a randomized trial of the EORTC cooperative group of radiotherapy. *Radiother Oncol* 1992;25(4):231–41.
10. Pinto LHJ, Canary PCV, Araujo CMM, et al. Prospective randomized trial comparing hyperfractionated versus conventional radiotherapy in stages III and IV oropharyngeal carcinoma. *Int J Radiat Oncol Biol Phys* 1991;21:557–62.
11. Datta NR, Choudhry AD, Gupta S. Twice-a-day versus once-a-day radiation therapy in head and neck cancer. *Int J Radiat Oncol Biol Phys* 1989;17:132.

8 Adenoid Cystic Carcinoma of the Parotid Gland

Robert J. Schweitzer

A locally aggressive neoplasm with a systemically indolent but often fatal course

CASE PRESENTATION

This 58-year-old woman was first examined by an otolaryngologist for a right preauricular painless mass of about 20 years' duration. One year before she had a bilateral rhytidectomy by a plastic surgeon. In the last 6 months there was increasing weakness of the musculature of the eyelid, face, and mouth on the right side with the appearance of a grape-sized second mass in the tail of the right parotid.

On physical exam there were two contiguous mobile masses in the right preauricular area measuring about 4.1 cm ∞ 2 cm, extending from the zygoma down to the lobe of the ear. There was no redness or fixation of the overlying skin. She was unable to close her right eye and there was 60% loss of function of the buccal branches of the facial nerve on the right. No adenopathy was noted. Clinical staging was T3b N0 M0.

Needle aspiration was consistent with adenoid cystic carcinoma (Fig. 8–1). Chest roentgenogram was negative for metastases. Computed tomography (CT) scan revealed an irregular subcutaneous soft tissue density involving the superficial lobe of the parotid and contiguous with the masseter muscle. There was no adenopathy (Fig. 8–2). At the time of surgery, the patient's mass was explored through the prior facelift incision. At the bifurcation of the facial nerve, the superior branches were noted to be hyperemic and surrounded by the tumor mass. Frozen section of the nerve showed perineural involvement with tumor. The main trunk had a similar hyperemic

appearance and was divided at the stylomastoid foramen. No microscopic sections were obtained of the proximal nerve segment, nor was any attempt made to dissect the intraosseous portion of the nerve. The inferior portion of the parotid gland, which contained a 1-cm nodule, was removed as a separate specimen. The upper portions of the superior lobe of the parotid were dissected off the zygoma, removing a small portion of the masseter muscle that adhered to the tumor. The remaining parotid and deep lobe were then removed and the superficial temporal artery was ligated. A node along the exterior jugular vein was removed and found to be negative for tumor.

Postoperatively, the patient was presented to the Bay Area Tumor Institute Tumor Board held at Summit Medical Center for discussion as to future course of action.

TUMOR BOARD DISCUSSION

Moderator: Robert J. Schweitzer, M.D., Surgical Oncologist

Gary Shrago, Radiologist, described the CT scan, stating there was a right-sided subcutaneous soft tissue density mass in front of the right tragus overlying the zygomatic arch and proceeding inferiorly in continuity with the superficial lobe of the parotid gland, as well as the retromandibular extension of the gland. A portion of the superior temporal artery was directly involved, and the mass was contiguous with masseter muscle. No obvious adenopathy was noted (see Fig. 8–2).

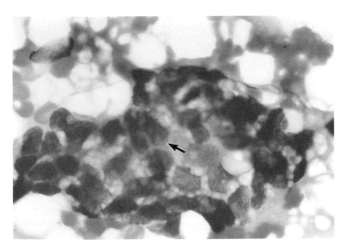

FIG. 8–1. Fine-needle aspiration of right parotid gland. Shown are numerous cells in a small cohesive group. Note the large, isomorphic nuclei, nuclear molding, and even nuclear outlines characteristic of basaloid cells (*arrow*). Pseudocystic spaces containing muco-substance are present.

Question

Do you see the facial nerve on the scan?

Dr. Shrago: We do not see the facial nerve. With tumors like this, when knowledge of nerve involvement preoperatively is important, the fat saturation technique using magnetic resonance imaging (MRI) will demonstrate nerve involvement. This has definite advantages in this situation over CT scan.

Dr. Diane Salyer, Pathologist, projected the needle aspiration slide showing groups of cells that have dark nuclei (see Fig. 8–1). The nuclei seemed to be molding, and there were pseudo-cystic spaces containing pink muco-substance. Given the location, this was consistent with adenoid cystic carcinoma of the parotid.

Question

How reliable is needle aspiration with this tumor as compared to other parotid neoplasms?

Dr. Salyer: Most pathologists experienced with fine-needle aspiration consider the salivary gland to be difficult because the underlying lesions are so facultative and so diverse in appearance. If you have a scant number of cells that do not have this particular appearance, it could be very difficult. In this slide there is truly molding and a differential in nuclei size and density, indicating it is a malignant neoplasm and not a cellular pleomorphic adenoma. The pink material is subtle, but suggestive of the amorphous material that exists in adenoid cystic cancers.

This section shows a cross section of the upper bifurcation of the facial nerve. The tumor has infiltrated the perineural spaces, which is a characteristic appearance for adenoid cystic carcinoma. There is no other neoplasm in the salivary gland that is so neurotrophic. This section shows a smaller branch of the facial nerve with actual infiltration of the nerve itself (Fig. 8–3). This section from the superficial lobe of the parotid shows entire replacement by a nest of tumor cells (Fig. 8–4). At first glance you would think it is an adenocarcinoma and you can see what looks like abortive luminal spaces. This is a so-called cribriform pattern. Some of the pink amorphous material associated with it, in fact, looks like cystic spaces, but it is a reduplication of the basilar laminar material. It is not true inspissated secretions. In some sections the neoplasm extends extremely close to the deep margins of dissection, so that involvement at this point could not be ruled out.

The inferior portion of the gland was submitted separately, containing a 1-cm nodule that was composed entirely of tumor. There were several benign lymph nodes associated with it. Because this nodule was far distant from the primary tumor, and because these tumors do not

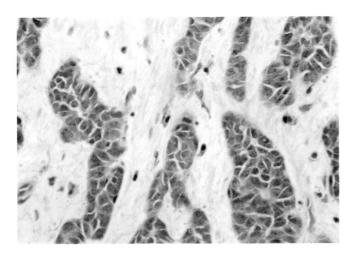

FIG. 8–2. CT axial image showing the tumor involving the superficial lobe of the parotid and abutting against the masseter muscle.

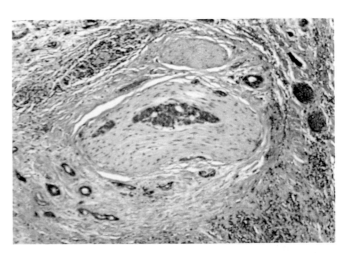

FIG. 8–3. Nerve fibers showing actual invasion by tumor.

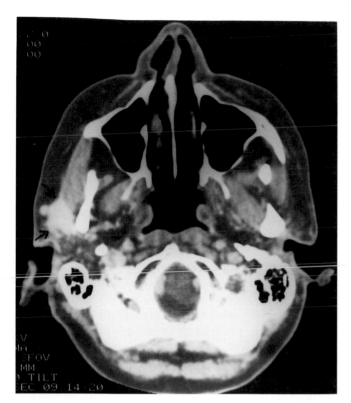

FIG. 8–4. Tumor from parotid gland resection. Note the tubuloglandular infiltrative pattern of compact, uniform cells. Mitotic figures (not seen here) are very scant, and true lumena are inconspicuous.

ordinarily have multicentric origin, this was interpreted as a lymph node completely effaced by tumor cells. These tumors do not routinely spread to lymph nodes but can do so with reports varying from 3% to 20%. Usually it spreads by contiguity along nerves and by hematogenous metastasis.

Question

Is this the solid or cribriform type?

Dr. Salyer: Like most salivary gland tumors, it has a spectrum of growth pattern that can be confusing sometimes in subclassifying them. This tumor is particularly distinctive because of small dark cells and the basilar laminar appearance, so that cytologically it always looks the same, but actually there are a variety of patterns. It can grow as a solid pattern, and that can be called solid adenoid cystic. It can actually form rather cysticlike spaces that contain abortive mucinous material. This is often called the cribriform pattern. Although the solid types are said to have a more ominous prognosis, it has not been demonstrated convincingly that pattern is related to prognosis. Prognosis is related more to staging and nerve involvement.

Pathologic stage was T3b N1 M0. The pathologic grade was II and the histologic pathology was adenoid cystic carcinoma.

Dr. John Salzman, Radiotherapist, stated that postoperative radiation would be started as soon as the wound is healed, giving at least 6,000 rads to achieve local tumor control. The field would include the stylomastoid foramen and intraosseous portions of the nerve, as well as the upper echelon of lymph nodes in the neck. In view of no other palpable disease, the lower neck would not be routinely treated. A wedged pair of photons would be used to obtain depth and also supplement that with electrons of appropriate energy. With this approach, we would hope to achieve local control recognizing, however, that there is a risk of distant metastases. With residual facial nerve involvement the outlook must remain guarded.

Dr. Englebrecht, Radiotherapist, stated it was their perception that adenoid cystic cancers are more radiosensitive than some of the other tumors, although it is not always radiocurable. In one large series reported, the local recurrence rate of adenoid cystic cancer was about 10%, which is a rate about one half to one third of what other malignant salivary gland tumors might have with similar postoperative radiation. In another article there were no local recurrences after surgery and radiation, but distant metastases often developed. In another, where only biopsy was done and no surgical resection was attempted, the tumor was treated with radiation only and 50% of those had long-term local control. So we believe it is relative radiosensitive, but one of the challenges to obtain adequate margins of radiation is to encompass all perineural spread. The radiation therapy is an important component to complement the surgical removal.

Question of Dr. Robert Schweitzer

Would some of the surgeons comment on the surgical procedure as to its adequacy and whether additional surgery might be indicated at this point?

Dr. Lionel Schour, Surgical Oncologist: There is a role for further surgery with this patient. One can use microscopic techniques, resecting the facial nerve back into the temporal bone in order to achieve tumor free margins. She started with a nerve paralysis so one is not worried about paralyzing the nerve. It is always desirable to document nerve involvement at the most proximal extent of the resection. This was not done by the surgeon. Also, it is desirable where possible not to remove the tumor in separate sections but to remove en bloc if possible. At the initial surgery possibly a more extensive local resection might have obtained more adequate margins on all aspects of the tumor, and a more adequate and thorough evaluation of the nodal status in the upper neck might have been done. There was probable spread to a lower parotid node. A lymphadenectomy with removal of nodes, at least in the upper neck, would have been indicated at that time.

Question of Dr. Laurie Schweitzer

How far would you chase the disease involving the facial nerve in its intraosseous portion?

Dr. Laurie Schweitzer, Head and Neck Surgical Oncologist: The nerve is already paralyzed, which simplifies the situation if you're going to follow the nerve in the mastoid up into the middle ear in the labyrinthine section of the nerve. Chances are the involvement is only in the mastoid portion of the nerve. With the intraparotid nodes containing tumor, I would certainly be interested to know what is going on in the rest of the neck. If further surgery is not contemplated, certainly the primary nodal depots should be included in the radiation field. There was no pain involved in her original symptoms, which is somewhat encouraging, indicating no sensory nerves are involved. Pain is not uncommon with adenoid cystic cancers.

Dr. Jai Balkissoon, Surgical Oncologist: I am also greatly concerned about local control here. Ideally, a more extensive local tumor and regional node removal might have been considered. I think the patient deserves a reoperation just to make sure there is no gross disease left behind locally and to follow the nerve up as far as you can, thereby doing the best cancer operation possible. In terms of the neck, I might even consider doing a neck dissection, at least removing nodes in the upper neck to be sure there is no involvement. Definitely I would give the patient postoperative radiotherapy to the primary area and the upper nodal areas.

Dr. Robert Schweitzer, Surgical Oncologist: I think the radiotherapist would agree with you. The point of treating microscopic disease when it is minimal gives a better chance for local control than if one has gross residual disease either in a local area or regional lymph nodes. Would chemotherapy have a role to play here?

Dr. David Pfister, Medical Oncologist: A number of agents have been used with recurrent or metastatic adenoid cystic cancer, including platinum, 5-fluorouracil, adriamycin, methotrexate, cytoxan, and vincristin, but the effect is always temporary. I would agree that a cancer operation had not been done—that's the most important thing.

Dr. Norman Cohen, Medical Oncologist, stated that he agreed with Dr. Pfister that the various agents can cause some response. The important thing to recognize is that this disease is going to recur in most patients. In review of the literature, the chance of recurrence based on the different histologic patterns varies, ranging from 100% recurrence with the solid to about 60% recurrence if it is a cribriform pattern. Not all will agree with that. The mortality again cited 30% at 5 years and 60% at 15 years. It is difficult to assess the role of adjuvant therapy because people recur 10 to 20 years later, whereas most of the adjuvant studies look at 2-, 3-, 4-, or 5-year intervals. So the long-term studies are not available. At U.C.S.F. several patients were treated in a neoadjuvant fashion using platinum and 5-FU without any effect or shrinkage on the primary, or increased survival after surgery and radiation. Should these patients get adjuvant therapy? They seem to be ideal candidates for this because most will develop distant metastases. I am not aware of any group that has studied this in a systematic way with a large number of patients to demonstrate the effect of adjuvant therapy on long-term survival. Theoretically, the patients who have a tumor that is responsive, and with micrometastases, adjuvant therapy is appropriate. So if you can present these data to a patient, and say there is every reason to give chemotherapy, and it's tolerable chemotherapy, it should be done, but it would almost have to be considered investigational.

In a small group of 10 patients Dr. Schweitzer referred to me over the last 14 years, we have used adjuvant chemotherapy using a combination of a variety of agents. I did not use platinum in this group because at that time we were more concerned with the toxicity. Only one person of this group developed pulmonary metastasis. I think patients like this are primary candidates for adjuvant therapy, but it has to be made clear to the patient that it is for investigative purposes.

Dr. Larry Strieff, Medical Oncologist: The urge to treat far exceeds the documented value of that treatment in terms of chemotherapy. As Dr. Cohen says, it's a bad disease that you wish you could have some impact on in the metastatic setting, but that does not necessarily translate into long-term benefit. It would take at least 10 to 20 years to follow up on people given adjuvant chemotherapy. Giving aggressive chemotherapy, without any established series to show a benefit, is difficult and is a hard sell for some people. I am thinking of this woman now who has had a facelift and now has lost her facial function and I wonder how she would take to losing her hair. As I said, it might be a hard sell.

Dr. Robert Schweitzer: This is one of the problems of the hard sell because over the years it has been difficult to get medical oncologists to give chemotherapy because of this hard sell, and the fact that you are using toxic drugs. There is no protocol for adjuvant therapy for adenoid cystic carcinoma even though it has such a high incidence of distant metastasis. We must try to interest large groups of surgeons who see these lesions, like the Society of Head and Neck Surgeons, to formulate some protocol for adjuvant therapy so that we can achieve data as to its effect on preventing metastatic disease occurring after many years.

Question for Dr. Jai Balkissoon

Would you resect a metastasis in the lung or liver if it were locally feasible?

Dr. Jai Balkissoon: Many of these tumors are slow growing. Sometimes people can live for many years with metastatic disease. With careful selection, resection of metastases might be of some value.

Dr. Jeff Demanes, Radiotherapist, stated that brachytherapy is effective therapy for both adenoid cystic and squamous carcinoma involving the head and neck region. Intraosseous extension and bone destruction, however, interfere with the applicator placement, affect radiation dose distribution, and limit the benefits. However, in a different location a combined program of external radiation and complex interstitial implantation is indicated for gross carcinoma. Microscopic residual disease after surgical removal with tumors in any location is often treated with intracavitary methods. We now employ a state-of-the-art computer base "high dose rate" remote after loading the system that completely eliminates radiation exposure to medical personnel, provides geometric optimization of the implant radiation dose, and frequently allows therapy to be given on an outpatient basis.

Dr. Robert Schweitzer: In summary, we have a woman with adenoid cystic carcinoma of the parotid that extends to deep margins, has perineural spread along the facial nerve to its point of division at the stylomastoid foramen, and has known metastasis to an intraparotid lymph node.

Recommendations were made to consider further surgery and follow with postoperative radiation to the primary area and neck. Adjuvant chemotherapy should be considered for this setting in the future in an effort to minimize distant metastasis.

I thank you all for your contributions.

Immediate Follow-Up

The patient refused surgery and adjuvant chemotherapy. Radiation therapy was given to the primary site and upper neck.

COMMENTARY by Don R. Goffinet

This woman, in otherwise good health, was found to have two contiguous mobile masses in the right preauricular area, as well as partial facial nerve paralysis. A total parotidectomy was performed, but tumor cells were noted at the deep resection margin as well as in the perineural lymphatics of the facial nerve. A separate portion of the inferior parotid gland, which contained a 1-cm nodule, was resected and this lesion was felt to be a lymph node completely replaced by neoplasm. The facial nerve was not reconstructed. The patient subsequently refused a repeat resection.

Salivary gland neoplasms comprise less than 5% of all head and neck malignancies, whereas adenoid cystic carcinoma, which makes up less than 10% of such tumors, is the most common cancer of the minor salivary and submandibular glands (1). These neoplasms can also arise in the parotid gland, although muco-epidermoid carcinomas are most common in this site. Adenoid cystic carcinomas have a long natural history (5-, 10-, and 15-year survival rates of 60, 50, and 30%, respectively) (Table 8–1). Because distant metastases can occur many years after

diagnosis, 20- to 25-year survival without evidence of disease is rare. The risk of cervical lymph node metastases at presentation is approximately 15% to 25% (2); in the present case, an intraparotid lymph node was apparently directly invaded by the tumor. Perineural lymphatic spaces are also commonly invaded by adenoid cystic carcinomas.

Indications for postoperative irradiation of malignant salivary gland tumors include the finding of involved surgical margins, perineural lymphatic infiltration, lymph node involvement, recurrences, or invasion of skeletal muscle or osseous structures (3). The prognosis is worse for patients whose adenoid cystic carcinomas are larger than 4.0 cm, involve bone, perineural lymphatics, facial nerve, or have a solid rather than glandular histology (4–12). The use of adequate sized (> 8 ∞ 8 cm) radiation ports is also important in obtaining optimal local control (13). The patient in this case presentation not only had an involved surgical margin, but also perineural extension along the facial nerve. Postoperative radiation therapy is definitely indicated in this situation and should be carefully planned to include the parotid resection bed, while treating deeply enough medially to include the deep resection margin (near the mid-line of the oropharynx) (Fig. 8–5). A limited CT scan obtained during treatment planning is useful in allowing precise localization of the treatment volume and in optimizing the radiation beam angles. A treatment plan is derived that includes not only the resection site but also the intraosseous path of the facial nerve beyond the stylomastoid foramen to the base of the skull.

The most common radiation therapy technique after parotidectomy uses an isocentrically oriented beam pair. The superior beam margin is placed at or slightly above the zygoma; the posterior border is in the postauricular area; the inferior margin is at the level of the hyoid bone; and the anterior field edge is at the posterior margin of the masseter muscle. Because the surgical margins were involved in the patient under discussion, the total radiation dose to the parotid bed should be at least 6,000 cGy. Lower doses (4,500–5,000 cGy) can be delivered to the intraosseous facial nerve and the base skull. In the treatment planning process, the radiation dose to the optic chiasm, retinal arteries, retinae, brain stem, brain, and spinal cord should all be calculated so that they do not exceed approximately 4,500 cGy. A daily radiation dose of 180 to 200 cGy is used. After delivering 4,500 to 5,000 cGy to the entire tumor bed, the radiation field size is reduced and a treatment boost is given to the resection site so that the total dose is approximately 6,000 to 6,600 cGy. This boost may be given using either an ipsilateral photon beam or an electron beam, with the energy to be determined by the required treatment depth—usually 12 to 16 MeV.

Radiation therapy can be expected to reduce the risk of a local recurrence by approximately 50%. Because a lymph node was involved by carcinoma in this case and a neck resection was not performed, the remaining ipsilateral cervical lymph nodes should also be irradiated. The superior cervical lymph nodes to the level of the hyoid bone are included in the oblique portals; an anterior neck field, matched to the superior ports, should be added inferiorly (with spinal cord protection) to deliver 5,000 cGy at 180 to 200 cGy per day to a depth of 3.0 cm.

Carefully planned radiation fields increase the likelihood of preserving the function of the opposite parotid gland, and simulation and port radiographs will ensure that the beam does not exit through the contralateral eye. If the superior beam edge is too high and there is risk of the beam exiting through the opposite globe, the top of the field may be reduced and a superficial electron field used in its place. During treatment, incisional bolus must be used to obtain an adequate radiation dose at the skin surface. The photon beam should be approximately 4 MeV, preferably from a linear accelerator operating at an 80- to 100-cm source to skin distance. Dental care must be optimized and any

needed restorations performed before the start of the radiation therapy course. Prophylactic fluoride rinses should also be used daily. Hydrocortisone cream may be required to lessen radiation epidermitis. Eustachian dysfunction, serous otitis media, and temporomandibular joint fibrosis may also occur. Properly planned irradiation should not result in brain injury, myelitis, or visual deficits.

Photon radiation therapy alone for large salivary neoplasms is unlikely to be curative; combining total parotidectomy and postoperative irradiation is optimal therapy for high-grade malignant lesions (10,14). The best local control for advanced, unresectable salivary gland tumors appears to be obtained by neutron treatment. Excellent long-term control of massive lesions with neutron beam therapy has been reported (15).

Since 1972, the Stanford University Department of Radiation Oncology has delivered postoperative irradiation to

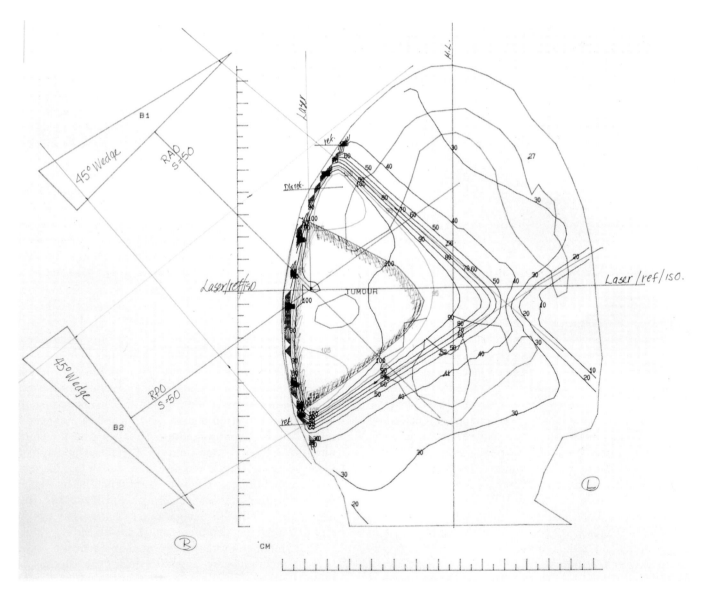

FIG. 8–5. Radiation dose distribution, right parotid region, for obliquely directed isocentric photon beam pair.

seven patients with adenoid cystic carcinomas of the parotid glands—six women (average age 28 years) and one man (age 67). Local control has been obtained in six of the seven patients, including two of three patients who had preoperative facial nerve involvement, with a mean follow-up period of 7 years. Radiation doses of 5,000 to 6,800 cGy to the tumor bed with oblique paired beams (as described above) and 5,000 cGy to the ipsilateral cervical lymph nodes were used. One patient succumbed to lung and liver metastases, and another has pulmonary metastases.

In summary, carefully planned postoperative radiotherapy results in improved local control of adenoid cystic and other salivary gland malignancies. Such treatments may be delivered safely, with minimal risk of dental, ocular, cerebral, or spinal cord injury.

REFERENCES

1. Fitzpatrick PJ, Theriault C. Malignant salivary gland tumors. *Int J Radiat Oncology Biol Phys* 1986;12(10):1743–7.
2. Bosch A, Brandenburg JH, Gilchrist KW. Lymph node metastases in adenoid cystic carcinoma of the submaxillary gland. *Cancer* 1980;45 (11):2872–7.
3. Guillamondegui OM, Byers RM, Luna MA, Chiminazzo H, et al. Aggressive surgery in treatment for parotid cancer: the role of adjunctive postoperative radiotherapy. *Am J Roentgenol Radium Ther Nucl Med* 1975;123(1):49–54.
4. Hamper K, Lazar F, Dietel M, Caselitz J, et al. Prognostic factors for adenoid cystic carcinoma of the head and neck: a retrospective evaluation of 96 cases from the German salivary gland registry. *J Oral Pathol Med* 1990;19:101–7.
5. Matsuba HM, Spector GJ, Thawley SE, Simpson JR, et al. Adenoid cystic salivary gland carcinoma: a histopathologic review of treatment failure patterns. *Cancer* 1986;57(3):519–24.
6. Matsuba HM, Thawley SE, Levine LA, et al. Adenoid cystic carcinoma of major and minor salivary gland origin. *Laryngoscope* 1984;94(10):1316–18.
7. Miglianico L, Eschwege F, Marandas P, Wilbault P. Cervico-facial adenoid cystic carcinoma: study of 102 cases. Influence on radiation therapy. *Int J Radiat Oncol Biol Phys* 1987;13:673–8.
8. Nascimento AG, Amaral ALP, Prado LAF, Kligerman J, Silveira TRP. Adenoid cystic carcinoma of salivary glands—a study of 61 cases with clinicopathologic correlation. *Cancer* 1986;57:312–9.
9. Santucci M, Bondi R. New prognostic criterion in adenoid cystic carcinoma of salivary gland origin. *Am J Clin Pathol* 1989;91(2):132–6.
10. Spiro IJ, Wang CC, Montgomery WW. Carcinoma of the parotid gland: analysis of treatment results and patterns of failure after combined surgery and radiation therapy. *Cancer* 1993;71(9):2699–2705.
11. Spiro RH, Huvos AG, Strong EW. Adenoid cystic carcinoma: factors influencing survival. *Am J Surg* 1979;138:579–83.
12. Weinstein GS, Conley JJ. Adenoid cystic carcinoma of the parotid gland: a review of surgical management with reference to the facial nerve. *Ann Otol Rhinol Laryngol* 1989;98(11):845–7.
13. Vikram B, Strong EW, Shah JP, Spiro RH. Radiation therapy in adenoid cystic carcinoma. *Int J Radiat Oncol Biol Phys* 1984;10:221–3.
14. North CA, Lee DJ, Piantadosi S, et al. Carcinoma of the major salivary glands treated by surgery or surgery plus postoperative radiotherapy. *Int J Radiat Oncol Biol Phys* 1990;18:1319–26.
15. Buchholz TA, Shimotakahara SG, Weymuller EA, et al. Neutron radiotherapy for adenoid cystic carcinoma of the head and neck. *Arch Otolaryngol Head Neck Surg* 1993;119:747–52.

EDITORIAL BOARD COMMENTARY

The initial priority in the management of this tumor is local control following surgical oncologic principles to achieve negative margins and using postoperative adjuvant radiation therapy. If local control can be achieved, the problem of a high systemic recurrence rate over a long period of time needs to be addressed with improved adjuvant therapies.

TABLE 8-1. *Adenoid Cystic Carcinoma of the Head and Neck*

Author & Reference Number	Number of Patients	Surgery	Surgery & XRT	XRT	LN +	NED	LOCAL CONTROL
Bosch, et al 1980 (2) (submaxillary gland)	10	6	4	0	4 (40%)	4 (mean follow up 5 yrs.)	
Hamper, et al 1990 (4) (All H & N sites)	74	all	?	?	5.4%	15 (20.3%) (7–22 yrs.)	
Matsuba, et al 1986 (5)	71	19	47	12		Actuarial 5 yr. Survival 65%	XRT alone 30% 5 yr., 25% 10 yr., Surgery alone 45% 5 yr., 25% 10 yr., Surgery & XRT 85% 5yr., 65% 10 yr.
Matsuba, et al 1984 (6)	76	24	36	16			Surgery – 25% 10 yr. Surgery & XRT – 83% 10 yr.
Miglianico, et al 1987 (7) (All H & N sites)	102	38	43	11	11 (11%)	46.1% 5 yr. 36.5% 10 yr. 26.8% 15 yr.	55.5% 5 yr., 37.7% 10 yr. (all patients) 38 pts. Surgery alone 44% } 5yr. 21 pts. XRT alone 65.8% } 5 yr. 43 pts. Surgery – XRT 77.8%
Spiro, et al 1979 (11)	136 (no prior rx)	most			29 (21%)		
Spiro, Wang, Montgomery 1993 (10)	16		16				13/16 (81%)
Vikram, et al 1984 (13)	74	25		49 (rec. or unresectable)			XRT alone – 3/49 (6.5%) 5 yr. Surgery & XRT – 13/25 (52%)
Bucholz, et al 1993 (15)	34			neutrons			Actuarial 5 yr. – LC 76% Actuarial 5 yr. Local 63% + regional

LN: Lymph node involvement   NED: No evidence of disease   LC: Local control   REC: Recurrent   XRT: Radiation Therapy

9

High-Grade Mucoepidermoid Carcinoma of the Parotid Gland

Ronald H. Spiro

An aggressive parotid gland carcinoma with a confusing presentation

CASE PRESENTATION

E.S. was a 60-year-old man who was admitted with a 2-month history of swelling over the left side of his jaw. About 2 weeks before admission, this began to enlarge rapidly, associated with some pain that radiated up posteriorly behind the left ear. A local physician was consulted, who prescribed an antibiotic, but there was no improvement. Subsequently, he was referred to a dentist, and then an oral surgeon. After obtaining a negative panoramic roentgenogram, the patient was referred for a head and neck surgical opinion.

Patient was a diabetic of 5 years' duration, controlled on oral medication. He described numbness of the left side of his face present for several months, associated with occasional tingling in the lower extremities, which he related to his diabetes.

He was a well-developed, heavy-set, healthy-appearing white man who had obvious fullness of the left side of his face overlying the angle of the mandible that extended inferiorly into the upper left neck. An ill-defined mass was palpable in this area, which seemed fixed with respect to the deeper tissues. Facial nerve function was completely normal, but there was a broad area of hypesthesia involving the skin of the left cheek in areas supplied by the second and third divisions of cranial V (Fig. 9–1). The clinical impression was malignant parotid gland tumor.

Fine-needle aspiration biopsy was performed at the time of the initial visit. The official report read: "Suspicious cells present. Cannot classify further. Suggest

biopsy for definitive classification." Unofficially, the cytologist commented that the smear probably contained carcinoma cells with sarcomatous features (Fig. 9–2A). A computed tomography (CT) scan of the head and neck was performed the same day. The report described a $4 \times 4 \times 3$ cm heterogeneous infiltrating tumor largely within the submandibular triangle below the masseter muscle and angle of the mandible with infiltrating densities extending into the substance of the parotid gland, possibly indicating perineural spread. The mass was thought to be extraparotid in origin, and there were multiple densities within the gland considered to be either residual glandular tissue or metastatic intraparotid nodes. Several submandibular nodes anterior to the mass suggested metastatic spread. It was the radiologist's impression that this tumor was most probably a sarcoma arising in the masseter muscle; parotid neoplasm was considered unlikely (Fig. 9–3).

Because neither the FNAB or the CT scan seemed consistent with the clinical impression, a Tru-cut needle biopsy was performed 3 days later. This time the report read: "High grade carcinoma, largely composed of poorly differentiated mucin-producing adenocarcinoma with small foci of squamous differentiation (poorly differentiated mucoepidermoid or adenosquamous carcinoma)" (Fig. 9–2B).

The patient was admitted to Memorial Sloan Kettering Cancer Center 10 days after his initial visit. The next day he had a left subtotal parotidectomy, sacrificing the lower division of the facial nerve and excising the underlying masseter muscle down to the periosteum of the mandible

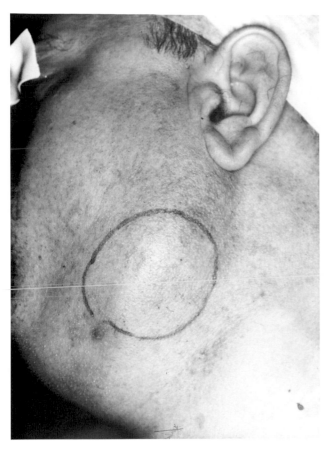

FIG. 9–1. Five-cm firm mass, somewhat fixed, overlying the angle of the left mandible and extending into the upper neck. Discolored area anterior to the mass marks the site where a Tru-cut needle biopsy was taken.

inferiorly. The left submandibular gland was excised in continuity with the tumor, as well as the upper deep chain of jugular lymph nodes (Level 2) (Fig. 9–4). Recovery was uneventful, and he was discharged on the eighth postoperative day with mild lower facial asymmetry.

The pathology report was high-grade mucoepidermoid carcinoma involving the parotid gland and adjacent fibroadipose tissue. Perineural invasion is noted. Surgical margins clear. Metastatic carcinoma was present in one Level 2 lymph node (Fig. 9–2C).

Postoperative radiation therapy was delivered in a hospital within his community. He received a total dose of 5,440 rads using a 15 MeV linear accelerator over a period of 7 weeks. The portals included the parotid gland and upper half of the ipsilateral neck, as well as the base of the skull, and the calculated dose to the parotid gland was 6,000 rads.

The patient was followed in his community and had no problems until 2 months later, when a routine CT scan showed an enlarged, necrotic lymph node in the left neck at the level of the cricoid cartilage.

Examination confirmed the presence of a 3-cm mass that seemed to be just below the skin tanning, which marked the inferior border of the previous neck radiation portal (Fig. 9–5).

Shortly thereafter, a completion left radical neck dissection was performed. He was discharged 6 days later and the pathology report was metastatic mucoepidermoid carcinoma with extracapsular extension. An additional 5,000 rads was delivered to the left lower neck and supraclavicular area over a 5-week period.

He remained disease-free in the head and neck area, but developed chest pain 8 months later. Chest radiographs showed a destructive lesion in the right 6th rib, associated with a sizable soft tissue mass. Question was also raised about a possible right upper lung nodule. Needle aspiration biopsy of the rib lesion performed elsewhere confirmed the presence of metastatic mucoepidermoid carcinoma. He received palliative chemotherapy elsewhere, deteriorated rapidly, and died 2 months after the onset of his chest pain. No autopsy was performed, but the cause of death was disseminated mucoepidermoid carcinoma, most extensively involving ribs and peritoneum. There was no clinical evidence of recurrence in the primary site or the neck.

COMMENTARY by William R. Panje

A rapidly enlarging salivary gland mass with pain and nerve dysfunction (facial nerve paresis/trigeminal or cervical cutaneous hypesthesia) strongly suggests a malignant salivary gland neoplasm. Fine-needle biopsy and CT scan with infusion should be performed on such suspicious salivary gland masses as a routine diagnostic evaluation. Because clinical examination alone can often be misleading, any additional testing that can improve the physician and surgeon's diagnostic specificity before embarking on definitive treatment in most cases improves the overall management of the patient. Even though in this case the fine-needle aspiration biopsy (FNA) was inconclusive, the clinical suspicion (sensitivity) was so high for a malignancy that a repeat FNA might be considered or a CT scan could be done. The FNA results often depend on adequacy of the sampling technique and the experience of the cytopathologist. Some well respected pathologists are vehemently opposed to FNA because in most but not all cases a definitive biopsy (sialadenectomy) will be subsequently performed regardless of a prior FNA. I, as well as other clinicians, disagree with this because the FNA will in many instances confirm one's suspicion and encourage a more specific evaluation, e.g., bone/gadolinium scans to determine metastasis from the parotid. Magnetic resonance angiography to determine hemangioma or carotid body tumor, technetium 99 to evaluate a Warthin's, mammography for possible metastatic breast cancer, CT/MRI scan for deep lobe parotid mass, schwannoma of IX–XII cranial nerves, or metastatic cervical adenopathy. In addition, in

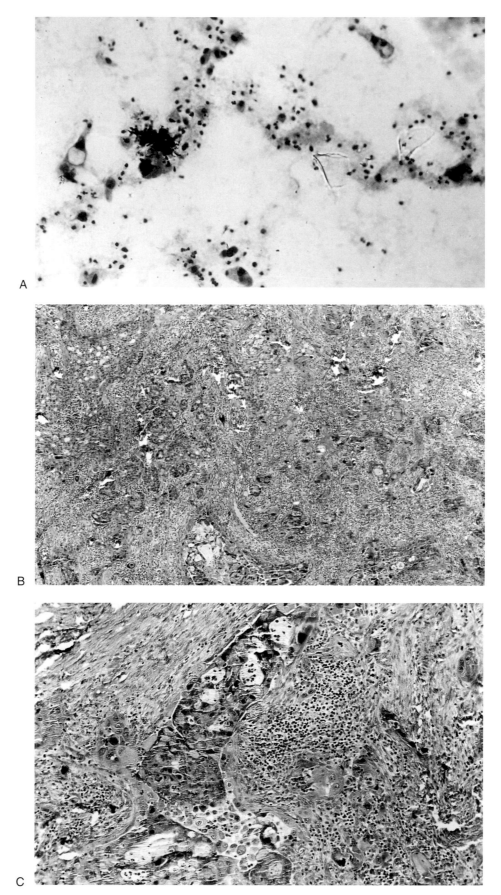

FIG. 9–2. A: FNAB showing scattered malignant cells. Carcinoma was favored over sarcoma. (Pap smear ×400.) **B:** Core biopsy (Tru-cut) showed a diffusely infiltrating, poorly differentiated, mucin-producing adenocarcinoma with squamous features, surrounded by lymphoid infiltrate. (H&E ×100.) **C:** Representative section from the surgical specimen showing a poorly differentiated mucoepidermoid carcinoma without special microscopic pattern formation. (H&E ×60.)

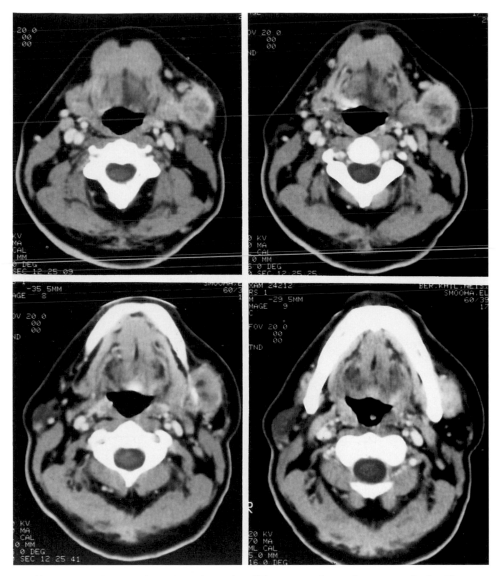

FIG. 9–3. Representative axial sections from the CT scan performed preoperatively. The mass was thought to be extraparotid in origin and parotid neoplasm was considered unlikely.

other less obvious cases than this one the FNA might suggest a malignancy, thus allowing the surgeon and his team to be better prepared preoperatively, but of more importance the patient may be better informed as to what to expect from the operation. Awakening with a facial paralysis and partial temporal bone resection after a 6-hour operation when it was thought that a 1-hour procedure would just "get rid of the lump" frequently produces an angry and distrustful patient.

Similarly, I think the CT scan with infusion provides useful information for diagnosis and subsequent treatment. Despite the radiologist's misleading impression in this case, personal review of the CT scan as well as a reading of the description indicate evidence of perineural involvement with extension into the parotid gland and cervical metastasis. These findings were confirmed at the

time of the surgery. This emphasizes the importance of the surgeon reviewing the actual tests including cytology, scans, roentgenograms, etc., rather than just reading reports. In this particular case I may have also obtained an MRI and a bone scan preoperatively.

The MRI would have possibly allowed better resolution of the perineural extension along the trigeminal cervical cutaneous, facial, and/or hypoglossal nerves. Again, the more complete the diagnostic preoperative evaluation, the better the surgeon can be prepared. Facial and/or hypoglossal nerve grafting at the time of the excision usually provides for excellent return of function in 2 to 4 months after the operation. Although the surgeon felt in this case that the facial nerve deficit was mild, a professional person who deals with the public for a living may find this same result catastrophic to

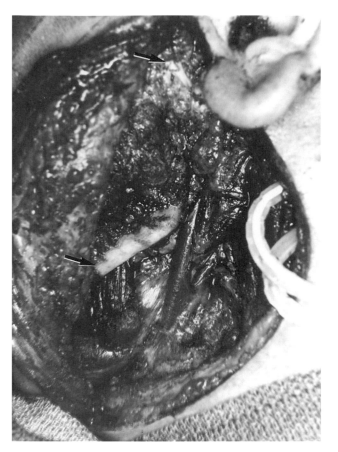

FIG. 9–4. View of the operative field after near-total left parotidectomy. The *upper arrow* points to the upper division of the facial nerve, which was preserved. The *lower arrow* shows where a portion of the masseter muscle was included with the specimen, including the underlying periosteum of the mandible. The submandibular gland and upper deep jugular lymph nodes were also removed with the specimen.

their work and life, regardless of the neoplasm's biologic activity.

A bone scan in this patient may have identified bone invasion or a larger area of mandibular periosteum involvement requiring a marginal (inferior) mandibulectomy and/or larger area of periosteum removal. If this neoplasm had been located more posteriorly, proximate to the external auditory canal and the mandible condyle, the need for an external temporal bone resection, including a condylectomy, may have been needed.

I agree with the concept of tailoring the operative procedure to the extent of disease. In this particular case my "tailoring" would have included intraoperative confirmation of perineural spread (biopsy of distal branches V2, 3, and cervical cutaneous nerves as well as frozen section analysis of the parotid specimen as well as any suspicious cervical nodes) and subsequent resection as necessary. Nodal dissection would have included levels I, II, and III as well as the accessory chain—probably a modified neck dissection.

Neck dissections are in general not indicated for parotid malignancy because there is usually less than a 15% incidence of ipsilateral nodal spread. However, the finding of a positive ipsilateral node either from a CT scan, FNA, or intraoperative biopsy with evidence of a parotid gland malignancy indicates a very aggressive neoplasm, suggesting the need for a more extensive neck dissection.

I am not a radiation oncologist, but as a co-member of a multidisciplinary head and neck oncology team (surgeons, radiation therapists, hematology/oncologist, etc.), the suggestion on my part would have been for much more aggressive adjunctive therapy. Once a cervical node is involved with cancer, the spread into adjacent lymph nodes becomes relatively disorganized at times, even skipping node levels. In this case the findings of perineural invasion, lymph node metastasis, and a high-grade mucoepidermoid carcinoma would have required large field radiation to include the skull base (V2, V3 extension) and at least complete ipsilateral anterior and posterior necks. Currently, we would have given simultaneous chemotherapy and radiation therapy.

Salivary gland neoplasm management presents a host of possibilities. The case in point reveals two acceptable ways

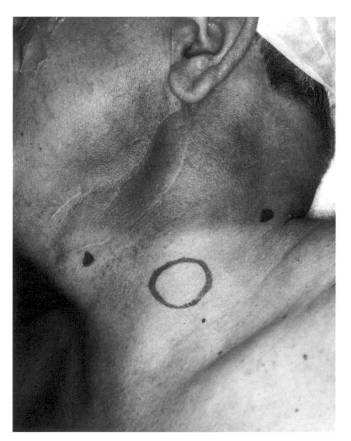

FIG. 9–5. A 3-cm clinically positive lymph node just inferior to the portal used to deliver postoperative radiotherapy to the neck. The lower half of the neck was not treated.

of approaching diagnosis and treatment. The final outcome in this specific case probably would have been the same regardless of either approach followed. However, low-grade malignancies, larger benign neoplasms, or deep lobe tumor may present an extremely different sequence of events for you, the surgeon, and the patient. Unlike Dr. Spiro, most of you have managed only a few parotid neoplasms and are at risk for unexpected complications, mental anguish, and "hassle" if and when you deal with a recurrence, especially for a benign neoplasm; the removal of the lateral lobe of the parotid when the neoplasm is really in the deep lobe; a positive margin found out 5 days after the operation; permanent facial nerve paralysis after removal of a benign neoplasm; a permanent facial paralysis when you know the facial nerve was intact intraoperatively; a sialocele that you convert into a salivary fistula; a Frey syndrome or an anesthetic ear the patient was not told about preoperatively and they had a benign tumor. Remember, the better prepared you and the patient are before the operation, the better postoperative result regardless of the outcome.

REFERENCE

1. *Comprehensive Management of Head and Neck Tumors, vols. I–III,* Thawley SA, Panje WR, eds. Philadelphia: WB Saunders; 1987.

EDITORIAL BOARD COMMENTARY

The three important points illustrated in this case included: 1) clinical judgment is at least as important as fine-needle aspiration biopsy and CT (and the latter can be even misleading, as shown in this case); 2) adjunctive radiation therapy must be as good as the surgery; and 3) distant dissemination can occur despite local control and remains an unresolved problem despite promising results from chemotherapy for local control.

High-grade mucoepidermoid carcinoma requires aggressive surgery and radiation therapy. It seems likely in this case that the outcome was dictated more by the biology of the tumor than the specific treatment given.

10

Squamous Cell Carcinoma of the Ear with Clinically Positive Parotid Nodes

Willard E. Fee, Jr.

A delay in diagnosis because of the common confusion of keratoacanthoma and squamous cell carcinoma

CASE PRESENTATION

This 53-year-old male personal injury attorney first presented to his family physician with a painful draining left ear. His past history was essentially noncontributory and he was treated with topical otobiotic drops initially, with resolution of his pain and drainage, but a 5-mm erythematous raised lesion was noted at the junction of his concha and external auditory canal. He was referred to a plastic surgeon for excision, which was accomplished, and the initial pathology demonstrated keratoacanthoma. The surgical wound was not closed, but left to heal secondarily. A small amount of purulent secretion developed during the healing phase and the patient was begun on dicloxacillin. Six weeks after the initial excision, the wound was healing slowly and by 10 weeks postoperatively, the wound had completely healed. Three months after the original surgery, the patient developed a small abscess in the postauricular area, which was incised and drained. A culture showed *Staphylococcus aureus* (coagulase positive). One week later, he developed a preauricular swelling and was again begun on dicloxacillin, which produced resolution of his cellulitis and a decrease of his pre- and postauricular swelling. Granulation tissue was noted in the posterior inferior cartilaginous portion of his ear canal and a biopsy showed invasive squamous cell carcinoma.

Five months later, the patient was referred to the Stanford Head and Neck Tumor Board, where the above history was noted. During childhood, he received radiation treatments (source and number unknown) for acne. He had lived in California all his life and had moderate sun exposure. He smoked a pipe, approximately five bowls per day for the last 20 years. He consumed approximately two mixed drinks and four glasses of wine per month. His only medication has been Kenalog lotion for chronic scalp dermatitis.

Physical exam on presentation revealed granulation tissue of the posterior inferior cartilaginous external auditory canal extending 3 mm onto the concha. There was moderate edema of the cartilaginous portion of the ear canal, but the bony canal and tympanic membrane appeared normal. The inferior aspect of the ear showed mild edema with erythema and it was slightly tender. There was a 2 × 1.5 cm postauricular lesion that was draining clear, watery fluid. A 2.5-cm firm preauricular lesion was noted that was freely mobile and nontender (Fig. 10–1). Facial nerve function was completely intact. Oral cavity, oropharynx, and larynx were normal and, specifically, there was no bulge to the lateral pharyngeal mucosa. Examination of the neck revealed a 1-cm left jugulo-digastric node, but was otherwise negative. An audiogram showed bilateral symmetrical high frequency sensorineural hearing loss with normal discrimination on speech testing. Acoustic reflexes were present bilaterally. His facial skin showed mild acne scarring, but was otherwise free of lesions. The remainder of his general physical examination was within normal limits.

Our pathologists concurred with the referring pathologist that the most recent biopsy of the left external canal showed morphologic features of a moderately well differentiated invasive squamous cell carcinoma. In retrospect,

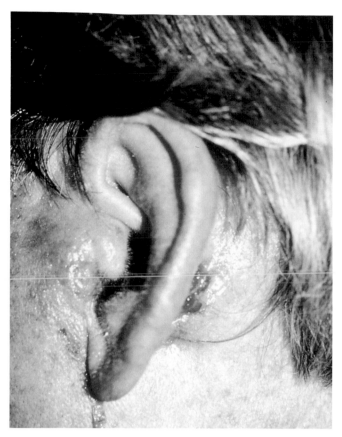

FIG. 10–1. Lateral view of the patient showing a preauricular mass just anterior to the tragus and a postauricular mass with granulation tissue. Exudate is seen exiting the external canal onto the lobule of the ear and upper neck skin.

the original lesion was believed to represent a well differentiated squamous cell carcinoma (Fig. 10–2).

Computed tomography (CT) scan showed moderate thickening of the inferior aspect of the pinna and extensive soft tissue induration that enhances in the preauricular and postauricular areas. There is clouding of the mastoid air cells adjacent to the external canal, but no bony erosion is identified. The middle ear space appears normal and no intracranial abnormalities are noted. There is extensive induration in and about the external auditory canal. Small soft tissue densities (probable retention cysts) are noted in the left sphenoid (Fig. 10–3) and are also seen in the antrum on other cuts.

Sadly, this is yet another case of a suspected keratoacanthoma that turned out to be a squamous cell carcinoma. The differential diagnosis can be an exceedingly difficult one, both pathologically and clinically. However, any keratoacanthoma that does not resolve completely by 6 weeks is best considered a well differentiated squamous cell carcinoma and treated appropriately. Squamous cell carcinoma of the external ear canal requires, at the least, a modified temporal bone resection followed by postoperative radiation therapy. If the middle ear space is involved, a total temporal bone resection is the treatment of choice, although we have had success with a modified temporal bone resection followed by drill out of the remaining temporal bone. The latter, although offering about the same chance of cure as a total temporal bone resection, produces significantly less morbidity and no operative mortality in contrast to a total temporal bone resection, where the operative mortality ranges between 5% and 10%. This patient will require a modified neck dissection (sparing the XIth nerve, if possible) plus a near total parotidectomy (sparing the superior portion of the deep lobe of the parotid). The best reconstruction for this patient is either a pectoralis major myocutaneous flap or a trapezius myocutaneous flap in view of the need to bring in bulk after his resection. The upper third of the auricle can be saved and should be inset into the temporal line so that the patient can retain support for wearing glasses in the future.

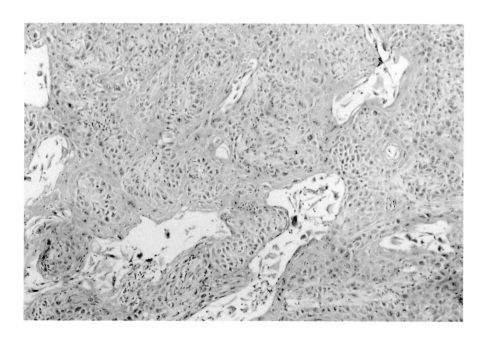

FIG. 10–2. Photomicrograph at 100× power, Hematoxylin and eosin stain of a frozen section of the ear canal lesion just before the patient's surgery showing a moderately differentiated squamous cell carcinoma.

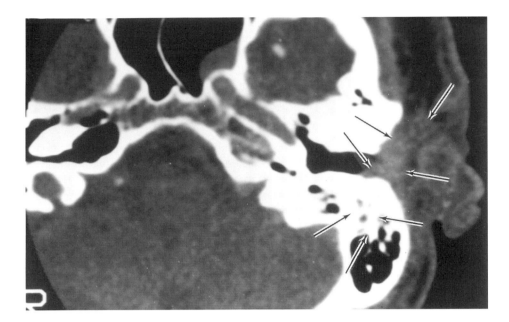

FIG. 10–3. CT scan of the patient's left temporal bone at the inferior aspect of the ear canal. The tumor is outlined by *arrows* and can be seen extending anteriorly to the cartilaginous ear canal into the soft tissues around the parotid gland. Posteriorly, the mastoid air cells near the tumor are opacified, although the superior aspect of the mastoid, middle ear space, and superior bony canal were free of disease. A probable retention cyst is present in the left sphenoid.

Additionally, this remaining appendage can be used to support an ear prosthesis.

Permission should be obtained to resect the facial nerve if that appears grossly involved, with immediate reconstruction by either a greater auricular nerve from the opposite neck or a sural nerve graft if more than 10 cm of the nerve needs to be resected.

Postoperative radiation therapy should be undertaken because of the high risk of local recurrence.

The patient underwent a left subtotal auriculectomy, modified temporal bone resection, radical neck dissection, and left pectoralis major myocutaneous flap reconstruction. The XIth nerve could not be saved because tumor was seen to be infiltrating the posterior belly of the digastric and the anterior, upper part of the trapezius muscle. Tumor extended to the facial nerve, but did not involve the facial nerve as it exited from the stylomastoid foramen. The facial nerve was identified and decompressed from its horizontal portion in the mastoid to the stylomastoid foramen. A superficial parotidectomy and partial deep lobe parotidectomy were performed. Tumor was eroding through the mastoid tip into the mastoid air cells. Grossly, all margins were deemed to be negative and this proved to be correct on permanent section (Fig. 10–4).

Postoperatively, the patient recovered uneventfully; his facial nerve function was 100%. He then received 5,000 rads to his temporal bone via the left anterior oblique and left posterior oblique fields in 25 treatments over 42 days; 5,000 rads was given to the left neck and supraclavicular area via an anterior field via 25 treatments over 42 days.

He tolerated the radiation well. Over the ensuing 5½ years, he had several basal cell carcinomas, squamous cell carcinomas, and actinic keratoses that were removed from

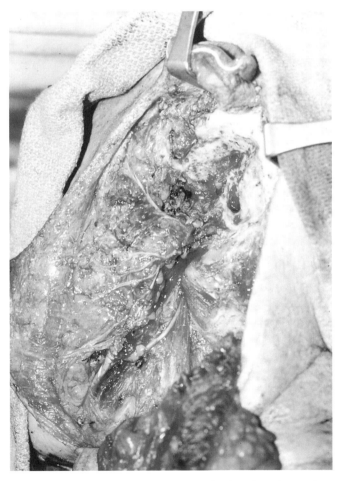

FIG. 10–4. Intraoperative photograph showing the patient after neck dissection, near total parotidectomy, and modified temporal bone resection. At the inferior aspect of the incision is a pectoralis major myocutaneous flap awaiting to be sewn into the defect.

his face and trunk by the Dermatology Service. Five and a half years after his resection, he developed a subcutaneous nodule in the left upper chest that was removed and reported as metastatic squamous cell carcinoma. He was referred back to our service for a wide local excision and flap reconstruction, which was performed uneventfully. He is 8½ years after his initial surgery (Fig. 10–5). Postoperative CT scan with soft tissue and bony windows are shown in Figures 10–6 and 10–7. He remains free of disease.

COMMENTARY by John G. Batsakis

It is cases such as this that add fuel to the controversy surrounding keratoacanthoma, a cutaneous lesion that always requires circumspection by pathologists and clinicians. The literature concerning keratoacanthoma offers little help. Antipodal statements that the solitary form of keratoacanthoma is a squamous cell carcinoma are aligned against detailed clinicopathologic studies that justify keratoacanthoma as a cutaneous pseudomalignant neoplasm (1–3).

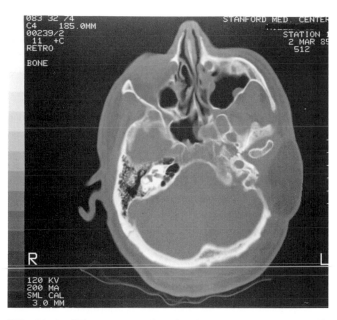

FIG. 10–6. CT scan 5 months after the original resection with soft tissue windows. The temporal bone lateral to the cochlear is absent on the left. Retention cysts are seen in the left sphenoid and antrum.

When one uses keratoacanthoma as a diagnostic term, one is describing a self-healing lesion of the skin that is mainly on sun-exposed areas of elderly people. Most keratoacanthomas occur on the face, forearms, or hands. Up to 80% of solitary keratoacanthomas are said to occur in the head and neck, particularly on the cheeks, nose, and

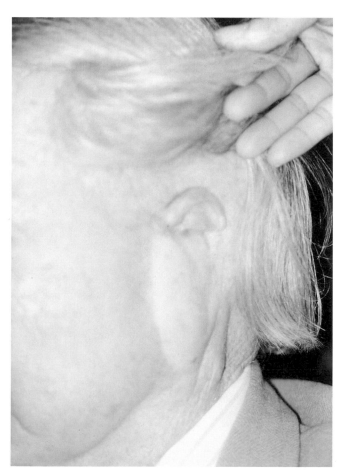

FIG. 10–5. Oblique field of the patient 8½ years after his resection.

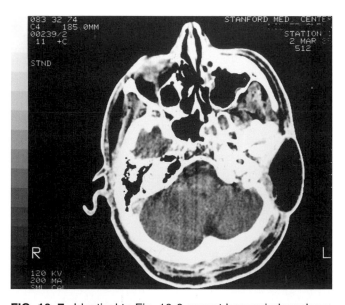

FIG. 10–7. Identical to Fig. 10-6 except bony windows have been used in the CT scan technique. The pectoralis major myocutaneous flap shows clearly as the darkened void on the scan.

lips. Besides the usual solitary form, keratoacanthoma also exists in several morphologic or syndromic forms (2).

In bona fide keratoacanthomas, there is an evolution through clinicopathologic stages: proliferative, mature, and resolving. The lesion usually reaches its full size within several weeks. Involution begins after a few months, with time from origin to spontaneous resolution usually taking 4 to 6 months (2). Some persist for a year or longer.

In its classic mature form, keratoacanthoma presents with a flasklike configuration of cells with a lateral collar and an abrupt marginal lipping that is well demarcated. There are no aberrant cytologic features except a mild hyperchromatism and an increased mitotic activity in the basilar layer.

The foregoing gives an impression of relative ease of diagnosis—not so! Reed (4) has indicated the lesions manifest a continuous histologic spectrum from the cytologically benign to the cytologically malignant. Schwartz (2) states that the only true test of distinction between a keratoacanthoma and squamous cell carcinoma is spontaneous resolution. So much for reliance on histopathology! Compounding already ambiguous histopathologic criteria are reports of perineural invasion and intravascular extension in keratoacanthomas, dismissed as "an alarming but benign phenomenon" (3,5).

It is my practice, espoused also by Hodak et al. (1), to regard solitary keratoacanthoma as a squamous cell carcinoma with a distinctive clinical and histopathologic appearance and as a tumor that, although capable of com-plete resolution without therapy, requires complete surgical removal. Punch or shave biopsies are never appropriate means to confirm a clinical diagnosis of keratoacanthoma.

If the solitary cutaneous keratoacanthoma is such a controversial lesion, where does the oral version stand (6)? It, like its counterpart in the skin, is to be regarded as well differentiated squamous cell carcinoma.

REFERENCES

1. Hodak E, Jones RE, Ackerman AB. Solitary keratoacanthoma is a squamous cell carcinoma: three examples with metastases. *Am J Dermatopathol* 1993;15:332–42.
2. Schwartz RA. Keratoacanthoma. *J Am Acad Dermatol* 1994;30:1–19.
3. Cooper PH, Wolfe JT. Perioral keratoacanthomas with extensive perineural invasion and intravenous growth. *Arch Dermatol* 1988;124:1397–401.
4. Reed RJ. Actinic keratoacanthoma. *Arch Dermatol* 1972;106:858–64.
5. Calonje E. Wilson James E. Intravascular spread of keratoacanthoma. An alarming but benign phenomenon. *Am J Dermatopathol* 1992;14:414–7.
6. Whyte AM, Hansen LS, Lee C. The intra-oral keratoacanthoma: a diagnostic problem. *Br J Oral Maxillofac Surg* 1986;24:438–41.

EDITORIAL BOARD COMMENTARY

Despite the delay in diagnosis, this patient had comprehensive pretreatment staging and well planned radical surgery with postoperative radiation therapy—optimal management for this tumor.

11 Merkel Cell Tumor of the Eyelid

John E. Schiller

A locally aggressive malignant skin tumor of neuroendocrine
origin requiring radical surgery and adjuvant
radiation therapy

CASE PRESENTATION

Dr. Kersey: Dr. Friedrich Merkel was a German anatomist and physiologist in the late 1800's who discovered a cell under the microscope that later proved, as he theorized, to be a neurotactile cell. In 1972, Dr. Toker, a dermatologist, published an article in the *Archives of Dermatology* about a malignancy felt to be derived from this particular cell. It has variously been called trabecular carcinoma, small cell carcinoma of the skin, and neuroendocrine carcinoma of the skin, and felt to derive, as I mentioned, from the neuroendocrine cell.

Dr. DuBois: This patient is a 75-year-old woman who presented with a red, elevated nodular lesion of her right lower eyelid. This was biopsied and the pathology report at that time suggested a possible metastatic adenocarcinoma but, on further review, I think all the pathologists concurred it was a Merkel cell tumor. She was admitted to Penrose Hospital, where a wide excision was performed on the right lower eyelid and the right cheek area and reconstructed with a split-thickness skin graft. Peripheral margins were all read as free of tumor, but there was concern about the deep margin being involved. The pathology, at that time, was consistent with a Merkel cell tumor. Later that month, she was admitted to the hospital for cellulitis of the graft area and there was some concern that there might be recurrent tumor, even at 3 weeks postoperative. She was readmitted approximately 6 weeks after her original surgery for sepsis secondary to a urinary tract infection. She had a host of other problems, including diabetes, pulmonary disease, and a neurogenic bladder. Three months after the original excision, the patient was admitted to the hospital for a canthoplasty to protect the cornea, but at that time reevaluation revealed locally recurrent tumor. The area was widely re-excised and reconstructed with a split-thickness skin graft. A tarsorrhaphy was performed at the same time. The pathology report at the reexcision revealed all the margins positive for tumor. We were obviously dealing with a very aggressive tumor. The right eye was enucleated and postoperative radiation therapy given. Figure 11–1 illustrates local recurrence after the original excision and split-thickness skin graph.

Dr. Kersey: I do not think that there were any pertinent radiographic studies done for this particular patient at that time, but I have asked Dr. Borgstede to make some comments about what imaging studies for this entity might be useful.

Dr. Borgstede: As Dr. DuBois mentioned, this is a very aggressive neuroendocrine tumor that can spread both locally, hematogenously, and lymphatically. I was able to find six articles that report a total of 11 cases, in which a variety of imaging studies were used to evaluate those patients, including nuclear medicine imaging, with gallium or MIBG, ultrasound, computed tomography (CT), and plain films. Based on the histologic features of this tumor, I would recommend a magnetic resonance image (MRI). There was some controversy for evaluation of distant disease, whether an MIBG scan, which is used in other neuroendocrine tumors, for example, carcinoids and pheochromocytomas, or gallium scan for distant metastases, would be of value. I think it depends on the presence of norepinephrine and its precursors that might be elaborated by the tumor. If those are elaborated, the MIBG scan would be good, otherwise the gallium scan would be of value.

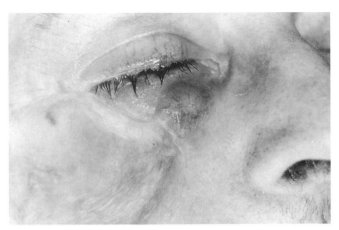

FIG. 11–1. Photograph of patient shows recurrent Merkel cell tumor of the eyelid (nodule below the eye).

Dr. Mayes, Pathologist: This is a section from the initial wedge biopsy showing a small blue cell tumor that fills the dermis and spares the epidermis (Fig. 11–2). Before 1972, when Toker first described Merkel cell carcinoma, these tumors were usually signed out as either lymphoma, metastatic small cell undifferentiated carcinoma, or melanoma. Melanoma is the easiest to rule out as it nearly always shows prominent involvement of the epidermal/dermal junction. This patient's tumor, on the other hand, shows no involvement of the epidermal/dermal junction or adnexal structures. Ruling out lymphoma is more difficult. The high power features show a dense population of small cells with smooth, dark chromatin, prominent nuclear molding, very little cytoplasm, and numerous mitoses (Fig. 11–3). The only lymphomas that would resemble this would be lymphoblastic lymphoma or small, noncleaved cell lymphoma. Immunohistochemistry was helpful in this case in making this distinction. Markers of lymphoid differentiation were all negative, whereas markers of neuroendocrine differentiation, including neuron-specific enolase and markers of epithelial differentiation such as cytokeratin, were positive. The morphologic and immunohistochemical features are diagnostic of a small cell undifferentiated carcinoma or neuroendocrine carcinoma. The fact that this neuroendocrine carcinoma is primary to the skin, and therefore a Merkel cell carcinoma, is really a clinical and not a pathologic determination. Neuroendocrine carcinomas are morphologically indistinguishable regardless of their site of origin (e.g., lung, bladder, parotid gland, or, in this case, the skin). Despite the name, the histogenesis of Merkel cell carcinoma is uncertain. Normal Merkel cells are located in the epidermis and are found primarily in the fingertips and the hands. Merkel cell carcinomas, by contrast, occur exclusively in the dermis and occur on sun-exposed skin, mostly around the face. The suggestion that Merkel cell carcinomas arise from Merkel cells is still, at this point, speculative. After biopsy, the patient was sent here for resection. The resection specimen showed tumor extend-

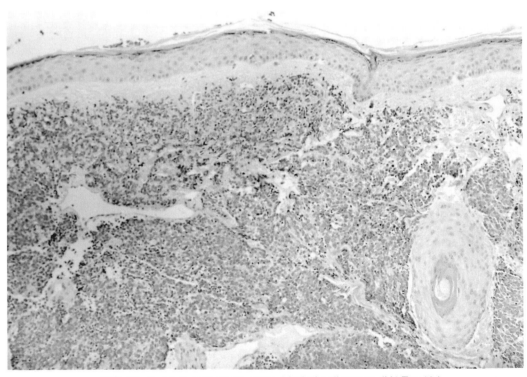

FIG. 11–2. Histopathologic slide, Merkel cell tumor. (H&E × 40.)

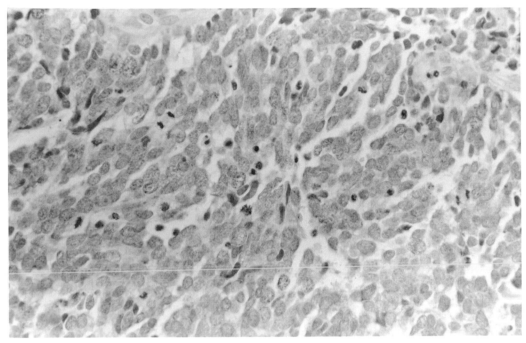

FIG. 11–3. Histopathologic slide, Merkel cell tumor. (H&E × 250.)

ing to the deep margin. The tumor was subsequently re-excised and showed a large bulk of tumor, which is surprising considering the tiny focus of marginal positivity present in the first resection specimen. At this point, the eye was enucleated. There was no evidence of tumor in the orbital contents. Finally, the third and final re-excision again showed extensive bulky tumor and, again, the deep margin was positive. Despite their morphologic similarities, neuroendocrine carcinomas of the skin behave differently from those at other sites, especially lung. Unlike oat cell cancers of the lung, the Merkel cell carcinoma tends to recur locally before metastasizing. The overall cumulative mortality at about 50% is considerably better than that of small cell undifferentiated carcinomas at other sites, such as lung.

Dr. Kersey: As the pathologist mentioned, most of these tumors do occur in the head and neck area and, if you pool the collective series, about 60% of patients do, in fact, present in the head and neck area. The vast majority of the remainder are on the extremities; this rarely occurs on the trunk. Since 1972, the natural history of this tumor has been better understood and more cases have been accrued. There is at least a 70% to 75% local recurrence rate with surgery alone. These tumors require wide surgical excision and postoperative adjuvant radiation therapy, including the regional nodes. The patient under discussion underwent radiation therapy after three surgical procedures, but it recurred again locally thereafter. It was at that point, with the patient in a nursing home, that she elected to have no further therapy. We do not know the exact cause of death, whether it was local

disease only, or whether she had metastatic disease. These tumors, in addition to recurring locally, do in fact metastasize, and there is a potential for systemic treatment as well.

Dr. Schiller: Being a small round cell tumor reminiscent of lymphoma, these small cell carcinomas were originally thought to be very sensitive to radiation. Should radiation doses be quite moderate or, because there may be problems with local control, should you use a very high dose of radiation?

Dr. Kersey: Of most of the patients that have been studied, there have been only two to three infield recurrences after doses of approximately 5,000 cGy. Recurrences have been observed just outside the radiation field. The recommendation from centers such as M.D. Anderson is to administer 4,500 cGy to 5,000 cGy after wide local excision. The field should include the local area as well as the ipsilateral neck. Chemotherapy may or may not play a meaningful role.

Dr. Martz: The same type of chemotherapy that has been useful for small cell carcinoma of the lung may be useful for Merkel cell tumors. I had another patient with a Merkel cell tumor who underwent wide local excision of her tumor with clear margins and no evidence of metastatic disease. We treated her with cisplatin and VP16. She continues to do well without any evidence of recurrence at this point. I think one could develop a case for this in an adjuvant setting.

Dr. Kersey: I believe the recommendation is that if there is definite evidence of nodal metastases or, obviously, if there is known metastatic disease, then certainly chemotherapy is recommended. It is still debatable whether adjuvant therapy should be used.

Dr. Anderson: The other patient described by Dr. Martz had the primary tumor on the buttock. Does this imply a different biologic behavior depending on primary site? Were wider surgical margins more readily obtainable on the buttocks than in the head and neck area?

Dr. Kersey: We have had only a limited number of cases in our institution. This is a rare disease, with many unknowns.

COMMENTARY by Ramon M. Esclamado

The patient discussed is a 75-year-old woman with Merkel cell carcinoma of the right lower lid. Initial treatment consisted of a wide excision of the skin of the right lower eyelid and cheek and reconstruction with a skin graft. Although the peripheral margins were free of tumor, there was concern about a positive deep margin. Approximately 3 months later, the patient developed a local recurrence; this was treated with a wide reexcision and split thickness skin graft. All the margins of the reexcised specimen were involved with tumor. Orbital exenteration was performed and was followed by definitive radiation. Six months later she developed another local recurrence, which was uncontrolled with additional surgery and radiation.

The case presentation is an excellent illustration of the highly aggressive nature of Merkel cell carcinoma. This is an unusual neuroendocrine carcinoma of the skin, originally described by Toker in 1972 (1). Numerous articles have been subsequently published; this has allowed a clearer understanding of the natural history of this disease. Recently, enough experience and follow-up data have been accrued to allow formulation of rational therapeutic strategies.

Merkel cell carcinoma is a dermal-based tumor, believed to be neuroendocrine in origin and most likely arising from a neural crest cell or from an ill-defined popluripotential epidermal stem cell (2). Histologic identification by light microscopy is difficult because this can resemble other neoplasms such as lymphomas, metastatic small cell carcinoma from the lung, melanoma, or poorly differentiated squamous cell carcinoma. Additional techniques used to establish the diagnosis include immunocytochemical staining for neuron-specific enolase (3) and electron microscopic findings of neurosecretory granules (2).

Rice and colleagues (4) recently reviewed 600 cases of Merkel cell carcinoma reported in the literature. The head and neck was most commonly involved, with 321 cases reported and 47% of these involved the cheek and eyelids. The mean age at presentation was 72 years, and there was essentially an even gender distribution. The mean size of the primary lesion was 2.0 cm. Of the 89 patients available for analysis, 11% presented with clinically palpable nodal disease, 7% had local recurrences, 48% had regional metastases, 21% had both local and regional metastasis, and 28% developed distant disease. Survival data showed that 27% were dead of their disease in an average of 16 months and 49% had no evidence of disease at an average follow-up of 22 months; however, 22% of these patients had a follow-up of less than 12 months. Six percent were alive with disease, and 18% were dead of other causes.

In a series of 29 patients reported by Goepfert and co-workers (5), it was found that 25% of patients developed local recurrence. Palpable regional lymphadenopathy was present in 45% of patients, and 83% of patients with primary lesions measuring less than 2 cm in diameter developed regional metastasis during the course of their disease. Some distant metastases occurred in 48% of patients, and most commonly occurred in conjunction with recurrent disease above the clavicle. They also reported a 75% failure rate in untreated necks, and multiple nodes were involved with metastatic tumor in 5 of 14 neck dissection specimens. Survival outcomes showed 58% of patients had no evidence of disease for 2 years, and 21% for 5 years.

It is generally agreed that Merkel cell carcinoma is a radiosensitive tumor (6,7). Morrison and colleagues (6) reported only 4 of 37 patients treated initially by surgery alone were locally or regionally controlled, whereas only 1 of 31 irradiated patients developed an in-field local or regional recurrence. There were three marginal recurrences. The role of chemotherapy is, as yet, undefined. Typically, drugs that are active against a small cell carcinoma of the lung are recommended in the treatment of unresectable Merkel cell disease. The experience by Feun et. al. (8) showed that 2 of 13 patients had prolonged, complete responses of 4 and 10 years; however, in the other patients, once there was disease progression, their course was usually quite rapidly fatal.

Based on these and others' experience, it is generally accepted that treatment for Merkel cell carcinoma should include wide excision of the primary lesion when feasible, along with careful frozen section control and re-excision of any positive margins. Therapeutic dissection of the involved regional nodes is indicated for clinically palpable disease. Elective treatment of draining nodes is recommended for N0 disease. Because radiation therapy is routinely recommended in adjuvant fashion to reduce the locoregional recurrence rate, elective neck dissection is not absolutely indicated, but left to the philosophy of the surgeon. Adjuvant chemotherapy is not proven, but clearly plays a role for unresectable or distant disease. Before managing recurrent local regional disease, it is important to rule out distant metastases with appropriate imaging of the head, brain, lungs, abdomen, and skeletal survey. Recurrent disease is usually managed with surgery and radiation therapy for locoregional control if there is no distant metastasis. Prognosis of this group of patients is uniformly poor. Based on the above discussion, an alternative approach to the case presented is as follows.

After primary excision of the initial primary lesion, an early re-excision to obtain a clear margin should be performed and followed by adjuvant radiation therapy. The radiation ports should include the primary site, as well as the ipsilateral parotid and cervical nodes inferiorly to the clavicle. Because there was no clinically palpable disease, performance of a parotidectomy and neck dissection is controversial and depends on one's treatment philosophy. At the time of the first local recurrence, distant metastatic work-up should be performed before attempted surgical salvage, which included orbital exoneration. If the metastatic work-up was negative, the patient may have benefited from regional lymphadenectomy, including parotidectomy at the time of salvage procedure for the local recurrence.

REFERENCES

1. Toker C. Trabecular carcinoma of the skin. *Arch Dermatol* 1972; 105:107–10.
2. Tang CK, Toker C. Trabecular carcinoma of the skin. *Cancer* 1978; 42:2311–21.
3. Gu J, Polak JM, VanNoorden S, et al. Immunostaining of neuron specific enolase as a diagnostic tool for Merkel cell tumors. *Cancer* 1983; 52:1039–43.
4. Rice RD Jr, Chonkich GD, Thompson KS, Chase DR. Merkel cell tumor of the head and neck: 5 new cases with literature review. *Arch Otolaryngol Head Neck Surg* 1993;119:782–6.
5. Goepfert H, Remmler D, Silva E, Wheeler D. Merkel cell carcinoma (endocrine carcinoma of the skin) of the head and neck. *Arch Otolaryngol* 1984;110:707–12.
6. Morrison WH, Peters LJ, Silva EG, et al. The essential role of radiation therapy in securing locoregional control of Merkel cell carcinoma. *Int J Radiat Oncol Biol Phys* 1990;19:583–91.
7. Coltar M, Gates, JO, Gibbs FA Jr. Merkel cell carcinoma: combined surgery and radiation therapy. *Am Surgeon* 1986;52:159–64.
8. Feun LG, Savarag N, Leghass, et al. Chemotherapy for metastatic Merkel cell carcinoma: review of the MD Anderson Hospital's experience. *Cancer* 1988;62:683–5.

EDITORIAL BOARD COMMENTARY

This aggressive tumor requires a wide surgical excision with confirmation of clear margins, regional node dissection for clinically suspicious nodes, and postoperative radiation therapy to include the regional nodes. Consideration can be given to elective node dissection. The role of chemotherapy requires more study and has not been accurately defined.

12 Basal Cell Carcinoma of the Nasal Labial Fold

John E. Schiller

Surgical excision or radiation therapy?

CASE PRESENTATION

Dr. Koehn, dermatologist: This is a 70-year-old white woman who initially had a skin cancer of the right nasal labial fold removed by curettment and electrofulguration about 12 years ago. Within the past 2 to 3 years it had recurred. On examination, she had a 2.0 × 1.0 cm fibrotic and translucent plaque of the right nasal labial fold extending onto both the cheek and the nasal ala (Fig. 12–1). Past medical history was otherwise unremarkable, and physical examination was negative.

Dr. Hughes, dermatologist: If biopsy showed this lesion to be a morpheaform or infiltrative type of basal cell carcinoma, if the lesion had clinically ill-defined borders, or if there was a history of recurrence after treatment, I would recommend microscopically controlled excision (Mohs') or consider radiation treatment if, for some reason, the patient could not tolerate surgery.

If the biopsy showed a nodular type basal cell carcinoma and the borders were clinically well defined, I would excise the lesion with 2- to 3-mm margins, confirming clear surgical margins histologically. Removal of this lesion by curettage and electrodesiccation, or by cryosurgery, are also options, but because skin cancers in this anatomic area are more prone to recurrence, I would not use either of these methods in this case.

Dr. Lewis, dermatologist: If the edges were distinct, I would undercut the lesion with a 2-mm margin. The resulting defect would be treated by means of electrodesiccation with curettage for additional assurance. If the edges were indistinct, the patient would be referred for plastic surgery, Mohs', or radiotherapeutic consultation.

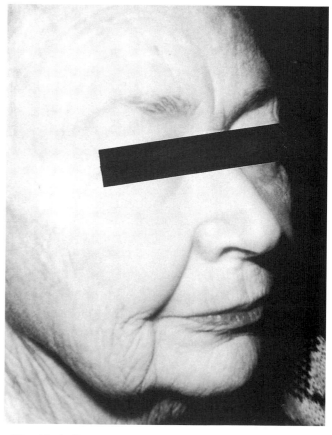

Fig. 12–1. Seventy-year-old woman with a 2.0 × 10.0-cm fibrotic and translucent plaque of the right nasal labial fold.

Dr. Koehn: The patient underwent Mohs' micrographic excisional surgery. The tumor proved to be penetrating and there was full thickness extension through the entire nasal ala. Final defect size was 2.3 × 1.5 cm (Fig. 12–2). Because of the aggressive nature of this tumor, the defect was allowed to heal by second intention. Six weeks later the excision site had healed remarkably well with minimal deformity of the nose (Fig. 12–3).

Pathology: Multiple sections show a centrally ulcerated multifocal basal cell carcinoma. Cords and nests of neoplastic epithelium display peripheral palisading of the epithelial cells. These freely infiltrate the dermis center of the specimen (Fig. 12–4).

Comments: Cancers of the nasal labial fold are typically quite aggressive and penetrating. There is unusual likeliness of recurrence after surgical or radiation therapy. Because of the embryologic fusion plane of the nasal and labial anlage, neoplasms in this location often extend unexpectedly deep. Slender strands of skin cancer cells are not readily detected by gross visualization or palpation. For all these reasons, Mohs' micrographic excisional surgery is the procedure of choice for cancer of the nasal labial crease.

Dr. Schiller, radiation oncologist: The use of radiation therapy for basal cell carcinomas usually yields excellent results. Radiation, specifically, should be the treatment of choice in areas where a surgical excision would require a graft closure, or an excision would change function, such as in areas about the eyelid, ear, or as in this particular patient, the nose. By using fractionated radiation, the cosmetic result should be very acceptable to excellent. However, the cosmetic result does depend on the amount of destruction associated with the tumor and the fractionation of the radiation treatment. Our particular approach is to use radiation doses of approximately 4,500 cGy given daily over a 3-week period. The equipment used should be a filtered superficial X-ray source, such as 120 KVP X-rays or low energy electrons with bolus. The local control with this method of management is very high and local recurrence or failure approximates those of a surgical resection, which is approximately 5%.

This patient's relatively small lesion could be treated quite well with radiation with an expected excellent cosmetic result. Tumors of a larger size may require a somewhat different technique regarding dose and time; however, despite the presentation, complete cure with radiation and reasonable cosmetic result is the expectation.

COMMENTARY by Jatin P. Shah

The patient presented in this discussion has recurrent basal cell carcinoma in the nasolabial fold area. Clinical presentation shows recurrence of tumor in a fibrotic scar that may lead the clinician to underestimate the surface extent of this lesion. If indeed the clinical assessment of

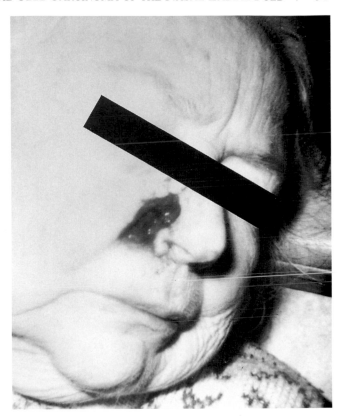

Fig. 12–2. Patient underwent Mohs' micrographic excisional surgery with final defect of 2.3 × 1.5 cm.

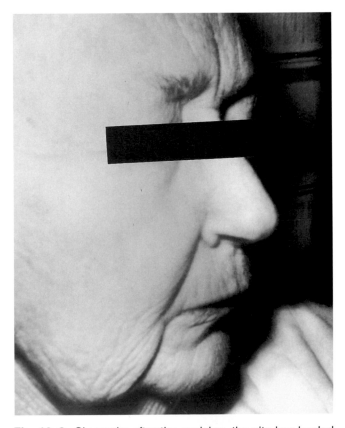

Fig. 12–3. Six weeks after the excision, the site has healed remarkably well.

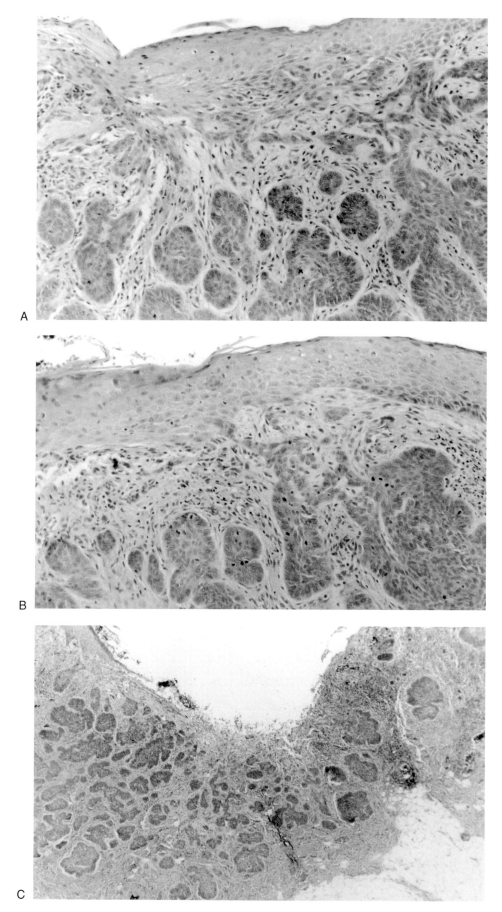

Fig. 12–4. A: Origin of neoplastic epithelial cords from the basal aspect of the epidermis. **B:** Cords of invasive carcinoma display peripheral palisading, increased mitatic activity, and fibrous reaction. **C:** Centrally ulcerated invasive basal cell carcinoma with fibrotic response.

the surface extent as well as the depth of penetration of this lesion is not adequate, then clearly micrographic surgery with histologic control for adequacy of lateral and deep margins is the therapeutic modality of choice for maximizing the chance for cure and reducing the chances of recurrence to a minimum. On the other hand, if the lesion is well demarcated and is felt to be easily assessable by clinical examination, then surgical excision with frozen section control of the margins of the surgical specimen would be the most expeditious way of treating this lesion. This surgery can be safely performed on an outpatient basis under local anesthesia.

Repair of the surgical defect in this area requires some discussion. If, indeed, the surgical defect is along the nasolabial skin crease as is seen in this patient, then adequate mobilization of the soft tissues with primary repair will provide an excellent cosmetic result. On the other hand, if the surgical defect is of such dimension that primary closure is not feasible, then a nasolabial flap repair provides an excellent aesthetic result. The repair of the surgical defect in a single-staged operation should be the ultimate goal in contrast to leaving the surgical defect open with the increased morbidity of the open wound for several weeks until the wound heals by secondary intention.

Skin graft in this region is not acceptable for aesthetic reasons. In a 70-year-old woman, there should be plenty of excess soft tissue and skin available to provide for a primary closure by mobilization and appropriate placement of the incision or the use of a nasolabial flap. The procedure of surgical resection and reconstruction is accomplished in a single-staged procedure with histologic control for complete excision of the recurrent lesion.

External irradiation can indeed control basal cell carcinoma in this location and the early aesthetic result would be quite good. However, whenever there is underlying cartilage beneath the skin lesion, the long-term results of radiotherapy are less than desirable. Cartilage atrophy with fibrosis and a puckered scar are usually seen, leading to a cosmetically unacceptable result. In addition to this, one cannot be absolutely certain in a patient in whom there is recurrent lesion in a fibrotic scar without any epidermal component regarding complete eradication of the lesion because the scar in the field of radiotherapy will always remain suspect for residual tumor. For these reasons, radiotherapy is not recommended as definitive treatment for this patient. Clearly, micrographic resection with histologic control of margins and immediate repair remains the ideal and most expeditious means of treatment in this elderly woman.

EDITORIAL BOARD COMMENTARY

This case illustrates an unresolved controversy between disciplines in the absence of prospective trials. The data suggest equivalent results with surgery or radiation therapy. As discussed by the contributors, treatment should be carefully tailored to the patient's individual needs and wishes.

13

Papillary Thyroid Carcinoma with Tracheal Invasion

Orlo H. Clark

Not all thyroid cancers are harmless

CASE PRESENTATION

This 44-year-old Caucasian woman was admitted with a chief complaint of hemoptysis of 14 months' duration. Other than a history of intermittent sinusitis and mild asthma, she had been in excellent health. Two years previously she was noted by her family physician to have a small nodule in the upper right portion of her thyroid gland. Subsequent evaluation 1 month later by an endocrinologist revealed a "0.5 to 0.75 cm firm but not hard, movable right anterior cervical lymph node that did not move appreciably with swallowing." Fourteen months before admission she presented to her family physician because of sinusitis and bronchitis. She stated that she had blood-streaked sputum twice. Her upper respiratory symptoms disappeared until 4 months before admission, at which time she complained of vague intermittent pains in her right ear, right maxillary sinus, and right side of her neck. She also complained of near constant postnasal drip, with occasional blood-tinged yellow mucus in the morning. Physical examination revealed mild tenderness over the right lobe of her thyroid gland. She had a sinus series and was referred to an otolaryngologist, who treated her for "reflux pharyngitis" with diet and H2 blockers. A chest radiograph and PPD for tuberculosis were negative. Her symptoms seemed to improve, but 2 months before admission her upper respiratory symptoms became more severe. She saw an allergist, who referred her to a pulmonologist. At bronchoscopy she was found to have a "broad-based, cauliflower-like mass within her upper trachea causing about 35% obstruction of the tracheal lumen." Biopsy revealed papillary thyroid carci-

noma. The patient denied any history of exposure to radiation. She had a maternal grandmother with a goiter but no family history of thyroid cancer. She had intermittent hoarseness without dysphasia and her only medication was Synthroid 0.125 mg/day. Past medical history revealed that she had been a nonsmoker for 14 years and drank only minimal amounts of alcohol.

Physical examination revealed a healthy-appearing Caucasian woman with normal vital signs. Positive physical findings were confined to the neck, where she had a firm to hard mass in the right lobe of her thyroid gland with what appeared to be several adjacent cervical lymph nodes that did not move with deglutition. There was also a delphian lymph node just cephalad to her cricoid cartilage that did move with swallowing. Indirect laryngoscopy revealed normally mobile vocal cords bilaterally.

Preoperative laboratory tests revealed a sensitive TSH level of 1.7 (normal = 0.3–5.0 mU/L); Hct 32 (normal = 36–46%); calcium 9.3 (normal = 8.4–10.2 mg/dL); thyroglobulin 12.3 (normal = 0–40 ng/L). A magnetic resonance image (MRI) revealed tumor extensions through the proximal trachea on the right, anteriorly and laterally (Fig. 13–1). The chest radiograph was normal.

At operation, an invasive thyroid tumor with desmoplastic reaction was present in the lower portion of the right lobe of the thyroid gland with up to 1 cm cervical lymph nodes extending inferiorly into the substernal space along the trachea. Some of these nodes were calcified. There was also a 1.5-cm delphian lymph node in the cricothyroid membrane. The thyroid tumor was invading through the trachea on the right. The left thyroid lobe appeared normal. Right upper and both left-sided parathy-

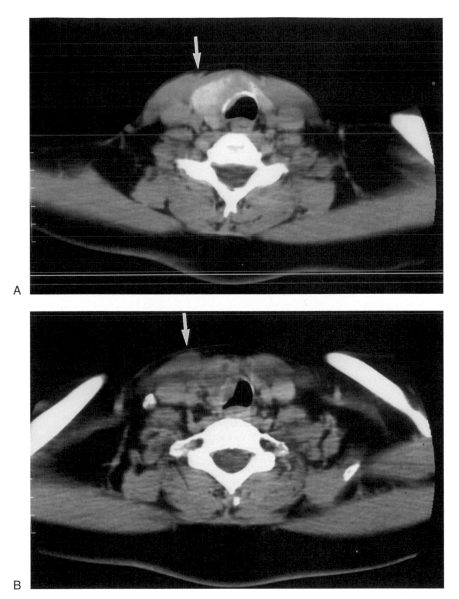

FIG. 13–1. MRI scan revealed an enlarged right thyroid lobe (**A**) with tracheal invasion. **B:** Note the flattening and invasion through the right wall of the trachea.

roid glands were in their usual position. They were identified and preserved. Both recurrent laryngeal nerves were also identified and preserved. After total thyroidectomy, the trachea was separated from the esophagus using sharp and blunt dissection. The recurrent nerves and parathyroid glands were mobilized laterally from the trachea. The trachea just distal to the cricoid cartilage was transected and a 4-cm segment of proximal trachea was removed. The oral tracheal tube was seen in the center of the trachea. The thyroid-hyoid ligaments and muscle were divided to "drop the larynx" and to prevent tension on the anastomosis that was done using 3-0 Maxon suture. The tracheal margins were free of tumor both by frozen and subsequent permanent section. The wound was closed in the usual fashion, and the patient was extubated without difficulty.

Pathologic examination revealed a papillary carcinoma infiltrating through the tracheal cartilage (Fig. 13–2) with superior and inferior resection margins free of neoplasm both microscopically and grossly (Fig. 13–3), metastatic thyroid cancer in 1/1 right mediastinal nodes and in 6/9 right central neck nodes, multifocal microinvolvement of the left lobe, and papillary carcinoma involving the right lobe and isthmus.

Postoperatively, the patient was taken to the intensive care unit. Serum calcium level fell from 9.3 to 8.4 mg/dL, and serum phosphorus increased from 3.5 to 3.9 mg/dL. The patient's voice was slightly lower pitched than preoperatively but without hoarseness, and it took several days for her to swallow without difficulty. She was discharged on her fifth postoperative day on cytomel (25 mg/bid). A postoperative radioiodine scan at 3 months, discontinuing

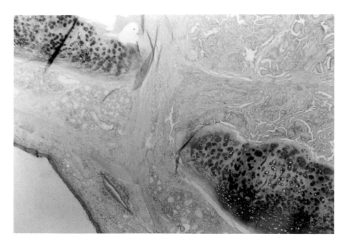

FIG. 13–2. Histologic examination revealed papillary thyroid carcinoma infiltrating the trachea.

cytomel for 2 weeks, revealed no uptake above background. She, however, was treated with 100 mCi of radioactive iodine. Her voice and swallowing are now normal.

The patient would be considered to have a Class 3 tumor by the DeGroot classification because of local invasion. By the classifications of age, grade, extent, size (AGES) or age, metastases, extent, and size (AMES), she would be considered to be at relatively low risk. She would also be at low risk with the TNM (primary tumor, lymph node, distant metastasis) classification because she is less than 45 years of age with a papillary thyroid cancer.

In summary, this 44-year-old Caucasian woman had a 2-year history of a thyroid nodule and a 14-month history

of hemoptysis. Evaluation preoperatively with MRI scanning and direct laryngoscopy and biopsy revealed an invasive papillary thyroid cancer. After total thyroidectomy and tracheal resection she appears to be free of disease. Preoperative discussions before treatment concerning the most appropriate treatment included (a) external radiation with or without chemotherapy, (b) laser resection of the intratracheal mass and total thyroidectomy with postoperative treatment with radioactive iodine or external radiation, and (c) total thyroidectomy with tracheal resection and lymph node resection. We elected to do the latter because we felt it was the treatment that was most likely to result in a tumor-free state and was associated with fewer long-term sequelae. Treatment included a total thyroidectomy, tracheal resection, and central neck dissection. The patient currently appears to be disease-free by radioiodine scanning and by serum thyroglobulin levels.

COMMENTARY by Oliver H. Beahrs

This case of a papillary adenocarcinoma of the thyroid gland is an interesting one and is a clinical presentation that is occasionally seen. It does illustrate nicely why a thyroid nodule, especially in a pediatric patient or a younger person, should always be considered with some suspicion of being malignant and removed. Approximately 50% of such nodules in the first group will prove to be cancers, and 10% to 20% of the cases in the older group. With regional lymphadenopathy being present, the likelihood of thyroid cancer becomes much greater. A patient of 44 has a life expectancy of another 40 or more years. Potential hazards to health should be treated when known to be present.

In this particular case, the occurrence of hemoptysis naturally requires evaluation. Bronchoscopy, which was indicated and done easily, established the diagnosis because of full-thickness invasion of the tracheal wall by a cancer and tumor mass extending into the lumen of the trachea.

Although most papillary cancers of the thyroid can be treated safely by conservative surgical procedures, partial, subtotal, or total thyroidectomy, with or without regional node dissection depending on specific findings clinically or grossly at the time of the operation, this woman's cancer cannot and requires more defined surgical considerations. However, because of the known "relatively benign" biologic behavior of papillary adenocarcinoma of the thyroid, it can still be treated more conservatively than a squamous cell adenocarcinoma of the head and neck region, which often requires a wide resection of the anatomic site of origin (e.g., larynx) and wide resection of regional nodal metastasis (e.g., radical neck dissection).

The alternatives to treatment in this case are appropriate. External radiation with or without chemotherapy does

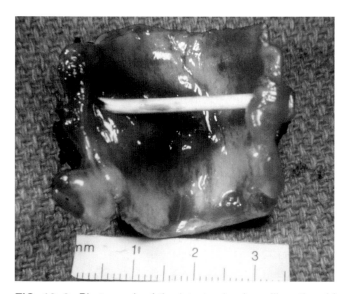

FIG. 13–3. Photograph of the intratracheal papillary thyroid cancer that obstructed about 35% of the tracheal lumen.

not seem reasonable if the findings indicate that appropriate surgery most likely would be definitive. To remove the intratracheal mass separately from the thyroid, the site of the primary tumor, without the intervening tracheal tissue, would unlikely be curative, even though radiation therapy was used as an additive measure. Because the lesion is reported to be a (pure?) papillary adenocarcinoma, it is unlikely that radioactive iodine would be of benefit.

The appropriate approach to the treatment of this case was what was done—a total thyroidectomy with resection of the involved trachea and removal of appropriate regional lymph nodal groups—in this case those in the central compartment. The surgery could have been extended to a right modified neck dissection had the findings indicated.

Fortunately, at least three parathyroid glands were identified and preserved. This was appropriate, and in treating papillary cancers, preservation of parathyroid tissue should always be attempted. Also, with tracheal preservation, the recurrent laryngeal nerves should be identified and preserved unless one or both are found to be involved by tumor. In this case, bilateral vocal cord function was normal and both nerves found to be free of tumor and preserved.

In this case, it was deemed possible to resect a full segment of trachea and re-establish continuity by a direct anastomosis. This naturally is preferable if technically feasible. Other measures that could be considered might be partial resection of the wall of the trachea, which would leave the defect open and require a temporary tracheostomy to be closed at a secondary operation. Rarely are cases so extensive as to require resection of the upper trachea and larynx with a permanent tracheostomy. This should be done only when the findings indicate that extensive surgery is essential to make the operation definitive.

With total thyroidectomy, thyroid hormone replacement therapy is essential. Periodic radioisotope scanning and always careful physical examination of the neck are important follow-up procedures.

EDITORIAL BOARD COMMENTARY

Although thyroid carcinoma is much less common than benign thyroid nodules, the combination of a solitary thyroid nodule, palpable surgical lymph node, and a history of hemoptosis should arouse suspicion for carcinoma of the thyroid gland.

14

Anaplastic Thyroid Cancer

Ashok R. Shaha

A disease in search of more effective treatment

CASE PRESENTATION

A.B., a 58-year-old black woman was admitted to the outside hospital with a large mass in the central compartment of the neck and with difficulty in breathing. The patient had noticed swelling in her neck over the past 2 years and was evaluated outside. A diagnosis of nodular goiter was made and the patient was given suppressive therapy. Over the past 3 months, the mass in the neck had been increasing rapidly in size and the patient had developed increasing difficulty in breathing and hoarseness, and noted enlarged nodes in the left neck. She also noted difficulty in swallowing and had considerable difficulty lying down in bed. A Tru-cut needle biopsy was performed, which was suspicious for malignant tumor, but the exact nature of the malignancy was not defined. Her chest roentgenogram at admission revealed diffuse pulmonary metastases. At this time she was transferred to Memorial Sloan-Kettering Cancer Center for further evaluation and management. The patient was born and brought up in South Carolina and has not been outside the United States. There is no family history of thyroid disease or history of radiation in the past. Past history included hysterectomy and hypertension, treated with Procardia.

At the time of her admission to Memorial, she appeared to be her stated age. There was mild stridor. The clinical examination of the head and neck revealed a large, firm mass measuring approximately 12 × 10 cm, which appeared to be fixed to the central compartment involving both lobes of the thyroid gland (Fig. 14–1). The lower extent of the mass extended behind the clavicles. In the lateral portion of the neck there were multiple metastatic lymph nodes. The trachea could not be evaluated because of fixation of the mass in front of the trachea. The neck skin was stretched and shiny. The examination of the oral cavity was normal. The examination of the larynx showed a paralyzed left vocal cord, considerable displacement of the larynx, and a narrow glottic chink. The patient was admitted to the hospital for further evaluation and management.

On admission, the patient had a roentgenography of the chest and a computed tomography (CT) scan of the neck, which revealed a large mass involving the thyroid with tracheal compression (Figs. 14–2, 14–3). The chest roentgenogram revealed bilateral pulmonary nodules. A fine-needle aspiration was suspicious for carcinoma of the thyroid, but the diagnosis of anaplastic thyroid cancer was not made on needle aspiration. The blood chemistry and thyroid function tests were within normal limits. A clinical diagnosis of carcinoma of the thyroid (specific type to be determined) was made. Clinical staging was T3 N1 M1, stage IV.

Two days after admission, the patient had considerable difficulty in breathing, could not lie down, and had bouts of severe stridor. At that time she was brought to the operating room and, after smooth induction of general anesthesia with the endotracheal tube, the neck was explored. After making the skin incision and raising the flaps, it was apparent that this was a large, solid, firm mass involving the thyroid, which was adherent to the trachea with multiple metastatic nodes in the lateral neck. The tumor could not be separated from the surrounding structures and was invading the strap muscles. A generous biopsy of this mass was taken and was reported on frozen section as anaplastic thyroid cancer. Because of the considerable difficulty that the patient had in breathing, the central portion of the thyroid mass was excised and a tracheostomy was performed (Figs. 14–4, 14–5). The patient recovered from the surgical procedure and had no further difficulty in breathing.

68

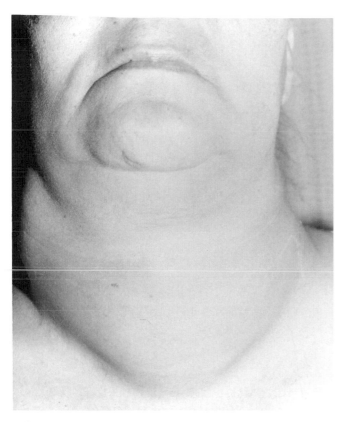

FIG. 14–1. Clinical presentation of anaplastic thyroid cancer.

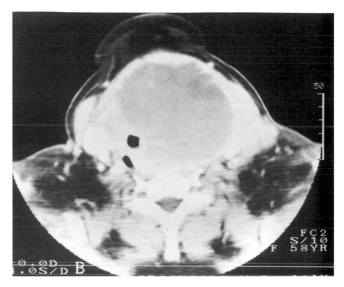

FIG. 14–2. CT scan of the neck showing a large thyroid mass with invasion of the muscles and displacement of the trachea and esophagus.

She was started on protocol of combination therapy including adriamycin, 10 mg/m² per week with radiation therapy. She was given 4,350 cGy by 6 MV photons in 30 fractions over a month. At the time of her discharge there was minimal response to the thyroid tumor. However, the patient did not have further difficulty in breathing. She was fed via a nasogastric feeding tube.

Approximately 4 weeks after discharge, the patient developed deteriorating pulmonary status and was admitted to another hospital with pulmonary failure and died approximately 1 week later.

TUMOR BOARD DISCUSSION

The case was presented to the tumor board and the participants included the pathologist, medical oncologist, radiation oncologist, and surgeons. The histology revealed a giant and spindle cell tumor with invasion of the surrounding muscles and soft tissues of the neck. Immunoperoxidase stains were performed, which were positive for keratin and vimentin. However, the tumor was negative for carcinoembryonic antigen (CEA), calcitonin, synaptophysin, and thyroglobulin. Anaplastic thyroid cancers can be divided into three groups: small cell variant, anaplastic thyroid cancer developing from previously known well differentiated thyroid cancer, and giant and spindle cell tumor. This patient's tumor belonged to the third category

of giant and spindle cell variety, which generally grows rapidly and invades surrounding structures (Figs. 14–6, 14–7).

The case was also discussed by the medical oncologist and radiation oncologist, who felt that the previously used protocol at Memorial Sloan-Kettering Cancer Center of adriamycin with external radiation therapy would be most beneficial.

However, there was also discussion regarding the advanced nature of the disease and a uniformly fatal outcome in anaplastic thyroid cancer of this magnitude.

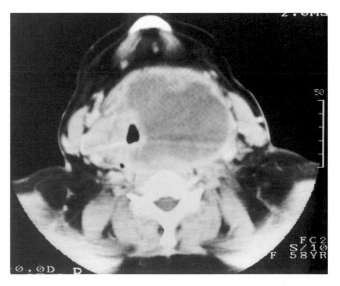

FIG. 14–3. CT scan showing tracheal displacement and esophageal compression.

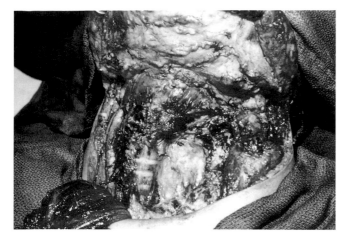

FIG. 14–4. Intraoperative photograph showing thyroid mass in the left neck with removal of isthmic tumor and exposure of the trachea.

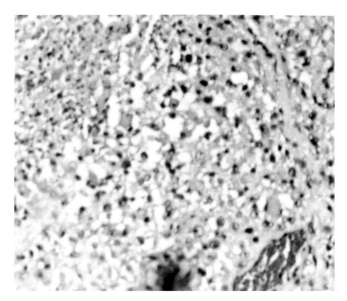

FIG. 14–6. Photomicrograph showing giant cells with focal necrosis. (H&E × 200.)

The surgical exploration was indicated in this case because of the unavailability of the prior diagnosis of anaplastic thyroid cancer and the acute airway distress that the patient was experiencing. Even though tracheostomy is generally not recommended in anaplastic thyroid cancer because the tumor invariably grows in the tracheostomy site, it was indicated in this case because of acute airway distress. The eventual demise of the patient in this case was clearly related both to the local extension of the disease and pulmonary metastasis with pulmonary failure. The average survival in patients with such advanced disease is only a few months. The giant and spindle cell variant proliferates rapidly with invasion of the trachea and esophagus. The eventual demise is mostly due to airway distress or cachexia and inanition. Further clinical trials with combination chemotherapy and altered fractionation of radiation therapy are indicated.

COMMENTARY by Oliver H. Beahrs

The record of the case of anaplastic thyroid cancer as presented by Dr. Shaha is a typical one of this disease. The past history is brief, but it does present several pertinent points. One is the presence of what was considered to be an adenomatous goiter present for at least 2 years, showing significant growth in the most recent 3-month period. Along with the increasing size of the lesion, the patient noticed difficulty swallowing, difficulty breathing, hoarseness, enlarged lymph nodes in the left neck, and evidence of diffuse pulmonary metastasis. These findings are pathognomonic of anaplastic cancer of the thyroid gland.

When seen at Memorial Sloan-Kettering Cancer Center, mild stridor was also present and the lesion was considered to be fixed to adjacent tissues in the midportion of the neck. On laryngoscopic examination, there was paralysis of the left vocal cord, which is further indication of a malignant lesion. Although other tests could be done and were performed, they do not contribute to the suspicion that an anaplastic cancer is present. Even though the needle biopsy was not successful in establishing the histologic diagnosis, there was no alternative, because of the suspicion of cancer and the clinical findings, except to proceed with the surgical approach in dealing with this lesion.

It is correctly staged as a stage IV lesion, as would be true for all anaplastic cancers. The surgical treatment was appropriate: exploration, debulking of the lesion, and the establishment of a tracheostomy. In the presence of what was diagnosed, a spindle cell anaplastic cancer of the thyroid gland, the only alternative is radiation therapy which, unfortunately and by far in most cases, has little effect. It

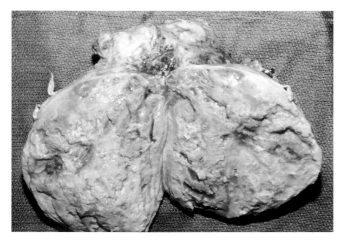

FIG. 14–5. Specimen of anaplastic thyroid tumor involving the isthmus. The picture shows only a third of the entire tumor.

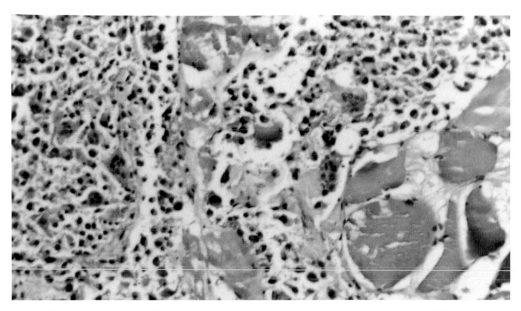

FIG. 14–7. Tumor with giant cells and osteoclasts invading the muscle. (H&E × 300.)

is highly unlikely that chemotherapy would contribute to the therapy.

The anaplastic carcinomas as a group have an entirely different clinical history than those of the other three types of cancers, that is, papillary, follicular, and medullary adenocarcinomas. This lesion grows rapidly and has a short life history, causing symptoms of dyspnea, hoarseness, vocal cord paralysis, and extension into other structures of the neck. It spreads early to the regional lymphatics and distantly most frequently to the lungs. In a very few number of patients, resection can be carried out with the hope of cure. In these instances, an extensive thyroidectomy should be done as consistent with the findings. As a rule, however, debulking of the lesion and freeing up the trachea can be accomplished along with a tracheostomy to protect the airway. Even though the patient is not having difficulty breathing, if there is residual tumor present, it is good to establish the tracheostomy to protect and maintain the airway during radiation therapy and thereafter.

Of interest in this type of cancer is the occurrence of mixed papillary adenocarcinoma along with anaplastic carcinoma, which suggests that a papillary carcinoma left alone long enough will undergo malignant transformation into an anaplastic carcinoma. In the study of some specimens removed in the course of surgery, pure papillary carcinoma can be found intermixed with highly anaplastic carcinoma. Anaplastic cancers represent less than 10% of other cancers of the thyroid, and its biologic behavior, as indicated above, is much more aggressive than the other three types which, as a group, are fairly well differentiated and usually have a long life history and a satisfactory survival rate when surgically treated. Most patients with anaplastic carcinoma die within 6 months. Only a rare case will survive beyond 12 months.

Because of the risk of this disease or the presence of one of the other types of cancers of the thyroid, any nodule in the thyroid gland, when known to be present, should be considered with some suspicion.

15

Medullary Carcinoma of the Thyroid Gland and Bilateral Pheochromocytomas —Multiple Endocrine Neoplasia 2A Syndrome

Courtney M. Townsend, Jr.

Molecular genetics testing can now identify family members who are gene carriers

CASE PRESENTATION

This 43-year-old woman was admitted to a local hospital with severe hypertension and left occipital cerebral vascular accident. During her work-up she was found to have significant elevations of both plasma epinephrine and norepinephrine. She was transferred to University Hospitals, where a computed tomography (CT) scan revealed bilateral adrenal masses most consistent with bilateral pheochromocytomas. The patient underwent bilateral adrenalectomy and had a satisfactory postoperative course. The patient had a negative family history for MEN syndrome, but the presence of bilateral pheochromocytomas was highly suggestive for (almost diagnostic of) multiple endocrine neoplasia (MEN) type 2A. Blood studies revealed increased basal and pentagastrin-stimulated calcitonin blood levels (120 pg/mL and 323 pg/mL, respectively—upper limit normal <100 pg/mL).

The patient had a history of asthma. She had a history of pregnancy-induced hyperthyroidism (Graves' disease) treated with propylthiouracil many years before admission. She has had no recurrence of symptoms. Her thyroid function studies are normal. Past surgical history included a total abdominal hysterectomy. She denied tobacco or ethanol use. Medications included Florinef, Cortef, albuterol, and theophylline. Family history was negative.

Blood pressure was 130/70, pulse 100, respiration 20, temperature 37°C, height 5'6", weight 130 pounds. The thyroid was not enlarged and contained no masses. There was no lymphadenopathy in the neck. The chest was clear. The remainder of the physical examination was normal: WBC 9,000, Hgb 14.6 g/dL, Hct 43.4%, Na 139 Meq/L, CI 104 Meq/L. CO 22 Meq/L, BUN 16 mg/dL, Cr 0.6 mg/dL, Glucose 100 mg/dL, ionized calcium 4.96, urinalysis clear, basal calcitonin 110 pg/mL (nl <100), pentagastrin-stimulated level 393 pg/mL at 10 min, CEA 1.6 ng/mL, chest roentgenogram was clear.

TUMOR BOARD DISCUSSION

Because of the history and the positive calcitonin simulation tests, it was felt that thyroid scan and CT scan were not required. It was decided that she should undergo elective total thyroidectomy. The pentagastrin-stimulated calcitonin was less than 1,000 pg/mL; it was felt that this represented early disease confined to the gland and the decision was made not to perform lymph node dissection at the time of thyroidectomy because there were no masses palpable in the neck. However, provision was made that if enlarged nodes were noted during the operation, a central node dissection would be carried out.

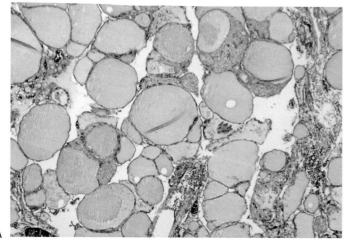

A

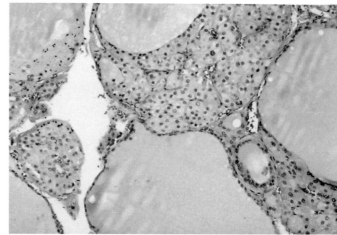

B

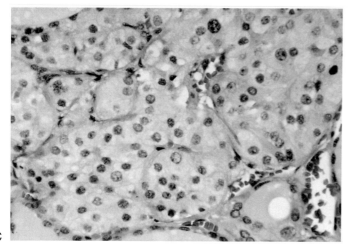

C

FIG. 15–1. **A:** C-cell hyperplasia could be seen throughout both lobes of the gland. (H&E, ×10.) **B:** Higher power view of C-cell hyperplasia surrounding follicles. (H&E, ×40.) **C:** The hyperplasia C-cells are of uniform size, possess bland cytoplasm, and show no mitotic activity. (IT&E, ×100.)

There were many small fine granules (½–1mm) visible on the cut surfaces of both lobes and the isthmus. There was one 8-mm nodule in the left lobe. There was no extracapsular extension. Both C-cell hyperplasia and medullary thyroid cancer were present throughout the gland (Fig. 15–1). The gross nodule was composed of mixed cellularity (Fig. 15–2). There was no vascular, lymphatic, or capsular extension.

The patient underwent a total thyroidectomy and parathyroid biopsy 8 months after bilateral adrenalectomy. The parathyroid showed a mild hyperplasia. No lymph nodes were noted and there were no gross abnormalities found in the capsule of the thyroid; therefore, she did not have cervical lymph node dissection. Her postoperative course was uneventful. She remained afebrile, eating and talking well, the ionized calcium remained within normal limits, and she was discharged home on postoperative day 2. Follow-up examinations will be conducted at regular intervals. She will have calcitonin levels measured every 4 months for the next 2 years. Because she was found to have mild hyperplasia, her calcium will also be monitored at regular intervals and, if she develops hypercalcemia, will undergo multiglandular parathyroidectomy.

COMMENTARY by Samuel A. Wells, Jr.

This 43-year-old woman first presented with hypertension and bilateral pheochromocytomas. After bilateral adrenalectomy, she returned 7 months later and was found to have an increased serum calcitonin level after the intravenous administration of pentagastrin. She is now admitted for total thyroidectomy.

It is of great interest that she has no family history of either thyroid disease or pheochromocytomas. On physical examination, she had no evidence of thyroidomegaly and there were no palpable lymph nodes in the neck.

Her laboratory data showed a normal serum calcium concentration. Her basal serum calcitonin level was 110 pg/mL (nl <100 pg/mL). After the administration of intravenous pentagastrin, her peak plasma calcitonin level was 393 pg/mL.

The patient underwent a total thyroidectomy and parathyroid biopsy. Pathologic exam showed bilateral medullary thyroid carcinoma. The parathyroid biopsy showed mixed hyperplasia.

The patient almost certainly has MEN 2A. There was no mention of the characteristic phenotype so typical of

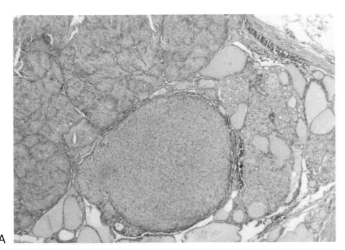
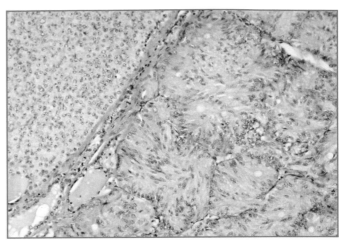

A

B

FIG. 15–2. A: Nodules of hyperplasia C cells and medullary carcinoma could be seen. (H&E ×10.) **B:** Nodular C-cell hyperplasia is more cellular and medullary cancer pattern is further dedifferentiated. (H&E × 40.)

patients with MEN 2B, and because there were pheochromocytomas present, the patient certainly does not have the familial non-MEN medullary thyroid carcinoma. Patients with MEN 2A frequently have hyperparathyroidism. The patient is being appropriately monitored for this.

Patients such as this often present as the index case of a large kindred with MEN 2A. It would be imperative that her kindred members be screened for the presence of medullary thyroid carcinoma, pheochromocytomas, and hyperparathyroidism. Virtually all patients with MEN 2A have medullary carcinoma, approximately half have pheochromocytomas, and less than half have hyperparathyroidism. The medullary carcinoma can be diagnosed by the administration of provocative agents. In our hands, the best provocative test has been the combined infusion of calcium and pentagastrin (1). Higher peak plasma calcitonin levels occur after the administration of these agents than after the administration of either pentagastrin alone or calcium alone.

One can readily tell whether a patient has been cured after thyroidectomy by measuring plasma calcitonin levels after the administration of calcium and pentagastrin in the postoperative period. Normal plasma calcitonin levels in the stimulated state indicate that there is no residual medullary thyroid carcinoma.

With the recent advances in molecular genetics testing, it is now possible to identify affected individuals at risk by genotyping large kindreds with markers that flank the predisposition gene for MEN 2A. This gene is located on chromosome 10. Very recently, two groups (2,3) have identified mutations in the RET proto-oncogene, and it indeed appears likely that this gene is the causative agent for MEN 2A and perhaps the related syndromes segregating medullary thyroid carcinoma. This abnormality is detected in all cells of the body and can readily be identified in white cells. This observation will markedly alter the method of diagnosis and screening of patients at risk, and will help detect family members who are gene carriers as well as those who are not.

REFERENCES

1. Wells SA Jr, Baylin SB, Linehan WM, et al. Provocative agents and the diagnosis of medullary carcinoma of the thyroid gland. *Ann Surg* 1978;188:139.
2. Mulligan LM, Kwok JBJ, Healey CS, et al. Germline mutations of the RET proto-oncogene in Multiple Endocrine Neoplasia Type 2A (MEN 2A). *Nature* 1993;363:458–60.
3. Donis-Keller H, Dou S, Chi D, et al. Mutations in the RET proto-oncogene are associated with MEN 2A and FMTC. *Hum Molec Genet* 1993;2:851–6.

SECTION II

Esophagus

16

Resectable Adenocarcinoma of the Esophagus Arising in a Barrett's Esophagus

Robert J. Ginsberg

Transhiatal esophagectomy without thoracotomy or combined abdominal and thoracic resection and anastomosis?

CASE PRESENTATION

D.S. is a 74-year-old white man who presented with a 1-month history of progressive dysphagia. Initially, he noticed difficulty with solids but more recently noticed dysphagia localized to the midchest, even with liquids. Twenty-four years ago, he had significant symptoms of reflux disease, was diagnosed as having a hiatus hernia, and underwent a transabdominal Nissen fundoplication. Apparently he was found to have an "ulcer" within his esophagus. Since that time, other than the occasional symptom of heartburn, he has been without upper abdominal symptomatology. Specifically, he denied anything but the occasional episode of heartburn easily controlled by antacids. He denied hematemesis or melena.

His past health was unremarkable other than one episode of renal colic. There is no history of cardiovascular disease. He was a 30 pack/year smoker but discontinued the habit 25 years ago. He was a social drinker. His family history was remarkable only in that one sibling died of cancer of unknown site.

Physical examination demonstrated a healthy white man appearing younger than his stated age. Complete physical examination failed to reveal any abnormalities. Specifically, there was no cervical lymphadenopathy, hepatomegaly, or other abdominal problems. Rectal examination was negative with negative occult blood.

Routine hematologic and biochemical survey was within normal limits other than a hemoglobin of 12.5 g. A barium swallow and upper gastrointestinal series was performed, which demonstrated a significant esophageal stricture at the level of the inferior pulmonary vein, below which was a large hiatus hernia. Clips were present, indicating previous surgery around the hiatus (Fig. 16–1).

An upper gastrointestinal endoscopy was performed. The esophagus was normal until 30.0 cm from the incisors, where a short stricture was identified (Fig. 16–2). The mucosa was markedly friable. The scope could be easily passed through the stricture into a large hiatus hernia whose mucosa was perfectly normal. The stomach and proximal duodenum were normal. Multiple brushings and biopsy specimens were taken from around the stricture and proximally in the esophagus. The stricture was then dilated gently after a guidewire had been passed, using fluoroscopic control. A 16-Savary bougie was easily passed.

The biopsy specimens demonstrated adenocarcinoma within a Barrett's esophagus. Further investigations included a CT scan of the chest and abdomen as well as an esophageal ultrasound for staging. The former investigation demonstrated a tumor within the esophagus without extension beyond its walls, located at and around the inferior pulmonary vein (Fig. 16–3). The esophageal ultrasound demonstrated a lesion at 30.0 cm extending

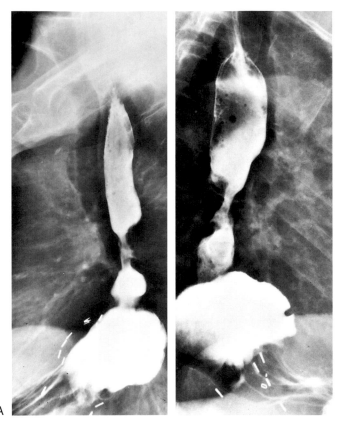

A

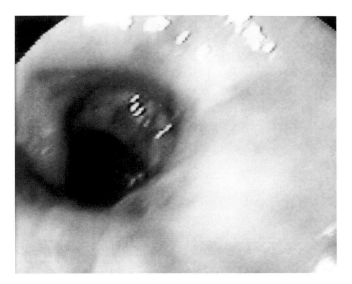

FIG. 16–2. Endoscopic view of the stricture.

FIG. 16–1. A: Barium swallow demonstrating a narrow stricture of the lower third of the esophagus above a hiatus hernia. Surgical clips indicate previous antireflux surgery. **B:** More detailed view of the stricture demonstrating ulceration, which suggests at least a T3 tumor.

B

through the muscle wall of the esophagus. Paraesophageal lymph nodes in the area appeared enlarged (Fig. 16–4). Intra-abdominal lymph nodes (left gastric and celiac) appeared normal. He was clinically staged T3 N1 M0, stage III.

Further investigations included an electrocardiogram and pulmonary function studies. These were all within normal limits.

The patient's history and findings were presented at Tumor Board. He was felt to be eligible for a nationwide intergroup esophageal carcinoma study (INT113) randomizing patients to immediate surgery with no adjuvant therapy versus induction chemotherapy (5-fluorouracil plus cisplatin ×3) followed by surgery and then two courses of similar chemotherapy. The patient was informed of this protocol and advised of ultimate surgery. The risks and benefits of the randomized protocol were explained. The possible benefits of chemotherapy were outlined. After much thought, the patient and his family elected not to be randomized to this protocol, electing surgical treatment alone for therapy.

The patient underwent an uncomplicated Ivor-Lewis esophagectomy. A complete abdominal and intratho-

racic lymph node dissection was accomplished with the esophagectomy. A sizable portion of lesser curvature of the stomach was removed with the esophageal specimen. A gastric tube was transplanted to the right chest, anastomosing the gastric tube to the esophagus, high in the right chest, using a two-layer hand-sewn anastomosis.

The patient's postoperative course was relatively unremarkable, except that he developed a supraventricular arrhythmia (atrial fibrillation) that required digitalization. At 1 week, a barium swallow was performed, demonstrating an intact anastomosis with good outflow through the pylorus (a pyloromyotomy had been performed at the

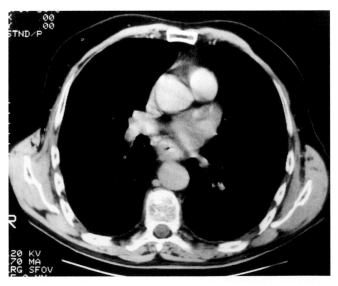

FIG. 16-3. CT scan at the level of the inferior pulmonary vein demonstrating full thickness involvement of the esophagus.

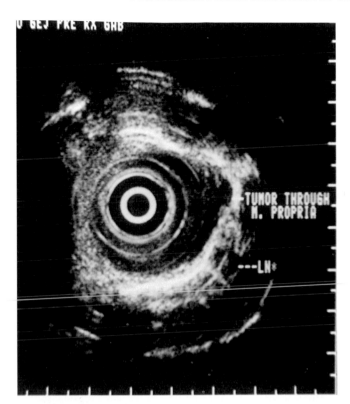

FIG. 16–4. Endoscopic ultrasound indicating tumor penetrating through the muscular propria

time of surgery) (Fig. 16–5). The patient was discharged on the 13th postoperative day, swallowing well and eating solid foods.

Pathologically, the specimen revealed an adenocarcinoma arising in Barrett's epithelium (Fig. 16–6). The primary tumor measured 3.5 × 4.5 cm and extended through the muscle wall (Fig. 16–7). All resection margins were negative. All lymph nodes were examined and failed to contain tumor. The final pathologic staging was T3 N0, stage IIA.

The patient was re-presented at Tumor Board. Neither radiation oncology nor medical oncology physicians felt that adjuvant therapy was indicated because the patient had had a complete resection. It was felt that there was no evidence that either modality improved survival.

The patient was seen 1 month after surgery. He was eating and swallowing well. The patient continued to do well, eating and swallowing well, and maintaining his weight within 10% of his preoperative weight. Nine months after his surgery, he began experiencing low back pain. A bone scan was performed, which demonstrated multiple areas of radioisotope uptake in his lumbar spine. Because of significant pain, his lumbar spine was irradiated. The patient continues to eat well and is now asymptomatic 1 year after surgery, with probable bony metastases to his lumbar spine.

COMMENTARY by Mark B. Orringer

The case under consideration is illustrative of the current "epidemic" of esophageal adenocarcinoma occurring in North America and Europe. At many of the major centers in the United States, adenocarcinoma now constitutes approximately two thirds of the esophageal cancers treated, in contrast to squamous carcinoma, which was the dominant histological finding until the past decade. Although esophageal adenocarcinoma may arise from the esophageal submucosal glands, rests of ectopic gastric mucosa, or an upgrowth of a gastric adenocarcinoma of the cardia, in most cases being seen in this country, adenocarcinoma arises in Barrett's mucosa associated with long-standing gastroesophageal reflux. Barrett's mucosa occurs predominantly in Caucasians, and in men more often than women by a ratio of at least 4:1. The history in these patients is remarkably similar. Years of symptomatic gastroesophageal reflux are recalled by the patient who comments that in recent years the degree of heart-

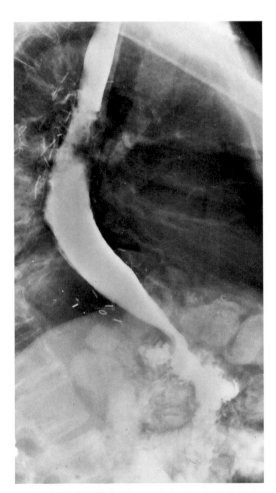

FIG. 16–5. Postoperative barium swallow on day 7 demonstrates a widely patent anastomosis in the upper thorax with good emptying of the gastric tube into the pylorus, which has now been mobilized to the hiatus.

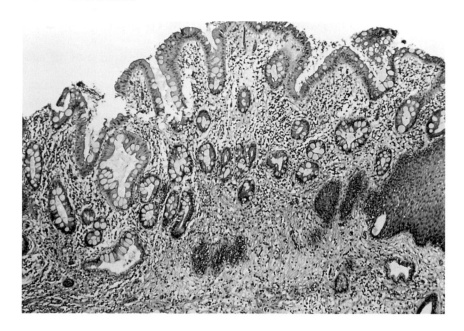

FIG. 16–6. Squamocolumnar junction of the esophagus demonstrating the Barrett's epithelium.

burn he has had has been relatively minor or absent. It is during this time that the normal esophageal squamous mucosa has been replaced by metaplastic columnar epithelium, which is not acid-sensitive and is therefore associated with far less heartburn and indigestion. Finally, dysphagia is noted as adenocarcinoma develops within the metaplastic Barrett's mucosa.

The patient who develops Barrett's mucosa has a greater degree of lower esophageal sphincter incompetence than the patient with gastroesophageal reflux but no Barrett's mucosa. Reflux symptoms in this patient population may be more refractory to medical therapy and justify an antireflux operation. It must be emphasized, however, that Barrett's mucosa per se is not an indication for

antireflux surgery because surgical correction of gastroesophageal reflux does not result in significant regression of the Barrett's mucosa, and surveillance esophagoscopy with biopsy is warranted even if the patient's reflux has been controlled. The primary indications for antireflux surgery in the patient with Barrett's mucosa include persistent reflux symptoms despite an intensive antireflux medical regimen, or the presence of ulcerative esophagitis that does not respond to medical therapy. Barrett's mucosa must be carefully biopsied to provide adequate sampling of the abnormal mucosa. This may necessitate three biopsies around the circumference of the esophagus at 3-cm intervals from the anatomic esophagogastric junction up to the abnormal squamocolumnar epithelial

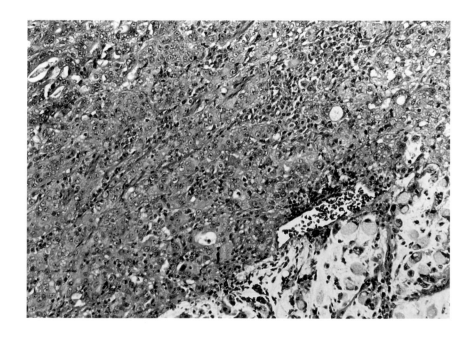

FIG. 16–7. Poorly differentiated adenocarcinoma arising in the Barrett's esophagus and invading muscle inferiorly.

junction. The presence of severe dysplasia within the Barrett's mucosa (it may be necessary to have two independent pathologists make this determination) warrants an esophagectomy rather than an antireflux procedure because of the potential for the development of adenocarcinoma.

In the patient who presents with dysphagia and an esophageal stricture, as was the case in this patient, two questions about the stricture must be answered: is the stricture benign or malignant, and can the stricture be dilated? Every esophageal stricture should be both biopsied and brushed for cytologic evaluation because the combination of brushing and biopsy establishes a diagnosis of cancer in 95% of patients in whom it is present. The value of esophageal ultrasound in the staging of these tumors is still not clearly established. I do not personally use esophageal ultrasonography in the assessment of our patients preoperatively because 95% of our patients with esophageal cancer deemed to be operative candidates have had tumors that can be resected with a transhiatal esophagectomy, and it is difficult for me to judge how ultrasonographic findings would alter this approach. The finding of enlarged lymph nodes with either a CT scan or ultrasonography does not prove that the lymph nodes contain tumor, and this is well illustrated in this case presentation in which the tumor was staged preoperatively with esophageal ultrasonography as T3 N1 M0 but proved to be T3 N0 at operation.

Multimodality therapy of esophageal carcinoma is now in vogue, even though most current information regarding the efficacy of this approach comes largely from uncontrolled pilot studies. In the reported University of Michigan experience, preoperative multidrug chemotherapy (5-FU, cisplatin, and MGBG) resulted in no improved survival when compared with historic controls. On the other hand, using combined chemotherapy (5-FU, cisplatin, and vinblastin) plus radiation therapy (4,500 rads given as 150 cGy bid) before esophagectomy, we have found that esophageal adenocarcinomas respond just as well as squamous carcinomas. Approximately 25% of patients so treated are complete responders (T0 N0 tumors in the resected specimen), and complete responders appear to have the best 5-year survival. Confirmation of these data derived from phase II trials awaits completion of the current phase III prospective randomized trials comparing surgery alone with combined chemotherapy and radiation therapy before esophagectomy now underway at the University of Michigan.

The surgical approach to adenocarcinoma of the distal esophagus is controversial. Those who regard such tumors as being primarily of gastric origin feel compelled to resect the proximal half of the stomach to obtain a better margin. This approach commits the surgeon to an intrathoracic esophagogastric anastomosis for reconstruction. In our experience, however, in most patients with adenocarcinoma of the distal esophagus and cardia, resection of the proximal stomach 4 to 6 cm distal to gross tumor can be achieved while still preserving the highest point along the greater curvature of the stomach, which is needed for construction of a cervical esophagogastric anastomosis after a transhiatal esophagectomy without thoracotomy. Transhiatal esophagectomy is particularly applicable in these patients because the abnormal esophagus with its contained tumor is readily mobilized under direct vision through the diaphragmatic hiatus, and the transhiatal resection involves mobilization of an otherwise normal intrathoracic esophagus. Furthermore, the necessity for a thoracotomy and intrathoracic esophagogastric anastomosis as required for the Ivor-Lewis approach used in the patient under consideration carries the potential for greater morbidity and mortality. There is an additional consideration that favors routine use, wherever possible, of a cervical esophagogastric anastomosis in these patients. Resection of the lower esophageal sphincter and construction of an intrathoracic esophagogastric anastomosis is invariably associated with gastroesophageal reflux, the degree being determined by the level of the anastomosis: low intrathoracic esophagogastric anastomoses are almost always associated with the development of reflux esophagitis, whereas those at the apex of the chest and in the neck are seldom associated with reflux. This is more than a theoretic problem because recurrent esophageal stricture and dysphagia within 1 year of an intrathoracic esophagogastric anastomosis may be due either to recurrent tumor or the development of a reflux stricture, and the differentiation between the two may be extremely difficult and constitute a challenging clinical problem. Although some argue that failure to resect the proximal half of the stomach results in a less than adequate cancer operation in these patients, in my experience, lower esophageal adenocarcinomas tend to metastasize more toward regional lymph nodes and proximally rather than along lymphatics within the wall of the stomach distally. Few of our patients have developed recurrence within the intrathoracic stomach, which has been "tubed" to preserve the entire greater curvature length, and death from distant metastatic disease is far more likely than tumor recurrence in the intrathoracic stomach. The course of the patient under discussion illustrates this well, metastases to the spine becoming evident within 1 year of the operation. I believe that most patients in whom preservation of the greater curvature is possible by dividing the stomach 4 to 6 cm beyond grossly palpable tumor are better served by a cervical esophagogastric anastomosis. This achieves the greatest esophageal margin of resection and minimizes the potential for suture-line tumor recurrence, a well documented problem after an intrathoracic esophagogastric anastomosis.

I emphasize the need for a gastric drainage procedure (my preference is a pyloromyotomy) in every patient undergoing an esophagectomy. Although division of the vagus nerves does not result in delayed gastric emptying and pylorospasm in every patient, this is a disastrous complication when it does occur, and a recent prospective randomized study from Hong Kong leaves little question that it is better to operate defensively and do a gastric drainage procedure at the time of esophagectomy than to wait and see if a problem with gastric emptying occurs. I also favor routine use of a feeding jejunostomy tube in all patients undergoing esophageal resection or bypass. The feeding tube can be used postoperatively to augment nutrition until oral intake is adequate but, even more important, it allows the patient to ambulate unencumbered by intravenous lines and bottles, and thereby enhances recovery. In the event of an anastomotic leak, it provides a far better means of alimentation than can be provided with intravenous parental nutrition.

In summary, patients with resectable adenocarcinomas of the esophagus, defined as those without evidence of distant metastatic disease or obvious local invasion that precludes resection, are best treated with an esophagectomy. In the University of Michigan experience, a transhiatal esophagectomy without thoracotomy is the procedure of choice, is associated with the least morbidity and mortality, and offers survival that is at least as good as that obtained after standard transthoracic resection. A cervical esophagogastric anastomosis is the safest esophageal anastomosis. Preoperative radiation therapy and chemotherapy for esophageal adenocarcinoma, just as for squamous cell carcinoma, results in complete remission in approximately 25% of patients, and this group appears

to have considerably improved survival. Prospective, randomized phase III trials are needed to prove definitively the value of preoperative radiation therapy and chemotherapy before esophagectomy, which has been suggested by the preliminary pilot studies reported.

SELECTED READINGS

1. Finley RJ, Inculet RI. The results of esophagogastrectomy without thoracotomy for adenocarcinoma of the esophagogastric junction. *Ann Surg* 1989;21:535–43.
2. Fok M, Cheng SWK, Wong J. Pyloroplasty versus no drainage in gastric replacement of the esophagus. *Am J Surg* 1991;162:447–52.
3. Forastiere AA, Gennis M, Orringer MB, et al. Cisplatin, vinblastine, and mitoguazone chemotherapy for epidermoid and adenocarcinoma of the esophagus. *J Clin Oncol* 1987;5:1143–9.
4. Forastiere AA, Orringer MB, Perez-Tamayo C, Urba SG, Zahurak M. Preoperative chemoradiation followed by transhiatal esophagectomy for carcinoma of the esophagus: final report. *J Clin Oncol* 1993;11: 1118–23.
5. Orringer MB. Transhiatal esophagectomy without thoracotomy for carcinoma of the thoracic esophagus. *Ann Surg* 1984;200:282–8.
6. Orringer MB, Marshall B, Stirling MC. Transhiatal esophagectomy for benign and malignant disease. *J Thorac Cardiovasc Surg* 1993; 105:265–76.

EDITORIAL BOARD COMMENTARY

Both surgical approaches described for this disease are acceptable. In light of the lack of proven benefit for a wide nodal resection, the surgeon's choice of procedure is likely experience-driven.

17

Carcinoma of the Cervical Esophagus

Francis G. Duhaylongsod, Anna L. Vaughn, and Walter G. Wolfe

*Is combined chemoradiation and surgery too much therapy
to swallow?*

CASE PRESENTATION

A 70-year-old white woman was referred to our hospital for evaluation and treatment of a partially obstructing malignant neoplasm of the cervical esophagus.

The patient had epigastric burning for 2 years for which she underwent an upper gastrointestinal barium study notable only for the presence of a small hiatal hernia. Six months before admission she began experiencing fullness in her throat. The next month, while undergoing a cataract extraction, she noted that the sensation of fullness had increased. Over the course of the next few months this progressed to mild dysphagia with large food boluses, and eventually into definite dysphagia with increasingly smaller quantities of food. One month before entry she began to have episodic postprandial regurgitation of solid food. She had no difficulty swallowing liquids.

Three weeks before admission she was seen by her personal physician and scheduled for prompt esophagoscopy. Because of an obstructing mass, the endoscope could not be advanced beyond the cervical esophagus. Tissue biopsy specimens obtained at endoscopy revealed a moderately differentiated invasive squamous cell carcinoma. A barium swallow documented an irregular lesion of the cervical esophagus with luminal narrowing (Fig. 17–1). The study also confirmed a small hiatal hernia. Because of significant dysphagia, the patient underwent dilation of the stricture using 7- and 9-mm Savary-Gilliard dilators passed over a guidewire followed by a 30-, 32-, and 34-French Maloney dilator. Esophagoscopy was again attempted; this time the entire esophagus was visualized and the tumor extent confirmed. The stomach and duodenum were normal. After her esophageal dilatation she was able to swallow without dif-

ficulty. Computed tomography (CT) of the neck, chest, and upper abdomen demonstrated a mass in the lower cervical esophagus beginning at the level of C5 and manifested by asymmetric thickening of the esophageal wall with extension to and mild compression of the posterior wall of the trachea at the level of T1. No evidence of adenopathy or distant metastases was present.

The patient was a housing supervisor for a local college and retired at age 67. She was diagnosed with anemia 20 years earlier, for which she was prescribed iron. Subsequent hematologic studies have not revealed anemia. A hysterectomy and appendectomy were performed 20 years earlier for leiomyomas. In addition, she had a previous hemorrhoidectomy and left wrist fracture. She has required no medications.

The patient's mother died of chronic obstructive lung disease, and her father and one brother from a myocardial infarction. Another brother died of cancer of unknown type. A widow of 25 years, she has three healthy children. There was no personal history of alcohol or tobacco abuse, previous dysphagia or esophageal reflux, lye ingestion, chills, sweats, weight loss, fatigue, hematemesis, hemoptysis, or melena.

Her temperature was 36.5°C, her pulse was 72, and her respirations were 16. The blood pressure was 152/80. Her weight was 54.4 kg, and her height was 160 cm. On physical examination, the patient was a thin woman in no acute distress. The head was normal. The left eye was status postcataract extraction with lens implantation. Oropharyngeal examination was negative. The trachea was in the midline. The neck showed no adenopathy, thyromegaly, or other masses. The lungs were clear and the heart was normal. Breast examination was negative. There was no

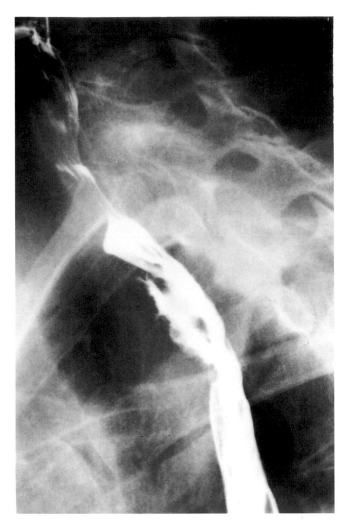

FIG. 17–1. A 70-year-old white woman with a 6-month history of progressive dysphagia. The initial barium swallow performed at an outside hospital revealed marked mucosal irregularity and luminal narrowing of the cervical esophagus.

supraclavicular, axillary, or inguinal adenopathy. The abdomen was normal with no hepatosplenomegaly, masses, or evidence of ascites; there was a well-healed midline abdominal scar. Rectal examination was negative; a stool specimen gave a test negative for occult blood. Neurologic examination was normal except for slight weakness in her left forearm, the site of her previous fracture; there was no hoarseness. The urine was negative. The hematologic and blood chemical values were normal. An electrocardiogram revealed a normal sinus rhythm, with minor, nonspecific ST-segment and T-wave abnormalities. Radiographs of the chest revealed normal lung fields and mediastinum. An endoscopic examination of the esophagus and upper airway showed the carcinoma to be 17 cm from the incisors, and no involvement of the larynx. The clinical TNM stage was IIA, T3 N0 M0.

At Tumor Conference, members of thoracic surgery, medical oncology, and radiation oncology reviewed in detail the pertinent history, physical examination, and diagnostic evaluation. In view of the generally poor prognosis of esophageal cancer and the persisting controversy concerning its appropriate management, different treatment options were discussed, including supportive therapy alone, palliative chemotherapy, and a potentially curative combination of chemotherapy, radiation, and resection. All participants agreed that the patient's desire for cure, her favorable performance status and freedom from other chronic illnesses, and the absence of clinical nodal and distant metastases favored consideration for combination chemotherapy and irradiation followed by surgical resection (1–3). The chemotherapy protocol included cisplatin (20 mg/m^2 per day) and VP-16 (60 mg/m^2 per day) intravenously for 5 consecutive days delivered every 4 weeks for three cycles. Concurrent with the second cycle of chemotherapy, the patient would begin radiation therapy to the cervical esophagus, upper mediastinum, and supraclavicular areas delivered in 25 fractions over 5 weeks (4,500 rads). After completion of chemotherapy and irradiation, the patient would be restaged. If the patient was judged inoperable because of metastatic disease or otherwise refused surgery, consideration was given to extending the total radiation dose another 1,500 rads. Alternatively, if the patient remained a surgical candidate, operation was scheduled for 3 to 4 weeks after radiation and chemotherapy were completed. Because this patient had a low cervical lesion, where it was clear that the stomach must be brought to the neck to insure an adequate proximal margin, she was a good candidate for transhiatal esophagectomy with cervical esophagogastrostomy. Since 1985, our published experience with combination chemotherapy and radiation followed by surgical resection for the treatment of squamous cell carcinoma of the esophagus has included 72 patients treated with esophagogastrectomy (2). Toxicity from irradiation and chemotherapy included leukopenia, thrombocytopenia, renal insufficiency, and radiation-induced esophagitis. In general, there was a dramatic reversal of pretherapy catabolism and wasting, with improvement in the patient's ability to swallow as well as appetite for food. Overall operative mortality was 5%, and 5-year survival for squamous cell carcinoma was 25% (2). Notably, 40% of patients were found to have no evidence of microscopic disease in the esophagectomy specimen, and this was associated with a remarkable 40% 5-year survival (2).

The patient received the first course of cisplatin, 30 mg, and VP-16, 100 mg, during her initial hospitalization. She tolerated the first cycle of chemotherapy well, but experienced severe nausea, vomiting, weight loss (-3.8 kg), and mild leukopenia while at home. The second cycle included cisplatin and a 50% reduced dose of VP-16 in an effort to avoid severe leukopenia. Radiation therapy was initiated and tolerated by the patient without difficulty. With appropriate medication at home her nausea and vomiting were lessened, and her weight loss was improved by eating several small meals each day combined with Ensure supplementation. The third cycle of chemotherapy included cisplatin and VP-16 at the reduced dose. Radiation therapy was completed simultaneously with the final cycle of chemotherapy, after receiving a total of 4,500 rads. Increasing complaints of dysphagia prompted a barium swallow study, which showed an area of smooth narrowing in the cervical esophagus at about the C6-C7 level (Fig. 17–2). After reviewing the patient's physical examination and pertinent radiologic studies we advised readmission in 4 weeks for surgical resection.

One week before the proposed date of operation, the patient was seen in surgery clinic for routine preoperative consultation. Physical examination revealed a 7.5 × 7.5-mm tender, subcutaneous nodule in the right neck. An excisional biopsy revealed well differentiated squamous cell carcinoma. Because of evidence of metastatic disease and the low likelihood that surgical resection would afford meaningful survival benefit, the operation was canceled. The patient underwent a barium swallow and CT of the neck, and her case was re-presented at Tumor Conference. The barium study showed a tight focal stricture with mild progression compared to the previous study; however, it was unclear whether this represented tumor or was secondary to radiation changes (Fig. 17–3). The neck CT revealed thickening of the proximal esophageal wall,

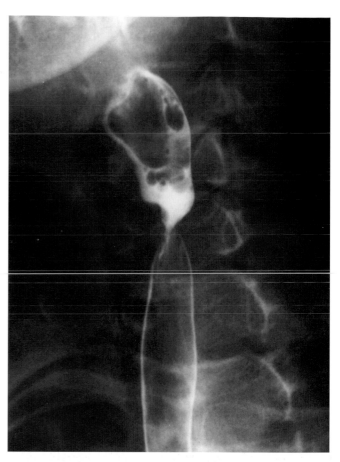

FIG. 17–3. After a biopsied subcutaneous nodule in the neck revealed squamous cell carcinoma, a barium swallow was performed showing a tight focal stricture with mild progression compared with the previous study (see Fig. 17–2). It was unclear whether this represented increased tumor growth or was secondary to radiation changes.

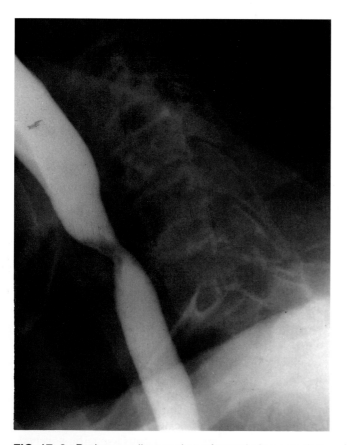

FIG. 17–2. Barium swallow study performed after completion radiation therapy and chemotherapy showing an area of smooth narrowing in the cervical esophagus at about the C6-C7 level.

extending approximately 5 to 6 cm, several small (<1 cm) cervical nodes adjacent to the carotid bundle, absence of mediastinal adenopathy, and several 2- to 3-mm peripheral pulmonary nodules in the left upper lobe, lingula, and right lower lobe, the significance of which was uncertain. Consensus was obtained in favor of supportive therapy alone, with repeated esophageal dilatations as necessary for dysphagia. Radiation and chemotherapy would be held in reserve for symptoms of metastatic disease.

One week after the positive biopsy, the patient was admitted to the hospital for esophageal dilatation. Despite previous irradiation to the cervical esophagus, the procedure was well tolerated with clear improvement in the patient's ability to swallow. Because of its proximal location, the tumor was too high to stent and unsuitable for laser debulking. Once home, she experienced a dramatic improvement in appetite, energy level, and weight gain. Bimonthly clinic visits over the next year failed to disclose progression of her disease. In fact, apart from mild arthritic pain complaints involving both shoulders, she continued to progress surprisingly well, maintaining a good appetite, stabilization of her weight, and excellent performance status. Semiannual physical examinations and chest radiographs have remained negative for evidence of recurrent disease. Currently, she is alive and well with only occasional mild dysphagia 7 years after her diagnosis of cervical esophageal carcinoma.

REFERENCES

1. Wolfe WG, Burton GV, Seigler HF, Crocker IR, Vaughn AL. Early results with combined modality therapy for carcinoma of the esophagus. *Ann Surg* 1987;205:563–71.
2. Wolfe WG, Vaughn AL, Seigler HF, Hathorn JW, Leopold KA, Duhaylongsod FD. Survival of patients with carcinoma of the esophagus treated with combined-modality therapy. *J Thorac Cardiovasc Surg* 1993;105:749–56.
3. Herskovic A, Martz K, Al-Sarraf M, et al. Combined chemotherapy and radiotherapy compared with radiotherapy alone in patients with cancer of the esophagus. *N Engl J Med* 1991;326:1593–8.

COMMENTARY by Lawrence R. Coia

The authors present a 70-year-old woman with a squamous cell carcinoma of the cervical esophagus for whom the treatment plan was chemoradiation followed by esophagectomy. However, because of what appeared to be progressive cancer following chemoradiation, esophagectomy was not performed. Remarkably, apart from occasional mild dysphagia, she remains alive and well 7 years after diagnosis of cervical esophageal cancer. This case illustrates several important considerations in the evaluation, management, and follow-up of esophageal cancer.

First, it is interesting to note the possibility that the patient may have had Patterson-Kelly (also called Plummer-Vinson) syndrome, which is characterized by iron deficiency, anemia, esophageal webs, and cervical or upper thoracic esophageal cancer, often arising in women of Scandinavian descent. The patient had no cigarette smoking or alcohol abuse history, each of which are independent risk factors for squamous cell carcinoma of the esophagus. She did have a history of anemia 20 years prior, for which she was prescribed iron. Her ancestry was not described.

Evaluation of the patient included esophagoscopy, barium swallow, CT scan of the neck, chest, and upper abdomen along with careful physical examination with attention to the head and neck. Upper airway endoscopy was performed as well; however, it was not stated whether bronchoscopy was performed. Patients with squamous cell carcinoma of the esophagus should have a bronchoscopy for two reasons: (a) to rule out second primary lung cancer, and (b) to determine if there is invasion of the trachea or bronchi. In this patient, CT scan suggested involvement of the posterior tracheal wall. Unfortunately, CT scan is not accurate in determining extraesophageal extension of disease. Extraesophageal extension is characterized by loss of fat plane between the esophagus and surrounding normal

structures. Unfortunately, many patients with esophageal cancer have poor nutrition and their periesophageal fat planes are not always readily seen on CT scan. A better study for evaluating depth of penetration of tumor into or through the esophageal wall is endoscopic ultrasound with an overall accuracy in T-staging of 85% (1,2). However, the 4-cm rigid tip and 13-mm diameter of the ultrasound probe limits passage through sonotic areas in about 25% of patients. This patient had an obstructing lesion that allowed complete esophagoscopy only after dilatation and, therefore, the patient may not have been a candidate for endoscopic ultrasound.

The present dilemma in staging esophageal cancer is well illustrated by this case. The patient was staged as T3 N0 M0 (stage IIA) using the 1992 AJCC staging system, yet this staging system is most accurately applied only to patients who have had esophagectomy as initial management because it is based on depth of wall penetration (T) and nodal involvement (N), both of which are best determined by pathologic review of the specimen. As stated earlier, CT scan is inaccurate for assigning "T" and "N," although it is useful in determining the presence or absence of distant metastases (M). Endoscopic ultrasound often is not performed because of lack of availability or inability to pass the probe through the lesion. The length of the tumor on endoscopy or barium swallow is of prognostic importance for patients managed with radiation or chemoradiation, yet tumor length is not part of the present staging system and is often not reported, as in this case. In the 1983 AJCC staging system, this patient's cancer would have been considered stage II because of obstruction. Without an appropriate staging system for patients managed with chemotherapy or radiation (alone or combined) as initial treatment, it is useful to record all available evaluative information, including factors shown to be important in the 1983 AJCC staging (length, obstruction, circumferential involvement, etc.). Other important considerations are sex (women do better than men), performance status, and degree of weight loss.

Regarding management of esophageal cancer, the group at Duke have been among the leaders in the use of chemoradiation followed by esophagectomy. The Duke investigators report a 25% 5-year survival, a 40% complete pathologic response rate, and a 40% 5-year survival for those patients who have had a complete pathologic response (3). These results are excellent and comparable to, if not better than, most series using preoperative chemoradiation (4). One must consider that a reasonable, if not superior, alternative is to use chemoradiation alone with surgery only for salvage. A large study from Fox Chase Cancer Center indicates that chemoradiation (5-FU, mitomycin, and 60 Gy) can result in a 60% local freedom from relapse, a 29% 5-year cause-specific survival, and a low treatment-related mortality (less than 2%)(5). An Intergroup study has confirmed the superiority of chemoradiation over radiation alone and has demonstrated a 25% 5-year survival with chemoradiation (5-FU, cisplatin, and 50 Gy)(6).

Cervical esophageal cancer is uncommon and results of treatment are often grouped with cancers of the head and neck. There are several approaches to the management of cervical esophageal cancer specifically. The curative surgical resection of cervical esophageal cancer requires a cervical or total esophagectomy with or without en bloc laryngopharyngectomy. The extent of dissection, the use of bilateral elective neck dissection, and the need for routine dissection of the mediastinal nodes are areas of controversy. In general, operative mortality following esophagectomy for cervical esophageal cancer has been relatively high (>20%), and 5-year survival ranges from 12% to 27% (7). There is relatively little information regarding the use of chemoradiation alone for the treatment of cervical esophageal cancer. Coia et al. reported five patients with cervical esophageal cancer treated with chemoradiation alone with outcomes similar to 52 patients with cancer of the thoracic esophagus, with one of five patients surviving more than 5 years (8). Santoro et al. treated 27 patients with combined chemoradiation with excellent results (9). Overall survival was 37%, with a median follow-up of 43 months.

Follow-up for esophageal cancer poses some interesting problems. Stricture following radiation or chemoradiation is not uncommon, occurring in up to two thirds of patients. The etiology of the stricture is often difficult to determine, with roughly half caused by recurrent tumor and half by radiation fibrosis (10). If no gross tumor is present on endoscopy, there may be little to distinguish tumor recurrence from fibrosis. Fibrotic strictures always occur within the radiation field and the distal extent usually corresponds to the bottom of the radiation field. Dilatation is successful in restoring swallowing function in most patients with benign fibrotic stricture. Results of endoscopic biopsy of the esophagus postradiation or chemoradiation may not correspond with the findings at esophagectomy or with clinical course. Patients who have a complete endoscopic response with negative biopsy postchemoradiation will be found to have residual cancer in the esophagectomy specimen in at least half the cases. On the other hand, a positive endoscopic biopsy does not necessarily mean progression will ensue. We have observed one patient with positive esophageal biopsy 2 years after completion of chemoradiation who refused salvage esophagectomy and remains alive and disease-free 7 years later. The Duke investigators present a simi-lar but not identical problem, namely a positive neck biopsy and suspicious stricture at the primary site postchemoradiation. Given the excellent outcome, one must agree that observation alone, rather than attempts at radical surgery, was appropriate for this patient.

Clearly, we need better predictors to determine which patients would be aided by esophagectomy postchemoradiation. We recommend chemoradiation alone for patients with squamous cell cancer of the esophagus with esophagectomy offered only to those who fail in the esophagus without other sites of failure. Patients with only local failure constitute only 10% of definitively treated patients. Small studies suggest biologic markers such as PCNA, EGFR, and TGA-alpha may be useful in predicting survival following chemoradiation with or without esophagectomy (11,12). Finally, regimens such as the excellent Duke regimen of chemoradiation followed by esophagectomy should be compared to surgery alone or chemoradiation alone in a Phase III study.

REFERENCES

1. Lightdale CJ (ed). Endoscopic ultrasonography. *Gastrointest Endosc Clin North Am* 1992;2:557–69.
2. Botet JF, Lightdale CJ, Zauber PG, et al. Pre-operative staging of esophageal cancer: comparison of endoscopic and US and dynamic CT. *Radiology* 1991;181:419–25.
3. Wolfe WG, Vaughn AL, Seigler HF, et al. Survival of patients with carcinoma of the esophagus treated with combined-modality therapy. *J Thorac Cardiovasc Surg* 1993;105:749–56.
4. Coia LR, Sauter ER. Esophageal cancer. *Curr Prob Cancer* 1994;18: 189–248.
5. Coia LR, Engstrom P, Paul A. Non-surgical management of esophageal cancer: Reports of a study of combined radiotherapy and chemotherapy. *J Clin Oncol* 1987;5:1783–90.
6. Herskovic A, et al. Combined chemotherapy and radiotherapy compared with radiotherapy alone in patients with cancer of the esophagus. *N Engl J Med* 1992;326:1593–8.
7. Mendenhall WM, Sonbeck MD, Parsons JT, et al. Management of cervical esophageal carcinoma. *Semin Radiat Oncol* 1994;4:179–91.
8. Coia LR, Engstrom P, Paul A. Long-term results of infusional 5-FU, mitomycin-C and radiation as primary management of esophageal carcinoma. *Int J Radiat Oncol Biol Phys* 1991;20:29–36.
9. Santoro A, Bidoli P, Salvini, et al. Larynx preservation with combined chemotherapy plus radiotherapy in squamous cell carcinoma of the upper esophagus. *Proc Am Soc Clin Oncol* 1993;12:279(abstr 899).
10. O'Rourke IC, Tiver L, Bull C, et al. Swallowing performance after radiation therapy for carcinoma of the esophagus. *Cancer* 1988;61: 2022–6.
11. Mukaida H, Toi M, Hirai T, et al. Clinical significance of the expression of epidermal growth factor and its receptor in esophageal cancer. *Cancer* 1991;68:142–8.
12. Sauter ER, Coia LR, Eisenberg BL, Hanks GE. Transforming growth factor alpha expression as a potential survival prognosticator in patients with esophageal adenocarcinoma receiving high-dose radiation and chemotherapy. *Int J Radiat Oncol Biol Phys* (in press).

18 Carcinoma of the Esophagus and Asynchronous Carcinoma of the Tonsil

Andre A. Abitbol

Aerodigestive cancer can occur in high-risk patients—careful follow-up is very important

CASE PRESENTATION

A 55-year-old man was initially seen in July 1987, with a 4-month history of dysphagia and odynophagia associated with some mild retrosternal discomfort and a 5-lb weight loss. The patient smoked two to three packages of cigarettes per day for 40 years and had a history of chronic ethanol abuse (usually a six-pack beer daily). An esophagram showed a 9-cm ulcerated lesion in the mid- and lower-third of the esophagus (Fig. 18–1). A chest roentgenogram showed upper lung bullous disease. A computed tomography CT scan of the chest showed a thickened walled esophagus compatible with carcinoma arising immediately below the level of the carina without evidence of hilar, mediastinal, or celiac adenopathy (Fig. 18–2). A magnetic resonance image (MRI) of the chest revealed a 10×4 cm posterior mediastinal mass involving the esophagus. Endoscopy revealed an ulcerated lesion measuring 8 cm in length, partially obstructing the lumen of the middle and lower third of the esophagus. Biopsy showed squamous cell carcinoma. Complete blood count revealed Hgb 12.6; Hct 36.3; WBC, 5,800; platelets 551,000. Chemical examinations revealed hyponatremia and hypoalbuminemia. The rest of the findings were within normal limits.

Physical examination in September 1987 revealed a middle-aged man who appeared thin and in excellent condition with good performance status. The physical examination was otherwise unremarkable. The patient was initiated on constant infusion 5-fluorouracil (1,000 mg/m^2 per 24 hr $\times$ 96 hr) and cisplatin (100 mg/m^2) for one cycle before initiation of radiation therapy. He received radiation therapy combined with 5-FU (1000 mg/m^2 24 hr $\times$ 96 hr) and cisplatin (1,000 mg/m^2) for two additional cycles. Treatment was delivered using AP/PA technique to a field measuring 14×7 cm, which received 3,060 cGy (180 cGy fraction; 5 fractions/week), 10 MV photons, followed by three-field (AP, LPO, RPO) technique (14×6 cm), delivering 1,440 cGy (180 cGy fraction; 5 fractions 1 week). The patient was treated and completed the course of radiation therapy and chemotherapy uneventfully. The WBC nadir was 2,100; the platelet count nadir was 242,000. The patient's dysphagia and appetite improved, and his weight returned to normal. Follow-up MRI showed the paraesophageal mass to be smaller than at the time of initiation of radiation therapy. Follow-up esophagoscopy 2 months after therapy was negative and follow-up esophagram was entirely negative (Fig. 18–3). He continued to do well after treatment and gained weight.

In January 1989, 2 years and 4 months after completion of radiation therapy, 5-FU, and cisplatin, he felt some discomfort on yawning in the area of the right tonsil with some mild associated pain on swallowing. His appetite was stable. Clinical examination revealed an ulcerated mass in the right tonsillar fossa. Biopsy showed squamous cell carcinoma. MRI of the head and neck showed a 1.5-cm right tonsillar lesion without associated adenopathy. Esophagram in September, 1989, and previous follow-up endoscopy did not show evidence of recurrence of the esophageal lesion. The

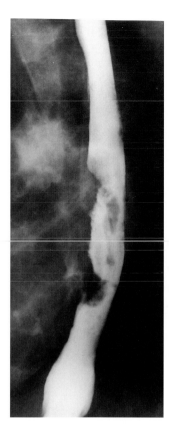
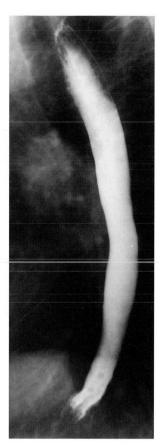

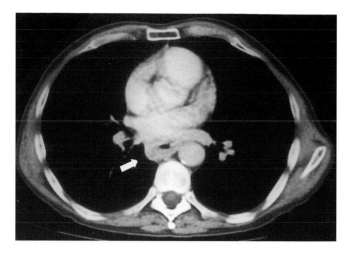

FIG. 18–2. CT scan of the patient. The esophageal lumen contains air and there is gross thickening of the esophageal wall conforming to the known cancer.

FIG. 18–1. (Left) Ulcerating carcinoma of the middle third of the esophagus. This type of lesion represents the classic Carmen-Kirkland complex, i.e., a central ulceration surrounded by rolled tumor margins. This is essentially pathognomic of malignancy.

FIG. 18–3. (Right) Posttherapy esophagram. No residual tumor is shown.

patient was referred for radiation therapy and received definitive radiotherapy directed to the oral pharynx. He received a total dose of 6,660 cGy in 37 sessions, which was completed on March 30, 1990, using 6 MeV photons, 180 cGy per fraction. The initial field used (parallel opposed) delivered 1,980 cGy and followed by right anterior obliques and right posterior oblique field to a total dose of 6,660 cGy. He had complete resolution of the mass in the right tonsillar fossa, has been followed for 1½ years since completion of radiation therapy to the tonsillar region, and remains free of disease. He no longer smokes or abuses alcohol. After the diagnosis of his tonsillar lesion and completion of radiation therapy, the patient has been maintained on Accutane by his medical oncologist. He tolerates the Accutane quite well. He is alive and well 6 years after treatment for the T2 N0 M0 squamous cell carcinoma of the esophagus and 3½ years after treatment for the T1 N0 M0 squamous cell carcinoma of the tonsil.

COMMENTARY by Joseph LoCicero III

As this case illustrates, many problems remain in the diagnosis and management of cancer of the esophagus. We will concentrate on two issues: accurate assessment, which is linked to precise prognostication, and choice of the most efficacious treatment.

Pretherapy staging is considered standard practice with many other tumors. An example is lung cancer, which involves assessment, often direct, of tumor size and extent as well as invasive sampling of mediastinal nodes. Because of the completeness of staging, tailored therapies now can be offered. It also facilitates systematic evaluation on a national scale of experimental multimodal approaches to locally advanced disease.

In contradistinction, pretherapy evaluation of esophageal cancer remains imprecise and sporadically applied. The three major methods used in this case were contrast esophagram, endoscopy, and computed tomography. The contrast esophagram evaluates only mucosal abnormalities. In some advanced cases, additional information may be inferred. Akiyama and associates (1) noted that axis deviation of the barium stream often indicated unresectability, but little else can be determined. Endoscopy affords direct visualization and guided biopsy of the mucosal aspects of the cancer. However, squamous cancer of the esophagus spreads submucosally. Miller in 1962 (2) and Wong in 1987 (3) demonstrated that more than one fourth of tumors extended from 3 to 6 cm and 10% extended 10 cm cephalad. This is not always appreciated at endoscopy; thus, treatment planning may be inadequate. CT scanning, often considered the definitive noninvasive study, is only 88% accurate in assessing direct tumor extension (4). A large nationwide study by the Radiologic Diagnostic Oncology Group demonstrated that the CT scan is little better than a coin flip when evaluating nodal involvement (5). However, it remains a sensitive and standard test for distant metastases to areas such as brain, lung, and liver.

Endoscopic ultrasound (EUS), a newer, promising noninvasive modality, should be an important pretherapy staging tool. EUS is useful not only for tumor invasion but also for lymphatic involvement. Lightdale and Botet (6) report 92% accuracy for tumor invasion and 88% accuracy for nodal involvement. It is also excellent for following up tumor regression during nonoperative therapies (7). The major drawbacks to ubiquitous implementation of this technology are the initial expense, the steep observer learning curve, and the inability to assess obstructing cancers that do not permit proper placement of the scope.

Laparoscopy and thoracoscopy are quite accurate in defining the T and N stages of esophageal malignancies. However, both procedures are time-consuming and require a general anesthetic (8). Several groups are assessing the usefulness of these technologies as major pretherapy staging tools.

Although the exact esophageal staging algorithm remains to be codified, it is clear that future studies on outcome must clearly define all aspects of the tumor at the beginning of treatment. As with other major thoracic malignancies, pretherapy staging should become commonplace.

Although constantly challenged, operative extirpation remains the prime treatment for squamous cell carcinoma of the esophagus. Among those treating early cancers of the esophagus, Huang and colleagues (9) reported a low surgical mortality rate (<1%) and a striking 5-year survival of 81%, whereas Akiyama and associates (10) report 54% (10). In this country, survival rates are lower, reflecting the later stage at the time of diagnosis. Orringer et al. (11) reported a 27% 5-year survival among 417 patients, and Vignewaran et al. (12) a 31% 5-year survival among 100 patients.

The type of resection is less important than completeness of the esophageal resection and accurate staging. Because squamous cancer tends to spread submucosally, a generous cephalad margin is necessary, which may be accomplished by either a transhiatal esophagectomy or an Ivor-Lewis approach. Putnam and colleagues (13) showed that a variety of surgical approaches performed in a residency training program on 248 patients did not affect morbidity and mortality. The quality of life for resected patients is good, with most (70%) reporting good alimentary comfort (14). Major symptoms of discomfort include early satiety, dysphagia, and dumping.

Radiation therapy is the most common alternative to an operation. However, most series report a 5-year survival of less than 20%. Because some of the patients in these series were not surgical candidates because of comorbidity or extensive disease, advocates of radiation therapy suggest that direct comparison to surgery is not fair. However, Wolfe and colleagues (15) recently presented a series of 49 patients with squamous cell cancer of the esophagus who were scheduled for operation but refused following combined radiation and chemotherapy. Again, overall survival was 20%. Still, the greatest experience comes from Asia. Yang and associates analyzed 1,136 5-year survivors of radiation therapy (16). Most long-term survivors received high radiation doses (50–80 Gy). The most important factors were a lesion less than 5 cm long, an upper third lesion, and demonstrated radiation sensitivity. Of these long-term survivors, 404 died. Local control remained a significant problem with recurrence or lymph node involvement in 50% of these individuals.

Several studies have shown improved survival with a multimodality approach. Nygaard et al. reported a Scandinavian three-armed trial with the best results in patients receiving 35 Gy of radiation followed by surgery (17). However, Wolfe and associates noted only 40% of the resected specimens were "sterilized" by radiation and chemotherapy (14). Again, this suggests that, in the long run, radiation and chemotherapy without resection will have a significant failure rate for this disease.

REFERENCES

1. Akiyama H, Kogure T, Itai Y. The esophageal axis in its relation to the resectability of carcinoma of the esophagus. *Ann Thorac Surg* 1972; 176:30–3.
2. Miller C. Carcinoma of the thoracic esophagus and cardia. *Br J Surg* 1962;49:507–16.
3. Wong J. Esophageal resection for cancer: the rationale of current practice. *Am J Surg* 1987;53:18–21.
4. Thompson WM, Halvorsen RA, Foster WL Jr, et al. Computed tomography for staging esophageal and gastroesophageal cancer: a re-evaluation. *Am J Radiol* 1983;141:951–65.
5. Webb WR, Gatsonis C, Zerhouni EA, et al. CT and MR imaging in staging of non-small cell bronchogenic carcinoma: report of the Radiologic Diagnostic Oncology Group. *Radiology* 1991;178: 705–12.
6. Lightdale CJ, Botet JF. Esophageal carcinoma: pre-operative staging and evaluation of anastomotic recurrence. *Gastrointest Endo* 1990;36: 11–4.
7. Rice TW, Boyce GA, Sivak MV. Esophageal ultrasound in the preoperative staging of carcinoma of the esophagus. *J Thorac Cardiovasc Surg* 1991;101:536–9.
8. LoCicero J. Laparoscopy/thoracoscopy for staging II: pretherapy nodal evaluation in carcinoma of the esophagus. *Semin Surg Oncol* 1993;9:56–8.
9. Huang GJ, Shao L, Zhang D, et al. Diagnosis and surgical treatment of early esophageal carcinoma. *Chin Med J* 1991;94:229.
10. Akiyama H. Principles of surgical treatment for carcinoma of the esophagus: analysis of lymph node involvement. *Ann Surg* 1981;194: 438–44..
11. Orringer MB, Marshall B, Stirling MC. Transhiatal esophagectomy for benign and malignant disease. *J Thorac Cardiovasc Surg* 1993; 105:265–9.
12. Vigneswaran WT, Trastek VF, Seigler HF, et al. Extended esophagectomy in the management of esophageal carcinoma of the upper thoracic esophagus. *J Thorac Cardiovasc Surg* 1994;107:901–6.
13. Putnam JB, Seull DM, McMurtrey MJ, et al. Comparison of three techniques of esophagectomy within a residency training program. *Ann Thorac Surg* 1994;57:319–25.
14. Collard JM, Otte JB, Reynaert M, Kestenes PJ. Quality of life three

years or more after esophagectomy for cancer. *J Thorac Cardiovasc Surg* 1992;104:391–4.

15. Wolfe WG, et al. Survival of patients with carcinoma of the esophagus treated with combined modality therapy. *J Thorac Cardiovasc Surg* 1993;105:749–53.

16. Yang AY, Gu XZ, Zhao S, et al. Long-term survival of radiotherapy for esophageal cancer. Analysis of 1136 patients surviving for more than five years. Internat *J Radiol Oncol Biol Physiol* 1983;9:1769–74.

17. Nygaard K, Hagen S, Hansen S, et al. Preoperative radiotherapy prolongs survival in operable esophageal carcinoma: a randomized multicenter study of preoperative radiotherapy and chemotherapy—the second Scandinavian trial in esophageal cancer. *World J Surg* 1992;16:1104–10.

EDITORIAL BOARD COMMENTARY

This case illustrates the importance of careful follow-up to detect new primary aerodigestive tract cancers in high-risk patients.

19

Resectable Squamous Cell Carcinoma of the Mid-Esophagus

Carolyn E. Reed

Surgery: When? Anything else?

CASE PRESENTATION

M.H., a 47-year-old black man, presented to his local physician in December 1986 with a 1-month history of dysphagia and weight loss of 17 lbs. He described difficulty swallowing mainly solid foods, a sensation of food sticking just below the sternal notch, and occasional regurgitation. He denied a change in appetite, cough, shortness of breath, hemoptysis, hematemesis, or change in bowel habits.

The patient had a 10-year history of heavy alcohol ("moonshine") abuse that was discontinued in 1975. He drank an occasional beer since then. He denied tobacco use. He had a history of seizures in the past, thought to be secondary to alcohol, hypertension, hyperlipidemia, and recurrent rectal fistulas. He was disabled secondary to partial blindness and retired from working in a textile mill.

Physical examination was unremarkable. His lungs were clear and his cardiovascular examination was normal. He had no cervical or supraclavicular lymphadenopathy. Abdominal examination revealed no masses or tenderness and normal liver span. Rectal examination revealed heme-negative stools.

Laboratory data revealed a normal SMA-7, WBC 11.6, Hct/Hgb 37.5/12.6, and normal platelet count. Chest roentgenogram was normal. A barium swallow and upper gastrointestinal series were obtained. There was a 5- to 7-cm long irregular narrowing in the midthoracic esophagus with shelving proximally and distally and irregularity of the mucosa, strongly suggestive of carcinoma of the esophagus (Fig. 19–1). There was no abnormality seen in the stomach or duodenum. The patient was then referred to the Veterans Hospital.

Esophagoscopy was performed and revealed exophytic circumferential tumor from 30 to 35 cm. The stomach was normal. The biopsy specimen was positive for poorly differentiated squamous cell carcinoma. Bronchoscopy revealed slight extrinsic compression of the left mainstem bronchus but no endobronchial disease. Computed tomography (CT) of the head, chest, and abdomen was performed. The computed tomogram showed a 7- to 8-cm thickened midesophagus with increased tissue density in the subcarinal region representing either extension of tumor through the wall of the esophagus or adenopathy. There was no evidence of liver metastases or celiac axis lymphadenopathy on the abdominal computed tomogram. Esophageal endoscopic ultrasonography was not available.

Additional laboratory data included normal liver function tests. Pulmonary function tests revealed an FVC of 4.10 (90% of predicted). FEV_1 of 3.31 (99% of predicted), and MVV of 90% of predicted. A room air blood gas showed a pH 7.37, pCO_2 39, HCO_3 22, 97% Hgb sat.

Tumor Board Assessment

At the time of evaluation, an institutional protocol was in effect. Patients with locoregional squamous cell carcinoma of the esophagus were randomized to surgery alone versus preoperative chemotherapy and hyperfractionated radiotherapy (RT) followed by surgery. Review of the chest CT scan at the Tumor Board meeting resulted in

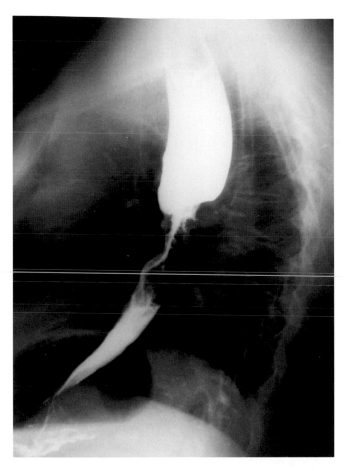

FIG. 19–1. Upper gastrointestinal series showing irregular narrowing in the midthoracic esophagus, strongly suggestive of carcinoma.

comments regarding the possibility of tumor involvement of the left mainstem bronchus. Another participant believed that it was more probable that subcarinal lymph nodes were involved with tumor. The surgeon commented on the inaccuracy of the CT scan in determining the depth of wall penetration and in assessing regional lymph node metastases. A member of the Tumor Board asked if magnetic resonance imaging (MRI) would be helpful, but most felt that MRI added little to CT for staging esophageal cancer. (Today endoscopic ultrasonography would have been added to the staging evaluation to assess better the depth of tumor invasion and detect abnormal regional lymph nodes.)

The patient's performance status was noted to be good and he was tolerating soft foods. He had no medical contraindications to surgical resection.

It was the opinion of the Tumor Board that the patient's tumor was potentially resectable and he should be offered admission into the randomized institutional protocol. The tumor was clinically staged as probable T3 N1 M0 (stage III).

The patient was randomized to receive neoadjuvant therapy followed by surgery. He was admitted to the medical oncology service and underwent chemotherapy consisting of cisplatin (5 mg/M^2 per day by constant infusion days 1–5 and 8–12), etoposide (VP-16) (100 mg/M^2 on days 1, 3, 5), and concurrent radiation therapy (1.2 Gy tid days 1–5 and 8–12) to a total dose of 36 Gy. He tolerated the therapy well with moderate esophagitis being his major complaint. Repeat CT scan of the chest and upper abdomen was read as showing only thickening of the middle esophagus.

The patient was readmitted to the surgical service 4 weeks after the completion of neoadjuvant therapy. Laboratory data were within normal limits and his weight was stable.

On February 27, 1987, he underwent thoracic esophagectomy, cervical esophagogastrostomy, pyloroplasty, and jejunostomy. The patient was first explored via a right posterolateral thoracotomy. There was a large bulky tumor mass beginning at the carina and extending approximately 6 cm distally. There was a great deal of fibrosis around the mass. Upon dissection, it became apparent that there was dense tissue extending directly from the region of the tumor to the aorta. Frozen section of this tissue was read as connective tissue scarring. It was therefore decided to proceed with esophagectomy, and the thoracic esophagus was mobilized with a wide dissection of posterior mediastinal periesophageal tissue. Subsequent abdominal exploration of the abdomen was negative for tumor, and the mobilized stomach was brought up through the posterior mediastinum and anastomosed (one-layer hand sewn) to the cervical esophagus via a left neck approach.

The patient's postoperative course was complicated by the onset of bilateral pneumonia with an adult respiratory distress syndrome (ARDS)-like picture requiring reintubation on postoperative day (POD) 3. Sputum cultures were unrevealing, and he was maintained on triple antibiotics and ventilator support. He gradually improved and finally extubated on POD #19. A gastrografin study followed by barium had been negative for an anastomotic leak. A chest and abdominal CT scan were consistent with bilateral necrotizing pneumonitis. The patient's nutrition was maintained by jejunostomy tube feedings. After extubation, the patient made rapid progress, increased his oral diet, and was discharged 12 days later.

Tumor Board Reassessment

Final pathologic findings revealed well-differentiated squamous cell carcinoma in the esophagus extending into the muscularis but not through the wall to the deep margin (Fig. 19–2). The proximal and distal margins were free of tumor. One of the distal periesophageal lymph nodes was

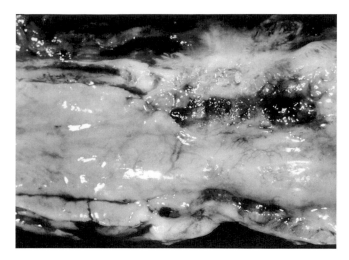

FIG. 19–2. Well differentiated squamous cell carcinoma of the esophagus extending into the muscularis.

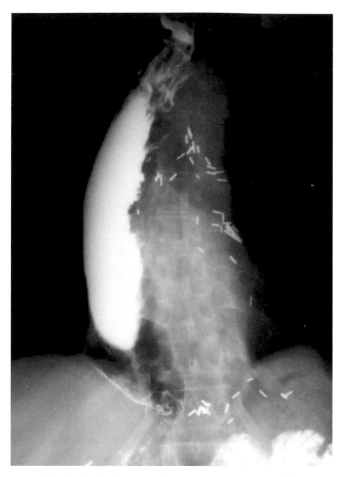

FIG. 19–3. Barium swallow, 2 years postoperative.

replaced with fibrotic tumor. Subcarinal and celiac lymph nodes were negative.

The patient was pathologically staged as T2 N1 M0 (stage IIB). A discussion ensued regarding the efficacy of postoperative adjuvant therapy. The radiotherapists believed that the patient would not benefit from RT because little further aid could be given. The pathologist commented that the fibrosis and foreign body giant cells seen in the specimen indicated that there was a pathologic response to the neoadjuvant treatment. After some debate, the medical oncologists elected to follow the patient.

The patient was seen in follow-up in the thoracic clinic at 3-month intervals until February of 1989. The patient adjusted his diet to small feedings and maintained his weight. He denied dysphagia or regurgitation. A barium swallow in 1989 is shown in Fig. 19–3.

The patient has been followed up at 6-month intervals since 1989 and remains alive and free of disease.

COMMENTARY by Mark B. Orringer

This case report illustrates well the current approach to resectable esophageal squamous carcinoma. The patient under consideration was typical in that he was black (in the United States the incidence of esophageal carcinoma in blacks is approximately 14 per 100,000 population as opposed to 7 per 100,000 in whites), and he had a history of alcohol abuse, which, like tobacco usage, is a well established etiologic factor in esophageal carcinoma. Worldwide, 95% of esophageal carcinomas are squamous cell carcinomas, and 5% are adenocarcinomas. In North American and Western European countries, however, there has been a recent and dramatic reversal in this ratio; esophageal adenocarcinoma arising in Barrett's mucosa now constitutes at least 50% to 60% of esophageal can-

cers being treated. As illustrated in this case presentation, the evaluation of dysphagia in the adult warrants two basic studies: a barium swallow and esophagoscopy. It is worth emphasizing that an "upper GI series" does not include detailed views of the esophagus; and if this test alone is ordered in the radiographic evaluation of the patient with dysphagia, an esophageal tumor will be missed. It is best to obtain both a barium swallow (to assess esophageal pathology) and an upper gastrointestinal series (to assess the suitability of the stomach as a possible esophageal substitute) in the evaluation of the patient with dysphagia. At esophagoscopy, abnormal mucosal lesions should be both biopsied and brushed for cytologic assessment because the combination of esophageal biopsy and brushings establishes the diagnosis of carcinoma in 95% of the patients who have this tumor.

Once the diagnosis of esophageal cancer is established, the therapeutic options are relatively limited, and the prognosis remains among the worst of all visceral malignancies, with 5-year survival historically seldom exceeding 10%. The 1-month history of dysphagia in the patient under consideration would imply relatively early detection of the tumor. Unfortunately, the development of esophageal cancer is insidious, and the flexible, muscular esophageal wall can adapt to partial obstruction, so that by the time the patient begins to experience dysphagia, the esophageal cancer has likely been present for 12 to 18 months. The extensive mediastinal lymphatic drainage of the esophagus is responsible for the predilection of this tumor for metastasis, and approximately 75% of esophageal cancers are incurable at the time of diagnosis either by virtue of locoregional lymph node invasion, direct extension to adjacent vital organs, or distant metastatic disease. Ninety-five percent of patients with esophageal cancer present with dysphagia, and whether or not cure is possible, they are desperately in need of palliation of their impaired swallowing, which not only interferes with normal nutrition but also creates the potential for pulmonary complications because of aspiration.

The three available modalities of therapy for esophageal carcinoma vary significantly in their effectiveness. Radiation therapy alone is the least morbid, but unfortunately relieves dysphagia in less than 25% of patients who have obstructing circumferential carcinomas. Chemotherapy alone has shown little evidence of significant benefit. Esophageal resection and reconstruction, because it provides the most effective relief of dysphagia as well as the potential for occasional cure, has been the traditional approach to the patient with resectable esophageal cancer. As illustrated by the case under consideration, however, the morbidity of the traditional transthoracic esophageal resection may be considerable in the patient whose nutritional and pulmonary status have been compromised by impaired swallowing. Therefore, before undertaking an esophageal resection for carcinoma, it is important to stage the tumor to insure that a major operation is not being undertaken in a patient with only a few months to live. For example, if a patient with esophageal carcinoma has a liver metastasis or metastasis to celiac axis or retroperitoneal lymph nodes, he has stage IV disease, which carries an average life expectancy of only 6 months and, therefore, in my opinion, precludes esophageal resection.

Staging of esophageal carcinoma begins with a careful history and physical examination. The finding of a hard, supraclavicular lymph node warrants a fine-needle aspiration biopsy, which, if positive for carcinoma, rules out esophagectomy as a therapeutic option. Recent neurologic symptoms or bone pain justify a brain and bone scan, although these studies are not obtained routinely in patients with esophageal carcinoma. By far, the CT scan has been one of the most useful tools for staging esophageal cancer. Its value in this regard, however, has been overemphasized in a number of reports. The CT scan is an excellent means for suggesting distant organ or lymph node (celiac axis or retroperitoneal) metastasis, but as a general principle, a CT-guided fine-needle aspiration of most abnormalities detected with the scan is warranted to prove that the abnormality is in fact due to carcinoma.

Despite published reports that contiguity of an esophageal tumor with the adjacent aorta is an excellent predictor of the nonresectability of the tumor, we have repeatedly found that contiguity as demonstrated by CT scan is not synonymous with invasion—many tumors felt to be unresectable on the basis of the CT scan prove to be resectable at operation. It is also important when using the CT scan as a means of assessing liver metastases from esophageal carcinoma to use a bolus infusion technique for imaging the liver because hepatic metastases may be missed with the standard CT scan. Finally, regarding staging, every upper- and middle-third esophageal carcinoma warrants a bronchoscopy to rule out tracheobronchial invasion by the tumor, which might preclude resection.

The patient with esophageal carcinoma is typically elderly and may have associated cardiorespiratory disease resulting from tobacco or alcohol usage. Preoperative assessment therefore often includes functional cardiac scans to demonstrate ischemia and pulmonary function tests to allow assessment of operative risk. Oral hygiene should be optimized and carious teeth either extracted or repaired preoperatively because the morbidity of an esophageal anastomotic leak may be directly related to the character of swallowed bacteria from the mouth. In recent years, esophageal ultrasonography has been added to the staging armamentarium, as this study allows better assessment of the depths of tumor invasion and the presence of abnormal regional lymph nodes adjacent to the esophagus. Esophageal ultrasonography requires that the esophageal probe be able to cross through the malignant stenosis for imaging, and this may be impossible with a high-grade stenosis. I have not used esophageal ultrasonography in my practice because most tumors that have been deemed to be nonresectable on the basis of barium swallow and CT scan findings have in fact been resectable at operation, and I am unconvinced that the findings of ultrasonography would alter my operative approach in these patients.

The case presented is an excellent illustration of the current approach to esophageal carcinoma using preoperative neoadjuvant therapy in a protocol setting. The surgical and oncologic literature contain data from a number of phase II trials incorporating chemotherapy and radiation therapy either before or after surgery. Thus, the current information regarding the efficacy of these multimodality treatments comes largely from uncontrolled pilot studies that frequently suggest improved survival over single-modality treatment. It must be realized, however, that these approaches remain investigational at the present time. In a number of series, including those reported from the University of Michigan, multimodality therapy has resulted in a pathologic complete response (T0 N0 M0 status) in approximately one quarter of the patients, and in this group, survival appears to be enhanced considerably. In our series, for example, our patients rendered completely tumor-free by preoperative radiation therapy and chemotherapy had a median survival duration of 70 months, and 60% were alive at 5 years. These encouraging results have justified our current phase III trial, prospectively comparing multimodality therapy with surgery alone. It bears emphasis that in approximately three quarters of patients so treated, complete eradication of the tumor is not achieved, and esophagectomy remains an integral part of the treatment plan so that the true impact of the therapy on the tumor can be assessed with pathologic examination of the specimen. Until nonresectional therapy can offer complete eradication of tumor in most of the patients so treated, esophagectomy is the "gold standard" for determining the efficacy of therapy. There is a current disturbing trend among oncologists to treat these patients with radiation therapy and chemotherapy alone, dispensing with esophagectomy. This has resulted in a growing number of patients presenting with recurrent tumor in an irradiated esophagus, which is far more difficult to resect several months after completing a full course of radiation therapy.

Comment on the operative approach used here is also warranted. During the past 15 years or so, the technique of transhiatal esophagectomy without thoracotomy has emerged as a valuable alternative to standard transthoracic esophagectomy. Avoidance of a thoracotomy has lessened the physiologic impact on an already debilitated patient, and the routinely used cervical esophagogastric anastomosis has virtually eliminated mediastinitis and sepsis associated with an intrathoracic esophagogastric anastomotic leak. In the patient under consideration, because of the proximity of tumor to the carina and airway, there is natural concern that transhiatal resection of the tumor without a thoracotomy may be fraught with more danger than would be the case if resection were performed transthoracically under direct vision. In our experience with transhiatal esophagectomy without thoracotomy in more than 500 carcinomas of the intrathoracic esophagus, one third of which were either upper or middle-third tumors, transhiatal resection has been possible in 97% of patients in whom it has been attempted, only 3% of our patients requiring a thoracotomy for resection of their tumors. Clearly, resection of middle-third esophageal tumors using the transhiatal approach is more difficult from a technical standpoint than resection of distal or upper-third tumors, and the surgeon should have a considerable experience with the transhiatal technique of esophagectomy before resecting the type of middle-third tumor that this patient had. Little is lost beginning the operation with an upper abdominal incision, mobilizing the stomach, carrying out a gastric drainage procedure, a Kocher maneuver, and inserting a feeding jejunostomy tube (the latter being routine in all our patients undergoing esophageal replacement or bypass). The transhiatal mobilization can then be begun, and if in the surgeon's estimation tumor fixation precludes continuing this approach, the abdominal incision can be closed and a thoracotomy carried out to allow completion of the esophagectomy. Regardless of the technique of esophagectomy, transhiatal versus transthoracic, a cervical esophagogastric anastomosis has emerged as the safest esophageal anastomosis because an anastomotic leak in the neck generally results in a transient cervical salivary fistula that heals spontaneously within 7 to 10 days and is associated with virtually no mortality. This is in sharp contrast with a intrathoracic esophagogastric anastomotic leak, which results in mediastinitis and which is fatal in 50% of patients with this complication. The postoperative respiratory distress and need for prolonged mechanical ventilatory assistance described in this patient is common after a combined thoracic and abdominal operation in a debilitated patient with esophageal cancer. The pain of a combined thoracic and abdominal approach results in splinting and secondary atelectasis and pneumonia, which are rarely encountered after a transhiatal resection. The resulting one-month hospitalization after esophagectomy described in the patient under consideration contrasts sharply with the average 10-day hospitalization after transhiatal esophagectomy and a cervical esophagogastric anastomosis, which we have described.

Finally, the discussion at the Tumor Board reassessment about the need for postoperative adjuvant therapy was interesting. There are currently no objective data showing improved survival with the addition of postoperative radiation therapy and/or chemotherapy in this patient population and, philosophically, I have difficulty recommending such treatment. The patient presents with dysphagia and survives an extremely difficult course of multimodality therapy that enables him to swallow comfortably. Further chemotherapy only increases patient discomfort and morbidity without clear survival advantage, and until the value of such an approach is demonstrated in a controlled prospective fashion, there seems little justification for it, even in patients with residual tumor in the resected specimen. Even in our patients whose resected esophagus contained some residual tumor after preoperative chemo- and radiation therapy, a 32% 5-year survival contrasted sharply with the average survival of only 14 months in our historic controls treated with esophagectomy alone. This case demonstrates the gratifying long-term survival that may be achieved now in selected patients with esophageal carcinoma that only a few years ago was regarded as being a hopelessly incurable disease, for which only palliation was the goal of therapy.

SELECTED READINGS

1. Finley RJ, Inculet RI. The results of esophagogastrectomy without thoracotomy for adenocarcinoma of the esophagogastric junction. *Ann Surg* 1989;21:535–43.
2. Fok M, Cheng SWK, Wong J. Pyloroplasty versus no drainage in gastric replacement of the esophagus. *Am J Surg* 1991;162:447–52.

3. Forastiere AA, Gennis M, Orringer MB, et al. Cisplatin, vinblastine, and mitoguazone chemotherapy for epidermoid and adenocarcinoma of the esophagus. *J Clin Oncol* 1987;5:1143–9.

4. Forastiere AA, Orringer MB, Perez-Tamayo C, Urba SG, Zahurak M. Preoperative chemoradiation followed by transhiatal esophagectomy for carcinoma of the esophagus: final report. *J Clin Oncol* 1993;11: 1118–23.

5. Orringer MB. Transhiatal esophagectomy without thoracotomy for carcinoma of the thoracic esophagus. *Ann Surg* 1984;200:282–8.

6. Orringer MB, Marshall B, Stirling MC. Transhiatal esophagectomy for benign and malignant disease. *J Thorac Cardiovasc Surg* 1993; 105:265–76.

EDITORIAL BOARD COMMENTARY

Despite clinical trials involving multimodality approaches, surgery to obviate dysphagia remains the optimal conventional treatment choice.

SECTION III

Stomach

20

Adenocarcinoma of the Cardia with Positive Celiac Nodes and Involvement of the Distal Pancreas and Splenic Hilum

Herbert C. Hoover, Jr.

Is bigger surgery better? Does multimodality therapy help?

CASE PRESENTATION

A 72-year-old white woman was referred to the Surgical Oncology Service with a 6-week history of epigastric pain and an approximately 10-lb. weight loss. The patient denied any nausea, vomiting, or hemachezia. Her health had previously been good, and her only medication was Pepsid at 40 mg/day. Her only prior operations had been three cesarean sections, and a thyroidectomy for a benign tumor in 1955.

Examination revealed a healthy appearing lady, who was well preserved for her stated 72 years of age. She had no cervical adenopathy. Her lungs were clear. The abdominal exam was benign, including a rectal exam with brown guaiac negative stool.

An upper gastrointestinal series revealed an ulcerative lesion in the cardia with posterior penetration (Fig. 20–1). A chest roentgenogram was unremarkable. An abdominal CAT scan showed no hepatic metastases. There was a thickness in the posterior cardia of the stomach, with extension down into the distal pancreas and toward the splenic hilum (Fig. 20–2). Her CEA was normal at less than 0.5. Her liver and renal function tests were normal. Hematocrit value was 37.3, with a white blood count of 6,100. The patient underwent an esophagogastroscopy, which showed a large ulcerating tumor posteriorly in the cardia that started just beyond the esophagogastric junc-

tion with extention down the cardia toward the greater curvature. The distal body of the stomach, as well as the antrum and duodenum, were normal. Endoscopic biopsy specimens revealed poorly differentiated infiltrating adenocarcinoma.

Because of the tumor location and the patient's body habitus, it was decided to perform a left thoracoabdominal approach for the esophagogastrectomy. Abdominal exploration revealed a firm tumor mass in the stomach cardia extending up to the esophageal hiatus and down into the tail of the pancreas and hilum of the spleen. There were enlarged lymph nodes down to the origin of the left gastric artery and onto the body of the pancreas. The distal stomach and the rest of the abdominal contents were normal. A radical esophagogastrectomy was performed with an en bloc resection of the distal 5 cm of the esophagus, the spleen, and distal third of the pancreas. The pancreatic cut edge was oversewn with mattress sutures of 3-0 silk. The left gastric lymph nodes were the only apparent lymph nodes enlarged. Frozen section margins of the esophageal and gastric walls were negative. A pyloric fracture was performed over a large Hagar dilator through the stomach. The duodenum was Kocherized and an end-to-side esophagogastrostomy to the anterior-remaining antrum was performed. A needle catheter jejunostomy was performed before closing. There was less than one unit of blood loss, and none was replaced.

101

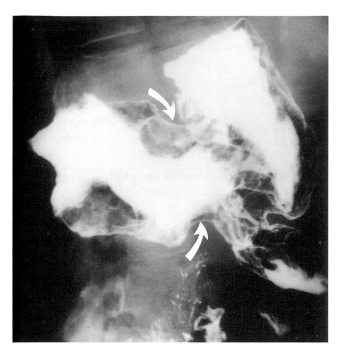

FIG. 20–1. Lateral spot film demonstrating posterior mass with large ulcer bed (arrows).

Pathologic examination of the specimen revealed a moderately well-differentiated adenocarcinoma invasive through the gastric wall (Fig. 20–3), with extension into the distal pancreas and splenic hilum. Three of 29 periesophageal and perigastric lymph nodes contained metastatic carcinoma. The esophageal and distal gastric margins were free of tumor. The patient had an unremarkable recovery. A barium swallow on the seventh postoperative day revealed a patent anastomosis without evidence of leakage.

The patient's case was discussed at the Multidisciplinary Tumor Board meeting. Postoperative chemotherapy with a platinum-based regimen was recommended, but the patient decided not to have any adjuvant therapy. She was followed up without additional therapy and did reasonably well until she was admitted with a left axillary mass 6 months later. This approximately 1.5-cm. rounded mass in the left posterior axilla was totally excised under local anesthesia and proved to be metastatic moderately differentiated adenocarcinoma consistent with the gastric primary. Three months later, she presented with a mass in the soft tissue of the right chest wall. This was again excised under local anesthesia and proved to be metastatic adenocarcinoma with similar histologic structure. At this point, she was complaining of severe epigastric pain, and a CAT scan was performed. This revealed nothing suggestive for recurrence within the abdomen. Upper endoscopy had to be performed again, and it showed just some mild gastritis with no signs of recurrent tumor. Because of unremitting pain, refractory to increasing nar-

cotics, she underwent a percutaneous celiac ganglion block, and also had an epidural catheter placed for pain control. None of these methods of pain control proved to be successful. Therefore, because of unremitting crampy abdominal pain suggestive of small bowel obstruction, she was examined 14 months after the intestinal operation. She was found to have metastatic gastric cancer to the proximal jejunum with dilation of the proximal bowel to 2 to 3 times normal. A resection of this obstructing segment was preformed with an end-to-end anastomosis. The patient's pain syndrome improved markedly postoperatively. Again, she was offered chemotherapy, but she decided against it. Six months later, she underwent excision of metastases from her right and left chest walls and left axilla under local anesthesia. Her condition gradually deteriorated, and she was placed in a nursing home. After diagnosis, she died of progressive disease in 27 months. There was no autopsy.

COMMENTARY by Murray F. Brennan

The case is well described. The decision to make a thoracoabdominal incision in a 72-year-old woman with weight loss (a known poor prognostic factor [1]) and a cardiac lesion might have been avoided. The patient, at the time of operation, was technically incurable, with a T4 lesion invading into the pancreas; one might have considered a more remote node biopsy confirming N2 disease and a more limited procedure (2). The extent of the node dissection is not described.

Postoperative chemotherapy was advised, but the patient declined and developed, as would be expected,

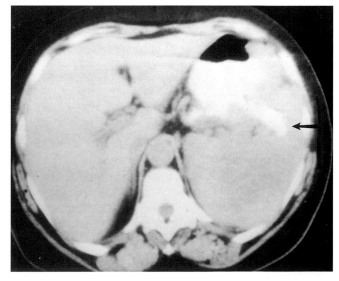

FIG. 20–2. Computed tomographic scan demonstrates large ulcerating gastric cancer with mass invading the spleen (arrow).

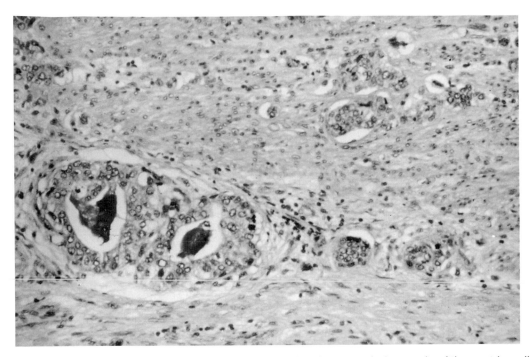

FIG. 20–3. Infiltrating gastric adenocarcinoma penetrating the muscularis propria of the gastric wall.

systemic metastasis within 6 months. Within 2 years the patient died of progression of disease.

This case raises some important issues:

The patient was incurable by any surgical procedure at the time of operation, and there are no data to support improved survival by extended dissection and resection of adjacent organs for T4 lesions. No evidence exists to suggest that more extensive operations are better palliation. Although extended surgical operations for advanced gastric cancer may relieve symptoms, they have not resulted in improved long-term survival.

The patient was offered postoperative chemotherapy, but no evidence exists that adjuvant chemotherapy for advanced gastric cancer has improved outcome and should be considered investigational.

Overall, the case illustrates the need for different approaches for advanced gastric cancer. Although surgery remains the primary modality, few if any patients with advanced gastric cancer are cured by operation. Adjuvant chemotherapy for "curative" resections has not improved survival (3). Current studies that explore the use of preoperative chemotherapy based on endoscopic ultrasound evaluation of T-stage are one alternative (4, 5).

REFERENCES

1. Fein R, Kelsen DP, Geller N, et al. Adenocarcinoma of the esophagus and gastroesophageal junction: prognostic factors and results of therapy. *Cancer* 1985;56:2512–8.
2. Smith JW, Shiu MH, Kelsey L, Brennan MF. Morbidity of radical lymphadenectomy in the curative resection of gastric carcinoma. *Arch Surg* 1991;126:1469–73.
3. Hermans J, Bonenkamp JJ, Boon MC, et al. Adjuvant therapy after curative resection for gastric cancer: meta-analysis of randomized trials. *J Clin Oncol* 1993;11:1441–7.
4. Lightdale CJ, Botet JF, Kelsen DP, et al. Diagnosis of recurrent upper gastrointestinal cancer at the surgical anastomosis by endoscopic ultrasound. *Gastrointest Endosc* 1989;35:407–12.
5. Botet JF, Lightdale CJ, Zauber AG, et al. Preoperative staging of gastric cancer: Comparison of endoscopic US and dynamic CT. *Radiology* 1991;181:426–32.

21

Carcinoma of the Stomach, Linitis Plastica Type

Gaylord T. Walker

The dilemma of local and regional control

CASE PRESENTATION

A 48-year-old black woman was referred to the gastroenterology service in April, 1991, with a 9-month history of nonspecific abdominal pain and early satiety associated with significant weight loss. The pain was aggravated by hunger and alleviated by eating. She could not quantify her weight loss but noted that her clothing sizes had changed. She denied change of bowel habits and blood in her stool. She had had no abdominal surgery. She had a 4-year history of diabetes treated with oral hypoglycemics and a 7-year history of hypertension. Medications included glipizide (Glucotrol) 5 mg qAM, hydrochlorothiazide 50 mg bid, propranolol 40 mg bid, and hydralazine 50 mg qAM. She denied alcohol use and smoked a half pack of cigarettes daily. Family history was remarkable only a grandfather who died of colon cancer.

The patient was 5′ 9″ tall and weighed 55 kg. Her blood pressure was 120/70 and her other vital signs were normal. Physical examination was remarkable for stigmata of moderate weight loss. All nodal basins were negative. The abdomen had a vague epigastric fullness but no distinct mass. Pelvic and rectal examinations were normal, and the stool was negative for occult blood.

Upper gastrointestinal endoscopy on April 17, 1991 revealed a submucosal mass effect extending from antrum proximally into the body of the stomach, predominantly along the lesser curvature. The antrum appeared rigid and the mucosa endoscopically appeared intact (Fig. 21–1). Endoscopic biopsies demonstrated chronic gastritis with some atypia. She underwent repeat endoscopy 1 week later. Repeat biopsies demonstrated infiltrating poorly differentiated adenocarcinoma.

She was mildly anemic with a Hgb of 9.5 g and a Hct of 29% with normal indices. Serum chemistries were normal. The remainder of her clinical evaluation included a chest film and electrocardiogram, which were normal.

This patient was initially presented to the Tumor Board on April 25, 1991, at which time she was clinically staged as a T3 NX M0, poorly differentiated diffuse adenocarcinoma of the stomach. Consensus opinion was to proceed directly to surgical exploration.

She underwent surgical exploration on April 26, 1991, after mechanical bowel preparation. Examination under general anesthesia revealed an ill-defined mass in the upper abdomen. At exploration there was a firm diffuse neoplasm in the antrum that extended through the posterior wall of the stomach along the greater curvature and invaded the distal tip of the pancreas. Gross surgical findings were consistent with the clinical diagnosis of gastric carcinoma of the linitis plastica type. There were several firm lymph nodes suspicious for metastatic disease along the greater curvature and in the splenic hilum. There was no evidence of hepatic or peritoneal metastases. A radical total gastrectomy with distal pancreatectomy and splenectomy was performed. Alimentary continuity was re-established with a stapled anastomosis to a retrocolic Roux-en-Y esophagojejunostomy. Oophorectomy and feeding jejunostomy completed the surgical procedure. Operative time was 4 hours, blood loss was 400 mL, two units of red cells were transfused.

104

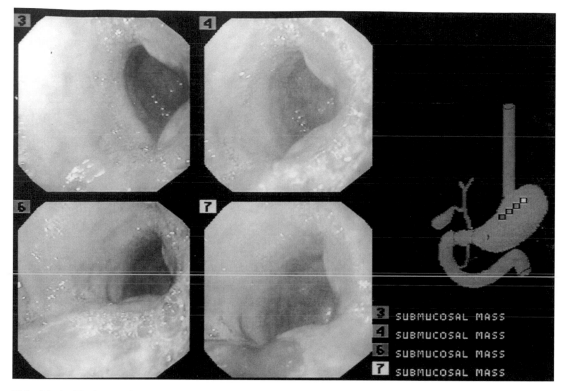

FIG. 21–1. Endoscopic appearance of the distal stomach showing the neoplasm in the foreground and the pylorus in the background. The posterior wall of the stomach is rigid, with a submucosal mass effect.

Pathologic examination of the specimen revealed a diffuse neoplasm invading through the serosa of the stomach. Microscopically, this was a poorly differentiated adenocarcinoma with extensive perivascular invasion and local invasion of the pancreas at the splenic hilum. Eighteen of 38 lymph nodes were positive for metastatic carcinoma (Figs. 21–2, 21–3, and 21–4). All surgical margins were microscopically free of disease. Pathologically, this was staged as a T4 N2 M0 stage IIIB carcinoma of the stomach.

The patient had a relatively unremarkable convalescence. Her recovery was complicated by atelectasis on the second postoperative day and delirium on the seventh postoperative day; both responded promptly to conservative management. She was again presented at Tumor Board on May 9, 1991. The medical oncology service noted that she would be a candidate for the upcoming SWOG 9008 protocol. This randomized prospective study of surgery alone versus surgery with adjuvant chemotherapy (5-FU and Leucovorin) and radiotherapy was not activated until August 1, 1991. Off protocol, no adjuvant therapy was recommended. She was discharged on May 19, 1991.

The patient did well for 4 months, at which time she presented with increased difficulty swallowing. Upper gastrointestinal endoscopy was performed and was unremarkable except for the expected postoperative findings.

An upper gastrointestinal series with a small volume of barium was performed on August 13, 1992. This study demonstrated a widely patent esophagojejunal anastomosis (Fig. 21–5) and high-grade partial obstruction of the proximal small bowel. Surgical re-exploration was recommended, but the patient initially refused. She was treated with nasogastric decompression and intravenous fluids with little improvement. After several days of nonoperative therapy, the patient consented to surgery and underwent re-exploration on August 16, 1991. The operative findings included extremely dense adhesions to the anterior abdominal wall and of all viscera. Three enterotomies were made during the tedious dissection. Many of the adhesions had a fibronodular character suspicious of recurrent tumor; however, all frozen sections were reported negative for malignancy. Complete exploration of the small bowel was judged imprudent because of the extremely difficult nature of the dissection. A dilated segment of proximal jejunum, confirmed endoscopically, was anastomosed to a loop of collapsed intestine, and all enterotomies were carefully closed. She did well for 8 days but then developed evidence of progressive intra-abdominal sepsis. She was emergently re-explored on August 24, 1991, and found to be leaking from one of the enterotomy closures. As all three enterotomies were in a relatively short length of intestine, this segment was resected and a stapled anastomosis performed. The

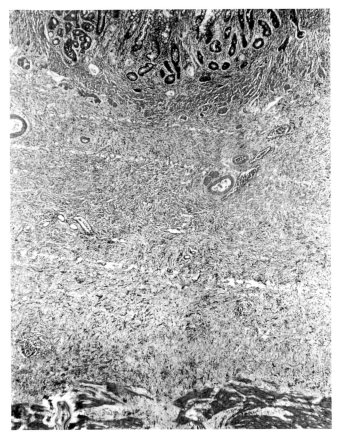

FIG. 21–2. Photomicrograph demonstrating thickening of the gastric wall with inconspicuous infiltrating neoplastic cells grouped in small cords. The muscularis propria is apparent at the bottom of the micrograph.

patient was again presented to Tumor Conference on August 29, 1991. Interestingly, recurrent carcinoma could not be identified on any of the material submitted from these two operations, even in retrospect.

Total parenteral nutrition and broad-spectrum antibiotics were administered. On September 3, 1991, the tenth postoperative day, she developed a high output enterocutaneous fistula. On September 12, 1991, the patient was entered on an investigational protocol of somatostatin analog for treatment of enteric and pancreatic fistula. The fistula output decreased immediately and dramatically to 300 mL daily and diminished further to less than 30 mL daily over the next 10 days. An upper gastrointestinal series on September 24, 1991 showed no evidence of enterocutaneous fistula and transit of contrast into the colon. The patient slowly improved and was discharged on October 8, 1991, after 56 days in hospital.

She did well for approximately 7 months before developing, on May 6, 1992, a spontaneous enterocutaneous fistula to the upper aspect of the midline incision. Biopsies of the wound demonstrated infiltrating adenocarcinoma. The patient was again presented at Tumor Confer-

ence on May 7, 1992. Medical oncology service offered the opinion that chemotherapy would have a low response rate and would be relatively contraindicated in the presence of an enterocutaneous fistula. The consensus opinion was that supportive care only was indicated unless a palliative operation was required. An upper gastrointestinal series on May 8, 1992, demonstrated a widely patent anastomosis but no progression of contrast beyond dilated proximal small intestine. Endoscopy on May 11, 1992, was unchanged from previous studies. On May 14, 1992, the patient underwent surgical exploration to close the enterocutaneous fistula and relieve her small bowel obstruction. This procedure was abandoned because the attempt to enter her free abdominal cavity was unsuccessful because of the presence of massive peritoneal carcinomatosis. The patient was discharged on May 18, 1992, for terminal care at home with intravenous fluids and narcotics. She expired on June 1, 1992. Permission for autopsy was not granted.

COMMENTARY by Harold J. Wanebo

The initial diagnosis of early gastric cancer and linitis plastica is problematic, especially in the United States and other Western countries. Although the early recognition of a stomach lesion may be demonstrated by a barium study,

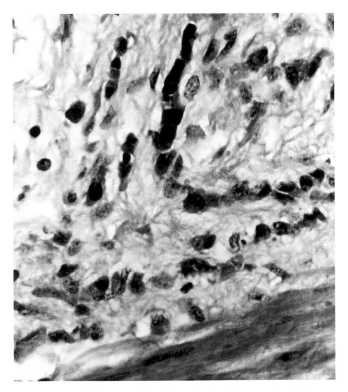

FIG. 21–3. High magnification photomicrograph of tumor cells infiltrating the muscularis propria of the stomach.

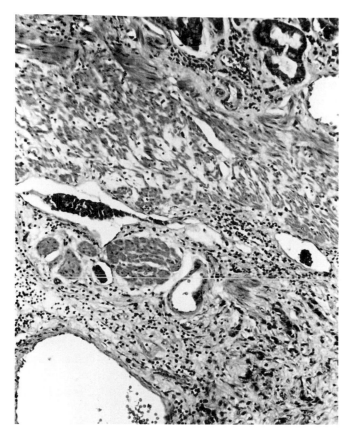

FIG. 21–4. Photomicrograph demonstrating extensive infiltration of the submucosa of the stomach by tumor cells and tumor emboli within lymphatics.

frequently the follow-up endoscopy fails to confirm the presence of a carcinoma. This case epitomizes this problem. The initial biopsies demonstrated a chronic gastritis with some atypia. Fortunately, the gastroenterologist did not accept this as the answer and performed more biopsies that subsequently were shown to confirm an infiltrating adenocarcinoma. This emphasizes the need to aggressively biopsy and rebiopsy gastric lesions to avoid missing a carcinoma. In the event the follow-up biopsy was negative, it would have been prudent to have treated this patient for the gastritis or possible ulcer disease for a defined period of time, that is, 4 to 6 weeks, and then to re-endoscope and rebiopsy. This patient was clinically staged as a T3 NX M0, poorly differentiated diffuse adenocarcinoma of the stomach. The Tumor Board decision was to proceed with resection. This is certainly logical even if it means performing a palliative resection if disease extends beyond the primary site. In this patient, the gross surgical findings were consistent with the clinical impression of linitis plastica and there were also several enlarged suspicious nodes along the greater curative and in the splenic hilum, although the liver and the rest of the peritoneal cavity appeared clear. One consideration before undertaking this exploration in a very high-risk patient might have been the

possibility of doing a laparoscopic staging and then considering preoperative therapy if the disease is locally extensive. With the laparoscope, one can certainly assess the peritoneal cavity, the liver, and the celiac axis nodes and have a reasonable visualization of the gastroesophageal junction nodes and gain an impression of the extent of tumor in the stomach. The presence of locally extensive disease or metastatic disease involving the nodes might prompt consideration of giving aggressive chemotherapy or combining radiation with chemotherapy before surgery for locally advanced disease.

At the time of the exploration, a radical total gastrectomy with distal pancreatectomy and splenectomy were performed. The question of removing the spleen should be addressed. It would be ideal if the resection could be carried out with preservation of the spleen because it would reduce the potential increased risk for infection with encapsulated organisms. The addition of splenectomy electively does not add to the curative potential of the resection (1). However, if the distal pancreas is resected along with the splenic artery and the short gastric vessels, it is unlikely the spleen will survive, and one is compelled to resect it. The importance of obtaining a satisfactory anastomosis should be noted. If a curative resection is done, one should attempt to achieve a clear or

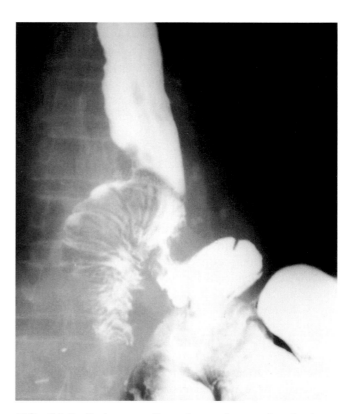

FIG. 21–5. Barium swallow 4 months postgastrectomy demonstrating a widely patent anastomosis and rapid transit of contrast into dilated proximal small bowel.

tumor-free margin. If the gastroesophageal junction is involved, this may require either a left or right thoracotomy. Obviously, in a patient in whom a palliative resection is being considered, this would not be necessary and one can do the resection through the hiatus.

The removal of the ovaries in those patients who are very high risk for metastases to the ovary (Kruckenberg tumor) is certainly of value, because the metastases to these organs are symptomatic and can manifest similar findings to primary ovarian cancer with metastases into the peritoneal cavity. The formation of a feeding jejunostomy tube is essential in these patients to ensure adequate postoperative nutritional support. The operative time was a respectable 4 hours and the blood loss was a very respectable 400 cc. The one area that was not addressed in the presentation is the type of node dissection performed. In general, an R2 dissection is recommended by Japanese and many Western authors, in which the second echelon of nodes that drain into the stomach are removed. This usually includes gastric bed nodes: perigastric nodes and removal of the lymph nodes along the left gastric artery to celiac axis and along the hepatic arteries to the hilum of the liver (N2 nodes) (1–4). There is controversy about this recommendation. The randomized Capetown trial showed no benefit of R2 versus R1 gastrectomy (although the patient numbers in this trial were very small) (5). Because this is a high-risk patient, no matter what operation was done, one need not equivocate about the need to perform an R2 or even an R3 node dissection. Operative design here was determined by the presence of bulk nodal metastases along the lesser curvature and in the splenic hilum. Although "radical gastrectomy" was used (perhaps because of the removal of the distal pancreas and the total stomach), this term is ill-defined and usually reserved to describe the extent of resection regarding the nodal structures, not the removal of contiguous organs. Although an extended resection with removal of associated organs may be needed to achieve local control, any effect on distant disease or survival is speculative (2).

Although all surgical margins were microscopically free of disease (which is the major element in ensuring local control), the extensive nodal metastases described and the poorly differentiated morphology make it unlikely that long-term control will be achieved. The patient was considered for the adjuvant protocol of the Intergroup Study, which consists of adjuvant chemotherapy 5-fluorouracil (5-FU) and leucovorin plus radiation therapy, but this protocol was unavailable at the time and there was no in-house protocol for adjuvant therapy. Considering that this patient had a stage IV (T4 N2 M0) cancer with an estimated survival in the 3% to 4% range (6), she would have merited a protocol comparable to the treatment arm of the Intergroup SWOG study. However, treatment off-study, despite the compelling individual situation, is not rational because no adjuvant therapy, even for patients as high-risk as this, has ever been shown to be of benefit.

This patient's course was predictable. In 4 months, she had difficulty in swallowing, but there was nothing demonstrated by upper gastrointestinal endoscopy; small bowel series showed a patent anastomosis but a high-grade partial obstruction of the proximal small bowel. When this patient was finally explored, there were the expected dense adhesions, many of which had a fibronodular character suspicious for recurrence, but were reported as negative. The numerous enterotomies involved attests to the difficulties of this re-exploration and the surgeons were fortunately able to do a decompressing jejunal bypass. Despite the negative biopsies for tumor, the presentation remains highly suspicious for carcinoma. Seven months later, the woman did return with the redevelopment of fistula, and biopsies at that time finally confirmed infiltrating adenocarcinoma.

This case presents the expected findings and outcome for this type of high-risk gastric cancer. In patients with stage III and IV disease, the median survival is 13 months in resected patients (7). The question of whether a more extended lymphadenectomy would be of value is unanswered. Although there is no proof from Western trial data (5), the data from Japan suggests that there is improved survival overall in patients with the R2 and possibly R3 dissection. Several Japanese studies suggest that removing the nodes that are one echelon beyond the level of the most distal metastases, that is, the extragastric nodes (N2 nodes), if the Level I perigastric nodes are involved, is of benefit especially if the N2 nodes are negative. The question of whether removal of the next echelon of nodes (an N3 node dissection) is of benefit is a matter of controversy, and there is no randomized data to support such an approach. However, many Japanese series have reported a survival rate of as high of 39% in patients with metastases to regional nodes (8).

In a retrospective study of 367 patients with gastric cancer with invasion of the gastric serosa, reviewed by Kaibara, there was no survival difference in the patients having dissection of the nodes at levels 1, 2, and 3 (50%) versus 1 and 2 (49.4%). Among their patients, 19 of 160 patients had metastases to Group 3 nodes and, of these, only 5 survived (about 25%). In three of the patients the nodes were in the hepatoduodenal ligament (4). They recommended that in patients with advanced gastric cancer who had serosal invasion and nodal metastases, a Level I and 2 node dissection should be performed along with dissection of nodes in the hepatoduodenal ligament. In this particular patient, my preference would be to do a full R2 node dissection (including the hepatoduodenal nodes and periesophageal nodes at the level of the diaphragm) and perhaps to sample the nodes at the root of the mesentery and at the level of the diaphragm, and to mark the high risk sites with clips. I would have added the radiation and the chemotherapy as described in the Intergroup/SWOG protocol.

REFERENCES

1. Douglass HO Jr. Potentially curable cancer of the stomach. *Cancer* 1982;50:2582–9.
2. Maruyama K, Okabayashi K, Kinoshita T. Progress in gastric surgery in Japan and its limits of radicality. *World J Surg* 1987;11:418–25.
3. Kodama Y, Sugimachi K, Soejima K, et al. Evaluation of extensive lymph node dissection for carcinoma of the stomach. *World J Surg* 1981;5:241–8.
4. Kaibara N, Sumi K, Yonekawa M, et al. Does extensive dissection of lymph nodes improve the results of surgical treatment of gastric cancer. *Am J Surg* 1990;159:218–21.
5. Dent DM, Madden MV, Price SK. Randomized comparison of R1 and R2 gastrectomy for gastric carcinoma. *Br J Surg* 1988;75:110–2.
6. Wanebo HJ, et al. Cancer of the stomach: patient care study by the American College of Surgeons. *Ann Surg* 1993;218:583–92.
7. Stern JL, Denman S, Elias EG, et al. Evaluation of palliative resection in advanced carcinoma of the stomach. *Surgery* 1975;77:291–8.
8. Maehira Y, Okuyama T, Moriguchi S, et al. Prophylactic lymph node dissection in patients with advanced gastric cancer promotes increased survival time. *Cancer* 1992;70:392–5.

22 Gastric Lymphoma

Martin S. Karpeh, Jr.

Surgery, if and when!

CASE PRESENTATION

M.G. is a 33-year-old man who, in August 1990, presented to his local doctor with complaints of intermittent epigastric pain over the prior 6 months. He reported occasional nausea that was exacerbated by cigarette smoking. The patient also reported a 20-pound weight loss as well as anorexia, malaise, and easy fatigability since the onset of his epigastric pain. He denied any fevers, chills, or night sweats and he also denied any history of hematemesis or melena.

His symptoms prompted an evaluation by a gastroenterologist, who ordered an upper gastrointestinal series, which demonstrated an infiltrative process in the gastric antrum (Fig. 22–1). This was followed up by an upper endoscopy, which revealed a 6-cm ulcer on the posterior wall of the gastric antrum. The lesion was biopsied and proved to be a large cell lymphoma. His staging work-up consisted of a chest X-ray, which was normal, and a computed tomography (CT) scan of the chest, abdomen, and pelvis, which showed marked thickening of the gastric antrum with questionable extension into the pancreatic head (Fig. 22–2). There was also a question of anterior mediastinal adenopathy on chest CT. Subsequent gallium scan and bone scan were both negative. Past medical history is significant for congenital hypertrophic pyloric stenosis treated surgically. He reported that he took Zantac for stomach pain. He reported no allergies.

The patient is employed as an electrician. He is married with no children. He admits to a 20-pack per year smoking history and moderate alcohol intake. His family history is negative for cancer.

On physical examination, his temperature was 36.4°C with a blood pressure of 120/80, pulse 68, respiration 20, weight 60 kg. His otoloaryngologic exam was normal. The neck was supple with no evidence of adenopathy and no masses. His chest exam showed clear lungs with equal breath sounds. Cardiac exam revealed a regular rate and rhythm with no murmurs or gallops. On examination of the abdomen, he was noted to have a flat abdomen with a well healed transverse right upper quadrant incision. He had normal bowel sounds with no tenderness, no masses, and no organomegaly. His genitalia were normal, with two descended testicles and no masses. On rectal exam he had normal tone with no masses and stool that was guaiac negative. The extremities showed no evidence of cyanosis, clubbing, or edema. He had no evidence of adenopathy. His neurologic exam was grossly intact.

His initial blood work showed a hematocrit of 38.2 with a white blood count of 9.5. His lactic dehydrogenase (LDH) level was 166 with normal liver function studies. Bilateral bone marrow biopsies demonstrated normal marrow.

The patient has a diffuse large cell lymphoma, which is the most common histopathology seen in lymphomas of the stomach. Given the locally advanced disease at presentation, he was staged as a II$_E$B by the Ann Arbor classification. These lymphomas are of intermediate grade by the Working Formulation and can behave in an aggressive manner with median survival measured in months. The 20-pound weight loss reported by this patient is a poor prognostic feature, which by the National Cancer Institute's staging scheme would make him a stage III lymphoma.

The treatment of choice for advanced stage aggressive lymphomas is combination chemotherapy with radiation or surgery reserved for poor responders. However, lymphomas of the stomach treated with chemotherapy carry the unique associated risk of bleeding or perforation.

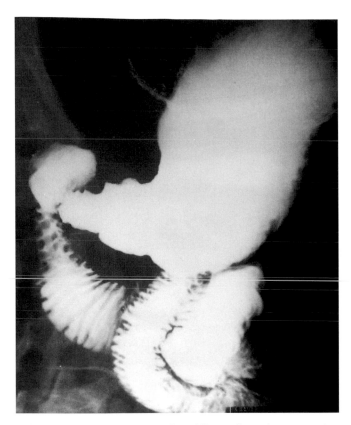

FIG. 22–1. Prone right anterior oblique view, demonstrating the patient's barium-filled stomach, which abruptly narrows at the gastric antrum. The mucosal outline of the antrum is irregular and did not distend on multiple views during the study.

These complications are often fatal in this group of patients. Discussions regarding the treatment of this patient centered on the risk/benefit ratio of primary chemotherapy, preserving the stomach and avoiding the potential morbidity of gastrectomy versus resecting the stomach to avoid the potential of a gastric perforation in an immunocompromised patient. Because of the young age of the patient and the presence of the gastric ulcer, the decision was made to resect the involved stomach, recognizing the need for subsequent systemic treatment.

The patient was admitted to the hospital on April 9, 1990, and operated on the next day. Operative findings showed significant enlargement of both the left gastric, portal, and hepatic arterial nodes, which were considered surgically unresectable. In addition, he had a number of firm enlarged nodes in the mesentery but no other significant periaortic or iliac adenopathy. The liver and spleen both appeared normal. The remainder of the small bowel and colon were normal. The appendix was essentially normal, although in its midportion it felt quite firm. The exact nature of this was unclear. He underwent a distal subtotal gastrectomy with biopsy of portal and mesenteric lymph nodes as well as of the liver. He also underwent an incidental appendectomy. His gastrectomy removed approxi-

mately 40% of the distal stomach and he was reconstructed with an antecolic isoperistaltic gastrojejunostomy.

The final pathology showed malignant lymphoma diffuse large cell type with transmural involvement. Ten regional nodes were positive for lymphoma (Fig. 22–3). All the margins were negative. Malignant lymphoma was present in three portal lymph nodes. The mesenteric lymph node, appendix, periappendiceal lymph nodes, and liver biopsy were also negative for lymphoma. Immunohistochemical stains were positive for LCA and L-26, consistent with a B-cell origin.

He was started on ProMACE-CytaBOM chemotherapy. The treatment period was 6 months and ended in October 1990, at which time all residual evidence of disease had regressed. His follow-up consisted of regular visits at 4-month intervals. In September 1991, a palpable left axillary lymph node and left inguinal lymph node were found on physical exam. This was in association with a viral-type illness. His adenopathy resolved without treatment and he was felt to still be free of disease. In June 1992, he developed epigastric tenderness and early satiety. His work-up at that time included a CT scan (Fig. 22–4), upper gastrointestinal series, and upper endoscopy. An ulcer was located in the remaining stomach, which a biopsy later demonstrated to be recurrent diffuse large cell lymphoma.

In August 1992, the patient was started on CHOP chemotherapy. He was readmitted in September 1992 because of 8 days of vomiting and early satiety. An upper gastrointestinal barium swallow and endoscopy ruled out a mechanical obstruction. Over the subsequent 4 weeks he continued to exhibit progressive symptoms of gastric outlet obstruction. On October 18, 1992, he underwent an abdominal CT scan to evaluate his response to therapy.

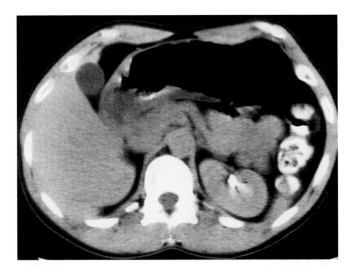

FIG. 22–2. Initial upper abdominal CT scan, demonstrating marked thickening of the gastric wall and a mass in the prepyloric region of the stomach.

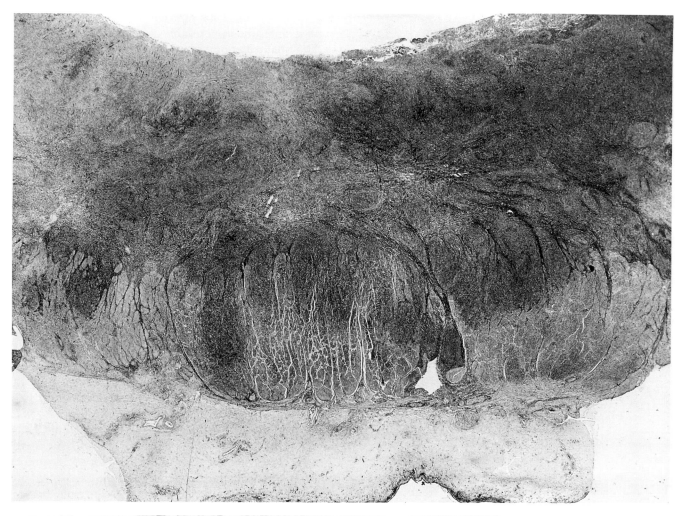

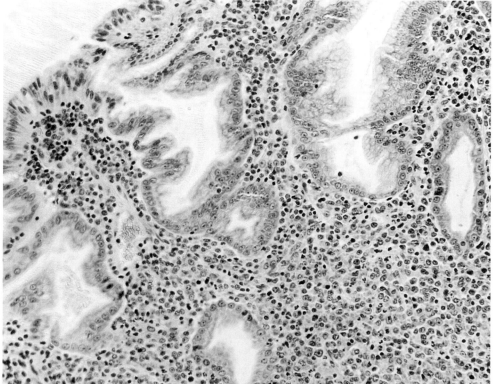

FIG. 22–3. A: Malignant lymphoma of the stomach, diffuse large cell type. The tumor involves the entire thickness of the gastric wall with mucosal ulceration. Massive nodal involvement accompanied this lesion (*low power*). **B:** Malignant lymphoma of the stomach. Note the large lymphocytes with prominent nucleoli (*high power.*)

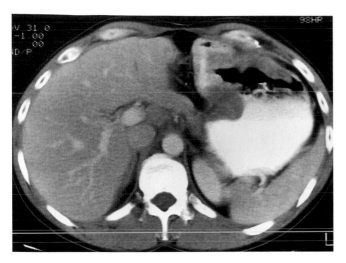

FIG. 22–4. Abdominal CT scan of the upper abdomen. Note the contrast-filled gastric remnant with significant thickening along the lesser curve.

This showed a questionable lesion in the left lobe of the liver (Fig. 22–5). An ultrasound confirmed the presence of a solid lesion. An upper endoscopy was repeated, which grossly appeared normal; however, biopsies later proved to be positive for lymphoma.

On November 5, 1992, he underwent re-exploration with resection of his gastrojejunostomy and reconstruc-

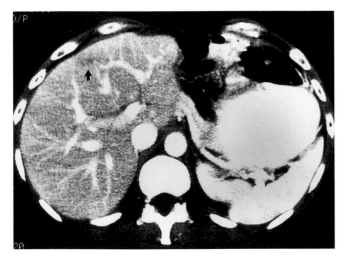

FIG. 22–5. Contrast-enhanced upper abdominal CT scan demonstrating resolution of the mural thickening of the stomach and a low attenuated lesion in the segment IV of the liver. (*Arrow* marks lesion.)

tion with a Billroth II type repair. The pathology demonstrated no residual lymphoma. The intraoperative biopsy of the liver showed benign liver tissue.

He is now being considered for bone marrow transplant protocol and was admitted February 19, 1993, to begin investigational chemotherapy.

COMMENTARY by Murray F. Brennan

This patient, with an extensive diffuse large cell lymphoma, presents the classic enigma of whether or not, in a patient with clinically advanced intra-abdominal lymphoma, surgical resection should be part of the initial therapy. This debate remains unresolved, although increasingly, surgical procedures are being reserved for those patients with apparently localized intra-abdominal disease.

The patient was operated on, on the assumption that the treatment with chemotherapy might result in perforation, obstruction, or bleeding. This controversy remains, but it is clear that many patients can be treated with primary radiation therapy and chemotherapy, reserving surgical procedures for the subsequent complications of the disease. Although perforation is the most feared complication in gastrointestinal lymphoma treated aggressively with chemotherapy, perforation is possible before chemotherapy, and therefore chemotherapy alone cannot be blamed as the sole precipitating factor.

The present case highlights the difficulties of determining whether or not to begin with a surgical procedure, given the presence of a positive diagnosis and extensive intra-abdominal disease. With significant antecedent weight loss and extensive noncontiguous intra-abdominal disease, the present patient might, in retrospect, have been treated initially with chemotherapy and radiation therapy as the primary modality, reserving operation for the complications of the disease.

SELECTED READINGS

1. Kemeny MM, Brennan MF. The surgical complications of chemotherapy in the cancer patient. *Curr Probl Surg* 1987;24:607–75.
2. Talamonti MS, Dawes LG, Joehl RJ, Nahrwold DL. Gastrointestinal lymphoma: a case for surgical resection. *Arch Surg* 1990;125:972–7.
3. Frazee RC, Roberts J. Gastric lymphoma treatment: medical versus surgical. *Surg Clin North Am* 1992;72:423–31.
4. Gobbi PG, Dionigi P, Barbieri F, Corbella F, et al. The role of surgery in the multimodal treatment of primary gastric non-Hodgkin's lymphomas. *Cancer* 1990;65:2528–36.

23

T3 N1 M0 Adenocarcinoma of the Antrum of the Stomach

Murray F. Brennan

Endoscopic ultrasound prompted investigational neoadjuvant therapy in this high cancer-risk patient

CASE PRESENTATION

A 44-year-old woman presented with epigastric pain. There is no other contributing information. Endoscopy and endoscopic ultrasound (Fig. 23–1) show an infiltrating T3 N1 lesion of the antrum. Computed tomography (CT) scan is negative for nodal or metastatic disease and confirms the antral enlargement (Fig. 23–2). She is referred for surgical opinion.

The patient received two cycles of preoperative FAMTX (5 fluorouracil, adriamycin [doxorubicam] methotrexate) over 2 months, without major morbidity. At operation she had an extensive local antral lesion adherent to the mesocolon and the pancreatic capsule. There were multiple enlarged matted nodes on the lesser curvature adjacent to the tumor. Biopsy of some peritoneal plaques, suspicious for tumor, were negative for tumor on frozen section. She underwent an extended distal gastrectomy with R2 nodal dissection and removal of the anterior leaf of the mesocolon and the pancreatic capsule. A peritoneal infusaport was placed for postoperative chemotherapy. The margins of resection were negative at frozen and permanent section.

In pathologic review she had a poorly differentiated ulcerated gastric adenocarcinoma extending through the gastric wall into perigastric adipose tissue (pT3). Nineteen lesser curvature nodes were negative for tumor and only 1 of 20 greater curvature nodes contained metastatic adenocarcinoma. The mesenteric plaques did not contain tumor.

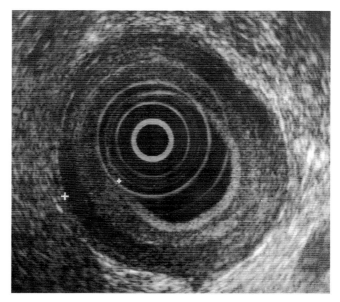

FIG. 23–1. An infiltrating T3 N1 lesion of the antrum is shown with endoscopic ultrasound.

She had an uneventful postoperative course and received her first course of intraperitoneal cisplatin and intravenous 5-fluorouracil before discharge. She had three courses of postoperative therapy over the ensuing 3 months and the port was removed. She is alive and well, without evidence of disease 15 months after operation.

114

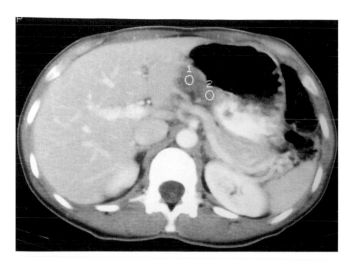

FIG. 23–2. CT scan confirms the antral enlargement.

TUMOR BOARD DISCUSSION

The standard approach to this problem would be gastric resection encompassing all tumor with intraoperative confirmation of negative margins, and the only debate would be the extent of the nodal dissection. However, with the advent of endoscopic ultrasound, where significant accuracy can be obtained as to the T stage of the lesion, consideration of preoperative protocols in high-risk patients can be obtained. The surgical procedure is designed to remove the local lesion completely. In our institution, the patient would get an R2 regional node dissection (1) (Fig. 23–3) based on the site of the lesion. We have previously shown (2) that the morbidity from regional node dissection is no greater than for more conservative operations for gastric cancer. Operative mortality for extended node dissection for distal antral lesions should be <2% (2). The benefit beyond accurate staging of the regional node dissection remains unproven. Current prospective randomized studies are underway to answer this question. If cytologic-positive disease is found at laparotomy, resection would be considered only as a palliative procedure.

In a prior study, we have shown that endoscopic ultrasound can accurately predict the T stage of a tumor; is less accurate in predicting N stage, and only of limited value in determining the presence of metastases (3). For both T and N stage, endoscopic ultrasound is superior to a CT scan (4). As N stage can be based only on inhomogeneity and size, accurate determination of pathologic involvement of nodes by endoscopic ultrasound is not possible. Nevertheless, it is known that increasing nodal size is accompanied by increasing frequency of metastasis (5). For example, in nodes <3 mm, the incidence of metastatic involvement for gastric cancer is 5.4%, and for nodes >2 cm, the incidence is 83%.

We have shown that patients with endoscopic T3 stage lesions, in the absence of any staging information, have a 75% chance of tumor recurrence within 2 years (6). For patients with T3 lesions, this is a justification to consider protocols in addition to surgical resection alone. Prior studies have shown that the regimen of FAMTX is superior in response and has decreased toxicity when compared with the EAP (etoposide, adriamycin [doxorubin] cisplatinum) regimen in advanced disease (7) and a prospective study of preoperative chemotherapy has been initiated, using FAMTX for all patients with T3 stage lesions or greater. This patient would be considered for an investigative preoperative chemotherapeutic regimen followed by a surgical resection.

In summary, this woman, with a poor prognostic gastric adenocarcinoma (undifferentiated bulky lesion) considered T3 by endoscopic ultrasound, underwent an investigational program of preoperative intravenous chemotherapy followed by postoperative intravenous and intraperitoneal chemotherapy. Such a protocol remains investigational and should be applied only to high-risk patients in an investigational setting. Morbidity of such a program is acceptable but can be accompanied by peritoneal "cocoon" formation, requiring reoperation.

REFERENCES

1. Smith J, Brennan MF. Surgical treatment of gastric cancer. Proximal, mid, and distal stomach. *Surg Clin North Am* 1992;72:381–99.
2. Smith JW, Shiu MH, Kelsey L, Brennan MF. Morbidity of radical lymphadenectomy in the curative resection of gastric carcinoma. *Arch Surg* 1991;126:1469–73.
3. Lightdale CJ, Botet JF, Kelsen DP, Turnbull AD, Brennan MF. Diagnosis of recurrent upper gastrointestinal cancer at the surgical anastomosis by endoscopic ultrasound. *Gastrointest Endosc* 1989;35:407–12.
4. Botet JF, Lightdale CJ, Zauber AG, Preoperative staging of gastric cancer: comparison of endoscopic US and dynamic CT. *Radiology* 1991;181:426–32.
5. Noguchi Y, Imada T, Matsumoto A, Coit DG, Brennan MF. Radical surgery for gastric cancer: a review of the Japanese experience. *Cancer* 1989;64:2053–62.
6. Smith JW, Brennan MF, Botet JF, Gerdes H, Lightdale CJ. Preoperative endoscopic ultrasound can predict the risk of recurrence after operation for gastric carcinoma. *J Clin Oncol* 1993;11:2380–85.
7. Kelsen D, Atiq OT, Saltz L, et al. FAMTX versus etoposide, doxorubicin, and cisplatin: a random assignment trial in gastric cancer. *J Clin Oncol* 1992;10:541–8.

COMMENTARY by David C. Hohn

The case presented by Dr. Brennan delineates most of the current issues concerning the management of locally advanced gastric cancer. The absence of benefit from postoperative adjuvant chemotherapy (1) provides the rationale for investigation of alternative chemotherapeutic treatment strategies.

Because of the cost and potential morbidity of aggressive treatment protocols and the poor prognosis, thorough

Gastric Lymphadenectomy

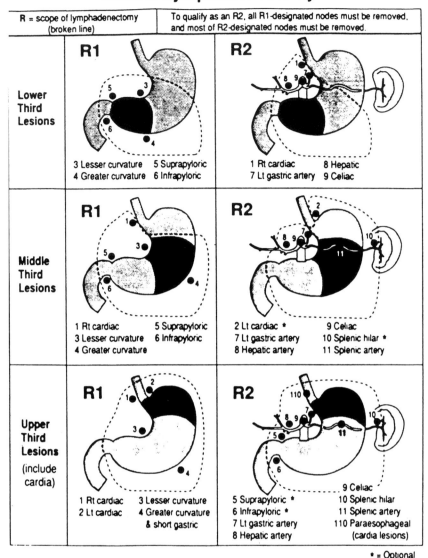

| R = scope of lymphadenectomy (broken line) | To qualify as an R2, all R1-designated nodes must be removed, and most of R2-designated nodes must be removed. |

Lower Third Lesions

R1
3 Lesser curvature   5 Suprapyloric
4 Greater curvature   6 Infrapyloric

R2
1 Rt cardiac   8 Hepatic
7 Lt gastric artery   9 Celiac

Middle Third Lesions

R1
1 Rt cardiac   5 Suprapyloric
3 Lesser curvature   6 Infrapyloric
4 Greater curvature

R2
2 Lt cardiac *   9 Celiac
7 Lt gastric artery   10 Splenic hilar *
8 Hepatic artery   11 Splenic artery

Upper Third Lesions (include cardia)

R1
1 Rt cardiac   3 Lesser curvature
2 Lt cardiac   4 Greater curvature
& short gastric

R2
5 Suprapyloric *   9 Celiac
6 Infrapyloric *   10 Splenic hilar
7 Lt gastric artery   11 Splenic artery
8 Hepatic artery   110 Paraesophageal
(cardia lesions)

* = Optional

FIG. 23–3. Extents of R1 and R2 lymph node dissections for proximal, mid, and distal gastric lesions. (From Smith et al., *Arch Surg* 1991;126:1469–73. Copyright © 1991, American Medical Association.)

pretreatment staging is important. There is increasing consensus that endoscopic ultrasound provides accurate thickness staging of T2 and T3 gastric cancers and is superior to CT scanning in this regard. Tio and co-workers (2) reported a 5% to 8% error rate for pathologic T2 and T3 lesions, although 25% of T1 lesions were overstaged and 40% of T4 lesions were understaged. We concur that endoscopic ultrasound does not accurately predict nodal involvement. Thus, the only currently justifiable reason to use endoscopic ultrasound is for selection of cases for investigational neoadjuvant chemotherapy trials. Patients being considered for an initial surgical approach are adequately evaluated with conventional endoscopy and an abdominal CT scan to screen for metastatic disease that might preclude laparotomy.

The role of peritoneal laparoscopy and cytology also deserve comment. We are not aware of studies that definitively show that cytologic positivity is independently predictive of a poor prognosis in the absence of other evidence of carcinomatosis. We have included routine preoperative laparoscopy with cytologic washing as a part of our initial evaluation for gastric neoadjuvant trials and have encountered patients with positive cytologies in the absence of gross intraperitoneal disease. A few of these patients have been treated with neoadjuvant chemotherapy and gastric resection and have achieved disease-free survival of 2 or more years. Although a positive peritoneal cytology found after neoadjuvant treatment may well predict poor prognosis, one might question whether the tumor cells are viable and whether postoperative chemotherapy (particularly intraperitoneal chemotherapy) might not still be effective in controlling peritoneal implantation and growth. We believe that the cost and morbidity of combined modality approaches, such as those used in this case, warrant use of laparoscopy for staging before institution of chemotherapy. We currently administer up to five courses of neoadjuvant chemotherapy, so we routinely place a jejunal feeding tube during the initial laparoscopy and administer jejunal feedings for the duration of treatment. Responding patients frequently demonstrate improved appetite and may not require tube feedings.

We concur fully with Dr. Brennan's comments regarding the use of regional (R2) node dissection for gastric cancer and await the results of the European randomized trial of regional node dissection.

Although T3 lesions have a high likelihood of intraperitoneal failure, prolonged intraperitoneal chemotherapy administered via an injection port must be questioned. Intraperitoneal catheters quickly become walled off by adhesions after they are placed, resulting in the "cocoon" formation to which Dr. Brennan alludes. As a result, uniform intraperitoneal drug distribution may be achievable only for a few days after catheter placement.

Intraperitoneal hyperthermic chemotherapy administered at the time of surgery has been employed by Koga (3) and by Fujimoto (4) with a reported 47% 2-year survival in patients with peritoneal metastases. This approach is currently being investigated at M.D. Anderson Cancer Center by Mansfield and associates.

The poor results achieved with surgery alone and surgery plus adjuvant chemotherapy in patients with T3 gastric cancers justify trials combining neoadjuvant chemotherapy, surgery, and postoperative intraperitoneal chemotherapy. Because of cost, complexity, morbidity, and uncertain benefit, these approaches should be considered investigational.

REFERENCES

1. Hermans J, Bonenkamp JJ, Boon MC, et al. Adjuvant therapy after curative resection for gastric cancer: meta-analysis of randomized trials. *J Clin Oncol* 1993;11:1441–7.
2. Tio TL, Coene PPLO, den Hartog Jager FCA, Tytgat GNJ. Preoperative TNM classification of esophageal carcinoma by endosonography. *Hepato-gastroenterology* 1990;37:376–81.
3. Koga S, Hamazoe R, Maeta M, Shimizu N, Murakami A, Wakatsuki T. Prophylactic therapy for peritoneal recurrence of gastric cancer by continuous hyperthermic peritoneal perfusion with mitomycin C. *Cancer* 1988;61:232–7.
4. Fujimoto S, Shrestha RD, Kokubun M, et al. Positive results of combined therapy of surgery and intraperitoneal hyperthermic perfusion for far-advanced gastric cancer. *Ann Surg* 1990;212:592–6.

24

T4 N1 M0 Stage IIIB Gastric Cancer

Angelos A. Kambouris and Frank R.I. Lewis, Jr.

Is extended lymph node dissection beneficial to the patient?

CASE PRESENTATION

A 60-year-old white woman presented to the medical service because of vomiting small amounts blood over a 2- to 3-week period, associated with indigestion. She was known to have had peptic ulcer disease in the past but had no recent symptoms. Investigation 1 year previously for fecal occult blood included an upper gastrointestinal series that was negative, a barium enema that was negative, and a proctosigmoidoscopy that showed a small hyperplastic rectal polyp. The polyp was removed. Upper gastrointestinal radiographs at this time showed a large tumor mass in the antrum of the stomach compatible with carcinoma (Fig. 24–1). A gastroscopy was performed and showed a 7-cm tumor mass with irregular margins and ulcerated base occupying the antrum of the stomach (Fig. 24–2). A biopsy showed adenocarcinoma. Physical examination showed an obese white woman in no apparent distress and with no abnormal physical findings in the abdomen. Laboratory evaluation showed an Hgb level of 12.8 g/%, all liver function tests and electrolytes within normal limits, and a normal chest radiograph.

With a histologic diagnosis of adenocarcinoma of the stomach and no evidence of disseminated disease, the patient was advised to undergo surgical resection. At operation, she was found to have a large tumor mass in the distal part of the stomach with puckering of the tissue around the serosa of the lesser curvature and a small wad of omentum tucked onto that mass. Several enlarged lymph nodes were palpated. A radical subtotal gastrectomy was performed, encompassing 80% of the stomach, with the greater and lesser omentum in continuity, the supra-and subpyloric lymph nodes, and all the lymph nodes along the celiac axis and the lesser curva-

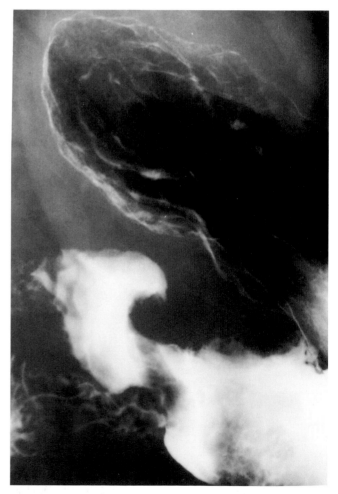

FIG. 24–1. Radiograph showing carcinoma of the gastric antrum.

118

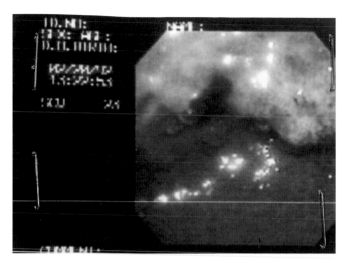

FIG. 24–2. Gastroscopic photograph of bleeding carcinoma.

ture up to the esophageal hiatus (R2 resection). A Billroth II reconstruction was performed. The margins of resection were clear on frozen section intraoperatively. The final histopathologic report showed a 12 × 9 cm ulcerated antral carcinoma penetrating through the serosa and involving the adjacent soft tissues, a 3 × 4 × 3.5 cm mass of matted lymph nodes, and 18 identifiable lymph nodes near the stomach as well as in omental and other locations. Two of the 10 lymph nodes adjacent to the tumor mass were found to contain metastases and all were within 3 cm of the tumor. Microscopic examination showed adenocarcinoma of the antrum, well to moderately differentiated, diffuse type with infiltrating borders, penetrating to the surrounding tissues (pT4 N1 M0), stage IIIB. The margins of resection were clear (Fig. 24–3).

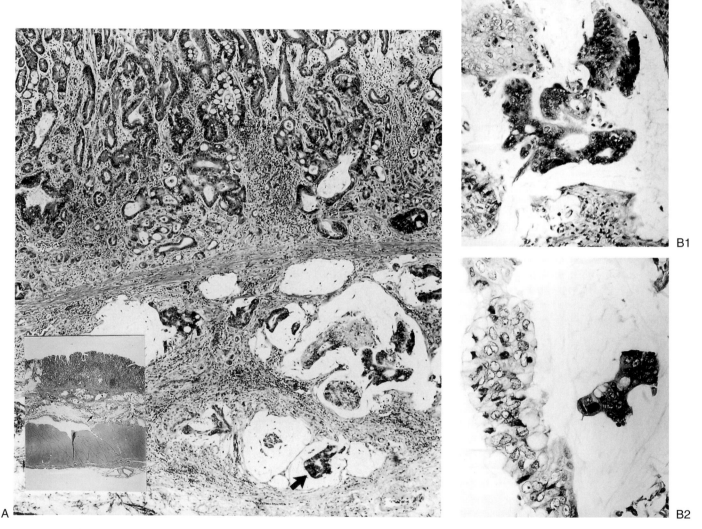

FIG. 24–3. A: Magnification showing infiltrating mucinous gastric carcinoma involving mucosa and submucosa (*arrow*). (Magnification ×10.) Insert: Full thickness of gastric wall with carcinoma (*arrow*). (Magnification ×2.5). **B:** Adenocarcinoma cells in mucin. (Magnification ×100 [B1] and ×200 [B2].)

After an uneventful recovery, the patient was discharged on the eighth postoperative day. Consultations were then obtained with medical and radiation oncologists. The medical oncologist assessed the postoperative status of the patient as being performance status 0-1. The findings of her gastric cancer were reviewed and the risk of recurrence was explained. The patient and family were informed of the "absence of proven efficacy for adjuvant chemotherapy, of the availability of National Clinical Trials of observation versus combined adjuvant radiation and chemotherapy, and of the risks associated with the adjuvant treatment." The radiation oncologist reviewed the information and discussed with the patient and family the risks of local regional recurrence and offered the choice of participating in a National Clinical Trial or proceeding with combined radiation therapy and chemotherapy, which is the accepted "standard" treatment among most radiation oncologists around the country. The patient opted for chemoradiation therapy. She received 4,500 cGy at 180 cGy per fraction, in conjunction with chemotherapy (5-fluorouracil) 500 mg/m^2 bolus on days 1 to 3 of week 1 and 4 while on radiotherapy, and 500 mg/m^2 intravenous bolus on days 1 to 5 every month for six cycles. Clinical and laboratory evaluations at the completion of chemotherapy showed no metastasis; a computed tomogram (CT) of the abdomen was negative and the carcinoembryonic antigen (CEA) level was 3.8. The patient tolerated the treatment with minimal discomfort, lost approximately 12 pounds, and had anemia with hemoglobin levels between 9 and 10 g/%. Six months after completion of adjuvant therapy, endoscopy showed mild gastritis; a biopsy was negative for recurrence. The CEA level remained at 3.9. All liver function tests were normal. She is currently 52 months postoperation and 46 months postcompletion of adjuvant therapy, has gained 40 pounds, and works full-time with no symptoms. Her current follow-up program is at 3-month intervals for physical examination, CEA, and basic biochemical tests, annual chest radiographs, and annual upper endoscopy.

COMMENTARY by Glenn D. Steele, Jr.

This case brings up several interesting points. First, the data from several Northern European trials looking at extent of gastric resection for advanced but resectable gastric adenocarcinomas and subsequent outcome are still in analysis. However, there is preliminary published work showing that there may be a significant increase in morbidity as the extent of resection increases without any near or long-term gain for the patient. In addition, the ability of the surgeon to do the precise node dissection as R1 versus R2 versus R3 nodes is questioned when the pathologic examination of the tissue block is analyzed. A small point, which is of recent note, concerns the fact that description of resections as "R" has now been changed by the Japanese as well as the European groups to "D," so that R1 versus R2 versus R3 is now referred to as D1 versus D2 versus D3.

At present, most resections in North America are designed to encompass a tumor, to describe adequately the regional node basins that are removed for accurate staging, and to obtain tissue clear of microscopic invasion for adequate anastomoses in both the proximal and distal resection margins.

A second major question that this presentation brings up is the legitimacy of any adjuvant therapy, whether it be pre- or postoperatively defined. Currently, with the single exception of an older gastrointestinal tumor study group, postoperative adjuvant chemotherapy trial, there have been no appropriately designed, prospective multi-institutional studies showing benefit to patients who are given postoperative adjuvant chemotherapy or chemoradiation therapy. Therefore, despite the statement that radiation oncologists consider postoperative radiation or chemoradiation standard therapy for patients at high risk for recurrence after gastric surgery, at present the appropriate considerations are inclusion into adjuvant therapy trials or careful follow-up after adequate surgery alone.

Finally, the question of designing follow-up is important. CEA is mentioned, as are other biochemical tests, and one should keep in mind that in the setting described in this case report, if tumor occurrence is defined, options are limited to palliation. Therefore, follow-up design should be stringently limited to the search for symptoms that might be palliated, unless of course the patient is part of a formal trial and disease-free, and overall survival is being assessed.

SECTION IV

Pancreas

25

Stage III Adenocarcinoma of the Head of the Pancreas

Troy G. Scroggins, Jr., Edwin Beckman, and Roger Tutton

Is adjuvant therapy appropriate?

CASE PRESENTATION

E.H. is a 64-year-old man who presented to an outside hospital in April 1993 with a 2- to 3-week history of persistent epigastric pain, described as a constant nonradiating ache within the midepigastric region. The pain was neither exacerbated nor relieved by eating. Initially, an upper gastrointestinal and ultrasound of the gallbladder were performed. Both tests were essentially normal except for a small hiatal hernia seen on the upper gastrointestinal study.

The patient had a history of peptic ulcerative disease and was subsequently started on Tagamet and Toradol for pain. The patient's pain was partially relieved but, within days of starting the Tagamet, he re-presented to his physicians with jaundice. Laboratory examination revealed a SGOT/AST of 407 U/L, a SGPT/ALT of 8/94 U/L, an alkaline phosphatase of 475 U/L, and a total bilirubin of 10.6 mg/dL. The patient's amylase was elevated at 138 U/L. A hepatitis profile was negative. A computed tomography (CT) scan of the abdomen revealed a slightly prominent common bile duct. Liver and pancreas were both well visualized and felt to be normal. There were no other abnormalities noted. At endoscopy, esophagitis was present with a linear ulcer at the gastroesophageal junction. The stomach was normal. There were multiple superficial ulcers present in the duodenal bulb. The second part of the duodenum was normal. At endoscopic retrograde cholangiopancreatography (ERCP), there was swelling noted at the ampulla of Vater, along with a pinpoint narrowing of the common bile duct in the region of

the head of the pancreas. The report notes that it was not possible to pass a guided wire into that area. The proximal common bile duct was dilated to the pancreatic head and there were no stones noted. There was narrowing of the pancreatic duct in the region of the pancreatic head. Biopsies were not performed at the time of ERCP. The patient was referred to the Ochsner Clinic for further work-up and management.

On May 5, 1993, the patient was evaluated at the Ochsner Clinic. Physical examination revealed an obviously jaundiced, well developed, well nourished man in no acute distress. His neck was without any cervical or supraclavicular adenopathy. The lungs were clear to auscultation bilaterally. The abdomen was soft, nontender, and without palpable masses or hepatosplenomegaly. There was no evidence of ascites. Extremities were within normal limits and there was no axillary or inguinal adenopathy.

A repeat CT scan of the abdomen with targeted pancreatic images was obtained on May 10, 1993. Again the liver and spleen enhanced homogeneously. There was evidence of dilation of some of the intrahepatic biliary ducts. Contrast medium from the patient's prior ERCP was noted within the gallbladder and the dilated common bile duct (Fig. 25–1). The maximum diameter of the common bile duct was 1.2 cm. In the region of the head of the pancreas, there was a hypodensity measuring approximately 1 × 2.5 cm (Fig. 25–2). The pancreatic duct was also dilated, but the mass in the head of the pancreas did not involve either the splenic or mesenteric veins. The portal vein also appeared uninvolved. The remainder of the CT scan was normal without any evidence of periaor-

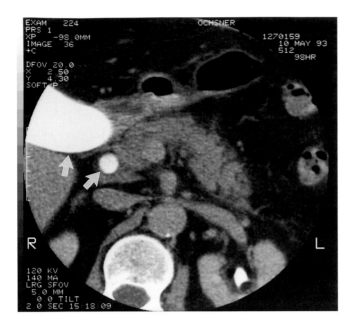

FIG. 25–1. *Arrows* point to contrast in the gallbladder and common bile duct.

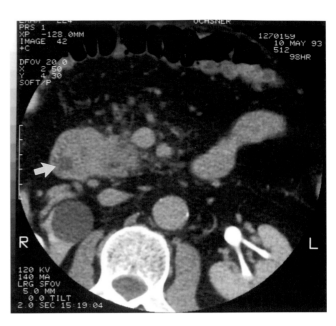

FIG. 25–2. *Arrow* points to the hypodensity in the head of the pancreas.

tic adenopathy. Overall, the CT was felt to be consistent with a small tumor in the head of the pancreas. Posteroanterior and lateral chest roentgenograms were normal. A CA 19-9 was markedly elevated at 4575 U/mL.

The gastroenterologist was reluctant to perform another ERCP because there were difficulties encountered during the first procedure. The CT scan indicated that the lesion was resectable. After discussion with the patient and his family, the decision was made to offer the patient exploratory laparotomy with possible pancreatic resection, if this proved to be pancreatic cancer.

On May 11, 1993, the patient was taken to the operating room for exploratory laparotomy and biopsies. Diffuse thickening of the pancreas with edema was noted, suggesting a subacute pancreatitis. There was a discrete indurated area noted in the head of the pancreas. Tru-cut needle biopsies of this area returned positive for adenocarcinoma. Peripancreatic nodes were then excised and sent for frozen section. These were negative for tumor involvement. The decision was made to proceed with a pylorus-preserving Whipple procedure (pancreaticoduodenectomy). The patient was reconstructed with a hepaticojejunostomy, a pancreaticojejunostomy, and a duodenojejunostomy. The patient tolerated the procedure well. Postoperatively, he did well and was ambulating by day 3. The patient's jaundice abated and his transaminases were within normal limits.

Pathologic examination revealed a moderately differentiated adenocarcinoma, consisting of irregular, intermediate, and large glands. Carcinoma is found principally at the junction of the head of the pancreas and

duodenum, with tumor present within the muscularis and submucosa of the duodenum (Fig. 25–3). There was also invasion of the carcinoma into the peripancreatic adipose tissue (Fig. 25–4). The actual carcinoma was found to be greater than 2.5 cm in its greatest dimension, but less than 4.5 cm. There were areas of chronic and acute pancreatitis but no other foci of tumor were noted within the pancreas. Metastatic carcinoma was noted in one of three periduodenal lymph nodes, but not identified in any of seven peripancreatic lymph nodes.

The patient was last seen at the Ochsner Clinic in October 1993. Physical examination was negative with no evidence of disease. The patient was gaining weight and tolerating a normal diet. He is scheduled for a repeat follow-up exam in 4 months.

Discussion at Tumor Board

Surgeon: This patient's pathologic stage is T2 N1 M0, which is stage III disease. Historically, these patients have a dismal prognosis and the question is whether to offer this patient adjuvant therapy. The tumor has been totally resected with negative margins and 1 of 10 lymph nodes were involved.

Radiation oncologist: Although the disease has been totally resected, we would recommended that the patient receive a course of postoperative radiotherapy to the tumor bed and remaining pancreatic tissue. We would normally recommend that this radiotherapy be delivered along with concomitant 5-fluorouracil. Our recommen-

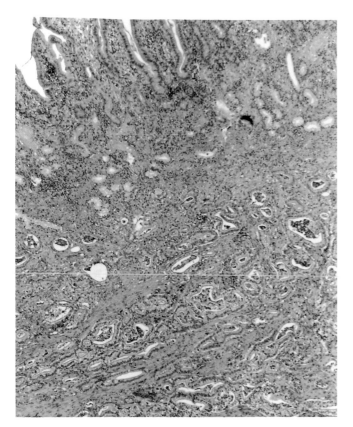

FIG. 25–3. Tumor infiltrating into the muscularis and submucosa of the duodenum.

dations are based on results of a randomized protocol from the Gastrointestinal Tumor Study Group, which randomized patients to receive surgery alone or surgery followed by chemotherapy and irradiation for resectable adenocarcinoma of the pancreas. The study showed a significant improvement in median survival in those patients who received adjuvant radiotherapy and chemotherapy. The median survival of this group was 21 months versus 11 months in those patients who received no further therapy. There was also a significant improvement in the 2-year survival.

Medical oncologist: We agree with offering the patient adjuvant combined modality therapy. The addition of chemotherapy to irradiation depends on the patient's performance status, but typically we have treated these patients with 5-fluorouracil at doses of 500 mg/m^2 intravenously daily for 3 days at the beginning of radiation therapy, repeating this course approximately 3 weeks later. Consideration can also be given to treating the patient with 5-fluorouracil 500 mg/m^2 weekly after his radiotherapy for up to 1 year. The patient's chance for long-term survival is still limited but, I would agree that from the available data, survival appears to be significantly improved with the addition of adjuvant therapy.

Surgeon: In the surgical literature there are retrospective reviews that report median survivals in the 15- to 20-

month range. These patients received no adjuvant therapy and the results are very similar to those reported by the Gastrointestinal Tumor Study Group in patients who received adjuvant therapy. On review of these studies, it is difficult to get a clear idea of the pathologic stage of patients after surgery. The reports that do separate survival by stage, such as those from Harvard Medical School, concur that in pathologic stage III disease survival is relatively short with surgery alone. I agree that this patient would be an excellent candidate for adjuvant therapy.

Radiation oncologist: Our normal course of irradiation would consist of 45 Gy to the tumor bed and remaining pancreatic tissue in 1.8-Gy fractions along with concomitant 5-fluorouracil. Note that in some of the recent Radiation Therapy Oncology Group protocols for unresectable disease, prophylactic liver irradiation is recommended. It will be interesting to see if this contributes to patients' local control or alters the pattern of recurrence.

Surgeon: This patient lives in Mississippi, so we will plan to make the appropriate contacts to facilitate his adjuvant therapy.

The patient subsequently received combined modality therapy with irradiation consisting of 50.4 Gy given to the pancreatic bed at 1.8 Gy per day along with 5-fluorouracil at 500 mg/m^2 for two courses during his irradiation. The patient tolerated his chemotherapy and irradiation well. He completed irradiation on August 6, 1993, and subsequently resumed a course of chemotherapy with 5-fluorouracil and leucovorin according to his outside medical oncologist. This decision to continue his chemotherapy was based on an elevated CA 19-9 of 139 in July 1993.

COMMENTARY by John L. Cameron

This patient with adenocarcinoma of the pancreas presented in a fairly typical fashion. He did not present with painless jaundice, but actually had epigastric pain as his initial symptom. This is much more common than is generally accepted. When he became jaundiced, he had what I feel is the appropriate first test. When a patient presents with obstructive jaundice and is suspected of having a periampullary cancer, a CT scan should be obtained. This not only allows one to confirm the diagnosis by seeing dilated biliary radicals within the liver and a dilated extrahepatic biliary tree, but also usually allows one to identify a periampullary mass. This confirms the diagnosis of a periampullary malignancy in the appropriate setting, and I do not believe further diagnostic studies are necessary. Furthermore, the CT scan is an excellent initial staging tool because one can determine whether liver metastases are present, lymphadenopathy in the peripancreatic region can often be detected, and usually one can get some idea as to whether or not the superior mesenteric vein, portal vein, and celiac axis and/or the superior mesenteric artery are involved in the tumor mass.

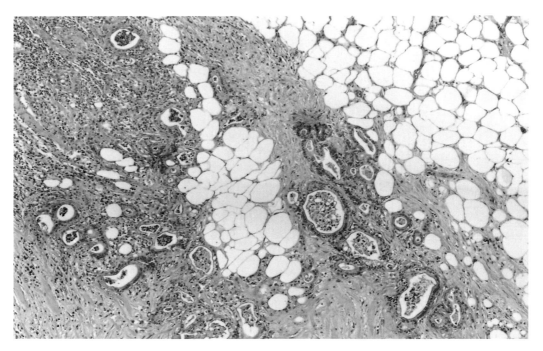

FIG. 25–4. Tumor invading the peripancreatic adipose tissue.

After a CT scan suggests the diagnosis, and shows no reason for unresectability, I feel visceral angiography should be performed as a further staging procedure. I believe patients who present with obstructive jaundice who are not candidates for a Whipple procedure, and who do not have duodenal obstruction, should be palliated nonoperatively either percutaneously or endoscopically. Therefore, I believe that further staging with angiography is appropriate, to avoid unnecessary laparotomies in some patients. If visceral angiography demonstrates that the celiac axis and its branches, the superior mesenteric artery, and the portal and superior mesenteric veins are not occluded or severely encased, I believe one should proceed with laparotomy.

It is not clear to me in the present case report why the patient had a second CT scan performed. In an era where we are trying to eliminate medical expenses, I believe the first CT scan should have been adequate for a preoperative work-up. In addition, I do not believe cholangiography should be performed endoscopically or percutaneously, unless there is a reason to expect delay until laparotomy for a potentially curative resection. If a patient wants surgery delayed for a week or two to get his or her affairs in order, or there are other medical reasons for delay, then I believe an endoprosthesis should be inserted endoscopically, or a biliary stent percutaneously. Otherwise, I see absolutely no reason to perform an endoscopic or percutaneous cholangiogram. Furthermore, in the case presentation it was suggested that a second ERCP was contemplated at the Ochsner

Clinic, and not performed only because of the difficulty of the first procedure. Again, I would question the need for a first, or a second, ERCP.

I would agree that pylorus preservation is appropriate for a patient undergoing a pancreaticoduodenectomy for a carcinoma of the head of the pancreas. Several years ago it was questioned whether or not the margins would be appropriate if one were to perform a pylorus-preserving procedure in the face of pancreatic cancer. I think that question has been answered, and unless a positive margin is obtained at the duodenum, I think there is no need to add a hemigastrectomy. I would question the intraoperative biopsy, however. I think most experienced pancreatic surgeons now proceed on the basis of the clinical presentation, the imaging studies, and the operative findings, without performing an intraoperative biopsy. In a particularly small pancreatic cancer, a positive biopsy is often impossible to obtain. Does one then not proceed with a Whipple procedure? The answer to that is no. A procedure that will not influence the surgeon's decision should be abandoned. I certainly put intraoperative biopsy in that category. I think intraoperative biopsy is necessary only if the lesion proves to be unresectable. In that case, a positive biopsy is necessary so that the radiotherapist and medical oncologist have confirmation of the neoplasm.

Our data demonstrate that by univariate analysis, size of the tumor, lymph node involvement, and histologic evidence of vessel invasion are all predictive in terms of long-term survival. Histologic grade and nerve involvement have not been. Of these factors, the most predictive has been the presence or absence of positive nodes. I certainly agree that the presence of positive nodes markedly decreases the chances of prolonged survival. However, in our data there is still an 8% likelihood that a patient will survive 5 years in the face of positive nodes. Thus, the finding of a positive node intraoperatively, if it is within the resection specimen, should not preclude resection.

I concur with the use of adjuvant therapy for all patients who undergo pancreaticoduodenectomy for carcinoma of the head of the pancreas. The Gastrointestinal Tumor Study Group has clearly demonstrated, and a subsequent study confirmed, that adjuvant therapy can effectively prolong survival. Our data demonstrate that 5-year survival in the absence of positive nodes is in the range of 40%. Although a substantial improvement over a decade or two ago, this still means that well over half the patients with negative node status will not survive long term. Thus, adjuvant therapy is clearly indicated in both node-positive and node-negative patients. The Gastrointestinal Tumor Study Group adjuvant regimen is a modest regimen that I am certain can be improved on. If one is involved in a multicenter trial looking for an improved adjuvant therapy, I think that is appropriate. Without access to a prospective randomized study, however, I think the Gastrointestinal Tumor Study protocol should be used.

SELECTED READINGS

1. Cameron JL, Pitt HA, Yeo CJ, Lillemoe KD, et al. One hundred and forty-five consecutive pancreaticoduodenectomies without mortality. *Ann Surg* 1993;217:430–5.
2. Cameron JL, Crist DW, Sitzmann JV, Hruban RH, et al. Factors influencing survival after pancreaticoduodenectomy for pancreatic cancer. *Am J Surg* 1991;161:120–4.
3. Crist DW, Sitzmann JV, Cameron JL. Improved hospital morbidity, mortality, and survival after the Whipple procedure. *Ann Surg* 1987;206:358–65.
4. Lillemoe KD, Sauter PK, Pitt HA, Yeo CJ, Cameron JL. Current status of surgical palliation of periampullary carcinoma. *Surg Gynecol Obstet* 1993;176:1–10.

EDITORIAL BOARD COMMENTARY

The author and the discussant comprehensively describe the problem of adenocarcinoma of the head of the pancreas.

The issues that remain controversial would be the routine use of angiography as proposed by Dr. Cameron and the preoperative use of laparoscopy.

With the current state of high quality helical CT scan, most patients no longer, in our opinion, need angiography. Laparoscopy is evolving as an efficient, rapid diagnostic tool that can avoid unnecessary laparotomy for the unresectable patient thought to be resectable on preoperative helical CT scan. With the development of laparoscopic ultrasound, refinements in laparoscopic diagnosis should be such that most patients deemed resectable after this procedure will proceed to potentially curative resection.

26

Zollinger-Ellison Syndrome

John N. Tasiopoulos, Mick Meiselman, Gene Chiao, Robin Levy, and
Stephen F. Sener

Where's the gastrinoma?

CASE PRESENTATION

A 41-year-old black woman was admitted with a 14-year history of treatment for peptic ulcer disease, using cimetidine, ranitidine, and famotidine. Persistent epigastric pain led to evaluation at our institution, and omeprazole, 20 mg per day, was prescribed. There was no family history of ulcer or parathyroid or pituitary disease.

Upper gastrointestinal endoscopy revealed diffuse bulbar ulcerations. A fasting serum gastrin level, performed with an antibody that recognized both the G-7 and G-34 forms of gastrin, was 324 pg/mL (normal <100 pg/mL). A secretin stimulation test had a baseline serum gastrin level of 327 pg/mL, which increased to 528 pg/mL and 474 pg/mL at 5 and 10 minutes after stimulation. Serum liver enzymes and calcium level were within normal limits.

Abdominal ultrasound, abdominal computed tomography (CT) scan with oral and intravenous contrast, and celiac-superior mesenteric artery angiogram did not reveal the location of the primary tumor. No metastatic disease in liver or lymph nodes was identified. Repeat upper gastrointestinal endoscopy failed to identify a primary tumor within the duodenal wall.

The patient's history and work-up were presented at our institutional Tumor Board. No consensus was reached during the discussion, which was centered around whether a pancreatectomy should be done to excise an occult tumor, if no primary or metastatic disease were found during exploration of the abdomen. Options for acid-reducing procedures that might be employed were also discussed.

The patient then had an exploratory laparotomy, done with the aid of intraoperative ultrasound. The duodenum

and pancreas were entirely mobilized and explored by manual palpation and ultrasound. Exploration of the "gastrinoma triangle" revealed only biopsy-proven reactive lymph nodes along the distal common bile duct and gastroepiploic artery. The duodenal wall was explored through a generous pyloroplasty, using a rigid operative endoscope and bimanual palpation. The primary tumor was not located, and there was no evidence of metastatic disease upon further exploration of the abdomen. Because the patient's ulcer disease had not reached intractability with medical therapy, a gastrectomy was not done. A truncal vagotomy and Heineke-Mikulicz pyloroplasty were performed. Biopsy of the gastric antrum, looking for G-cell hyperplasia, showed chronic superficial gastritis. Because no primary or metastatic disease was found, the surgical oncologist was unwilling to accept the postoperative morbidity or the operative mortality risk associated with a pancreatectomy.

Two weeks after the procedure, the patient had recurrent epigastric pain, fever, and diarrhea. Another upper gastrointestinal endoscopy finally revealed an 0.8-cm submucosal nodule in the first portion of the jejunum. Biopsies were consistent with a neuroendocrine tumor. The endoscopy was repeated, and an India ink tattoo was placed adjacent to the tumor. An attempt to obliterate the tumor was done with a cautery forceps. Fasting serum gastrin levels done 2, 3, and 8 weeks after the endoscopic obliteration were 228, 249, and 227 pg/mL, respectively.

With the persistent elevation of the fasting serum gastrin levels, the patient was re-explored. There was no metastatic disease found in the liver or peritoneal cavity. The intramural nodule and the India ink tattoo were found 10 cm distal to the ligament of Treitz. Resection of the proximal jejunum and clinically N0 regional lymph nodes along the superior mesenteric artery showed a neuroendocrine carcinoma with four histologically positive nodes (Fig. 26–1). Lymph nodes sampled in the small bowel mesentery distal to the node resection and along the superior mesenteric artery proximal to the node resection did not have metastatic tumor. Stains of the tumor were strongly positive for gastrin and negative for vasoactive intestinal peptide and serotonin.

The patient recovered and has done well, without complications from the vagotomy and pyloroplasty. Fasting serum gastrin levels done at 1, 4, and 12 months after the second operation were 44, 45, and 66 pg/mL, respectively.

COMMENTARY by Courtney M. Townsend, Jr.

This case nicely demonstrates three important principles in managing patients with Zollinger-Ellison syndrome (ZES). They are: (a) all patients with ZES, in the absence of widespread metastatic disease, should undergo operation to search for and resect all tumor possible; (b) the vast majority of patients with ZES, whether sporadic or familial, who are cured have ectopic "or extrapancreatic gastrinoma"; and (c) widespread search beyond the gastrinoma triangle is required at operation when no obvious tumor is found.

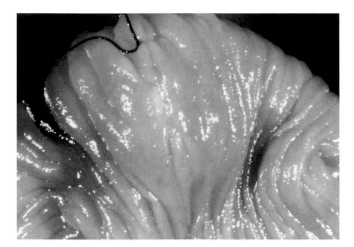

FIG. 26–1. Resection of proximal jejunum, demonstrating intramural gastrinoma and India ink tattoo.

The question of what to do when no tumor is found still is one that bedevils those of us who care for patients with ZES. It is clear that blind pancreatectomy is not indicated, but less clear is what should be done to the stomach. ZES is the only syndrome caused by endocrine tumors of the pancreas in which the patient can be completely cured of symptoms of hormone excess even in the presence of unresectable tumor by removal of the end organ—the stomach. Total gastrectomy in these patients is not fraught with the same terrible sequelae that may occur in patients who have total gastrectomy for gastric adenocarcinoma. Total gastrectomy is still an option that must be considered. In this patient, because the symptoms were managed easily with relatively standard doses of Omeprazole, and there were not significant debilitating symptoms present, the truncal vagotomy and pyloroplasty may well have provided significant palliation for a long period of time. However, the only way to assure patients completely that they will never have symptoms of acid hypersecretion is to perform total gastrectomy. There are reported incidents of breakthrough using the more powerful proton pump blockers than had been thought previously. The medicine must be taken daily and is expensive. Medicine not taken is no better than no medicine being available.

The attempts at obliteration by endoscopic techniques of nodules thought to be gastrinoma should not be performed. These patients require a proper operation to remove tumor and regional lymph nodes. This is well illustrated by the current case in which the small nodule in the jejunum was associated with four lymph nodes that contained metastatic deposits. This patient is cured, and that would not have been possible if endoscopic obliteration of the jejunal nodule had been carried out. The patient should have periodic secretin provocation because it is not uncommon for patients to have normal serum gastrin at times and yet have elevated gastrin after secretin provocation. This patient is a wonderful example of a patient with sporadic ZES cured by surgical resection of tumor who will not require life-long antisecretory medication.

EDITORIAL BOARD COMMENTARY

The authors and discussant appropriately raise most issues. One entity not discussed is the use of preoperative endoscopic ultrasound, which has proved highly efficient in localizing duodenal lesions situated in the submucosa.

27
Unresectable Adenocarcinoma of the Head of the Pancreas

John P. Hoffman and Pasha Agarwal

To treat or not to treat

CASE PRESENTATION

This 71-year-old woman presented to her doctor with weakness, nausea, and painless jaundice in August 1991. She had lost 15 pounds in 1 month.

Initial laboratory studies revealed a blood sugar of 606 mg%, total bilirubin of 16.2 mg%, and direct bilirubin of 11.9 gm%. The alkaline phosphatase was 393 units (37–107), SGOT was 127 units (12–45), and a GGT was 1,829 units (8–69). The lipase was 284 units (7–60) and the amylase was 29 (34–122). Prothrombin time was 12.6 s, white blood count was 6,100/mm³, and Hmb was 12.7 g/dL. Previous laboratory tests had been drawn in July 1991; these had all been within normal limits except for a mildly elevated blood sugar. The patient had developed diabetes mellitus 2½ years previously and was under good control until recently, with 2.5 mg of oral Micronase daily. There was no family history of pancreatic cancer. She was a nonsmoker and took only occasional alcohol.

A computed tomography (CT) scan revealed a 3.5-cm mass in the head of the pancreas and dilated intrahepatic bile ducts (Fig. 27–1). An ERCP revealed a partially obstructed pancreatic duct and a completely obstructed intrapancreatic common bile duct (Fig. 27–2). An attempt at endoscopic biliary stenting was unsuccessful. On October 11, 1991, she underwent percutaneous transhepatic cholangiography and a percutaneous transhepatic stent placement (Fig. 27–3).

The patient's blood sugars were controlled with intermittent doses of regular insulin and Micronase. There was a transient rise in lipase to 625 units after her percuta-

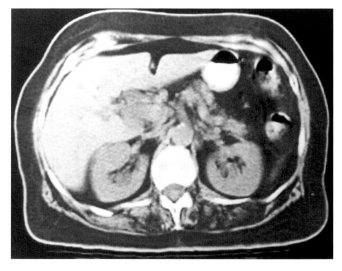

FIG. 27–1. CT scan at presentation showing mass in head of pancreas.

neous stent placement. The CEA was 53 ng/mL and the CA 19-9 was 116,240 units/mL.

A CT scan of the lungs, abdomen, and pelvis revealed no extrapancreatic metastases, so the patient was considered for treatment with preoperative chemotherapy and radiotherapy. Therefore, a percutaneous, CT-directed fine-needle biopsy of the mass in the pancreas was performed and the diagnosis of adenocarcinoma was made (Fig. 27–4).

She was discharged home 2 days after her stent placement, only to be readmitted 4 days later with shaking

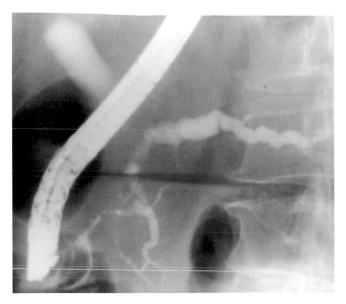

FIG. 27–2. ERCP showing dilated pancreatic and bile ducts.

chills and weakness. Biliary cultures grew out *Klebsiella pneumoniae.* The biliary stent was shown to be completely obstructed and it was therefore exchanged for a larger (10 F) stent, which again allowed free drainage into the duodenum. Five days later more fever was noted and another tube check revealed the stent again to be occluded. The tube was again exchanged. She was treated with Ceftriaxone, 1 g intravenously daily, and eventually was able to undergo capping of the stent.

Treatment was begun with Mitomycin-C, 19 mg (10 mg/m²) intravenously over 2 hours and 5-fluorouracil (5-FU), 1,900 mg (1,000 mg/m²) in 1,000 mL of 0.45% sodium chloride over 24 hours, repeated for a total of 96 hours. This was given in concert with radiation therapy in 180-cGy fractions to the pancreatic cancer and a surrounding area of 3 cm. The therapy was tolerated well and she was discharged home after six treatments, 2 weeks after her admission for the cholangitis. Discharge medications included Micronase 2.5 mg daily, MS-Contin 30 mg po bid, Zantac 150 mg po bid, Viokase two tablets with meals, and Reglan 10 mg po 10 minutes before meals.

She was readmitted 2½ weeks later with dehydration and weakness after having received 12 more radiotherapy treatments. Her appetite had decreased such that she had lost another 12 pounds in the interim. Total parenteral nutrition was established. Radiotherapy was continued, as was her next cycle of chemotherapy, which consisted of 5-FU, 1,740 mg daily over 96 hours. The radiotherapy was completed in 37 days. At 3,960 cGy, there was a reduction in the fields to 2-cm margins around the tumor for the last six treatments. During this hospitalization, the patient developed more nausea, diarrhea, and depression, which only partially responded to antidepressant therapy. In view of the continued nausea,

a CT of the brain was performed, which revealed no metastases.

Although an upper gastrointestinal series was normal, the patient was essentially unable to eat because of her nausea, even after radiotherapy had been completed. Therefore, a percutaneous endoscopic gastrostomy was placed and tube feeding was begun with Osmolite HN. One month after the previous exchange, the biliary stent was again exchanged and the patient was discharged on tube feedings and neural protamine Hagedorn (NPH) insulin at 10 units daily.

She was readmitted 8 days later, 5 weeks after the completion of her radiotherapy, for an exploratory celiotomy. The intent was to perform a resection if there were no metastatic disease. A repeat CT scan of the chest, abdomen, and pelvis revealed no change in the size of the pancreatic tumor and no metastases. The CA 19-9 had fallen to 670 units/mL and the CEA to 3.6 ng/mL. A celiac and superior mesenteric artery (SMA) arteriogram revealed no encroachment of tumor on either the superior mesenteric and hepatic arteries, nor on the portal and superior mesenteric veins (Fig. 27–5).

The patient was taken to surgery on January 7, 1992, where a 4-mm nodule was noted in segment 2 of the liver. This was biopsied and shown to contain a moderately differentiated metastatic adenocarcinoma (Fig. 27–6). The remainder of the peritoneal cavity contained no gross metastatic disease. The tumor in the pancreas was approx-

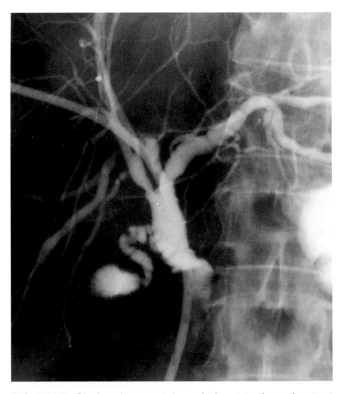

FIG. 27–3. Cholangiogram taken during transhepatic stent placement.

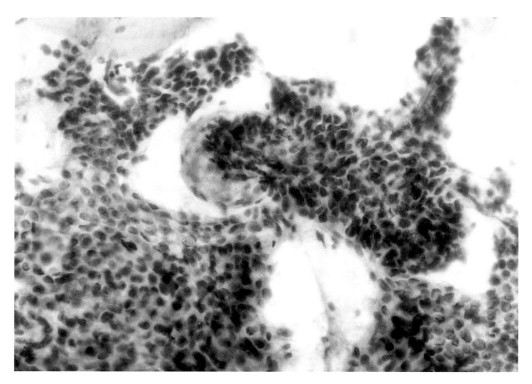

FIG. 27–4. Fine-needle aspiration sample from CT-directed biopsy of pancreatic head mass. (Original magnification ×200.) Moderately differentiated adenocarcinoma.

imately 4 cm in diameter and mobile. It was decided to perform an internal bypass. The gallbladder was removed and a retrocolic side-to-side choledochojejunostomy was performed. The previous biliary stent was intubated with a wire and replaced with a new 12-mm Cook biliary

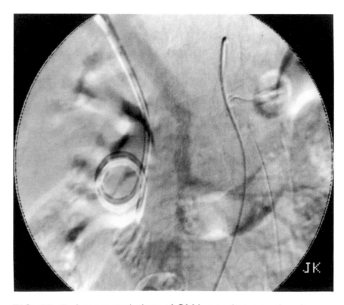

FIG. 27–5. Late portal view of SMA arteriogram showing no encroachment of tumor upon veins.

catheter that was then placed through the anastomosis as a stent. Postoperative complications included a partial distraction of the biliary stent 1 week after surgery. This required replacement under fluoroscopic control. The patient also had Candida recovered from her blood cultures and, therefore, her venous port was removed and replaced with a temporary catheter through which she received a 10-day course of amphotericin-B. Her biliary stent was removed 3 weeks postoperatively after a widely patent choledochojejunostomy was demonstrated by cholangiogram. She was discharged 3½ weeks after surgery on tube feedings at home and 18 units of NPH insulin daily. In 3 weeks her nausea had disappeared and she was able to eat normally. Therefore, her percutaneous endoscopic gastrostomy (PEG) tube was removed. She began to gain weight and was seen by a medical oncologist in March for a discussion regarding treatment options. The CA 19-9 had become elevated to 3,186 units/mL in mid-February. The CEA had risen to 21 ng/mL and the CA 19-9 to 4,813 units/mL on March 6.

The medical oncologist suggested possible treatment with 5-FU and leucovorin. She declined the offer in March because she was feeling so well. By April, she noted increasing fatigue and pains in her joints. In view of her increasing weakness, 5-FU and leucovorin were again offered. This regimen was begun at a dose of 425 mg/m^2 of 5-FU daily for 4 days along with leucovorin at 20 mg/m^2, also for 4 days. The only complication was that of

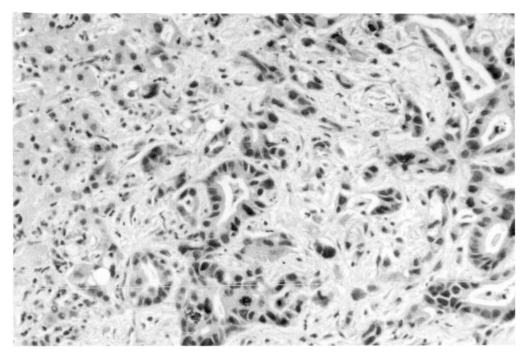

FIG. 27–6. Liver biopsy showing normal hepatocytes and metastatic adenocarcinoma. (Original magnification ×200.)

mouth ulcers. Her diabetes had come under better control after the chemotherapy had been initiated. She was given her second course of chemotherapy in late May, with the observation that her energy and appetite had both improved. Nevertheless, the markers had continued to rise (CEA 123.6 ng/mL, CA 19-9 26,828 units/mL). A CT scan revealed widespread hepatic metastases (Fig. 27–7).

No change was noted in the primary tumor in the pancreas. The patient returned 1 month later, feeling well and able to eat normally. However, she had continued to lose weight, from 158 pounds in March down to 134 pounds in May. She elected to receive Mitomycin C at 10 mg/m². This was given in July and again 4 weeks later. Despite therapy, the CA 19-9 rose to 45,238 units/mL and the

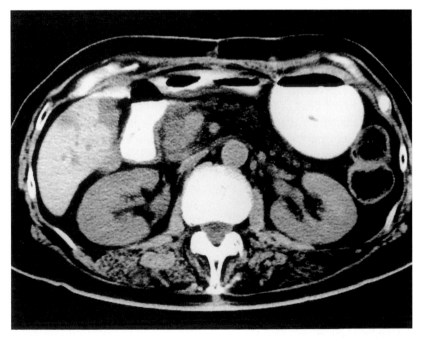

FIG. 27–7. CT showing hepatic metastases and no change in size of pancreatic mass.

CEA 292 ng/mL on July 29. She was readmitted 1 week later with intractable nausea. Radiologic studies revealed a fecal impaction. With rehydration and cathartics, she was enabled to eat normally and left the hospital in 5 days. A call from the patient's daughter 2 weeks later revealed that she had no more appetite and did not wish to take any more medication. She died at home on August 30, 1992, 1 year from the onset of her obstructive jaundice.

COMMENTARY by A. R. Moossa

The management of this patient was based on two reasonable clinical assumptions: (a) the patient's cancer was confined to the local-regional area of the head of the pancreas at the time of presentation, and (b) preoperative chemotherapy and radiotherapy would "downstage" the disease and provide a more effective surgical extirpation with a higher chance of cure. Unfortunately, the patient developed metastatic disease that was identified when she was explored 5 months later. Let us consider some of the issues in more detail.

The relationship of the recent onset of diabetes mellitus and the pancreatic cancer is receiving renewed interest by many investigators. It has been postulated that there are two types of diabetes mellitus in pancreatic cancer: (a) a group of individuals in whom the hereditary type of diabetes mellitus is present for a long time, and this may be a possible risk factor in the development of pancreatic cancer; and (b) a subset of patients in whom the hyperglycemia is of much shorter duration and is probably a consequence of the pancreatic cancer.

It is impossible in this case to evaluate any causal relationship between the glucose intolerance and the pancreatic cancer because there is uncertainty regarding the exact duration of the in situ phase of human pancreatic cancer and the hyperglycemia.

When a 71-year-old woman who is a nonsmoker and only occasionally drinks alcohol develops obstructive jaundice, and a CT scan reveals a mass in the head of the pancreas and dilated intrahepatic bile ducts, the diagnosis is obvious. Should an ERCP be routinely performed? This author believes that it should not because of the risk of introducing infection into an obstructed ductal system. However, if endoscopic stenting for biliary drainage is planned, as it was in this case, then it is appropriate to perform an ERCP.

Unfortunately for the patient, the endoscopic biliary stenting was unsuccessful. On October 11, she underwent percutaneous transhepatic cholangiography and percutaneous transhepatic stent placement. There was an inordinately long interval between the ERCP and the percutaneous stent placement, and this is not explained. During that time, the patient's liver function can deteriorate.

It is important to appreciate that this woman developed all the septic complications of biliary stenting. The stent had to be changed repeatedly under antibiotic cover before the patient could be started on the combination of chemotherapy and radiotherapy.

Of note is that the serum level of two tumor markers, CEA and CA 19-9, were both grossly elevated. Statistically, these elevations are associated with a poor prognosis.

Percutaneous CT-directed fine-needle biopsy of the mass in the head of the pancreas was performed and confirmed the diagnosis of adenocarcinoma. This obsession with obtaining a tissue diagnosis before treatment is worrisome. What other condition could have presented all those clinical and radiologic findings? The pancreas and peripancreatic tissues share a rich network of vascular and lymphatic plexuses. Common sense dictates that unnecessary needling for diagnosis has a risk of disseminating the cancer, although this is rarely reported in the literature. Recent data from the Massachusetts General Hospital show conclusively that percutaneous biopsy of pancreatic cancer increases the incidence of positive cytology from peritoneal washings.

Both chemotherapy and radiotherapy have systemic effects on the patient, leading to further decrease in appetite and oral intake. Because the patient continued to lose weight, it was appropriate to start total parenteral nutrition. The patient continued to have nausea and depression. A CT scan of the brain was performed to rule out cerebral metastases. This author has to confess that he has never seen brain metastases from a pancreatic cancer in isolation without obvious metastases elsewhere. It was also clinically sound, because an upper gastrointestinal series was normal, to perform a percutaneous endoscopic gastrostomy to provide the patient with an enteral feeding route while the chemotherapy and radiotherapy treatment were completed.

Unfortunately, by the time the patient was explored 5 months after presentation, she had a metastatic nodule in the liver. This was appropriately biopsied and proved to be metastatic adenocarcinoma. Accordingly, the plan for resection was abandoned and a biliary-enteric diversion was performed to relieve the patient from any type of stent. Whether a gastrojejunostomy should have been performed prophylactically at the time, in case the patient later developed gastric outlet obstruction, is debatable and is a "judgment call" on the part of the surgeon. Because the intention was to continue treating the patient with multiple chemotherapy postoperatively, this author would have personally performed a gastrojejunostomy. Be that as it may, the patient had a stormy postoperative course that necessitated replacement of the biliary stent and treatment of Candida sepsis. She remained in-hospital for 3½ weeks after surgery! Further treatment with chemotherapy was delayed largely because of the patient's decision. Nonetheless, 3 months after the operation, it was clear that the patient's disease had evolved into an accelerated tempo, based on her symptoms and on the increasing levels of her tumor markers. She succumbed, like most patients with pancreatic cancer, from widespread metastatic disease within the abdomen.

An alternative approach to such a patient would have been to perform an abdominal operation, at the time of presentation, without prior ERCP, percutaneous stenting, or percutaneous biopsy. If the tumor were resectable, either a Whipple resection or a total pancreatectomy (the patient was already diabetic) would have been performed. The tumor would thus have been staged pathologically, with emphasis on peripancreatic extension and lymph node invasion. Postoperative adjuvant therapy in the form of chemotherapy or radiotherapy could then have been given. The patient was a good operative risk and, in retrospect, this approach could have avoided many of the septic complications associated with the stenting.

EDITORIAL BOARD COMMENTARY

Drs. Hoffman and Agarwal provide the appropriate spectrum of approaches to adenocarcinoma of the pancreas. Salient points are made by both authors. In no other disease are we more in need of improved management plans. The morbidity of unsuccessful therapy, either surgical, chemotherapy, or radiation, is very significant. The present case illustrates all the potential complications of aggressive, nonsurgical treatment. The way in which the case was approached seems to assume local unresectability which, by description, was not so even at the time of operation 4 months after diagnosis; the tumor did appear to be resectable, but it was the presence of metastasis that precluded it.

Our approach would have been directed at avoidance of transhepatic stenting, given the number of studies that have shown that the morbidity of such an approach exceeds any significant benefit. A laparoscopy performed at the time of diagnosis may well have determined the presence of metastatic disease for which no conventional therapy has been proven to have any benefit, and the 4 months of ineffective therapy might well have been avoided. Certainly, a laparoscopy before the final operation would have avoided further surgical morbidity. We trust that the option of supportive care only was suggested at each stage of this woman's course.

28

Ductal Adenocarcinoma of the Tail of Pancreas

David B. Gough and Jon A. van Heerden

A tumor with little respect for prompt diagnosis or diligent surgery

CASE PRESENTATION

A 64-year-old obese woman with a known history of alcohol abuse was investigated for a 1-month history of vague dyspepsia. An ultrasound examination demonstrated multiple gallstones and a mass in the pancreas (Fig. 28–1). Computed tomography (CT) confirmed a 5.5-cm, mixed solid/cystic lesion in the tail of the pancreas with no evidence of invasion of adjacent structures or metastases either regionally or distally (Fig. 28–2). The patient was evaluated for general anesthesia by obtaining an electrocardiogram, a chest roentgenogram, and routine hematologic and biochemistry examinations, all of which were normal. Pulmonary function studies (FVC, FEV, $FEV_1/FVC\%$, and FEF) were in all instances greater than 85% of that expected for the patient phenotype. Serum albumin was normal and there had been no evidence of recent weight loss. Discussion with the patient and her relatives of the risks, benefits, and likely outcome of surgery included the possibility of a nonresectable situation, the relatively poor survival associated with pancreatic cancer in general, and the theoretical increased risk of pneumococcal infection if a splenectomy were to be performed in association with pancreatic resection. After these discussions, it was decided to proceed to operation.

Blood was cross-matched for possible transfusion, the patient's gastrointestinal tract was prepared with a "Go-Lytely" preparation, and a pneumococcal vaccine was administered. Under general anesthesia, a nasogastric tube and urethral catheter were passed, and the peritoneal cavity was entered through an upper transverse epigastric incision. A large mobile lesion was noted in the tail of the pancreas, which did not invade the stomach or the large bowel mesentery. No evidence of local or distant tumor spread was encountered. Gallstones were noted in a subacutely inflamed gallbladder. The gastrocolic omentum was divided, exposing the pancreas in the floor of the lesser sac. By incising the peritoneum along the inferior aspect, the pancreas was mobilized. The splenic artery was isolated, doubly ligated, and transected close to its origin. The body of the pancreas was circumvented and transected with electrocautery anterior to the superior mesenteric vein. The splenic vein was then doubly ligated and the pancreas was dissected off the posterior abdominal wall. By freeing the avascular lateral, superior, and inferior attachments of the spleen, en bloc removal of the spleen, tail of the pancreas, and splenic artery and vein with adjacent nodes was accomplished. The stump of the pancreas was oversewn with two layers of interrupted silk sutures and an omental plug was attached to the raw area. The main pancreatic duct was carefully searched for but was not visualized. A cholecystectomy was then performed in routine fashion, doubly ligating the cystic duct stump. A Jackson-Pratt suction drain was placed in the pancreatic bed. No blood was transfused. A somatostatin analog (octreotide) was infused intravenously (150 g/q6h) during the procedure and administered subcutaneously for 5 days afterward.

Histologic examination of the resected specimen (Fig. 28–3) revealed a grade III mucin-producing adenocarci-

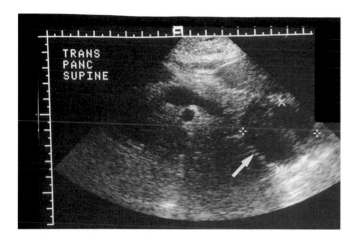

FIG. 28–1. Ultrasound (transverse view) shows a 5.5-cm mixed solid/cystic lesion in the tail of the pancreas.

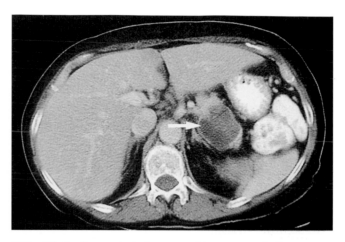

FIG. 28–2. Computed tomographic scan of the upper abdomen illustrating a 5.5-cm partially solid lesion in the tail of the pancreas. No evidence of local spread is apparent.

noma (8×6×4 cm). Excision margins were clear and multiple nodes were free of metastatic tumor (Fig. 28–4).

Postoperatively, urine output was maintained above 35 mL/hour. A nasogastric tube was kept in place for 2 days and daily drainage from the tube and abdominal drain was documented. On the fourth postoperative day, less than 100 mL issued from the abdominal drain. It was removed 9 days after surgery when 24-hour drainage was approximately 20 mL. There were no postoperative complications.

External beam irradiation and chemotherapy (5-fluorouracil) were advised after surgery, but the patient refused. The patient was scheduled for CT evaluation in 6 months. Although this follow-up examination suggested liver metastases, CT-guided biopsy failed to provide histologic confirmation. The patient died 8 months after surgery with suspected liver metastases.

The world-wide incidence of pancreatic cancer is increasing, although recent studies estimate the incidence in the United States (9/100,000) to be relatively static (1). Although associated with significant mortality in previ-

ous decades (>20%), pancreatic surgery, particularly of the tail, can now be performed with minimal mortality (<5%) (2), although morbidity remains high (30%) (3).

In this patient, two important decisions had to be addressed when the ultrasonographic findings were disclosed: (a) was this lesion a cancer, and (b) if so, would operative intervention benefit the patient? Even with modern technology, to determine with absolute confidence that a partially solid pancreatic lesion is not malignant is impossible without surgical biopsy. To determine resectability is sometimes as difficult. In general terms, lesions of the pancreatic body present late because symptoms often imply invasion of the celiac plexus and cause pain or, by their bulk, produce obstruction of the gastrointestinal tract. For this reason, resectability is frequently lower than with lesions in the head of pancreas, which often present earlier with obstructive jaundice. For all lesions in the pancreas, resectability may be as low as 5% (4). This woman could be described as one of the more fortunate because her tumor was detected in an accidental

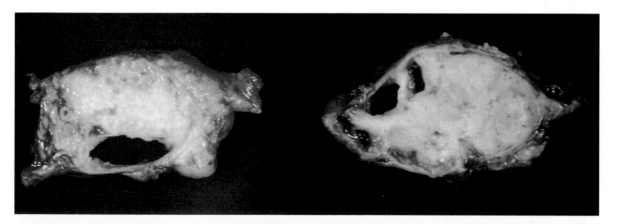

FIG. 28–3. Cut sections of the distal pancreas show complete effacement of the lobular architecture of the pancreas by grey-white glistening tissue with cysts up to 1.8 cm in diameter.

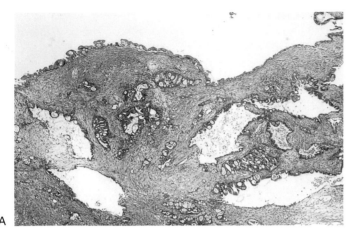

A

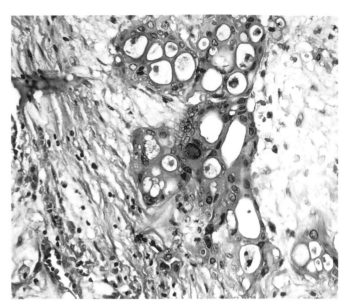

B

FIG. 28–4. **A:** Histologic sections show an infiltrating adeno-carcinoma associated with the production of mucin-filled cysts of varying sizes (*left*). **B:** Detail (*right*) showed large intracyto-plasmic mucin vacuoles and marked nuclear atypia indicative of malignancy.

fashion. As the ability to categorically deny the presence of cancer would be impossible, the major thrust of further investigation was to determine operability.

The differential diagnosis entertained at the time of presentation included benign or malignant neoplasms of the pancreas and, in view of the history of alcohol abuse and the ultrasound findings, a complex pseudocyst of the pancreas was also a possibility. At this stage, options for further evaluation included tumor markers, needle biopsy, CT, upper gastrointestinal series, endoscopic retrograde cholangiopancreatography (ERCP), angiography, and magnetic resonance imaging (MRI).

Tumor markers such as CEA or Ca 19-9 are thought to be 85% specific at best (5) and, therefore, as suggested above, a negative result would not have altered management. Although fine-needle aspiration of the pancreas might confirm malignancy, a negative result does not exclude malignancy. Moreover, the patient would have been subjected to an added risk of tumor spread or intraperitoneal seeding of malignant cells if this course were followed (6,7). In general, our surgical philosophy is to consider percutaneous aspiration biopsy only in those instances where operative intervention is not a consideration. Because a positive result from either tumor markers or aspiration cytology would not preclude surgery, these tests were not performed, but thought was given instead to tests that might delineate tumor extent and resectability.

If liver metastases had been evident or if extrapancreatic involvement had been demonstrated, then surgery might not have been appropriate because cure would not have been possible (8). Unlike carcinoma of the pancreatic head, the need for palliation of incipient bile duct or gastric outlet obstruction is not usually a consideration in lesions of the pancreatic tail. Therefore, "palliative

surgery" in the case of advanced disease is rarely a consideration. This makes reliable preoperative staging a vital component of preoperative evaluation.

ERCP has proved useful in establishing a diagnosis of pancreatic cancer but is of little value in outlining tumor extent (9). An upper gastrointestinal series might hint at tumor extent, but would yield far less staging information than either CT, ultrasound (US), or MRI. MRI has not been found superior to CT in delineating pancreatic cancers (10), and although US is sometimes useful in pancreatic cancer, its use depends too much on the quality of instrumentation and ability of the observer to be uniformly reliable (11). Selective angiography is sometimes helpful in the investigation of tumors of the head of pancreas indicating inoperable mesenteric or portal vein involvement or superior mesenteric artery encasement. However, in tumors of the tail, it does not provide further useful additional information in comparison to CT (8). CT therefore remains the gold standard of pancreatic imaging and was our method of further evaluation.

Laparoscopy, often an important preliminary step before major gastrointestinal surgery and an increasingly important adjunct to staging of gastrointestinal malignancies, was not performed in this case. Some studies, however, would suggest that the incidence of intraperitoneal and liver metastases is sufficiently common to make this a useful procedure in evaluating patients in whom CT shows a potentially resectable lesion (12).

The only treatment offering potential cure for a patient with pancreatic cancer is surgery. As there is a considerable possibility that a decision not to proceed might be taken after the abdomen was opened in our patient (90%) (8) and as the chances of long-term cure are slim (30% 5-year survival at best if lesions <2 cm) (13), it was important to discuss fully the options, risks, and probable outcome with the patient and responsible relatives. Furthermore, laparotomy in an obese elderly patient is not without risk. Therefore, appropriate evaluation of functional status, particularly of respiratory function and nutritional state, was appropriate. To this end, pulmonary function studies were performed and indicated reasonable respiratory function as did assessment of nutritional status.

Although the risk of infection after splenectomy in adults is controversial (14), we believe that the risk/benefit ratio is low enough to recommend routine pneumococcal vaccination. Although this is ideally performed 6 weeks before surgery, from a practical standpoint this usually occurs a few days before surgery. Preparation of the gastrointestinal tract was also performed to reduce the possibility of contamination from intestinal flora; if resection of adjacent involved viscera was necessary, that is AJCC stage II (Table 28–1).

Although a midline incision gives reasonable access to the pancreas, in this patient's case, a transverse epigastric incision was chosen. This incision provides suitable access to the pancreas and spleen and is associated with fewer postoperative wound problems, for example, dehiscence and herniae. Evidence of intraperitoneal, liver, omental, colonic, or nodal involvement would have reduced the likelihood of cure and would have altered our decision to proceed. It is suggested that only AJCC stage I and II tumors will benefit from surgical resection (8).

The surgical options for tumors of the pancreatic tail are few: total pancreatectomy, distal pancreatectomy, or distal pancreatectomy with splenectomy. As total pancreatectomy or radical regional resection does not confer survival benefit and is associated with significant morbidity (15), we opted for a less radical procedure. We feel that the theoretical risks of infection after splenectomy in adults do not outweigh the potential gain of a better "cancer operation" when the spleen and tail of the pancreas are resected en bloc. Furthermore, we feel

that splenectomy facilitates distal pancreatectomy. Insofar as possible, we avoid transfusion in cancer surgery, and there is some evidence to suggest this strategy to be appropriate in light of reports that note that administration of blood during surgery for pancreatic cancer adversely affects survival (16).

Although some would argue that the celiac plexus should be injected for control of pain, or potential pain, during surgery for pancreatic carcinoma (17), this procedure is not without risk. Furthermore, our patient did not have or develop associated back pain with her tumor, and in our experience, radiologic injection of the celiac plexus is possible, if required. Because deep venous thrombosis (DVT) is a recognized risk in elderly obese patients undergoing surgery, and particularly in those with pancreatic cancer, a mechanical device ("thrombo-guards") performing pneumatic compression of calf and thigh muscles during surgery was employed and early ambulation in graduated compression stockings encouraged in an effort to reduce the risk of DVT after surgery.

No form of treatment is superior to surgery in resectable pancreatic cancer (8). The role of adjuvant therapy in this type of tumor is less clear. There is no definite evidence of benefit derived from intraoperative radiotherapy for pancreatic cancer in randomized trials (18), and because there are potential complications, intraoperative radiotherapy was not used.

Other possibilities for adjuvant therapy in pancreatic cancer include hormonal manipulation, cytokine therapy (interleukin-2, IL-2), somatostatin, chemotherapy, and external beam irradiation. Of these, combination adjuvant radiation and chemotherapy (5-FU and DXT) were advised because this regimen has been shown to have a slightly beneficial effect on patient longevity (19). Although it has been documented that some pancreatic tumors possess hormone receptors, and in some animal models of pancreatic cancer gonadotrophin agonists appear to confirm survival benefit, no evidence for survival benefit with hormonal manipulation has been demonstrated in humans (20). Similarly, theoretical advantages associated with somatostatin inhibition of cholecystokinin in pancreatic tumor promotion have not translated to survival advantage in humans (21) and, certainly, the diarrhea associated with prolonged high-dose somatostatin administration makes this a difficult treatment option for patients. Cytokine therapy (e.g., IL-2) is associated with considerable toxicity but has been used in animal models of pancreatic cancer and has been suggested to offer limited benefit. Again, this form of adjuvant therapy has not been demonstrated to offer survival advantage in humans.

Follow-up for any cancer is important from two aspects: to identify recurrence if treatment options exist and to be able to give accurate prognostic information to patients and relatives. In relation to pancreatic cancer, the former is less important because no therapy has had

Table 28–1. *AJCC staging of carcinoma of the pancreas*

Stage	TNM description
I T1–2 N0 M0	No direct extension and no regional noda linvolvement
II T3 N0 M0	Direct extension into adjacent tissue but no lymph node involvement
III T1–3 N1 M0	Regional lymph node involvement with or without adjacent tissue involvement
IV T1–3 N0–1 M1	Distant metastatic disease present

T1 indicates no direct extension beyond pancreas, T1a that the lesion is less than 2 cm in diameter, T1b that the lesion is more than 2 cm in diameter.

T2 indicates limited direct extension into adjacent bile duct, stomach, or duodenum.

T3 indicates that there is advanced local extension.

N0 indicates no nodal involvement.

M0 indicates no metastases.

worthwhile impact on pancreatic cancer recurrence. CT is the radiologic investigation of choice and should be performed at intervals of 3 to 6 months. Tumor markers such as CA 19-9 may in the future give added information but, at this stage, are thought to be useful only in those patients in whom evidence of CA 19-9 has disappeared after resection. Further modification of techniques for tumor DNA analysis may lead to more accurate assessment of recurrence risk because it has been shown, as in other tumors, that nondiploid lesions are subject to a higher risk of recurrence (22).

In summary, although this woman presented in a rather fortuitous fashion and was managed with best available treatment, her outcome was typical for patients with pancreatic cancer who, in most cases, fail to survive for even 1 year after surgery.

REFERENCES

1. American Cancer Society. *Cancer facts and figures 1991.* Atlanta: American Cancer Society; 1991.
2. van Heerden JA. Pancreatic resection for carcinoma of the pancreas: Whipples versus total pancreatectomy—an institutional experience. *World J Surg* 1984;8:880–8.
3. Trede M, Schwall G. The complications of pancreatectomy. *Ann Surg* 1988;207:39–47.
4. Connolly MM, Dawson PJ, Michelassi F, Moosa AR, Lowenstein F. Survival in 1001 patients with carcinoma of the pancreas. *Ann Surg* 1987;206:366–73.
5. Steinberg W. The clinical utility of the CA 19-9 tumor associated antigen. *Am J Gastroenterol* 1990;85:350–5.
6. Rashleigh-Belcher HJC, Russell RCG, Lees WR. Cutaneous seeding of pancreatic carcinoma by fine needle aspiration biopsy. *Br J Radiol* 1986;59:182–3.
7. Weiss SM, Skibber JM, Mohiuddin M, Rosato FE. Rapid intraabdominal spread of pancreatic cancer. *Arch Surg* 1985;120:415–6.
8. Warshaw AL, Fernandez-del Castillo C. Pancreatic carcinoma. *N Engl J Med* 1992;326:455–65.
9. Michelassi F, Erroi F, Dawson PJ, et al. Experience with 647 consecutive tumors of the duodenum, ampulla, head of pancreas and distal common bile duct. *Ann Surg* 1989;210:544–54.
10. Steiner E, Stark DD, Hahn PF, et al. Imaging of pancreatic neoplasms: comparison of MR and CT. *AJR* 1989;152:487–9.
11. Balthazar EJ, Cahko AC. Computed tomography of pancreatic masses. *Am J Gastroenterol* 1090;85:343–9.
12. Warshaw AL, Gu Z-Y, Wittenberg J, Waltman AC. Preoperative staging and assessment of resectability of pancreatic cancer. *Arch Surg* 1990;125:230–3.
13. Tsuchiya R, Noda T, Harada M, et al. Collective review of small carcinomas of the pancreas. *Ann Surg* 1986;203:77–81.
14. Singer DB. Postsplenectomy sepsis. *Perspect Pediat Pathol* 1973;1:285–311.
15. van Heerden JA, ReMine WH, Weiland LH, McIlrath DC, Ilstrup DM. Total pancreatectomy for ductal adenocarcinoma of the pancreas. *Am J Surg* 1981;142:308–11.
16. Cameron JL, Crist DW, Sitzman JV, et al. Factors influencing survival after pancreaticoduodenectomy for pancreatic cancer. *Am J Surg* 1991;161:120–5.
17. Sarr MG, Cameron JL. Surgical management of unresectable carcinoma of the pancreas. *Surgery* 1982;91:123–33.
18. Dobelbower RR Jr, Konski AA, Merrick HW III, Bronn DG, Schifeling D, Kamen C. Intraoperative electron beam radiation therapy (IOE-BRT) for carcinoma of the exocrine pancreas. *Int J Radiat Oncol Biol Phys* 1991;20:113–9.
19. Gastrointestinal Tumor Study Group. Further evidence of effective adjuvant combined radiation and chemotherapy following curative resection of pancreatic cancer. *Cancer* 1987;59:2006–10.
20. Conn PM, Crowley WF. Gonadotrophin-releasing hormone and its analogues. *N Engl J Med* 1991;324:93–103.
21. Smith JP, Solomon TE, Bagheri S, Kramer S. Cholecystokinin stimulates growth of human pancreatic adenocarcinoma SW-1990. *Dig Dis Sci* 1990;35:1377–84.
22. Allison DC, Bose KK, Hruban RH, et al. Pancreatic cancer cell DNA content correlates with long term survival after pancreaticoduodenectomy. *Ann Surg* 1991;214:648–56.

COMMENTARY by John L. Cameron

The diagnosis and management of this 64-year-old woman with carcinoma of the body of her pancreas, as described by Drs. Gough and van Heerden, were carried out in an expeditious and exemplary fashion. In treating this disease there are few options, and thus in most institutions the management would have been similar to that carried out at the Mayo Clinic. It is interesting that this patient was a woman because with carcinoma of the head of the pancreas there is a male predominance. However, with carcinoma of the body and tail of the pancreas, in a series of 113 patients reported in 1992 from The Johns Hopkins Hospital, the disease was more common in women.

Most patients with carcinoma of the body of the pancreas present with abdominal pain, as did the patient discussed above. However, weight loss is also a common feature, being present in more than half of such patients. It is not clear to me why this patient had an ultrasound examination first. In my experience, for any patient over the age of 60 years, CT scan is to be preferred as the first test rather than ultrasound. If ultrasound is the first study, then generally patients are going to require both examinations, as did this patient. In most institutions I do not believe pulmonary function studies would be part of a routine preoperative evaluation. Only if pulmonary symptoms were present would arterial blood gases or pulmonary function studies be determined. In addition, "Go-Lytely" would not be administered in many hospitals, as it is usually indicated for colonic bowel preparation. The ingestion of "Go-Lytely" is not a pleasant experience, and if not clearly indicated is to be avoided.

The operative procedure as described by Drs. Gough and van Heerden was interesting in that they divided the neck of the pancreas first, and then mobilized the gland from neck to body to tail. I believe most surgeons would have mobilized the spleen out of the retroperitoneum, divided the vasa brevia and omental attachments, and then dissected the tail and the body of the pancreas out of the retroperitoneum, dividing the neck of the pancreas only at the end of the dissection. The administration of the somatostatin analog octreotide, although theoretically attractive, is probably an unnecessary expense. Clinically relevant pancreatic-cutaneous fistulas rarely result after distal pancreatectomy for a carcinoma of the body or tail when the remaining head and its ductal system are normal. Furthermore, the use of a nasogastric tube for 2 days after surgery is a practice that probably would be avoided in most institutions. For most abdominal surgery, nasogastric suction is not only unnecessary but is a substantial patient inconvenience and can increase the incidence of respiratory complications.

It is unknown whether or not adjuvant therapy is effective in prolonging survival after resection of a carcinoma of the body or tail of the pancreas as it clearly is for carcinoma of the head of the pancreas. However, we would agree that adjuvant therapy should be recommended.

I would disagree with the authors that celiac plexus injection with 50% alcohol should be avoided because the procedure carries risks. In a prospective randomized study carried out at The Johns Hopkins Hospital, this procedure was found not only to be effective for pain relief in patients with carcinoma of the pancreas, but actually resulted in prolongation of survival in those patients who preoperatively presented with pain. In addition, the procedure was carried out with virtually no risk.

The course of this patient postoperatively, unfortunately, was typical of patients with carcinoma of the body and tail of the pancreas. In the series of 113 patients with carcinoma of the body and tail of the pancreas reported from The Johns Hopkins Hospital in 1992, only 9 patients (8%) were resectable. Of these nine patients, one survived for 6 years, and a second is alive 3 years after surgery.

After preoperative staging, only 62 patients were operated on, 9 were resected, and among those patients only 2 survived long term. The median survival of patients not operated on was 2 months. For those patients explored and only biopsied, the median survival was 4 months. For those patients who were operated on and biopsied and a palliative bypass carried out, the median survival was 6 months. For those patients undergoing resection, median survival was 7 months.

In summary, the presentation, management, and course of the patient presented by Drs. Gough and van Heerden were unfortunately typical of patients with carcinoma of the body and tail of the pancreas. Although one might argue with minor points in the diagnostic work-up and operative management of this patient, basically it was carried out in a standard fashion that represents current state of the art. Unfortunately, the current state of the art is totally inadequate and is not likely to improve until a tumor marker is found in stool or blood that allows earlier detection of this lethal neoplasm.

SELECTED READING

1. Nordback IH, Hruban RH, Boitnott JK, Pitt HA, Cameron JL. Carcinoma of the body and tail of the pancreas. *Am J Surg* 1992;164:26-31.

29

Malignant Islet Cell Carcinoma of the Pancreas

Michael J. DeMeure and James R. Wallace

Is postoperative adjuvant chemotherapy needed?

CASE PRESENTATION

This 30-year-old Caucasian man was in his usual state of good health until 4 months ago when he experienced an episode of hematemesis. An esophagogastroduodenoscopy demonstrated gastritis. He had no further problems until immediately before this admission, when he developed hematemesis and melena. He also began to have sharp, colicky upper abdominal pain that subsequently became dull and constant. His vomitus had initially been bloody but then became clear and bile-tinged. His past medical history is remarkable only for an elective right inguinal hernia repair and a right rotator cuff tear. His current medications are ranitidine and occasional acetaminophen. He is not allergic to any medications. He does not smoke and drinks one or two beers weekly. He is employed as an electronics technician. His family history is notable only in that his father has peptic ulcer disease.

Initial physical exam showed him to be hemodynamically stable. He had no rashes. His heart and lung exam were normal. His jugular veins were not distended, and he had no discernible adenopathy. His abdomen was neither tender nor distended. The spleen was enlarged with the tip easily palpable below the left costal margin. The stool was guaiac- positive for occult blood.

Admission laboratory data showed a hematocrit value of 36%. His platelet count was 201,000/cm³. The serum electrolyte levels were normal with a blood urea nitrogen of 9 mg/dL and a creatinine level of 0.9 mg/dL. The serum glucose level was 101 mg/dL. The serum amylase was 45 IU/L. A liver enzyme panel consisting of serum bilirubin,

alkaline phosphatase SGPT, and GGT was normal. A urine analysis was normal. The chest radiograph and electrocardiogram were normal.

Endoscopic evaluation of the upper gastrointestinal tract now showed erosive esophagitis and gastric varices. A computed tomographic (CT) scan of the abdomen and pelvis demonstrated a large 7 × 8 cm mass in the region of the tail of the pancreas (Fig. 29–1). It appeared to have a necrotic center. The splenic vein was occluded and gastric varices were noted. There was evidence of diffuse fatty infiltration of the liver but no focal

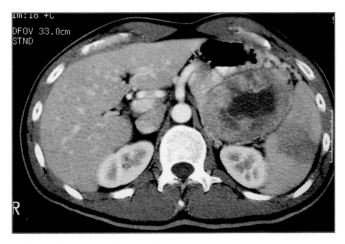

FIG. 29–1. A CT scan showing a large 7 × 8 cm mass located in the tail of the pancreas that consists of a very thickened wall and low density center presumably representing necrosis. Large perigastric varices are seen.

lesions. There was no evidence of enlarged lymph nodes in the retroperitoneum.

Preoperative serum gastrin, glucagon, insulin, and chromogranin A levels were normal. Pneumococcus, H. influenzae and meningococcus vaccines were administered days before operation. A bilateral subcostal incision was made. A thorough exploration of the abdomen showed only a large mass in the tail of the pancreas. There was no evidence of masses within the liver. There were no gallstones. The stomach was smooth, with no masses, but there were varices present in the short gastric vessels. The spleen was enlarged to about three times its normal size. The colon and pelvis were normal. Upon entering the lesser sac, the posterior wall of the stomach was noted to be free from the pancreatic mass. The mass encompassed the distal half of the tail of the pancreas, was hard, and was intimately involved with the hilum of the spleen. The spleen and tail of the pancreas were removed en bloc. The pancreatic duct was identified and oversewn. The capsule of the pancreas was approximated with interrupted sutures. Frozen section of the specimen performed during the operation demonstrated an islet cell tumor with a clear surgical margin at the pancreatic border. Postoperatively the patient did well, except for a prolonged ileus. He was maintained on nasogastric suction until 2 weeks after his operation, at which time the patient was able to eat and was discharged.

A firm mass measuring $11.0 \times 6.5 \times 3.0$ cm was present in the submitted tail of the pancreas. This mass abutted the splenic hilum. The cut surface had a homogeneous, fish-flesh, tan appearance. Microscopy showed nests and balls of tumor cells divided by thin, fibrous septa (Fig. 29–2). These cells are characterized by ample amounts of eosinophilic cytoplasm and vesicular nuclei with clumped chromatin. Scattered mitotic figures were seen. Sections through the splenic vein showed a large tumor thrombus composed of the same malignant cells, extending up to the venous ligature. Immunohistochemical staining for glucagon was positive in the cytoplasm of the cells. Staining, however, for insulin, gastrin, chromogranins, and pancreatic polypeptide was negative. The spleen was not invaded by the tumor and was otherwise normal. The final diagnosis is, therefore, a malignant pancreatic glucagonoma. Without residual disease, radiation therapy was believed to be of no benefit and was not recommended.

In general, islet cell carcinomas are quite indolent, requiring months to years to recur, at which time the lesions may be surgically resectable. The evaluation by Medical Oncology centered on three points: first, the patient is quite young, desirous of beginning a family, and is concerned about potential gonadal toxicity should adjuvant chemotherapy be recommended. Additional concerns with adjuvant chemotherapy include the possible late complications. Patients have received adriamycin and DTIC as part of the

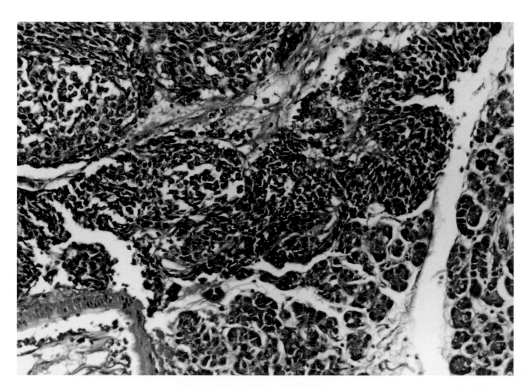

FIG. 29–2. A histologic section through the pancreatic tumor shows nests and balls of tumor cells divided by thin fibrous septae. These cells are characterized by ample eosinophilic cytoplasm and vesicular nuclei with clumped chromatin. Scattered mitotic figures are seen.

ABVD chemotherapy regimen for Hodgkin's disease since approximately 1970. Thus, there is an almost 25-year follow-up on such patients. To date, those patients have not had an increased risk of secondary malignancies or early onset of cardiac disease. The fact that the ABVD regimen relatively spares the gonads in terms of toxicity is one of the many reasons why this regimen has essentially replaced the original MOPP regimen for Hodgkin's disease. No one yet, however, has lived for 30 or 40 years after such a treatment regimen. Streptozocin carries the risk of renal and pancreatic islet damage. The risk of pancreatic islet cell damage is approximately 10%, and can be monitored with serial glucose testing. Short-term renal complications exist, so renal function is monitored by serial blood tests and urinalysis. Although there have been some late renal complications from a variety of nitrosourea-containing regimens, this has not been observed with streptozocin, perhaps because it has been used in few situations in which long-term survival is anticipated. Finally, the best chance for cure is to eradicate potential microscopic disease immediately because, should he relapse, the chances of long-term disease control are limited.

The consensus opinion was to treat with chemotherapy based on the analogy with breast cancer. It is now clear that adriamycin plus DTIC gives a response rate of more than 30% in islet cell tumors. Streptozocin alone historically gave a response rate of somewhere between 15% and 30%. Adjuvant chemotherapy was first demonstrated to be effective in breast cancer patients using melphalan alone, a drug that has about a 20% to 25% response rate in breast cancer. Modern chemotherapy regimens for breast cancer have a much higher level of antitumor activity and a correspondingly improved efficacy rate in preventing relapse of early-stage breast cancer. It seems that the scientific observation and differential analogy are valid. Following this line of reasoning, the patient was referred for sperm banking to allow for the possibility of chemotherapy-induced sterility. In the meantime, the patient and his wife will pursue starting a family and we anticipate beginning adjuvant chemotherapy 8 to 12 weeks after operation.

The patient is now 9 months from his operation and is doing well. Postoperative serial measurements of serum glucagon and chromogranin A levels have been normal.

He has resumed work as an electrician for the past 7 months and his wife is now 10 weeks pregnant.

COMMENTARY by Murray F. Brennan

The present case appropriately represents a rather classic presentation of a malignant islet cell tumor. Large cystic lesions in the distal pancreas are usually islet cell tumors with central necrosis, although cystadenomas or cystadenocarcinomas can present in similar fashion. The gastric varices and splenic vein obstruction would suggest a malignant lesion. There was no clinically significant endocrine dysfunction and a normal blood glucose.

The operative approach, I would have thought, was appropriate and the splenectomy certainly justified. We would have considered pneumococcal prophylaxis in a young man, given either more than 1 week before the procedure or at the time of his follow-up visit.

One might debate the diagnosis of malignant glucagonoma in this patient. Diagnosis is based on immunohistochemical representation of marked glucagon staining on the resected specimen. Some clinicians reserve the functional title for those who have clinical function or markedly elevated serum markers. In this case, serum markers were not available preoperatively and, rather surprisingly, given the selective staining of the tumor for glucagon, no postoperative baseline level was obtained, which would be an excellent marker for subsequent recurrence. The patient had none of the sequelae of extensive glucagon production such as glucose intolerance, marked hypoaminoacidemia, or desquamating skin rash.

A further issue of considerable debate was the decision to treat this patient with adjuvant chemotherapy. Malignant islet cell tumors are notoriously variable in their clinical course, some being cured in a first operation, others with metastatic disease that is indolent, and others with aggressive metastatic dissemination. The value of chemotherapy in this situation is certainly unproved and an alternative would have been to follow the patient conservatively. Treatment would then be reserved for recurrent disease.

SECTION V

Bile Duct

30

Papillary Cholangiocarcinoma (Klatskin Tumor)

Leslie H. Blumgart

Can surgery cure? Does anything else help?

CASE PRESENTATION

An otherwise healthy 56-year-old white man presented with painless jaundice. The patient's history dates back to 6 years before this presentation, when he had an episode of pruritis and jaundice accompanied by a total bilirubin of 5.8, alkaline phosphatase of 163 U/L (nl 0–115), SGOT 50 U/L, and SGPT 114 U/L. Before this first episode, he had no history of fatty food intolerance, abdominal pain, weight loss, or prior jaundice. The patient does not smoke and rarely drinks alcohol. No history exists of hyperlipidemia, prior blood transfusions, or hepatitis. An abdominal ultrasound at that time demonstrated a contracted gallbladder with no stones, and no dilated extra- or intrahepatic bile ducts. An abdominal computed tomography (CT) scan showed the pancreas to be normal, and again the liver had no dilated ducts or other abnormalities. Endoscopic retrograde cholangiopancreatography (ERCP) was performed and showed a normal pancreatic duct and a normal common bile duct, without stones or dilatation; notation was made, however, of the fact that there was no visualization of the bile ducts in the left lobe of the liver beyond the main left hepatic duct. His clinical course at the time of this original event was one of gradual resolution of his jaundice and pruritis over 2 months, with the bilirubin level dropping to 2.1 and alkaline phosphatase becoming normal. No further testing was done, and the patient was lost to follow-up for 6 years.

The patient proceeded to do well until 3 months before this admission, when he noted, while overseas, the onset of a sudden "flu-like" illness accompanied by some nausea and rigors. One month later the patient noted himself to be jaundiced again, but because the previous attack many years prior had subsided spontaneously, he deferred medical advice for several weeks until pruritis developed. Upon seeking attention, he was found to be clinically jaundiced, with a serum total bilirubin of 8.8 mg/dL (nl 0–1.0), alkaline phosphatase of 461 U/L (nl 0–115), AST 255 U/L, and ALT 463 U/L; his prothrombin time and PTT were normal, CBC normal, and platelet count normal. Antismooth muscle antibody was weakly positive at the 1:20 range; a full hepatitis panel was negative. Serum iron and iron-binding levels were nonspecifically mildly elevated and possibly consistent with some type of hepatic inflammatory process. A serum protein electrophoresis was normal.

The radiologic evaluation at this second presentation consisted of a right upper quadrant ultrasound, which showed a somewhat thickened gallbladder wall but without stones, and some mild dilatation of the intrahepatic bile ducts; a CT scan of the liver showed no abnormality. Because of the concern of the chronic elevation of serum liver function studies over the years, a percutaneous right lobe of liver biopsy was done before evaluation at our institution, ostensibly to rule out chronic hepatitis; the biopsy showed normal liver cells, with no evidence of fatty change, cirrhosis, or malignancy. This was followed by an ERCP showing abrupt cessation of dye flow in the common hepatic duct, just proximal to the takeoff of the cystic duct; a percutaneous transhepatic cholangiography showed an obstruction of the right and left hepatic ducts, along with a 4-cm obstructed segment of common hepatic duct (Fig. 30–1). At this point, an 8F ring biliary drainage catheter was placed percutaneously through the hepatic

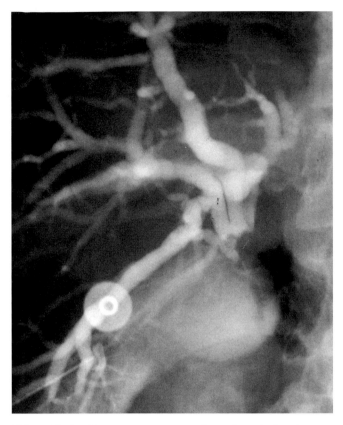

FIG. 30–1. Percutaneous transhepatic cholangiogram demonstrates the right and left hepatic ducts to be obstructed as well as the common hepatic duct.

duct obstruction and into the duodenum for internal biliary drainage; the patient was now referred to our institution.

Further investigation at our institution consisted of celiac, left gastric, and superior mesenteric arteriography; tube study of the indwelling biliary-duodenal catheter; and dynamic CT portography. The arteriogram demonstrated an aberrant right gastric artery arising from the left hepatic artery, otherwise standard arterial anatomy; the venous phase showed severe compression of the left portal vein with patency of the main portal vein branch and anterior impression on the right main portal vein branch (Fig. 30–2). The contrast injection through the indwelling biliary drainage catheter showed a papillary-appearing, expansile filling defect of the proximal left hepatic duct with extension into the proximal common hepatic duct; no filling defects were seen in the right hepatic duct (Fig. 30–3). Dynamic CT portography of the liver demonstrated the entire left hepatic lobe to be diffusely atrophic, with dilated intrahepatic bile ducts that appeared to be compressed adjacent to each other (Fig. 30–4). Moreover, a soft tissue mass was present within the proximal left hepatic duct and the proximal common hepatic duct, corresponding to the filling defects seen on the cholan-

giogram; this mass demonstrated compression on both the right and left portal vein branches.

At this point, the clinical impression was one of a high bile duct carcinoma (cholangiocarcinoma) of the papillary type, which is generally associated with a more favorable prognosis than the usual sclerosing type. The patient was taken to the operating room and explored through an abdominal chevron incision with a vertical upper midline extension. Findings at the time of exploration included gross atrophy of the left lobe of the liver involving segments II, III, and IV, along with hypertrophy of the remaining segments. The gallbladder was modestly distended, and there was no obvious lymphatic nodal involvement. The left hepatic duct, the common hepatic duct, and the upper common bile duct were distended by a soft papillary tumor that had multiple sites of origin ("papillomatosis"); however, the origin of the right hepatic duct appeared to be free of tumor. During the dissection of the portal and hilar vessels it became apparent that they were free of tumor invasion and, in particular, the left branch of the portal vein was compressed, but not invaded. Therefore, a complete resection was performed in the form of excision of common bile duct including cholecystectomy and left hepatic lobectomy (segments II, III, IV) with excision of confluence of bile duct en bloc. Intrahepatic Roux-en-Y hepaticojejunostomy to the

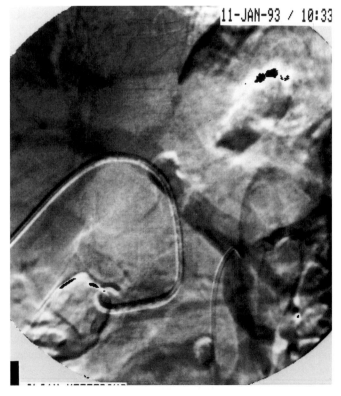

FIG. 30–2. Portal venous phase of the arteriogram shows the left portal vein to be severely compressed by tumor; the main portal vein and right portal branch appear uninvolved.

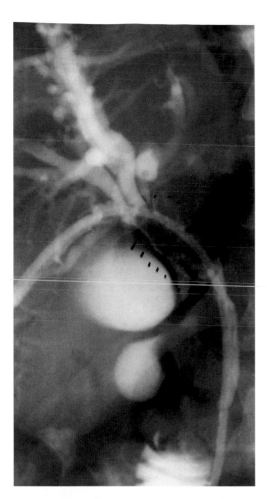

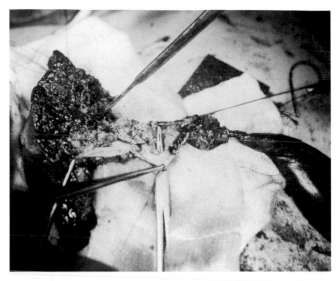

FIG. 30–5. The resected specimen is shown, consisting of attached gallbladder (*far right*), common hepatic duct, right hepatic duct margin (shown with hemostat going through its orifice), left hepatic duct, and left lobe of liver (segments II, III, IV). The resected left lobe of the liver is severely atrophic because of long-standing biliary obstruction. Note the papillary-appearing, bulging tumor as it extends throughout the left hepatic duct (from the hemostat up to the cut edge of the hepatic parenchyma).

FIG. 30–3. Injection of the indwelling biliary-duodenal stent demonstrates a papillary-appearing, expansile filling defect of the proximal left hepatic duct, with extension into the common hepatic duct (outlined by *black marks*).

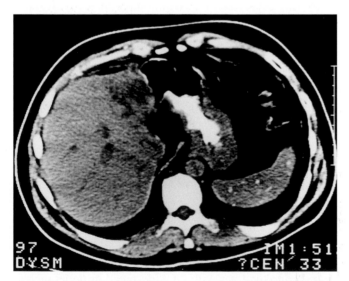

FIG. 30–4. Dynamic CT scan of the liver shows dense atrophy of the entire left lobe of the liver, consistent with long-standing left hepatic bile duct obstruction by tumor; the intrahepatic ducts of the left lobe proximal to the obstruction are markedly dilated.

remaining four hepatic ducts (two right sectoral ducts and two caudate ducts) was performed. Figure 30–5 shows the resected specimen with the bile duct opened and the papillary-appearing tumor filling the left hepatic duct. The total blood loss for the operation was 630 cc, with 315 cc occurring during the hepatic parenchymal transection; no transfusions were required. Postoperatively, the patient's course was unremarkable, and he was discharged to home on the tenth postoperative day tolerating a normal diet, and with a serum bilirubin level that was normal.

The final histologic report demonstrated that the tumor was a multifocal papillary adenocarcinoma of the bile duct ("cholangiocarcinoma") extensively involving the intraparenchymal biliary system and common hepatic duct, with focal involvement of the left hepatic duct (Fig. 30–6). There were several microscopic foci of stromal invasion present; however, the invasive component was limited in scope and did not extend completely through the fibrous tissue surrounding the biliary system at any point (Fig. 30–7); additionally, there was neither involvement of the liver parenchyma nor extrahepatic extension present. The gallbladder, cystic duct, and resected portion of the right hepatic duct were negative for tumor, and the distal bile duct margin was free of tumor as well. The resection was considered curative with all margins negative, and no adjuvant radiation or chemotherapy was recommended at the Tumor Board conference.

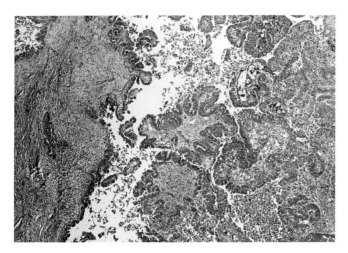

FIG. 30–6. Low-power photomicrograph shows the bile duct wall (*left*) lined by neoplastic epithelial cells that form papillary fronds filling the lumen (*right*).

COMMENTARY by John W. Braasch

This most interesting case of a Klatskin tumor illustrates the short- and long-term results of unilobar hepatic duct obstruction. At first there is brief cholangitis and jaundice, then return to normal liver function as the contralateral lobe takes over bilirubin metabolism and infection subsides, and finally lobar atrophy and contralateral lobar hypertrophy (1,2).

Klatskin tumors in general are adenocarcinomas more than 95% of the time. These tumors are most often located in the common hepatic duct or the right and left extrahepatic ducts. They frequently are associated with the presence of gallstones (3). However, the preoperative diagnosis of Klatskin is at times followed by the finding of a benign tumor, a localized sclerosing cholangitis, or nonspecific fibrous constriction in the region of the common hepatic duct or bifurcation (4). Occasionally, stones have eroded from the gallbladder onto or into the bile ducts to produce imaging similar to Klatskin tumors (Mirrizi syndrome).

Staging of Klatskin tumors can be accomplished using ultrasound, CT, arteriography, portal ultrasound, portal venography, cholangiogram by percutaneous or endoscopic means, or percutaneous cholangioscopy (5–7). These methods can outline the extent of gross tumor but cannot tell with assurance the depth of infiltration or the presence of nodes too small to be imaged by ultrasound or CT. Only percutaneous cholangiography with multiple biopsies can indicate multicentric disease with any semblance of surety (6). Location staging of the tumor in the biliary system has been reported by Bismuth (7). Stage I involves the common bile duct; stage II, the common hepatic duct; stage III, the common hepatic duct and either right or left hepatic ducts; and stage IV is diffuse. Obviously, the lower stages are more favorable.

Cytologic differences in adenocarcinomas are important. In one study, long-term survival occurred only in patients with moderately well differentiated tumors (8). As illustrated in this case, papillary tumors may have a long natural history. Their favorable aspects are that they do not tend to invade the wall of the duct but, on the other hand, are more likely to be multicentric (9).

The ideal treatment of Klatskin tumors is resection for cure. Negative margins, a lack of multicentricity, papillary histology, a lower grade of malignancy, or a lack of invasion portends a longer survival. There is some evidence that 5-year survival with a large majority of these favorable aspects might approach 20% to 30% of cases (10–14). This resection might include either of the two liver lobes and its accompanying hepatic duct with, possibly, a segment or two removed from the preserved lobe (10). Routine resection of the caudate lobe has been proposed by Nimura and others (10) because of a very high proportion of involvement of the caudate ducts by tumors in the Klatskin position. More extensive resections have been proposed to remove parts of the portal venous system supplying a remaining lobe or even portions of the arterial supply (15,16). It seems likely that these aggressive approaches might be indicated in only a few cases in which there is favorable histologic finding and the extended resection was necessary to obtain clear margins.

The question of liver transplantation arises. Transplantation seems logical for tumor stage II carcinomas restricted to the liver without widespread or nodal metastases and not suitable for partial liver resection because of the lobes and segments involved. The experience with transplantation is not extensive (17–19) but supports its use in highly selected cases. The major problem with the

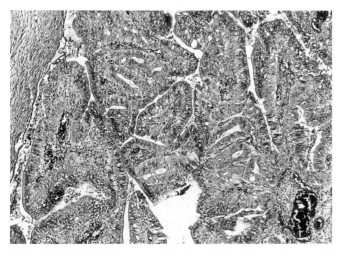

FIG. 30–7. At higher magnification, this photomicrograph demonstrates that each papilla consists of an inflamed fibrovascular core lined by a single layer of columnar cells, with features of malignancy including nuclear atypia and pseudostratification.

indications for transplantation is recognizing microscopic spread outside the liver preoperatively or at laparotomy.

The best palliation seems to be resection with proximal anastomosis of the biliary system or amputation of the biliary ducts above the tumor and proximal anastomosis to the jejunum, although a blinded prospective trial has not been suitably organized (3). Other procedures for palliation include intubation carried out either retrograde via an endoscope or percutaneously through the liver. The obstructed biliary ducts may be dilated and stents may be placed, which range from Silastic to newer metal expandable types (11, 20). Stenting is useful in patients with lesser survival times because plugging and migration of stents may be a multiple recurring problem for longer surviving patients. Adjuvant chemotherapy does not have an adequate track record and the same may be said for external radiation or brachytherapy delivered by percutaneous intraductal stents (3).

To return to the management of this case, the imaging work-up was very appropriate. The surgical resection was most satisfactory except that excision of the caudate lobe might have been considered as a routine measure. The prognosis in this case is good, but not uncommonly there is recurrence of postoperative tumor in the sixth through the tenth postoperative years.

REFERENCES

1. Braasch JW, Whitcomb FF Jr, Watkins E Jr, et al. Segmental obstruction of the bile duct. *Surg Gynecol Obstet* 1972;134:915–20.
2. Longmire WP Jr, Tompkins RK. Lesions of the segmental and lobar hepatic ducts. *Ann Surg* 1975;182:478–95.
3. Stain SC, Baer HU, Dennison AR, Blumgart LH. Current management of hilar cholangiocarcinoma. *Surg Gynecol Obstet* 1992;175:579–88.
4. Wetter LA, Ring EJ, Pellegrini CA, Way LW. Differential diagnosis of sclerosing cholangiocarcinomas of the common hepatic duct (Klatskin tumors). *Am J Surg* 1991;161:57–63.
5. Looser C, Stain SC, Baer HU. Staging of hilar cholangiocarcinoma by ultrasound and duplex sonography: a comparison with angiography and operative findings. *Br J Radiol* 1992;65:871–7.
6. Nimura Y. Staging of biliary carcinoma: cholangiography and cholangioscopy. *Endoscopy* 1993;25:76–80.
7. Bismuth H, Nakache R, Diamond T. Management strategies in resection for hilar cholangiocarcinoma. *Ann Surg* 1992;215:31–8.
8. Ross AP, Braasch JW, Warren KW. Carcinoma of the proximal bile ducts. *Surg Gynecol Obstet* 1973;136:923–8.
9. Tompkins RK, Johnson J, Storm FK, Longmire WP Jr. Operative endoscopy in the management of biliary tract neoplasms. *Ann J Surg* 1976;132:174–82.
10. Nimura Y. Hepatectomy for proximal bile duct cancer. In: *Surgical disease of the biliary tract and pancreas. Multidisciplinary management*, Braasch JW, Tompkins RK, eds. St. Louis: Mosby Year Book; 1994.
11. Baer HU, Stain SC, Dennison AR et al. Improvements in survival by aggressive resections of hilar cholangiocarcinoma. *Ann Surg* 1993;217:20–7.
12. Pinson CW, Rossi RL, Extended right hepatic lobectomy, left hepatic lobectomy and skeletonization resection for proximal bile duct cancer. *World J Surg* 1988;12:52–9.
13. Cameron JL, Pitt HA, Zinner MJ, et al. Management of proximal cholangiocarcinomas by surgical resection and radiotherapy. *Am J Surg* 1990;159:91–8.
14. Tompkins RK, Saunders K. Roslyn JJ, Longmire WP Jr. Changing patterns in diagnosis and management of bile duct cancer. *Ann Surg* 1990;211:614–21.
15. Tsuzuke T, Ogata Y, Iida S, et al. Carcinoma of the bifurcation of the hepatic ducts. *Arch Surg* 1983;118:1147–51.
16. Lygidakis NJ, van der Heyde MN, van Dongen RJAM, et al. Surgical approaches for unresectable primary carcinoma of the hepatic hilus. *Surg Gynecol Obstet* 1988;166:107–14.
17. O'Grady JG, Polsen RJ, Rolles K, et al. Liver transplantation for malignant disease. Results in 93 consecutive patients. *Ann Surg* 1988;107:373–9.
18. Haug CE, Jenkins RL, Rohrer RJ, et al. Liver transplantation for primary hepatic cancer. *Transplantation* 1993;53:376–82.
19. Pichlmayr R, Weimann A, Steinhoff G, Ringe B. Chirurgische eingriffe bei proximalen gallenwegstumoren. *Chirurg* 1992;63;539–47.
20. Adam A, Chetty N, Roddie M, et al. Self expandable stainless steel endoprostheses for the treatment of malignant bile duct obstruction. *Am J Roentgenol* 1991;156:321–5.

31 Gallbladder Cancer

Stephen F. Sener, Richard H. Larson, and Janardan D. Khandekar

*Does any tumor-directed therapy make a difference once
the gallbladder has been removed?*

CASE PRESENTATION

A 39-year-old black woman presented at another hospital with a 2-month history of intermittent epigastric pain. The pain occurred 2 hours after eating and was accompanied by nausea. The patient was admitted for medical evaluation with severe pain in the epigastrium radiating across the abdomen to the back and right shoulder. She was vomiting relentlessly.

Her past medical and family history were unremarkable, except that the patient had been treated for about 1 year for iron-deficiency anemia with oral iron supplements.

At the time of admission, the initial laboratory data revealed a white blood cell count of 8,400 and a Hmb of 7.8 g/dL. The liver function profile showed a total bilirubin (0.2–1.3) of 2.1 mg/dL, alkaline phosphatase (50–136) of 233 U/L, LDH (100–225) of 800 U/L, SGOT (5–35) of 646 U/L, SGPT (7–56) of 462 U/L, and serum amylase (30–110) of 46 U/L.

An ultrasound showed thickening of the gallbladder wall, cholecystolithiasis, and a bile duct of 1.1 cm diameter. Choledocholithiasis was not seen.

An open cholecystectomy and common bile duct exploration were done. At operation, the findings were consistent with acute cholecystitis—a firm gallbladder was packed with stones. The surgeon did not see gross infiltration of the liver bed by tumor. The slightly dilated bile duct was explored after an operative cholangiogram showed obstruction to contrast dye at the ampulla of Vater. No bile duct stones were found. After a Bakes dilator was passed into the duodenum, an 18-F T tube was placed in the common bile duct.

Microscopic examination of the gallbladder revealed cholecystitis and a poorly differentiated primary adenocarcinoma infiltrating the entire thickness of the wall, with invasion of serosa and subserosal fat. Perineural invasion was also noted.

Further staging evaluation revealed a CEA level of 0.7 (<3.0) ng/mL. A computerized tomogram (CT) did not demonstrate lymphadenopathy, primary tumor extension into liver, or metastatic disease. A chest roentgenogram showed normal results.

The patient recovered well and was asymptomatic when her case was presented at our hospital Tumor Board 2 months after cholecystectomy. The consensus opinion was that the patient be reoperated on for operative staging and treatment and have postoperative external beam radiation with sensitizing doses of 5-fluorouracil (5-FU).

At reoperation in our hospital, no metastatic disease was identified. Specifically, there was no ascites, peritoneal seeding, omental seeding, obvious tumor in the liver bed, or liver metastases. Portal vein–hepatic artery lymphadenectomy demonstrated histologically uninvolved nodes. Hepatic resection of the gallbladder fossa (Couinaud IV–V) revealed poorly differentiated adenocarcinoma. There was no gross invasion of the hepatic parenchyma, and resection margins were free of tumor (Fig. 31–1). The limits of resection were marked with surgical clips to outline the radiation field.

Five weeks after lymphadenectomy-hepatectomy, the patient started radiation-chemotherapy, consisting of 5-fluorouracil, 1,000 mg/day for 3 days, by bolus systemic intravenous infusion during the first and last 3 days of radiation treatments. The dose of radiation was 5,000

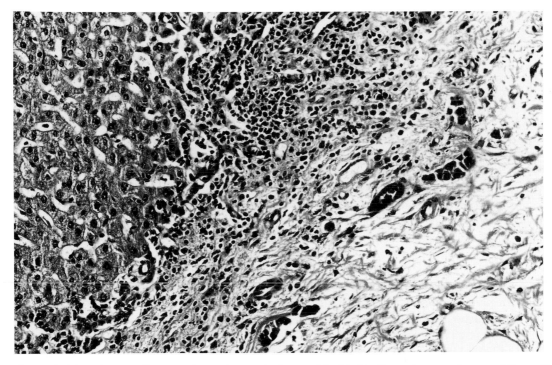

FIG. 31–1. Hepatic resection specimen demonstrating residual infiltrating adenocarcinoma of the gallbladder surrounded by inflammatory response in the gallbladder bed (*right*) approaching hepatic parenchyma (*left*) (×200).

cGy, delivered in anterior and lateral opposed fields at 200 cGy/day for 25 days. The adjuvant therapy was delivered without dose or treatment schedule modification.

The patient was well and disease-free for 16 months, when she presented with a gastric outlet obstruction and obstructive jaundice. Upper gastrointestinal endoscopy with retrograde cholangiopancreatography (ERCP) demonstrated a mass in the lateral duodenal wall, which, on microscopic examination, revealed recurrent adenocarcinoma. The proximal bile duct was not able to be cannulated during the procedure because of a distal common bile duct stricture. A CT scan demonstrated the mass in the subhepatic space, invading the duodenum. There was no evidence of hepatic metastases or other extrahepatic disease. The proximal biliary tree was dilated, as suggested by the ERCP. Celiac-superior mesenteric artery angiogram demonstrated the mass, but there was no invasion or distortion of portal vein identified.

The patient was returned to the operating room to bypass the biliary and gastrointestinal obstructions. At the time of laparotomy, the only tumor found was an unresectable local recurrence of the primary cancer, extending from the lateral duodenal wall up into the Couinaud IV hepatic segment and into the central portion of the liver. A T tube was placed in the proximal common bile duct, and a posterior retrocolic loop gastrojejunostomy was done. A feeding jejunostomy tube was also inserted.

The patient had a prolonged postoperative hospital course lasting 6 weeks, during which she developed a lateral duodenal fistula with sepsis. Percutaneous drainage, hyperalimentation, antibiotics, H_2 blockers, and somatostatin analog were ultimately able to control the fistula.

Approximately 3 months after the bypass operation, the patient felt well enough to receive four weekly intravenous bolus injections of 5-FU 1,000 mg, and leucovorin, 400 mg. However, within 2 months the patient presented with a complete right transverse colon obstruction. At this time, a CT scan revealed significant ascites and advanced local recurrence of cancer involving the colon, duodenum, subhepatic space, and liver. There was no evidence of metastatic disease in liver or gross disease elsewhere in the abdominal cavity. No further interventions other than comfort measures were thought appropriate by patient and treating physicians, and the patient expired in the care of the hospice unit.

The disease-free survival time from cholecystectomy to bypass for local recurrence was 16 months, and the total survival time was 23 months.

COMMENTARY by John W. Braasch

Unfortunately, this case of gallbladder carcinoma is all very typical. This is a tumor that is difficult to prevent, to recognize preoperatively, and to treat appropriately, and about which it is difficult to obtain meaningful data for its future management.

Carcinoma of the gallbladder (adenocarcinoma in 95% of cases) is a rare tumor, most common in women and usually (85–90%) associated with cholelithiasis (1,2), as was the case with this patient. Carcinoma is not considered common enough to warrant cholecystectomy as a preventative measure in all patients with cholelithiasis. However, in patients with pedunculated polyps larger than 1 cm in diameter and in patients with smaller sessile polyps (3,4), cholecystectomy is indicated because carcinoma is present in many lesions of this nature. Also, an association exists with porcelain gallbladder and carcinoma, which indicates prophylactic cholecystectomy (5).

It has been suggested (6) that abnormal configurations of the pancreatic and bile duct junctions are associated with carcinoma of the gallbladder as well as with choledochocyst. It is not certain whether the risk of carcinoma of the gallbladder is high enough in these patients with abnormal junctions to warrant prophylactic cholecystectomy.

Ultrasonography (7), computed tomography (8), and magnetic resonance imaging (MRI) (9) are capable of recognizing local thickening of the gallbladder wall and the possibility of the presence of carcinoma. The expense of mass screening of all patients with gallstones by imaging at 6-month intervals seems prohibitive. Doing the same for symptoms would have saved only 2 months of cancer growth before exploration in this patient.

No blood tests are specific and sensitive enough to provide early warning, although the serum levels of alpha-fetoprotein have been reported (10) to be elevated in the presence of carcinoma of the gallbladder.

In summary, no readily available and common indications exist for early surgery for carcinoma of the gallbladder. For this reason, it is common for the diagnosis to be made first in the pathology laboratory, as was the case with the patient under discussion.

Five-year survival after cholecystectomy depends mainly on tumor grade and extension (1). When confined to the mucosa, it approaches 100%. With penetration of the muscularis, it is about 80%, and with involvement of the serosa, it plummets to about 15%. With lymph node and liver involvement, it is 5% or less (11). The overall median survival is about 6 months because most patients are not treated until extension of disease has occurred.

To improve this dismal survival rate, more extensive surgery, at times preceded and followed by radiation and chemotherapy, has been suggested and carried out. These operations have included wedge resection of the gallbladder bed (liver segments IV and V) coupled with lymph node dissection of the hepatoduodenal ligament into the hilus of the liver. Others have carried out more significant lobar hepatectomy and even pancreatoduodenectomy in conjunction with lymph node dissection of the hilus, which permits a more complete node dissection.

In one study (12) of 25 patients who had extension of the tumor only into the muscle layer and had a lymph node dissection and excision of the liver bed, 36% had positive nodes and 41% had liver extension. The patient under consideration had serosal invasion and therefore was in an advanced category (the most common).

The question arises whether right extended hepatectomy with pancreatoduodenectomy, which permitted meticulous dissection around the great vessels and in the duodenohepatic ligament, should have been performed in this patient who had serosal involvement. In 1990, Donohue et al. (13) found no overall survival advantage between cholecystectomy and cholecystectomy plus wedge resection of the liver bed and node dissection. However, this group stated that a radical procedure might benefit individual patients. In 1994, Nakamura et al. (14) found that seven patients with Nevin stage 5 disease who had hepatopancreatoduodenectomy had a significantly improved survival time and quality of life compared with 34 patients who had palliative procedures only. In 1994, Chijiiwa and Tanaka (15) reported a somewhat more optimistic experience. In 32 patients, after extended cholecystectomy plus en bloc lymph node dissection, the actual 5-year survival rate was 53%. This group of patients included five with stage I, four with stage II, and 23 with stage III or IV disease. Of patients with stage III disease with pN1a node metastases (hepatoduodenal ligament), 50% survived 5 years. Of patients with pN1b-positive nodes or distant metastases, no patient survived more than 3 years. In this latter group, pancreatoduodenectomy was not of value.

Even more optimistic was the 1992 report of Shirai et al. (16), who applied a variety of resective procedures designed to encompass all tumor, with varying success. In 20 patients with negative nodes (mostly T2 lesions), the actual 5-year survival rate was 85%. Surprisingly, in 20 patients with positive nodes (mostly T2 lesions), the 5-year survival rate was 45%. Included in these 40 patients were 26 patients whose operative procedures included pancreatoduodenectomy.

The results of chemotherapy (17) (intra-arterial mitomycin), using historical control subjects, did not show much difference between the two groups, a result that is typical of other reports.

The use of intraoperative radiation and/or postoperative radiotherapy (18) has not been shown to be effective. Studies on the use of radiotherapy and chemotherapy are difficult to interpret because of the scarcity of cases, the variety of stages presented, and the variety of operative procedures used. However, it seems likely that none of these adjuncts has been or will be proved beneficial using the currently available equipment and drugs.

REFERENCES

1. Henson DE, Albores-Saavedra J, Corle D. Carcinoma of the gallbladder: histologic types, stage of disease, grade, and survival rates. *Cancer* 1992;70:1493–97.
2. Cubertafond P, Gainant A, Cucchiaro G. Surgical treatment of 724 carcinomas of the gallbladder: results of the French Surgical Association survey. *Ann Surg* 1994;219:275–80.
3. Kozuka S, Tsubone M, Yasui A, Hachisuka K. Relation of adenoma to carcinoma in the gallbladder. *Cancer* 1982;50:2226–34.
4. Ishikawa O, Ohhigashi H, Imaoka S, et al. The difference in malignancy between pedunculated and sessile polypoid lesions of the gallbladder. *Am J Gastroenterol* 1989;84:1386–90.
5. Cornell CM, Clarke R. Vicarious calcification involving the gallbladder. *Ann Surg* 1959;149:267–72.
6. Kimura K, Ohto M, Saisho H, et al. Association of gallbladder carcinoma and anomalous pancreaticobiliary ductal union. *Gastroenterology* 1985;89:1258–65.
7. Lu MD, Hirata T, Nishihara K, Yamasaki K, Nakayama F. Improved delineation of the gallbladder wall with ultrasonography: its value in assessment of the depth of carcinoma invasion. *J Clin Ultrasound* 1991;19:471–7.
8. Kumar A, Aggarwal S. Carcinoma of the gallbladder: CT findings in 50 cases. *Abdom Imaging* 1994;19:304–8.
9. Sagoh T, Itoh K, Togashi K, et al. Gallbladder carcinoma: evaluation with MR imaging. *Radiology* 1990;174:131–6.
10. Brown JA, Roberts CS. Elevated serum alpha-fetoprotein levels in primary gallbladder carcinoma without hepatic involvement. *Cancer* 1992;70:1838–40.
11. Ogura Y, Mizumoto R, Isaji S, Kusuda T, Matsuda S, Tabata M. Radical operations for carcinoma of the gallbladder: present status in Japan. *World J Surg* 1991;15:337–43.
12. de Aretxabala X, Roa I, Burgos L, et al. Gallbladder cancer in Chile: a report on 54 potentially resectable tumors. *Cancer* 1992;69:60–5.
13. Donohue JH, Nagorney DM, Grant CS, Tsushima K, Ilstrup DM, Adson MA. Carcinoma of the gallbladder: does radical resection improve outcome? *Arch Surg* 1990;125:237–41.
14. Nakamura S, Nishiyama R, Yokoi Y, et al. Hepatopancreatoduodenectomy for advanced gallbladder carcinoma. *Arch Surg* 1994;129:625–9.
15. Chijiiwa K, Tanaka M. Carcinoma of the gallbladder: an appraisal of surgical resection. *Surgery* 1994;115:751–6.
16. Shirai Y, Yoshida K, Tsukada K, Muto T, Watanabe H. Radical surgery for gallbladder carcinoma: long-term results. *Ann Surg* 1992;16:565–8.
17. Makela JT, Kairaluoma MI. Superselective intra-arterial chemotherapy with mitomycin for gallbladder cancer. *Br J Surg* 1993;80:912–5.
18. Todoroki T, Iwasaki Y, Orii K, et al. Resection combined with intraoperative radiation therapy (IORT) for stage IV (TNM) gallbladder carcinoma. *World J Surg* 1991;15:357–66.

SECTION VI

Liver

32 Liver Metastases from Colorectal Cancer

Robert S. Warren

Surgery is the only treatment with curative potential—but only a few patients will be cured

CASE PRESENTATION

J.F. is a 40-year-old hardware engineer with possible hepatic metastases from a primary colorectal cancer. Nineteen months ago the patient underwent a routine physical examination. The blood work demonstrated a microcytic anemia and the stool guaiac was positive. A colonoscopy revealed a mass in the transverse colon and biopsy demonstrated a moderately well-differentiated adenocarcinoma. No other lesions were identified in the colon. A chest roentgenogram and abdominal computed tomogram (CT) were normal and the carcinoembryonic antigen (CEA) value was 12.3 g/L. An extended right hemicolectomy was performed. There was no evidence of extracolonic disease at surgery but 4 of 14 lymph nodes in the specimen were found to contain carcinoma.

Postoperatively, the patient received adjuvant chemotherapy consisting of 5-fluorouracil (5-FU) and levamisole over a period of 12 months. The CEA value normalized after his colectomy and remained in the normal range throughout the 1-year course of adjuvant chemotherapy. Three months ago, the CEA value as well as liver function tests were normal, but 2 weeks ago the CEA was found to have increased to 16 g/L. A second determination showed a value of 18 g/L.

Over the past 6 months, J.F. has felt well. His appetite has been excellent and his weight has been stable. He returned to work 2 months after his colectomy and has had no difficulty with the exception of occasional fatigue. He has had no change in his bowel habits and denies abdominal pain or other gastrointestinal symptoms. His only medication is Metamucil, one tablespoon daily. Past medical history is significant for an appendectomy at age 12, but he had no other medical or surgical illnesses. He has no known allergies. He does not smoke, uses alcohol occasionally, and has never used intravenous drugs.

Physical examination reveals a somewhat overweight gentleman who is well developed and appears healthy. His blood pressure is 140/98; pulse is 80; respirations are 12 per minute. Examination of the head and neck is normal. The lungs are clear to auscultation and percussion. Cardiac exam demonstrates a regular rate and rhythm without murmurs or gallops. The abdomen is soft and nontender. There is a well healed midline incision. The liver edge is palpable at the right costal margin and is smooth. The spleen is not palpable. Rectal exam reveals a normal prostate and no palpable mass. The stool is brown and heme-negative.

The hematocrit value is 40.2%, the white blood cell count 8,200 cells/ L, and the platelets 220,000 cells/L. Urinalysis is negative. Liver function tests reveal a total bilirubin of 0.8 mg/dL (nl 0.1–1.2), an alkaline phosphatase of 96 (nl 36–122), and an AST of 23 (nl 12–42). The prothrombin time is 11.0 s (normal 10.3–13.3). Electrolytes and renal function are normal.

A diagnostic work-up for presumed recurrence of his colon cancer was instituted. Colonoscopy demonstrated a normal-appearing ileocolonic anastomosis. No new mucosal abnormalities were identified. A computed tomographic scan of the thorax revealed mild bilateral pleural thickening without pleural effusion. The lung parenchyma showed focal areas of scarring, but there were no parenchymal lung lesions suggestive of metastases. However, the chest CT scan, which extended into the upper abdomen, demonstrated two low density areas within the liver consistent with metastases.

A magnetic resonance image (MRI) of the abdomen was obtained. This revealed the liver to be normal in size and shape. There was a 3-cm lesion in the anterior segment of the right lobe that was hyperintense on T2-weighted images (Fig. 32–1) and hypointense on T1-weighted images (Fig. 32–2). A second similar size lesion was identified peripherally in segment 8 of the liver. No other focal lesions were identified. The gallbladder, bile duct, pancreas, spleen, adrenals, and kidneys were within normal limits. There was no evidence of adenopathy within the porta hepatis, at the celiac axis, or elsewhere in the retroperitoneum.

In summary, the patient is a 40-year-old man, who was admitted 18 months after colectomy for an AJCC stage III carcinoma of the colon, with a rising CEA and radiographic evidence of two metastases to the right lobe of the liver.

TUMOR BOARD CONFERENCE

The following points were discussed at the Tumor Board.

Is the patient resectable and can he be cured? Hepatic metastasectomy is curative in a small but significant fraction of patients with metastatic colon cancer to the liver. Numerous retrospective studies have reported 5-year survival rates of 25% to 35% in such patients. Indications for

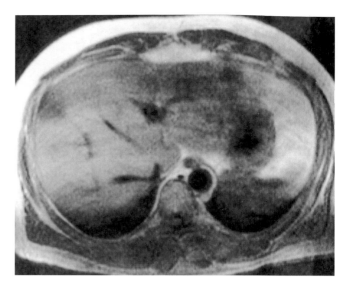

FIG. 32–2. MRI of the abdomen (T1-weighted image). The same lesion depicted in Fig. 32–1 is hypointense on the T1-weighted image.

hepatic resection for metastatic colon cancer have evolved over the past several years. Generally agreed on criteria for consideration of liver resection include patients with three or fewer tumors and the absence of radiographic evidence of extrahepatic disease. The goal is to render the liver free of tumor with a 1-cm margin of normal liver parenchyma. This may be accomplished either by anatomic or nonanatomic resections of the liver metastases, as long as sufficient hepatic parenchyma remains after resection. The magnitude of the resection is dictated by the number, size, and location of the tumors. The presence of cirrhosis or advanced age of the patient may limit the capacity to regenerate and consequently may render the patient unresectable. Fortunately, hepatic metastases rarely develop in the cirrhotic liver. This patient is a young man without a significant drinking history and should be an excellent candidate for a major liver resection. His tumors involve segments 5 and 8. These could be removed by segmental resections or, more likely, a right hepatic lobectomy. At laparotomy, any suspicious lymph nodes in the hepatoduodenal ligament, along the hepatic artery or at the celiac axis, would be biopsied. After this, intraoperative ultrasound is routinely used to identify and biopsy small liver lesions not seen preoperatively.

This patient has no pathologic diagnosis of metastasis. Is a CT-guided biopsy needed before surgery? This patient has an elevated CEA and radiographic evidence of resectable liver metastases. The abdominal CT at the time of his colectomy was normal. A preoperative histologic diagnosis of metastatic carcinoma would not alter our therapy. A negative biopsy would not rule out metastasis

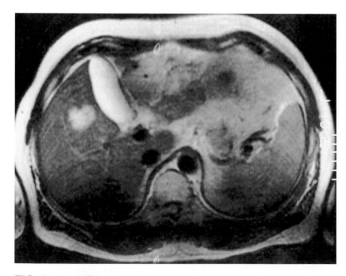

FIG. 32–1. MRI of the abdomen (T2-weighted image). There is a 3-cm hyperintense lesion in the anterior segment of the right lobe.

and would consequently not alter the plan for exploratory laparotomy with liver biopsy.

This patient has two tumors seen on MRI. If the number and location of metastases is critical in determining resectability, what is the best imaging modality to detect hepatic metastases? Conventional CT scan with IV contrast and MRI are comparable modalities in imaging hepatic metastases. Each has a sensitivity of approximately 85% with a somewhat lower specificity. CT arterial portography (CTAP), however, has become the single imaging modality of choice at this institution for identifying small lesions within the liver. Although the specificity for small lesions is not great, we believe that the CTAP will help direct the surgeon during intraoperative ultrasonography to identify and biopsy small hepatic lesions at the time of laparotomy. I would not, however, add a CTAP in this patient because the MRI is of good quality.

Would a bone scan be helpful in this patient? Bony metastases are uncommon in metastatic colon cancer. Approximately 10% of patients with advanced disease have skeletal metastases at autopsy. In patients with a low volume of metastatic tumor in the liver and no symptoms of bone disease, the false-positive rate of a bone scan exceeds the true positive rate. Thus, without bony symptoms, I would not perform a bone scan.

If you find no evidence of nodal or other extrahepatic disease at laparotomy but the intraoperative ultrasound identifies two or three additional lesions in the liver that on biopsy reveal metastatic cancer, what alternatives to liver resection would you consider? Should we encounter too numerous metastases to justify resection, we have two alternative therapies that are being carried out on a protocol basis. The first consists of cryoablation of the tumors or a combination of resection of the superficial lesions and cryoablation of the deep parenchymal tumors. This is an evolving modality and the long-term efficacy of cryoresection is essentially unknown. Early studies indicate that cryoablation for hepatic metastases from colorectal cancer is indeed effective at controlling the tumors that are frozen. But, because this modality has been used in patients with multiple hepatic tumors, our concern is that other microscopic metastases within the liver that are undetectable by any imaging modality will lead to failure to control disease within the liver. Consequently, our protocol combines cryoresection with adjuvant liver-directed chemotherapy through an implantable hepatic artery infusion pump. Our experience with this approach is too early to evaluate in terms of its efficacy. An alternative is to deliver chemotherapy regionally through the hepatic artery infusion pump alone, without cryoresection. We are studying the combination of intra-arterial fluorodeoxyuridine and 5-FU plus systemic leucovorin in a phase II protocol. Criteria for entrance into this study consist of unresectable disease confined to the liver with a sufficiently large number of tumors (seven or more) that preclude cryoresection.

What are the options for systemic therapy in this patient should he be found to have unresectable disease and declines to participate in protocols of regional chemotherapy or cryosurgery? This patient has developed hepatic metastases in the face of 5-FU–based adjuvant chemotherapy. The standard systemic therapy consists of 5-FU modulated by leucovorin, but the anticipated objective response rate in someone who has received 5-FU previously is probably in the 20% range. Other modulators of 5-FU, such as alpha-interferon or N-(phosphonacetyl)-L-aspartate (PALA), are probably no better. Mitomycin C is a less attractive second choice with a response rate of approximately 20%. This patient could also be considered for phase I trials of experimental therapeutic agents. An additional option would be to undergo no therapy because the patient is asymptomatic and the prolongation of survival in patients with advanced colorectal cancer using any regimen of systemic chemotherapy is marginal.

If the recurrence rate after liver resection for colon cancer metastases is 65% to 75%, is there a role for adjuvant chemotherapy after liver resection? There is no demonstrable benefit of chemotherapy after attempted curative liver resection for colorectal metastases, although this question has not been examined adequately in clinical studies. Approximately half of those patients who fail after liver resection recur in the remaining liver as the first site; the remainder recur in the lung, lung plus liver, or at other sites. It is tempting to treat patients with either adjuvant liver-directed chemotherapy or with a combination of regional and systemic therapy, but this should be undertaken as an experimental protocol that should include a no-treatment control arm. A large fraction of the patients we see with resectable liver metastases have failed systemic 5-FU–based chemotherapy given either for metastatic disease or as an adjuvant after their colon primary resection, as is the case with J.F. In these patients, it is difficult to argue that any available chemotherapeutic regimen is likely to be effective as an adjuvant after hepatic resection.

The patient underwent exploratory laparotomy with the intent to perform a hepatic resection. No extrahepatic disease was encountered. Intraoperative ultrasound examination revealed the two previously identified tumors in segments 5 and 8. In addition, a 5-mm lesion superficially in the left lateral segment was identified and biopsied by wedge resection. Pathologic examination revealed this to be a hemangioma (Fig. 32–3). A Tru-cut biopsy of the tumor in segment 5 was performed, which revealed metastatic adenocarcinoma. The lesion in segment 8 was superficial and had a gross appearance of a metastasis. A right hepatic lobectomy was performed. The closest margin of resection was 1.4 cm. The two identified lesions each measured 3 cm in greatest dimension and demonstrated well differentiated adenocarcinoma with mucin deposition and necrosis,

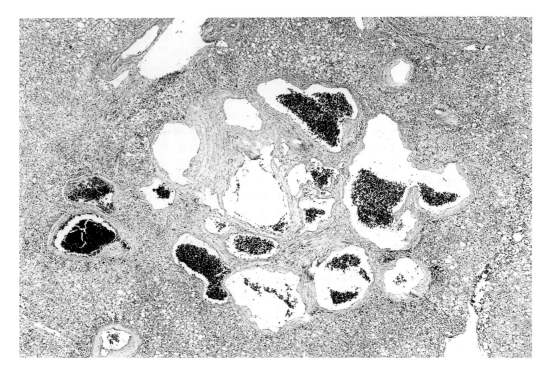

FIG. 32–3. Hemangioma of the liver.

consistent with metastases from a colonic primary (Fig. 32–4). No other lesions were seen on serial section of the right lobe of the liver. Estimated blood loss was 1,850 mL. Two units of packed RBCs were transfused. Closed suction drains were placed under the right diaphragm and at the porta hepatitis.

Postoperatively, the patient did well initially. There was no evidence of bile leak. Bowel function returned by postoperative day 5, but just before planned discharge on postoperative day 9, the patient developed abdominal distention and nausea. Plain films of the abdomen revealed a partial small bowel obstruction. This was treated by naso-

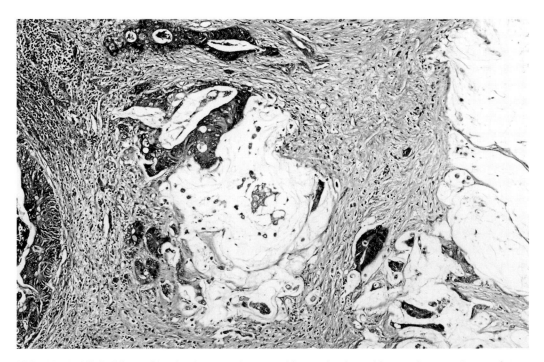

FIG. 32–4. Well-differentiated adenocarcinoma with mucin deposition and necrosis consistent with metastasis from a colonic primary.

gastric intubation and intravenous fluids. With this management, the small bowel distension resolved and normal bowel function returned. The patient was discharged on postoperative day 13, taking a regular diet. He has been followed with serial liver function tests, chest roentgenogramy, and CEA determinations and remains disease-free 6 months after liver resection.

COMMENTARY by James H. Foster

This case raises many important questions about the diagnosis and management of liver metastasis in patients who have undergone bowel resection for carcinoma: how best to find such metastases? What is the natural history of patients without treatment? Are there effective therapies other than resection? Can resection be done safely? Is a survival benefit achieved by resection? And, what are the selection criteria that predict favorable outcome? Twenty-five years of increasing experience with resection have provided data that bring us close to some answers.

The educated surgeons' hands are the best and most cost-effective detector of liver metastasis. Intraoperative ultrasonography may add a few percentage points to sensitivity, but the great advantage suggested in some publications is largely due to the relative insensitivity of the unskilled hand. Careful bimanual evaluation of the liver at the time of bowel resection should spare the patient much of the cost and distress of preoperative and postoperative imaging. Remember, though, that all liver nodules in patients with bowel cancer are not necessarily metastatic disease. Needle biopsy confirmation should be done in most instances. If the liver is clear at the primary laparotomy, how should the patient be followed? More of that below.

Suture line recurrence of colon carcinoma is rare. Disease usually goes to lymph nodes and liver and less often to lungs, rarely to bone. In asymptomatic patients a conventional CT with intravenous contrast is perhaps the most effective imaging method: to find metastatic lesions, to define the relationship of such lesions to the critical inflow and outflow vessels of the liver, and to appreciate mesenteric, para-aortic, and hilar nodal disease. Enthusiasts tout the superiority of MRI, dynamic CT, CT arterial portography, etc. Any clinical advantage to the patient of these expensive new technologies has yet to be proved. Because extrahepatic disease, even if resectable, is a contraindication to liver resection for metastatic colorectal cancer, and because chest CT is much more sensitive than conventional chest roentgenograms in showing small metastatic foci, candidates for liver resection should all undergo chest CT preoperatively. I would agree with Dr. Warren that in this setting, needle biopsy confirmation of the metastatic nature of the new liver lesions was not needed because the old CT scan had been normal.

In such a patient as the one under consideration, what would have happened if we did nothing? The experience from the Mayo Clinic provides perhaps the best answer. It is clear that with earlier diagnosis of liver metastasis, survival without treatment of patients with limited disease is now on the average of 18 months to 2 years. Perhaps as many as a quarter of the patients will live 3 years without therapy, but very few will live 5 years.

What about other therapeutic options for asymptomatic patients with colorectal secondaries in their liver? No clear survival advantage has been demonstrated for any nonoperative therapy when compared with supportive therapy alone. Although the use of intra-arterial infusions, the addition of leucovorin to 5-FU, and perhaps the use of local treatments of tumor nodules such as cryotherapy or alcohol injection may increase response rate (i.e., transient reduction in tumor size), that response has not translated into a consistent increase in patient survival. Toxicity, cost, and patient distress are markedly increased by all these measures. Thus, their use for an asymptomatic patient can hardly be justified outside of a properly controlled experimental protocol, yet they are recommended more often than not, probably because of both our presumption that it is better to do something than nothing and our assumption that the patient will want something done and under our current insurance programs can ignore the cost thereof. My experience would suggest otherwise. If various options are thoroughly explained to the patient, and if the morbidity, survival, and cost are thoroughly discussed by a trusted surgeon, the rare good-risk patient with resectable liver metastases will elect resection rather than chemotherapy because only it offers a chance for cure. Most asymptomatic patients with nonresectable disease will choose to wait for the occurrence of symptoms before undertaking morbid, noncurative measures. This shared decision for observation requires only lengthy discussion between the patient and his surgeon, who must be fully informed about all the various treatment options.

If no treatment is the best therapy for the asymptomatic patient with unresectable colorectal liver secondaries, the only rationale (from the patient's point of view) for follow-up examinations is to discover resectable disease. The CEA-directed second-look procedure experience suggests that cure rarely follows resection of recurrent extrahepatic disease. Only the patients with limited liver disease apparently benefit. Therefore, if a patient is not a candidate for liver resection, or if the patient has known extrahepatic recurrence, it makes little sense to look for liver involvement.

An argument could be made for a CEA determination every 6 months for 3 years and for a single abdominal CT scan 2 years after bowel resection in the asymptomatic patient. The value of repeat colonoscopy is largely in finding second primary lesions rather than discovering suture line recurrence.

Finally, if we're lucky enough to find a favorable patient such as our 40-year-old hardware engineer, should we recommend resection? We know now that 25% of such patients will live 5 years after liver resection, but we have also learned that 40% of those 5-year survivors will eventually succumb to disease. Only resection provides a hope of cure, a hope shared by all those resected until recurrence eventually is detected in 70% to 85%. Operative mortality after elective liver resection is in the range of 2% in experienced hands and morbidity is low and transient. Remember that resection provides a 100% "complete remission" in chemotherapy terms.

So, for medical and humanistic reasons, I commend the surgeon for his aggressive approach to this patient. More extensive liver involvement, underlying systemic or hepatic nonmalignant disease states, and advanced age increase the risk and reduce the benefit of such heroic measures. It may be that the long-term survivors would have fared as well without resection and that biology rather than surgery should claim the credit, but with our present state of ignorance/knowledge it would seem that we should continue to recommend resection for selected patients.

EDITORIAL BOARD COMMENTARY
by Glenn D. Steele, Jr.

Innumerable institutional prospective studies now show that intraoperative ultrasound is more sensitive than even the most talented surgeon's palpation of the liver. The resolution capacity for tumors in the depths of the right lobe is approximately 3 to 4 mm and no one who I know has the ability to palpate such small lesions, particularly when they are at the junction of the hepatic veins and the cava or in the caudate lobe. Knowing about these before doing a resection is much more rational than finding out about them in the middle of or at the conclusion of the parenchymal finger fracture. In addition, application of the intraoperative ultrasound technique through a per-cutaneous laparoscopic approach may save many patients with unsuspected profuse disease in the liver from unnecessary or unhelpful laparotomies.

Dr. Foster's joining cryosurgical ablation, or even alcohol injection, with other categories of regional or systemic chemotherapy, is unwarranted. Cryosurgical ablation has come to be seen as an option (in some cases) to resection. Tumor control results are no better but certainly no worse. The collected series of David Morris, T.S. Ravikumar, and our own, which now includes more than 250 patients, show a pattern of failure and disease-free survival superimposable on the experience of the prospective multi-institutional study of resectional surgery for isolated liver metastases from colon and rectum carcinoma—Gastrointestinal Tumor Study Group 6584 (GITSG) study. However, in the cryosurgical ablation experience of the three authors noted above, there have been no deaths and the median length of stay is approximately one third that of the resection patients.

I am in full agreement with both Drs. Foster and Warren that even though most patients who undergo successful resection of their isolated metastases will eventually recur (shown by both the extended GITSG follow-up as well as David Nagorney's follow-up of the Adson, Mayo Clinic series of liver resection patients), they do live longer than any of the nonresected patients in natural history studies of comparable stage liver metastasis. Select populations of patients with four or fewer asymptomatic metastatic lesions isolated to the liver have a median survival of 18 to 24 months without any treatment, but all die within 5 years. In the resection and cryoablation experience, all successfully treated patients achieve a "complete response" and median survival is greater than 30 months. A number are still alive after 10 years. In other words, all of us agree that in this select group of patients, removal or complete destruction of isolated liver metastases is still the only rational approach with curative intent.

33

Hepatoma in a Cirrhotic Liver

Glenn D. Steele, Jr. and Keith Stuart

Does surgery cure? How often? Any other options?

CASE PRESENTATION

The patient was a 66-year-old man without significant past medical history who initially presented with severe hematemesis. Questioning revealed a 40-year history of heavy drinking, primarily red wine. He had noted several days of black, tarry stools but had deferred evaluation until he saw blood in his vomitus.

Physical exams showed an older man in no acute distress. Otolaryngologic examination was unremarkable, and fundi were benign. The oropharynx was without lesions, and there was no lymphadenopathy. The lungs were clear, and a cardiac exam was unremarkable. The abdomen was soft and nontender. The liver edge was palpable 3 cm below the right costal margin. This was ballottable. The spleen was not palpable. There was gross ascites evident with moderate abdominal distention, a palpable fluid wave, and a positive fluid shift. Extremities showed 2+ pitting edema to the knees bilaterally. Skin was anicteric but showed multiple small spider hemangiomata. Palms were erythematous but showed no sign of Dupuytren's contracture.

Immediate upper endoscopy demonstrated multiple esophageal and gastric varices. The former were successfully injected with sodium morrhuate, but the latter were not amenable to sclerotherapy. The patient received multiple transfusions and was eventually stabilized during an admission to the intensive care unit, receiving intravenous pitressin and nitroglycerin to reduce portal venous pressure.

After discharge he stopped drinking, but over the following 2 years he had five recurrent episodes of variceal bleeding, requiring multiple sclerotherapy injections. Simultaneously, he developed progressive ascites. He had

two episodes of spontaneous bacterial peritonitis and required several therapeutic paracenteses. A combination of spironolactone and furosemide was unable to control his ascites, so he was judged to be a candidate for a central shunt to decrease his portal pressure.

The patient was taken to the operating room, where a portal-renal shunt was performed. The left renal vein was anastomosed to the posterior aspect of the portal vein, creating a side-to-side portacaval shunt. At the time of surgery a 4-cm lesion on the anterior aspect of the liver was noted. This had not been seen on preoperative studies. Biopsy of this showed well differentiated hepatocellular carcinoma with clear cell features (Fig. 33–1). This was believed to be unresectable because of the degree of his cirrhosis. Postoperative staging showed no evidence of metastatic disease.

Two months after recovery from his operation, the patient was readmitted for treatment of his hepatoma. Because surgery was not an option and external beam radiation or systemic chemotherapy have little efficacy, he elected to undergo chemoembolization of his tumor. This involved intra-arterial instillation of chemotherapy (doxorubicin) mixed with ethiodol (an oil-based contrast agent that is selectively retained within tumor tissue). This is immediately followed by Gelfoam particle embolization, leading to excellent retention of high doses of doxorubicin within the tumor and the creation of arterial insufficiency to the lesion (Fig. 33–2). He underwent treatment with this in March 1991 and was discharged within 6 days. He tolerated the procedure well, although he developed fevers to 101°F without any evidence of infection, and increased ascites and edema, requiring treatment with diuretics.

One month later he was fully asymptomatic, and at 3 months his computed tomography (CT) scan showed a

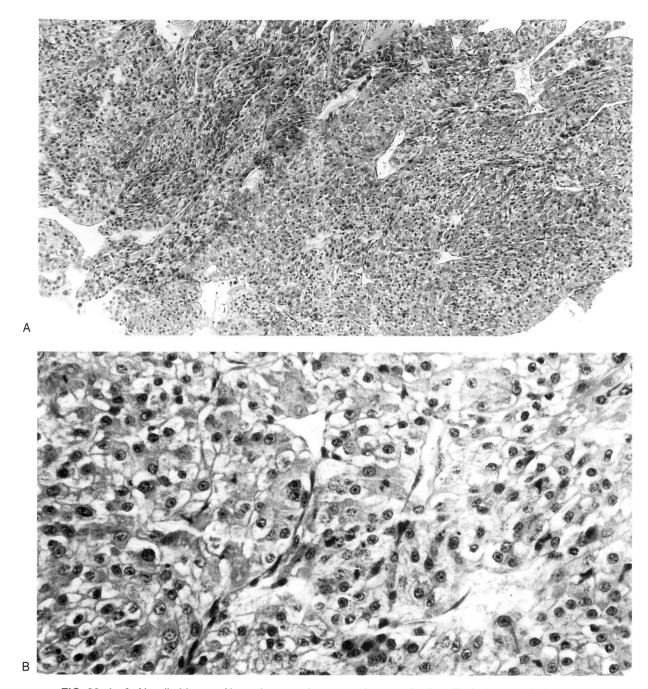

FIG. 33–1. A: Needle biopsy of hepatic mass demonstrating neoplastic cells that resemble hepatocytes arranged in a trabecular pattern (H&E stain). **B:** High magnification demonstrating round tumor cells with a single large nucleolus and focal clear cell change in cytoplasm. A prominent sinusoidal network is present around the tumor cells. Bile pigment was noted in scattered tumor cells (H&E stain).

47% reduction in the cross-sectional area of the tumor (Fig. 33–3). His bilirubin had fallen from 2.8 to 1.5 mg/dL, and his albumin was stable at 2.6 g/dL. Alpha-fetoprotein (AFP) was not elevated. He continued to do well, remaining asymptomatic without abdominal pain, bleeding, ascites, jaundice, fatigue, or anorexia. Of note, he developed insulin-dependent diabetes within 6 months after the procedure.

Eleven months afterward, in February 1992, he developed increasing jaundice, with bilirubin rising to 10.2 mg/dL and AFP up to 118 ng/mL. His liver edge had enlarged to 5 cm below the right costal margin, but a CT scan showed no change in the size of the lesion that had been treated. However, diffusely abnormal hepatic parenchyma was noted, consistent with diffuse tumor infiltration (Fig. 33–4). He underwent chemoemboliza-

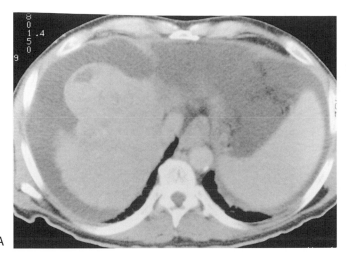

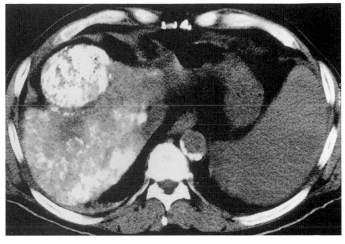

A   B

FIG. 33–2. A: CT scan before chemoembolization, demonstrating extensive ascites and a large extruding mass in the anterior right hepatic lobe. **B:** Nonenhanced CT 1 day after chemoembolization, showing retention of high-contrast ethiodol with doxorubicin within the tumor, along with some nonspecific distribution within the remainder of the right lobe. (Note the resolution of ascites after successful functioning of the portacaval shunt.)

tion again at this time, and again tolerated the procedure well except for moderate right upper quadrant pain and worsening ascites and edema. He was successfully treated with diuretics. However, although his bilirubin came down to 6.4 mg/dL and his AFP fell to 63 ng/mL, he did not have any significantly prolonged improvement in his liver function tests. Therefore, 2 months later, he was given a systemic treatment with 5-Fluorouracil (5-FU) and leucovorin. Systemic doxorubicin, which has a marginally better response rate, was not used because of his elevated bilirubin levels. He received treatment with this for several weeks, but his liver function tests did not significantly improve. He developed fatigue, cachexia, and

hematemesis and was admitted to the hospital, where he was found to be bleeding once again from esophageal and gastric varices. This could not be controlled, and he became encephalopathic, expiring with exsanguination and hepatic failure.

COMMENTARY by James H. Foster

One must admire the heroic efforts made by this patient's doctors to control the growth of an incurable tumor. Over the past three decades we have learned that dearterialization of primary liver cancer (PLC), more

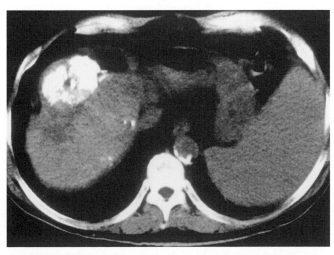

FIG. 33–3. Nonenhanced CT at 3 months, demonstrating a 47% reduction in tumor dimensions.

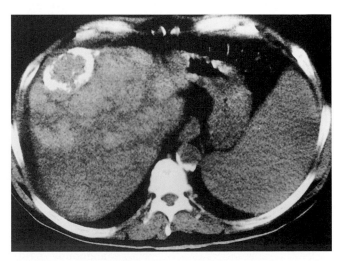

FIG. 33–4. Nonenhanced CT scan at 11 months, showing viable tumor growth within the treated lesion, as well as extensive infiltrative disease throughout the hepatic parenchyma.

discrete embolization, hyperthermia, and intra-arterial perfusion with currently available agents are not effective by themselves in increasing survival or even palliation. When we combine such ineffective measures, are we really adding whole numbers or multiplying fractions? Perhaps such efforts are justified at a limited number of centers specializing in innovative treatments, but a few words of caution are needed.

At enormous cost—in dollars and in patient days away from home—the growth of an asymptomatic tumor was possibly slowed for a few months. What would have been this patient's fate if the tumor had not been discovered, or had been found and not treated?

Years ago it was clear that patients with untreated PLC died rapidly, averaging only 6 months of survival after diagnosis. However, that was when diagnosis was made only when the tumors were large and/or widespread. The experience of the Shanghai group with subclinical carcinoma is instructive (1). Although their 5-year survival after resection of small, asymptomatic PLC is high, 10-year survival drops off sharply. Thus, true cure may be rare indeed, but the natural history and progression may be better than suspected. Persistence, recurrence, or multifocal origin seem to be the rule when PLC occurs in a cirrhotic liver. That may be even more true of Western patients. Although a few of my own cirrhotic patients have lived for a year or two after resection of small PLC, all have eventually succumbed to their disease, as did all who survived resection in a national survey (2). Now that I refuse tumor resection to asymptomatic cirrhotic patients, I have watched several such patients live several years without treatment.

Should we use other therapies if resection is not chosen? The results of a prospective trial comparing various imaginative interventions for PLC that demonstrated that none was superior to supportive care alone are sobering (3). Newer technologies and knowledge have resulted in recent trials with cryosurgery, intratumor alcohol injections, radioimmunotherapy with targeted antibodies, and biologic therapies including cytokines, lymphokine-activated killer cells (LAK) cells, and adoptive immunotherapy. Chemoembolization using anticancer agents combined with lipoidal has been pioneered in Asia and Europe at several centers. Occasionally, it will result in impressive tumor shrinkage but will the patient benefit? I am reminded of the spectacular reduction in large head and neck cancers that followed arterial infusion of methotrexate 30 years ago—a treatment long since given up after adequate controls and prolonged follow-up could demonstrate no lasting advantage.

The progression of liver failure in patients without tumors but with advanced cirrhosis is variable. We have all seen patients live 10 years or more, even after the onset of bleeding varices and ascites. A pneumonia, the flu, a medication change, or some other stress may tip a delicate balance toward metabolic failure, reversible or otherwise. How many days did we subtract or how many did we add to this patient's ledger with our multiple anesthesia and interventions? Have we increased the patient's antitumor immunocompetence or reduced it? Did this patient die of tumor or liver failure? Did he die because of his disease or because of his treatment?

Those answers are not available for this patient or any other single patient. My own bias is clear, but it will also remain unproved until proper trials are done comparing treated patients with those who receive no treatment, patients who have similar disease burden and liver injury. In the meantime, most of us treating patients with unresectable PLC will serve them better by focusing on adding to the number of comfortable days at home rather than on reducing tumor size. It is the nature of our profession to want to do something positive for our patients and the nature of the surgeon to want to attack the disease, but if we truly want medicine to be more scientific, we must not let technology run too far ahead of proven results.

REFERENCES

1. Tang ZY, Yu YQ, Zhou XD, et al. Surgery of small hepatocellular carcinoma. *Cancer* 1989;64:536–41.
2. Foster JH, Berman MM. Primary epithelial cancer in adults. In: *Major Problems in Clinical Surgery, Solid Liver Tumors*, vol XXII. Philadelphia: WB Saunders; 1977.
3. Lai ECS, Choi TK, Tong SW et al. Treatment of unresectable hepatocellular carcinoma: results of a randomized controlled trial. *World J Surg* 1986;10:501.

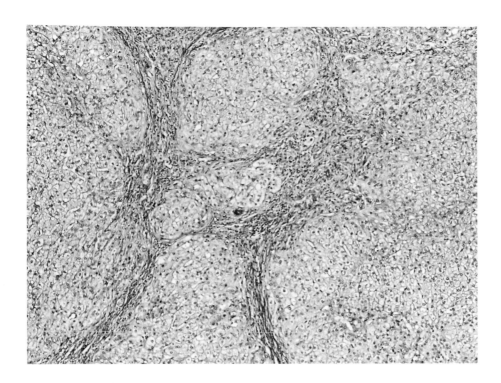

FIG. 34–4. Microscopically, the tumor consists of variably sized nodules of disorganized hepatocytes separated by tracts of fibrous tissue containing proliferating bile ductules. The fibrous tissue is infiltrated by chronic inflammatory cells.

as 20% of hepatocellular carcinomas will present with AFP levels within the normal range (2). In the fibrolamellar variety of hepatocellular carcinoma, the incidence of normal AFP is thought to be even higher; most patients show no circulating levels of this marker (1). In a recent study, one marker that has been found to be useful has been neurotensin (3). This marker is also by no means found universally in fibrolamellar hepatocellular carcinomas. Therefore, if the clinical picture is suspicious for a malignant process, such as was suggested by the rapidly growing nature of the tumor in the current case, then additional investigative procedures must be pursued.

In the investigation of hepatic masses, the most commonly used modality is CT. The difficulties in distinguishing between FNH and fibrolamellar hepatocellular carcinoma by CT was discussed above. In our hands, a diagnostic modality of choice in the evaluation of hepatic lesions remains angiography. Visceral angiography is capable of diagnosing hemangiomas. In addition, the vascular pattern noted on angiography often distinguishes adenoma, FNH, and malignant lesions (4).

The use of percutaneous needle biopsies is controversial. The possibility of spreading tumor by percutaneous needle aspiration has been demonstrated for a variety of tumor types (5). In addition, the possibility of significant bleeding in cases of percutaneous biopsies of hemangiomas or adenomas (6) has been appreciated. In our opinion, there is little role for percutaneous needle biopsies in the management of solitary hepatic masses. Clearly, a hepatic mass with radiologic appearance of a neoplasm in a patient with a high circulating level of AFP, or in a patient with a history of colon cancer and a rising CEA level, requires no needle biopsies. In the current case of

rapidly enlarging hepatic masses, despite negative tumor markers, needle biopsies were also unnecessary. The rapidly expanding nature of the current tumor, as well as the symptomatology produced by the tumor, represented sufficient indications for surgical exploration and resection, whether the lesion was benign or malignant. On exploration, the tumor had the characteristic gross appearance of a FNH and a resection was performed.

REFERENCES

1. Soyer P, Roche A, Levesque M, Legmann P. CT of fibrolamellar hepatocellular carcinoma. *J Comput Assist Tomogr* 1991;15:533–8.
2. Kew MC. Alpha-fetoprotein. In: *Modern trends in gastroenterology,* Read AE, ed. London: Butterworths; 1975:91–114.
3. Collier NA, Bloom SR, Hodgson HJF, Weinbren K, Lee YC, Blumgart LH. Neurotensin secretion by fibrolamellar carcinoma of the liver. *Lancet* 1984;1:538–40.
4. Blumgart LH. *Surgery of the liver and biliary tract.* New York: Churchill Livingstone; 1988.
5. Quaghebeur G, Thompson JN, Blumgart LH, Benjamin IS. Implantation of hepatocellular carcinoma after percutaneous needle biopsy. *J Roy Coll Surg Edinb* 1991;36:127.
6. Shortell CK, Schwartz SI. Hepatic adenoma and focal nodular hyperplasia. *Surg Gynecol Obstet* 1991;173:426–31.

COMMENTARY by Glenn D. Steele, Jr.

The most important aspect of this case is to make absolutely certain that a young, otherwise healthy individual does not pass from the stage of curable to incurable by ignoring or misdiagnosing a fibrolamellar hepatocellular carcinoma (1,2). The differential diagnosis, which includes FNH, hepatic adenoma, and rarer entities such as choledochal cysts with or without intestinal metaplasia (3), are all approached by numerous diagnostic tests. Arguments in favor of CT scan, dynamic CT scan, MRI, and even in the case of FNH versus hepatic adenoma versus hepatocellular carcinoma, the technetium sulfur colloid 99 liver spleen scan (4), have been made. Needless to say, specificity and sensitivity comparisons based on prospective, randomized trials are absent, and the diagnosis of a solitary lesion in a noncirrhotic liver, particularly in a young woman, demands that the surgeon prove that whatever the lesion is, it not be ignored to the point of incurability.

Although one can be nihilistic about hepatocellular carcinomas in general, particularly those that appear in a cirrhotic liver (5), the single exception of the fibrolamellar variant especially in young women may present a more optimistic possibility of cure and, thus, the attempt to completely resect is always justifiable.

If the panoply of noninvasive diagnostic tests still leave a definitive diagnosis to be desired, what then should the approach to histology be? Although Blumgart and his colleagues argue that percutaneous needle biopsy may spread the liver tumor, especially when the tumor is an hepatocellular carcinoma, this is rarely the weak link in diagnosis or therapy of any of these disorders. More often, the primary problem is that the lesion is not representatively sampled and, therefore, no definitive histologic diagnosis is made or, worse, a hypervascular lesion is biopsied that leads not only to lack of diagnosis but to an acute abdominal emergency. Particularly in the case of FNH versus hepatocellular carcinoma of the fibrolamellar variant, definitive histologic diagnosis on the basis of a core needle may be difficult to impossible even without any of the above complications.

In the case summarized by Blumgart and colleagues, there are compelling reasons to move straightaway to operation. First is the symptomatology which, of course, mandates an attempt at palliation (often almost as important a goal as cure). And second, the liver mass was increasing in size and perhaps in multicentricity. Having agreed with the need for a laparotomy, perhaps one could add some recent data in which laparoscopic staging, and a translaparoscopic ultrasonography (evaluating the tumor's presence and location in the liver and performing a laparoscopic-directed biopsy), could have obviated the need for a full laparotomy. Such an approach in preliminary, single institution studies has begun to show a significant effect on clinical decision making (6). In addition, one can quibble about why a birth control history was not included because this might imply adenoma as a preferential diagnosis (7).

The major question that I have concerning this case, however, is the decision to perform a so-called left trisegmentectomy after the histologic diagnosis of FNH was made. It is very rare (8) that such lesions cause symptoms. Therefore, our advice has been to leave FNH alone once it is definitively diagnosed.

Finally, although in the setting that Dr. Blumgart and colleagues find themselves, left trisegmentectomy may be routine with a very low probability of complications or even mortality, it is rarely done as an anatomic procedure and, most likely, would not be a physiologically cost-effective approach in the routine primary or secondary surgery environment. First, if most FNH patients do not present with symptoms, there would be no benefit in doing any procedure except what was necessary to make a definite diagnosis. Second, if this had turned out to be an hepatocellular carcinoma, particularly one with multicentricity, the need to do a large, nonanatomic resection would not have been a good prognostic sign. Most often, there is an inverse correlation between extent of hepatic resection necessary for either primary or secondary cancer and the patient's ultimate survival, in addition to the increased probability of acute morbidity and mortality. One additional technical point is the option of cryosurgical ablation (9), which might have allowed a segmental resection of the larger lesion and a freeze of the smaller in this case. The major attraction is decreased morbidity with no difference in outcome if performed correctly.

If this patient had been found to have an hepatic adenoma, then the explanation for the rapid growth and the symptomatology would be both more intuitive and more concerning because the next probable event would have been either an intratumoral bleed or extrahepatic tumor expansion and peritoneal bleed. For both those reasons, the justification for palliative as well as preemptive resection would have been much more straightforward than with the FNH diagnosis.

REFERENCES

1. Soreide O, Czerniak A, Bradpiece H. Bloom S, Blumgart L. Characteristics of fibrolamellar hepatocellular carcinoma: a study of nine cases and a review of the literature. *Am J Surg* 1986;151:518–23.
2. Craig JR, Peter RL, Edmondson H, Omata M. Fibrolamellar carcinoma of the liver: a tumor of adolescents and young adults with distinctive clinico-pathologic features. *Cancer* 1980;46:372–9.
3. Case Records of the Massachusetts General Hospital (Case 52-1988). *N Engl J Med* 1988;319:1718–25.
4. Welch TJ, Sheedy PF II, Johnson CM, et al. Focal nodular hyperplasia and hepatic adenoma: comparison of angiography, CT, ultrasound, and scintigraphy. *Radiology* 1985;156:593–5.
5. McDermott WV Jr, Jenkins RL, Cady B, Steele G Jr. Primary and metastatic cancer of the liver. In: *General surgical oncology*, Steele G Jr, Cady B, eds. Philadelphia: WB Saunders; 1992:185–94.
6. Babineau TJ, Lewis WD, Jenkins RL, Bleday R, Steele G Jr, Forse RA. The role of staging laparoscopy in the treatment of hepatic malignancy. *Am J Surg* 1994;167:151–5.
7. Knowles DM II, Casarella WJ, Johnson PM, Wolff M. The clinical, radiologic, and pathologic characterization of benign hepatic neoplasms: alleged association with oral contraceptives. *Medicine (Balt)* 1978;57:223–7.
8. Kerlin P, Davis GL, McGill DB, Weiland CH, Adson MA, Sheedy PF II. Hepatic adenoma and focal nodular hyperplasia: Clinical, pathologic, and radiologic features. *Gastroenterology* 1983;84:994–1002.
9. Ravikumar TS, Kane R, Cady B, Jenkins R, Clouse M, Steele G Jr. A five-year study of cryosurgery in the therapy of liver tumors. *Arch Surg* 1991;126:1520–4.

35

Hepatoma in a Young Woman

Harold O. Douglass, Jr.

Anything but surgical resection here?

CASE PRESENTATION

Right subcostal pain associated with profuse diarrhea developed in a 22-year-old woman 2 years before her first admission at this center. This was treated with lamb, rice, and water by her personal physician. The pain persists and is aggravated by twisting her torso to the right and left. Episodic diarrhea lasting 4 to 5 days occurs about every 3 weeks. Between bouts of diarrhea, she is intermittently constipated, moving her bowels only every 2 to 3 days. However, for the past 2 weeks, she has had diarrhea. Stools are black or tan on occasion. During the week before admission, her urine was light brown on one occasion.

She now has constant right upper quadrant pain with intermittent exacerbation. During these times, she describes the pain as "burning" and feeling like a "stone." Four months before this admission, she was told of liver enlargement and a radionuclide liver scan showed the liver to extend 4 cm below the costal margin.

She took oral contraceptives (0.5 mg norgestrol and 0.05 ethinyl estradiol) daily for 8 years (from age 13 until she was 20).

At the age of 4 years, a tumor developed on her left lower eyelid that was locally excised but recurred 2 months later. Further excision demonstrated a malignant schwannoma invading the orbit, and a left orbit exenteration was performed. There has been no further recurrence.

A tonsillectomy was performed at age 16 years.

The patient had a good appetite. She had chronic right frontal headaches. There was occasional facial blushing. Retinal hemorrhage 1 year before this admission was treated conservatively. Intermittent pain in the right eye with photophobia was noted, with conjunctivitis 6 months later. There were complaints of floating scotomata and

dental caries. Approximately once each month she had an episode of epistaxis and had two bouts of hematemesis (not treated) 2 months before coming to this center.

She stopped smoking because she became short of breath. She used to smoke one pack daily for 8 years.

Menarche was at age 12. Menstrual periods are regular at 28-day intervals, except when "under stress." She had no pregnancies.

She drank one six-pack of beer daily beginning about the time she started to smoke, but reduced her intake to three to four six-packs per week after the first year. Two years before admission, she stopped all intake of ethanol-containing fluids.

She had no allergies and took no medications.

The patient was born 2 months premature, with placenta previa, delivered via cesarean section, with a birth weight of 6½ lbs. There was initial formula intolerance, but after a change in formula, feeding was satisfactory.

There was no family history of cancer, heart disease, or neurologic problems. Her father and maternal grandfather consumed excessive amounts of alcohol.

The abdomen was obese without palpable masses. The liver span was 10 cm, including 7 cm below the right costal margin at the midclavicular line, 5 cm below margin, 1.5 cm lateral to the midline. The liver edge was hard and moved with respiration. No pararectal masses were palpated.

Initial laboratory studies included urine pH 5.0, negative for protein, glucose; hemoglobin 11.5 g/dL, hematocrit 35%, platelets $488 \times 10^3/mm^3$, WBC $7.6 \times 10^3/mm^3$, prothrombin time 10.8 s (control 12 s), partial thromboplastin time 37 s (control 35 s); and bilirubin, alkaline phosphatase, AST, and LDH all within normal limits. There were no electrolyte or renal chemistry abnormalities. Hepatitis antigen was nonreactive and the α-fetoprotein was detectable. Serum protein electrophoresis showed slight elevation of the α-2 and β-globulins. The serum amylase was 365 μ/100 mL (normal less than 200).

On admission, an ultrasound showed multiple echogenic areas in an enlarged liver. The chest roentgenogram was not remarkable. An arteriogram showed a vascular "football-sized mass" in the right lobe of the liver supplied by the celiac, right hepatic via the superior mesenteric and collateral gastroduodenal arteries (Fig. 35–1), with a tumor blush. The portal vein was displaced superiorly, and the right kidney was displaced inferiorly. Computed tomography (CT) of the head showed no evidence of local recurrence of the schwannoma.

Because of the presence of a liver mass with facial flushing and apparent intensifying diarrhea, evaluation for a possible neuroendocrine tumor was undertaken but found to be negative. Although hepatic adenoma or hepatoma seemed the most likely diagnosis, the remote possibility of metastatic disease from the orbital malignancy excised many years earlier would require at least a review of the histopathologic material from the excision of that malignancy. Review confirmed malignant schwannoma.

A right hepatic lobectomy with cholecystectomy was performed via a thoracoabdominal approach. The postoperative course was complicated only by transient bile leakage around the intra-abdominal sump drains.

Grossly, the tumor measured 18 × 13 × 10 cm, separated from the normal liver by a fibrous capsule that circumscribed the tumor (Fig. 35–2, Fig. 35–3). The thickness of the intact liver margin around the tumor was 3 cm or more. The cut surface of the tumor was dark brown and

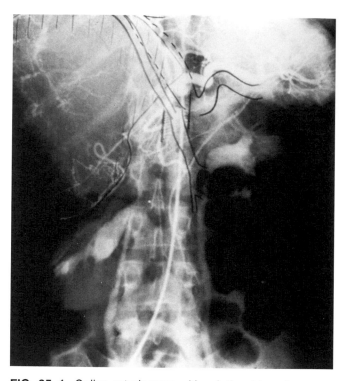

FIG. 35–1. Celiac arteriogram with relationships of venous phase and superior mesenteric arteriogram drawn on film. Note aberrant right hepatic artery as first branch on the right side of the superior mesenteric artery.

had a homogeneous appearance in color and consistency but was softer than the surrounding normal liver. Microscopically, the tumor was composed of polygonal cells with abundant cytoplasm in which bile pigment could be recognized. Many areas were well differentiated and suggested an adenoma. In other areas, nuclei were variable in

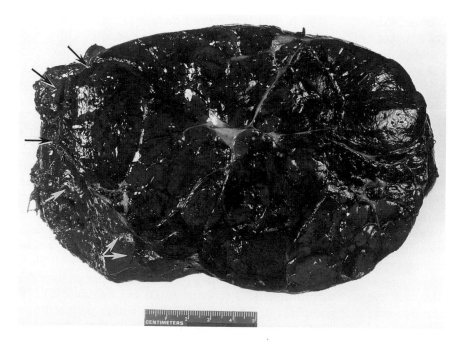

FIG. 35–2. Gross specimen of right lobe of liver (rotated left to right) showing fibrous "capsule" and margin of healthy liver.

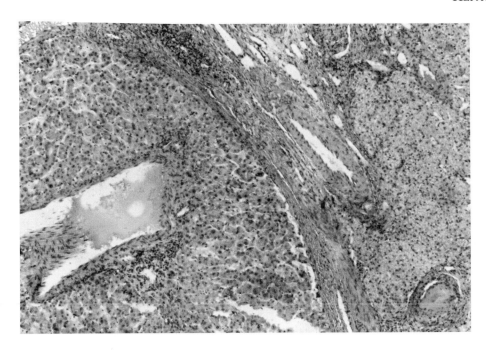

FIG. 35–3. Photomicrograph of tumor margin and "capsule," oriented as in Fig. 35–2.

size and shape (Figs. 35–4, 35–5) Some cells were multinucleated and a few mitoses were identified.

Although there is no evidence that adjuvant therapy is of any value in the treatment of patients with hepatomas, postoperative chemotherapy was offered to this patient. She chose to receive treatment. Four years later, she became pregnant and delivered a normal, healthy child. A subsequent pregnancy was also carried to term with the delivery of a healthy child. Eleven years postoperatively, a small incisional hernia was identified and repaired. Thirteen years postoperatively, a complete new orbital prosthesis was fabricated.

COMMENTARY FROM WEEKLY CANCER CONFERENCES

Although uncommon in the United States, hepatoma is a major cause of cancer-related death world-wide. Most are associated with cirrhotic changes in the liver resulting from hepatitis B infection. In the United States and Europe, the cirrhotic liver in which hepatomas develop is often of nutritional etiology (i.e., Laennec's cirrhosis). Histologically, hepatomas associated with cirrhosis tend to be poorly to moderately differentiated.

FIG. 35–4. Well-differentiated area showing bile canniculi, some containing bile pigment.

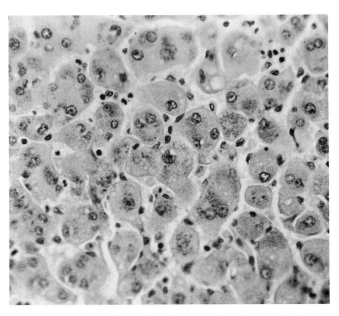

FIG. 35–5. Less-differentiated area showing variation in nuclear size, multinucleated cells, and loss of orientation around bile canniculi.

This patient had a history of a moderate alcohol intake but not stigmata of cirrhosis and had no evidence of prior hepatitis B infection. In the noncirrhotic liver, α–fetoprotein serves as a marker of hepatoma in 60% or more of patients, particularly if the tumor is well differentiated. Unfortunately, tumor markers were absent in this patient.

A variant hepatoma, fibrolamellar hepatoma, is sometimes seen in young women. This tumor has well-defined borders. When completely resected with a 2-cm margin of normal liver, the cure rate is high. Other well-differentiated tumors, particularly if surrounded by an apparent fibrous capsule, also have a good prognosis when resected en bloc with a 2- to 3-cm rim of normal liver, as was the case in this patient.

A large solitary hypervascular tumor in an otherwise normal liver should immediately suggest the likelihood of hepatoma. Large benign adenomas, particularly when there has been a history of hormone use, should also be considered.

Before considering resection of a hepatoma, a search for metastatic disease in celiac and periaortic lymph nodes, lungs, and bone should be undertaken. The presence of ascites, even in small amounts, suggests a poor prognosis. If the ascites is bloody, the outlook is grim.

There is no evidence that any adjuvant therapy is of benefit to patients with hepatoma. Radiation therapy is valuable for the relief of pain from bone metastases, but has no other role in the treatment of patients with hepatoma outside of an organized experimental protocol.

COMMENTARY by Paul H. Sugarbaker

I read with great interest the unusually successful result that was achieved with this young woman. Her disease process was considerably different, in my opinion, from most patients with hepatoma. Her symptoms were long standing and she had complained of pain for 2 years in her right upper abdomen. This implies a slow growth of this malignancy. Also, the histopathology showed many well-differentiated areas. Often, hepatomas show bizarre cells, many mitoses, necrosis, and all the histopathologic features associated with an extremely rapidly progressing tumor.

Apparently, Dr. Douglas proceeded with his operation without a percutaneous biopsy. I completely agree with this approach. Percutaneous biopsy of liver tumors before surgery is usually meddlesome, does not change the surgical approach, and can be associated with considerable morbidity. Of greatest worry is the intra-abdominal dissemination of cancer cells that may result from needle disruption of the capsule of a cancerous process. Whether the tumor is primary or metastatic, percutaneous needle biopsy is rarely indicated. Surgical exploration is the diagnostic procedure of choice.

The preoperative arteriogram was interesting. It did suggest that this was a malignant process. The need of a preoperative arteriogram in patients with liver tumors has been questioned by many. Our group rarely performs preoperative arteriography in patients with liver tumors. A possible exception to this is the need for arteriography if a pump or a port is to be considered if the lesion is unresectable. Few surgeons use regional chemotherapy with liver tumors at this point in time.

Our own routine for workup of a suspect hepatoma is the CT portogram (1–3). We believe that it is important to assess the number of lesions in the liver and the relationship of the liver tumor to the liver vasculature and to rule out the presence of tumor in the portal vein. The most accurate examination for all three objectives is CT portography.

Our surgical approach would be through a midline abdominal incision. With the use of self-retraining retractors, the thoracoabdominal approach is rarely required. Our use of this incision is limited to those patients in whom we cannot separate tumor mass from the diaphragm. Even in this situation, crossing the costal margin is rarely required. The margin of normal liver was very adequate (4). Large tumors should have 2 cm of normal liver between the specimen and the margin of excision. In smaller tumors a narrower margin is acceptable (5–8).

It's interesting that this patient did receive postoperative chemotherapy. We do not treat primary tumors with systemic chemotherapy because the responses are so very low. It seems unlikely that chemotherapy would effectively treat micrometastatic disease from hepatoma.

Often, high-grade hepatomas are marginally resectable because of tumor involvement of portal structures. In this situation, intra-arterial chemoembolization treatments have been used successfully to shrink a tumor before its resection (8). Although not shown in a randomized control study, these chemoembolization procedures may also effectively palliate and prolong the survival of patients with unresectable hepatoma.

A final comment about the ruptured hepatoma. This is not an uncommon situation and may be seen in up to 30% of the lesions. If the tumor is resectable from the liver, we have used intraperitoneal adriamycin and cisplatin to eliminate micrometastatic disease on peritoneal surfaces. Although no randomized control studies are available, long-term success has been achieved in these patients. Before this time, ruptured hepatoma was an universally fatal disease process.

REFERENCES

1. Reining JW, Dwyers AJ, Miller DL, Sugarbaker PH. Liver metastasis detection: comparative sensitivities of MR imaging and CT scanning. *Radiology* 1987;162:43–7.
2. Nelson RC, Chezmar JL, Sugarbaker PH, et al. The ability of CT during arterial portography to preoperatively localize focal liver lesions to specific liver segments. *Radiology* 1990;176:89–94.
3. Sugarbaker PH, Nelson RC, Murray DR, et al. Liver computerized tomography for hepatic resection: a segmental approach. *Surg Gyne-*

col Obstet 1990;171:189–95.

4. Sugarbaker PH. Rule of the least margin: Rationale for surgical treatment planning in gastrointestinal cancer. *Reg Cancer Treat* 1991; 4:116–20.

5. Sugarbaker PH, Leighton SB. Hepatic parenchymal suction dissector. *Surg Gynecol Obstet* 1986;163:267–9.

6. Hughes KS, Simon R, Sugarbaker PH, et al. The Hepatic Metastases Registry: resection of the liver for colorectal carcinoma metastases: a multi-institutional study of patterns of recurrence. *Surgery* 1986;100: 278–84.

7. Sugarbaker PH. Transverse hepatectomy, en bloc resection of liver segments 4b, 5 and 6. *Surg Gynecol Obstet* 1990;170:250–2.

8. Sugarbaker PH, Steves MA. A cytoreductive approach to treatment of multiple liver metastases. *J Surg Oncol* (in press).

9. Sugarbaker PH, Ryan AM. Treatment of peritoneal carcinomatosis. A manual for physicians and nurses (in progress).

SECTION VII

Duodenum

36

Duodenal Cancer Treated by a Whipple Procedure

Murray F. Brennan

Laparoscopic staging accurately identified resectability

CASE PRESENTATION

G.D. is a 51-year-old man who presents with right upper quadrant epigastric pain of 4 months' duration. He was treated initially with antacid medications, with mild relief. However, the pain continued and ultrasound demonstrated a dilated common bile duct and a dilated gallbladder. There was no evidence of any stone disease. He then underwent an upper gastrointestinal series with some suggestion of an intrinsic mass in the duodenum. This was followed by endoscopy, which revealed a tumor in the second portion of the duodenum, partially obstructing the ampulla of Vater. Biopsy specimens were obtained and were consistent with a moderately differentiated adenocarcinoma. A computed tomography (CT) scan was subsequently obtained, revealing no evidence of liver metastasis or other metastatic disease or adenopathy.

He was referred for definitive treatment. On review of systems, he had had minimum weight loss, and on physical examination the only abnormality was a palpable gallbladder. Laboratory tests revealed an elevated LDH, AST, and alkaline phosphatase, and a markedly elevated GGT. His bilirubin was 1.9 mg%.

At presentation at the weekly Tumor Board, the discussion centered on the following issues:

1. What is the appropriate treatment for this man?
2. Are any other investigations indicated or justified?
3. Is this tumor an ampullary or duodenal carcinoma? And, if so, how would it be expected to behave?
4. If a duodenal carcinoma, could a more limited resection than a pancreaticoduodenectomy be performed?
5. What is the preferred management?

He was admitted and underwent a laparoscopy, laparotomy, and conventional pancreaticoduodenectomy. No disease was encountered on laparoscopy, which was performed using three ports, the two superior ports placed in the line of the subsequent bilateral subcostal incision. Laparoscopic ultrasound was not performed. At operation, a large mass involving the duodenum, extending into the head of the pancreas, with a dilated but not obstructed common bile duct, was found. After pancreaticoduodenectomy, he had an uneventful recovery, with some ileus lasting approximately 5 days. He was discharged on the ninth postoperative day.

Pathology revealed an extensive invasive, poorly differentiated adenocarcinoma arising in the nonampullary duodenal mucosa, measuring 3.5 × 5 cm, extending into the periduodenal soft tissue and into the pancreas. The margins of resection were negative and 24 examined regional nodes were negative for tumor. No adjuvant therapy was given, and he remains alive and well without symptoms 1 year later.

It is now clear from several studies that duodenal adenocarcinoma behaves much more like gastric adenocarcinoma than does conventional pancreatic adenocarcinoma (1). The patients, therefore, can be considered for approaches similar to that for gastric cancer. Postoperatively, no adjuvant therapy has been shown to change the outcome of gastric adenocarcinoma, and therefore none would be used, although this has been debated by some (2). The patient with node-negative duodenal cancer would be expected to have a good long-term survival exceeding 70% (1–4).

Laparoscopy was used in this case as part of an investigative protocol to try to eliminate unnecessary major explorations for pancreatic, gastric, or duodenal adenocarcinoma. The presence of metastatic disease in a patient who was not obstructed would clearly preclude embarking on further major resection. Without obstruction, no palliative procedure need be performed, certainly not by open operation.

The extent of laparoscopy continues to be of some debate. In the main, laparoscopy is performed using two or occasionally three ports, predominantly to identify liver or peritoneal metastasis and to examine various degrees of local invasion or metastasis. In pancreatic adenocarcinoma, the advent of the laparoscopic ultrasound probe has allowed us to use a more aggressive and extensive laparoscopy dissection and Doppler ultrasonography to determine whether or not the superior mesenteric vein or artery or the celiac artery are involved, issues not easily appreciated in conventional screening laparoscopy. Current programs examining the use of instant cytopathology attained at the time of laparoscopy await confirmation.

REFERENCES

1. Brennan MF. Duodenal cancer. *Asian J Surg* 1991;13:204–9.
2. Barnes G Jr, Romero L, Hess KR, Curley SA. Primary adenocarcinoma of the duodenum: management and survival in 67 patients. *Ann Surg Oncol* 1994;1:73–8.
3. Rotman N, Pezet D, Fagniez PL, et al. Adenocarcinoma of the duodenum: factors influencing survival. *Br J Surg* 1994;81:83–5.
4. Delcomre R, Thomas JH, Forster J, Hermreck AS. Improving resectability and survival in patients with primary duodenal carcinoma. *Am J Surg* 1993;166:626–31.

COMMENTARY by Glenn D. Steele, Jr.

The case described by Dr. Brennan was discussed rationally and handled appropriately. Indications for doing large procedures (even palliative) in patients with duodenal and ampullary carcinoma are quite different from when the same procedures are being considered in patients with ductal pancreatic cancer. Even if the duodenal carcinoma described in this case were found at laparoscopic exploration to have periduodenal nodal involvement, there still would be a good justification for pancreaticoduodenectomy because the latency of disease recurrence after complete clearance of gross disease is greater than in pancreatic cancer. Furthermore, the ability to preempt duodenal obstruction and/or bleeding often justifies the bigger operation, even when the goal is known to be palliation.

Although the Tumor Board apparently addressed the question of a more limited resection, the matter was not discussed in detail. The decision to perform a pancreaticoduodenectomy is evidence enough that a more limited resection in this patient was certainly not considered optimal. More generally, limited resections for duodenal carcinomas are probably, at this time, never justifiable, and for ampullary cancers, other than adenomatous polyps of the ampulla, more limited resections, even if technically feasible, should be considered deviations from standard and potentially curative care.

My only quibble in the care of this patient was with the application of laparoscopy as part of the preoperative staging. I think that without clinical evidence of extensive peritoneal spread, this patient was going to need a biliary, if not gastrointestinal, bypass and in light of the liberal indications for pancreaticoduodenectomy, even in the presence of N1 disease for patients with duodenal cancer, an argument could be made to move immediately to full laparotomy. Nevertheless, Dr. Brennan mentions that laparoscopy was a part of an experimental procedure. With that specific justification, it's hard to be overly critical of its application.

37

The Carcinoid Syndrome: Carcinoid of the Ileum with Liver Metastases

Mark S. Talamonti, Michael Lyster, Al B. Benson III

Octreotide and chemoembolization produced excellent palliation

CASE PRESENTATION

J.D.A. is a 69-year-old man who presented with complaints of cutaneous flushing and occasional dizziness. These problems began approximately 7 months before this initial evaluation. Since that time, he additionally noted increasingly frequent and severe episodes of diarrhea, an intermittent rash on multiple areas of his body, and occasional dyspnea. He has a history of coronary artery disease and chronic stable angina; and initially, he ascribed these symptoms to his cardiac medications, which included digoxin and a calcium channel blocker. With progression and increasing severity of his symptoms, he sought evaluation. His past surgical history is significant for coronary artery bypass surgery and bilateral carotid endarterectomies 5 years ago. He also has a history of emphysema with a greater than 90-pack-year smoking history.

Physical examination revealed an alert man in no acute distress. At the time of his initial examination, the patient began to develop cutaneous flushing; and during that episode, his blood pressure was 140/95 with frequent ectopy noted on palpation of his radial pulse. His head and neck examination was normal except for intermittent and frequent facial flushing. His neck was supple and free of lymphadenopathy, and his lungs were clear bilaterally. Cardiac examination revealed an early grade II/VI systolic murmur and a decrescendo grade II/VI diastolic murmur. The patient's rhythm was regular but frequent ectopy was noted. The abdominal exam was without evidence of tenderness or frank hepatosplenomegaly although the liver edge was palpable just below the costal margin. His stools

were guaiac-negative. An electrocardiogram revealed variable periods of atrial flutter and fibrillation.

These signs and symptoms were believed to be consistent with a possible diagnosis of the carcinoid syndrome, and a 24-hour urine collection was performed for 5-hydroxyindoleacetic acid levels (5HIAA). Urine 5HIAA levels were markedly elevated with 75 mg in the first 24-hour collection (normal range 2-8 mg/24 hours). A second assay was performed and again confirmed elevated levels of urine 5HIAA. Pancreatic polypeptides were normal and biochemical analysis for pheochromocytoma was unremarkable.

The patient was then referred to surgical oncology section for further management. The patient's clinical presentation and biochemical studies were consistent with a diagnosis of the carcinoid syndrome. A computed tomography (CT) scan of the abdomen was performed and revealed bilobar liver metastases and suggestion of a 3-4 cm mass in the right lower quadrant. Upper and lower endoscopic exams were normal. A barium enema was within normal limits and an upper gastrointestinal barium study and small bowel series were performed. This latter study revealed a lesion in the distal ileum, approximately 10 cm proximal to the ileocecal valve, consistent with a primary midgut tumor. Echocardiography revealed poor left ventricular function and a 30% to 45% reduction of the expected ejection fraction. Additionally, there was significant mitral and aortic regurgitation. Although carcinoid disease affects the tricuspid valve and right-sided structures, no abnormalities of these valves were identified. Ultrasound-guided needle biopsy of the largest liver lesion provided histologic confirmation of metastatic carcinoid consistent with a small bowel primary (Fig. 37–1)

IMPRESSION

In summary, this patient is a 69-year-old man who presented with the symptoms of cutaneous flushing, diarrhea, occasional dizziness, and intermittent dyspnea. Physical examination was remarkable for frequent ectopy, an early systolic murmur, and a decrescendo diastolic murmur. Biochemical characterization included urinary 5HIAA levels that were markedly elevated. Anatomic localization studies included upper and lower bowel contrast roentgenography and computed tomography. These studies demonstrated extensive liver involvement with metastatic disease and the localization of the primary midgut tumor to the distal ileum measuring approximately 3-4 cm in size. Ultrasound-guided liver biopsy confirmed the diagnosis. It should be noted that the patient did not have any symptoms such as bleeding or obstruction related to the presence of the primary tumor.

MANAGEMENT

Because of the patient's distinctive symptoms and progressive severity of his problems, octreotide blockade was initiated. Octreotide is the somatostatin analog that currently provides the most effective means of managing the symptom complex associated with malignant carcinoid syndrome. The mechanism of action results from inhibition of the release of bioactive mediators from the meta-

static lesions. Octreotide also possesses potent pro-absorptive actions in the gastrointestinal tract, which may diminish the secretory diarrhea of the carcinoid syndrome (1). Therapy was initiated with a starting dose of 100 DK subcutaneously administered twice a day. It produced clear symptomatic improvement within 72 hours. The daily dose was then increased to 200 DK b.i.d. and the patient had nearly complete relief from cutaneous flushing and a significant reduction in his diarrhea and dyspnea.

Treatment options for the primary carcinoid tumor and the liver metastases were then discussed at the multimodality tumor conference. An important factor in the consideration of this patient's treatment planning was his past history of coronary and carotid vascular disease and emphysema. Laparotomy for the purposes of primary tumor resection and debulking of the liver metastases was discussed. Patients with nonmetastatic primary midgut tumors should undergo resection to avoid the complications of bleeding and bowel obstruction. Most common in the ileum or right colon, these tumors should be resected together with the regional lymph node drainage. The cure rate is high for those patients in whom all visible malignant disease can be resected (2). These data raise the question of aggressive surgical resection of the primary lesion and the metastases. Several surgical series have demonstrated an extended survival with resection of the primary and metastatic tumors (3–7). Experience from the Mayo Clinic has suggested that curative surgery should be considered in all patients with completely resectable metastatic disease (2). Unfortunately, only 10% to 25% of patients with hepatic metastases may be curable with a formal hepatic resection. The extent of our patient's liver disease precluded any attempt

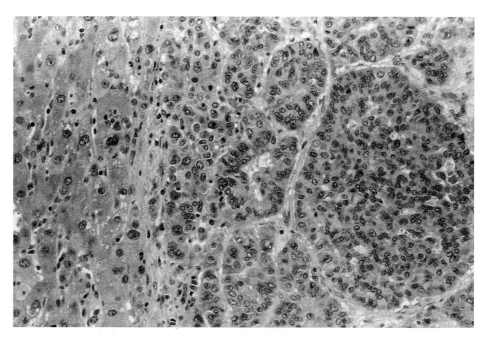

FIG. 37–1. Metastatic carcinoid tumor in the liver from a primary ileal tumor. On the left is normal liver and on the right is a carcinoid lesion showing an insular pattern, consistent with a mid-gut primary (x200).

at curative resection. Experience from other institutions has suggested that debulking of hepatic metastases may substantially palliate systemic symptoms of the carcinoid syndrome. The duration of effective palliation is usually brief, and substantial morbidity may be associated with partial hepatectomy for the purpose of cytoreduction.

Because of the diffuse liver involvement that precluded curative resection and his medical problems that made aggressive cytoreductive surgery extremely problematic, other treatment options were considered. In addition, nearly complete symptomatic relief had been achieved with octreotide blockade and therefore surgical exploration for the purposes of debulking the liver metastases and resecting an otherwise asymptomatic primary tumor was not deemed in the best interest of this high risk patient. Systemic chemotherapy with streptozocin, doxorubicin, chlorozotocin, DTIC, and 5-FU has demonstrated response rates of approximately 20%, yet these regimens still have only limited long-term efficacy in patients with metastatic carcinoid tumors (2). Interruption of the hepatic arterial blood supply as a form of metastatic treatment has been proposed in the past. Ischemic treatment of metastatic carcinoid tumors is possible because these tumors are primarily supplied by the hepatic artery. Hepatic parenchyma can thus remain perfused via portal vein flow despite hepatic arterial occlusion. The ligation of the hepatic artery as a method of devascularization does not seem to be effective because extensive anastomotic recirculation is rapidly developed after hepatic artery ligation with no significant or prolonged tumor ischemia. In contrast, peripheral intrahepatic arterial embolization has been shown to be extremely effective in symptomatic patients with liver metastases from carcinoid tumors. Embolization of distal hepatic artery branches provides more precise and prolonged ischemia with less damage to normal hepatic parenchyma compared with major vessel ligation.

Recent published reports suggests the efficacy of a combination of chemoembolization and octreotide blockade in unresectable or poor-risk patients (8,9). Our current institutional protocol involves the use of hepatic artery chemoembolization. Several institutions have demonstrated significant symptomatic improvement with an improved median survival time after peripheral hepatic artery embolization in patients with metastatic carcinoid tumors. Chemoembolization is the concurrent intra-arterial administration of a collagen particle with chemotherapeutic agents. The collagen is minimally antigenic and does not significantly bind to chemotherapeutic agents. Administered intra-arterially, it penetrates to the precapillary sphincter and then fills the vascular space in a retrograde fashion. Regional drug delivery is therefore enhanced by flow arrest. The combination of regional delivery of chemotherapeutic agents and vascular interruption is thought to improve the response rate and the duration of response to therapy. Our current protocol utilizes an embolic suspension containing Angiostat colla-

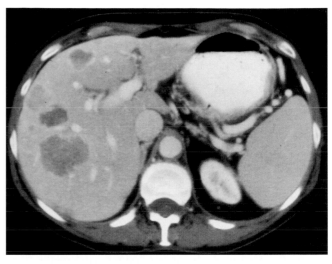

FIG. 37–2. Computed tomography scan with contrast enhancement of large, bilobar hepatic metastases from primary mid-gut tumor.

gen, 10 mg/mL, and cisplatin 10 mg/mL, mitomycin C 3 mg/mL, and doxorubicin 3 mg/mL. It is administered up to a maximum dose of 8.75 mL under continuous fluoroscopic monitoring. Subsequent embolizations are carried out at 4-week intervals if clinically indicated. Thus, our final treatment recommendation to this patient was to maintain octreotide blockade with frequent monitoring of his 5HIAA levels and to initiate hepatic artery chemoembolization. The patient underwent his first two embolizations without any significant complications. Serial CT scans have been performed; and after two embolizations, the scans have demonstrated a decrease in the size of the liver metastases (Figs. 37–2 and 37–3). There is no evidence of other distant metastases. His symptoms remain well controlled with octreotide blockade.

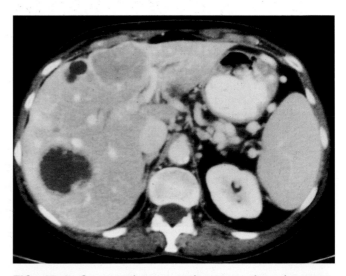

FIG. 37–3. Computed tomography scan after chemoembolization. Note tumor regression of the right lobe lesions after embolization. There has been progression of the lesion in the left medial segment that had not yet been treated.

REFERENCES

1. Hurst RD, Modlin IM. Future prospects for somatostatin analogs. *Contemp Oncol* 1991;1:27–32.
2. Moertel CG. An odyssey in the land of small tumors. *J Clin Oncol* 1987;5:1503–22.
3. Ahlman H, Schersten T, Tisell LE. Surgical treatment of patients with the carcinoid syndrome. *Acta Oncologica* 1987;28:403–7.
4. McEntee GP, Kvols LK, et al. Cytoreductive hepatic surgery for neuroendocrine tumors. *Surgery* 1990;12:1091–96.
5. Makridis C, Oberg K, Juhlin C, et al. Surgical treatment of mid-gut carcinoid tumors. *World J Surg* 1990;14:377–85.
6. MacGillivray DC, Synder DA, Drucker W, et al. Carcinoid tumors: the relationship between clinical presentation and the extent of disease. *Surgery* 1991;110:68–72.
7. Soreide O, Berstad T, Bakka A, et al. Surgical treatment as a principle in patients with advanced abdominal carcinoid tumors. *Surgery* 1992;111:48–54.
8. Basson MD, Ahlman H, Wangberg B, et al. Biology and management of the midgut carcinoid. *Am J Surg* 1993;165:288–97.
9. Hajarizadeh H, Ivancev K, Mueller CR, et al. Effective palliative treatment of metastatic carcinoid tumors with intra-arterial chemotherapy/chemoembolization combined with octreotide acetate. *Am J Surg* 163;479–83.

COMMENTARY by Dr. John H. Donohue

The management of patients with carcinoid syndrome must be divided into two components: 1) treatment of the systemic effects of the tumor and 2) therapy directed at controlling the neoplasm's growth. Although the clinical manifestations of the carcinoid syndrome can be abrogated, at least temporarily, in most patients, the extent of metastatic tumor limits the effective options for primary tumor control.

This patient is typical for carcinoid syndrome given the symptoms of flushing, diarrhea, and dyspnea (these occurred in 73%, 65%, and 8% of 91 patients presenting at the Mayo Clinic) (1), a primary ileal tumor, and the extensive hepatic metastases. His medical history is notable for significant peripheral atherosclerosis and coronary artery disease. The latter problem, rather than his metastatic carcinoid disease, is the cause for his valvular heart disease, because right-sided valvular lesions (pulmonary stenosis and tricuspid regurgitation) are the result of carcinoid syndrome.

Patients with metastatic carcinoid tumors who are asymptomatic or have mild complaints related to their disease are usually managed conservatively. When significant symptoms occur, the management of carcinoid syndrome is best achieved with octreotide, a somatostatin analog (2). Although occasional patients experience regression of their tumor with octreotide, stabilization of tumor growth is more common and seen in up to 50% of patients (3). Interferon has shown some promise in relieving tumor symptoms and controlling tumor growth (4) although it has no apparent advantage over octreotide. Symptoms of bowel obstruction or ischemia resulting from mesenteric fibrosis were not apparent in this patient but are indications for surgical exploration. Patients with recurrent symptoms despite escalating doses of octreotide (doses up to 500 mg t.i.d.),

patients with more advanced metastatic disease, or patients with anaplastic tumors (improved responses have been seen with etoposide and cisplatin [5]) require more aggressive treatment.

In carefully selected patients cytoreductive surgery should be considered. In a minority of patients, all gross disease can be removed and occasional patients remain disease-free for years. For most patients, surgical resection is palliative and is only of value when the vast majority (>90% tumor volume) can be excised (6). Because hepatic metastases are preferentially perfused by the hepatic artery, combination therapies combining interruption of the hepatic artery with chemotherapy have been used to increase the lackluster results of chemotherapy alone (1,7). Hepatic artery ligation (8), intermittent pneumatic occlusion (9), and embolization (7,10) have all been used as means to interrupt the vascular inflow to the tumor. The last approach has several advantages including avoidance of an operation and the fact that embolization can be repeated on multiple occasions. Using an alternating chemotherapy regimen of doxorubicin plus dacarbazine and streptozocin plus 5-fluorouracil, a median duration of response of 24 months has been achieved in combination with hepatic artery occlusion (1).

Given the patient's medical status, lack of symptoms from his primary tumor and the extent of his hepatic metastases, the approach of octreotide plus hepatic artery embolization and regional chemotherapy is the most efficacious option for this man. He will likely enjoy symptomatic relief for months, if not longer, and have a reasonable duration of survival. Although treatable and controllable, patients with carcinoid syndrome are rarely, if ever, curable.

REFERENCES

1. Moertel CG. An odyssey in the land of small tumors. *J Clin Oncol* 1987;5:1503–22.
2. Kvols LK, Moertel CG, O'Connell MJ, et al. Treatment of malignant carcinoid syndrome: evaluation of a long acting somatostatin analog. *N Engl J Med* 1986;315:663–6.
3. Saltz L, Trochanowski B, Buckley M, et al. Octreotide as an antineoplastic agent in the treatment of functional and nonfunctional neuroendocrine tumors. *Cancer* 1993;72:244–8.
4. Moertel CG, Rubin J, Kvols LK. Therapy of metastatic carcinoid tumor and the malignant carcinoid syndrome with recombinant leukocyte A interferon. *J Clin Oncol* 1989;7:865–8.
5. Moertel CG, Kvols LK, O'Connell MJ, Rubin J. Treatment of neuroendocrine carcinomas with combined etoposide and cisplatin. Evidence of major therapeutic activity in the anaplastic variants of these neoplasms. *Cancer* 1991;68:227–32.
6. McEntee GP, Nagorney DM, Kvols LK, et al. Cytoreductive hepatic surgery for neuroendocrine tumors. *Surgery* 1990;108:1091–6.
7. Kvols LK. The carcinoid syndrome: a treatable malignant disease. *Oncology* 1988;2:33–9.
8. Moertel CG, May GR, Martin JK, et al. Sequential hepatic artery occlusion (HAO) and chemotherapy for metastatic carcinoid and islet cell carcinoma (ICC). *Proc ASCO* 1985;4:80.
9. Persson BG, Nobin A, Ahren B, et al. Repeated hepatic ischemia as a treatment for carcinoid liver metastases. *World J Surg* 1989;13:307–12.
10. Ruszniewski P, Rougier P, Roche A, et al. Hepatic arterial chemoembolization in patients with liver metastases of endocrine tumors. A prospective phase II study in 24 patients. *Cancer* 1993;71:2624–30.

SECTION VIII

Small Bowel

38 Leiomyosarcoma of the Small Bowel

John H. Donohue

Complete surgical resection is the only effective treatment,
but wasn't enough in this case

CASE PRESENTATION

A 44-year-old man was referred for evaluation and treatment of an abdominal mass noted by his local physician. This business manager had complained of abdominal pain during the last 6 months. Because the discomfort was initially in the epigastrium, histamine receptor type II blockers were prescribed for alleged peptic ulcer disease. During the last 3 months, the pain localized in the lower abdomen, was exacerbated by vigorous activity such as jogging, and was accompanied by pressure on the bladder. The patient denied changes in his bladder and bowel function, as well as weight loss, fatigue, fever, and night sweats.

The patient's previous medical history was unremarkable. He had bilateral inguinal hernia repairs as an infant but no illnesses, hospitalizations, or allergies. He was on no medications. His parents died in their 50s of a heart attack (father) and alcoholic cirrhosis (mother). There was no family history of cancer.

On physical examination, the patient appeared trim and healthy, with unremarkable vital signs. Pertinent negative findings included the absence of peripheral adenopathy, hepatomegaly, or splenomegaly, and normal testicular and rectal examinations. There was a large abdominal mass that measured 15 to 20 cm in diameter filling the lower abdomen to the level of the umbilicus. This was firm and moved slightly with compression.

Preoperative laboratory included a hemoglobin of 14.7 g/dL, white blood cell count of 6.8×10^9/L with normal differential, platelet count of 304×10^9/L, normal serum electrolytes, albumin of 4.0 g/dL, glucose 86 mg/dL, alkaline phosphatase 196 U/L, AST 27 U/L, total bilirubin 0.4 mg/dL, and creatinine of 1.1 mg/dL. Chest radiograph and computed tomography (CT) were within normal limits. An abdominal CT scan with oral and intravenous contrast done before referral showed a large, partially cystic mass in the pelvis and lower abdomen, probably originating in the left iliac region (see Figs. 38–1, 38–2). Although the findings were nonspecific, a retroperitoneal sarcoma was suspected radiographically.

The differential diagnosis preoperatively included retroperitoneal or visceral sarcoma, lymphoma, and mucocele. After obtaining informed consent and performing a bowel prep, the patient underwent abdominal exploration through a midline incision. The mass was found to arise from the distal jejunum and to be adherent to the left pelvic sidewall and lateral aspect of the sigmoid mesocolon, such that the sigmoid colon was displaced to the right. There were no peritoneal implants of tumor, retroperitoneal or mesenteric adenopathy, or evidence of hepatic metastasis on inspection.

The mass was mobilized, taking a rim of sigmoid colon mesentery and pelvic side wall, including a segment of the left vas deferens, where the mass was adherent. A 10-cm segment of jejunum and adjacent mesentery was excised with the tumor, after which a primary end-to-end anastomosis was performed. The specimen weighed 1,405 grams and the tumor measured $20 \times 15 \times 10$ cm (Fig. 38–3) Histologically, the tumor was a cystic grade 2 leiomyosarcoma entirely exoenteric in its growth. The margins of resection were grossly and microscopically clear of involvement. Using the American Joint Committee on Cancer Staging criteria, this sarcoma represented pathologic stage IIB (Gr 2, T2, N0, M0) disease.

The patient's postoperative recovery was unremarkable, and he left the hospital 8 days after the operative pro-

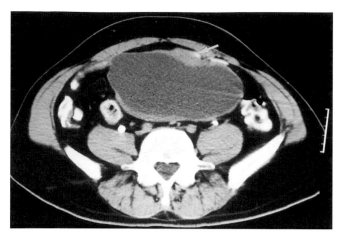

FIG. 38–1. Preoperative CT scan of the lower abdomen showing a large cystic mass with involvement of contrast-filled intestine (*arrow*).

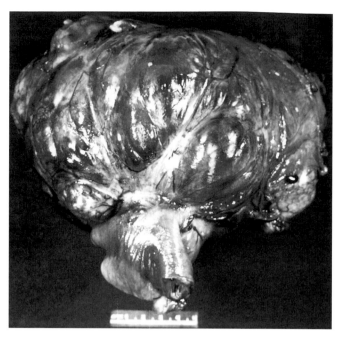

FIG. 38–3. Operative specimen photographed showing a large exoenteric mass (superiorly) and the involved portion of jejunum (inferiorly).

cedure. No adjuvant radiation or chemotherapy was recommended. The patient returned for follow-up 3 months later with no new complaints. A CT scan of the abdomen, chest radiograph, and blood tests were unremarkable except for postoperative changes.

Six months after resection, the patient returned for a second follow-up visit. Although the patient was still asymptomatic, and blood tests and chest roentgenogram showed normal results, three new low-density lesions were seen in the liver on abdominal CT scan (Fig. 38–4). Hepatic ultrasound confirmed these as hypoechoic solid masses typical for metastases but found no additional tumors. Because of the rapid recurrence of disease and multiple hepatic metastases, no immediate surgical intervention was recommended.

Instead, the patient returned for a third CT scan 6 weeks afterward, which showed multiple bilobar hepatic metastases. There was no evidence of intra-abdominal recurrence or pulmonary metastasis on roentgenography. The patient had remained asymptomatic with stable weight and normal activity. The options of no treatment or combination chemotherapy were discussed with the patient, who wished to pursue further treatment nearer to home.

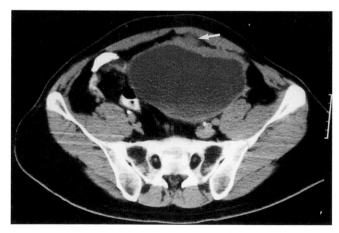

FIG. 38–2. Preoperative CT scan of the pelvis showing the mass with abutment on the left iliopsoas muscle and possible impingement on the anterior abdominal wall (*arrow*).

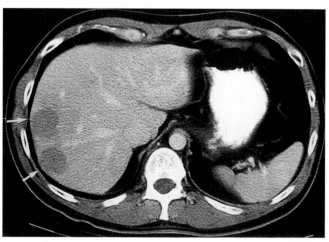

FIG. 38–4. Postoperative CT scan showing new hepatic metastases in the lateral aspect of the right lobe of liver (*arrows*).

COMMENTARY by Murray F. Brennan

This case is consistent with a leiomyosarcoma of the small intestine. The important features of the presentation are the careful examination of the testes in an asymptomatic, relatively midline mass in a young man. Germ cell tumors (prognostically the most favorable diagnosis) must not be missed. If there is any question, then testicular ultrasound and serum markers for germ cell tumors would also be performed. In the present case, however, the CT scan did not suggest a germ cell lesion, given the anterior and cystic nature of the lesion and the lack of retroperitoneal involvement.

No other tests were indicated or necessary. Preoperative biopsy was appropriately avoided in this patient because complete resection was possible. The operation was appropriately performed and no gross disease was left behind. Histopathologically, the lesion was characterized as a cystic leiomyosarcoma of intermediate grade. The probability of metastasis would be likely, and of all lesions, an intermediate grade visceral leiomyosarcoma of large size is least predictable for risk of metastasis.

Metastasis rapidly occurred in the liver and from that point any further treatment would be considered purely investigational. In a young man, unproven investigational possibilities such as hepatic embolization, intraperitoneal or intrahepatic chemotherapy, or systemic chemotherapy would all be considered, but with no evidence at present that survival would be improved. In summary, for visceral leiomyosarcomas, the major determinant of prognostic outcome is the initial complete resection of the tumor, followed by the histologic grade of the lesion.

SELECTED READINGS

1. Bevilacqua RE, Rogatko A, Hajdu SI, Brennan MF. Prognostic factors in primary retroperitoneal soft tissue sarcoma. *Arch Surg* 1991; 126:328–34.
2. Jaques DP, Coit DG, Hajdu SI, Brennan MF. Management of primary and recurrent soft tissue sarcoma of the retroperitoneum. *Ann Surg* 1990;212:51–9.

SECTION IX

Appendix

39 Pseudomyxoma Peritonei

William E. Burak, Jr. and William B. Farrar

*Keep after this peritoneal-based indolent disease surgically
to achieve long-term survival*

CASE PRESENTATION

A 73-year-old white man was in his usual state of normal health until 6 months before admission when he was found to be anemic. Further workup was refused at that time. During the following months, he had right-sided abdominal pain requiring hospitalization. At the time of admission, the patient described the pain as dull, constant, and nonradiating. He denied constipation, obstipation, genitourinary symptoms, or weight loss. No upper gastrointestinal symptomatology or history of abdominal distension could be elicited. His past medical history was significant for non-insulin–dependent diabetes mellitus (25 years) and hypertension for 2 years. The patient underwent a transurethral resection of his prostate 3 years before admission for benign prostatic hypertrophy. Medications at the time of admission included an antihypertensive agent and an oral hypoglycemic.

A family history of leukemia (mother) and lung cancer (sister) was obtained. Alcohol and tobacco use was denied by this retired welder.

Physical examination revealed a man of stated age in no acute distress. Vital signs were normal, sclera anicteric, and no cervical adenopathy was noted. Lungs were clear to auscultation and his heart was without murmurs or gallops. Abdominal examination revealed mild right lower quadrant tenderness, but no masses could be appreciated. The liver was palpable approximately 3 cm below the costal margin and was felt to have a smooth edge. There was slight abdominal distension, but shifting dullness and a fluid wave were absent. Digital rectal examination was unremarkable and stool was heme-test negative. No extremity edema was present.

Laboratory values included a hemoglobin of 11.1 g and hematocrit of 34.1%. Electrolytes, coagulation profile, and liver function tests were all in the normal range. A serum carcinoembryonic antigen (CEA) level was obtained and found to be 73.2 (normal 0-5). Urinalysis was without abnormalities. Subsequently, colonoscopy was performed, which revealed 2 small polyps (3 mm) in the cecum and a 1- cm villoglandular rectal polyp. No other masses or lesions were identified. An esophagogastroduodenoscopy was then undertaken and found to be unremarkable. Following this, a CT scan of the abdomen and pelvis revealed the presence of a large amount of loculated ascitic fluid, with density greater than water. "Scalloping" of the liver by this fluid was clearly seen. Collections were present in the perihepatic and pelvic region as well as in both paracolic gutters (Fig. 39–1) Computed tomography–guided aspiration of this perihepatic fluid revealed mucoid material with cytologically atypical cells, which together are suggestive of pseudomyxoma peritonei.

At this point, the patient was taken to the operating room where he underwent an exploratory laparotomy with the tentative diagnosis of pseudomyxoma peritonei. Multiple diffuse, mucinous masses were found involving the omentum, pelvis, right and left paracolic gutters, and perihepatic area. When the appendix was identified, it appeared that the tip was thickened and involved in the mucinous process. Omentectomy, appendectomy, cholecystectomy, liver biopsy, and resection of all visible disease were undertaken. The patient experienced an uneventful recovery and was discharged on the eighth postoperative day.

Pathologic results revealed a well-differentiated papillary mucinous adenocarcinoma in the lumen of the appen-

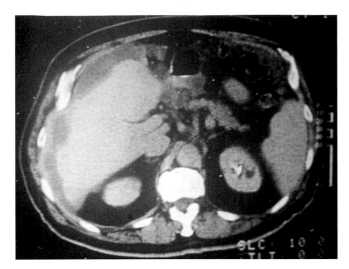

FIG. 39–1. Computed tomography scan of the abdomen from initial presentation. Note the "scalloping" of the liver parenchyma.

dix (Fig. 39–2) The appendix surface was covered by abundant masses of mucin, and focal tumor cells were seen. The multiple mucinous masses demonstrated focal areas of tumor cells (glandular epithelium) among huge masses of mucin. The liver parenchyma was also coated with tumor implants and mucin. A pathologic diagnosis of grade 1 mucinous adenocarcinoma of the appendix with widespread peritoneal dissemination was reported. After discharge, the patient was lost to follow-up until he presented 3 years later with a 4-month history of progressive abdominal distension and dyspnea. A second abdominal CT scan revealed recurrence of numerous large, loculated intra-abdominal masses consistent with recurrent pseudomyxoma peritonei (Fig. 39–3). A large left hydrothorax was also present, which yielded 3,200 mL of straw-colored

fluid with benign cytology when aspirated. The pleural effusion rapidly reaccumulated, necessitating placement of a chest tube. After this, a thoracic CT scan was done that revealed multiple left-sided pleural-based lesions thought to be pseudomyxoma peritonei (Fig. 39–4). With extra-abdominal disease present, a decision against resection of his intra-abdominal tumor was made; and the patient was discharged after removal of the chest tube. The patient expired 18 months later. The exact cause of the death was never documented, but thought to be related to intestinal obstruction.

DISCUSSION

Surgical Oncologist: Pseudomyxoma peritonei was described by Werth in 1884 as massive amounts of mucinous ascites found in association with benign ovarian neoplasms (1). This definition has evolved to include peritoneal implants of mucin, columnar epithelium, and various amounts of free mucin, associated with benign, borderline, and malignant mucinous neoplasms most often originating in the appendix or ovary (2). The patient presented here had a well-differentiated mucinous adenocarcinoma of the appendix, as is frequently seen. The etiology appears to be related to malignant obstruction of the appendiceal lumen (3,4,5), although there have been reports of pseudomyxoma peritonei originating from rupture of benign cystadenomas (6). It appears that the peritoneal cavity "reacts" to some irritating agent or tumorigenic stimulus causing widespread mucinous change throughout the abdomen (2).

Abdominal distention, dyspnea, and dyspepsia are common presenting symptoms, with anorexia and weight loss the late findings (6). Abdominal pain is also seen in 50% of patients, while 13% were entirely asymptomatic

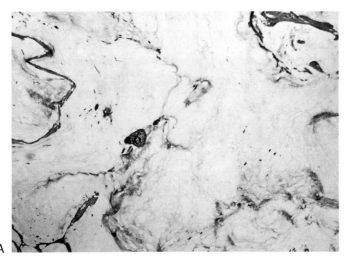

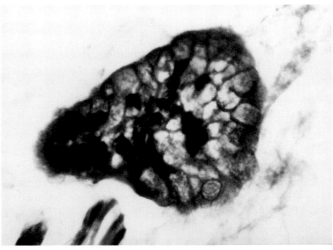

FIG. 39–2. A: Pseudomyxoma peritonei with small aggregate of tumor cells. B: Detail of neoplastic cells with bland nuclei and cytoplasmic mucin. (Hematoxylin and eosin 125X [A], 1200X [B]).

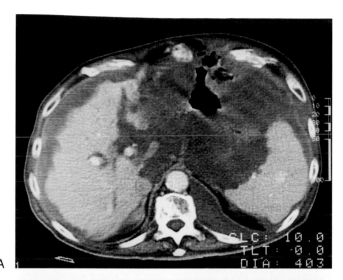

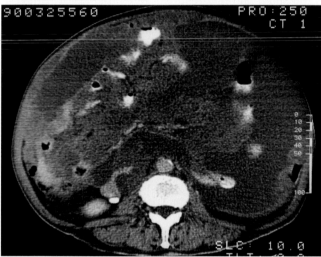

FIG. 39–3. Abdominal CT scan revealing recurrent pseudomyxoma peritonei.

in one series (7). The clinical presentation of the patient presented today is consistent with these findings.

The diagnosis of pseudomyxoma peritonei can be made in several ways. Frequently, it is initially discovered at laparotomy and can be mistaken for carcinomatosis. However, these implants are gelatinous and do not invade visceral organs, making it distinct from typical carcinomatosis. Computed tomography of the abdomen was used in this case and has traditionally been helpful in making the original diagnosis and evaluating the extent of the disease. "Classic" findings include ascites with attenuation values greater than water, low-attenuation soft tissue masses with internal mottled densities, distinctive rimlike calcifications, and compression of abdominal viscera without direct invasion (8). A more specific sign found in patients with pseudomyxoma peritonei is scalloping of the hepatic margin from extrinsic compression of the liver by fluid-filled ascitic spaces containing gelatinous material (8,9,10). The ultrasound findings of numerous thick-

walled intraperitoneal septate cysts, with associated peritoneal liver scalloping, also suggests the diagnosis (11).

Paracentesis has been used as a preoperative diagnostic tool with some success. The thick gelatinous nature of the ascites often precludes aspiration, however when successful, cytologic evaluation may be helpful and has certain characteristics (12).

Surgery remains the primary treatment for patients with pseudomyxoma peritonei. The initial operation consists of a thorough exploration to identify and resect the primary tumor. Because the origin is usually appendiceal, appendectomy should be performed; but, often, the appendix is surrounded by diffuse tumor requiring a right hemicolectomy. In female patients, bilateral oophorectomy should also be undertaken, as the ovaries can be the source of pseudomyxoma peritonei, and if not, they frequently harbor metastases. All gelatinous implants should be removed, which can be done without much technical difficulty because of the lack of visceral invasion of this neoplasm. Omentectomy should also be performed as the omentum is generally involved in the diffuse process. Because of the widespread nature of this disease, the surgeon is not able to obtain wide surgical margins and simple removal of all gross implants is all that is possible. Some authors have suggested irrigating the peritoneal cavity with 5% dextrose, a mucolytic agent (13,14).

Medical Oncologist: To get a better understanding of the treatment options for pseudomyxoma peritonei, one must examine the histology and behavior of the disease. It is generally believed that pseudomyxoma peritonei of appendiceal origin arises from low-grade mucinous adenocarcinomas or cystadenocarcinomas (3,4,6,7,15). The histologic characteristics include a monotonous sheet of mucinous material within which a curvilinear strand of epithelium can be seen. The strands of epithelium are usu-

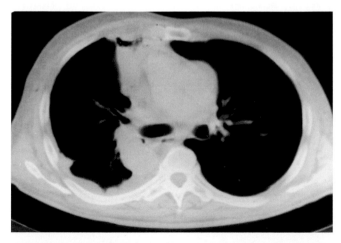

FIG. 39–4. Computed tomography of the thorax with multiple pleural based lesions in the left posterior and medial hemithorax.

ally a single layer thick and well differentiated. Cellular and nuclear architecture are similar to that of normal colonic epithelium. Although mucin-containing vacuoles are frequent, there is no evidence of invasion seen (16).

The pattern of spread of true pseudomyxoma peritonei is unique in that it usually remains contained in the peritoneal cavity and does not possess the ability to metastasize to distant sites (7). Transdiaphragmatic migration of tumor cells is the mechanism believed to be responsible for pleural involvement seen in advanced cases, as in the case presented. The pathogenesis of local spread is controversial, with some authors attributing it to metaplasia of the peritoneal cells in response to a stimulus from the mucinous fluid (17); however, most favor implantation of cells from the primary site. Local recurrences are extremely common and patients can survive for prolonged periods as this is a very indolent disease. Visceral invasion is rarely seen and death is generally a result of intestinal obstruction and loss of gut function on the basis of peritoneal implants. Five year survival rates have been quoted as ranging from 54% to 75%, with ten year survival being 18% to 60% (7,18).

It is difficult to recommend treatment for a disease as uncommon as pseudomyxoma peritonei because prospective, randomized studies are not available for analysis. The literature contains retrospective series and case reports which are inconsistent and in some cases, contradictory. As mentioned previously, surgery remains the mainstay of treatment for primary disease and recurrences, often out of necessity due to complications such as intestinal obstruction. Similarly, the use of chemotherapy has not been studied in a randomized, prospective fashion. Sugarbaker et al. report encouraging results with the combined use of cryoreductive surgery and postoperative intraperitoneal chemotherapy with 5-FU and Mitomycin C, however the follow-up was short at the time these results were published (16). Systemic chemotherapy after surgery traditionally has been used in hope of prolonging survival; however, results are not conclusive. Historically, 5-FU has been the drug of choice for appendiceal mucinous adenocarcinoma and pseudomyxoma peritonei. Although some believe it may favorably impact survival (7,15), others argue, pointing out that no prolongation of life has been documented, attributable to chemotherapy (2,18). Until prospective trials can be undertaken, this issue remains unresolved and chemotherapy cannot be recommended in the adjuvant setting. Patients with recurrent, unresectable disease are generally considered candidates for systemic chemotherapy, but again, prolongation of survival has yet to be demonstrated.

Radiation Oncologist: Radiation therapy has been used with success as an adjuvant therapy in patients with large-bowel adenocarcinomas, namely rectal. Improved local control rates can be achieved in this setting, as has been documented (19). The patterns of spread of pseudomyxoma peritonei makes it theoretically difficult to treat with radiation, as the field would have to include the entire abdomen. Additionally, the malignant cells, being very well differentiated and not dividing rapidly, are not ideally sensitive to this mode of treatment. Because of these characteristics, there has been an overall lack of enthusiasm for the therapeutic use of radiation in this group of patients.

In a review of 38 patients with pseudomyxoma peritonei at M.D. Anderson Hospital, 8 patients received postoperative radiation therapy, 2 with intraperitoneal gold, 3 with mid-abdominal radiation (3,000 R), and 3 with strip abdominal radiation (3,000 R) (7). A 75% 5-year survival rate was obtained in this group of patients, compared with 44% in patients treated with chemotherapy alone. Although these differences are not statistically significant, the authors suggest a benefit. This group of patients is too small and the treatment too variable for firm conclusions to be drawn.

At this time there is no role for radiation therapy in the treatment of pseudomyxoma peritonei.

SUMMARY

Pseudomyxoma peritonei, arising from mucinous adenocarcinomas of the appendix is a relatively uncommon and indolent disease with 5 year survival rates of 50% to 75%. Systemic metastases are extraordinarily rare with most patients succumbing to the effects of intra-abdominal recurrences and intestinal obstruction. Surgery remains the mainstay of treatment with the goal being resection of all gross disease. Adjuvant chemotherapy and radiation have not proven to be of benefit in these patients. The indolent nature of this disease often justifies repeat laparotomies and resection as no other treatment modality has been found to be effective.

REFERENCES

1. Werth R. Pseudomyxoma peritonei. *Arch Gynecol Obstet* 1884;24:100–18.
2. Mann WJ, Wagner J, Chumas J, Chalas E. The management of pseudomyxoma peritonei. *Cancer* 1990;66:1636–40.
3. Grodinsky M, Rubnitz AS. Muocele of the appendix and pseudomyxoma peritonei: a clinical review and experimental study, with case report. *Surg Gynecol Obstet* 1941;73:345–54.
4. Cheng K. An experimental study of mucocele of the appendix and pseudomyxoma peritonei. *J Pathol Bacterol* 1949;61:217–25.
5. Woolner LB. Carcinoma of the appendix: comments on pathology. *Proc Mayo Clinic* 1953;28:17–20.
6. Landen S, Bertrand C, Maddern GJ, et al. *Surg Gynecol Obstet* 1992;175:401–4.
7. Fernandez RN, Daly JM. Pseudomyxoma peritonei. *Arch Surg* 1980;115:409–14.
8. Lee H, Agha F, Wentherbech, Boland R. Pseudomyxoma peritonei: radiologic features. *J Clin Gastroenterol* 1986;8:312–16.
9. Mayes GB, Chuang VP, Fisher RG. CT of pseudomyxoma peritonei. *AJR* 1981;136:807–8.
10. Yeh H, Shafir MK, Slater G, et al. Ultrasonography and computed tomography of pseudomyxoma peritonei. *Radiology* 1984;153:507–10.

11. Hopper KD. Ultrasonic findings in pseudomyxoma peritonei. *South Med J* 1983;76(8):1051–2.
12. Costa M, Oertel YC. Cytology of pseudomyxoma peritonei: report of two cases arising from appendiceal cystadenomas. *Diagn Cytopathol* 1990;6(3):201–3.
13. Piver MS, Lele SB, Pastner B. Pseudomyxoma peritonei: possible preventions of mucinous ascites by peritoneal lavage. *Obstet Gynecol* 1984;64:959–65.
14. Haid M, Bowie L, Kim D, et al. Peritoneal washing therapy for pseudomyxoma peritonei. *South Med J* 1981;74(8):913–15.
15. Novell R, Lewis A. Role of surgery in the treatment of pseudomyxoma peritonei. *J R Coll Surg Edin* 1990;35:21–4.
16. Sugarbaker PH, Kern K, Lack E. Malignant pseudomyxoma peritonei of colonic origin. *Dis Col Rectum* 1987;30(10):772–79.
17. Sandenbergh HA, Woodruff JD. Histogenesis of pseudomyxoma peritonei: review of cases. *Obstet Gynecol* 1977;49:339–45.
18. Smith JW, Kemeny N, Caldwell C, et al. Pseudomyxoma peritonei of appendiceal origin: The Memorial Sloan-Kettering Cancer Center experience. *Cancer* 1992;70(2):396–401.
19. Gastrointestinal Tumor Study Group: Prolongation of the disease free interval in surgically treated rectal carcinoma. *N Engl J Med* 1985; 312:1465–72.

COMMENTARY by Lee E. Smith

Pseudomyxoma peritonei is a rare condition that has been found in less than 1 in 10,000 surgical procedures. Ordinarily, these tumors are of ovarian or bowel origin. This condition is found in association with either benign or low-malignant potential neoplasms from ovarian teratoma, ovarian fibroma, uterine carcinoma, adenocarcinoma of the bowel, adenocarcinoma of urachal cyst, mesenteric cyst of the umbilicus, carcinoma of the common duct and tumor of the fallopian tube (1). Growth is slow and may be fatal after a long course entailing several operations. Obviously, a high-grade malignancy denotes a worse prognosis.

As the second surgical commentator, I have had the opportunity to read the commentary of a surgical oncologist, a medical oncologist, and a radiotherapeutic oncologist. What has been said is a textbook approach and points out the usual method for treatment of this disease. On the other hand, I have chosen to discuss some of the current literature that has been reported to have theoretic value in dealing with this rare disease. Seldom do physicians and surgeons have the opportunity to see a large number of these patients; therefore, randomizing or modifying treatment to several treatment groups is unlikely.

These low-grade or benign type tumors spread directly through the peritoneal cavity when cells float free and implant on the surfaces of the peritoneum and viscera. From these points, the abnormal cells produce the mucin that gives this disease its name. Current thinking on this subject addresses the concept that superficial abnormal cells may be directly attacked by an intraperitoneal approach. Clearly, it is not expected that the removal of all these abnormal cells is possible. Therefore, adjunctive tumorcidal agents are used.

Surgery to remove the tumor cells is termed cytoreductive surgery. This includes excision of the omentum and adnexa. Local destructive techniques for superficial implants may be directed at any involved surface, which may include visceral surfaces or peritoneal sidewalls. The type of technology used varies with the surgeon. Recently, the Argon beam coagulator has been used to destroy the superficial cells (2). The choice of the Argon beam coagulator is rational because the beam spreads over the tissue surfaces giving a homogeneous distribution of energy and a uniform depth of energy penetration. An eschar is created that is about 2.5 mm deep when a 130-watt setting is used. For fear of perforation, power setting is decreased to the 40-watt level when bowel surfaces are treated. Another instrument used is the ball-tipped electrocoagulation probe (3). This probe may be used to electrocoagulate directly on implants, or it may be used for dissection of peritoneal surfaces.

In general, these treatment methods are imperfect in achieving total cytoreduction; thus, additional chemotherapy may be useful in killing the residual cells. Because these are superficial cells readily accessible via the intraperitoneal space, introduction of chemotherapeutic agents into the cavity makes sense. Usually, a catheter for lavage is left in place at the end of the cytoreductive surgery. Often 5-fluorouracil is one of the selected agents because it is known to be effective against adenocarcinoma (4,5). Mitomycin C has been used in combination as a second agent (5).

Immunotherapy for pseudomyxoma peritonei has been suggested with the use of a streptococcal preparation, OK-432 (6). This is also used as an adjunct to surgical cytoreduction, which includes bilateral oophorectomy and omentectomy. Immunotherapy is begun with intraperitoneal administration at surgery. Then, intramuscular doses are given twice a week. These cases are few, but the early results are promising.

An entirely different approach is taken by a group at the National Cancer Institute who use photodynamic therapy (7). In this case, dihematoporphyrin ethers are injected intravenously 48 to 72 hours before laparotomy. This chemical circulates and binds selectively to cancer cells; hence, they are rendered light-sensitive and cells exposed to light are destroyed. At the time of laparotomy, a red light is delivered to all peritoneal surfaces using a special Argon pumped dye laser. Energy levels at the 0.2 to 3.0 J/cm^2 delivered. This is a time-consuming procedure to direct light, which reaches onto all affected surfaces. Solutions that transmit light into crevices and around corners may be of value and speed up the procedure. The use of a dilute lipid emulsion has been found to diffuse the light evenly around the surface of the cavities. The light is expected to penetrate approximately 5 mm. The destruction of tumor cells is a function of exposing the light to the surfaces that are involved. The complications are a result of the photosensitivity imparted for weeks after the injection. This technique has promise and is specific in its action on tumor cells that take up the hematoporphyrin ether.

The treatment modalities included in this discussion are innovative and rational; yet, because the number of available cases to define their efficacy is so small, the best approach will evade us for years. The concept of surgical cytoreduction is central to all of these adjuvant therapies.

REFERENCES

1. Kahn MA, Demopoulos RI. Mucinous ovarian tumors with pseudomyxoma peritonei: a clinicopathological study. *Int J Gynecol Pathol* 1992:11(1):15–23.
2. Huff T, Brand E. Pseudomyxoma peritonei: treatment with the Argon beam coagulator. *Obstet Gynecol* 1992;80(3):569–71.
3. Sugarbaker PH, Kern K, Lack E. Malignant pseudomyxoma peritonei of colonic origin. Natural history and presentation of a curative approach. *Dis Colon Rectum* 1987;30(10):772–779.
4. Nast MF, Kemp GM, Given FT Jr. Pseudomyxoma peritonei: treatment with intraperitoneal 5-fluorouracil. *Eur J Gynaecol Oncol* 1993; 14(3):213–17.
5. Sugarbaker PH, Landy D, Jaffe G, Pascal R. Histologic changes induced by intraperitoneal chemotherapy with 5-Fluouracil and mitomycin C in patients with peritoneal carcinomatosis from cystadenocarcinoma of the colon or appendix. *Cancer* 1990;1:1495–501.
6. Fukuma K, Matsuura K, Shibata S, Nakahara K, Fujisaki S, Maeyama M. Pseudomyxoma peritonei: effect of chronic continuous immunotherapy with a streptococcal preparation, OK-432 after surgery. *Acta Obstet Gynecol Scand* 1986;65(2):133–7.
7. Sindelar WF, DeLaney TF, Tochner Z, Thomas GF, Dachoswki LJ, Smith PD, Friauf WS, Cole JW, Glatstein E. Technique of photodynamic therapy for disseminated intraperitoneal malignant neoplasms. Phase I study. *Arch Surg* 1991;126(3):318–24.

SECTION X

Colon

40

Adenocarcinoma of the Cecum, T3 N1 M0 (Stage III)

Terence N. Moore and James Eastman

Surgery plus chemotherapy or radiotherapy as well?

CASE PRESENTATION

G.D. was a 63-year-old white man who saw his family physician in November 1987 for anemia. He had gone to the blood bank to make a donation and the anemia was found. His family physician noted occult positive stool and referred the patient to a gastroenterologist. The patient had no symptoms of diarrhea or other changes in bowel habits. There was no change in caliber of stool and no mention was made of alteration of stool color. There was no abdominal mass and neither the patient nor his physician could palpate a mass. Colonoscopy was recommended and performed on November 30, 1987. This revealed a large, ulcerated friable lesion near the cecum. Biopsy via colonoscopy revealed an adenocarcinoma. His metastatic work-up included a normal chest roentgenogram. Blood studies revealed normal liver enzymes and kidney function. On December 1, 1987, an exploratory laparotomy was performed and a "baseball-size" lesion was noted in the cecum that grossly appeared to extend into the retroperitoneum. The liver, gallbladder, and pancreas were normal to palpation. There was no gross adenopathy. A right hemicolectomy was performed with an end-to-end ileocolonic anastomosis successfully completed. The patient recovered uneventfully and was discharged to home on iron supplement. His CEA titer was 0.96.

The hemicolectomy specimen of December 1, 1987, included 8 cm of ileum and 24 cm of cecum and ascending colon. In the cecum, immediately beyond the ileocecal junction was a 5×4 cm deeply ulcerated firm tumor that occupied 50% of the circumference of the bowel. No other lesion was noted. The margins of resection were clear, but on gross section tumor was noted to extend through the muscularis propria into pericolonic fat.

Histopathologic examination revealed an infiltrating, moderately differentiated colonic adenocarcinoma with tumor extending through the muscularis propria into pericolonic fat and to just below the serosa (Figs. 40–1, 40–2). The margins of resection were clear. One of 16 pericolonic lymph nodes contained tumor.

The patient's problem was presented to the Tumor Board. It was noted that in stage III lesions, chemotherapy with 5-fluorouracil (5-FU) is often of benefit. Because the tumor was tethered to the retroperitoneal tissues and had positive nodes, the question of radiation therapy was raised. The radiation oncologist felt that these two factors significantly increase the chances of local recurrence of disease. Although there is not extensive data in the literature regarding irradiation of colonic neoplasms, the data available do indicate that those tumors of the cecum, ascending colon, and descending colon that penetrate positively and invade or potentially invade the retroperitoneal tissues have a significant chance of local recurrence, which can be substantially decreased by postoperative treatment to the tumor bed and surrounding tissues. Also, in this instance, the presence of a positive node also enhances the chance of local recurrence. Although local radiation therapy decreases the chances of local tumor recurrence in such cases, there are no firm data indicating that it increases the overall survival rate because there may be intraperitoneal spread of tumor by the operative procedure or distant metastatic disease.

The patient was treated postoperatively with 5-FU chemotherapy but was not referred to the radiation oncol-

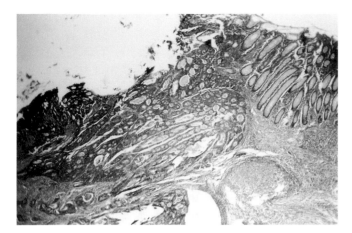

FIG. 40–1. Infiltrating adenocarcinoma (*left*) in the wall of the cecum.

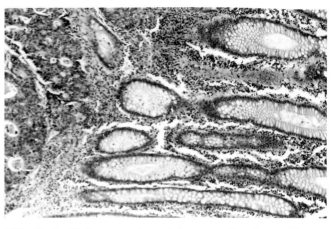

FIG. 40–2. High power view of the tumor interface with normal cecum.

ogist for treatment to the tumor bed or lymph node drainage area.

Nine months later, in August 1988, the patient was found to have a stage C adenocarcinoma of the prostate. Because of the high chance of recurrence of his cecal lesion, approaching 60%, and the low chance of survival from it, the decision was made to treat the prostatic tumor palliatively. The patient was given 1,500 Roentgens in-air to each breast with 140 KV, 20 ma radiation with 0.2 mm of added Cu filtration as prophylaxis against breast enlargement from the subsequent delivery of diethylstilbestrol as hormonal palliation.

By March 1990 the patient had developed symptomatic abdominal metastasis. He had been on and off chemother-

apy for the cecal metastasis and had been changed from diethylstilbesterol to leuprolide acetate in an attempt to control the prostatic malignancy.

By March 1991 there had been progression of liver metastasis such that the patient had significant liver pain. He also had lytic, painful metastatic disease to the left hip for which a course of palliative radiation was given.

On July 23, 1991, the patient presented to radiation oncology with a 10-cm midanterior abdominal wall mass below the umbilicus. A CT scan (Fig. 40–3) revealed multiple abnormalities including small periaortic lymph nodes and anterior abdominal wall mass involving the left rectus muscle measuring 9.5 × 7.9 cm, a right paracolic mass 4 cm in diameter, and a 3.4 × 2.1 erosive lesion in

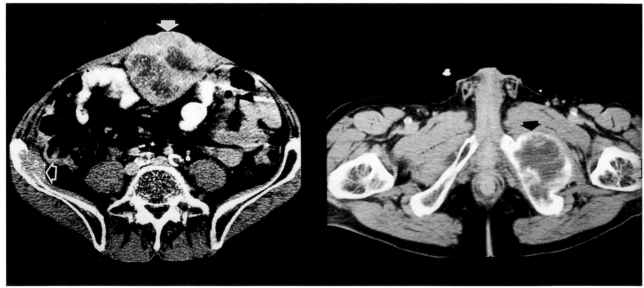

A   B

FIG. 40–3. CT scans of the lower abdomen and pelvis. **A:** There is a 9.5 × 7.9 cm mass involving the left rectus muscle (*white arrowhead*) and an erosive lesion in the right iliac wing *(open arrowhead)*. A 4-cm right pericolic mass and small periaortic lymph nodes were also present in other sections. **B:** An expansile mass is present in the left inferior pubic ramus (*black arrowhead*).

the right iliac wing. Also present was a 7.5 × 6.2 cm mass in the left inferior pubic ramus.

Radiation was given to the right iliac crest and abdominal mass. Thirty Gray was delivered to the abdominal lesion in 12 fractions over 19 elapsed days with right and left anterior oblique portals using 60° wedges treating with 4 MV X-rays. The right hip lesion was also treated.

The patient developed intractable nausea and vomiting and was admitted to the hospital on August 2, 1991. He died of abdominal dissemination of cecal carcinoma on September 5, 1991, at home with hospice care.

COMMENTARY by Glenn D. Steele, Jr.

The patient, with a T3 N1 adenocarcinoma of the cecum, was diagnosed and resected correctly. Current issues concerning applicability of laparoscopic staging or even laparoscopic-assisted colectomy would not be pertinent in this patient with a large cecal primary. In fact, even if the primary were mobile, until laparoscopic-assisted colectomy is compared formally to conventional resection of colonic and rectal lesions, the technique should not be applied outside of a trial setting. As to the tethering of the lesion and implications concerning radiation therapy, I agree completely with the conclusions of the Tumor Board. Despite several institutional studies, particularly at the Massachusetts General Hospital, and at the Mayo Clinic, there has never been any evidence that radiation therapy, even for T4 lesions, changes the abdominal or systemic disease recurrence, although it has conceptual appeal. Numerous attempts at accruing patients in multi-institutional national trials to address this question in patients specifically with T4 N0 disease have not been enthusiastically supported.

My only quibble is with the systemic therapy given. As of 1990, there was consensus that for patients with stage III colon cancer, 5-FU and levamisole postsurgical resection would be standard therapy. The use of 5-FU alone is not appropriate. Recent evidence suggests that even patients with stage II colon cancer but with bad prognostic variables, including aneuploid cytology, perforation, and obstruction, might also be legitimate candidates for 5-FU and levamisole. Recent trials in which leucovorin is combined with 5-FU without levamisole should be mature in several years, with presumed modification of the present systemic chemotherapy recommendations.

Finally, follow-up in most patients (obviously not in this patient with the more pressing prostatic carcinoma) should be determined by attention to symptoms of recurrence and to a screening for metachronous colorectal cancers or precancers through periodic colonoscopy. Extensive biochemical and radiologic follow-up to find early asymptomatic recurrence should be limited to patients on trials in which disease-free survival is one of the endpoints being assessed.

41 Carcinoma of the Colon with Liver Metastasis

LaSalle D. Leffall, Jr.

Simultaneous primary and metastatic tumor resection or sequential surgery? Systemic therapy after?

CASE PRESENTATION

This 69-year-old woman was admitted with a dull midabdominal ache relieved by bowel movements, hematochezia described as maroon blood mixed with stools, and intermittent diarrhea. She denied weight loss. Her past medical history was significant for diverticulitis, hysterectomy performed at age 42 years for symptomatic fibroids, and an appendectomy at age 41 years. Her family history was unremarkable.

On physical examination, her pulse was 82, blood pressure 130/90, T 98.1, and R 20. Her only significant findings were a midline scar, hemorrhoids, and yellow stool, which was guaiac positive. Her electrolytes and hematologic studies were normal. The patient underwent a barium enema, which revealed an annular carcinoma of the sigmoid colon (Fig. 41–1). She then underwent colonoscopy, which confirmed a constricting lesion 25 cm from the anal verge and a sessile polyp in the distal transverse colon. Colonoscopic biopsy revealed invasive, moderately differentiated adenocarcinoma of the sigmoid colon and tubular adenoma of the transverse colon.

The patient underwent an extended left hemicolectomy with primary anastomosis and en bloc resection of a segment of ileum adherent to the tumor. On exploration, she was noted to have a hard mass deep in the lateral segment of the left lobe of the liver that clinically was thought to represent metastatic disease. Pathologic evaluation of the surgical specimen revealed a villous adenoma of the left colon with early malignant changes and a well-differentiated adenocarcinoma of the sigmoid colon with invasion of the muscularis, T2 N0 M1, stage IV (Fig. 41–2). The margins of resection were free of tumor. The resected small bowel showed no malignant involvement.

A subsequent computed tomography (CT) scan of the abdomen did not confirm a metastatic lesion in the left lobe of the liver but did reveal a cyst in the medial segment of the left lobe (Fig. 41–3).

The patient's case was discussed in Tumor Board. The recommendation was for re-exploration with segmental resection of the lateral segment of the left lobe. An hepatic arteriogram was not indicated. Three weeks after her previous procedure, she underwent resection of the lateral segment of the left lobe of the liver with a margin of resection of 3 cm (Fig. 41–4). The deeply located nodule proved on pathologic study to be metastatic moderately differentiated adenocarcinoma of the colon (Fig. 41–5). Three nodules were identified, the largest of which measured 3 × 4 cm. Her pre- and postoperative carcinoembryonic antigen (CEA) levels were 3.24 and 2.9 ng/mL, respectively.

Two years after her initial procedure, the patient underwent a colostomy for stool incontinence resulting from spinal stenosis at the T12 level with paraplegia. No evidence of recurrence was found. A CT scan performed before the colostomy did not reveal evidence of liver metastasis (Fig. 41–6).

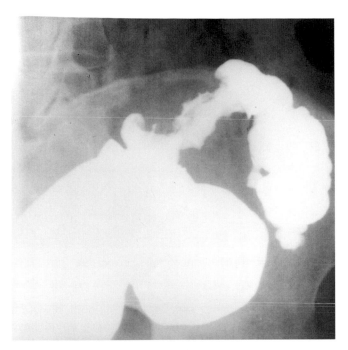

FIG. 41–1. Single contrast barium enema reveals a constricting lesion of the sigmoid colon.

COMMENTARY by Robert J. Mayer

This 69-year-old woman developed abdominal pain, altered bowel habits, and hematochezia leading to the detection of a sigmoid carcinoma that had spread in a radiographically occult manner to the liver. Both the primary tumor and the liver metastases were resected, no chemotherapy was administered, and the patient remains well 2 years after the completion of these procedures. The case history illustrates several important points regarding the management of patients with colorectal cancer.

There was nothing in this patient's medical history that placed her at increased risk for the development of a large bowel cancer (1). She lacked a family history for cancer or polyps and also was free of any prior episodes of colitis. Diverticulitis has not been shown to be a causative factor. The presenting symptoms of altered bowel habits and visible blood in the stool occur more frequently in the presence of cancers in the descending or sigmoid colon or the rectum than in more proximal locations, where anemia or obstruction without hema-

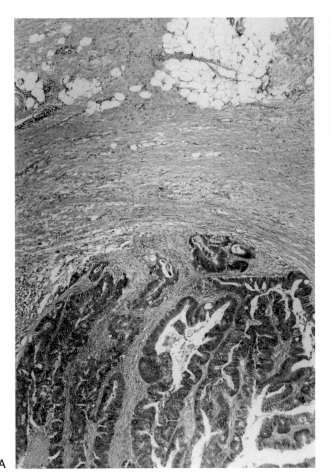
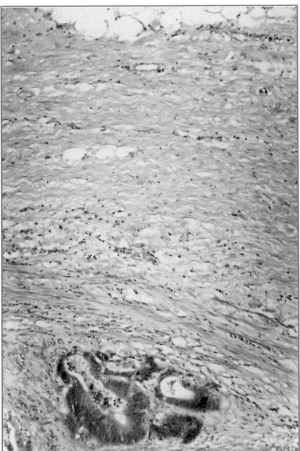

FIG. 41–2. A,B: Photomicrographs demonstrating a well-differentiated adenocarcinoma extending into the inner muscle layer, T2 (**A**, lower power; **B**, high power).

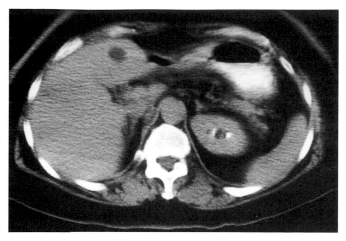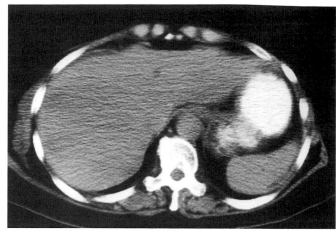

A

B

FIG. 41–3. CT scans reveal a cyst in the medial segment of the left lobe **(A)**, but no metastatic foci **(B)**.

tochezia are more frequent. When a barium enema demonstrated the annular lesion in the sigmoid, a colonoscopy was correctly requested because approximately 25% of individuals with a neoplasm in one part of the large bowel will have a synchronous lesion elsewhere (2). Indeed, a tubular adenoma of the transverse colon was identified and was (presumably) removed endoscopically.

The patient underwent a left hemicolectomy, at which time the sigmoid lesion was found to be adherent to a segment of the ileum, which was also removed. There was no evidence of spread to lymph nodes and the resection margins were clear. As is frequently observed, the sigmoid tumor was found to have arisen from a villous adenoma; approximately 25% of villous adenomas harbor malignancy, and a villous histology in an adenomatous polyp predicts a greater likelihood of cancer than does a tubular adenoma such as was found in this patient's transverse colon (3). At the time of surgery, a hard mass was palpated in the left lobe of the liver but, wisely, the surgeon elected not to attempt an hepatic

resection at the same time as the sigmoid resection because the probability of complications would have been increased. One wonders, however, why a needle biopsy of the liver mass was not performed. The case history described the patient as having a T2 N0 M1 malignancy because the tumor itself invaded only into the muscularis of the sigmoid. However, more information regarding such a staging would seem indicated in view of the adherence of the tumor mass to the terminal ileum, raising the question as to whether a T4 N0 M1 designation might not have been more appropriate. Such a distinction is particularly relevant in view of data suggesting that patients with a T4 lesion have a greater chance of experiencing a local-regional recurrence (4), leading to an ongoing intergroup randomized, controlled trial assessing the value of local radiation therapy following the resection of these intraperitoneal lesions (5).

Understandably, some degree of uncertainty was expressed by the Tumor Board, which discussed future management for this patient. The absence of a liver biopsy in the setting of a patient thought to have a T2 N0 lesion and a

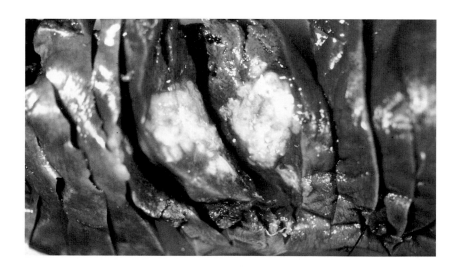

FIG. 41–4. Resected specimen of the lateral segment of the left lobe of liver.

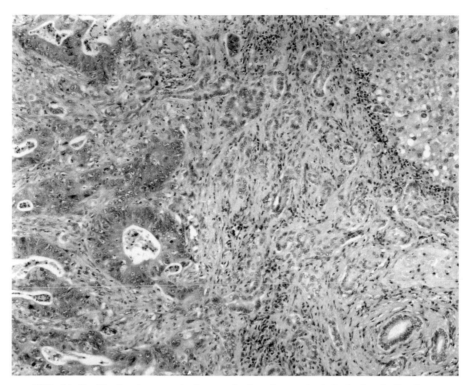

FIG. 41–5. Photomicrograph demonstrating the metastatic lesion in the liver.

normal CEA level (3.24 ng/mL) undoubtedly made some physicians wonder whether a liver metastasis was really present. Although the CEA titer is an imperfect tumor marker, it is rarely normal in the presence of liver metastases (6). This ambiguity was compounded by a CT scan that revealed only a benign-appearing cyst. Many might have argued that the presence of a definite metastasis should have been documented by the hepatic angiogram, which would also have provided anatomic information to guide a surgeon, should a resection have been contemplated. Curiously, the Tumor Board believed that such a

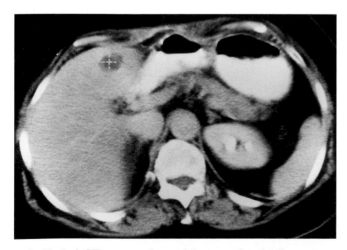

FIG. 41–6. A CT scan performed 2 years after the liver resection reveals no evidence of metastasis and an unchanged cyst in the medial segment of the left lobe.

procedure "was not indicated." Additionally, others might have suggested that the best outcomes for patients who undergo hepatic resections for metastatic colorectal cancer occur when such tumor spread is documented more than 1 year after the removal of the primary tumor. A multi-institutional study indicated the most favorable outcomes from such a procedure to occur in patients in whom more than 1 year had elapsed after the original operation with such individuals having had node-negative disease, only one or two liver metastases, and with there being no evidence of any extrahepatic spread (7). In such a setting, approximately 25% to 30% of patients have experienced long-term benefit. Data regarding the resection of synchronous hepatic metastases are even more anecdotal (8). Nonetheless, this patient did undergo such a resection, and the lateral segment of the left lobe, containing three nodules, was removed. One presumes that an intraoperative ultrasound was carried out because such a procedure is far more sensitive in detecting the presence of otherwise occult lesions and could be helpful in confirming that the metastatic disease was restricted to this single segment of the left lobe (9).

Should this patient have received postoperative adjuvant therapy? Put another way, are there data to justify the use of adjuvant therapy for patients who have undergone the resection of a stage IV colon cancer? This is a controversial area in which there is general agreement that the risk for recurrence is high, but no objective information that the use of preventative chemotherapy will reduce the likelihood of relapse. Several ongoing randomized trials are currently addressing this issue. For a clinical setting such as this, such studies are comparing the use of intra-arterial hepatic chemotherapy accompanied by systemic chemotherapy to a nontreatment control (Eastern Cooperative Oncology Group) or the use of systemic 5-fluorouracil (5-FU), levamisole, and leucovorin to 5-FU and levamisole (North Central Cancer Treatment Group). Without participation in one of these clinical experiments, the present standard of care would not favor adjuvant treatment, but close observation for 2 to 3 years with quarterly CEA titers and periodic CT scans.

REFERENCES

1. Mayer RJ. Tumors of the large and small intestine. In: *Harrison's Principles of Internal Medicine*, 13th ed, Isselbacher KJ, ed. New York: McGraw Hill; 1994:1424–31.
2. Achkar E, Carey W. Small polyps found during fiberoptic sigmoidoscopy in asymptomatic patients. *Ann Intern Med* 1988;109: 880–3.
3. Shinya H, Wolff WI. Morphology, anatomic distribution and cancer potential of colonic polyps. An analysis of 7000 polyps endoscopically removed. *Ann Surg* 1979;190:679–83.
4. Willett C, Tepper JE, Cohen A, et al. Local failure following curative resection of colonic adenocarcinoma. *Int J Radiat Oncol Biol Phys* 1984;10:645–51.
5. Intergroup Protocol 0130. Phase III study of radiation therapy, levamisole and 5-fluorouracil vs 5-fluorouracil and levamisole in selected patients with completely resected colon cancer. Martenson JA and Willett C, study chairs.
6. Mayer RJ, Garnick MB, Steele GD, Zamcheck N. Carcinoembryonic antigen (CEA) as a monitor of chemotherapy in disseminated colorectal cancer. *Cancer* 1978;42:1428–33.
7. Hughes KS, Rosenstein RB, Songhorabodi S, et al. Resection of the liver for colorectal carcinoma metastases. A multi-institutional study of long-term survivors. *Dis Colon Rectum* 1988;31:1–4.
8. Cady B, Stone MD. The role of surgical resection of liver metastases in colorectal carcinoma. *Semin Oncol* 1991;18:399–406.
9. Cady B, Stone MD, McDermott WV, et al. Technical and biological factors in disease-free survival after hepatic resection for colorectal cancer metastases. *Arch Surg* 1992;127:561–9.

42

Perforated Cecal Cancer with Psoas Abscess

Edward M. Copeland III

Preoperative or postoperative systemic and regional
therapy with "adjuvant" surgery

CASE PRESENTATION

The patient is a 54-year-old man with a 3-week history of right lower quadrant pain and intermittent fever. A decrease in appetite and diarrhea had led to progressive weakness over the prior 2-month interval. Ten days before admission, a right flank and contiguous right lower quadrant mass appeared and was accompanied by temperature elevation to 104°F with night sweats. There was no family history of colorectal cancer.

On physical examination, positive findings were limited to the abdomen and flank. Bowel sounds were present and normal. The right flank was extremely tender. There was a 10 × 10 cm tender mass palpable in the right lower quadrant; otherwise, the abdomen was soft and non-tender. Rectal examination revealed the right lower quadrant mass. Hemoccult was trace positive. The differential diagnosis in order of probability was appendiceal abscess, cecal diverticulitis with abscess, perforated cecal carcinoma with abscess, regional enteritis with abscess, and right-sided ulcerative colitis. Distant possibilities were lymphoma and tuberculous peritonitis. An ameboma was unlikely because the patient had not been outside of the United States in the recent past.

Admission laboratory values were hematocrit of 35.4%, white blood count of 11,600/mm³ with 11% band forms, alkaline phosphatase of 141 IU/L (nl 30–120), SGPT of 48 IU (nl 0–40), SGOT of 31 IU/L (nl 0–40). Electrolytes and renal profile were within normal limits. Urinalysis was negative, and urine culture grew no organisms.

The patient was placed on intravenous (i.v.) ampicillin, gentamicin, and clindamycin, and was allowed clear liquids by mouth. Chest roentgenogram and electrocardiogram were within normal limits. Computed tomography (CT) of the abdomen and pelvis using i.v. and oral contrast enhancement was done (Fig. 42–1). The study demonstrated extensive thickening of the cecum and proximal ascending colon, which appeared circumferential in extent. There was an associated phlegmonous mass in the right lower quadrant that extended into the retroperitoneum. There was evidence of a fluid collection in the retroperitoneum that appeared to be multiloculated. This collection extended into the right psoas muscle and tracked inferiorly into the pelvis. No lymphadenopathy or hepatic abnormalities were identified. The differential diagnosis by CT scan was, once again, carcinoma of the colon with abscess formation, diverticular abscess, Crohn's disease, and periappendiceal abscess as the most likely explanations for these radiographic findings.

Because the patient had normal bowel sounds and a soft abdomen, his bowel was cleansed with an oral polyethylene glycol preparation and he underwent colonoscopy the day after admission. An exophytic, polypoid mass immediately proximal to and somewhat surrounding the ileocecal valve was identified. Multiple biopsies revealed an adenocarcinoma.

The patient improved symptomatically and exploratory laparotomy was contemplated for the third day after admission. A large psoas abscess was identified by CT scan, so the anticipated operation was an exploratory

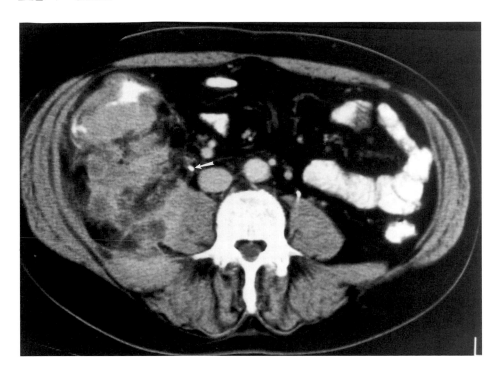

FIG. 42–1. CT scan with intravenous and oral contrast that reveals a large lesion of the cecum containing multiple areas of loculated fluid and air with involvement of the right psoas muscle. Both ureters are identifiable. The right ureter *(arrow)* is displaced anteriorly and medially off the psoas muscle and appears to be partially involved with the phlegmonous process.

laparotomy with either right hemicolectomy or bypass combined with drainage of the abscess.

At the time of operation, a very large cecal mass firmly affixed to the retroperitoneal structures over the right psoas muscle was identified. Although the inferior aspect of the cecum was mobile, there was no plane along the ascending colon between the underlying kidney and ureter. Extirpation of the right colon would have required a right nephrectomy in an infected field. Consequently, the most prudent choice of operation at this point was to exclude the perforated cecal mass from the gastrointestinal tract by doing an ileotransverse colostomy. The omentum was mobilized from the transverse colon, which was then divided between two rows of staples. The terminal ileum was identified just proximal to the ileocecal valve and, in a similar manner, was divided between two rows of staples. The proximal portion of the divided ileum was anastomosed to the distal end of the divided transverse colon in a functional end-to-end manner using stapling techniques. A separate incision was made in the right upper quadrant of the abdomen and the proximal portion of the divided transverse colon was brought out through this opening and later, after the abdominal wall closure, was matured as a colonic mucous fistula. Because the cecal lesion was not obstructing, the distal transected ileum was left closed by the staple line rather than bringing it to the skin as a mucous fistula. The defunctionalized segment of right colon containing the carcinoma was adequately vented through the mucous fistula created with the proximal divided transverse colon.

With the abdominal cavity still open, the psoas abscess was located by probing with a long spinal needle percuta-neously through the right flank. Once pus was obtained, a separate muscle-splitting right flank incision was made over the spinal needle and into the psoas abscess. Multiple loculations were encountered and were broken up with a finger. Two suction catheter drains were placed into the abscess cavity, which was packed with iodine-impregnated gauze.

The abdominal cavity was irrigated with a large amount of warm normal saline solution. Using a clean set of instruments, the fascia was closed with a running polyglyconate synthetic suture and strengthened on several occasions with interrupted polyglyconate sutures. The skin and subcutaneous tissues were left open and packed with a fine mesh gauze. The mucous fistula was matured by removing the staple line with electrocautery and sewing the free edge of the colon to the skin using interrupted chromic catgut sutures. Culture of the purulent material from the abscess cavity grew a pure colony of *Escherichia coli* sensitive to all antibiotics tested. The patient's recovery was uneventful and he was discharged on the 12th postoperative day.

Flank and midline incision wounds healed rapidly by secondary intention. Six days postdischarge a repeat CT scan of the abdomen and pelvis showed better delineation of the relationship between the cecal mass and the urinary tract. The mass penetrated Gerota's fascia and appeared to invade the lower pole of the right kidney. The retroperitoneal abscess had resolved.

Because of the extensive nature of the right colon cancer, external beam radiation therapy was recommended. The mass was so large that it excluded the small bowel from the right side of the abdominal cavity and 4,500 cGy in 4½ weeks was delivered through anterior and posterior portals with no discernible injury to the liver or small bowel.

After a rest period of 4½ weeks after completion of radiation therapy, the patient was readmitted to undergo a definitive resection of the right colon carcinoma. The carcinoembryonic antigen (CEA) serum level was 7.8 ng/mL preoperatively and the alkaline phosphatase, SGPT, white blood count, and hematocrit had returned to normal ranges.

At the time of admission, the patient was a healthy-appearing 54-year-old man. The mass in the right lower quadrant and right flank was still palpable but nontender. The patient was given magnesium citrate by mouth for bowel preparation.

At operation, multiple intra-abdominal adhesions were lysed by sharp dissection and the mucous fistula was dissected free of the abdominal wall. The terminal ileal stump was identified and the distal cecum was mobilized. At this juncture, the large cecal mass invaded the psoas muscle. The right ureter ran through the center of this indurated mass and the inferior pole of the right kidney appeared invaded by the malignant process. Consequently, the kidney, ureter, right colon, and a portion of the psoas muscle were mobilized en bloc. The duodenum was mobilized by using a Kocher maneuver and retracted medially. The renal artery and vein were readily identifiable and doubly clamped, divided, and ligated. The specimen was removed without injury to the duodenum. The midline wound was closed with an interrupted polyglyconate suture and the skin was closed with staples. The fascia in the ostomy site was reapproximated with polyglyconate suture and the skin was packed open. The patient tolerated the procedure quite well with a 1,200-cc blood loss.

The pathology specimen contained the entire right colon, right kidney, and a portion of right ureter and right psoas muscle. The kidney and ureter were attached by periuretered fat to a retrocecal mass measuring $11 \times 7.5 \times 3.5$ cm in size. The cecum appeared separate from the underlying mass but contained an ulcer crater 4.8×2.5 cm in size on the posterior wall just above the ileocecal valve. The ulcer and associated mass appeared to invade the full thickness of the cecal wall. Microscopically, the cecum contained a moderately differentiated adenocarcinoma that invaded into the muscularis propria of the cecum but did not extend into the pericolic fat. Extensive necrosis, fibrosis, and chronic inflammation of the pericolic fat and psoas muscle were present. There was no identifiable tumor in the right kidney or ureter. No lymph nodes were identified in the specimen.

The patient's CEA level fell to 1.4 ng/mL postoperatively and he had an uneventful recovery.

It is now 5 years since the patient's colon resection and he is free of disease by physical examination, abdominal CT scan, colonoscopy, and CEA level.

TUMOR BOARD DISCUSSION

This patient's cecal cancer perforated into the psoas muscle and, therefore, penetrated through the entire muscle wall of the cecum and into the pericolic fat. Yet, on final pathology report, the tumor appeared to be contained within the muscularis propria of the cecum with no evidence of penetration into the pericolic fat or into the kidney. When administered with regularity, preoperative radiation therapy for rectal cancer will result in downstaging of the disease and, occasionally, a rectal cancer can be totally obliterated by preoperative radiation therapy, particularly when combined with 5-fluorouracil (5-FU). Multiple reports have identified preoperative radiation therapy with or without 5-FU, resulting in marked regression of a rectal carcinoma (1–3). It would appear that preoperative radiation therapy worked in a similar fashion in this patient. The set of anatomical circumstances at the initial operation allowed for diversion of the fecal stream with an ileotransverse colostomy and decompression of the defunctionalized right colon via a mucous fistula. The small bowel was eliminated from the radiation field simply by the size of the cecal mass, and no acute or chronic radiation enteritis occurred from this therapeutic dose of radiation therapy. Because the right colon specimen contained no lymph nodes, the assumption must be made that they were obliterated by either the radiation therapy or by the fibrosis pursuant to the inflammation from the psoas abscess.

Therapeutic doses of preoperative external beam radiation therapy with or without 5-FU have not been used often for adenocarcinoma of the abdominal colon. In fact, one of the indications for intraoperative radiation therapy is residual disease on the psoas muscle, abdominal wall, or pelvic side wall after abdominal colectomy for carcinoma. The success obtained in this patient with external beam radiation therapy to a total dose of 4,500 cGy in 4½ weeks might indicate an expanded role for radiation therapy in the treatment of large, bulky adenocarcinomas of the abdominal colon, to include those lesions that impinge on structures not readily sacrificed such as the duodenum and kidney. Down-staging of the disease might well lead to a decrease in local recurrence as well as an increase in survival, as has occurred with the use of preoperative radiation therapy for carcinoma of the rectum (4–6). Likewise, adjacent organs might be spared resection.

Another interesting aspect of this case that should not be overlooked was the drainage of the psoas abscess through a separate incision in the flank. The intra-abdominal cavity was never contaminated by purulent material. Postoperative recovery after the initial operation was straightforward and reoperation was not fraught with multiple adhesions often seen from generalized peritonitis. Likewise, opening into the abscess cavity transperitoneally would have exposed the peritoneal cavity to the potential of seeding of tumor cells within it. Defunctionalizing the right colon eliminated the possibility of an enterocutaneous fistula through the flank wound and allowed the abscess cavity to heal rapidly. Neoadjuvant therapy could begin quickly.

REFERENCES

1. Mendenhall WM, Bland KI, Copeland EM, et al. Does preoperative radiation therapy enhance the probability of local control and survival in high-risk distal rectal cancer? *Ann Surg* 1992;215(6):696–706.
2. Mohiuddin M, Marks G. High dose preoperative irradiation for cancer of the rectum, 1976–1988. *Int J Radiat Oncol Biol Phys* 1991; 20(1):37–43.
3. Kodner IJ, Shemesh EI, Fry RD, et al. Preoperative irradiation for rectal cancer: improved local control and long-term survival. *Ann Surg* 1989;209(2):194–9.
4. Stockholm Rectal Cancer Group. Preoperative short-term radiation therapy in operable rectal carcinoma. *Cancer* 1990;66:49–55.
5. Gérard A, Buyse M, Nordlinger B, et al. Preoperative radiotherapy as adjuvant treatment in rectal cancer: final results of a randomized study of the European Organization for Research and Treatment of Cancer (EORTC). *Ann Surg* 1988;208(5):606–14.
6. Reis Neto JA, Quilici FA, Reis JA, Jr. Comparison of nonoperative versus preoperative radiotherapy in rectal carcinoma: a 10-year randomized trial. *Dis Colon Rectum* 1989;32(8):702–10.

COMMENTARY by Christopher G. Willett

The case presentation by Dr. Copeland of a 54-year-old man with a perforated cecal carcinoma with psoas abscess highlights two controversial points in the current management of patients with colorectal cancer: (a) the use of adjunctive irradiation in colon carcinoma, and (b) the selection of preoperative irradiation versus postoperative irradiation. In the case of this patient, Dr. Copeland and colleagues successfully used a strategy of full-dose preoperative irradiation (45 Gy) of an advanced cecal carcinoma with localized perforation into the psoas to permit tumor regression and facilitate a curative resection. Five years after surgery, this patient is disease-free without treatment-related morbidity.

A major goal in the management of colon carcinoma in the 1990s will be an improved patient selection for adjuvant treatment. Distant metastases often develop in patients with advanced (stages IIB and III) colon tumors. Because of the documented benefit of 5-FU and levamisole in patients with AJCC stage III tumors (1), the thrust of present clinical investigations has been in examining adjuvant chemotherapy treatment. Prospective studies are evaluating levamisole, leucovorin, and 5-FU in various doses, combinations, and modes of administration (bolus vs. infusion), as well as interferon and autologous vaccines in the adjuvant setting.

In contrast, there has been little systematic examination of the role of radiation therapy for patients with colon carcinoma, unlike the situation for patients with rectal carcinoma. This is largely attributable to the perception by many oncologists that colon carcinoma (as opposed to rectal cancer) is much more likely to recur systemically than locally, so local treatment offers little survival benefit. Although distant metastases occur frequently in patients with advanced colon tumors, there are also subsets of patients especially at risk for local failure. Gunderson et al. found that among 91 patients with stages C1-3 colon carcinomas who required reoperations, 48% had local recurrences (2). Duttenhaver et al. reported local failure rates of 10% in patients with stages A, B1, B2, and C1 tumors, but it was at least 30% for stages B3, C2 and C3 lesions (3).

Although tumor stage is an important predictor of local recurrence for both rectal and colon carcinomas, anatomic location is a critical factor for colon tumors as well. For ascending and descending colon cancers (relatively immobile bowel), a wide radial resection margin may be difficult to achieve because of retroperitoneal extension. On the other hand, a wide circumferential margin is usually possible for tumors of the sigmoid and transverse colon (mobile bowel), so the risk of local failure is minimal. The likelihood of local recurrence for tumors in the cecum and proximal and distal portions of the transverse and sigmoid colon (partially mobile bowel) is variable. For patients with more advanced tumors having not only transmural invasion but also adherence to adjacent structures (with and without lymph node involvement), local failure rates exceed 30% (4). For patients undergoing resection of carcinomas with tumor-associated perforation, the incidence of local failure can be up to 50% (5).

To summarize, local failure is an important consideration for patients with colon tumors in locations where a wide radial resection margin is difficult to achieve and for patients with tumors invading transmurally to involve adjacent structures. Adjuvant radiation therapy should be considered for these patients.

In this case presentation, the tumor of a 54-year-old man invaded into the retroperitoneum and psoas muscle with an associated perforation and abscess at the tumor site, which extended into the retroperitoneum and pelvis. Given the extensive local invasiveness of this tumor, the likelihood of achieving a wide retroperitoneal soft tissue margin with an initial surgical approach would be minimal, and the subsequent risk of local failure high. To improve local control in this high-risk setting, Dr. Copeland and colleagues opted for a course of full-dose preoperative irradiation (45 Gy) rather than postoperative irradiation. For this patient, preoperative irradiation can be favored for many reasons. First, a high-dose preoperative regimen sterilizes a large percentage of tumor cells and may minimize the risk of tumor implantation in the peritoneal cavity after a "marginal" resection has been performed. Second, partial regression obtained from external beam radiation therapy may allow a complete gross resection to be performed. For patients with unresectable rectal cancer, the use of full-dose preoperative irradiation converts 48% to 64% of patients to a resectable status, thus allowing a complete gross resection (6).

Third, these large tumors usually displace abdominal and retroperitoneal viscera to a degree that radiosensitive organs such as the small bowel can be effectively excluded from the preoperative radiation therapy field. Because of reduction of normal tissue irradiation by the tumor's displacement of viscera outside the radiation field, it is usually feasible to deliver a full course of treatment with excellent tolerance, which may not be possible postoperatively.

Available information evaluating combinations of irradiation and surgery for treatment of colon carcinoma are limited to retrospective studies suggesting benefit to subsets of patients with colon carcinoma receiving postoperative irradiation (7). A randomized prospective intergroup trial combining postoperative irradiation with 5-FU and levamisole versus 5-FU and levamisole for patients with B3 and C3 tumors and certain C2 lesions with gross penetration into the retroperitoneum has been recently initiated. Unfortunately, there are little data examining the results of preoperative irradiation and surgery for colon cancer. As this case has illustrated, judicial selection of preoperative irradiation may yield benefits to selected patients with colon cancer.

REFERENCES

1. Moertel CG, Fleming TR, MacDonald JS, et al. Levamisole and fluorouracil for adjuvant therapy of resected colon carcinoma. *N Engl J Med* 1990;322:352–8.
2. Gunderson LL, Sosin H, Levitt S. Extrapelvic colon—areas of failure in a reoperation series: implications for adjuvant therapy. *Int J Radiat Oncol Biol Phys* 1984;11:731–41.
3. Duttenhaver JR, Hoskins RB, Gunderson LL, et al. Adjuvant postoperative radiation therapy in the management of adenocarcinoma of the colon. *Cancer* 1986;57:955-63.
4. Willett CG, Tepper JE, Cohen AM, et al. Failure patterns following curative resection of colonic carcinoma. *Ann Surg* 1984;200:685–90.
5. Willett CG, Tepper JE, Cohen AM, et al. Obstructive and perforative colonic carcinoma. Patterns of failure. *J Clin Oncol* 1984;3:379–84.
6. Willett CG, Shellito PC, Tepper JE, et al. Intraoperative electron beam radiation therapy for primary locally advanced rectal and rectosigmoid carcinoma. *J Clin Oncol* 1991;9:843–9.
7. Willett CG, Fung CY, Kaufman DS, et al. Postoperative radiation therapy for high-risk colon carcinoma. *J Clin Oncol* 1993;11:1112–7.

43

Sigmoid Colon Carcinoma with Multiple Synchronous Adenomatous Polyps

Michele D. Davis and L. Peter Fielding

Subtotal colectomy: when? Adjuvant therapy: for whom?

CASE PRESENTATION

A 48-year-old Caucasian woman presented with crampy abdominal pain and a change in stool caliber, but no history of passage of bright red blood per rectum, melena, or weight loss. Hypertension was well controlled with daily hydrocholorothiazide, and she had a total abdominal hysterectomy 8 years before for benign disease. Her maternal grandmother died of metastatic colon cancer. The patient was a fit, well nourished woman with normal vital signs and unremarkable physical examination except for guaiac-positive stool. Laboratory tests were normal (WBC 8,500/µL; hemoglobin 12.3 g/dL; hematocrit 36%; serum alkaline phosphatase 80 IU/L; carcinoembryonic antigen (CEA) assay 3.0 ng/dL). Barium enema revealed a moderately large, nonobstructing tumor in the midsigmoid colon, with no other abnormality. Colonoscopic examination confirmed a large polypoid lesion at the midsigmoid with five polyps in the transverse and right colon ranging in size from 0.4 to 1.3 cm. The polyps were removed by snare excision and sent with biopsy specimens from the sigmoid tumor for histopathology. The tumor was a moderately differentiated adenocarcinoma; two of the polyps (one each in the transverse and right colon) contained foci of carcinoma in situ (Haggitt level 2), and other lesions were benign adenomatous polyps. Abdominal computed tomography (CT) scan showed the sigmoid colon lesion without evidence of local spread or lymph node enlargement and an equivocal lesion in the left lobe of the liver.

TUMOR BOARD DISCUSSION

Conventional staging for colorectal cancer has focused on the assessment of anatomic tumor spread after operative intervention (1–3), and the TNM system recommendations of the American Joint Committee on Cancer (AJCC) have been accepted in North America (4).

The CT scan may be useful to detect hepatic metastases, but the accuracy of this investigation varies between 73% and 94% (5). This test is more reliable in detecting recurrence after resection (6). However, many "equivocal" lesions eventually declare themselves as secondary hepatic tumors (7) and, therefore, the CT scan result is relevant in this patient.

Evaluation using intrarectal ultrasound would not help this patient, but instrumentation allowing endoluminal ultrasonic evaluation for colonic tumors has recently become available. Although early experience with ultrasound to determine the depth of primary tumor invasion has shown promise, assessment of paraintestinal lymph node involvement has not been successful (8). Evaluation with radiolabeled antitumor antibody preoperatively detected with external scanning devices or intraoperatively using a handheld gamma counter (RIGS) may become a valuable tool (9,10).

Liver function tests and CEA levels are not specific for metastatic disease (11), but the size and grade of the tumor are of prognostic significance (12) and often correlate with the preoperative CEA level. Furthermore, elevated preoperative CEA correlates with poorer prognosis in these patients (13).

Patients with carcinoma of the large bowel should undergo preoperative (and if necessary perioperative) colonoscopy to delineate synchronous lesions (benign or invasive tumors) before surgical resection of the primary tumor. What options for surgical resection are there in this patient in light of the presence of the primary tumor in the sigmoid colon with several polyps in the colon?

The presence of more than one neoplasm raises questions about the length of colon to be resected. The importance of benign polyps and their malignant potential in the adenoma-carcinoma sequence is well recognized (14,15). Polyps with carcinoma in situ (malignant cells superficial to the muscularis mucosa) are adequately treated by complete endoscopic polypectomy when this can be shown histologically. The relative risk of metastatic potential in these lesions is low, probably because of the absence of lymphatics superficial to the muscularis mucosa (16–18). Haggitts classification of the level of invasion for pedunculated polyps is as follows: level 0—carcinoma in situ (above muscularis mucosa); level 1—invades muscularis mucosa but limited to polyp head; level 2—invades polyp neck; level 3—invades polyp stalk; level 4—invades submucosa of bowel wall below polyp and above muscularis propria.

It is helpful to mark the site of the polyp removal by injecting some sterile India ink into the submucosal plane (19); with clear margins, the rate of recurrent metastatic disease is about 7%. However, if resection margins are actually involved or nearly involved, then the rates of tumor recurrence are 48% and 23%, respectively (20). Therefore, patients with Haggitt level 1 or 2 lesions may be treated by endoscopic polypectomy alone (21) (except those with identified vascular invasion or poorly differentiated lesions), whereas patients with Haggitt levels 3 or 4 invasion should have formal resection.

The correlation of tumor grade in a polyp with tumor recurrence shows that poorly differentiated lesions are at much higher risk of recurrence than with well or moderately differentiated lesions (16,18,21,22). Therefore, formal segmental resection is usually indicated for poorly differentiated polyps even if apparently "complete" resection has occurred, unless co-morbid disease precludes surgery.

This patient underwent snare polypectomy for five polyps in the right and transverse colon, two of which had foci of carcinoma in situ. Should we conclude that this patient requires no further surgical treatment for these polyps apart from the resection for the sigmoid adenocarcinoma?

There are a number of surgical options. This patient has a mucosa that forms adenomatous growths with malignant potential. Therefore, it would be reasonable to advise a subtotal colectomy with ileorectal anastomosis (23) because considering the age of the patient, additional tumors are likely during her lifetime. In addition, tumor surveillance is simplified because of the extent of the resection. However, if the patient were 25 to 30 years older, most surgeons would feel more comfortable with a resection of the sigmoid lesion and primary anastomosis, leaving the right and transverse colon in situ.

If a subtotal colectomy is being considered, some consideration should also be given to gut function and continence. Under these circumstances, a subtotal colectomy, sparing the cecum and the ileocecal valve by fashioning a cecorectal anastomosis, should be considered.

The patient undergoes resection and is noted to have no evidence of metastatic disease, either in the liver (by palpation or intraoperative ultrasonography) (24) or metastasis to the peritoneum. There is a 5-mm area of ulceration at which the tumor has eroded the visceral peritoneum, but no contiguous involvement of adjacent organs or structures. Of 15 lymph nodes, 5 are positive for moderately differentiated adenocarcinoma. What adjuvant therapy, if any, should be offered to this patient?

This patient has a T4 N2 M0 sigmoid tumor (stage III, Dukes C2) with a 5-year survival rate of approximately 30%. Therefore, adjuvant chemotherapy should be given because the presence of the tumor on the surface of the specimen and in lymph nodes demonstrates that the patient is at high risk of dying of her disease, and this risk can be reduced by adjuvant chemotherapy.

Although there is some controversy about adjuvant chemotherapy for colon cancer, this patient should be treated with a regimen containing 5-fluorouracil (5-FU) (25,26). This controversy concerns whether additional agents, such as levamisole, should be added to the 5-FU. In 1989, the NCI Consensus Development Conference on Adjuvant Therapy for Patients with Colon and Rectal Cancer recommended that all patients with stage III, Dukes' C cancer receive adjuvant chemotherapy using 5-FU and levamisole or be enrolled in an alternative investigational protocol (27). There are many such clinical trials that involve varying doses of 5-FU with or without alpha-interferon, levamisole, and/or leucovorin.

Two other forms of adjuvant therapy should be considered in this patient: because the tumor was on the peritoneal surface of the bowel, the high rate of intraperitoneal recurrence may be reduced by the intraperitoneal instillation of 5-FU in the perioperative period (28); and pre- and postoperative portal vein infusion with 5-FU and heparin may also improve 5-year survival rates (29).

Because it is possible that systemic and intraportal 5-FU act to improve patient survival through different mechanisms, it would be reasonable to suggest that all patients undergoing resective surgery should have intraportal infusion, and those patients with stage III tumors found at histopathology should then proceed to a 1-year treatment of cycled systemic 5-FU and levamisole.

About 40% of patients undergoing "curative" resection for colorectal cancer will develop a tumor recurrence (30). Although many recurrent tumors are deemed unresectable at the time of detection, most practitioners continue avid patient follow-up in the hope of finding a recurrence or a metachronous lesion at a "curable" stage. This patient has a high chance of recurrent disease because of the multiple neoplasms, the involvement of several lymph nodes, and the presence of tumor on the surface of a specimen. Therefore, postoperative surveillance is necessary.

Reasonable surveillance strategies include routine laboratory investigation, history and physical examination and stool hemoccult testing at 3-month intervals for 2 years and then two to three yearly thereafter; CEA levels, colonoscopy, or barium enema and chest roentgenogram and CEA levels at 3-month intervals for 2 years and then annually; and colonoscopy or barium enema at the first-year anniversary date and then, if clear, at 2- to 3-year intervals thereafter. Although CEA-directed second-look procedures were thought to be beneficial in treating patients with recurrent disease, there is no overall benefit to this approach.

The consensus conclusion for this 48-year-old woman is that she should undergo subtotal colectomy with cecorectal anastomosis followed by adjuvant chemotherapy using 5-FU and levamisole in cycled fashion for 1 year. This therapeutic approach should achieve (a) a potentially "curative" operative resection; (b) a reduced field of growth for neoplastic development; (c) improved large bowel function because of the retention of the ileocecal valve; and (d) an increased survivorship relative to surgery alone. In addition, there should be some consideration given to the use of peri- and postoperative intraportal intraperitoneal adjuvant chemotherapy with 5-FU and heparin.

REFERENCES

1. Dukes CE. The classification of cancer of the rectum. *J Pathol Bacteriol* 1932;35:323–32.
2. Chapuis PH, Dent OF, Newland RC, et al. An evaluation of the American Joint Committee pTNM staging method for cancer of the colon and rectum. *Dis Colon Rectum* 1986;29:6–10.
3. Zinklin LD. A critical review of the classification and staging of colorectal cancer. *Dis Colon Rectum* 1983;26:37–43.
4. American Joint Committee on Cancer. *AJCC Manual for Staging of Cancer*, 4th ed, Beahrs OH, Henson DE, Hutter RVP, Kennedy BJ, eds. Philadelphia: JB Lippincott; 1992:76–79.
5. Freeny PC, Marks WM, Ryan JA, Bolen JW. Colorectal carcinoma evaluation with CT: preoperative staging and detection of postoperative recurrence. *Radiology* 1986;158:347–53.
6. Beart RW Jr, O'Connell MJ. Postoperative follow-up of patients with carcinoma of the colon. *Mayo Clin Proc* 1983;58:361–3.
7. Findlay IG, McArdle CS. Effect of occult metastases on survival after curative resection for colorectal cancer. *Gastroenterology* 1983;85:596–9.
8. Boyce GA, Sivak MV Jr. New approaches to the diagnosis of malignant and premalignant lesions: colonoscopic endosonography and laser-induced fluorescence spectroscopy. *Semin Colon Rectal Surg* 1991;2:17–21.
9. Doerr RJ, Abdel-Nabi H, Krag D, et al. Radiolabeled antibody imaging in the management of colorectal cancer: results of a multicenter clinical study. *Ann Surg* 1991;214:118–24.
10. Nieroda CA, Mojzisik C, Sardi, et al. The impact of radio-immune guided surgery (RIGS) on surgical decision making in colorectal cancer. *Dis Colon Rectum* 1989;32:927–32.
11. Fletcher RH. Carcinoembryonic antigen. *Ann Intern Med* 1986; 104:66–73.
12. Arnaud JP, Koehl C, Adloff M. Carcinoembryonic antigen (CEA) in the diagnosis and prognosis of colorectal cancer. *Dis Colon Rectum* 1980;23:141–4.
13. Sener SF, Imperato JP, Chmiel JS, et al. The use of cancer registry data to study preoperative carcinoembryonic antigen level as an indicator of survival in colorectal cancer. *Cancer* 1989;39:51–7.
14. Tierny RP, Ballantyne GH, Modlin IM. The adenoma to carcinoma sequence. *Surg Gynecol Obstet* 1990;171:81–94.
15. Wolff WI, Shinya H. Definitive treatment of "malignant" polyps of the colon. *Ann Surg* 1975;182:516–25.
16. Haggitt RC, Glotzbach RE, Soffer EE, et al. Prognostic factors in colorectal carcinomas arising in adenomas: implications for lesions removed by endoscopic polypectomy. *Gastroenterology* 1985;89:328–36.
17. Fried GM, Hreno A, Duguid WP, et al. Rational management of malignant colon polyps based on long-term follow-up. *Surgery* 1984;96:815–21.
18. Conte CC, Welch JP, Tennant RE, et al. Management of endoscopically removed malignant colon polyps. *J Surg Oncol* 1987;36:116–21.
19. Poulard JB, Shatz B, Kodner I. Preoperative tattooing of polypectomy site. *Endoscopy* 1985;17:84–5.
20. Stein BL, Coller JA. Management of malignant colorectal polyps. *Surg Clin North Am* 1993;73:47–66.
21. Nivatongs S, Rojanasakul A, Reiman HM, et al. The risk of lymph node metastasis in colorectal polyps with invasive adenocarcinoma. *Dis Colon Rectum* 1991;34:323–8.
22. Williams CB, Geraghty JM. The malignant polyp: when to operate: the St. Mark's experience. *Can J Gastroenterol* 1990;4:549–53.
23. Brief DK, Brener BJ, Goldenkranz R, et al. Defining the role of subtotal colectomy in the treatment of carcinoma of the colon. *Ann Surg* 1991;213:248–52.
24. Charnley RM, Morris DL, Dennison AR, et al. Detection of colorectal liver metastases using intraoperative ultrasonography. *Br J Surg* 1991;778:45–8.
25. Levitan N. Chemotherapy in colorectal carcinoma. *Surg Clin North Am* 1993;73:183–98.
26. Moertel CG, Fleming TR, MacDonald JS, et al. Levamisole and fluorouracil for adjuvant therapy of resected colon carcinoma. *N Engl J Med* 1990;322:352.
27. NIH Consensus Conference. Adjuvant therapy for patients with colon and rectal cancer. *JAMA* 1990;264:1444–50.
28. Sugarbaker PH. Mechanisms of relapse for colorectal cancer: implications for intraperitoneal chemotherapy. *J Surg Oncol* 1991;2(suppl):36–41.
29. Fielding LP, Hittinger R, Grace RH, Fry JS. Randomized controlled trial of adjuvant chemotherapy by portal vein perfusion after curative resection for colorectal adenocarcinoma. *Lancet* 1992;340:502–6.
30. Sugarbaker PH, Gianola FL, Dwyer A, et al. A simplified plan for follow-up of patients with colon and rectal cancer supported by prospective studies of laboratory and radiologic test results. *Surgery* 1987;102:79–87.

COMMENTARY by Jerome J. DeCosse

The case presentation describes a relatively young woman with an invasive midsigmoid cancer and several dispersed colorectal adenomas that had been removed by endoscopy. The strategy and tactics of assessment are very appropriate. Only about 8% of all colorectal cancers in women occur under age 50 years. With her young age and a background of colorectal cancer in a grandmother, there is a suspicion of genetic risk; other first-degree relatives over age 30 years should be advised to have annual tests for fecal occult blood, and if over age 40 years, a colonoscopy may be merited.

Because the patient needs an operation, endoscopic ultrasound has little value. For the same reason, further preoperative evaluation of the equivocal CT scan findings in the left lobe is not warranted. Had a solitary metastasis been found in the left lobe of the liver in an otherwise curable patient, the left lobe should have been resected synchronously with curative resection of the primary sigmoid cancer.

The pathologist reported carcinoma in situ within two dispersed colorectal adenomas. These cancer cells are above the muscularis mucosa, have no life-threatening potential and, so long as excision was complete, do not require further treatment. These multiple adenomas are important because the patient is likely to develop another cancer elsewhere in the colon and confronts a lifetime of repeated colonoscopies.

Although the key issue here is the life-threatening cancer in the midsigmoid colon, for her protection, a subtotal or total colectomy is the operative procedure of choice. Many surgeons would perform an end-to-end colocolostomy at the pelvic brim or at the rectosigmoid junction. Although the references cited above are appropriate, the strategy of subtotal colectomy in a curable setting is not new: the concept was suggested 40 years ago (1). Evidence that retention of the ileocecal valve makes a difference in function seems marginal at best and adds to the complexity of the operation. After subtotal colectomy, the patient should resume acceptable gastrointestinal function. Particularly in a younger person such as this patient, increased ileal resorption during ensuing postoperative months usually eliminates requirements for any antidiarrheal medications. With rare exception, the patients are satisfied.

The patient's likelihood of cure approximates 50%. The most likely site for recurrence is the liver. Although adjuvant portal vein infusion has suggested survival benefit in some studies (2–4), none has shown a reduction in hepatic metastases; benefit, if any, from the chemotherapy appears to be systemic, not regional.

On histopathologic scrutiny, the patient was found to have a Dukes' C tumor. In this setting, a medical oncology consultation should be obtained for consideration of adjuvant chemotherapy. In the litigatious east, I am aware of malpractice actions that were initiated because this standard was not pursued.

The principles of postoperative follow-up are generally well described. Some of the suggested surveillance strategies may be too intense. This patient can be followed with rigid or flexible sigmoidoscopy. In those with an intact colon, most of us would request or perform a colonoscopy 1 year after primary resection, but much earlier if an obstructed tumor had been present. If the subsequent colonoscopy was negative for neoplasia, future endoscopies would be performed at biennial or triennial intervals. Although evidence for benefit is limited, patients should be encouraged to maintain a healthy lifestyle, namely, a low fat, fiber-enriched diet, reasonable physical activity, avoidance of obesity, and moderation in alcohol consumption.

REFERENCES

1. Lillehei RC, Wangensteen OH. Bowel function after colectomy for cancer, polyps, and diverticulitis. *JAMA* 1955;159:163.
2. Beart Jr RW, Moertel CG, Wieand HS, et al. Adjuvant therapy for resectable colorectal carcinoma with fluorouracil administered by portal vein infusion. *Arch Surg* 1990;125:897–901.
3. Wolmark N, Rockette H, Wickerham DL, et al. Adjuvant therapy of Dukes' A, B, and C adenocarcinoma of the colon with portal-vein fluorouracil hepatic infusion: preliminary results of national surgical adjuvant breast and bowel project protocol C-02. *J Clin Oncol* 1990;8:1466–75.
4. Fielding LP, Hittinger R, Grace RH, et al. Randomized controlled trial of adjuvant chemotherapy by portal-vein perfusion after curative resection for colorectal adenocarcinoma. *Lancet* 1992;340:502–6.

44

Malignant Degeneration and Stricture Formation in a Patient with a Long History of Chronic Ulcerative Colitis

James F. Evans and Robert Eyerly

This type of patient might have benefited from a surveillance program

CASE PRESENTATION

This 41-year-old female dietary aid at a nursing home and mother of three children was first seen at the Geisinger Clinic in consultation for the treatment of chronic ulcerative colitis. She was referred by her physician to the gastroenterology department because of a recent exacerbation of her symptoms. The original diagnosis had been made 17 years before this referral. Her chronic symptoms consisted primarily of diarrhea. Bleeding and colicky abdominal pain had been present, but had not been as prominent as the diarrhea. She had never had any extracolonic manifestations of the disease such as uveitis, arthritis, pericholangitis, or erythema nodosum. She presented to her physician at this time with a recent increase in the amount of rectal bleeding. Her prior treatment had consisted primarily of anticholinergic medication for symptoms. She had received occasional corticosteroids in the remote past. She had never been hospitalized. She had not been enrolled in a surveillance program for colon cancer. There was no family history of ulcerative colitis or colon cancer. The patient's past medical history was negative except for the present illness.

Physical examination at the initial office visit was normal with the exception of hemorrhoids and a stool that tested positively for blood. Office anoscopy revealed purulent mucous and mildly inflamed mucosa. Microscopic examination of the discharge revealed sheets of polymorphonuclear leukocytes. Laboratory evaluation revealed a hemoglobin of 12 g/dL. She was significantly iron deficient, with a serum iron of 43 (nl 60–135). Sedimentation rate was mildly elevated. Review of a barium enema performed 5 years before referral revealed pancolonic involvement.

Because of her exacerbation of symptoms, she was placed on Azulfidine EN-tabs, two po qid, Imodium, one capsule qid, and a low residue diet. Folic acid, ferrous gluconate, and vitamins were added to the regimen. With the latter regimen, she gained weight and the number of stools decreased from 10 per day to 3 per day. She had no hematochezia.

Two considerations mandated an immediate evaluation for colorectal adenocarcinoma. The first was a recent exacerbation of her symptoms, in this case, rectal bleeding. The second was her risk estimate. Based on Lennard-Jones' estimate for patients with pancolitis, a history in excess of 10 years, and onset before 40 years of age (1% per year), she was felt to have a risk in the range of at least 5% to 10%. A barium enema revealed a tubular, ahaustral colon (Fig. 44–1). There was evidence of ulceration and pseudopolyp formation. There was some mucosal irregularity at the hepatic flexure and a mass in the rectum associated with a stricture (Fig. 44–2). Colonoscopy to the cecum with multiple biopsies revealed extensive pathology. Active disease was present at numerous sites. Severe dysplasia was demonstrated at 30 and 55 cm from the anus. Carcinoma in situ was present at 58 cm. A large carcinoma was seen in the rectum, extending from 3 cm to 10

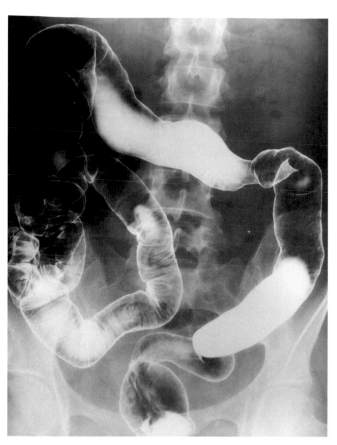

FIG. 44–1. Barium enema showing an ahaustral colon found in chronic ulcerative colitis.

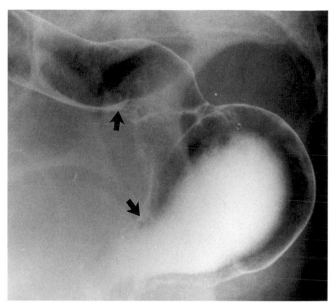

FIG. 44–2. Barium enema showing flat infiltrating tumor (arrows) with stricture formation on anterior wall of rectum.

cm above the dentate line. It appeared to be a deeply infiltrating tumor involving about one-half the circumference of the rectal wall. It was located anteriorly. A second, and clinically unapparent, adenocarcinoma was found on a random biopsy specimen at 58 cm. Serum carcinoembryonic antigen (CEA) was 1.7 ng/mL. Thorough evaluation for metastatic disease was negative.

The case was presented to the Surgical Oncology Multidisciplinary Tumor Conference. All consultants agreed that a total proctocolectomy with ileostomy was indicated. The construction of a continent pouch ileostomy was felt to be an option. The patient underwent a total proctocolectomy with Brooke ileostomy. A total abdominal hysterectomy/bilateral salpingo-oophorectomy, and partial vaginectomy were also performed to provide an adequate anterior margin. A "pelvic sling" of absorbable synthetic mesh was placed to keep the small bowel out of the pelvis in anticipation of postoperative external beam radiation therapy to the pelvis. The patient had an uneventful postoperative course.

The pathologist identified three colorectal cancers in the specimen. AJCC stage I cancers were found in the cecum (1.5 cm in diameter) and in the sigmoid colon (0.5 cm in diameter). Both these lesions were intermediate grade (Fig. 44–3). Thirty-one lymph nodes identified in the mesentery of the intra-abdominal colon contained no

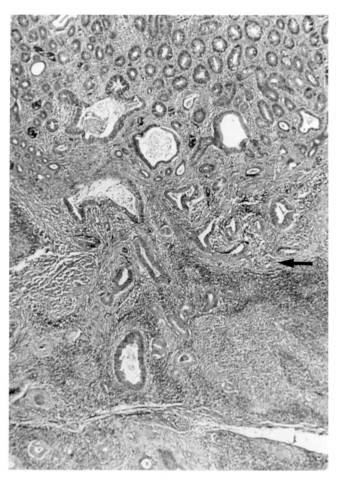

FIG. 44–3. In this random section from the ascending colon, malignant glands are more numerous in the lower mucosa (arrow indicates the muscularis mucosa) but are invading deeply into the submucosa in the lower part of the field. (H&E × 156).

tumor. The third cancer was in the rectum, extending from 3 to 10 cm from the anal verge. It completely penetrated the rectal wall to involve the muscle of the vaginal wall. One perirectal lymph node contained a metastasis (stage III). This lesion was high grade (Fig. 44–4).

All consultants felt that the risks of local pelvic recurrence and systemic recurrence were very high. The prognosis for the two adenocarcinomas of the colon was favorable because they were both T1 N0 intermediate-grade lesions. The rectal adenocarcinoma, however, was a high-grade, T3 N1 lesion. The incidence of locoregional recurrence for this lesion was estimated to be in the 40% range after surgery alone. Systemic dissemination was also felt to be a likely event. The expected 5-year survival with surgery alone was felt to be in the 35% to 40% range. Based on data from both the Gastrointestinal Tumor Study Group (GITSG) and the North Central Cancer Treatment Group (NCCTG), combination adjuvant therapy with both chemotherapy and radiation therapy was felt to be indicated. A "sandwich" technique of cytotoxic chemotherapy, followed by external beam radiation to the pelvis, followed by more chemotherapy was favored.

While awaiting the results of adjuvant therapy trials comparing various 5-fluorouracil (5-FU) combinations and using data on results in advanced disease, the chemotherapy regimen recommended was a combination of 5-FU and low-dose leucovorin. One or two courses before pelvic radiation therapy was recommended. A multiple field, 180 cGy/day, bladder-distended technique to a total dose of at least 5,000 cGy was recommended to follow the initial courses of chemotherapy. Three days of intravenous 5-FU given as a bolus at the beginning and end of radiation therapy was recommended as a "radiation potentiator." Additional 5-FU and leucovorin to complete 1 year of adjuvant therapy completed the recommended therapy. Therapy was complicated by diarrhea and mild cystitis.

The patient was followed up in the outpatient department at 3-month intervals. Approximately 11 months after the completion of all adjuvant therapy, she complained of mild colicky abdominal pain. CEA had risen from 0.7 to 3.3. These symptoms progressed to intermittent vomiting 2 months later. Upper gastrointestinal series and small bowel X-ray were normal. Physical examination revealed no signs of recurrence, but CEA had risen further to 8.4. She had also lost 20 lbs in several months. She was admitted to the hospital for further evaluation.

Several imaging tests were performed. Chest roentgenogram was normal. Bone scan was also normal. Intravenous

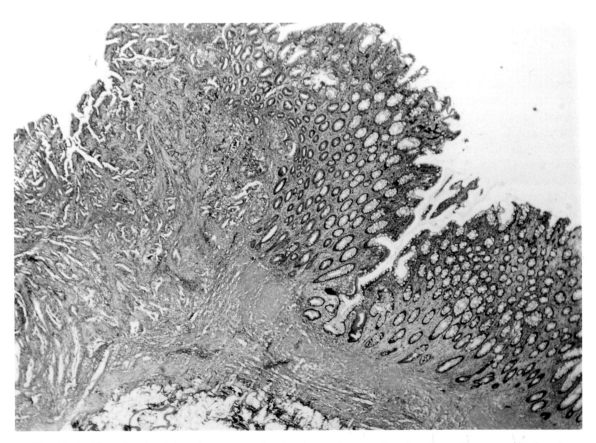

FIG. 44–4. Chronic glandular changes and a tendency to pseudopolyp formation representing the chronic ulcerative colitis are seen on the *right*. Carcinoma is seen on the surface and invading the submucosa on the *left*. The section is from the grossly-recognized rectal carcinoma. The muscularis propria was completely invaded. (HEE × 313).

pyelogram revealed an obstructed left ureter and a nonfunctioning left kidney. A computed tomography scan of the abdomen and pelvis revealed a presacral soft tissue mass without other abnormalities. Fine-needle aspiration cytology revealed malignant cells.

Exploratory laparotomy revealed metastatic tumor in the abdominal wall and diffuse tumor studding of the peritoneal surfaces below the pancreas. With palliative therapy only, the patient developed renal failure and died within 2 months of surgery. No post-mortem examination was performed.

This case demonstrates some of the difficulties that may be associated with the diagnosis of colon cancer in patients with panulcerative colitis of long duration. Compliance with surveillance may be limited. Dysplasia may or may not precede colon cancer. Cancer may be difficult to identify endoscopically, resulting in diagnosis at an advanced stage with accompanying poor prognosis. Because of these difficulties, prophylactic total proctocolectomy with ileoanal pouch reconstruction should be discussed with young patients who have diffuse colonic involvement with ulcerative colitis. Their cumulative risk, as reflected in this case, supports an aggressive preventive surgical approach to these patients.

COMMENTARY by George E. Block and Roger D. Hurst

This unfortunate patient belonged to a subset of patients with ulcerative colitis who are at high risk for the development of colorectal cancer. These patients may be identified by common clinical characteristics: chronicity (>8–10 years of disease), pancolitis (disease extending from the rectum well into the right colon), relative youth at the onset of colitis (1) (mean age 23 years) and, more recently, the presence of dysplasia (2) of the rectum or colon on random biopsy specimens.

To discover precancerous (dysplasia) and early cancers (in situ), a program of surveillance as advocated by Levin and others has become the standard of care for these high-risk patients (3).

The surveillance program consists of a yearly clinical examination and complete colonoscopy at least every 2 years. Data from Lennard-Jones'(4) series indicate the risk for developing cancer or high-grade dysplasia to be 13% at 25 years. Other series have found similar cancer risks, but there appears to be considerable variation.

This program of surveillance, although conceptually attractive and successful in some instances, has not universally resulted in the elimination of the cancer risk for colitic patients (5–8). The reasons for this are varied: patient and physician compliance decreases with time, carcinoma may develop de novo without pre-existing dysplasia, and, from a practical standpoint, most surveillance patients who undergo colectomy often have a multitude of other factors necessitating operation such as

macroscopic cancers, debilitating symptoms, strictures, etc. At the University of Chicago, screening for cancer in patients with ulcerative colitis was associated with an overall improvement in survival and a delay of the time of colectomy; however, improvement was not related to the anticipated benefits of an enhanced cancer-related survival (9).

Although the results of various prospective and retrospective studies regarding surveillance are in conflict (10–13), colectomy should be offered to the patient as a rational alternative to medical treatment in long-standing colitis, especially when complicated by dysplasia or stricture. Any operative procedure performed to eliminate the cancer risk in the colitic patient or to cure an already present cancer must remove the entire colon and rectum. Invasive tumors are often multifocal, carcinomas may develop in any retained segment of the rectum or colon and, because of chronic inflammation, macroscopic tumors are often not palpable at the time of exploration.

The choice operation to eliminate the cancer risk is a total colectomy, partial proctectomy, rectal mucosectomy, and ileoanal anastomosis of an ileal pouch. Total proctocolectomy and end-ileostomy is rarely necessary, and ileal–rectal anastomosis does not eliminate the cancer risk. Recently, particularly with the application of stapling devices, anastomosis of the ileal pouch is made either at the transition zone of the anal canal or above the dentate line. Studies from the Mayo Clinic (14) indicate the presence of inflamed rectal mucosa within 1 cm of the dentate line in 89% of the patients studied and rectal mucosa traversed half the length of the transition zone in 75% of the patients. Obviously, an anastomosis done at or above this point will leave rectal mucosa in place, which is theoretically at risk for malignant change in the future. If the operation is done to eliminate the cancer risk, any technique that involves leaving in place inflamed rectal mucosa must be viewed with caution at present.

The patient presented was an unfortunate individual who apparently did not receive appropriate examination such as rectal digital examination, rigid proctoscopy, or colonoscopy until the rectal cancer was advanced. The presence of an invasive low anterior rectal carcinoma eliminates the possibility of a sphincter-saving procedure. Indeed, the surgeons were correct in their aggressive approach to the patient, which included a partial vaginectomy and total hysterectomy. Because the cancer was locally advanced and a total proctectomy was necessary, a more extensive operative procedure should be considered. The addition of a wide pelvic lymphadenectomy including total mesorectal excision and removal of the obturator nodes has resulted in improved local recurrence rates and survival (15,16).

The use of adjuvant chemoirradiation therapy, although theoretically sound, was obviously inadequate to control this far advanced tumor. Postoperative irradiation may result in fewer local recurrences (17), but its influence on overall survival is, at best, inconclusive. Extended pelvic lymphadenectomy has yielded better results in selected series (18) than conventional operation supplemented by adjuvant chemoirradiation therapy. The use of adjuvant chemoirradiation therapy awaits further definition by prospective treatment protocols.

SUMMARY

The patient with chronic pancolitis is at risk for development of a carcinoma of the colon or rectum and this risk increases with time. A program of surveillance for dysplasia has not proven to give uniform protection for the patient with chronic pancolitis and the risk of a carcinoma developing after the onset of colitis is up to 20% at 40 years. Patients undergoing surveillance are still at risk for the development of cancer and consideration should be given to the operative removal of the colon and rectum.

If a "prophylactic" proctocolectomy is performed, retention of rectal mucosa or the transitional zone of the anal canal still places the patient at a theoretic risk for the development of carcinoma in later life.

If a macroscopic tumor is present, an appropriate lymphadenectomy should be performed with the colectomy. For large, invasive, and mucinous tumors of the rectum, an ileal–anal anastomosis is not feasible. These patients should undergo total proctocolectomy, supplemented by pelvic lymphadenectomy including obturator node removal. Adjuvant chemoradiotherapy is an attractive, but unproven, supplement to operation.

EDITORIAL BOARD COMMENTARY

Prospective, randomized clinical trials have demonstrated a statistically significant reduction in local recurrence and mortality in stage III rectal cancer patients treated with chemoradiation.

REFERENCES

1. Lashner BA, Silverstein MD, Hanauer SB. Hazard rates for dysplasia and cancer in ulcerative colitis. Results from a surveillance program. *Dig Dis Sci* 1989;34:1536–41.
2. Lennard-Jones JE, Morson BC, Ritchie JK, et al. Cancer in colitis: assessment of the individual risk by clinical and histological criteria. *Gastroenterology* 1977;73:1280–9.
3. Levin B, Lennard-Jones JE, Riddell RH, et al. Surveillance of patients with chronic ulcerative colitis. WHO Collaborating Center for the Prevention of Colorectal Cancer. *Bull WHO* 1991;69:121–6.
4. Lennard-Jones JE, Melville DM, Morson BC, et al. Precancer and cancer in extensive ulcerative colitis: findings among 401 patients over twenty-two years. *Gut* 1990;31:800–6.
5. Taylor BA, Pemberton JH, Carpenter HA, et al. Dysplasia in chronic ulcerative colitis: implications for colonoscopic surveillance. *Dis Colon Rectum* 1992;35:950–6.
6. Rutegard JN, Ahsgren LR, Janunger KG. Ulcerative colitis. Colorectal cancer risks in an unselected population. *Ann Surg* 1988;208:721–4.
7. Thirlby RC. Colonoscopic surveillance for cancer in patients with chronic ulcerative colitis: is it working? *Gastroenterology* 1991;100:570–2.
8. Woolrich AG, DaSilva MD, Korelitz BI. Surveillance in the routine management of ulcerative colitis: the predictive value of low grade dysplasia. *Gastroenterology* 1992;103:431–8.
9. Lashner BA, Kane SP, Hanauer SB. Colon cancer surveillance in chronic ulcerative colitis: historical cohort study. *Am J Gastroenterol* 1990;85:1083–7.
10. Rutegard J, Ahsgren L, Janunger KG. Ulcerative colitis. Mortality and surgery in an unselected population. *Acta Chir Scand* 1988;154:215–9.
11. Lashner BA. Recommendations for colorectal cancer screening in ulcerative colitis: a review of research from a single university-based surveillance program. *Am J Gastroenterol* 1992;87:168–75.
12. Langholz E, Munkholm P, Davidsen M, Binder V. Colorectal cancer risk and mortality in patients with ulcerative colitis. *Gastroenterology* 1992;103:1444–51.
13. Ekbom A, Helmick C, Zack M, Adami HO. Ulcerative colitis in colorectal cancer. A population-based study. *N Engl J Med* 1990;323:1228–33.
14. Ambroze WLJ, Pemberton JH, Dozois RR, et al. The histological pattern and pathological involvement of the anal transition zone in patients with ulcerative colitis. *Gastroenterology* 1993;104:514–8.
15. Michelassi F, Block GE, Vannucci L, et al. Five to twenty-one year follow-up and analysis of 250 patients with rectal adenocarcinoma. *Ann Surg* 1988;208:379–89.
16. Enker W, Laffer UT, Block GE. Enhanced survival of patients with colon and rectal cancer is based upon wide anatomic resection. *Ann Surg* 1979; 190:350–60.
17. Rosenthal SA, Trock BJ, Coia LR. Randomized trials of adjuvant radiation therapy for rectal carcinoma: a review. *Dis Col Rectum* 1990;33:336–43.
18. Koyoma Y, Moriya Y, Hojo K. Effects of extended lymphadenectomy for adenocarcinoma of the rectum. Significant improvement of survival rate and decrease of local recurrence. *Jpn J Clin Oncol* 1984;14:623.

45

Adenocarcinoma of the Stomach with Brain and Liver Metastases

Thomas A. Gaskin

*Is there ever any justification for palliative therapy when
there are no symptoms?*

CASE PRESENTATION

Dr. Jose Cusco (medical resident): This gentleman is a 64-year-old Caucasian male roofer who was admitted to the hospital 4 days ago after he presented to the emergency room with memory loss and subsequent inability to speak. He has been healthy all his life and does not avail himself of routine medical care of any sort.

Two to three weeks before his presentation to the emergency room, he began having episodes of vomiting, which was not projectile, and had lost approximately 5 lbs.

He had an episode of dizziness a year ago and had another episode of dizziness 3 days ago. He denied any abdominal pain. All this history was obtained from his wife because on his way home from work on the day before admission he had vomited several times, told his wife he was sick, and went to bed.

An hour later, however, he was unable to speak and she brought him to the emergency room. There is no significant past history. The following day, he was seen by neurology and by gastroenterology and had a number of studies performed.

Dr. William S. Blakemore (surgeon): I expect you are going to show us a chest radiograph and a computed tomography (CT) scan of the head.

Dr. Roy Gandy (surgeon): I'll bet he had a lot more studies than that done. I'd be surprised if that was all that he had.

Dr. Kerri Berthold (radiology resident): Dr. Gandy is right. I have a number of studies that were performed on

March 4, 1993; would you like to see his chest radiograph?

Dr. Blakemore: Yes, I would. Incidentally, does he smoke?

Dr. Rudy Navari (medical oncologist): He neither smokes nor drinks.

Dr. Blakemore: You said he worked as a roofer. Asphalt?

Dr. Navari: No, he almost exclusively installs red cedar shingle roofing. These are nailed. In recent years he has begun treating the shingles with a preservative after application but for most of his life there were no chemicals involved in the process at all.

Dr. Blakemore: I still expect we will see something on the chest radiograph.

Dr. Berthold: This is the admission EPA and lateral chest radiograph, and there is no evidence of any significant abnormality (Fig. 45–1).

Dr. Alton Baker (diagnostic radiologist): I reviewed these films last night and really there is no abnormality at all on them.

Dr. Blakemore: Well, the way this case presented, I was expecting to see evidence of small cell cancer with cerebral metastases.

Dr. Baker: Well, here is the CT brain scan from March 4, 1993. There are some low density lesions in the right frontal and left parieto-occipital regions (Fig. 45–2). The overall appearance of this is most like an infarction, but in my experience it would be unusual to have simultaneous infarctions in two separate vascular regions and, because

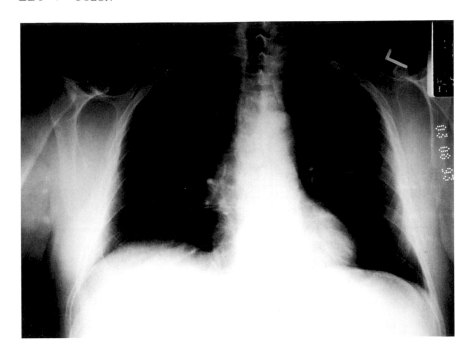

FIG. 45–1. Lateral chest radiograph showing no evidence of any significant abnormality.

of that, we thought that metastatic disease was more likely.

Dr. Navari: He had an abnormal electroencephalogram (EEG) and a normal carotid duplex examination. Why don't you show them the ultrasound now?

Dr. Berthold: This is the abdominal ultrasound that his internist ordered on the day of admission and it shows multiple lesions in the right hepatic lobe of low echogenicity and some with high echogenicity. There is a low echoic lesion involving the left kidney. We think that the low echogenic lesions probably are metastatic disease.

The smaller high echogenic lesions may be hemangiomata (Fig. 45–3).

Dr. Navari: Would anyone like to suggest where we go from here?

Dr. Kraig Knoll (surgical resident): How about a magnetic resonance image (MRI) brain scan and a CT scan of the abdomen?

Dr. Navari: Well, here is the MRI brain scan.

Dr. Baker: As you can see there are multiple masses supratentorially in both hemispheres. The largest one is present in the right occipital lobe. These lesions are in the

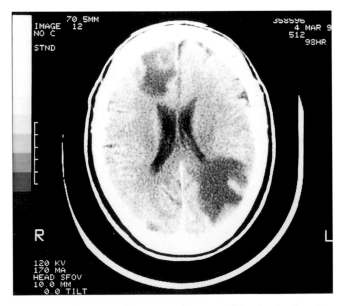

FIG. 45–2. Computed tomography scan of the brain showing low-density lesions in the right frontal and left parieto-occipital regions.

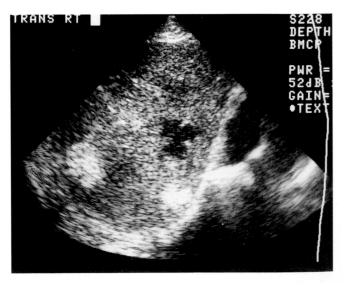

FIG. 45–3. Abdominal ultrasound. Multiple lesions in the right hepatic lobe of low echogenicity and some with high echogenicity are shown.

gray-white matter junctions and most likely represent metastases (Fig. 45–4). He has not had a CT scan of the abdomen yet.

Dr. Navari: He did have an esophagogastroduodenoscopy (EGD), which showed a fungating mass in the distal esophagus or upper fundus and a biopsy was taken.

Dr. Tom Gaskin (vascular surgeon): Was this done by the medical gastroenterology or by the surgical service? Is there another clue in the history that you have left out? I'm a little bit surprised that you went directly to endoscopy on his second day.

Dr. Navari: Actually, his admitting physician's initial impression was gastric cancer and it was he who requested the EGD almost simultaneously with ordering the head studies.

Dr. Gaskin: Did the gastroenterologist mention the extent of the lesion down the stomach and whether or not it was obstructing the esophagus and whether there was any infiltration of the esophagus and what the limits on that were?

Dr. Navari: He said that there was a fungating mass in the distal esophagus or upper stomach. He doesn't mention a hiatal hernia but he does mention a hernia sac.

Dr. Gaskin: I rest my case. By the way, how is the man doing at this point?

Dr. Navari: The aphasia resolved spontaneously. We started some Decadron on that day but his aphasia had begun to subside even before then.

Dr. Arthur Ludwig (pathologist): We received biopsy fragments from the stomach (Fig. 45–5) and from the distal esophagus (Fig. 45–6). I think that you can all appreci-

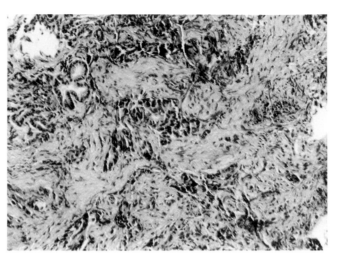

FIG. 45–5. Gastric adenocarcinoma: poorly differentiated microglandular structures within a reactive desmoplastic stroma within the gastric submucosa.

ate the chaotic gland formation. It is an infiltrating, poorly differentiated adenocarcinoma. On this fragment, you can see some esophageal mucosa so it is involving the distal esophagus somewhat.

Dr. John Pinkston (radiation oncologist): Are you fairly secure in your diagnosis? Could this be something other than a stomach cancer? I can't remember the last time that I have seen a gastric adenocarcinoma present with cerebral metastasis.

Dr. Navari: I can't recall the last time I have seen a gastric cancer with cerebral metastases at all, much less presenting with cerebral metastases.

Dr. Ludwig: Well, look again at this section here. This is a gastric carcinoma, at least it appears to be in the gastrointestinal tract. I think we can pretty well exclude lung and kidney as part of the differential.

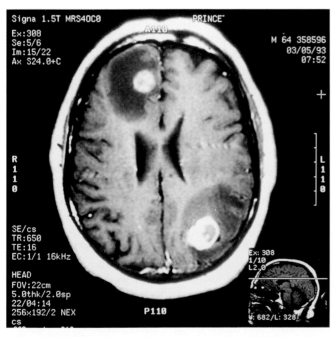

FIG. 45–4. MRI scan of the brain showing multiple masses supratentorially in both hemispheres.

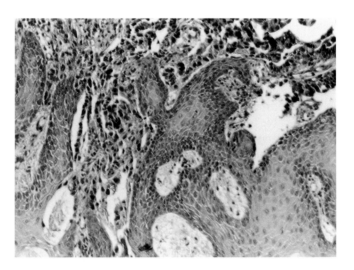

FIG. 45–6. Lower esophagus with poorly differentiated gastric adenocarcinoma infiltrating the lamina propria.

Dr. Navari: I did a very brief literature search because of this and gastric carcinoma rarely metastasizes to the brain, but it does occur.

Dr. Brian Larson (radiation oncologist): Do we have any other studies to review?

Dr. Navari: We have some other studies ordered but they are not available yet. I wanted to present this man to get some ideas about where to go. Dr. Larson, based on what we have already, do you think we need any additional studies? For instance, would you be willing to radiate his brain without a tissue diagnosis of his cerebral lesions?

Dr. Larson: Considering the extent of his metastatic disease in the liver and in the brain, I certainly wouldn't insist that we put him through a brain biopsy.

Dr. Navari: What kind of results can we expect from whole brain radiation?

Dr. Pinkston: I think we could get pretty fair palliation with whole brain radiation. I would not want to be pinned down on the duration of response, but I would expect that we could get pretty good short to intermediate control of the cerebral mets.

Dr. Navari: What about the primary lesion? How should that be treated?

Dr. Gaskin: I think it goes without saying that what we are interested in in this instance is palliation. We want him to be as comfortable as possible for as long as possible and for his final days to be as peaceful as possible. The reason I say that is that dying of esophageal obstruction or bleeding and vomiting from an uncontrolled tumor in the gastric fundus is not very pleasant. I would be surprised if anything we could do would control the hepatic metastasis. By the way, you never mentioned any laboratory work. What are his liver functions like?

Dr. Cusco: His bilirubin is 4 and alkaline phosphatase is 500.

Dr. Gaskin: My guess is that he will die from the hepatic mets, assuming that Drs. Pinkston and Larson can control his cerebral mets, so I don't want us to overlook some type of palliative procedure on his primary cancer.

Dr. Navari: We had fairly good results using 5-fluorouracil (5-FU) and leucovorin and platinol, both in terms of control of the primary tumor and the hepatic disease. Obviously, we don't expect any long-term control, but we might be able to do something.

Dr. Blakemore: Perhaps, Dr. Gaskin would like to say something about the role of the hepatic artery infusion pump controlling metastatic disease. We did some of the early work on this at Penn. I really have not kept up in the last couple years. All I know is that the early enthusiasm for it seems to have waned somewhat.

Dr. Gaskin: You are right. It is not applicable in this case. There is a diminishing role for hepatic artery infusion pumps. Resective therapy is generally preferred and is becoming increasingly common and increasingly safe and it is much more effective. About the best anyone

could do with the hepatic artery infusion pumps was to double life expectancy. It is attractive from a clinical kinetic point of view as a delivery system, but really has not lived up to its initial promise very well. Dr. Navari, what kind of control of the primary tumor can you expect with chemotherapy and perhaps the addition of radiation?

Dr. Navari: It is hard to say. I really believe that he will probably die of his metastatic disease before developing esophageal obstruction. If we got a really good response in the liver and a more incomplete response in the primary tumor, then we really could be faced with the possibility of someone who is debilitated by his treatment and then developed some obstruction.

Dr. Gaskin: That is the point I wanted to make. If he needs palliation of his primary tumor, it is better to do that initially rather than at the 11th hour. I would like to have some better definition of the primary tumor before giving too aggressive of a recommendation. I would like to go back and make sure I didn't say anything that might be construed unduly critical of our colleagues in gastroenterology. The point I wanted to make was that it really helps the surgeon to know some precise anatomic details about a tumor that may be treated surgically. It may take nothing more than a video tape of a portion of the examination so that it can be reviewed. The still pictures often are helpful but they do not tell the whole story. Laparoscopic staging is useful in upper gastrointestinal malignancies and some palliative procedure can be accomplished. Staging is not necessary here. We already have distant metastases, and palliative bypass and stenting could wait until symptoms developed.

Dr. Navari: Dr. Pinkston, I know that you have already seen the gentleman and have recommended a course of radiation therapy to him. My recommendation is for 5-FU, leucovorin, and platinol with or without primary radiation depending on what Dr. Pinkston thinks about that. Dr. Gaskin, we will talk to this man about a surgical consultation and you can review the studies with the gastroenterologist and see if he needs any palliative surgical treatment early on.

COMMENTARY by Murray F. Brennan

The present case report is interesting, as the authors provide the "real life" commentaries of a Tumor Board. The case is unusual, with the primary presentation of gastric adenocarcinoma as a brain metastasis. Delightfully, the chief of surgery goes directly "where the money might be" and looks for a chest radiograph and a CT scan of the head. Not surprisingly, the patient has many more investigations than that! With cost containment in mind, we identify that the patient had an EEG, carotid duplex, abdominal ultrasound, CT of the brain, chest radiograph, brain MRI, and esophagogastroduodenoscopy.

It is hard for this reviewer to think that surgery has anything to offer in this situation. The discussion centers on what degree of palliation one might get from the whole brain radiation. Then again, the patient's symptoms from his cerebral metastasis appear to be already resolved! The case is left up in the air. Rather surprisingly, no mention is made of doing nothing except relieving him of his symptoms, none of which appear to be very great.

I would have thought that the issue here would be what could be done to make the gentleman more comfortable? If vomiting is the problem, then endoscopic laser treatment would be the easiest way to relieve his symptoms if possible. Decadron appears to have resolved his aphasia, although that may have resolved spontaneously. I would have thought that the patient needed "a single doctor" who could discuss his prognosis, the limited therapeutic options, and involve the patient and his family in any decision making.

EDITORIAL BOARD COMMENTARY

In fact, the situation was discussed with the patient's family and he was referred for hospice care.

46 Familial Adenomatous Polyposis

Jerome J. DeCosse

Preemptive surgery: when and how?

CASE PRESENTATION

At Tumor Board in February 1993, a restorative proctectomy (ileoanal anastomosis with pouch) was recommended for this 37-year-old man. Both his troubled past history as well as events after the Tumor Board illustrate the natural history of familial adenomatous polyposis (FAP), and provide an opportunity to review the pathogenesis and management of this autosomal dominant disorder in the context of emerging knowledge.

In 1970, the patient, then 13 years old, underwent a screening sigmoidoscopy because his mother had died of colon carcinoma in the setting of FAP. Although asymptomatic, he was found to have rectal polyps. Surgery was recommended but declined. In October 1976, at age 19, rectal bleeding occurred. Rigid sigmoidoscopy showed the distal two thirds of the rectum spared of polyps, but an air-contrast barium enema examination revealed many polyps in the colon (Fig. 46–1). At that time, a total colectomy was performed, with construction of an ileorectal anastomosis 15 cm from the anal verge. The resected specimen harbored more than 700 polyps. Microscopic examination showed both adenomatous polyposis with marked focal atypia and multiple areas of early adenomatous change in flat mucosa. The patient was subsequently treated with frequent outpatient snare cautery or diathermy of recurrent rectal adenomas. In 1980, he required an exploratory laparotomy for an adhesive small bowel obstruction, but was then lost to follow-up.

The patient reappeared in late November 1992, complaining of persistent, red rectal bleeding. Examination of his calvarium and mandible demonstrated multiple osteomas. Rectal digital examination revealed several large,

easily palpated polyps; and proctosigmoidoscopy showed a large, pedunculated polyp about 8 cm from the anal verge. In January 1993, after unsuccessful attempts at outpatient removal of the polyp, the patient was admitted, and a midrectal tubular adenoma, measuring $3.2 \times 2.5 \times 1.5$ cm, was snared endoscopically in the operating room. Microscopic examination showed a tubular adenoma with marked focal superficial atypia. At least 15 to 20 additional polyps, some measuring up to 12 mm in diameter, were evident in the remaining rectum.

At this time, the patient was reviewed at Tumor Board. A restorative proctectomy was recommended because the rectal mucosa was carpeted with polyps and because future follow-up would likely be unsuccessful. An upper gastrointestinal endoscopy and a computed tomography (CT) scan of the abdomen and pelvis also were recommended.

The patient, however, refused an operation. After the polypectomy, rectal bleeding stopped and the patient was asymptomatic. Carcinoembryonic antigen was 2.0 µg/L. Because he was reluctant to undergo surgery, the patient was started on Sulindac 150 mg b.i.d. to control rectal polyps.

In late April 1993, the patient had a grand mal seizure. On examination, general weakness was present, but a sensory or motor defect was not found. A CT scan of the head demonstrated a 6-cm, left frontal lobe mass with mild ring enhancement and associated edema (Fig. 46–2). Proctosigmoidoscopy showed reduction in the size of rectal polyps. The patient was admitted and, on May 21, 1993, a frontal lobe, grade III oligodendroglioma (stage III B G3, T2, M0) was incompletely removed. At present, the patient is convalescing and neurologically intact. Radiation therapy has been initiated, but his prognosis is dismal.

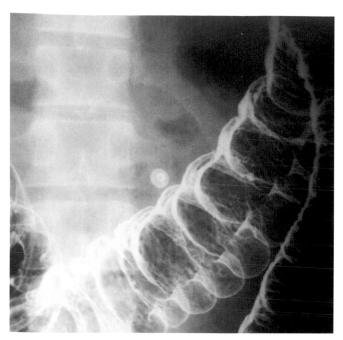

FIG. 46–1. An air-contrast view of the left transverse colon, showing numerous small sessile mucosal adenomas.

COMMENTARY by Jerome J. DeCosse and Glenn D. Steele, Jr.

The patient illustrates the complex problems encountered in the diagnosis and management of the polyposis patient. New information on the pathogenesis and treatment of FAP, however, is emerging to help with difficult decisions. The following comments based on the case presentation highlight these promising developments.

"His mother had died of colon carcinoma in the setting of FAP."

The gene for FAP was identified in 1987: it is located on chromosome 5q21 (1–3), and subsequent studies have confirmed the consistent absence of this sequence, called the APC gene, in affected persons. The deletion is presumed to result in loss of a suppressor gene. One allele is missing by inheritance, but the other allele must also be lost for phenotypic expression. Hence, inheritance is autosomal dominant at the cellular level, whereas expression is recessive at the molecular level. Linkage analysis, which requires more than one family member at risk, has been available for several years to identify affected persons. Recently, a polymerase chain reaction has been developed for direct detection of the mutation (4). This assay will likely become widely available during the next few years for presymptomatic detection and genetic counseling.

"The patient . . . underwent a screening sigmoidoscopy."

When a patient with FAP is detected, the physician is obligated to seek out other potentially affected relatives. In adolescents, screening should begin at about age 12 with flexible sigmoidoscopy. Unless rectal or sigmoid polyps are identified at that time, further evaluation by colonoscopy or barium enema roentgenography is unnecessary and only serves to drive youngsters away from future study. Phenotypic expression also may be detected by examination of the retina for presence of congenital hypertrophy of the retinal pigment, called CHRPE.

The importance of upper gastrointestinal endoscopy had not been widely recognized when the patient first presented himself in 1976. Because the patient with FAP is at substantial risk for periampullary carcinoma, endoscopy is important in preoperative evaluation and during subsequent follow-up. Patients with FAP typically have numerous small polyps in the stomach, but these are innocuous hamartomas. Duodenal polyps, however, are regularly adenomas, and adenomatous change in the pancreatic ampulla is consistently present.

"Examination of his calvarium and mandible demonstrated multiple osteomas."

Gardner syndrome, a term applied more commonly in this country, associates multiple colorectal adenomas with sebaceous cysts, lipomas, fibromas, desmoid tumors, and osteomas. Although it has been customary to distinguish Gardner syndrome (mesenchymal expression) from FAP (epithelial expression), the same gene locus is absent in both; therefore strengthening belief that this distinction

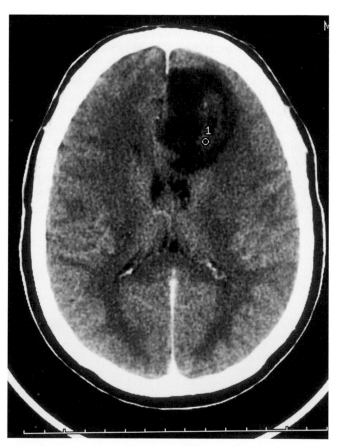

FIG. 46–2. CT scan of head reveals left frontal lobe mass with mild ring enhancement and associated edema.

should not be made. All FAP patients either have extra-colonic expressions or have the capacity for them.

"He required an exploratory laparotomy for . . . obstruction."

This was not a coincidence (5). The FAP patient is at increased risk for adhesion formation. This risk appears associated with the proclivity for desmoid disease, which manifests either as a discrete tumor or as desmoid fibro-plasia. The desmoid is a low-grade, nonmetastasizing fibrosarcoma that, in the patient with FAP, usually occurs in the mesentery, retroperitoneum, or abdominal wall, and can be life-threatening. Desmoids typically appear after operative intervention.

"A restorative proctectomy was recommended."

During the past decade, restorative proctocolectomy, that is, total removal of the colon and rectum with ileoanal anastomosis, preservation of sphincteric function, and construction of a pouch reservoir, has become a widely accepted initial operative procedure for colorectal poly-posis. All target colorectal mucosa is removed. A tempo-rary ileostomy is generally required. Operative mortality is acceptably low but morbidity is high: most patients have some fecal incontinence or sexual dysfunction, or both.

In other centers, particularly in Europe, the preferred, initial operative procedure is a total colectomy and ileo-rectal anastomosis performed at 12 to 15 cm from the anal verge. All agree that a total proctectomy is necessary if the rectum has many adenomas, if mid- or upper-rectal cancer is present, or if the patient is not amenable to regu-lar follow-up. Patients who have had an ileorectal anasto-mosis have a cumulative incidence of rectal cancer of 13% at 25 years (6).

"Sulindac . . . was started . . . to control rectal polyps."

After ileorectal anastomosis, most remaining rectal polyps diminish or disappear, a process called sponta-neous regression. Ultimately, rectal polyps recur. These rectal polyps are the setting for nutritional and pharmaco-logic efforts to maintain long-term regression. Sulindac, a prostaglandin synthetase inhibitor, has shown effective-ness in randomized trials (7).

"A frontal lobe glioma was removed."

Properly, this patient should now be subclassified as having Turcot's syndrome, a rare association with FAP. Turcot's syndrome was originally described as an associ-ation of colorectal adenomas with medulloblastoma in adolescence. Malignant gliomas are being encountered increasingly.

"His prognosis is dismal."

This patient's history reflects the difficulties and chal-lenges involved in caring for the polyposis patient. It may be argued that he should have had his rectum removed much earlier, and that he represents a failure of the acade-mic health care system to maintain follow-up. The patient, however, is not going to die from gastrointestinal cancer.

With reduction of risk by removal of the colon, the polyposis patient has survived to confront the life-threat-ening challenges of systemic disease. Patients who have had a colectomy and ileorectal anastomosis have a risk of dying from rectal cancer of 2% at 15 years of follow-up (6). The likelihood of dying from either upper gastroin-testinal cancer or desmoid disease is at least three times greater. Hence, long-term, general surveillance remains essential in this relatively young population.

REFERENCES

1. Herrera L, Karati S, Gibas L, et al. Brief clinical report: Gardner syn-drome in a man with an interstial deletion of 5q. *Am J Med Genet* 1986;25:473–6.
2. Bodmer W, Bailey C, Bodmer J, et al. Localization of the gene for familial adenomatous polyposis on chromosome 5. *Nature* 1987;328:614–6.
3. Leppert M, Dobbs M, Scambper P, et al. The gene for familial poly-posis coli maps to the long arm of chromosome 5. *Science* 1987;238:1411–3.
4. Anndo H, Miyoshi Y, Nagase H, et al. Detection of 12 germ-line mutations in the adenomatous polyposis gene by polymerase chain reaction. *Gastroenterology* 1993;104:989–93.
5. Sener S, Miller H, DeCosse J. The spectrum of polyposis. *Surg Gynecol Obstet* 1984;159:525–32.
6. DeCosse J, Bülow S, Neale K, et al. Rectal cancer risk in patients treated for familial adenomatous polyposis. *Br J Surg* 1992;79:1372–5.
7. Giardiello F, Hamilton S, Krush A, et al. Treatment of colonic and rec-tal adenomas with sulindac in familial adenomatous polyposis. *N Engl J Med* 1993;328:1313–6.

47

Exploratory Laparotomy in a Young Woman for a Right Ovarian Neoplasm: Metastatic Carcinoma from an Unrecognized Small Primary Cecal Cancer

Warren E. Enker

Plan your treatment for the most "treatable" disease

CASE PRESENTATION

S.D. is a 41-year-old premenopausal woman in good health. She presented in August 1987 with vague right lower abdominal discomfort and intermittent bloating. The patient denied any change in her bowel habits or any change in the appearance of her stool. She denied bleeding per rectum, but did have an intermittent history of bleeding per rectum in years past, attributed to hemorrhoids. She denied any obvious abdominal pain, but did have a vague history of right lower quadrant discomfort for the past 3 months. The discomfort bore no relation to meals, physical activity, or defecation. The patient denied any sense of incomplete defecation, any mucus production per rectum, or any change in appetite or weight.

The patient has a past history of scoliosis with repeated episodes of chronic low back pain. She has been treated as an outpatient on several occasions for acute urinary tract infections. The patient has never undergone any previous surgery and has never been admitted to a hospital for any major medical illness. She is not allergic to any medications and does not smoke now, but did smoke from age 18 to age 27. She does not drink.

The family history is significant for a sister who has ovarian cancer, and a maternal grandmother with colon cancer. The family history is also significant for diabetes mellitus.

Physical examination revealed a moderately overweight white woman, in no acute distress. There was no supraclavicular adenopathy. The liver was not enlarged to palpation or percussion. The abdomen was otherwise soft, flat, and nontender with no organomegaly or masses. The inguinal regions were normal. Digital/rectal examination was within normal limits. Bimanual vaginal examination revealed a vague sense of right adnexal fullness with tenderness.

Pelvic ultrasonography suggested a right adnexal mass, 4×6 cm in diameter, consistent with ovarian neoplasm. There was no visible ascites. Flexible fiberoptic sigmoidoscopy to 45 cm was within normal limits. A barium enema revealed no evidence of a colonic neoplasm. Visualization of both the terminal ileum and the appendix were noted; however, cecal filling was not optimal. CA-125 was 6 U/mL and carcinoembryonic antigen (CEA) was 12.6 ng/mL (nl 0–5). Preoperative blood tests revealed hemoglobin of 12.4, hematocrit of 37%, total bilirubin of 0.4 mg/dL (nl 0–1.0), SGOT 20 U/L (nl 10–37), LDH 151 U/L (nl 60–200) and alkaline phosphatase 112 U/L (nl 30–188). A repeat CA-125 was 12 U/mL (nl 0–35) and CEA was 1.2 ng/mL (nl 0–5).

A preoperative cervical pap smear was normal and the patient had a history of normal pap smears.

The patient was admitted to the hospital on November 10, 1987, and underwent a mechanical bowel prep with polyethylene glycol solution. On November 11, the patient underwent exploratory laparotomy through a lower midline incision. A 4 × 6 cm cystic and solid neoplasm of the right ovary was observed. There was no evidence of metastases to the peritoneal surfaces or the lining of the abdominal cavity, to regional or extraregional lymph nodes, to the liver, or to any other structures. Peritoneal washings ultimately demonstrated no evidence of tumor cells.

An area of induration was appreciated, incidentally, on the lateral posterior surface of the cecum. The cecum was, for the most part, intraperitoneal. Further palpation suggested the presence of a discrete mass, 3 cm above the appendix on the posterior lateral surface of the cecum.

A right salpingo-oophorectomy was performed, and the neoplasm was submitted for frozen section. Histopathology of the frozen section revealed metastatic adenocarcinoma in the ovary consistent with colonic origin. The fallopian tube was negative.

An intraoperative consultation from the Colorectal Service was obtained. Based on the intraoperative findings, the results of the frozen section, and an adequate mechanical bowel prep, a right radical hemicolectomy was performed with primary anastomosis. The ileocolic, right colic, and right branch of the middle colic vessels were isolated and divided at their origins from the superior mesenteric vessels. The right colon was generously mobilized away from the retroperitoneum and the duodenum. A primary stapled side-to-side (functional end-to-end) anastomosis was constructed.

A supracervical hysterectomy was performed without incident. The stump of the cervix was reperitonealized with a running absorbable suture. The patient's postoperative recovery was unremarkable.

The pathology consultation report revealed a specimen consisting of terminal ileum, cecum, and ascending and right transverse colon. The terminal ileum measured 16 cm in length and the colon measured 22 cm in length. The bowel was not dilated. The serosal surfaces were smooth. On opening the specimen along its antimesenteric border, normal mucosal folds were observed except in the cecum where a 3.5-cm shallow, well-circumscribed, but ulcerated carcinoma was present. Cutting through the lesion suggested the possibility of invasion into the pericolic fat.

Microscopic examination revealed adenocarcinoma of the colon, moderately well differentiated, penetrating full-thickness through the muscularis propria into the pericolic fat. A single focus of lymphatic invasion was noted immediately adjacent to the primary tumor. Metastatic adenocarcinoma was observed in a single mesenteric replaced lymph node with no remaining lymph node architecture observed. Sixteen negative regional lymph nodes were reported. There was no vascular or perineural invasion.

Permanent sections confirmed the presence of metastatic adenocarcinoma in the right ovary, consistent with colonic adenocarcinoma. The left ovary and tube revealed no evidence of neoplasm. The uterus was otherwise normal.

Medical oncology consultation was obtained and the patient's case was discussed in a multidisciplinary conference. Proponents of adjuvant chemotherapy pointed to the existence of a lymph node metastasis and of lymphatic invasion and an ovarian metastasis. Those who argued against the use of "adjuvant" chemotherapy pointed to the presence of metastatic disease in the ovary, with all known disease resected. Without evidence to support an impact of 5-fluorouracil–related chemotherapy in the prevention of recurrence after the resection of metastatic disease, adjuvant therapy was not recommended.

The patient underwent intensive follow-up, including serial physical examinations every 4 months, surveillance colonoscopy every year for the first 2 years followed by biannual examinations, serial CEA and LFTs determinations, and annual chest roentgenogram. The patient was last seen in follow-up in December 1992 and had no evidence of recurrence or of metastatic disease. Photomicrographs revealed the primary colon cancer with metastatic disease in the ileocolic mesentery and a focus of metastatic colonic adenocarcinoma within her ovary.

COMMENTARY by Ira J. Kodner

The pretreatment evaluation of this young woman with a family history of colon cancer and ovarian cancer requires a comment in that the patient with an elevated CEA, a suspicious family history, and especially one with symptoms and findings of pelvic tumor would indicate the need for complete colonoscopy for surveillance of the large intestine and rectum for cancer. Barium enema and flexible sigmoidoscopy is the second best; flexible sigmoidoscopy should never be considered as adequate screening in any high-risk patient. I would also suggest the advantage of computed tomography (CT) scanning in evaluation of a patient with pelvic tumor.

The relationship of the ovary to cancer of the colon and rectum presents an interesting surgical dilemma. Any consideration should deal with a clear distinction between prophylactic and therapeutic aspects of the surgery. This is especially true when the issue arises of removal of the ovary during surgery for known primary colorectal cancer. Is the ovary removed to prevent further metastasis, or is the ovary removed because there is a known high incidence of metastatic disease to the ovary? The consensus seems to be, from a limited number of studies, that if cancer has metastasized to the ovary, the prognosis is so poor that removal makes no long-term difference in survival. This existence of metastatic cancer to the ovary is a marker for hematogenous spread, and the thought that it would occur to just one ovary is wishful thinking.

In the postmenopausal woman having surgery for known colorectal cancer, the ovaries should probably be removed, if this does not add to the complexity of the surgical procedure, in order to reduce the risk of subsequent ovarian neoplasms that might be difficult to diagnose because of the changes in the tissue resulting from the colorectal surgical procedure.

In premenopausal women, our policy is to leave the ovaries in unless they have been radiated or the cancer is known to be of a very aggressive type, such as poorly differentiated with a high risk of hematogenous spread. If the ovaries have been radiated, as we do frequently in an institutional protocol in a preoperative fashion for rectal cancer, the ovaries will become nonfunctional and should be removed because of the risk of metastatic disease or subsequent primary ovarian cancer, perhaps even related to the radiation itself. It is also important for the surgeon to make a specific effort to keep the ovaries in the intraperitoneal position to maintain the fertility of the woman and prevent the "entrapped ovary" syndrome. This occurs when the rectum is removed and the ovaries fall into the cavity and become quickly excluded as extraperitoneal structures. This is especially important in young women having proctectomy for benign conditions such as inflammatory bowel disease.

Once a metastasis is found in the ovary during surgery, the ovary should be removed to lower the tumor burden. Although this means that the patient has hematogenous spread of the cancer, systemic chemotherapy should be reserved for patients with symptomatic disease requiring palliation. If local extension to the ovary occurs, wide en bloc resection should be undertaken and adjuvant radiation therapy to the tumor bed considered. Intraoperative radiation therapy or one of the various new forms of brachytherapy should be considered only in the context of a clinical trial.

SELECTED READINGS

1. Birnkrant A, Sampson J, Sugarbaker PH. Ovarian metastasis from colorectal cancer. *Dis Colon Rectum* 1986;29:767–71.

2. Boyce GA, Sivak MV Jr, Lavery IC, et al. Endoscopic ultrasound in the pre-operative staging of rectal carcinoma. *Gastrointest Endosc* 1992;38:468–71.

3. Fry RD, Fleshman JW, Kodner IJ. Cancer of colon and rectum. *Clin Symp* 1989;41:2–32.

4. Halpern SE, Dillman RO, Amox D, et al. Detection of occult tumor using indium 111–labeled anticarcinoembryonic antigen antibodies. *Arch Surg* 1992;127:1094–1100.

5. Heys SD, Eremin O. The relevance of tumor draining lymph nodes in cancer. *Surg Gynecol Obstet* 1992;174:533–40.

6. Kodner IJ, Fleshman JW, Fry RD. Anal and rectal cancer: principles of management. In: *Maingot's abdominal operations,* Schwartz SI, ed. Norwalk, CT: Appleton & Lange; 1989:1107–17.

7. Kodner IJ, Fry RD, Fleshman JW. Current options in the management of rectal cancer. In: *Advances in surgery,* Cameron JL, ed. St. Louis: Mosby-Year Book; 1990:1–38.

8. Kodner IJ, Fry RD, Fleshman JW. Current options in the management of rectal cancer. *Adv Surg* 1991;24:1–39.

9. Kodner IJ, Fry RD, Fleshman JW. Management of colon and rectal tumors. In: *Current surgical therapy,* Cameron JL, ed. Philadelphia: BC Decker; 1992:191–203.

10. Kodner IJ, Shemesh EI, Fry RD, et al. Preoperative irradiation for rectal cancer. Improved local control and long-term survival. *Ann Surg* 1989;209:194–9.

11. Krook JE, Moertel CG, Gunderson LL, et al. Effective surgical adjuvant therapy for high-risk rectal carcinoma (see comments). *N Engl J Med* 1991;324:709–15.

12. Matthews JM, Kodner IJ, Fry RD, Fazio VW. Entrapped ovary syndrome. *Dis Colon Rectum* 1986;29:341–3.

13. Mendenhall WM, Million RR, Pfaff WW. Patterns of recurrence in adenocarcinoma of the rectum and rectosigmoid treated with surgery alone: implications in treatment planning with adjuvant radiation therapy. *Int J Radiat Oncol Biol Phys* 1983;9:977–85.

14. Moertel CG. Accomplishments in surgical adjuvant therapy for large bowel cancer. *Cancer* 1992;70(suppl):1364–71.

15. O'Connell MJ, Gunderson LL. Adjuvant therapy for adenocarcinoma of the rectum. *World J Surg* 1992;16:510–5.

16. Orkin BA, Dozois RR, Beart RWJ, et al. Extended resection for locally advanced primary adenocarcinoma of the rectum. *Dis Colon Rectum* 1989;32:286–92.

17. Patanaphan V, Salazar OM. Colorectal cancer: Metastatic patterns and prognosis. *South Med J* 1993;86:38–41.

18. Syzek EJ, Bogardus CR, Jr. High dose rate sources in remote afterloading brachytherapy: implications for intracavitary and interstitial treatment of carcinoma. *J Okla State Med Assoc* 1990;83:541–5.

19. Talbot IC, Ritchie S, Leighton M, et al. Invasion of veins by carcinoma of rectum: method of detection, histological features and significance. *Histopathology* 1981;5:141–63.

SECTION XI

Rectum

48

Stage II Rectal Carcinoma

Steven J. Stryker

The best chance to cure is at the initial treatment:
"good" surgery, "good" adjuvant chemoradiation

CASE PRESENTATION

The patient is a 49-year-old man referred for counseling and management of a recently diagnosed rectal carcinoma. The patient was in good overall health until 6 months before diagnosis, when he began to notice infrequent blood streaks on stool. This continued, and began to occur more frequently over the 6 to 8 weeks before diagnosis. In addition, the blood was more easily visible and now mixed with the stool, as well as streaking the surface. He denies any other change in his bowel habit. Specifically, he denies any alteration of stool frequency or consistency, any urgency, tenesmus, or any pain with defecation. In addition, he denies any symptoms of anorexia, fatigue, weight loss, or bone pain. He gives no history of other prior gastrointestinal neoplasia and no other chronic medical illnesses. He has never had any surgical procedures and is currently on no medication. Of interest, his family history is strongly positive for colorectal cancer. His father was diagnosed with colon cancer at age 60 years and his mother was diagnosed with colon cancer at age 72 years. His maternal grandmother also was diagnosed with colon cancer in her mid-70s.

The patient had recently undergone a colonoscopy at an outside hospital as the initial diagnostic procedure. A 4-mm sessile polyp at the cecum was removed completely by hot biopsy forceps and proved to be a tubular adenoma on histologic evaluation. A 2 × 3 cm polypoid lesion with central ulceration was located in the upper rectum. Multiple biopsies of this latter lesion showed a grade II infiltrating adenocarcinoma. A computed tomography (CT) examination of the abdomen and pelvis and a chest radiograph were also obtained and showed no evidence of

metastatic disease. The primary lesion was not well demonstrated on CT scan.

At the time of referral, no other pertinent history was obtained. Physical examination was unremarkable. Specifically, there was no evidence of lymphadenopathy, abdominal mass, or organomegaly. Digital rectal examination was unremarkable. Rigid proctosigmoidoscopy was performed and showed a 2 × 3 cm ulcerating tumor involving approximately one third of the rectal circumference and located from 11 cm to 13 cm above the anal verge. Our diagnosis at this time is a grade II adenocarcinoma of the upper to middle third of the rectum with no evidence of metastatic disease.

Would an endorectal ultrasound be useful to further stage this lesion before treatment planning? The management of rectal carcinoma has evolved over the past century to the current situation where many therapeutic options are available, depending on characteristics of both the patient and the lesion itself. One of the key determinants is the accurate preoperative assessment of tumor penetration. Although we personally have found endorectal ultrasound to be most useful in treatment planning for carcinoma in the distal rectum, its value in more proximal lesions is still being investigated. In this patient, we ordered an endorectal ultrasound.

As previously mentioned, the outside chest radiograph was unremarkable. The CT scan showed no evidence of extensive locoregional disease and no metastatic disease. The endorectal ultrasound is an excellent means of determining depth of invasion of rectal tumors. Although somewhat less reliable in assessing perirectal lymph nodes, its sensitivity and specificity of 80% to 90% is clearly superior to CT assessment of perirectal nodal involvement (1). This patient's endorectal ultrasound showed a 2.5-cm long tumor with invasion deep into the muscularis propria throughout most of the extent of the lesion (Fig. 48–1). In one area, however, disruption of the echogenic serosal layer was suspected. No hypoechoic or enlarged lymph nodes suspicious for metastases were seen. Therefore, our endorectal ultrasonographic stage is T3 N0.

Is there a role for preoperative (neoadjuvant) radiation therapy, with or without chemotherapy, in this patient? Neoadjuvant radiation therapy given preoperatively has been used with increasing frequency in the management of patients with rectal carcinoma. Appropriate doses of radiation before surgery reduces the number of viable cancer cells, theoretically decreasing the chance of tumor spill during manipulations associated with rectal cancer removal. Although numerous studies have demonstrated a downstaging of the tumor with preoperative radiation therapy to the pelvis, the oncologic benefit to the patient is not clearly defined for all clinical situations. Certainly, patients initially staged as T4 with tethering or fixation to the bony pelvis are often considered unresectable at presentation, but can be converted to resectable with preoperative radiation therapy. Another clinical scenario in which we have seen reason to radiate preoperatively is the patient with a bulky tumor in the distal rectum. Since routinely radiating such patients over the past 6 years, our incidence of positive surgical margins has decreased. Hopefully, this

will translate into better local control when adequate numbers of patients so treated are available for analysis. Decreased pelvic recurrence after preoperative radiation therapy has been demonstrated in a randomized study by the European Organization for Research and Treatment of Cancer (EORTC) (2). Finally, many of our patients have been able to undergo sphincter-preserving procedures after down-staging bulky distal tumors with preoperative radiation with combined chemotherapy (3).

With respect to the current patient under discussion, I don't feel that preoperative radiation therapy would be necessary. When we do employ preoperative radiation therapy, we typically combine this with radiosensitizing doses of 5-fluorouracil (5-FU) administered intravenously.

With a localized cancer well above the level of the anal sphincter, there is currently no role for preoperative radiation therapy. Local ablation of rectal cancer is appropriate in a highly select group of patients. The advantages include lower perioperative morbidity and improved functional outcome, compared with more radical procedures. Tumors selected for this approach are typically well differentiated, 3 cm or less in diameter, and readily accessible in the distal half of the rectum. When these selection criteria are followed, survival is comparable to more radical extirpation (4). Our preferred technique is transanal full-thickness excision, although contact radiotherapy, electrofulguration, and laser ablation have also been used successfully. The role of adjuvant radiation

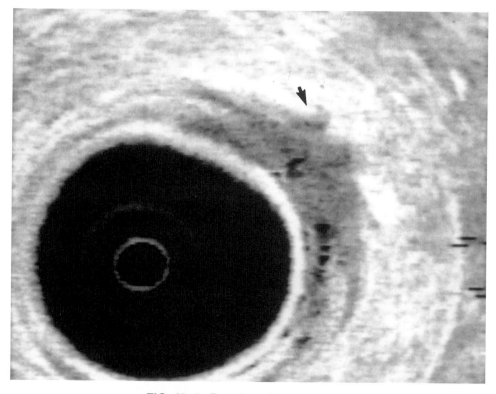

FIG. 48–1. Rectal carcinoma, stage II.

after transanal excision is currently being investigated. Although the patient under consideration has a tumor small enough to excise locally, the proximal location (distal margin 11 cm above anal verge) precludes conventional transanal excision. Newer instruments employing magnification optics (transanal endoscopic microsurgery, TEM) may be applicable, in the future, to lesions in this location (5).

An abdominal resectional approach is thus warranted in this patient. Because the tumor is located well proximal to the sphincter apparatus, a sphincter-saving approach is appropriate (low anterior resection or coloanal anastomosis). Nonetheless, certain oncologic principles must be strictly followed. A distal margin of at least 2 cm is required. A complete mesorectal excision has been shown to improve local control and usually can be accomplished with preservation of the autonomic nerves to the genitourinary system (6). Retrospective studies of extended lateral pelvic lymphadenectomy have failed to convincingly show benefit and are clearly associated with increased morbidity.

After a detailed discussion with this patient regarding treatment options and all pertinent perioperative risks, surgery was undertaken. Abdominal exploration revealed no evidence of metastatic disease. The tumor was readily palpated straddling the peritoneal reflection anteriorly at the midrectal level. The surface of the rectum was umbilicated by the tumor, but there was no visible extension to the free peritoneal surface. A nerve-sparing complete mesorectal excision and low anterior resection was performed, using a double-stapling technique flush with the puborectalis at the anorectal junction. The patient had an uneventful recovery and was discharged on the seventh postoperative day.

The specimen received consisted of a portion of colon and rectum measuring 26 cm in length. The intact specimen was inked circumferentially at the level of the palpated tumor. The opened specimen revealed a tumor measuring $2.4 \times 2.0 \times 0.5$ cm with central ulceration located 4 cm from the distal margin (Fig. 48–2).

Histologically, we observed a grade II adenocarcinoma extending through the muscularis propria into the perirectal fat (Fig. 48–3). The inked surgical margins circumferentially were all well clear of the lesion. The distal margin was separately examined and negative for involvement. Nine perirectal lymph nodes were identified and none showed metastatic disease.

This patient is considered stage II (T3 N0 M0). Is adjuvant chemotherapy and/or radiation therapy warranted? The inability to stage patients accurately with rectal cancer preoperatively has complicated prior attempts to select patients best suited for preoperative radiotherapy. In contrast, randomized prospective data exist, demonstrating the efficacy of adjuvant pelvic irradiation administered to T3 or N1-N2 (stage II or III) patients postoperatively. Until accurate preoperative staging techniques are more widely available, postoperative radiotherapy will continue to play a significant role in the treatment of rectal cancer.

A multicenter Danish study and the National Surgical Adjuvant Breast and Bowel Project (NSABP) both showed better local control for T3 or N1-N2 patients, but no survival advantage (7,8). The Gastrointestinal Tumor Study Group (GITSG) and, more recently, the North Central Cancer Treatment Group (NCCTG), showed survival advantage for these same T3 or N1-N2 rectal cancer patients receiving radiation therapy combined with 5-FU and methyl-CCNU (9,10). We would advise the patient

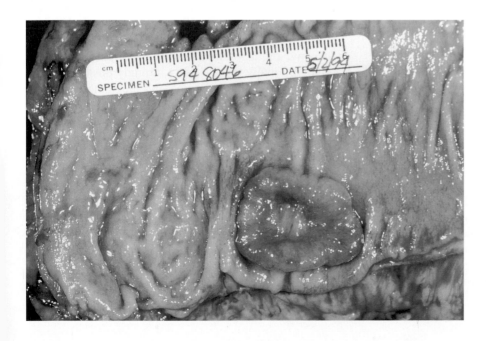

FIG. 48–2. Rectal adenocarcinoma.

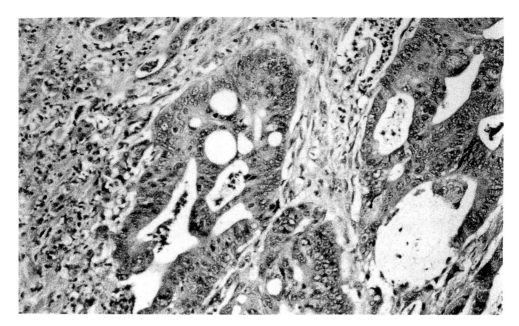

FIG. 48–3. Grade II adenocarcinoma.

being discussed (T3 N0 M0) to undergo 45 to 48 Gy pelvic radiation in 180-cGy fractions via three or four treatment ports to minimize irradiation of nearby viscera. We would like to initiate treatment within 35 days of surgery. And, finally, we would ask our medical oncology colleagues for their advice regarding chemotherapy.

A rationale for adjuvant chemotherapy relates to two distinct clinical settings. One is as a radiosensitizing agent in an individual who requires adjuvant radiation therapy. The other setting is when chemotherapy is administered to eliminate occult micrometastases in patients at high risk for subsequent clinical metastatic disease (N1). This latter indication for chemotherapy does not pertain to our current stage II patient (T3 N0 M0) and therefore will not be considered further.

If, indeed, this stage II lesion is rectal rather than colonic, I would certainly agree with pelvic radiotherapy combined with chemotherapy (9,10). I ask that this site of origin be clarified because many of the studies cited define the proximal rectal margin as being at the level of the peritoneal reflection.

The distal margin of the tumor was below the peritoneal reflection. Therefore, this malignancy should be classified as rectal in location.

Two adjuvant treatment options would be presented to this patient. First, the option of participating in a phase III clinical trial for stage II rectal cancer would be presented. Our institution is currently participating in ECOG trials, of which this patient would be eligible (e.g., ECOG 59304). If the patient refused a randomized trial or were ineligible for these trials, treatment with 5-FU (500 mg/m^2 per day, days 1–5, 29–33), along with pelvic radio-

therapy, would be offered. In consultation with the patient and his wife, he elected to enter ECOG 59304 and received preradiation, concomitant, and postradiation continuous infusion 5-FU.

The patient was evaluated with physical examination and proctoscopy 30 days postradiation and just before starting his last course of continuous infusion chemotherapy. He is working full-time and feeling well. He has two to four bowel movements each day with normal continence and only rare fecal urgency. Voiding and sexual function are normal. Examination of peripheral lymph nodes and his abdomen were both within normal limits. Proctoscopy to 15 cm showed no residual radiation proctitis and a normal-appearing anastomosis 5 cm above the anal verge.

He will be followed with physical examination, endoscopy, and laboratory studies as per protocol (every 4 months). Finally, because of a strongly positive family history of colorectal carcinoma and the somewhat early onset of this patient's malignancy, his four siblings and one child will be advised to undergo stool testing for occult blood and screening colonoscopy at regular intervals beginning somewhere around age 35 or 40 years.

REFERENCES

1. Wong WD, Orrom WJ, Jensen LL. Preoperative staging of rectal cancer with endorectal ultrasonography. *Perspect Colon Rectal Surg* 1990;3:315–34.
2. Gerard A, Buyse M, Nordlinger B, et al. Preoperative radiotherapy as adjuvant treatment in rectal cancer. *Ann Surg* 1988;208:606–14.
3. Stryker SJ, Kiel KD, Rademaker A, et al. Preoperative "chemoradiation" for stages II and III rectal carcinoma. *Arch Surg* 1996;131:514–9.
4. Biggers OR, Beart RW Jr, Ilstrup DM. Local excision of rectal cancer. *Dis Colon Rectum* 1985;29:374–7.

5. Buess G, Mentges B, Mawhecke K, et al. Minimal invasive surgery in the local treatment of rectal cancer. *Int J Colorect Dis* 1991;6:77–81.

6. Karanjia ND, Schache DJ, North WRS, Heald RJ. The close shave in anterior resection. *Br J Surg* 1990;77:510–2.

7. Balslev I, Pedersen M, Teglbjaerg PS, et al. Postoperative radiotherapy in Dukes B and C carcinoma of the rectum and rectosigmoid. A randomized multicenter study. *Cancer* 1986;58:22–8.

8. Fisher B, Wolmark N, Rockette H, et al. Postoperative adjuvant chemotherapy or radiation therapy for rectal cancer: results from NSABP Protocol R-01. *J Natl Cancer Inst* 1988;80:21–9.

9. Gastrointestinal Tumor Study Group. Prolongation of the disease free interval in surgically treated rectal carcinoma. *N Engl J Med* 1985; 312:1465–72.

10. Krook J, Moertel C, Gunderson L, et al. Effective surgical adjuvant therapy for high-risk rectal carcinoma. *N Engl J Med* 1991;324: 709–15.

COMMENTARY by Glenn D. Steele, Jr.

The case of this young patient was presented and discussed in such an optimal fashion that little is left to say in my commentary. I have no disagreements with the thinking on adjuvant chemotherapy and with the thinking on adjuvant radiation therapy. The only addition would be to mention that perhaps within the next few years application of blood testing for either germ-line or somatic mutations known to be associated not only with familial adenomatosis polyposis but with variations might explain inherited susceptibility such as this family represents. Molecular genetic analysis could supply an alternative in diagnostic screening to what currently is the correct recommendation but still somewhat empiric colonoscopic examination of first degree relatives at a relatively early age (somewhere between 30 and 40 years of age even if asymptomatic). Furthermore, the applicability of various sampling techniques to stool in "sentinel" patients such as this man could give us a more cost-effective option in following what obviously is a quite high risk for metachronous premalignant or malignant changes in the residual large bowel mucosa.

49

An Unresectable Cancer of the Rectum Without Demonstrable Distant Metastases

Paul H. O'Brien, John S. Metcalf, and Stephen I. Schabel

*"Unresectable" rectal cancer can be effectively palliated
and sometimes cured*

CASE PRESENTATION

The patient was a 65-year-old white man who came to the Medical University of South Carolina after noting a change in bowel habit with intermittent gross rectal bleeding over the previous 6 months. He became concerned when during the past month he had the feeling of incomplete evacuation. There was no associated weight loss or anorexia. On physical examination the patient, 5'11" and 200 lbs., had no family history of colorectal cancer or familial polyposis syndromes.

The most significant finding, on rectal examination, was a hard, fixed 6-cm mass that could be palpated and was attached to the posterior and left pelvic wall. The mass was not mobile by the initial and subsequent examiners. A flexible sigmoidoscopy revealed the cancer to be 7 cm in its greatest diameter and to encircle almost the entire rectum. Biopsies revealed moderately well-differentiated adenocarcinoma. A colonoscopy was performed; two small, less than 1-cm polyps were noted in the transverse colon. A CEA level was drawn, which subsequently came back 9 ng/mL. Normal levels in our laboratory are 1 to 5 ng/mL. A computed tomography (CT) scan of the upper abdomen to study the liver was completed without evidence of metastases, as indeed was a CT scan of the chest, which was free of metastases.

Pathology revealed a moderately differentiated mucinous adenocarcinoma invading into the muscularis propria. The intramucosal component of this tumor consisted of crowded, abnormally branched glands lined by columnar epithelial cells, the nuclei of which were stratified. When compared with the adjacent normal rectal mucosa, the population of goblet cells within the tumor is markedly diminished (Fig. 49–1). However, the invasive component assumes a different growth pattern with large pools of mucin-containing strips of neoplastic glandular epithelium, glandular structures, and small cell clusters (Fig. 49–2).

The inferior margin of the carcinoma was felt to be 5 cm from the anal sphincter. In our institution, when a cancer of the rectum is of this magnitude and is felt to be firmly fixed to the lateral and posterior pelvic wall, primary resection is not attempted.

This lateral film of a full column barium enema (Fig. 49–3) showed a long irregular stricture of the rectum narrowing the lumen of the rectum to only a few millimeters in a circumferential fashion. There is a wide space between the rectum and the sacrum. Even though no bony destruction is apparent on the plain films, a tumor of this size clinically likely has deeply invaded adjacent perirectal tissues. Both CT and magnetic resonance scanning are useful modalities in evaluating the extent of perirectal invasion, particularly in rectal cancers.

Radiation Therapy felt this patient was a good candidate for radiation treatment with 4,000 to 5,000 cGy with 5-fluorouracil (5-FU) given at a dosage of 15 mg/kg dur-

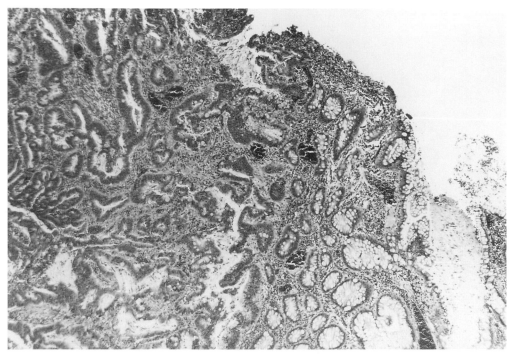

FIG. 49–1. An histologic section showing a markedly diminished population of goblet cells within the tumor.

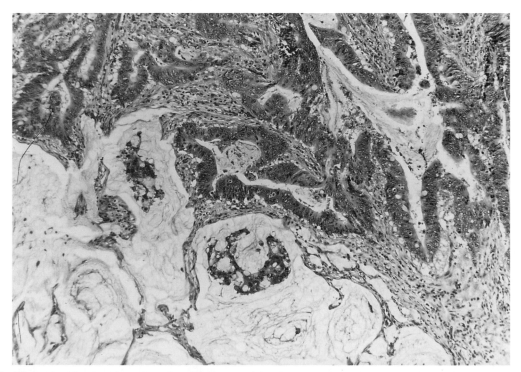

FIG. 49–2. An histologic section showing large pools of mucin-containing strips of neoplastic glandular epithelium, glandular structures, and small cell clusters.

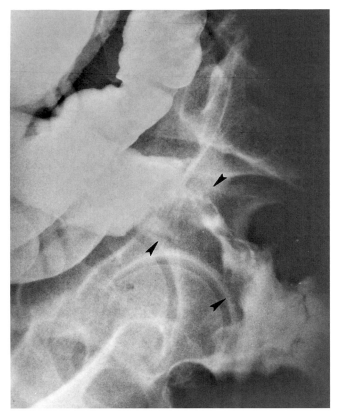

FIG. 49–3. This lateral film of a full column barium enema shows a long irregular stricture of the rectum *(arrows)* narrowing the lumen of the rectum to only a few millimeters in a circumferential fashion.

ing the first 3 days of treatment. This was acceptable to Medical Oncology. The final dose to be given to the patient was 4,500 cGy. During the second week of radiation therapy our patient's rectal discomfort and bleeding became worse. This was assumed to be proctitis complicated by the fecal stream. A sigmoid end colostomy and mucus fistula were generated surgically, which provided relief to the patient and permitted the continuation of the radiation therapy. An intestinal sling of Dexon mesh was placed to minimize radiation insult to the small bowel at the time of surgery.

Two weeks after termination of the radiation therapy, the patient was taken to the operating room and examined under anesthesia. There was a 50% reduction in the gross size of the tumor; however, the tumor remained firmly adherent to the posterior and lateral wall of the pelvis. The CEA level was 7 ng/mL.

At tumor conference a review of composite resections of posterior pelvic malignancies was discussed. The procedure was felt to be too extensive, and the resources for performing this procedure with an acceptable operative mortality and morbidity were not available. The patient was followed. He proceeded to do well for 19 months and then he began to lose his appetite, lose weight, and multi-

ple densities were noted in his liver on CT scan. The patient died 19 months postinitiation of palliative radiation therapy and chemotherapy. The patient did not develop severe pelvic pain during his terminal days.

COMMENTARY by Leonard L. Gunderson

The case for discussion was presented as an unresectable cancer of the rectum without demonstrable distant metastases. Although the patient's lesion appeared to be locally unresectable for cure by physical examination, both before and after pelvic irradiation plus 5-FU, on neither occasion was a pelvic plus low abdominal CT mentioned as a component of the workup. In a male patient, large lesions can appear immobile because of bulk and the limitation of an exam restricted to a single orifice (as opposed to the advantage of bimanual exam in female patients). Pelvic CT can confirm clinical fixation by demonstrating lack of a free space or fat plane between the lesion and the pelvic sidewall or presacrum. If a free space exists, then gross total resection of a primary lesion is probably feasible after preoperative irradiation plus chemotherapy despite apparent clinical fixation. The abdominal CT should not be restricted to the liver because the lower abdomen can be evaluated to rule out extensive nodal involvement along the course of the inferior mesenteric vessels or in the para-aortic region. A CT scan of the liver can be falsely negative in 10% to 15% of cases, so we also obtain liver function studies as a component of the workup. If either the alkaline phosphatase or lactic dehydrogenase (LDH) value is moderately elevated, we would obtain a second diagnostic imaging study of the liver before considering resection after preoperative irradiation.

Irradiation treatment factors are uncertain in this patient because the authors did not discuss dose per fraction, time factors, or field parameters (? entire true pelvis vs. tumor plus 2 cm, etc). We are left to assume the patient received 45 Gy in 25 fractions of 1.8 Gy. The duration of treatment interruption due to the temporary diverting colostomy is not mentioned. Was the 45 Gy delivered over 4, 6, 7, or 8 weeks? (This has implications with regard to treatment impact on tumor.) The placement of Dexon mesh at the time of colostomy was probably unnecessary for the adjuvant irradiation dose levels used in this patient and others with primary as opposed to recurrent lesions. However, this maneuver would have allowed delivery of an additional 15 to 20 cGy in 1.8- to 2.0-cGy fractions after the surgeons elected not to attempt resection, because dose limiting small bowel was now clearly outside the pelvis (i.e., achieve a total dose of 60 to 65 Gy within a reduced field).

In our institution, this patient would have been explored 3 to 5 weeks after completion of preoperative irradiation (45–54 Gy in 1.8-Gy fractions) plus 5-FU (plus leucovorin) if the additional studies we would have obtained at time of restaging demonstrated no evidence of extrapelvic disease. Although a repeat pelvic CT would have been part of the evaluation, lack of free space would not have negated an exploration and an attempt at gross total resection. This exploration would have been performed in a special operating room that contains a linear accelerator with electron capabilities. After resection, additional irradiation could then be given to the site of the initial fixation (positive or narrow margins pathologically) with intraoperative electrons via special lucite cylinders or by placement of hollow close-ended tubes for afterloading with Ir192. In this manner, pelvic control could be maximized with the inherent chance of decreasing the risk of distant metastases and improving survival. Node-positive patients are increasingly being considered for 6 to 12 months of postresection chemotherapy with 5-FU plus leucovorin or levamisole.

DISCUSSION OF PERTINENT LITERATURE

When external irradiation alone or in combination with immunotherapy or chemotherapy is used for patients with locally advanced colorectal cancers, local progression occurs in more than 90% of patients (1,2) and long-term survival is infrequent (2% 5-year survival in the PMH series). A randomized Mayo Clinic study suggested that 5-FU increased the benefit of irradiation with regard to median survival and relief of symptoms (3).

With lesions that are initially unresectable for cure because of disease fixation to surgically unresectable structures, cures have been obtained by combining moderate-dose preoperative irradiation with later resection (45–50 Gy in 1.8- to 2.0-Gy fractions over 4½–5 weeks). Survival results are not consistently better than irradiation alone, although local control is better (4–7). The incidence of pelvic relapse in patients resected after preoperative irradiation ranges from 36% to 76%. If the tumor is initially fixed to an unresectable structure (presacrum, pelvic sidewall), although 45 to 50 Gy may shrink tumor to the degree that a later resection is feasible in 50% to 90% of patients, viable cells may persist at the margins of initial adherence even if the pathologist has not identified positive margins.

If maximal resection is performed before external irradiation, local control and survival appear to correlate with the amount of residual disease (microscopic residual after gross total resection vs. gross residual after subtotal resection). In three published series (8–10), the local recurrence risk with gross residual was 50%, 52%, and 86% versus 15%, 30%, and 70% with microscopic residual (in the latter series [10], all patients had pathologic confirmation of positive resection margins).

When intraoperative irradiation (IORT) with electrons is combined with conventional treatment for locally advanced primary colorectal cancers, separate analyses

from Massachusetts General Hospital and Mayo Clinic suggest an improvement in both local control and survival (11–14). In an early Massachusetts General Hospital series, disease relapse within irradiation fields was 43% versus 0% for 17 non-IORT versus 16 IORT patients and 1- and 2-year survival was statistically better with IORT (11). An updated Massachusetts General Hospital analysis reports actuarial 5-year survival of 43% in 42 IORT patients (12). In a Mayo comparison of 17 non-IORT and 20 IORT patients, local control was 24% versus 80%, median survival 18 versus 37 months, and 3-year survival 24% versus 50% (13,14). The preferred sequencing of modalities in IORT-containing regimens is usually preoperative external irradiation plus chemotherapy followed by maximal resection and IORT (14,15). Several analyses have shown the advantage of achieving a gross total resection whenever such is safely feasible, even when IORT is a component of treatment (12,16).

Because systemic risks are also high with locally advanced colorectal cancers, the addition of chemotherapy to irradiation and resection has rationale. Randomized trials for metastatic colorectal cancer have demonstrated an advantage of 5-FU plus leucovorin over 5-FU alone with regard to median survival. Pilot trials have also demonstrated that the two-drug combination can be combined with irradiation with acceptable tolerance, thus starting effective local and systemic treatment simultaneously (17–19). Preliminary analyses combining 5-FU plus leucovorin with preoperative irradiation for fixed rectal lesions suggest a potential increase in resectability and complete pathologic response rates when compared with preoperative irradiation alone (17,18). The combination of preoperative irradiation plus chemotherapy (+ or ± IORT) could therefore potentially lead to improvements in the local and distant control as well as survival of locally advanced lesions as seen in adjuvant rectal postoperative studies (20–22).

REFERENCES

1. Cummings BJ, Rider WD, Harwood AR, et al. External beam radiation therapy for adenocarcinoma of the rectum. *Dis Colon Rectum* 1983;26:30.
2. O'Connell MJ, Childs DS, Moertel CG, et al. A prospective controlled evaluation of combined pelvic radiotherapy and methanol extraction residue of BCG (MER) for locally unresectable or recurrent rectal carcinoma. *Int J Radiat Oncol Biol Phys* 1982;8:1115.
3. Moertel CG, Childs DS, Reitemeier RJ, et al. Combined 5-fluorouracil and supervoltage radiation therapy of locally unresectable gastrointestinal cancer. *Lancet* 1969;2:865.
4. Stevens KR, Allen CV, Fletcher WS. Preoperative radiotherapy for adenocarcinoma of the rectosigmoid. *Cancer* 1976;37:2866.
5. Emami B, Pilepich M, Willet C, et al. Management of unresectable colorectal carcinoma (preoperative radiotherapy and surgery). *Int J Radiat Oncol Biol Phys* 1982;8:1295.
6. Dosoretz DE, Gunderson LL, Hoskins B, et al. Preoperative irradiation for unresectable rectal and rectosigmoidal carcinomas. *Cancer* 1983;52:814.

7. Mendenhall WM, Bland KI, Pfaff WW, et al. Initially unresectable rectal adenocarcinoma treated with preoperative irradiation and surgery. *Ann Surg* 1987;205:41.

8. Allee PE, Tepper JE, Gunderson LL, Munzenrider JE. Postoperative radiation therapy for incompletely resected colorectal carcinoma. *Int J Radiat Oncol Biol Phys* 1989;17:1171.

9. Ghossein NA, Samala EC, Alpert S, et al. Elective postoperative radiotherapy after incomplete resection of colorectal cancer. *Dis Colon Rectum* 1981;24:252.

10. Schild SE, Martenson JA, Gunderson LL, Dozois RR. Long-term survival and patterns of failure after postoperative radiation therapy for subtotally resected rectal adenocarcinoma. *Int J Radiat Oncol Biol Phys* 1989;16:459.

11. Gunderson LL, Cohen AM, Dosoretz DE, et al. Residual, unresectable or recurrent colorectal cancer: external beam irradiation and intraoperative electron beam boost + resection. *Int J Radiat Oncol Biol Phys* 1983;9:1597.

12. Willett CG, Shellito PC, Tepper JE, et al. Intraoperative electron beam radiation therapy for primary locally advanced rectal and rectosigmoid carcinoma. *J Clin Oncol* 1991;9:893.

13. Gunderson LL, Martin JK, Beart RW, et al. External beam and intraoperative electron irradiation for locally advanced colorectal cancer. *Ann Surg* 1988;207:52.

14. Gunderson LL, Dozois RR. Intraoperative irradiation for locally advanced colorectal carcinomas. *Perspect Colon Rect Surg* 1992;5:1.

15. Gunderson LL, Suzuki K, Devine RM, et al. IORT for locally advanced colorectal cancers—results and sequencing issues. *Proc 4th Int Symp IORT* Verlag Die Blaue Eule 1993;365.

16. Kramer T, Share R, Kiel K, Roseman D. Intraoperative radiation therapy of colorectal cancer. In: *Intraoperative radiation therapy*, Abe M, ed. New York: Pergamon Press; 1991;310.

17. Minsky BD, Cohen AM, Kemeny N, et al. Enhancement of radiation induced downstaging of rectal cancers by fluorouracil and high dose leucovorin chemotherapy. *J Clin Oncol* 1992;10:79.

18. Bosset JF, Pavy JJ, Hamers HP, et al. Determination of the optimal dose of 5-fluorouracil when combined with low dose d, l-leucovorin and irradiation in rectal cancer: results of three consecutive phase II studies. *Eur J Cancer* (in press).

19. Moertel CG, Gunderson LL, Mailliard JA, et al. Early evaluation of 5FU plus leucovorin (CF) as a radiation enhancer for locally unresectable, residual or recurrent gastrointestinal cancer. *J Clin Oncol* 1994;12:21.

20. Gastrointestinal Tumor Study Group. Prolongation of the disease-free interval in surgically resected rectal cancer. *N Engl J Med* 1985;312:1465.

21. Gastrointestinal Tumor Study Group. Survival after postoperative combination treatment of rectal cancer. *N Engl J Med* 1986;315:1294.

22. Krook JE, Moertel CG, Gunderson LL, et al. Effective surgical adjuavnt therapy for high risk rectal carcinoma. *N Engl J Med* 1991;324:709.

50 Rectal Adenocarcinoma

Robert W. Beart, Jr.

Do not sacrifice the chance for cure to save the sphincter

CASE PRESENTATION

This is a 56-year-old black man who presented with a 2-month history of intermittent bright red blood per rectum. He has noticed no significant change otherwise in bowel habits. He has had no history of prolapsing hemorrhoids or anal pain. He denies diarrhea or constipation. Otherwise, he has continued his active work as a computer operator and feels well. The remainder of his history was noncontributory.

The physical examination reveals a well-developed black man, appearing his stated age. No supraclavicular nodes were felt. His chest is clear to auscultation and percussion. The abdomen is soft and nontender without organomegaly. On digital rectal exam, he has a mass anteriorly that is not ulcerated or hard, the lower border of which begins below the level of the prostate gland anteriorly and extends about 4 cm proximal and is about 2 cm wide.

Proctoscopic examination identified a mass beginning at 7 cm above the verge anteriorly, extending for 4 cm and about 2 cm wide. The exam was otherwise negative.

A barium enema, chest roentgenogram, and electrocardiogram were normal. The hematocrit was 13.5 and WBC was 10,000. Stool for occult blood was positive.

TUMOR BOARD DISCUSSION

Radiation oncology: If a biopsy of this lesion proves to be a carcinoma, then preoperative radiation therapy should be considered. There is some evidence to suggest that this will help decrease postoperative recurrences. This is anecdotal, and there are no randomized prospec-

tive studies to support this position, but this therapy has gained some popularity.

Medical oncology: The patient at this point is not a candidate for additional chemotherapy. If he is judged to be a candidate for preoperative radiation, chemotherapy will add to the effectiveness of the radiation therapy. A combination of 5-fluorouracil (5-FU) and perhaps mitomycin or other chemotherapy may be considered. An ultrasound of the rectum may help with additional staging information.

Surgeon: This patient is a potential candidate for sphincter preservation. Staging information that should be obtained preoperatively includes a computed tomography (CT) scan of the abdomen and pelvis with contrast, flow cytometry, carcinoembryonic antigen, a biopsy, and transrectal ultrasound. If the tumor is well differentiated, no deeper than T2, and N0 based on ultrasound and CT scan, with a diploid flow cytometric pattern, then local excision is the procedure of choice. If, however, the tumor shows aneuploid or poorly differentiated features, then a lymphadenectomy needs to be carried out. A tumor that extends below the prostate gland, despite the fact that it is 7 cm above the anal verge, may require an abdominoperineal resection. Proctoscopic distance measurements can be misleading. A better guide to possibilities of resection are the anatomic relationships of the tumor. If the tumor is above the level of the prostate gland and not in continuity with the puborectalis muscle posteriorly, then excision by low anterior coloanal techniques is feasible. Lymphadenectomy will be comparable to that performed with an abdominoperineal resection. If, however, the tumor impinges on the puborectalis muscle or is below the level of the prostate gland, then it is difficult to do a wide resection and restore intestinal continuity. In that situation, an abdominoperineal resection will likely be necessary.

As requested at the Tumor Board, an ultrasound was done and showed the tumor to penetrate through the muscle wall, but without evidence of lymph node involvement. The CT scan demonstrated no lymph node involvement, CEA was 3.6, and flow cytometry was not available on the tumor. The tumor was a grade 2 adenocarcinoma on biopsy. Based on this information, a local excision was carried out. The pathology of the tumor demonstrated complete excision, but venous and lymphatic invasion were evident. Internal Medicine had little to add to the workup at this point. This is an unfavorable prognostic indicator and puts the patient at an increased risk for local and distal metastasis. Additional surgery should be considered.

If, however, the patient refuses additional surgery, which likely will require colostomy, then adjuvant radiation therapy should be considered. There is ample evidence to suggest that cure rates can be improved with this technique. Approximately 5,000 cGy should be given.

Chemotherapy should be given in addition to radiation therapy. Consideration should be given to long-term adjuvant therapy, much like we do for colon cancer, because these patients are at high risk to fail distantly.

It is the surgical department's recommendation that this patient have a lymphadenectomy, which likely will require an abdominal perineal resection. We agree with the radiation therapist that if the patient refuses this recommendation, then adjuvant radiation therapy should be offered as a second line of treatment. We agree that this should be combined with chemotherapy, and consideration should be given to a long-term chemotherapy regimen, because the patient is at high risk for distant recurrence.

COMMENTARY by Glenn D. Steele, Jr.

The nub of this case is the location and extent of the distal rectal adenocarcinoma. Undoubtedly, the correct recommendation for this patient is an abdominoperineal resection. This could have been done before an attempt at local excision because there was essentially no co-morbidity obviating the benefit of a full celeotomy. Only with tumors of smaller diameter have any institutional or multi-institutional studies shown benefit for local excision approaches to sphincter preservation. National trials are still under analysis in defining whether complete local excision (with sphincter preservation) combined with chemoradiation for T2 or early T3 lesions are, in fact, equivalent to abdominoperineal resection. For this patient, only if co-morbidity had been severe would a compromise with abdominoperineal resection be justifiable. And such compromise could create a situation that eventuates in regional disease recurrence, which for patients with rectal carcinoma represents a disastrous way of dying. Whether this particular patient has had compromise of his chance for cure because of the initial attempt at local excision after which presumably he will have an abdominoperineal resection, is an important but unanswerable question.

All the comments concerning preoperative radiation or chemoradiation in downsizing tumor are appropriate, but speculative. The real question is whether such downsizing of the tumor or downstaging of the tumor stage has any effect on increasing cure. No such proof is available from any institutional or multi-institutional trials. The present NSABP RO2 trial asking a similar question is presently accruing patients. A slightly different intergroup national trial is just now getting underway and answers concerning preoperative chemoradiation versus postoperative will not be in for a number of years.

SELECTED READINGS

1. Beynon J, Mortenson N, Rigby H. Rectal endosconography, a new technique for the preoperative staging of rectal carcinoma. *Eur J Surg Oncol* 1988;14:297–309.
2. Ellis L, Mendenhall W, Bland K. Local excision and radiation therapy for early rectal cancer. *Am Surg* 1988;54:217–20.
3. Coco C, Magistrelli P, Granone P, et al. Conservative surgery for early cancer of the distal rectum. *Dis Colon Rectum* 1992;35:131–6.
4. Moertel CG. Accomplishments in surgical adjuvant therapy for large bowel cancer. *Cancer* 1992;70:1364–71.
5. Krook J, Moertel C, Gunderson L. Effective surgical adjuvant therapy for high risk rectal carcinoma. *N Engl J Med* 1991;324:709–15.
6. Graham R, Garnsey L, Jessup J. Local excision of rectal carcinoma. *Am J Surg* 1991;160:306–12.
7. Biggers OR, Beart RW Jr, Ilstrup DM. Local excision of rectal cancer. *Dis Colon Rectum* 1986;29:374–7.

51

A Patient with Refractory Perineal/Pelvic Pain, Postabdominal Perineal Resection, Radiotherapy, and Chemotherapy

Harold J. Wanebo

Any treatment that will prevent or delay regional growth of advanced rectal cancer is of extreme benefit even if cure is rare

CASE PRESENTATION

A 53-year-old man presented to his primary care physician with blood in his stools and was found to have a rectal mass, which was also shown by barium enema. A colonoscopy confirmed a large mass of the rectum 10 cm from the anal verge. The remaining colon was free of disease. His chemistry profile was within normal limits. Magnetic resonance imaging (MRI) and computed tomography (CT) scan of the abdomen and pelvis did not reveal any metastatic disease. Preoperative carcinoembryonic antigen (CEA) was within normal limits. He underwent a low anterior resection with a primary anastomosis using the EEA stapler on April 7, 1987.

Pathologic examination revealed a moderately well-differentiated adenocarcinoma extending to the muscularis propria and into the subserosa; 12 lymph nodes were free of disease. The 10-cm proximal and 3-cm distal margins were reported to be clear. The intraoperative course was reported to be uneventful. However, on postoperative day 2 he started to have a low urine output, left lower quadrant pain, and fever. A CT scan of the pelvis showed a left lower quadrant collection (that was drained); he also was found to have a high creatinine and urea nitrogen

content. A urology consult was obtained. An intravenous pyelogram was performed and a small left ureteral leak identified. A left percutaneous nephrostomy tube was inserted and intravenous antibiotics were started. The patient did well and was discharged to home. He was readmitted electively 3 months later and taken to the operating room for exploration of the left ureter; a distal stricture was seen and he had a ureteral reimplantation. Since then, he was followed up by history and physical exam (including a digital rectal exam, stool guaiac testing, and serum CEA levels at 3-month intervals). A postoperative baseline CT scan of the abdomen and pelvis was obtained 2 months after the initial colectomy. He also had yearly colonoscopies and CT scans of the abdomen and pelvis and biyearly chest films.

In the summer of 1989, the patient complained of poorly defined nonradiating perineal and buttock pain. A CT scan of the pelvis revealed a 5 × 5 cm presacral mass with possible invasion of the bladder wall (Figs. 51–1, 51–2) Serum CEA was still within normal limits. Digital rectal exam showed a friable mass at the anastomosis, which was confirmed by colonoscopy. A CT scan of the chest was normal. A CT-guided biopsy of the presacral mass revealed adenocarcinoma. Bone scan was negative

251

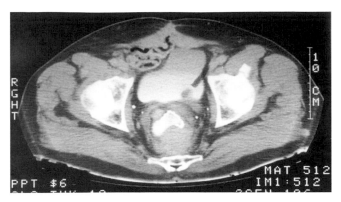

FIG. 51–1. CT scan of the pelvis showed a large presacral mass with extension to the posterior surface of the prostate and bladder. This was biopsied, showing an adenocarcinoma.

and cytoscopy revealed involvement of the posterior wall of the bladder. The patient was seen by medical and radiation oncology, and was presented to the Tumor Board.

TUMOR BOARD DISCUSSION

This is a patient who had a previous primary resection of a rectal cancer that was well differentiated and extended through the muscular coat, essentially a B2 cancer, but with negative nodes and adequate margins including a 3-cm distal margin. A decision was made at that time that the distal margin was adequate (these margins are now considered to be adequate and one does not need to obtain a 5-cm margin, as the results from even a 2-cm margin are considered adequate in most cases). The question of adjuvant therapy apparently was decided against, although some might consider adjuvant therapy for a B2 cancer of the rectum because there is still a 30% failure rate in some series. Although a major concern is with the Dukes C patients having nodal metastases, there is also concern about patients with Dukes B for local failure and there is consensus among many surgeons that postoperative chemoradiation for this group may be of benefit as well.

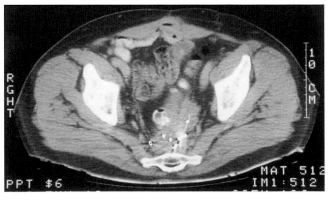

FIG. 51–2. CT scan in midpelvis, just below the level of the sciatic notch, showing a large presacral recurrence with prominent extension into the left side of the pelvis.

The patient had essentially done well and remained free of tumor for approximately 2 years except for the ureteral stricture problem, but the development of pain heralded a recurrence in early 1989, prompting workup that demonstrated an apparent suture line recurrence, which on CT was an obvious pelvic recurrence manifesting itself at the anastomotic line. At this point, the question of adding radiation and chemotherapy was discussed. It was pointed out that if the patient's tumor could not be re-resected, then perhaps palliative radiation and chemotherapy could be given. In the event that the tumor could be re-resected, then perhaps preoperative chemotherapy and radiation could be given followed by resection and adjuvant therapy. It was elected, therefore, to give this patient preoperative therapy and to re-evaluate and attempt an exenteration by abdominal sacral resection.

He received approximately 4,500 cGy of external beam radiation to the pelvis with chemosensitization (5-fluorouracil [5-FU] and cisplatin) over a 5-week period. He had some diarrhea and 5-pound weight loss that he regained. He was explored 4 weeks after completion of radiation therapy. He was found to have a large presacral mass originating from the rectum and involving the posterior wall of the bladder and sacrum. He underwent removal of the bladder, rectum, anus, and sacrum with creation of a permanent end sigmoid colostomy and bilateral ureteral insertion into a ileal pouch. The sacral resection was performed through the S1-S2 level. A pelvic node dissection was performed. Pathologic exam showed the presence of a large tumor involving the posterior wall of the bladder with extension into the sacrum. Histologic exam showed viable adenocarcinoma with invasion of the periosteum, but not into the bone of the sacrum. All the gross and microscopic margins of the tumor mass were clear of tumor. The nodes from the bilateral pelvic node dissection were negative for metastases. His postoperative course was uneventful except for weakness of left plantar flexion that improved on physical therapy.

Postoperatively, he was started on chemotherapy with 5-FU and leucovorin that he tolerated well. He was followed up at 3-month intervals with history, physical examination, and serum CEA; a CT scan of the abdomen and pelvis, and colonoscopy were performed every year. A delayed complication in the form of a stricture at the L ureter ileal junction developed 2 years later. This responded to an initial decompression by a PCN tube and the stricture was successfully dilated by percutaneous balloon ureteroplasty. The patient has been doing well since then. There is no evidence of disease 6 years since his initial colectomy and 4 years since his abdominal sacral resection.

COMMENTARY by Bernard Levin

The recurrence of a rectal cancer is a devastating event and special attention must be focused on symptoms, especially pain control. In the initial evaluation of a patient with pelvic recurrence after curative resection of rectal cancer, it is important to exclude widespread metastases in the abdomen and chest by CT scan if extensive surgical intervention is contemplated. Subsequently, as was done in this case, a multidisciplinary strategy must be constructed that will usually involve the radiation oncologist, surgical oncologist, and medical oncologist. Other members of the team may include a enterostromal therapist, especially as in this case where both an end colostomy and an ileal conduit have to be appropriately placed.

Chemoradiation therapy usually involving 5-FU with or without leucovorin, sometimes in combination with cisplatin, is being increasingly used. With radiation therapy alone, 80% to 90% of patients experience initial pain relief (1), but additional therapies are needed to achieve long-term benefit. Surgical resection and brachytherapy or intraoperative electron beam therapy are being increasingly used (2).

REFERENCES

1. Pacini P, Cionini L, Pirtoli L, et al. Symptomatic recurrence of carcinoma of the rectum and sigmoid: the influence of radiotherapy on the quality of life. *Dis Colon Rectum* 1986;29:865–8.
2. Kaufman N, Nori D, Shank B, et al. Remote after loading intraluminal brachytherapy in the treatment of rectal, rectosigmoid and anal cancer: a feasibility study. *Int J Radiol Oncol Biol Phys* 1989;7:663–8.

52

Rectal Carcinoma with Pulmonary Metastases

M. Margaret Kemeny

Surgery for primary and metastatic disease: When?
Systemic therapy: Why?

CASE PRESENTATION

A 68-year-old man began to note rectal bleeding. A workup for this problem led to a colonoscopy. On this examination a sessile lesion was seen in the rectum 6 cm from the anal verge. A biopsy revealed carcinoma, and an abdominal perineal resection was recommended. The patient refused this option. The patient had no history of loss of appetite, weight loss, cough, abdominal pain, or change in bowel habits.

Computed tomography (CT) scan of the abdomen and pelvis was normal. The patient's past medical history included adult-onset diabetes mellitus. He followed his blood glucose levels at home with a glucometer and took Micronase (2.5 mg) daily. Other medical problems included glaucoma, treated with Timoptic drops daily. The rest of his history was unremarkable. He had no history of prior operations or hospital admissions. There was no family history of cancer.

He was a retired aircraft designer. He used alcohol socially. He smoked up until 1967, but did not smoke at all after that time.

He underwent a transanal excision of the rectal lesion. Pathology revealed a cancer in a villous adenoma that infiltrated the mucosa and the muscularis propria but did not completely penetrate through the rectal wall. The tumor was a moderately differentiated adenocarcinoma with no evidence of vascular or lymphatic invasion (Fig. 52–1). The margins of the resected specimen were negative for tumor. Laboratory studies at the time included white blood count $8.3 \times 10^3/\mu L$, hematocrit 43.3%, hemoglobin 14.8 g/dL, platelets $298 \times 10^3/\mu L$, and creatinine 1.1 mg/dL. His electrolytes were all within normal limits. Serum alkaline phosphatase was 67 U/L (nl 36–137), LDH 143 U/L (nl 103–269), and carcinoembryonic antigen (CEA) 3.0 ng/mL. The postoperative course after the resection was uneventful. A subsequent CT scan of the chest revealed two lesions in the right lung.

Because of the suspicious CT scan, a fine-needle aspiration biopsy was done of the largest chest lesion. This showed adenocarcinoma, consistent with a metastasis.

A second biopsy of the lung lesion was done to rule out primary lung cancer because it was believed unusual for a T2 rectal lesion to have metastasized. This was reported as adenocarcinoma. It was agreed on that these were metastatic nodules, and that the patient should be started on chemotherapy.

Physical exam at that time revealed a thin man in no distress. His blood pressure was 130/80. He had no palpable adenopathy in the cervical area. Chest exam revealed lungs clear to percussion and auscultation. There were no murmurs or gallops on cardiac exam. He had no hepatosplenomegaly and no abdominal masses. The prostate was normal on rectal exam, and there were no rectal masses. Stool was guaiac negative. There were no focal neurologic findings.

Three months after the initial operation, a CT scan was done (Fig. 52–2), and the patient was started on monthly doses of mitomycin C 10 mg/M², 5-fluorouracil (FU) 850 mg, and leucovorin 100 mg all given intravenously over 1

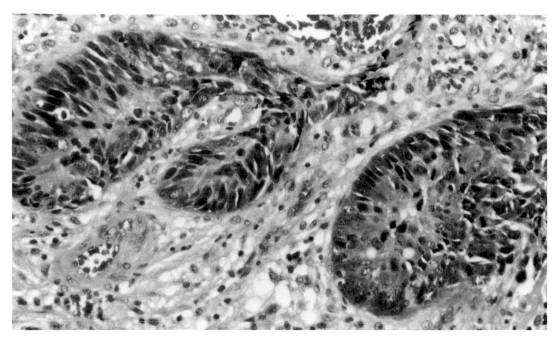

FIG. 52–1. Neoplastic glands composed of elongated cells with oval and "cigar-shaped" nuclei. The glandular lining cells show disarrangement and vary in size and shape. This microscopic appearance is consistent with histologic Grade II adenocarcinoma of the rectum. The background is highly vascular, inflammatory, and necrotic tissue (H&E × 350).

hour. Four months later he was admitted to the hospital for a deep venous thrombosis of the left lower extremity. He was treated with intravenous heparin and given another cycle of chemotherapy while hospitalized. He was discharged on coumarin. This thrombosis was the only problem he had with the chemotherapy.

He was followed up with CT scans of the chest, which showed initial regression (Figs. 52–3, 52–4). Six months later, a repeat CT scan showed some progression in the larger chest lesion from 1.9 cm × 1.6 cm to 2.2 cm × 1.8

cm. CEA remained constant at 2.9 ngn/mL. Because of the stable disease for 6 months and because of the fact that all the known metastatic disease was in one lobe of the lung, the patient was considered for a lung resection.

He was seen by a thoracic surgeon, who recommended a brain CT and bone scan. These tests were both performed and showed no disease.

Because he had disease that was slowly progressing while he was on optimal chemotherapy for rectal cancer, and because he had no other sites of disease, he was taken

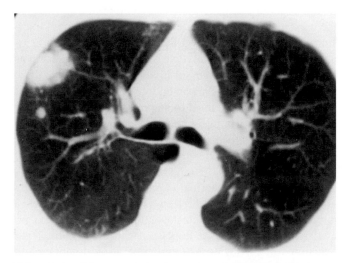

FIG. 52–2. CT scan of the lung done 6/12/91 showing two lesions in the upper lobe on the right side.

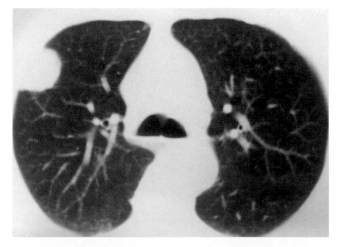

FIG. 52–3. CT scan of the lung done on 8/14/91 showing regression of the larger lesion in the right upper lobe.

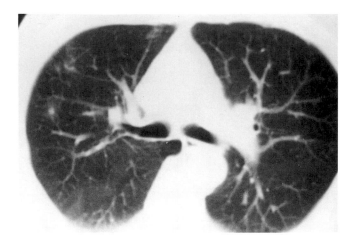

FIG. 52–4. CT scan of the lung done on 8/14/91 showing the smaller of the two metastatic lesions.

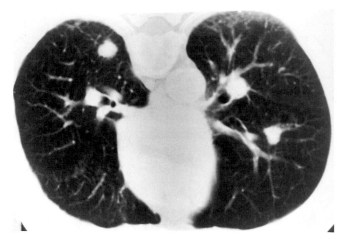

FIG. 52–6. CT scan of the lung done 12/28/92 showing multiple lung nodules in both lung fields.

to the operating room for a right upper lobectomy. At operation, two lesions were seen in the right upper lobe. Pathology revealed two metastatic adenocarcinomas (Fig. 52–5). All lymph nodes were negative.

He did well postoperatively. Chemotherapy was not restarted, and he was followed with liver function tests, CEA levels, and chest roentgenograms.

One year after thoracotomy, a chest radiogram revealed multiple pulmonary nodules. A CT scan of the chest showed multiple parenchymal lung nodules in both the left and right lung fields (Fig. 52–6).

The approach to this new problem was discussed at Tumor Board. Surgically, there was felt to be no further options. The radiation oncologist felt the disease was too diffuse for their modality. The medical oncologist felt there were two options. One would be to try a phase I/II drug if any were available. The other would be to start him on 5-FU, leucovorin, and alpha-interferon.

After researching, it was found that no phase I treatment was available for rectal cancer. The patient was then started on 5-FU, leucovorin, and alpha-interferon.

COMMENTARY by Alfred M. Cohen

This case history illustrates an unusually aggressive rectal carcinoma that represents a considerable problem in patient management. Biopsy of a sessile lesion in the middle to lower third of the rectum revealed carcinoma. An abdominoperineal resection was recommended but refused by the patient. Under these circumstances, other therapeutic options include low anterior resection with coloanal reconstruction, local excision, or fulguration. A transanal local excision was performed and, according to the case history, appropriately was a full-thickness excision. Pathology indicated a T2 NX MX grade II adenocarcinoma without any adverse prognostic factors such as vascular or lymphatic vessel invasion. Apparently, there were no areas of anaplasia on histology. The Astler-Coller system should not be used to stage such patients because the lymph node status is unknown. A transrectal ultrasound could have been performed preoperatively, but the accuracy in regard to determining lymph node positivity remains marginal.

Several published series of patients who have undergone radical surgery for T2 lesions indicate a 12% to 29% range of lymph node metastases (1–3). If there was no evidence of disease in the lungs, patients undergoing local excision for T2 lesions should receive adjuvant pelvic radiation therapy and 5-FU chemotherapy to maximize local control and survival (4–7).

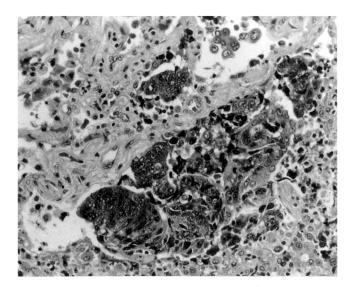

FIG. 52–5. Glandular neoplastic clusters in lung parenchyma consistent with metastatic colonic primary. Note the similarity of the adenocarcinoma to that of Fig. 52–1 (H&E × 350).

Patients with low rectal cancer are more likely to present with pulmonary metastases in the absence of hepatic metastases because of the direct vascular drainage through the hypogastric venous plexus in the lower half of the rectum. With a T2 moderately differentiated cancer, it is very unusual to have synchronous distal metastases and, despite the presence of two lesions, an effort was made to document metastatic disease versus synchronous primary lung cancer. The patient had been a smoker in the past but not in the prior 25 years. The major clinical decision at that time was whether to begin chemotherapy or to proceed directly to pulmonary resection. Before any resection for metastatic disease, a complete extent of disease workup to rule out another primary cancer is appropriate. The patient had a bone scan and a brain CT scan. An abdominal/pelvic CT scan, a careful rectal examination, and a repeat colonoscopy would have been appropriate before proceeding with pulmonary resection. The long-term follow-up of pulmonary resection for metastatic adenocarcinoma of the colon and rectum indicates a 20% long-term survival (8). As long as all disease can be resected, it does not appear to make any difference whether it was a single lesion or multiple lesions.

In this patient, whose disease could be encompassed by pulmonary lobectomy, I would have preferred to proceed directly with a resection.

However, after an interval of observation on systemic chemotherapy it was certainly appropriate to reassess the patient and proceed with pulmonary resection after a 6-month interval. Although the patient had only a 1-year disease-free survival off chemotherapy after his pulmonary resection, this was effective palliation.

The last feature of this case that warrants discussion is the use of salvage chemotherapy under these circumstances. The patient had already received 5-FU chemotherapy with some initial benefit. The likelihood of any secondary chemotherapy producing a meaningful remission is less than 10%, and prolongation in survival is slight. Entering patients into phase I trials is certainly appropriate. The use of alpha-interferon–containing chemotherapy with its toxicity (flu-like syndrome) is to be carefully considered (9). Without entering a research program, I would have strongly encouraged the patient to consider only supportive care. I would have also encouraged the surgeon to take over terminal care of the patient rather than continuing with multiple subsequent chemotherapy regimens off formal protocol of dubious clinical benefit.

REFERENCES

1. Brodsky JT, Richard GK, Cohen AM, et al. Variables correlated with the risk of lymph node metastasis in early rectal cancer. *Cancer* 1992;69:322–6.
2. Minsky BD, Mies C, Recht A, et al. Resectable adenocarcinoma of the rectosigmoid and rectum: 2. The influence of blood vessel invasion. *Cancer* 1988;61:1408–16.
3. Minsky BD, Rich T, Recth A, et al. Selection criteria for local excision with or without adjuvant radiation therapy for rectal cancer. *Cancer* 1989;63:1421–9.
4. Rich TA, Weiss DR, Mies C, et al. Sphincter preservation in patients with low rectal cancer treated with radiation therapy with or without local excision or fulguration. *Radiology* 1985;156:527–31.
5. McCready DR, Ota DM, Rich TA, et al. Prospective phase I trial of conservative management of low rectal lesions. *Arch Surg* 1989;124:67–70.
6. Minsky BD, Cohen AM, Enker WE, et al. Sphincter preservation in rectal cancer by local excision and postoperative radiation therapy. *Cancer* 1991;67:908–14.
7. Willett CG, Tepper JE, Donnely S, et al. Patterns of failure following local excision and postoperative radiation therapy for invasive rectal adenocarcinoma. *J Surg Oncol* 1989;7:1003–8.
8. McCormack PM, Burt ME, Bains MS, et al. Lung resection for colorectal metastases: 10-year results. *Arch Surg* 1992;127:1403–6.
9. Wadler S, Schwartz EL, Goldman M, et al. 5-Fluorouracil and recombinant alpha-2a-interferon: an active regimen against advanced colorectal cancer. *J Clin Oncol* 1989;7:1769–75.

53

Recurrent Rectal Cancer

Bruce Minsky

What are the goals of treatment?

CASE PRESENTATION

The patient is a 62 year-old man who, 2 years before presentation, underwent a low anterior resection for a T2 N0 M0 mobile adenocarcinoma located on the posterior wall of the rectum 8 cm from the anal verge. Review of the pathologic studies revealed moderately differentiated adenocarcinoma extending into but not through the muscularis propria. There was no evidence of colloid, lymphatic vessel invasion, or blood vessel invasion. Twelve mesorectal and pelvic lymph nodes sampled were negative for metastatic disease. The proximal and distal margins of resection were negative. The lateral margin was not assessed. Carcinoembryonic antigen (CEA) was 6.4 preoperatively and 1.1 postoperatively. The patient received no postoperative adjuvant therapy.

Although follow-up visits every 3 months were recommended, the patient did not return for follow-up. The patient subsequently presented with a 6-week history of sciatic-type pain radiating to both lower extremities. Relevant physical findings revealed a fixed, circumferential mass 3 cm from the anal verge extending proximally to 8 cm. Biopsy revealed recurrent adenocarcinoma consistent with the patient's prior rectal cancer. An abdominal/pelvic computed tomography (CT) scan confirmed a 5-cm rectal mass contiguous with but not invading the sacrum (Fig. 53–1). There was no evidence of adenopathy or liver metastasis. The remainder of the metastatic workup, including a chest radiography and liver function tests, was within normal limits. Preoperative CEA was 15.7.

The patient was enrolled on a phase I protocol of preoperative combined modality therapy. The preoperative segment of the protocol consists of 5-fluorouracil (5-FU) and leucovorin (LV) for one cycle. Pelvic radiation therapy (5,040 cGy at 180 cGy/day) began on day 8. A second cycle of 5-FU/LV was given concurrent with the fourth week of radiation. Four to 5 weeks after completion of radiation therapy, the patient underwent surgery and intraoperative radiation therapy (IORT). An additional six cycles of 5-FU/LV were delivered 4 to 5 weeks postoperatively.

At the time of operation, there was no evidence of tumor and the patient underwent an abdominoperineal resection. On pathologic examination there was a complete response. IORT with Iodine-125 brachytherapy was delivered to the tumor bed along the sacrum (Fig. 53–2). The minimum peripheral dose was 16,000 cGy. Postoperative CEA was 0.7. The patient received six cycles of postoperative 5-FU/LV and is alive and well 2 years after his abdominoperineal resection.

After the patient's initial surgery for a T2 N0 M0 adenocarcinoma of the rectum, he appropriately received no adjuvant therapy. The risk of local recurrence, depending on the series, is less than 10% (1). The use of postoperative adjuvant combined modality therapy in resectable rectal cancer should be limited to patients with T3 and/or N1,2 disease. Of note, the lateral (radial) margin of resection was not assessed. This margin may be responsible for a substantial number of local recurrences in patients undergoing potential curative surgery for rectal cancer (2).

Randomized trials of postoperative radiation therapy plus chemotherapy reveal a decrease in local failure (3) and increase in survival of patients with primary resectable rectal cancer (3–5). However, in patients with unresectable disease, it is more difficult to obtain these results.

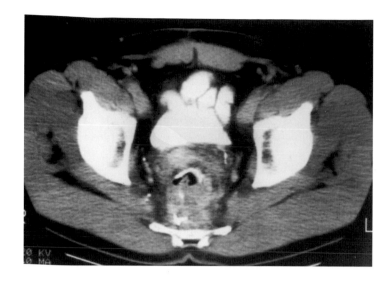

FIG. 53–1. Abdominal/pelvic CT scan reveals a 5-cm rectal mass contiguous with but not invading the

The standard approach to patients with unresectable rectal cancer is preoperative radiation therapy followed by surgery. The use of full-dose preoperative radiation therapy converts 48% to 64% of patients to a resectable status (6–9). However, despite a complete resection and negative margins, the local failure rate will vary, depending on the degree of tumor fixation, from 24% to 55%.

To improve the results of preoperative radiation, a number of approaches have been used. These include IORT and the addition of systemic chemotherapy. The primary advantage of IORT is that the radiation can be delivered to the site with the highest risk of local failure (tumor bed) while decreasing the dose to the surrounding normal tissues. IORT can be delivered by two techniques: electron beam and brachytherapy. At Memorial Sloan-Kettering Cancer Center (MSKCC), the IORT is delivered by brachytherapy (10).

The phase I/II nonrandomized trials from the Massachusetts General Hospital (11,12) and the Mayo Clinic (13) suggest that the addition of electron beam IORT to preoperative pelvic radiation in patients with unresectable rectal cancer improves local control compared with preoperative radiation therapy alone. The Radiation Therapy Oncology Group has an ongoing prospective phase III randomized trial in order to validate the phase I/II results.

Given the advantage of chemotherapy reported in patients with resectable rectal cancer in the postoperative adjuvant randomized trials (3–5,14), it is reasonable to combine 5-FU–based chemotherapy with radiation therapy in the preoperative setting.

This patient was treated on a MSKCC phase I protocol of preoperative 5-FU, high-dose LV, and sequential radiation therapy (15). Twenty patients (13 primary and 7 recurrent) have been enrolled. Six patients received IORT with brachytherapy. The pathologic complete response rate was 20%, and 89% underwent a complete resection with negative margins. These down-staging and resectability results were improved compared with a similar group of patients at MSKCC who received preoperative radiation therapy without chemotherapy (16). With a median follow-up of 3 years, the local failure rate was 26% and the overall 3-year actuarial survival was 69% (17). The cur-

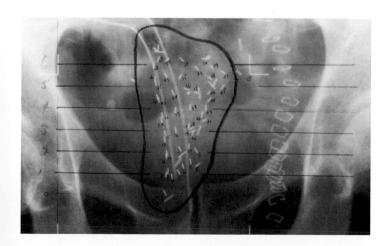

FIG. 53–2. Intraoperative radiation therapy with Iodine-125 brachytherapy delivered to the tumor bed. The minimum peripheral dose is 16,000 cGy.

rent approach at MSKCC for patients with unresectable rectal cancer is preoperative 5-FU, low-dose LV, and concurrent radiation therapy followed by surgery, IORT, and six cycles of postoperative 5-FU/LV (18).

REFERENCES

1. Minsky BD, Mies C, Recht A, et al. Resectable adenocarcinoma of the rectosigmoid and rectum: 1. Patterns of failure and survival. *Cancer* 1988;61:1408–16.
2. Quirke P, Durdey P, Dixon MF, et al. Local recurrence of rectal adenocarcinoma due to inadequate surgical resection. Histopathological study of lateral tumor spread and surgical excision. *Lancet* 1986;1:996–9.
3. Krook JE, Moertel CG, Gunderson LL, et al. Effective surgical adjuvant therapy for high-risk rectal carcinoma. *N Engl J Med* 1991;324:709–15.
4. Gastrointestinal Tumor Study Group. Prolongation of the disease-free interval in surgically treated rectal carcinoma. *N Engl J Med* 1985;312:1465–72.
5. Douglass HO, Moertel CG, Mayer RJ, et al. Survival after postoperative combination treatment of rectal cancer. *N Engl J Med* 1986;315:1294–5.
6. Dosoretz DE, Gunderson LL, Hedberg S, et al. Preoperative irradiation for unresectable rectal and rectosigmoid carcinomas. *Cancer* 1983;52:814–8.
7. Emami B, Pilepich M, Willett C, et al. Effect of preoperative irradiation on resectability of colorectal carcinomas. *Int J Radiat Oncol Biol Phys* 1982;8:1295–9.
8. Mendenhall WM, Bland KI, Pfaff WW, et al. Initially unresectable rectal adenocarcinoma treated with preoperative irradiation and surgery. *Ann Surg* 1986;205:41–4.
9. Minsky BD, Cohen AM, Enker WE, et al. Radiation therapy for unresectable rectal cancer. *Int J Radiat Oncol Biol Phys* 1991;21:1283–9.
10. Minsky BD, Cohen AM, Enker WE, et al. Intraoperative brachytherapy alone in incompletely resected recurrent rectal cancer. *Radiother Oncol* 1991;21:115–20.
11. Willett CG, Shellito PC, Tepper JE, et al. Intraoperative electron beam radiation therapy for recurrent locally advanced rectal or rectosigmoid carcinoma. *Cancer* 1991;67:1504–8.
12. Willett CG, Shellito PC, Tepper JE, et al. Intraoperative electron beam radiation therapy for primary locally advanced rectal and rectosigmoid carcinoma. *J Clin Oncol* 1991;9:843–9.
13. Gunderson LL, Martin JK, Beart RW. Intraoperative and external beam irradiation for locally advanced colorectal cancer. *Ann Surg* 1988;207:52–60.
14. Fisher B, Wolmark N, Rockette H, et al. Postoperative adjuvant chemotherapy or radiation therapy for rectal cancer: results from NSABP protocol R-01. *J Natl Cancer Inst* 1988;80:21–9.
15. Minsky BD, Kemeny N, Cohen AM, et al. Preoperative high-dose leucovorin/5-fluorouracil and radiation therapy for unresectable rectal cancer. *Cancer* 1991;67:2859–66.
16. Minsky BD, Cohen AM, Kemeny N, et al. Enhancement of radiation induced downstaging of rectal cancer by 5-FU and high dose leucovorin chemotherapy. *J Clin Oncol* 1992;10:79–84.
17. Minsky BD, Cohen AM, Kemeny N, et al. Efficacy of pre-operative 5-FU, high dose leucovorin, and sequential radiation therapy for unresectable rectal cancer. *Cancer* 1993(in press)
18. Minsky B, Cohen A, Enker W, et al. Pre-operative 5-FU, low dose leucovorin, and concurrent radiation therapy for rectal cancer. *Cancer* 1994;73:273–80.

COMMENTARY by Bernard Levin

This patient had undergone a low anterior resection for a mobile T2 N0 M0 adenocarcinoma 2 years before the current presentation with recurrent rectal cancer. Pathologic findings at the time of the initial resection were those of a moderately differentiated adenocarcinoma extending into but not through the muscularis propria.

The proximal and distal margins of resection were negative, but the (lateral) radial margin was not assessed. The decision to withhold postoperative adjuvant therapy was appropriate for the stage of the lesion, given that the actuarial survival for this group of patients is 79% (1).

The pattern of symptoms reported by the patient is typical. His subsequent management with preoperative chemoradiation on a phase I protocol, surgical resection, and intraoperative radiation therapy (brachytherapy) was effective. Preliminary data from Memorial Sloan Kettering Cancer Center presented by Dr. Minsky attest to the value of this approach in that 89% of patients underwent a complete resection with negative margins. Subsequent postoperative therapy with 5-FU and LV is reasonable, although specific data supporting this are not yet available.

I will focus primarily on the problem of local recurrence after resection of rectal cancer. Overall, the depth of intramural and extramural invasion and the presence of lymph node metastases are the principal risk factors for relapse (2,3). Gunderson and Sosin (4) evaluated the areas of relapse found at operation after curative resection of rectal cancer in 74 patients. Local pelvic metastases or periaortic node involvement were the sole source of failure in 48% of the 52 patients who relapsed.

In 1986, Quirke et al. (5) first drew attention to the importance of analysis of the lateral (radial) margin after curative rectal cancer surgery. They studied rectal cancers using transverse whole-mount cross-sections of resected specimens and demonstrated unsuspected carcinoma of the lateral margins of resection in 14 of 52 analyzed specimens. Of the 14 patients, 12 developed a local recurrence. Other pathologic factors (T status, N status, lymphatic vascular invasion, ploidy) and operative considerations have been reviewed in detail by Enker (6). In their prospective studies, Enker and colleagues have found that ploidy alone is of little significance in prognosis (7), but proliferative index may be of greater prognostic value. Patients with diploid tumors of low proliferative index appear to have cancers that are not particularly aggressive, whereas patients whose tumors are both aneuploid and of high proliferative index are more likely to have a poor outcome. Increasingly, molecular markers are being investigated and may be useful in a prognostic sense. Despite favorable histopathologic staging, the finding of molecular abnormalities such as allelic deletions of chromosome 17 (8) or chromosome 1 deletions (9) may be used to influence a decision concerning preoperative or postoperative therapy as well as subsequent chemotherapy. The incorporation of such studies into randomized cooperative group studies will be of inestimable value in the future (10).

REFERENCES

1. Paty PB, Enker WE, Cohen AM, et al. Treatment of rectal cancer by low anterior resection with colo-anal anastomosis. *Ann Surg* 1994;219:365–73.

2. Enker WE, Heilweil ML, Hertz REL, et al. En bloc pelvic lymphadenectomy and sphincter presentation in the surgical management of rectal cancer. *Ann Surg* 1986;203:426–33.
3. McDermott FT, Hughes ESR, Phil E, et al. Local recurrence after potentially curative resection for rectal cancer in a series of 1008 patients. *Br J Surg* 1985;72:34–7.
4. Gunderson LL, Sosin H. Areas of failure found at re-operation (second or symptomatic look) following "curative surgery" for adenocarcinoma of the rectum: clinicopathologic correlation and implications for adjuvant therapy. *Cancer* 1974;34:1278–92.
5. Quirke P, Dudley P, Dixon MF, et al. Local recurrence of rectal adenocarcinoma due to inadequate surgical resection. Histopathologic study of lateral tumor spread and surgical excision. *Lancet* 1986;1:996–96.
6. Enker WE. Operative considerations in rectal cancer. In: *The pelvic dissection in cancer of the colon, rectum, and anus*, Cohen AM, Winwer S, Friedman MA, Gunderson LL, eds. New York: McGraw-Hill; 1994:561–70.
7. Enker WE. Flow cytometric determination of tumor cell DNA content and proliferative index as prognostic variables in colorectal cancer. *Perspect Colon Rectal Surg* 1990;3:1–32.
8. Kern SE, Fearon ER, Tersmette KWF, et al. Allelic loss in colorectal carcinoma. *JAMA* 1989;261:3099–3103.
9. Laurent-Puig P, Olschwang S, Delattre O, et al. Survival and acquired genetic alterations in colorectal cancer. *Gastroenterology* 1992;102:1136–41.
10. Tempero M, Anderson J. Progress in colon cancer: Do molecular markers matter? *N Engl J Med* 1994;331:267–8.

SECTION XII

Anal Canal

54

Epidermoid Cancer of the Anal Canal

Herand Abcarian

A nonsurgical disease, for the most part!

CASE PRESENTATION

A 49-year-old Caucasian female school teacher was seen with complaints of anal pain and bleeding for approximately 9 months. The patient attributed her pain and sensation of swelling on the right side of the anal region to hemorrhoids and resorted to over-the-counter topical medications, oral analgesics, and warm baths, which alleviated her symptoms to some extent. She subsequently visited her obstetrician-gynecologist, who performed a rectal examination and diagnosed her condition as "ulcerated hemorrhoids" and further topical medication was ordered with minor symptomatic relief. The patient stated that her condition had worsened significantly with rapid enlargement of the area of swelling and ulceration during the last 3 months. Her bowel movements were regular but painful. Her past medical history revealed that she had no allergies, no previous medical illnesses, was a nonsmoker, and drank wine socially. She was gravida II, para II, and had a history of a total abdominal hysterectomy, bilateral salpingo-oophorectomy, cholecystectomy, and was on estrogen therapy to prevent osteoporosis. Her family history was remarkable in that her older sister had had surgery for colon cancer 5 years previously, and according to the patient she was cured of her disease.

Physical examination revealed a 6-cm long ulceration with indurated base, tender to touch on the right anterior quadrant of the anal canal extending to the perianal region (Fig. 54–1). At anoscopy, the indurated ulceration extended to 1 cm proximal to the dentate line on the right anterior quadrant encompassing about 60° of the circumference of the anal canal. Flexible sigmoidoscopy revealed no other pathology. The examination of both groins revealed no enlargement of lymph nodes and her physical examination was otherwise negative.

Examination under spinal anesthesia revealed an indurated ulceration extending proximal to the dentate line on the right anterior quadrant. Multiple biopsy specimens were taken from this area, and the patient was discharged on analgesics and sitz baths.

The pathology report was as follows: A $1.3 \times 1.2 \times 0.8$ roughly ovoid portion of soft tissue, firm and focally hyperemic, red and gray in color suggestive of mucosal surface was identified. The cut surface showed nodular gray-white thickening. On microscopy, the classical finding of basaloid (cloacogenic) carcinoma was identified (Fig. 54–2).

Four days postoperatively, the patient underwent additional workup including complete blood count, chest roentgenogram, and electrocardiogram all of which were normal. Chemistry panel revealed essentially no abnormality in her electrolytes, liver function tests, lipid profile, or fasting blood glucose level. Hemoglobin was 13.2, white count was 8,800 with normal differential and PT/PTT were within normal limits. A computed tomography (CT) scan of the abdomen and pelvis revealed that the solid organs and partially visualized pancreas were normal. There was no retroperitoneal mass or enlarged adenopathy seen in the pelvis or in the region of both groins.

With the diagnosis of a stage II epidermoid carcinoma (basaloid or cloacogenic type), a central line was inserted in the subclavian vein and the patient was begun on chemoradiation therapy (Nigro protocol). The patient received 15 mg/m^2 of mitomycin C as a bolus injection the first day and was begun on 1,000 mg/m^2 per day of 5-fluorouracil (5-FU) on a continuous infusion basis over

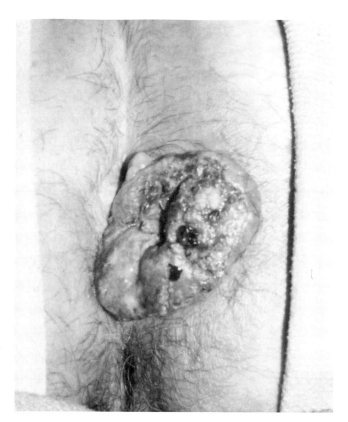

FIG. 54–1. View of the perineum with the patient in jack-knife position. A large ulcerated epidermoid (cloacogenic) carcinoma of the anal canal and perianal region is seen extending approximately 3 cm beyond the anal verge.

a 4-day period. On day 1, radiation therapy was started to the anal canal and retrorectal lymph nodes as well as both groins. The patient received fractionated doses of 200 cGy given on a daily basis for a total of 20 treatment days. A slightly larger dose of radiation therapy was prescribed because of the magnitude of the lesion, as the length of the lesion was slightly over 6 cm. Upon completion of 4,000 cGy, the patient was readmitted to the hospital, and 4 additional days of intravenous 5-FU of 1,000 mg/m² per day was administered on a continuous infusion basis.

The patient tolerated the chemoradiation very well. She had an episode of vaginitis and urinary tract infection during the radiation therapy. The urinalysis revealed 15 to 20 white cells and 4+ bacteria. Urine culture and sensitivity revealed over 100,000 *Escherichia coli,* which were sensitive to Ciprofloxin. She was placed for 1 week on 500 mg of Ciprofloxin twice a day with excellent resolution of her urinary tract infection, and a negative urine culture was obtained 10 days after the completion of antibiotic therapy.

The lesion had a remarkable regression during and after the chemoradiation. Eight weeks after the completion of the second course of chemotherapy, no tumor could be seen or felt in the anal and perianal regions (Fig. 54–3). The patient was taken to the operating room on an outpatient basis and an excision biopsy of the full length of the linear scar was performed down to the subcutaneous fat in the perianal region down to and including the circular muscle of the rectum and portion of the internal sphincter.

The pathology report indicated that the specimen from the right anterior anal wall consisted of elements of

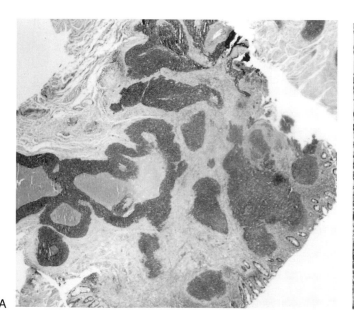

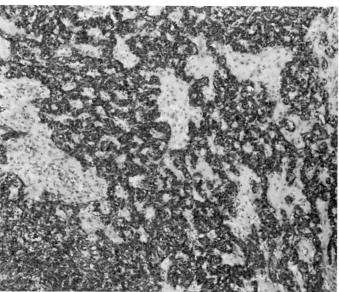

FIG. 54–2. Photomicrograph of anal biopsy revealing pallisading sheets of hyperchromatic cells typical of basaloid (cloacogenic) carcinoma.

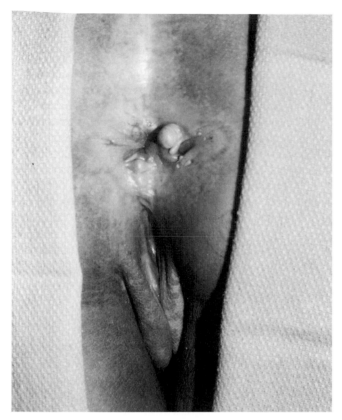

FIG. 54–3. View of the patient's perineum 8 weeks after completion of chemoradiation therapy. Note complete disappearance of the ulcerated lesion except for a small skin tag at the site of the previous lesion.

white and tan mucosa measuring 4.1 × 2.1 × 1.1 cm. The tan mucosa was edematous. There was suture marking the distal end. The specimen was serially sectioned and submitted as most proximal, midproximal, mid-distal, and most distal quarters. There was no evidence of carcinoma in any of the examined sections (Fig. 54–4).

The suture line on the right anterior anorectal quadrant healed per primam and, except for mild residual tenderness, the patient was asymptomatic 4 weeks later.

Follow-up in December 1989 was negative and the patient was placed on a follow-up regimen of physical examination and anoscopy every 3 months.

One year after initial surgery, the patient underwent anoscopy and a small mucosal lesion grossly resembling granulation tissue was seen measuring 1 cm in diameter in the right anterior quadrant at the apex of the surgical scar. A biopsy specimen was obtained from this lesion, and pathologic diagnosis confirmed granulation tissue at the anal wound site with no evidence of malignancy. Subsequent to this, the patient was continued on routine follow-up and had an unremarkable postoperative follow-up on every third month. The anal canal has remained normal, the patient has remained fully continent, and there has been no evidence of any groin nodes on subsequent examinations. The following year, during one of her follow-up examinations, the patient underwent a total colonoscopy, which was negative for neoplastic disease. It was recommended that the patient continue to be examined on a regular basis for her anal canal lesion every 3 months and fecal occult blood testing on an annual basis, all of which have been negative. The patient underwent a repeat surveillance colonoscopy because of her family history of colon cancer three years later, which again revealed a well-healed anal scar with no evidence of recurrence in the anal canal. Her groins have also remained negative. The plan is to follow her up with examination of the anal canal every 6 months, annual fecal occult blood testing, and repeat colonoscopy for surveillance of colon cancer every 3 to 5 years.

COMMENTARY by Victor W. Fazio

This case represents one of the great success stories of clinical research in recent times. Chemoradiation for invasive squamous cell carcinoma of the anal canal was used originally as preoperatively adjunctive therapy. Nigro et al. (1) observed that subsequent abdominoper-

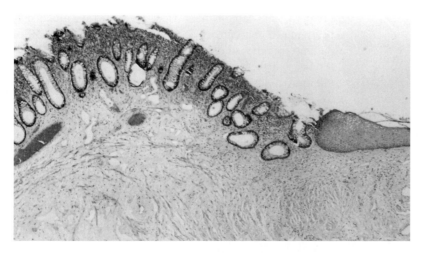

FIG. 54–4. Photomicrographs of anal biopsy at the site of cloacogenic carcinoma after chemoradiation. Normal mucosa and anoderm is seen with no residual carcinoma.

ineal rectal resection specimens usually did not show evidence of residual cancer. This led to the current treatment recommendation, namely, if clinical resolution of local anal canal cancer follows chemoradiation, then close follow-up only is recommended, reserving resective surgery for recurrence of the tumor.

Concerning the case under discussion, certain comments may be made:

Anal canal carcinoma is an uncommon condition, representing about 1% to 2% of large bowel malignancies. This condition is most common in women, and in patients in the sixth or seventh decade, typified by this case. The symptoms of pain and bleeding are classical, as is the finding of an anal canal ulcer. Unfortunately, the diagnosis is commonly delayed, symptoms being attributed to hemorrhoids, as was the case here. This serves notice on patients and physicians to have persistent symptomatology checked with rectal examination. This includes routine anoscopy and proctoscopy, if necessary, with anesthesia—should local pain preclude an adequate examination. Biopsy of a mass or indurated area is done especially if the lesion appears ulcerated. This patient had no predisposing conditions, such as condylomata, fistula, leukoplakia, human papilloma virus, or human immunodeficiency virus infection.

The physical findings of an ulcer in the anal canal is typical, although in this case, the tumor at 6 cm in longest dimension is bigger than the average of 3 to 4 cm reported in the literature. An important part of the assessment is that of a "good" examination. This commonly involves examination under anesthesia, as was the case here. This staging is not easily assessed on clinical grounds. One of the staging systems used to define local extent of tumor is as follows:

T1 tumor is limited to internal sphincter
T2 tumor involves external sphincter
T3 tumor extends to rectum or perianal skin.

Nodal assessment—short of biopsy excision—is apt to understage those with microscopic nodal disease, especially in inaccessible areas, such as the internal iliac chain. The staging system used by UICC classifies T1 lesions as less than 2 cm; T2 lesions are 2 to 5 cm in diameter with minimal infiltration; T3 are tumors greater than 5 cm; and T4 infiltrates muscle or bone. The importance of accurate staging is not clear at present as:

1. Some series report favorable outcomes even with advanced (T3) local lesions (2), although progressive penetration of tissue by tumor usually carries a proportionate adverse prognosis.
2. Chemoradiation is appropriate therapy in most circumstances, even for advanced lesions to "downsize" the local extent of disease. Notwithstanding, we will commonly augment clinical staging with CT scanning (as was done here) and with endoluminal ultra-

sound of the rectum and anal canal. Thus, comparisons of outcome with different treatment regimens may be made relative to the tumor stage.

Basaloid carcinoma was found on biopsy. These basaloid tumors (cloacogenic) arise from the anal transitional zone and account for 25% to 30% of all anal canal cancers (3). These lesions may exhibit changes similar to basal cell cancers of the skin, with nests of cells and an orderly palisading of cells at the periphery. The cloacogenic or transitional cell tumors appear more like the anoepithelium with indistinct borders and basal nuclei. Spread to lymph nodes occurs in 35% to 50% of cases—with involvement of nodes in the distribution of the lateral pelvic wall and superior hemorrhoidal vessels as well as inguinal nodes. Most epidermoid cancers of the anal canal (75 to 90%) have already penetrated to the anal sphincter.

The timing of treatment, chemotherapeutic agents, radiation dose, fractionation, and targeting used here was the same as used at our institution, although radiation doses to 4,500 cGy or higher may be used at other institutions. Opinion varies as to radiation dose, fractionation, and type of field, e.g., parallel opposed fields versus perineal boost via a perineal port. Most radiation treatments include inguinal and pelvic nodes. The specifics of chemotherapy are also somewhat different from one center to another, although the combination used in this case is the classical one. Leukopenia or thrombocytopenia occurs in 25% of patients within 3 weeks of treatment, but usually these effects are not severe. If proctitis or perineal dermatitis is severe, split-course therapy is advocated by Cummings et al. (4) and, indeed, is commonly used routinely by their group at Princess Margaret Hospital, Toronto. Treatment-induced damage to pelvic structures is rare. Anal stricture may occur with circumferential tumors that have been irradiated. Dilation is usually successful. However, high strictures in the rectum often require resective surgery. In Cummings' series, 8% of 73 patients required operation for treatment-related morbidity (5). The patient in this study was remarkably free of significant reactions.

In few situations is early follow-up of patients treated for cancer as important as in those with chemoradiation given for anal canal cancer. Because shrinkage and disappearance of the cancer occurs in about 60% to 80% of patients, one has to detect at an early stage those who will require further treatment, namely, surgery. Several authors advocate examination, under anesthesia, and an excision biopsy of the residual scar, or at least a "generous" biopsy, as was done in this case. This is likely to give the most complete information, on histologic review, of the status of the patient regarding local persistence of tumor. Other clinicians have expressed concern that such a sizable biopsy could result in a nonhealing actinic ulcer and have favored multiple Tru-Cut needle biopsies to minimize the risk of persistent ulceration, and to be certain to get to the full depth of the original lesion pretreatment. This issue remains unsettled, although several experienced clinicians contend that concerns of nonhealing biopsy wounds are excessive.

One authority (4), noted that after treatment the primary site is usually scarred with a rubbery feel. The scar is commonly extensive and choice of biopsy site is problematic. Thus, no biopsy is done in follow-up, unless a clinically suspicious area is noted.

How often should biopsies be done or should they be done at all after the first post-treatment check up? Again, there is no good information on this. Most clinicians will not do routine biopsies, but will do repeat examinations, under anesthesia if necessary, and biopsy if there is any appearance of change, e.g., nodularity, ulceration, induration, or ultrasound evidence of abnormality. Most recurrences will occur within the first 24 months of treatment. One could argue for extending the follow-up interval to semiannual after the first 2 years of follow-up. The colonoscopic surveillance plans performed in this patient's case is appropriate.

Clearly, this patient had a spectacular outcome. There was minimal side effect of therapy; major surgery was avoided. The patient was spared of having a colostomy and despite the advanced local nature of the ulcerated cancer, she is now more than 5 years out from therapy with no evidence of disease. In a collected series of 104 patients, Nigro et al. (1) reported a complete response to chemoradiation of 97 patients. Thirty-one underwent abdominoperineal resection (same as part of the protocol at that time) and there were 13 deaths from cancer with a 24- to 132-month follow-up. Cummings et al. (4) reported the outcome on 93 patients treated by different schedules of chemoradiation: The primary cancer was controlled in 79%; anorectal function was preserved in 76% overall, and in 94% of those whose primary cancer was controlled by chemoradiation. The actuarial 5-year cause-specific survival rate was 77%. These data compare more than favorably with survival rates of 50% to 60% with abdominoperineal resection. It can be fairly stated that chemoradiation is now the first-line therapy for epidermoid carcinoma of the anal canal. Details of optimal regimens need to be defined. For most patients, abdominoperineal resection of the rectum is reserved for salvaging cases in which local cancer persists after chemoradiation.

REFERENCES

1. Nigro ND, Vaitkevicius VK, Considine BJ. Combined therapy for cancer of the anal canal: A preliminary report. *Dis Colon Rectum* 1974;17:354.
2. Papillon J, ed. *Rectal and anal cancer: conservative treatment by irradiation—an alternative to radical surgery.* Berlin: Springer-Verlag; 1982.
3. Boman BM, Moertel CG, O'Connell MJ, et al. Carcinoma of the anal canal. A clinical and pathological study of 188 cases. *Cancer* 1984;54: 114–25.
4. Cummings BJ, Rotstein LE, Stern HS. Anal carcinoma. In: *Current therapy in colon and rectal surgery,* Fazio VW, ed. Philadelphia: BC Decker; 1990:64–7.
5. Cummings BJ. Current management of epidermoid carcinoma of the anal canal. *Gastroenterol Clin North Am* 1987;16:125–42.

SECTION XIII

Lung

55

Surgical Management of Small-Cell Carcinoma of the Lung and Related Cancers

John R. Benfield and Liisa Russell

Don't assume that all patients thought to have small-cell lung cancer really have it. Surgery is not always contraindicated in this family of neoplasms.

CASE PRESENTATIONS

The following two cases illustrate the considerations that govern decisions about the surgical management of patients with small-cell lung cancers (SCLC) and related neoplasms. This group of cancers has also been referred to as neuroendocrine tumors (1) or amine precursor uptake derivative (APUD) cancers (2).

Case 1

A 65-year-old Caucasian man with a 100+ pack per year smoking history developed a flulike syndrome in January 1992. He was otherwise asymptomatic. Past history included exposure to asbestos many years ago, while working as a mechanical supervisor.

The findings on physical examination included no peripheral lymphadenopathy and increased anteroposterior diameter of the chest. The heart was in regular sinus rhythm without murmurs, and the abdomen was without abdominal masses. Rectal examination was negative for occult blood in the stool.

Pulmonary function tests included FEV = 1.1 liters, FEV/FVC = 48%, paO_2 = 59, $paCO_2$ = 52, ph 7.40. Chest radiograph and computed tomography (CT) scan demonstrated a left upper lobe lesion without evidence of medi-

astinal lymphadenopathy (Fig. 55–1). Bone scan showed normal uptake.

Before referral, fine-needle aspirate had been done (Fig. 55–2). The interpretation before referral was "undifferentiated carcinoma with large- and small-cell components."

Preoperative impression: (a) undifferentiated carcinoma, upper lobe of left lung, with large and small-cell components: T2 N0 M0, and (b) respiratory dysfunction secondary to chronic obstructive pulmonary disease.

Operations: Wedge excision of left upper lobe mass and mediastinal exploration with video-assisted thoracotomy.

Postoperative diagnosis: Small-cell carcinoma with a large-cell undifferentiated component (Fig. 55–3).

Postoperative therapy: Five cycles of chemotherapy with carboplatinum and VP16 were delivered between May 27, 1992, and September 16, 1992. This treatment was well tolerated. No radiotherapy was given.

Follow-up: July 14, 1993, 19 months after diagnosis and 16 months after operation, the patient was free of recurrent disease or residual cancer.

Case 2

A 79-year-old Caucasian man was referred for evaluation of an asymptomatic left lung mass. Before referral, 1 year prior, fine-needle aspirate was interpreted as undif-

273

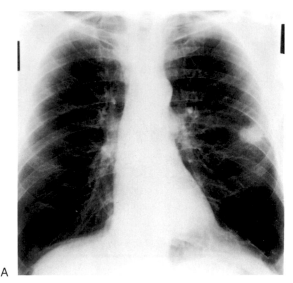

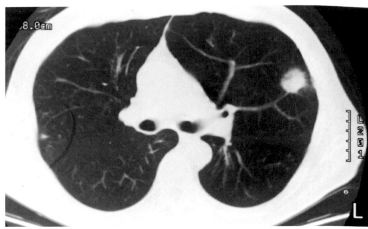

FIG. 55–1. A,B: Left upper lobe mass with irregular borders seen on chest radiograph and CT scan. A tiny peripheral lung nodule on the right that was judged to be a granuloma has remained stable throughout treatment and follow-up.

ferentiated small-cell carcinoma, and the patient had received treatment with chemotherapy that was only partially effective. Objective remission, short of 50%, occurred. The medical oncologist was dissatisfied with the result, and the question of precise diagnosis was raised.

Complete staging evaluation, including bone marrow aspiration, chest radiograph, and CT scan (Fig. 55–4) showed no evidence of disease outside the thorax or in the lymphatics.

Pre-operative impression: (a) possible SCLC (Kulchitsky cell carcinoma, grade III), or (b) possible atypical carcinoid Kulchitsky cell carcinoma (grade II).

Operation: Left pneumonectomy was accomplished.

Postoperative diagnosis: Kulchitsky cell carcinoma (KCC), grade II (atypical carcinoid), T2 N0 M0, stage I (Fig. 55–5).

Follow-up: Ten years after erroneous initial diagnosis of small-cell carcinoma of the lung and 9 years after pneumonectomy for removal of a stage I atypical carcinoid, the patient was free of carcinoma of the lung.

TUMOR BOARD DISCUSSION

Small-cell undifferentiated carcinoma of the lung has been considered a systemic disease by definition. Nonop-

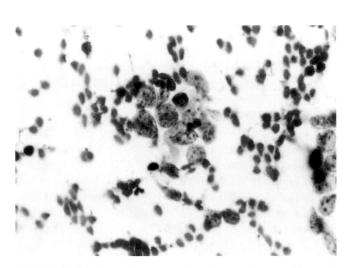

FIG. 55–2. High-grade neuroendocrine carcinoma with small and large cell component. This smear of a fine-needle aspiration biopsy of a lung mass contains highly atypical undifferentiated small and large tumor cells on a bloody and necrotic background. The nuclei are hyperchromatic and have coarsely granular chromatin (PAP × 625).

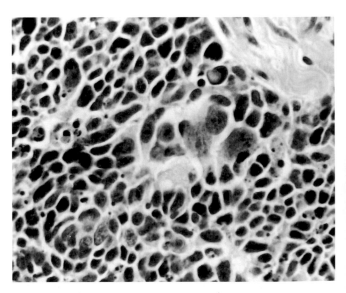

FIG. 55–3. High-grade neuroendocrine carcinoma with small and large cell component. A section of a wedge excision specimen shows a partly necrotic tumor comprising a dual population of small and large undifferentiated malignant cells. The small cells exhibit nuclear molding. Some of the large cells have nucleoli (H&E, × 625).

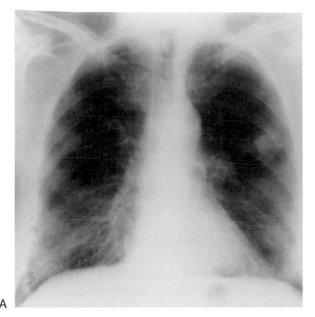

A

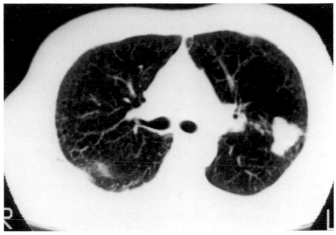

B

FIG. 55–4. A,B: Left lung mass with irregular borders seen on chest radiograph and CT scan. This tumor involved the upper and lower lobes, and removal required pneumonectomy. Pleural scarring on the right was from inflammatory disease that was arrested and has remained stable.

erative therapy has been the recommended treatment (3). There is growing evidence to indicate that resection of small-cell cancers is an important part of treatment, at least in selected cases (4,5). However, the role of resection in the treatment of SCLC remains controversial (3–6).

If one accepts that chemotherapy is the most effective treatment for systemic SCLC, and that the disease is usually systemic when the diagnosis is made, when and why should SCLC ever be resected? Case #1 is consistent with the experience of others (2,3) that certain patients with SCLC, or variations thereof, may be cured with resection

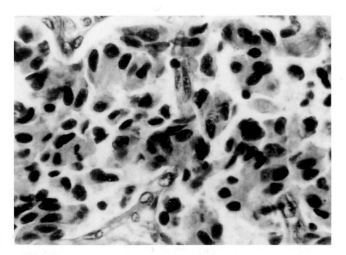

FIG. 55–5. KCC, grade 2 (atypical carcinoid). A section of a resected lung specimen shows tumor cells growing in a trabecular pattern. There is moderate anisonucleosis and nuclear pleomorphism as well as small focal necroses (H&E, ×625).

and chemotherapy. Case #2 shows that a definitive diagnosis of SCLC may be erroneously made if cytologic or biopsy samples are inadequate or suboptimal. These experiences contribute to the following viewpoint.

Precise and complete preoperative diagnosis and staging are crucially important as the basis for management decisions. Radiographic evidence of lymph node metastases may be erroneous, and therefore mediastinal biopsies are often recommended. SCLC should be resected at least under the following circumstances: (a) when it is encountered as an incidental, unexpected finding at thoracotomy; (b) when the preoperative diagnosis is in doubt, after complete staging evaluation that includes bone marrow aspirate, brain scan, bone scan, and mediastinoscopy; (c) when SCLC is apparently in stage I at the time of diagnosis, resections such as lobectomies or segmentectomies are indicated, if they can be done safely without significant risk to the patient and if they result in complete removal of all known cancer. Complete staging evaluation intraoperatively, that is, mediastinal node sampling, is required to make possible a rational decision as to whether or not to proceed with resection. Pneumonectomy is usually contraindicated if lymph node metastases are found at thoracotomy.

At the present time, elective pulmonary resection to treat SCLC with evidence of locoregional spread is contraindicated, except as part of approved research protocols. We believe that, without extrathoracic metastases, evidence of systemic disease requires proof of lymph node metastases.

There is evidence that SCLCs are biologically related to carcinoid tumors, and that these neoplasms arise from Kulchitsky cells, and that about 10% of patients with carcinoid tumors may develop SCLC (7). Therefore, we have adopted the term Kulchitsky cell carcinomas (KCC) to refer to this family of neoplasms. We refer to typical carcinoid as KCC, grade I, and to atypical carcinoid as KCC, grade II. Small cell carcinoma is referred to as KCC, grade III.

We have illustrated that the differentiation of KCC, grades II and III, may be difficult. Because KCC, grade II (atypical carcinoid) is curable with resection, it is important to remove cancers for which the diagnosis of SCLC is not totally conclusive. Current evidence suggests that KCC grade III may also be curable in about 25% of patients treated with a combination of resection and chemotherapy.

In summary, accurate diagnosis, insistence on histologic proof, and the combination of resection with chemotherapy in selected patients is our currently recommended approach for the treatment of SCLC. The KCC nomenclature is recommended as a reminder of potential diagnostic confusion between SCLC and atypical carcinoid, and as a reminder of the relationship between carcinoid (KCC, grades I and II) and small-cell undifferentiated carcinoma (KCC, grade III).

REFERENCES

1. Warren WH, Faber LP, Gould VE. Neuroendocrine neoplasms of the lung. *J Thorac Cardiovasc Surg* 1989;98:321–2.
2. DeCaro LF, Paladugu R, Benfield JR et al. Typical and atypical carcinoids within the pulmonary APUD spectrum. *J Thorac Cardiovasc Surg* 1983;86:528–36.
3. Cook RM, Miller YE, Bunn PA. Small cell lung cancer. Etiology, biology, clinical features, staging and treatment. *Curr Prob Cancer* 1993;17:69–144.
4. Ginsberg RJ. Operation for small cell lung cancer—where are we? *Ann Thorac Surg* 1990;49:692–3.
5. Salzer GM, Muller LC, Huber H, et al. Operations for N2 small cell lung carcinoma. *Ann Thorac Surg* 1990;49:759–62.
6. Bunn PA. Operation for stage IIIa small cell lung cancer? *Ann Thorac Surg* 1990;49:691.
7. Paladugu RR, Benfield JR, Pak HY, Ross RK, Teplitz RL. Bronchopulmonary Kulchitsky cell carcinomas: a new classification scheme for typical and atypical carcinoids. *Cancer* 1985;55:1303–11.

COMMENTARY by Robert L. Quigley

Neuroendocrine bronchopulmonary tumors arising from Kulchitsky cells have been classified into three groups: Group I = typical carcinoids, Group II = atypical carcinoids, Group III = small-cell lung carcinomas. Small-cell lung carcinoma (SCLC) accounts for 20% to 25% of all bronchogenic carcinoma and is associated with the poorest 5-year survival. SCLC has been further classified into three different histologic cell types: small-cell carcinoma, mixed small-cell/large-cell carcinoma, and combined small-cell carcinoma (1). Small-cell carcinoma comprises 90% of all cases.

Case #1 represents a 65-year-old man with a left upper lobe mass and severe pulmonary dysfunction. An FEV_1/FVC of less than 50% with significant CO_2 retention warrants more extensive pulmonary function testing, including, at the least, calculation of the diffusion capacity (<60% is associated with significant postoperative morbidity) (2). As indicated, a thorough and complete metastatic work-up is indicated, in part because of the working pathologic diagnosis, particularly since there is evidence that the tumor described here behaves more aggressively, is resistant to therapy, and has a worse prognosis (3). In addition, CT scan of the adrenal glands and liver could be considered.

Case #2 represents a 79-year-old man with a misdiagnosed left lung mass. One can only assume that before surgery the likelihood of the patient tolerating a pneumonectomy was determined with appropriate pulmonary function testing, including a demonstrable $FEV_1 > 2$ L. Because of his age, ventilation/perfusion scans would be indicated to determine expected loss of lung function. Expected loss of function can be calculated by:

$$\frac{\text{preoperative } FEV_1 \times \text{\# functional segments resected}}{\text{total \# segments in both lungs}}$$

As outlined, preoperative diagnosis and staging are critical in the management of SCLC. Although traditionally surgery has been limited to those cases of stage 1 disease (local), an incidental finding at thoracotomy, or an unclear diagnosis in the context of a negative metastatic work-up, Sugarbaker et al. have recently described several other indications (4). These include patients with regional disease achieving a complete response to chemotherapy (i.e., adjuvant surgical resection). Furthermore, they suggest surgery may be preferred over adjuvant radiotherapy because the latter necessitates lowering the total chemotherapy dose administered. Radical surgery including pneumonectomy is contraindicated for SCLC when positive mediastinal lymph nodes are encountered at thoracotomy. However, when the pathology represents atypical carcinoid (i.e., Group II), as was the diagnosis in the second case report, an aggressive approach is indicated, assuming adequate pulmonary function, as would apply to well differentiated carcinoma of the lung (5).

The optimal treatment of the nonresectable cases of SCLC is still somewhat controversial. Recently, the use of cisplatin and etoposide combinations, which are nontoxic to the cardiac/pulmonary/esophageal systems, has received appropriate attention (6). Clinical trials are still required to determine the ideal dose, volume, fractionation, and timing of radiation therapy for local control (7). It appears that prophylactic cranial irradiation is of benefit only to the subgroup of patients with limited staged disease in complete remission after chemotherapy (30–36 Gy in 2 Gy/day fractions) (8).

Therapeutic options of the future will include colony-stimulating factors, which will attenuate chemotherapy-induced myelosuppression and permit administration of planned chemotherapy doses (9). In addition, monoclonal antibodies to the ganglioside fucosyl-GM$_1$, a selective marker for SCLC, may have applications for radioimmunoimaging as well as in immunotherapy for SCLC (10).

REFERENCES

1. McCue PA, Finkel GC. Small-cell lung carcinoma. An evolving histopathological spectrum. *Semin Oncol* 1993;20(2):153–62.
2. Ferguson MK, Reeder LB, Mick R. Optimizing selection of patients for major lung resection. *J Thorac Cardiovasc Surg* 1995;109:275–83.
3. Hirsch F, Mattews M, Aisner S, et al. Histopathologic classification of small-cell lung cancer. Changing concepts and terminology. *Cancer* 1988;62:973–7.
4. Mentzer SJ, Reilly JJ, Sugarbaker DJ. Surgical resection in the management of small-cell carcinoma of the lung. *Chest* 1993; 103(suppl)(4):349S–51S.
5. Marty-Ané C-H, Costes V, Pujol JL, et al. Carcinoid tumors of the lung: do atypical features require aggressive management? *Ann Thorac Surg* 1995;59:78–83.
6. Turrisi AT III. Innovations in multimodality therapy for lung cancer—combined modality management of limited small-cell lung cancer. *Chest* 1993;103(suppl)(4):56S–9S.
7. Turrisi AT III. Incorporation of radiotherapy fractionation in the combined-modality treatment of limited small-cell lung cancer. *Chest* 1993;103(suppl)(4):418S–22S.
8. Abner A. Prophylactic cranial irradiation in the treatment of small-cell carcinoma of the lung. *Chest* 1993;103(suppl)(4):445S–8S.
9. Demetri GD. Impact of hematopoietic growth factors on the management of small-cell lung cancer. *Chest* 1993;103(suppl)(4):427S–32S.
10. Vangsted AJ, Zeuthen J. Monoclonal antibodies for diagnosis and potential therapy of small-cell lung cancer—the ganglioside antigen fucosyl-GM$_1$. *Acta Oncol* 1993;32(7/8):845–51.

EDITORIAL BOARD COMMENTARY

The classification of pulmonary neuroendocrine neoplasms is controversial and complex. Currently, the classification described by Travis et al. (1) is widely used. This divides these tumors into four groups: typical carcinoid, atypical carcinoid, large-cell neuroendocrine carcinoma, and small-cell carcinoma. Typical and atypical carcinoid occupy the low-grade, well differentiated end of the spectrum with the latter possessing more malignant histologic and clinical features. Small-cell carcinoma and large-cell neuroendocrine carcinoma represent the high-grade, poorly differentiated end of the neuroendocrine spectrum. Small-cell carcinoma is a distinct clinicopathologic entity with aggressive behavior and widespread metastases and characteristic cytologic features of scant cytoplasm, finely granular chromatin, inconspicuous nucleoli, and frequent mitoses. Large-cell neuroendocrine carcinoma is a large-cell, poorly differentiated carcinoma that shows neuroendocrine features by light microscopy, as well as by immunohistochemistry and electron microscopy. This tumor corresponds most closely to the intermediate-cell differentiated neuroendocrine carcinoma described by Gould et al. (2). Clinical experience with this tumor is limited.

REFERENCES

1. Travis WD, Linnolia RI, Tsoucos MG, et al. Neuroendocrine tumors of the lung with proposed criteria for large-cell neuroendocrine carcinoma. An ultra-structural immunohistochemical, and flow cytometric study of 35 cases. *Am J Surg Pathol* 1991;15:529–53.
2. Gould VE, Linnolia RI, Memoli VA, Warrow WH. Neuroendocrine cells and neuroendocrine neoplasms of the lung. *Pathol Annu* 1983; 18:287–330.

56 Mesothelioma

Charles A. Enke

A tricky disease

CASE PRESENTATION

R.M. is a 71-year-old man who presented with a several-month history of malaise and fatigue, followed by a 2-week history of increasing shortness of breath, dyspnea on exertion, and right pleuritic chest pain. His local physician obtained a chest roentgenogram, which demonstrated a moderately large right pleural effusion. His primary physician performed a thoracentesis, which produced 1,400 cc of bloody fluid. Cytology was felt to be consistent with either atypical mesothelial cells or a well differentiated mesothelioma.

Additional history was significant for a limited history of smoking that was discontinued 30 years ago. The patient also had a history of asbestos exposure during World War II when he worked salvaging naval ships destroyed at Pearl Harbor. The patient denied history of cough or hemoptysis. There was no history of tuberculosis exposure.

Physical exam demonstrated a 71-year-old Caucasian man in no acute distress. No adenopathy was identified. Pulmonary exam revealed dullness to percussion over the lower half of the right lung field. The lungs were otherwise clear. Abdominal exam revealed no organomegaly and no ascites. Examination of the extremities showed no clubbing, cyanosis, or edema.

He underwent a computed tomography (CT) evaluation of the chest and abdomen. The CT scan of the chest demonstrated bilateral pleural calcified plaques consistent with asbestosis (Fig. 56–1). There was a large right pleural effusion with associated pleural thickening, including the mediastinal pleura and diaphragm. There was atelectasis of the right lower and middle lobes. No mediastinal adenopathy was identified. The left thorax

was normal. The CT scan of the abdomen revealed no abnormalities.

Bronchoscopy demonstrated a normal left respiratory tree. No endobronchial lesions were seen on the right side. Compressive atelectasis of the right middle and lower lobes was identified. Bronchial washings were negative for malignancy. Thoracentesis was repeated, followed by biopsy of the right pleura using an Abram's pleural needle. Cytology demonstrated atypical mesothelial cells. Pleural biopsy was felt to be consistent with malignant mesothelioma (Fig. 56–2). The immunophenotype of this histologically and clinically malignant tumor is EMA pos, CK pos, CEA neg, Leu-M1(CD-15) neg, and is diagnostic of malignant mesothelioma in this setting. The patient had stage I disease (T2 N0 M0).

The patient was seen by the Medical Oncology Service, which recommended chest tube placement with sclerotherapy and treatment with MAID chemotherapy regimen (MESNA, adriamycin, ifosfamide, and DTIC). Sclerosis was successfully accomplished with bleomycin. The patient received three cycles of the MAID regimen and then had repeat CT studies, which demonstrated limited improvement of the compressive atelectasis and no evidence of recurrent pleural effusion. Disease remained limited to the right thorax. The patient's dyspnea resolved, as did the pleuritic chest pain. The patient received an additional three cycles of the MAID regimen, which was completed 5 months after diagnosis. The patient was followed up with no clinical change over the next 5 months. He then began to develop significant right pleuritic chest pain along with increasing dyspnea. A follow-up chest CT demonstrated progressive pleural-based disease and interval development of mediastinal adenopathy. Disease did not involve the left thorax or the

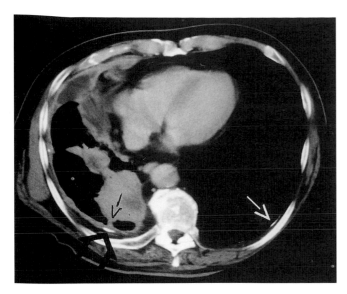

FIG. 56–1. Axial CT of the lower thorax reveals evidence of volume loss of the right lung associated with right lower lobe atelectasis. A focal fluid collection anteriorly is consistent with loculated pleural effusion. Pleural thickening containing calcification (*arrows*) is demonstrated compatible with asbestosis. (Courtesy of Kevin Nelson, M.D.)

abdomen. His pleuritic pain was poorly controlled with infusional morphine.

He was seen by the radiation oncologists, who recommended palliative radiation to the right thorax and mediastinum. A combination of 6-MV photons with lung blocking and electrons were prescribed to treat the pleural rind of tumor, yet spare uninvolved lung parenchyma. A total of 2,600 cGy of the prescribed 4,600 cGy had been delivered when the treatment was terminated because of rapid respiratory deterioration. The patient died shortly after of progressive disease 12 months after diagnosis.

The patient's case was presented to the Tumor Board post mortem. The surgical oncologist did not think that an extrapleural pneumonectomy was an option at presentation because of the involvement of the diaphragm and mediastinal pleura. Intrapleural phototherapy was also mentioned, although it was believed to be limited to pleural-based tumor less than 1 cm thick.

The medical oncologists present did not recommend bleomycin as a sclerosis agent because of concerns about restrictive lung disease development. The recommendation was for a maximum of three cycles of multiagent chemotherapy and then either surgery or radiation.

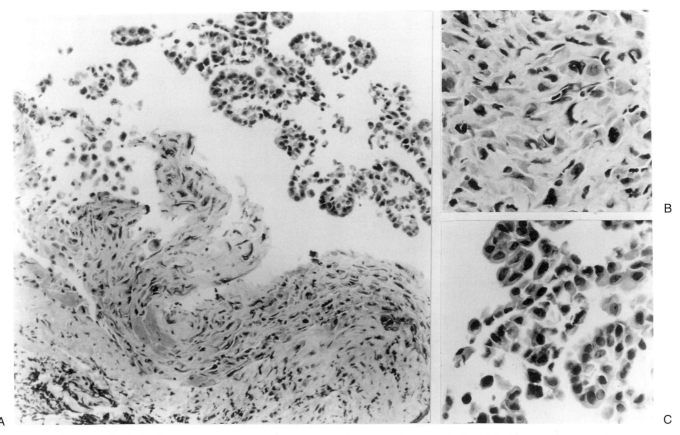

FIG. 56–2. A: Malignant mesothelioma infiltrating the parietal pleura. Note the biphasic pattern and the prominent papillary morphology of the surface tumor (H&E, ×125). **B:** High power view of the infiltrating portion of the tumor (H&E, ×500). **C:** Nuclear atypia in the papillary portion of the tumor (H&E, ×500). (*Mod Pathol* 1993;6:179–184. Courtesy of Mark Hapke, M.D.)

The radiation oncologists indicated that they would have recommended therapy earlier in this patient's disease course. The previous multi-institutional trial comparing radiation with or without low-dose adriamycin was discussed. It was suggested that there was no apparent benefit to adding low-dose adriamycin to radiation treatment. Even though radiation was not initiated until late in this patient's clinical course, it was suggested that his survival with initial chemotherapy was similar to those results reported in the radiation therapy literature.

COMMENTARY by E. Carmack Holmes

Pleural mesothelioma is an uncommon tumor with about 2,000 cases reported annually in the United States. It has, however, become a very important disease because of its association with industrial carcinogens, notably asbestos. The disease is found in Navy yard workers, asbestos factory workers, steampipe fitters, and other similar professions. Frequently, the exposure to asbestos can be 20 or more years before the onset of the malignancy. It has been reported that individuals with heavy exposure to asbestos have a 300-fold increase in the frequency of mesotheliomas. It has even been suggested that particles of asbestos carried home on the clothing of asbestos workers may pose a hazard for family members.

There is a benign form of mesothelioma. The two malignant forms comprise the fibrosarcomatous type and the epithelial type.

Malignant mesothelioma is a fatal disease, and attempts at effective treatment have, in general, been disappointing. The patients remain relatively asymptomatic until the disease is fairly advanced; therefore, the natural history is poorly understood. Malignant pleural mesothelioma tends to remain localized to the pleural space with progressive growth at that site but, eventually, mesothelioma can metastasize both to the regional lymph nodes and systemically.

Numerous attempts have been made to improve the therapy for patients with malignant pleural mesothelioma. Some have advocated radical extrapleural pneumonectomy, but many have discarded this procedure. Others feel that there is a role for extrapleural pneumonectomy in patients with more limited disease. However, there is no evidence that extrapleural pneumonectomy has a significant impact on overall survival (1). Another technique that has been employed is to perform a surgical pleurectomy without removing the lung. This can be followed by external beam radiation therapy or direct installation of chemotherapeutic agents into the pleural cavity (2).

Our approach to malignant mesothelioma consists of performing a thoracoscopy and confirming the diagnoses identifying the extent of disease. We investigated the use of installation of intrapleural cisplatin and cytosine arabinoside and have now abandoned this treatment. Instead, at the time of thoracoscopy, we insufflate talc to insure pleuradesis. Postoperatively, the trocar incision sites are irradiated to prevent local wound recurrence. Recurrence at thoracentesis sites and thoracotomy incisions are not uncommon, and these areas should be irradiated prophylactically to prevent soft tissue recurrence in these scars.

Chemotherapy for mesothelioma remains experimental. A number of different regimens have been evaluated, but none have been found to be superior to other chemotherapeutic modalities and, indeed, there is little evidence that chemotherapy improves survival. The hallmark of management is palliation, and radiation therapy can be used effectively to palliate chest wall pain.

The case presented is a typical example of the presentation of mesothelioma. The bloody pleural effusion and the CT scan findings are characteristic of mesothelioma. In this instance, a diagnosis was obtained without a thoracoscopy. Sclerosis was successfully and adequately accomplished with bleomycin. This patient probably did not benefit from chemotherapy. Unless there is a clinical protocol evaluating a chemotherapeutic regimen, we would not treat this patient with chemotherapy. Rather, we would use radiation therapy to palliate symptoms as they develop. This patient died of progressive disease 12 months after the diagnosis, which is the typical course that these patients have.

REFERENCES

1. Rush VW, Piantadosi S, Holmes EC. The role of extrapleural pneumonectomy in malignant pleural mesothelioma. *J Thorac Cardiovasc Surg* 1991;102:1–9.
2. Sugarbaker DJ, Heher EC, Lee TH, Couper G, et al. Extrapleural pneumonectomy, chemotherapy and radiotherapy in the treatment of diffuse malignant pleural mesothelioma. *J Thorac Cardiovasc Surg* 1991;102:10–5.

57 Pancoast Tumor

Joseph Miller

Shoulder pain in a smoker requires a chest roentgenogram

CASE PRESENTATION

The patient is a 67-year old man who presented to his family physician with left shoulder pain. He was referred to an orthopedist, who diagnosed bursitis of the left shoulder and treated it with cortisone. When symptoms persisted for 6 weeks, he again went to his internist who, at that time, did a routine chest roentgenogram. The chest radiograph showed a left apical mass. On further questioning, the patient described a dull pain in the left neck, arm, and shoulder. He had numbness and tingling into the distribution of the ulnar nerve to the level of the elbow. A review of systems was negative except for a 40 to 45-year smoking history of two packs per day.

Physical examination was negative except for hypertrophic pulmonary osteoarthropathy. There was no Horner's syndrome. Workup included a chest radiograph (Fig. 57–1), which showed a left apical density. The computed tomography (CT) scan showed a large left upper mass lying adjacent to the vertebral body of T1 and T2. An magnetic resonance image (MRI) (Fig. 57–2) showed the mass in the left upper lobe with no involvement of the subclavian artery or vein. Bone scan showed destruction of the first and second ribs. Fiberoptic bronchoscopy was nonremarkable. A fine-needle aspiration was performed and was positive for large-cell carcinoma of the lung.

Physiologically, the patient had good pulmonary function and underwent an exercise treadmill test for physiologic cardiac staging. The ETT was negative. The patient was diagnosed as having a classic Pancoast tumor and referred to the section of radiation oncology for preoperative radiation therapy. He received 3,000 Gy preoperatively according to the original criteria of Paulson and Wood. Three thousand rads were delivered in 300-rad fractions over 10 days. He was allowed a 2-week rest period and then readmitted.

He was taken to the operating room, where he underwent an en bloc left upper lobectomy with chest wall resection of the first, second, and third ribs along with the sensory division of the lower cord of the brachial plexus. He remained intubated 3 days postoperatively. The remainder of his postoperative course was uneventful. He was surgically dismissed on his 12th postoperative day. Two weeks later he returned and was doing quite well. He was then referred to radiation therapy for an additional 2,500 Gy.

The final pathology was a large-cell carcinoma of the lung with margins clear and all nodes negative. Pathologic staging was T3 N0 M0 stage IIIA (i.e., chest wall involvement).

On the basis of our experience, the expected 5-year survival is 30%.

TUMOR BOARD DISCUSSION

Pancoast tumor was originally described by Pancoast in 1936. Terminology should distinguish between Pancoast tumor, which is a tumor in the superior pulmonary sulcus associated with shoulder and arm pain versus Pancoast syndrome, which includes the same radiographic and clinical features of Pancoast tumor plus a Horner's syndrome. Classical symptomatology and radiographic findings consist of a density in the pulmonary sulcus with pain in the shoulder/neck/arm and is associated with symptoms of involvement of the C6-C7 nerve root. Before the report of Paulson in 1966, there was no significant reported 5-year survival. In 1966, Paulson presented data

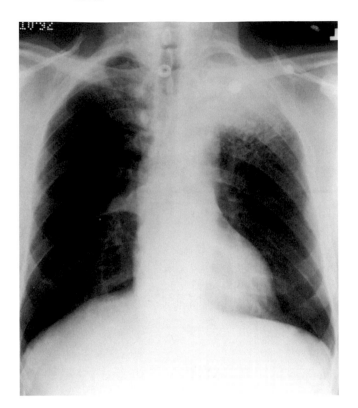

FIG. 57–1. Chest radiograph showing a left apical density.

on 17 patients treated with 3,000 rads preoperatively followed by en bloc resection of the upper lobe/first, second, and third ribs and sensory division of the ulnar nerve. They subsequently reported a 31% 5-year survival. We have basically followed the original protocol of 3,000 rads given preoperatively followed by surgical resection. For the past 15 years we have added an additional 2,500 rads postoperatively. In a previously reported series we had a 31% actuarial 5-year survival rate.

Preoperative evaluation should consist of a chest roentgenogram, CT scan, MRI of neck, brachial plexus, and vertebral bodies, bone scan, CT or MRI of brain, PFTs, and ETT. A diagnosis can generally be made by fine-needle aspiration.

Radiation therapy is given preoperatively to 3,000 rads. Some radiation therapists advocate 4,500 rads preoperatively. A delay of 2 weeks is given, followed by surgical resection. We have found it useful to leave the patient intubated for 3 days to allow the chest wall to stabilize, and this tends to prevent collapse of the remaining lung on the operated side. Although not advocated by all authors, we have found the addition of postoperative radiotherapy to decrease the chance for local recurrence. Extensive vertebral body involvement, involvement of the subclavian artery and vein, and extensive involvement of the brachial plexus is generally considered a contraindication to resection. The expected 5-year survival is 25% to 33%.

COMMENTARY by James D. Cox

The history of a left apical sulcus tumor in this 67-year-old man is a common one for this infrequent presentation of carcinoma of the lung. The vague discomfort leading to a tentative benign diagnosis and then discovery of the apical mass is common.

Apical sulcus tumors first characterized by Henry Pancoast in 1936 constitute approximately 3% of all carcinomas of the lung at the present time. Any histopathologic type can present in the apical sulcus. Adenocarcinomas and large-cell carcinomas, as in this case, are most frequent.

With current imaging approaches, the resectability of patients can usually be well assessed. The traditional approach to treatment was followed in this case with a brief course of preoperative radiation therapy followed by resection. This approach made good sense in the era when it was developed by Paulson. It was assumed that the surgical resection, complete or incomplete as it might be, was the only available treatment for such patients.

The work of Komaki and her colleagues at the Medical College of Wisconsin demonstrated the potential curability of patients with unresectable Pancoast tumors, opening the door for different approaches in planning overall management of these patients. The success of definitive radiation therapy is clearly related to the total dose that must be delivered to these large and invasive tumors. Therefore, it is important not to compromise the time-dose factors in radiotherapeutic management of patients with apical sulcus tumors by the split course, as was practiced in this case.

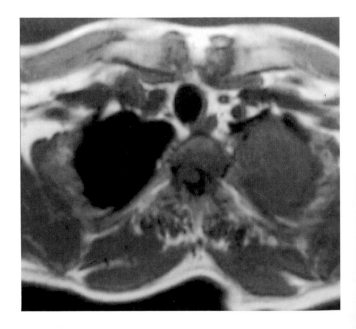

FIG. 57–2. MRI scan showing no involvement of the subclavian artery or vein.

In the case at hand, it is probable that no disadvantage of the preoperative irradiation occurred. There is certainly no evidence that there was any advantage to this treatment, although theoretically, there should be. If, however, the patient had proved not to have a resectable tumor, there was no possibility of doing the required high-dose continuous radiation therapy that might have offered him cure if unresectable.

In the case described, there was a period of approximately 40 days between the end of the preoperative radiation therapy and the resumption of irradiation postoperatively. With this great delay, the 25 Gy given postoperatively has little biologic effect and in many cases may actually be given to a tumor that is recurring if there is microscopic residual. In a study of definitive radiation therapy for non–small-cell carcinoma of the lung, interruptions of 5 days or more in a planned course of high-dose radiation therapy to the most favorable patients resulted in a much lower survival than those patients who completed the course of treatment without interruptions or delays.

At the University of Texas M.D. Anderson Cancer Center, the current approach to apical sulcus tumors is predicated on surgical resection without prior chemotherapy or radiation therapy. If the tumor is unresectable, definitive radiation therapy combined with chemotherapy can be used. If resection is completed successfully, postoperative radiation therapy with 1.2 Gy twice daily to a total dose of 69.6 Gy is accompanied by concurrent oral etoposide and cisplatin. This sequence of events gives the total group of patients with Pancoast tumors the greatest probability of cure.

SELECTED READINGS

1. Komaki R, Roh J, Cox JD, Lopes da Conceicao A. Superior sulcus tumors: results of irradiation of 36 patients. *Cancer* 1981;48:1563–8.
2. Komaki R. Prognostic factors of 85 patients with superior sulcus tumors (stage III) treated at M. D. Anderson Cancer Center, presented at the IASLC Workshop: controversies in staging and treatment of locally advanced NSC lung cancer, Bruges, Belgium, June 17–21, 1990.
3. Cox JD, Pajak TF, Asbell S, Russell AH, Pedersen J, Byhardt R, Emami B, Roach III M. Interruptions of high-dose radiation therapy decrease long-term survival of favorable patients with unresectable non-small cell carcinoma of the lung. *Int J Radiat Oncol Biol Phys* 1993;27:493–8.

EDITORIAL BOARD COMMENTARY

The case report describes destruction of first and second ribs on bone scan. Usually bone scans describe abnormal uptake, but seldom "destruction." The results of the pathology report do not include the histology of the ribs, which is needed for pathologic staging. The reason for a treadmill exercise test is not stated.

58

T3 N2 Adenocarcinoma of the Lung

Larry R. Kaiser, Angela B. Wurster, and Leslie A. Litzky

A high rate of failure despite vigorous efforts

CASE PRESENTATION

V.P. is a 48-year-old white man who initially presented to his local physician in September 1991 with severe right shoulder pain. This pain extended along the posterior aspect of his right shoulder and continued along the ulnar distribution of his right upper extremity. Additionally, he noted weakness in his right hand such that he was unable to use a nail clipper, but could button his shirt.

A chest radiograph revealed a right apical lung lesion (Fig. 58–1). A magnetic resonance imaging (MRI) scan of the spine was within normal limits. A computed tomography (CT) scan of the chest was performed and confirmed the presence of a 5-cm right upper lobe lesion with ipsilateral mediastinal and hilar adenopathy (Fig. 58–2). There was no involvement of the vertebral bodies, but a radionuclide bone scan showed increased uptake in the right first and second ribs compatible with direct extension of the primary tumor mass. A core-needle biopsy was successful in obtaining diagnostic material that showed the lesion to be a poorly differentiated adenocarcinoma. By clinical criteria, he was staged as T3 N2 M0 and further invasive staging procedures were not performed.

Chemotherapy with mitomycin, velban, and cisplatin was begun with the thought that the patient would proceed to resection after completion of three cycles. At the conclusion of the chemotherapy regimen he was seen by a surgeon, who felt the patient had not responded sufficiently to the preoperative regimen to warrant resection. The patient began a course of radiation therapy on February 3 and completed it on March 11, receiving a total of 5,040 cGy in 28 fractions. During this period he was able to maintain his weight and performance status.

He presented to our office for a second surgical opinion just before completing his course of radiation therapy. His major complaint was continued right shoulder pain as well as pain along the medial aspect of the right upper extremity. His past medical history was notable only for minor episodes of back pain. He denied any history of shortness of breath, cardiovascular disease, diabetes, or weight loss. During his military service in Korea 30 years previously, he sustained a gunshot wound to the abdomen that necessitated a laparotomy and bowel resection. The bullet traversed the liver and entered the right hemithorax for which a chest tube was placed, but a thoracotomy was not required. His medications at the time of his first visit included MS contin 30 mg b.i.d., prednisone 10 mg t.i.d., naprosyn 250 mg b.i.d., and ativan 1 mg as needed. He smoked two packs of cigarettes per day for 34 years and quit 1 year previously. He worked for 30 years as a plumber and stated that he was aware of prior asbestos exposure. His family history was remarkable in that his mother died of breast cancer.

On physical examination, he was a healthy-appearing, slightly obese white man, 5' 7" tall, 203 pounds. He had no evidence of a Horner's syndrome. There were no palpable cervical or supraclavicular lymph nodes. Inspection of the chest revealed his radiation therapy tattoos, a previous tube thoracostomy site on the right, and minimal skin tanning in the irradiated field. Auscultation of the chest demonstrated good air entry bilaterally with no crackles, wheezes, or bronchial breath sounds. His heart rate was regular at 80 beats per minute, with a normal S1 and S2, and no murmur was heard. Examination of the abdomen showed a well-healed midline incision, and no hepatomegaly or other masses. The right hand had dimin-

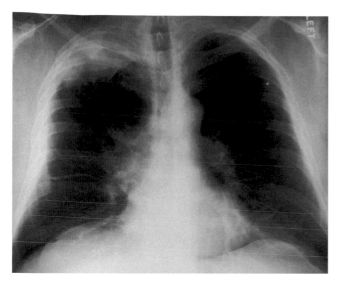

FIG. 58–1. Initial chest radiograph demonstrating the left apical lung mass with associated fullness of the right hilum and superior mediastinum.

ished grip strength and moderate weakness of the intrinsic muscles with no definite wasting of the muscles noted. No sensory loss could be demonstrated.

At the time of our consultation, a repeat CT scan of the chest was obtained, which demonstrated a partial response to the chemotherapy and radiation with a reduction in tumor size and mediastinal and hilar adenopathy (Fig. 58–3). A repeat chest radiograph was also consistent with a partial response to therapy (Fig. 58–4). We also obtained an MRI scan of the chest to assess further the proximity of the tumor to the brachial plexus, subclavian vessels, and vertebral bodies (Fig. 58–5). A full extent of disease workup was also repeated, which failed to demonstrate evidence of disseminated disease. Pulmonary function studies were normal.

On March 31, 3 weeks after completion of radiation therapy, the patient underwent flexible fiberoptic bronchoscopy and mediastinoscopy. No endobronchial lesions were noted and right level II (upper paratracheal), level IV (lower paratracheal), level VII (subcarinal), and left level IV lymph nodes were all negative for tumor. Two days later, a right upper lobectomy with resection of the chest wall and ribs 1 through 3 along with a mediastinal

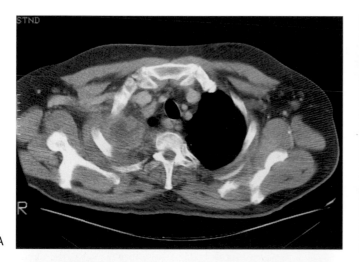

A

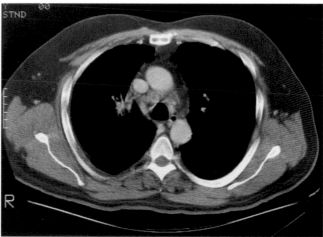

B

C

FIG. 58–2. A: Initial CT scan showing the right apical lung mass with probable involvement of chest wall. **B:** Right paratracheal adenopathy (1.5 cm) is seen adjacent to the superior vena cava. **C:** 2.5-cm subcarinal mass.

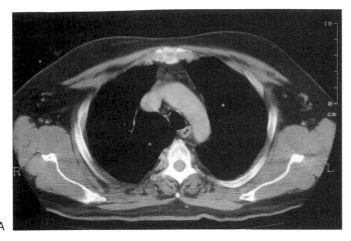

A

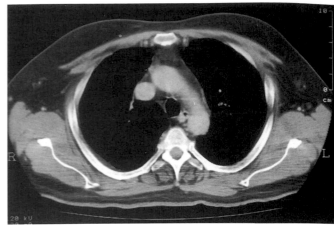

B

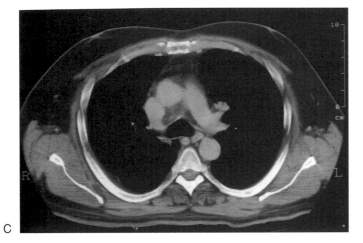

C

FIG. 58–3. A: CT scan performed after radiation therapy and chemotherapy demonstrating reduction in size of the previously seen paratracheal adenopathy. **B:** CT slice at the inferior border of the aortic arch showing no evidence of paratracheal adenopathy. **C:** A significant decrease in the size of the subcarinal adenopathy is also seen.

lymph node dissection was performed. The tumor involved the lower cord of the brachial plexus and it was necessary to take the T_1 nerve root. The C_8 nerve root was spared. The subclavian vessels were not involved. All resection margins were negative. Despite the intensive preoperative therapy, viable tumor was present in the resected specimen (Fig. 58–6). His course immediately after the operation was uneventful and he was discharged on the eighth postoperative day. He was begun on a program of physical therapy to improve the strength and coordination of the right hand. His grip strength was slightly diminished and fine motor tasks were difficult, as they had been preoperatively. He remained on MS contin for pain at the time of discharge.

At his first postoperative visit 3 weeks after discharge, the patient felt that both the pain and the strength in his right upper extremity were improved. His wound had healed nicely. He was re-evaluated by his radiation oncologist who, based on the completeness of the resection, recommended no further radiation therapy. Approximately 2 months later, he noted the onset of severe left hip pain that troubled him more than his right upper extremity symptoms and he was losing weight. On July 22 he was

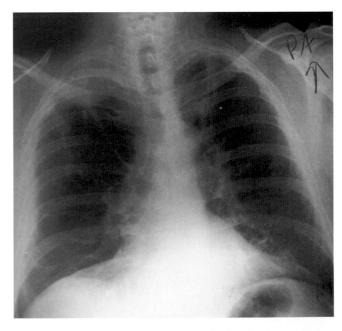

FIG. 58–4. Chest roentgenogram obtained after radiation and chemotherapy showing a decrease in the size of the primary lesion as well as the hilar fullness.

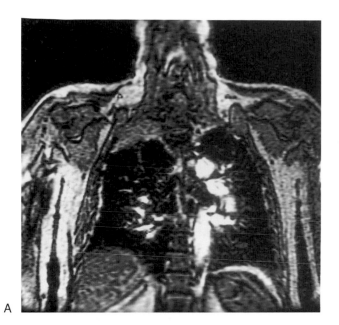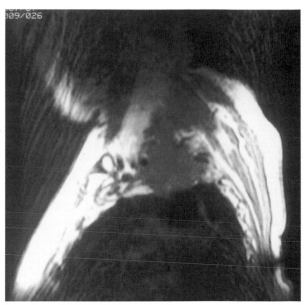

A   B

FIG. 58–5. Coronal (**A**) and sagittal (**B**) MRI images showing the apical lung lesion after the preoperative therapy. There was no evidence of vertebral body or subclavian vessel involvement.

noted to have a 5-cm left axillary mass as well as several subcutaneous nodules over the left upper quadrant of his abdomen, each measuring 2 to 3 cm in size. Needle-aspiration biopsy of the left axillary mass was positive for adenocarcinoma. He died on August 1 before the initiation of any further therapy.

COMMENTARY by Robert B. Livingston

The case presented is that of a middle-aged smoker who developed a superior sulcus tumor, accompanied by signs and symptoms indicative of brachial plexus involvement. He underwent noninvasive staging, which demonstrated

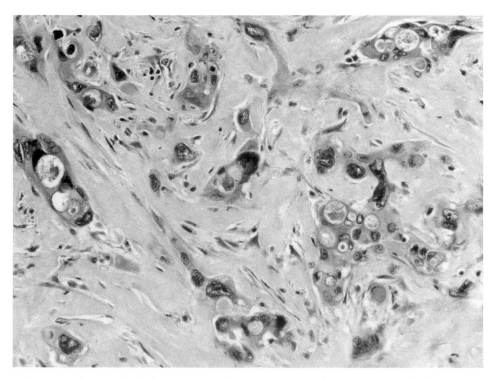

FIG. 58–6. Photomicrograph of the resected primary lung tumor demonstrating an infiltrating, poorly differentiated adenocarcinoma with a prominent desmoplastic response (H&E, ×200).

enlarged mediastinal nodes, including a 2.5-cm subcarinal mass. A radionuclide bone scan "showed increased uptake in the right first and second ribs compatible with direct extension of the tumor mass," and the tumor was deemed clinical T3 N2 M0 (clinical stage IIIA). He then received three cycles of "neoadjuvant" mitomycin, vinblastine, and cisplatin chemotherapy, but went on to radiation therapy rather than resection as the next step because he was felt to have an inadequate response. The radiation therapy was given to an unspecified treatment volume at 180 cGy per fraction to a total of 5,040 cGy. Because of persistent brachial plexus symptoms despite irradiation, the patient sought a second surgical opinion, which led to radiographic studies that demonstrated a partial response and no evidence of disseminated disease. After a negative mediastinoscopy, he underwent lobectomy with resection of the chest wall and ribs 1 through 3, plus a mediastinal node dissection and sacrifice of the T_1 nerve root to obtain negative resection margins. We learn that "viable tumor was present in the resected specimen," but not in the nodes, and apparently the ribs were uninvolved, because his postsurgical classification was T3 N0 M0. No more therapy was given and, unfortunately, within a few months he developed distant recurrence that proved to be rapidly fatal.

This patient did not have "standard" therapy for an operable superior sulcus tumor, which is generally considered to be preoperative irradiation followed by surgery (1). The decision not to follow this course of action may have been the presence of N2 nodes presumed pathologic by reason of size on his staging CT scan. Some would argue that he should have undergone mediastinoscopy to prove that these N2 nodes were positive, but a 2.5-cm nodal mass is very likely to be positive (2). MVP chemotherapy was given, probably based on the reports from the Memorial Hospital group that many patients with "IIIA, N2" disease by chest roentgenographic criteria can be made resectable using that regimen, and the favorable initial survival experience reported for this neoadjuvant approach (3). No resection was performed after completion of the MVP, however, because he was judged to have an inadequate response, presumably by radiographic criteria. This decision not to resect can be criticized, because by radiographic criteria he still had only a partial response when he was ultimately resected, after the completion of chest irradiation, and yet microscopically these enlarged nodal masses contained no viable tumor. We now know that "evident" persistent disease, by radiographic criteria after completion of neoadjuvant therapy, may often be a false positive (4).

Radiation therapy was conservative, presumably because of the prior exposure to MVP and some (justifiable) fear of a potential toxic interaction on lung tissue between mitomycin C and ionizing irradiation. However, the findings at subsequent surgical resection indicate that it and/or the chemotherapy was capable of sterilizing the nodal disease, an observation that has been made before with preoperative irradiation alone. Despite a very aggressive ultimate surgical approach, with a complex lobectomy and sacrifice of the T_1 branchial plexus root, this patient manifested hematogenous early dissemination and death, an event that remains common despite our best efforts. Adenocarcinoma of the lung usually fails at systemic sites rather than locally (5), and has become the most common histologic type in the United States among non–small-cell cancers (6).

Another approach with promising results for patients with "IIIA, N2" and even selected IIIB patients involves concurrent, combined cisplatin-etoposide chemotherapy and chest irradiation, followed by surgical resection (7). The Southwest Oncology Group has observed resectability in 73% of such patients, all of whom were surgically staged, and 2-year survival is in the range of 35% for both IIIA and IIIB. A large intergroup trial is now underway to compare this approach to more intensive chemotherapy and irradiation without subsequent resection because the contribution of the surgery to outcome in these patients remains problematic. That trial is aimed at "IIIA, N2" disease, excluding superior sulcus lesions, but a companion study for Pancoast tumors is under development.

REFERENCES

1. Paulson DL. The "superior sulcus" lesion. In: *Lung cancer,* Delarue NC, Eschapasse H, eds. Philadelphia: WB Saunders; 1985.
2. Holmes EC, Livingston R, Turrisi R. Neoplasms of the thorax. In: *Cancer medicine,* 3rd ed., Holland JF, Frei E, Bast RC, Kufe DW, Morton DL, Weichselbaum RR, eds. Philadelphia: Lea & Febiger; 1993.
3. Gralla RJ. Preoperative and adjuvant chemotherapy in non-small cell lung cancer. *Semin Oncol* 1988;15:8–12.
4. Taylor SG, Trybula M, Bonomi PD, et al. Simultaneous cisplatin fluorouracil infusion and radiation followed by surgical resection in regionally localized stage III, non-small cell lung cancer. *Ann Thorac Surg* 1987;43:87–91.
5. Matthews MJ, Kanhouwa S, Pickren J, et al. Frequency of residual and metastatic tumor in patients undergoing curative surgical resection for lung cancer. *Cancer Chemother Rep* 1973;4:63–7.
6. Vincent RG, Pickren JW, Lane WW, et al. The changing histopathology of lung cancer. *Cancer* 1977;39:1647–55.
7. Rusch VW, Crowley JJ, Lonchyna V, Livingston, RB, Benfield JR. Surgical resection of stage IIIA and stage IIIB non-small cell lung cancer after concurrent induction chemoradiotherapy. A Southwest Oncology Group trial. *J Thorac Cardiovasc Surg* 1993;105:97–106.

EDITORIAL BOARD COMMENTARY

The "final surgical staging" was not T3 N0 M0. Staging is established before definitive therapies. He was a clinical T3 N2 M0 (clinical stage IIIA), but pathologic staging cannot be established because pathologic staging cannot be made after chemotherapy and/or radiotherapy.

59

Bronchoalveolar Carcinoma

L. Penfield Faber

Learn from a classic case

CASE PRESENTATION

A 68-year-old Caucasian male patient presented to his local physician with a new onset cough productive of a thin, watery sputum. The cough was not purulent, and the patient denied any evidence of blood in the sputum. He complained of a mild lower chest pain that seemed to radiate laterally and to the right upper quadrant. He denied fever, weight loss, and any prior malignancy. He had stopped smoking 35 years ago. He denied any significant occupational exposure, including asbestos, and he worked as an accountant in an office setting. Physical examination revealed a healthy-appearing 68-year-old man who did not appear to be particularly ill. Examination of the head and neck revealed no palpable adenopathy. The contour of the chest was normal, and palpation did not elicit any chest pain. Coarse rales were heard in the right posterior lung base, and the remainder of the right and left lung fields were clear to auscultation. Heart tones were normal and examination of the abdomen was free of any significant findings.

A chest radiograph was obtained and identified an infiltrate in the right lower lobe (Fig. 59–1). A clinical diagnosis of pneumonitis was made and the patient was placed on broad-spectrum antibiotics. He presented to his physician 14 days later, stating that his cough was the same and the right lower chest discomfort was persisting. A repeat chest radiograph revealed similar findings and a bronchoscopy was recommended. This examination identified a normal-appearing tracheobronchial tree on both the right and left sides, and the orifice of the right lower lobe was patent without any evidence of neoplasm or obstruction. In view of the persistent infiltrate in the right lower lobe, a bronchial brushing and transbronchial biopsy were carried out. The bronchial brushing revealed cells consistent with a diagnosis of adenocarcinoma, and the transbronchial biopsy revealed a highly atypical glandular pattern that was suspicious for adenocarcinoma. A diagnosis of adenocarcinoma of the lung was entertained.

Discussant: How should clinical staging of this patient be carried out?

Thoracic surgeon: Bronchoscopy has established a diagnosis of carcinoma, and the next important step would be to obtain a computed tomography (CT) scan of the chest, liver, and adrenals. The CT scan includes the liver and adrenals to rule out metastasis to these organs, as they are a common repository for metastatic disease from lung cancer. It is important to evaluate the hilum and mediastinum for any lymph node enlargement. Cervical mediastinoscopy is indicated when mediastinal lymph nodes are greater than 1 cm in diameter, as the finding of metastatic carcinoma in mediastinal lymph nodes changes the clinical staging of the patient from a stage I or stage II to a stage IIIA. Positive mediastinal nodes would indicate consideration for neoadjuvant therapy or a decision that the patient is not an operative candidate. In this patient, the CT scan was negative for any involvement of the liver or adrenals, and mediastinal lymph nodes were not enlarged (Fig. 59–2). The bronchoscopic examination had revealed a normal right lower lobe bronchus, and the patient is a candidate for right lower lobectomy.

Discussant: There was no mention of bone scan or brain scan as part of the clinical staging program.

Thoracic surgeon: This patient had no evidence of central nervous symptomatology and did not complain of bone pain. It was thought that the infiltrate in the base of the right lower lobe was irritating the pleura and was a cause of the chest pain. If there was concern about any of

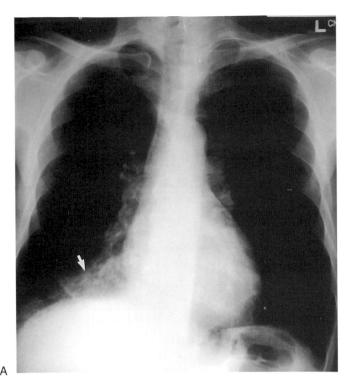

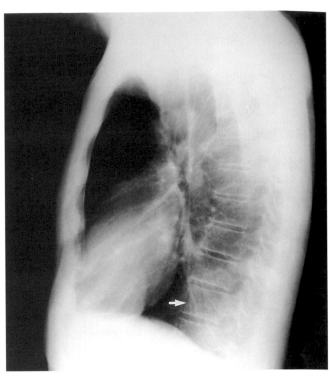

A

B

FIG. 59–1. A: PA film of the chest shows an infiltrate in the base of the right lower lobe. **B:** Lateral chest radiograph that also identifies the infiltrate.

the patient's pain being evidence of metastatic bone disease, then a bone scan should be obtained. In asymptomatic patients who have proven lung cancer, the incidence of unsuspected bone or brain disease is approximately 6% or 7%. One must consider the usefulness of these studies in relationship to this low yield. Therefore, these studies were not done on this patient.

The patient had a right thoracotomy, and careful evaluation of the entire lung revealed the right middle and right upper lobes to be entirely within normal limits. There was no palpable evidence of extension of the disease into the right hilum or the superior mediastinum. The base of the right lower lobe was consolidated and did not appear to be a masslike lesion as one customarily sees with bronchogenic carcinoma. A right lower lobectomy was carried out, along with an appropriate mediastinal lymphadenectomy.

Pathologist: A significant portion of the right lower lobe had a solid consistency with edema and gray discoloration. Histologic evaluation revealed the characteristic findings of a bronchioloalveolar carcinoma. Cuboidal or cylindrical cells line the alveolar septa and the basic pulmonary architecture was preserved (Fig. 59–3). The hilar (level 11), subcarinal (level VII), and mediastinal (levels II and IV) lymph nodes were all negative for any evidence of metastatic carcinoma. The pathologic diagnosis was bronchioloalveolar carcinoma.

Discussant: Was any postoperative adjuvant therapy recommended?

Oncologist: There is certainly no indication for radiation, as all of the regional lymph nodes are free of any evidence of metastatic carcinoma. Even though this diffuse type of bronchioloalveolar carcinoma may subsequently appear in other areas of the lung, there is no indication for postoperative chemotherapy.

Thoracic surgeon: The patient did well after the lobectomy, and the 6-month follow-up chest radiograph was satisfactory. He was referred back to his physician, and at 18 months after the surgical procedure, the patient again complained of cough. A chest radiograph revealed a patchy infiltrate in the right middle lobe, as well as a patchy infiltrate in the left upper lobe (Fig. 59–4). He had no fever and denied chest pain, hemoptysis, and weight loss.

Discussant: Is there any consideration that this is something other than recurrent bronchioloalveolar carcinoma?

Thoracic surgeon: It is well known that the diffuse type of bronchioloalveolar carcinoma is probably multicentric in origin, and it was clinically felt that the new infiltrates represented recurrence of the cancer. They again had the characteristic pattern of this type of cancer.

Discussant: Should bronchoscopy and clinical staging be repeated?

Thoracic surgeon: The infiltrate is not particularly sizable, and bronchoscopy by brushing and transbronchial

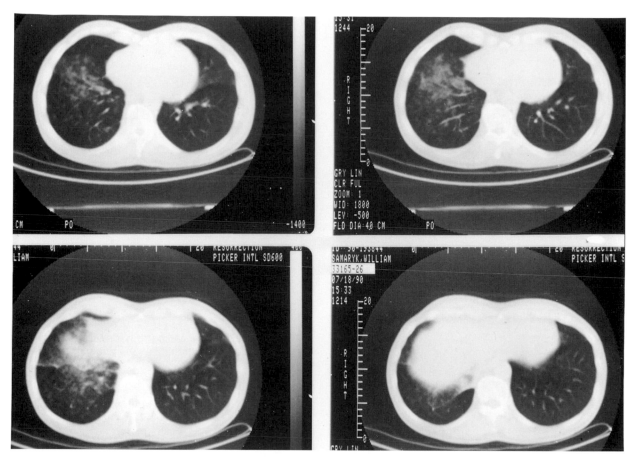

FIG. 59–2. CT scan depicts the parenchymal infiltrate in the base of the right lower lobe. Other cuts demonstrated no adenopathy.

techniques may not establish histologic confirmation of recurrent cancer. The sputum cytology might be helpful in this regard, but the clinical pattern is so classic that further studies were not carried out. The disease is certainly not resectable, and whether mediastinal lymph nodes are enlarged or not, it is not particularly important to the clinical management of this patient. Bronchioloalveolar carcinoma metastasizes late in its course to distant organs, and bone scan and brain scan would not be particularly helpful as long as he is asymptomatic in this regard.

Discussant: How should he be treated?

Medical oncologist: Chemotherapy is not particularly effective for bronchioloalveolar carcinoma. However, it would be appropriate to consider a trial of cisplatin and etoposide for this patient. He can be followed up with serial chest radiographs to determine if there is any clinical improvement. As the disease is now diffuse, pulmonary functions can also be monitored. This patient was managed with three cycles of chemotherapy. Unfortunately, his chest radiograph did not demonstrate any improvement, and because of some side effects from the chemotherapy, the patient elected not to proceed with any further treatment. He has had a surprisingly protracted

course after the clinical appearance of the recurrent cancer. Chest radiograph reveals worsening of the cancer (Fig. 59–5), and the patient requires continuous oxygen therapy for severe shortness of breath.

He remains alive 5 years after the right lower lobectomy.

COMMENTARY by E.C. Holmes

This patient presents in a typical manner for bronchoalveolar carcinoma (BAC). These patients frequently are diagnosed with pneumonia. This is particularly true for the diffuse BAC, which can involve an entire lobe. Clinical staging as performed in this case is appropriate. Indeed, metastases to the brain from bronchoalveolar carcinoma are much less common than for other types of non–small-cell lung cancer. Typically, bronchoalveolar carcinoma does not respond well to chemotherapy and, therefore, postoperative adjuvant chemotherapy is not recommended in these patients.

Recent studies at UCLA have indicated that over a period of 35 years, from 1955 to 1990, BAC rose from less than 5% to 24% of all lung cancer seen at UCLA

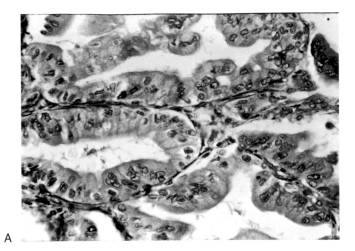

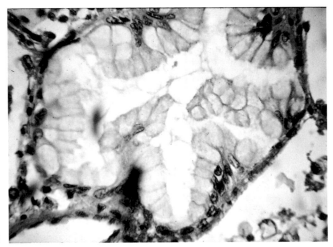

FIG. 59–3. A: A cuboidal and cylindrical pattern is noted in the cells lining the alveolar septa. **B:** Basic pulmonary architecture is preserved, but the alveolus is filled with the cancer cells.

($p<0.001$) (1). This increase occurred predominantly in women, and the male to female ratio was approximately 1:1. Clearly, the incidence of bronchoalveolar carcinoma is higher in the female population than in the male population. In contrast to other forms of lung cancer, bronchoalveolar carcinoma showed a high incidence of multifocality (25% vs. 5%, $p<0.001$). The mucinous subtype in this study was more strongly associated with diffused pulmonic involvement, and the sclerotic subtype was more strongly associated with multifocal involvement. At UCLA, BAC is now the most common type of lung cancer diagnosed, and is approximately equal in incidence to squamous carcinoma and other adenocarcinomas. A similar increase has been reported in Japan, and the sex distribution noted in the UCLA study has been confirmed by others (2). Also, it has been noted that BAC is not strongly associated with smoking. In the UCLA study, approximately 30% of the patients never smoked, and 30% smoked only intermittently or remotely.

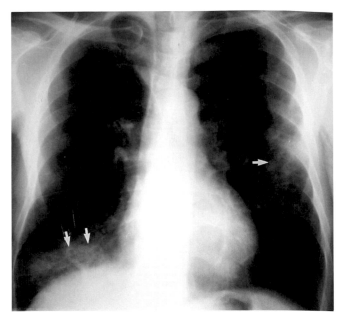

FIG. 59–4. PA chest radiograph identifies infiltrative cancer in the base of the right middle lobe and in the lateral left lung.

The Lung Cancer Study Group reviewed 235 patients with pure BAC (3). They also observed that bronchoalveolar carcinoma was common in patients who did not smoke. This study also showed that bronchoalveolar had a better overall survival than other forms of non–small-cell lung cancer, and

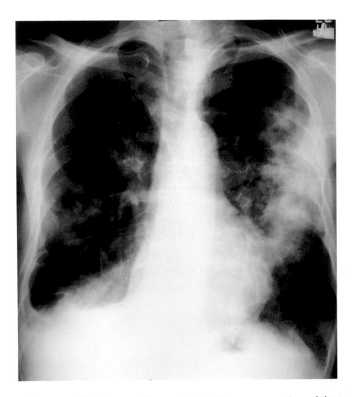

FIG. 59–5. PA chest radiograph identifies progression of the bronchioloalveolar carcinoma

had a significantly lower incidence of brain metastases. The Lung Cancer Study Group also observed that bronchoalveolar carcinoma occurs more frequently in those without a history of smoking than does adenocarcinoma.

BAC clearly is a unique subset of non–small-cell lung cancer. It closely resembles a retrovirally mediated endemic disease of sheep called "jaagsiekte" or sheep pulmonic adenomatosis, a disease that shares with its human counterpart a propensity for diffuseness and multifocality (4). Although there has never been direct evidence indicating a viral etiology for human BAC, occasional reports of sheep farmers developing the diffuse form of BAC and its histologic resemblance to "jaagsiekte" has raised the possibility of a viral origin for human BAC. The dramatic increase in incidence, the younger age distribution, the nearly 1:1 sex ratio distribution, and a high incidence of multifocality suggests the possibility of a virus-initiated or -promoted disease.

The multifocal nature of BAC was first described by Malassez in the 19th century (5). The basis of BAC multifocality has always assumed to be the tumor's inherent propensity for spreading along alveolar routes. Recent studies using molecular markers argue against this intrapulmonary aerosol/aspiration or lymphatic spread. These molecular studies provide evidence for a multicolonality as a basis for some cases of multifocal BAC.

These molecular studies strongly suggest that the multifocality of BAC is not due to direct spread, but to true multicentric origin of multicolonal tumors (6). Clearly, bronchoalveolar carcinoma is a unique type of lung cancer with distinguishing pathologic, biologic, epidemiologic and, perhaps, etiologic features that set it apart from all other forms of lung cancer. These unique characteristics of this tumor have certain implications for their management. Their overall good survival suggests that an aggressive surgical approach should be taken. The lack of high incidence of brain metastases indicates that these tumors do not have the same aggressive tendencies to disseminate as do other non–small-cell lung cancers, and the multifocality of these tumors suggests that parenchymal sparing procedures should be performed by the surgeon.

REFERENCES

1. Barsky SH, Cameron R, Osann KE, et al. Rising incidence of bronchoalveolar lung cancer and its unique clinico-pathological features. *Cancer* 1994;73:1163–70.
2. Ikeda T, Kurita Y, Inutsuka S, et al. The changing pattern of lung cancer by histological type. A review of 1151 cases. *Lung Cancer* 1991;7:157–64.
3. Grover F, Piantadosi S, The Lung Cancer Study Group. Recurrence and survival following resection of bronchoalveolar carcinoma of the lung—The Lung Cancer Study Group experience. *Ann Surg* 1989;209:779–90.
4. Bonne C. Morphological resemblance of pulmonary adenomatosis (jaagsiekte) in sheep and certain cases of cancer in the living man. *Am J Cancer* 1939;35:491–501.
5. Malassez L. Exaamin histologique d'un cas de cancer encephaloide du poumon. *Arch Physiol Norm Pathol* 1876;3:372.
6. Barsky S, Grossman D, Ho J, Holmes EC. The multifocality of bronchoalveolar lung carcinoma: evidence and implications of a multiclonal origin. *Mod Pathol* 1994;7:633–9.

60

Clinical T1 N0 M0, Stage I Non–Small-Cell Lung Cancer—Pathologic T2 N2 M0, Stage IIIA Adenocarcinoma of the Lung

Willard A. Fry

Unsettled controversies include preoperative staging with mediastinoscopy and the role of complete mediastinal lymph node dissection for unanticipated nodal disease

CASE PRESENTATION

The patient is a 49-year old Asian woman, a resident of the United States for 24 years, who presents with an indeterminate lung lesion of the left lower lobe of the lung. She has never smoked tobacco, and her spouse is a nonsmoker as well. She works as a hospital dietitian. She has had a nonproductive cough for 5 months. She is known to be tuberculin positive for many years. After returning from a trip to Taiwan, where traditional herbal medical treatment was employed with no improvement, she consulted a family friend and neighbor, who is also a physician, and a chest radiograph was performed (Fig. 56–1). She was referred to a pulmonologist upon receipt of the radiology report. Past medical history was unremarkable except for a hysterectomy done at age 43 for uterine fibroids and three cesarean sections for childbirth. She had sustained no weight loss, and her performance status was excellent. Physical examination was within normal limits. Her blood counts and chem 20 were normal, as was an electrocardiogram. Pulmonary functions revealed an FVC of 2.44 L (105% of predicted), an FEV_1 of 2.17 L, a

FEV_1/FVC ratio of 89%, and an MVV of 72 L/min (94% of predicted).

A computed tomography (CT) scan of the chest confirmed the mass lesion and showed no mediastinal lymphadenopathy (Fig. 60–2). Diagnostic bronchoscopy gave normal visual findings. Using fluoroscopic control, brushings were taken from a segmental bronchus of the left lower lobe leading to the lesion, and they were positive for adenocarcinoma. Thoracotomy was recommended, and the patient agreed.

At thoracotomy, performed through an axillary incision, the mass lesion was noted in the lower lobe. A left lower lobectomy was performed without difficulty. Lobar and segmental bronchopulmonary lymph nodes were excised with the specimen, en bloc, interlobar, hilar, aortic arch, tracheobronchial angle, and subcarinal lymph nodes were sampled according to the Lung Cancer Study Group protocol (Fig. 60–3). None was grossly suggestive for metastasis. The patient made an uneventful recovery.

The surgical pathologist reported that the lesion was indeed adenocarcinoma, measuring 3.5 cm in greatest dimension, and that there was evidence of lymphatic inva-

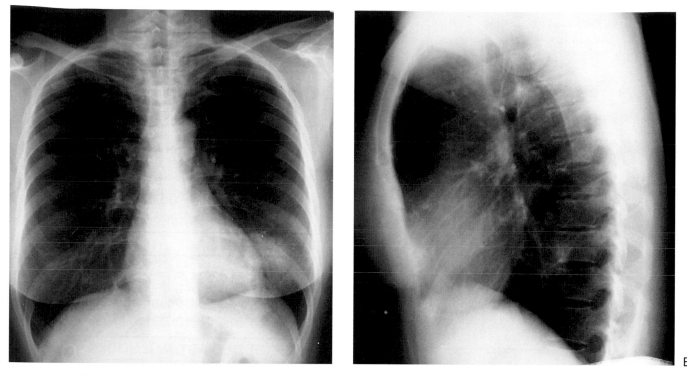

FIG. 60–1. PA and lateral chest radiograph demonstrate a mass lesion in the left lower lobe—very suspicious for cancer.

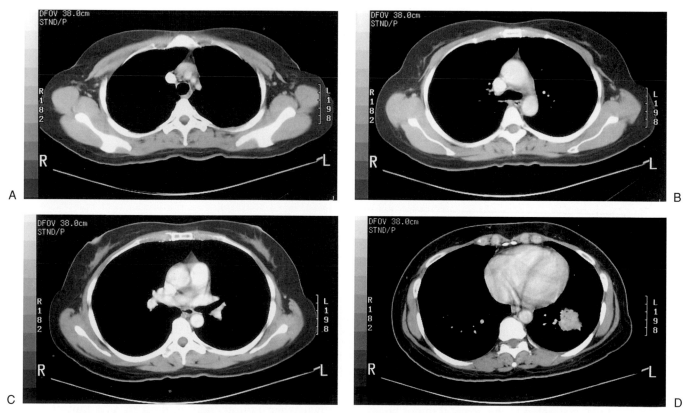

FIG. 60–2. CT of the lung and mediastinum shows no suggestion of mediastinal or bronchopulmonary lymphadenopathy. The lower lobe mass is appreciated.

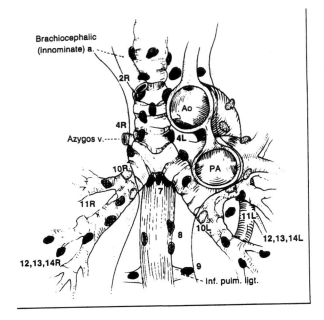

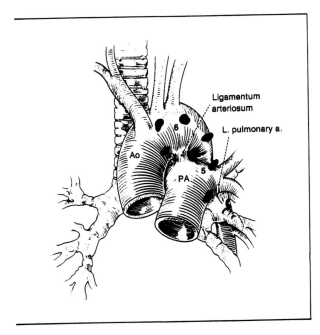

N₂ NODES

SUPERIOR MEDIASTINAL NODES

● **1** Highest Mediastinal

● **2** Upper Paratracheal

● **3** Pre- and Retrotracheal

◐ **4** Lower Paratracheal
(including Azygos Nodes)

AORTIC NODES

● **5** Subaortic (A-P window)

● **6** Para-aortic (ascending
aorta or phrenic)

INFERIOR MEDIASTINAL NODES

● **7** Subcarinal

◐ **8** Paraesophageal (below carina)

● **9** Pulmonary Ligament

N₁ NODES

○ **10** Hilar

◍ **11** Interlobar

● **12** Lobar

● **13** Segmental

● **14** Subsegmental

FIG. 60–3. Lymph node map for lung cancer staging. First proposed by Naruke, it has been approved by the UICC, EORTC, and American Joint Committee on Cancer.

sion in the surrounding lung parenchyma. The bronchial resection margin was free of tumor. However, lymph node metastasis was noted in one lobar node and in the subcarinal node, thus giving the pathologic stage of T2 N2 M0, stage IIIA.

The patient was presented to the hospital tumor board. The overall prognosis was felt to be extremely guarded—particularly with the positive subcarinal lymph node—and there was consensus that she was more at risk to get in

trouble with disseminated disease than with locoregional recurrence. The radiotherapists suggested that the patient might benefit from radiation therapy to the mediastinum. However, it was pointed out that five randomized clinical trials have failed to demonstrate an improvement in survival when radiotherapy is used in an adjuvant setting after complete resection of non–small-cell lung cancer. The radiotherapists pointed out that there is a documented decrease in symptomatic locoregional recurrence after adjuvant therapy and that none of the previous random-ized clinical trials had employed megavoltage radiation with linear accelerators.

The medical oncologists felt that the patient might con-ceivably be helped by adjuvant chemotherapy, particu-larly using a platinum-based regimen. They agreed that there is considerable controversy in the published litera-ture over the survival benefits of adjuvant chemotherapy for completely resected non–small-cell lung cancer.

The role of prophylactic cranial radiation (PCI) was raised. Our institution has been concerned with the late side effects of cranial radiation, and in the absence of clin-ical findings, no one was anxious to recommend PCI. One observer asked if a magnetic resonance image (MRI) of the brain had been performed. The answer was no, because

the patient was asymptomatic and it was felt that the test was too costly to perform on a random, routine basis.

The tumor board was reminded that there is an inter-group randomized clinical trial (0115) started by ECOG (ECOG 3590; Fig. 60–4). All patients receive postopera-tive mediastinal radiation (54 Gy) and half the group is assigned to receive four cycles of chemotherapy with platinum and VP-16. Those assigned to the "double treat-ment limb" are to have the therapies started concurrently.

The guarded prognosis and the lack of proven benefit of adjuvant therapy were presented to the patient and her family. They asked to take a copy of the protocol consent form home to discuss with their physician friend. The patient agreed to participate and was assigned to receive chemoradiation.

Schema

Stratification Factors

Nodal Status

N_1
N_2

Histology

Squamous
Other

Weight Loss in Previous 6 Months

< 5%
≥ 5%

Lymph Node Dissection

Sampling
Complete Node Dissection

R
A
N
D
O
M
I
Z
E

TRT[1]   50.4 Gy

TRT[1]   50.4 Gy

+

DDP + VP-16[2]

[1] Concurrent TRT   50.4 Gy/28 fractions/6 weeks
                       (1.8 Gy/day 5 days/week)

[2] Cisplatin (DDP)   60 mg/M^2 IV days 1, 29, 57, 85

    Etoposide (VP-16) 120 mg/M^2 IV days 1, 2, 3; 29, 30, 31;
                       57, 58, 59; 85, 86, 87

Begin within
24 hours of
initiation of TRT

FIG. 60–4. Schema for ECOG 3590. The randomization is done in the central office. The patient and/or the physician may not stipulate which treatment limb the patient should receive.

COMMENTARY by Robert J. Ginsberg

With increasing frequency we are seeing adenocarcinoma in nonsmoking Asian women. There is some epidemiologic evidence that this may be related to charcoal fumes in cooking areas without proper ventilation, which were common in China until very recently (1).

This patient presents with a solitary lesion in the left lower lobe. The standard preoperative investigation for a clinical stage I lung cancer includes those modalities that were used in this case. Routine screening for metastatic disease beyond a complete physical examination, routine blood work, and CT scan of the chest and upper abdomen is not cost-effective (2).

The role of preoperative mediastinoscopy in such an individual is controversial. Most surgeons feel that for clinical stage I lung cancer as demonstrated on CT scan (no mediastinal or hilar adenopathy), no preoperative mediastinoscopy is required. However, when a preoperative diagnosis of adenocarcinoma is present, and especially a T2 lesion, I prefer preoperative mediastinoscopy to identify occult N2 disease because recent reports have demonstrated improved results of treatment for stage IIIA (N2) disease using induction chemotherapy or chemoradiotherapy before surgery (3,4). It is well demonstrated and has been my own clinical impression that patients suffering from clinical stage I adenocarcinoma, especially larger tumors (T2), often have occult mediastinal lymph node metastases not demonstrated on CT scan.

Lymphatic drainage from left lower lobe tumors includes peribronchial, subcarinal and, ultimately, superior mediastinal lymph nodes. The latter lymph nodes are inaccessible by standard left thoracotomy. In this case, the fact that there were occult metastases present in the single sampled subcarinal lymph node makes one concerned that superior mediastinal disease may also have been present and remains undetected in this case. Had a mediastinoscopy demonstrated superior mediastinal lymph node involvement, it is unlikely that this patient would have been offered initial surgery, and if N3 disease were present (contralateral) at mediastinoscopy, most authorities would not treat by surgical resection, even after induction therapy, but would offer curative radiotherapy.

In this patient, a left lower lobectomy was performed and mediastinal lymph node sampling (one from each mediastinal area) was performed. No frozen section analysis was done of these mediastinal lymph nodes. This latter step is important because, if a positive mediastinal or even hilar node is found, there is fairly uniform opinion that a complete mediastinal lymph node dissection should be performed to ensure completeness of resection (5). Without frozen section analysis and with normal-appearing lymph nodes, Dr. Fry did not proceed with what I feel would have been optimum treatment for this patient—complete mediastinal lymph node resection. It is unknown whether or not persisting disease is present in the other subcarinal nodes or in unsampled superior mediastinal nodes.

When a complete resection is performed for lung cancer involving single station N2 disease, the results of surgery alone yield approximately a 30% 5-year survival (6). In this case, only single samples of mediastinal lymph node stations were examined and therefore the exact extent of mediastinal involvement is unknown. As well, without a complete mediastinal lymph node dissection or preoperative mediastinoscopy, it is unknown whether or not a complete resection has been performed. If more than one mediastinal lymph node station is involved with tumor, or an incomplete resection has been performed, the results of surgery with or without adjuvant treatment falls precipitously to below a 10% survival figure at 5 years (7).

The question of postoperative adjuvant therapy is well discussed in the presentation. Because of the suggested improved outlook with chemoradiotherapy (versus radiotherapy) in the postoperative setting for this stage of disease as demonstrated in a previous Lung Cancer Study Group Trial, the current NCI-funded Intergroup Trial is a worthwhile endeavor that should be supported by all thoracic surgeons and oncologists.

REFERENCES

1. Mumford JL, He XZ, Chapman RS et al. Lung cancer and indoor air pollution in Xuan Wei, China. *Science* 1987;235:217.
2. Maddaus M, Ginsberg RJ. Diagnosis and staging. In: *Thoracic surgery*, Pearson FG, Deslauriers, Ginsberg RJ, Hiebert CA, McNeally MF, Urschel HC, eds. New York: Churchill Livingstone; 1994:671–90.
3. Rosell R, Gomez-Codina J, Camps C, et al. A randomized trial comparing preoperative chemotherapy plus surgery with surgery alone in patients with non-small cell lung cancer. *N Engl J Med* 1994;330: 153–8.
4. Roth JA, Fossella F, Komaki R, et al. A randomized trial comparing perioperative chemotherapy and surgery with surgery alone in resectable Stage IIIA non-small cell lung cancer. *J Natl Cancer Inst* 1994;86:673–80.
5. Martini N, Ginsberg RJ. Techniques of lobectomy. In: *Thoracic surgery*, Pearson FG, Deslauriers, Ginsberg RJ, Hiebert CA, McNeally MF, Urschel HC, eds. New York: Churchill Livingstone; 1995:848–54.
6. Martini N, Flehinger BJ. The role of surgery in N2 lung cancer. *Surg Clin North Am* 1987;67:1037–49.
7. Watanabe Y, Hayashi Y, Shimizu J, Oda M, Iwa T. Mediastinal nodal involvement and the prognosis of non–small cell lung cancer. *Chest* 1991;1002:422–8.

SECTION XIV

Mediastinum

61 Recurrent Mediastinal Nonseminomatous Germ Cell Malignancy

Valerie K. Israel, Christy A Russell, Dechen Dolkar, and Oscar Streeter

Adequate initial chemotherapy is necessary before resecting residual tumor

CASE PRESENTATION

M.G. is a 22-year-old Hispanic man who initially presented to LAC/USC with palpable left supraclavicular lymph nodes and a $12 \times 16 \times 15$ cm anterior mediastinal mass with moderate pericardial effusion. His tumor markers were alpha-fetoprotein (AFP) 26,700 (nl <20), β-subunit of human chorionic gonadotropin (βHCG) <3 (nl <5), and lactate dehydrogenase (LDH) 233 (nl <300). Biopsy of a left supraclavicular lymph node revealed mature teratoma with metastatic yolk sac elements (Figs. 61–1, 61–2). The immunohistochemical stain was positive for AFP. Physical exam and ultrasound of the testes did not reveal any masses.

One week later, the patient was entered onto SWOG 8997 protocol and received five cycles of VIP ([etoposide 75 mg/m^2 + ifosfamide 1.25 g/m^2 + cisplatin 20 mg/m^2] daily for 5 days) every 21 days with resultant normalization of his AFP level and without complications. Although the preoperative AFP rose to 56, the patient underwent a thoracotomy and resection of residual tumor. Pathologic findings reported the residual mass as a mixed germ cell tumor: predominantly mature teratoma with a yolk sac component. One month later he received one cycle of postoperative VIP with an AFP equal to 105. The

patient was then lost to follow-up on his abrupt return to Mexico.

One year later he presented with a 4×7 cm left infraclavicular mass with an AFP equal to 5,700 and a βHCG <3. A computed tomography (CT) scan of the chest with contrast showed a large recurrent mediastinal mass invading the chest wall and a right adrenal mass (Fig. 61–3). An echocardiogram revealed a small pericardial effusion. A fine-needle aspirate of the chest wall mass revealed a germ cell tumor and the patient was referred to medical oncology and treated with BOP-VP chemotherapy (bleomycin 20 U/m^2 day 1, vincristine 2 mg day 1, cisplatin 60 mg/m^2 day 1, and etoposide 75 mg/m^2 days 1 and 2). He received nine cycles over 12 weeks: the first seven cycles were given weekly and the last two cycles every 2 weeks. He tolerated the chemotherapy well and had no complications. Bleomycin was not given with the last two courses because of a mild cough with a slight interstitial pattern on chest radiograph that warned of early bleomycin toxicity. The patient had a normal AFP during the last two cycles of chemotherapy. The patient has had normal tumor markers for the past 8 weeks.

A CT scan of the chest with contrast was repeated 3 weeks after the completion of BOP-VP, which showed minimal residual anterior mediastinal abnormality, yet it

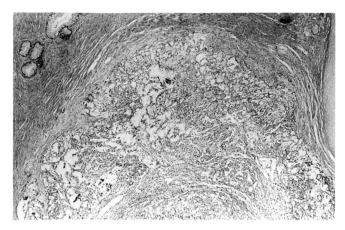

FIG. 61–1. Pathology of the initial biopsy showing mature teratoma with focus of yolk sac elements (×25).

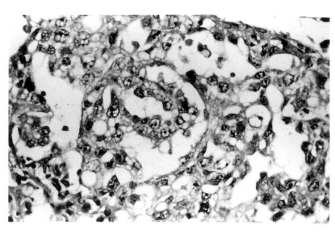

FIG. 61–2. Pathology of the yolk sac elements (×400); at the center is a Schiller-Dourall body.

was unclear if this represented mature teratoma, fibrosis, or immature elements (Fig. 61–4A). The right adrenal mass had resolved (Fig. 61–4B). The interstitial changes on chest roentgenogram and the patient's mild cough resolved. The patient was presented to Tumor Board by Medical Oncology for consideration and discussion of re-resection of residual mediastinal disease, surgical exploration of the area of the resolved right adrenal mass, the role of radiotherapy, and the role of further chemotherapy.

TUMOR BOARD DISCUSSION

The medical oncology staff critiqued the course of the patient: they stated that the biopsies of the supraclavicu-

lar lymph nodes on initial presentation and of the recurrent chest wall mass were not necessary to establish the diagnosis of a germ cell malignancy because of the elevated AFP, particularly in conjunction with a midline tumor in a young person. Medical oncology also noted that the elevated AFP level at the time of the mediastinal resection was most likely an oversight. Nonseminomatous germ cell patients should be rendered as free of viable tumor as possible, evidenced by normal tumor markers, before undergoing resection of residual masses. However, salvage surgery may be attempted if normal tumor markers cannot be achieved despite aggressive chemotherapy.

Recommendations by the thoracic surgeons were divided. One group felt that mediastinal re-resection

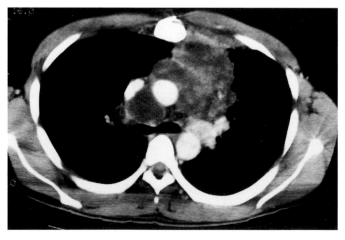

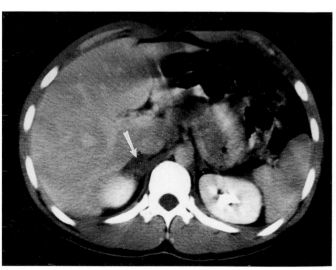

FIG. 61–3. CT scan with contrast demonstrating (**A**) large heterogeneous anterior mediastinal mass invading through the left chest wall and (**B**) a right adrenal mass (*arrow*); this scan was done when M.G. presented with recurrence and visible infraclavicular mass.

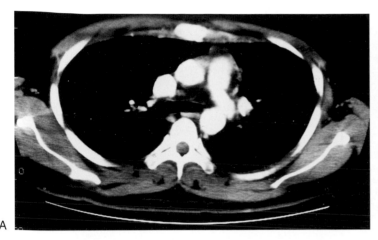
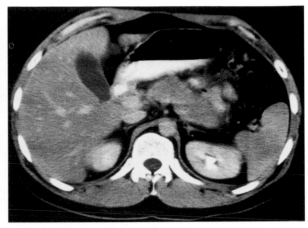

FIG. 61–4. CT scan with contrast showing (**A**) minimal residual anterior mediastinal tissue and (**B**) resolution of right adrenal mass; this scan was performed 11 weeks after treatment with BOP-VP and was unchanged from the scan done 3 weeks after chemotherapy (not shown).

would be contraindicated in all circumstances. The other group felt that the patient should be monitored with serial CT scans of the chest and adrenals and serum tumor markers every 3 months; then, if his mediastinal disease progressed and he was once again recaptured by chemotherapy, the residual disease could be resected at that time. Both groups believed that the right adrenal gland should not be explored.

The thoracic surgeons were reluctant to perform another mediastinal resection for two reasons. First, they stated that repeat mediastinal resections carry significant morbidity. However, they pointed out that the risk of lacerating the heart at repeat thoracotomy was decreased because the pericardium was not removed during the initial mediastinal resection. Second, it was unclear if the residual mass merely represented fibrosis, not requiring resection.

The recommendation of the thoracic surgeons to repeat mediastinal re-resection if the tumor progressed and once more responded to chemotherapy was accepted by the staff of Medical Oncology with certain concerns. The prognosis of the patient was compromised by the site of the primary and the optimal chance of cure occupied a narrow window. The patient was already unusual because his recurrence responded so well to retreatment with chemotherapy and his chances of having as good a response a third time were less than ideal.

The staff of Medical Oncology emphasized that germ cell tumors are different from other neoplasms. Resection of residual mass may provide surgical cure if the residual tissue consists of mature teratoma or may dictate the need for further chemotherapy if immature elements are identified. The decision to defer exploration of the right adrenal gland was more readily accepted: the mass had completely resolved and the literature does not contain data on the exploration of resolved adrenal masses. Further

chemotherapy without evidence of active disease was clearly not indicated. The patient had two cycles with normal serum tumor markers that were currently sustained for 8 weeks and there was no evidence of progressive disease on CT scans. Referral for bone marrow transplant was also suggested, although the published results for mediastinal germ cell cancers have been disappointing. Radiation Oncology felt that there was no role for mediastinal radiation in this setting.

Seven weeks after presentation to Tumor Board, the patient complained of headache, intermittent blurred vision, and left-sided weakness of the upper and lower extremities. Neurologic exam revealed a mild left facial droop, a positive Rhomberg, $^4/_5$ motor strength of the upper and lower left extremities, dysdiadokinesia of the left upper and lower extremities, and hyperesthesia of the left side of the body. The patient was immediately started on decadron and admitted to the hospital. An emergency magnetic resonance image (MRI) of the brain revealed at least seven parenchymal central nervous system lesions that enhanced with gadolinium and were consistent with metastases; the sites included a large bilateral frontoparietal, left occipital, two left cerebellar, a left thalamic, and right midbrain lesions; minimal edema was present (Figs. 61–5B,C). Serum AFP was 560. Whole brain radiotherapy (WBRT) was initiated the same day, and completed to a dose of 4,200 cGy with opposing lateral fields delivered on a 4-MV linear accelerator with the dose calculated to the D-mid depth. The first 10 fractions were given as 3 Gy each, with the remaining dose reduced to 2 Gy/day. Seventeen fractions were delivered over 23 days. The patient demonstrated marked gradual improvement of his symptoms, except for minimal residual complaints of left eye blurring, which improved with ophthalmic drops.

During radiotherapy the AFP continued to rise; 2 days before the end of WBRT the AFP was 2,780, and

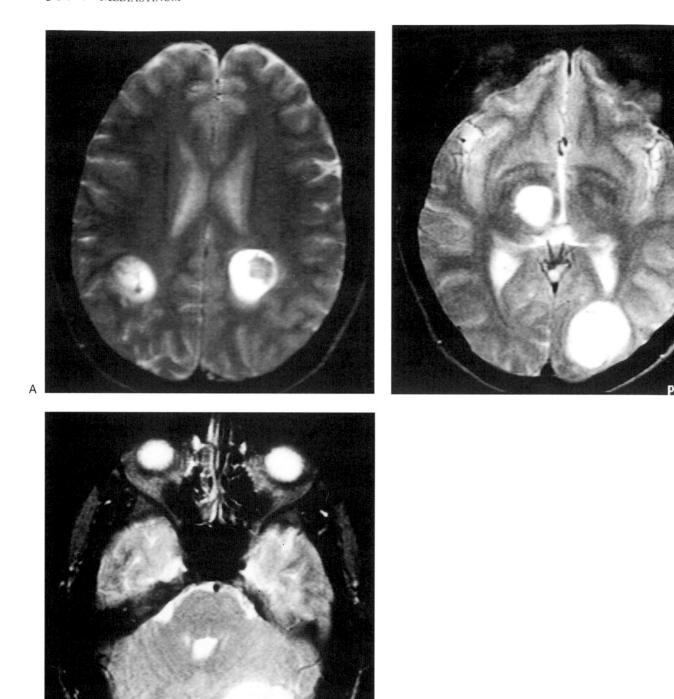

FIG. 61–5. A,B,C: MRI of the brain with gadolinium showing multiple enhancing lesions consistent with metastatic lesions.

11 days after the end of WBRT, AFP was 1,130. At this time it was felt that the increase in AFP may be due to destruction of central nervous system tumor cells and may not be from progressive disease in the mediastinum. Therefore, an AFP and CT scan of the chest and abdomen were repeated 2 weeks later (see Fig. 61–4): the anterior mediastinal disease was unchanged or slightly decreased and the AFP was 260. The patient has returned to Mexico and declines further follow-up.

COMMENTARY by Marc B. Garnick

Although germ cell tumors of the testis represent one of the most curable neoplasms that oncologists deal with in the 1990s, there are certain situations that represent significant therapeutic challenges. Anterior mediastinal germ cell neoplasms represent one such challenge. Unfortunately, despite significant improvements in many aspects of chemotherapy and surgical management, this disease still remains problematic. Whether the intrinsically less responsiveness of these tumors to treatment represents the large size they obtain before diagnosis, their anatomic location, or simply genetic differences in the molecular make-up remains to be determined. Nevertheless, the historic and current disappointing results demands novel and innovative approaches to treatment.

The initial approach of using VIP chemotherapy was reasonable. It is important to monitor the rate of decline of the biologic markers. We do not have the information in this case. If the markers do not fall on their biologic half-life (approximately 6 days for AFP and 1 day for HCG), a worse prognosis can be expected. The fact that the postchemotherapy, preoperative AFP was rising is most disturbing, and I, too, would have strongly considered additional chemotherapy before performing the initial thoracotomy. Time and time again, the presence of positive markers or, more importantly, rising markers in the postchemotherapy period, is usually associated with unresectable cancer, and always signifies the need for additional systemic chemotherapy.

Another approach at this time would have been to administer additional chemotherapy with agents to which germ cell tumors are known to respond, or to consider the patient for bone marrow transplant. If the markers normalize at that time, consideration for thoracotomy should be entertained. I must emphasize that the role of surgery in these cases is extraordinarily important—but it must be judiciously timed and used to get the greatest benefit.

I do not agree with the medical oncologist's assessment that a supraclavicular lymph node biopsy did not need to be performed. Although the diagnosis of germ cell cancer is indisputable based on the clinical and biochemical presentation, it is imperative to have a tissue diagnosis and actual pathologic cell type at the initiation of treatment because these cancers can undergo sarcomatous degeneration as well as being associated with hematologic malignancies (such as acute megakaryocytic leukemia) and other disorders of platelet function. One could argue that a baseline bone marrow evaluation should also have been considered at the onset.

Because I would not have performed the first thoracotomy when the AFP was rising, I would have strongly considered the thoracotomy after completion of the BOP-VP chemotherapy program. The single most important thing to manage at this time in the patient's course is avoiding complications associated with bleomycin pul-monary toxicity. The surgery should not be performed if there are any alterations on either chest radiograph or in pulmonary function testing that suggest bleomycin lung disease. These alterations must be resolved before performing any surgery in the bleomycin-treated patients. Intra- and postoperative precautions need to be taken. These include keeping the patient on the euvolemic to hypovolemic side, and keeping a close watch on the inspired oxygen concentration during the operation. Patients who are "wet," and given high inspired oxygen concentrations are the most likely to get into trouble with the rare, but devastating, ARDS-like picture that can accompany the postoperative surgical course in bleomycin-treated patients.

If residual cancer is found at the time of exploration, then additional chemotherapy must be administered. This could include two additional cycles of the BOP-VP chemotherapy, or any other chemotherapy to which the patient was responsive. If either teratoma or fibrosis was found, no additional chemotherapy is usually warranted. However, aggressive surgical approaches must be offered if, at some later time, radiographic abnormalities are demonstrated in the absence of positive tumor markers. The pathologist must also be diligent in searching for unusual elements, such as sarcomatoid features in the resected specimen. Also, the rare association of leukemia (which seems not to be secondary to the chemotherapy, but rather associated with the original cancer) needs to be watched for in the postoperative and postchemotherapy period. I agree, also, that at this time, there was no need to explore the adrenal gland, and that there was no role for radiation therapy.

The development of central nervous system metastases should come as no surprise in this case. In such high-risk patients, it is not unusual to obtain a baseline bone scan and radiologic evaluation of the central nervous system. Although bony abnormalities are unusual and tend to occur more often with seminomas, the presence of asymptomatic central nervous system disease is not at all uncommon in patients with extragonadal germ cell cancers. Such a finding demands urgent intervention with radiation treatment, and in selected cases, surgical resection of brain lesions. Long-term survival has been reported in selected patients with such aggressive treatment programs.

I think that the long-term prognosis for this patient is poor, and would consider him for additional investigational therapy if his tumor markers do not normalize over the next several weeks.

SELECTED READINGS

1. Bauer KA, Skarin AT, Balikian JP, Garnick MB, Rosenthal DS, Canellos GP. Pulmonary complications associated with combination chemotherapy programs containing bleomycin. Am J Med 1983;74:557–63.
2. Broun ER, Nichols CR, Kneebone P, et al. Long-term outcome of patients with relapsed and refractory germ cell tumors treated with

high-dose chemotherapy and autologous bone marrow rescue. *Ann Intern Med* 1992;117:124–8.

3. Garnick MB, Canellos GP, Richie JP. The treatment and surgical staging of testicular and primary extragonadal germ cell cancer. *JAMA* 1983;250:1733–41.

4. Garnick MB. Testicular cancer and other trophoblastic diseases. In: *Harrison's principles of internal medicine,* 13th ed, Isselbacher KJ, Braunwald E, Wilson JD, Martin JB, Fauci AS, Kasper DL, eds. New York: McGraw-Hill Book Co; 1994:1858–62.

5. Garnick MB. Urologic cancer. *Sci Am Med* 1993;IX:13–7.

6. Gonzalez-Vela JL, Savage PD, Manivel JC, Torkelson J, Kennedy BJ. Poor prognosis of mediastinal germ cell cancers containing sarcomatosis elements. *Cancer* 1990;66:1114–6.

7. Kantoff PW, Garnick MB. Late toxicities, long-term follow-up, less intensive treatment: leading issues in the therapy of testis cancer. *J Clin Oncol* 1988;6:1216–9.

8. Motzer RJ, Gulati SC, Mazumdar M, et al. Phase II trial of VAB-6+ high-dose carboplatin + etoposide with autologous bone marrow transplantation for poor risk germ cell tumor patients. *Natl Proc ASCO,* abstract 720, 1993.

9. Nichols CR, Hoffman R, Einhorn LH, Williams SD, Wheeler LA, Garnick MB. Hematologic malignancies associated with primary mediastinal germ cell tumors. *Ann Intern Med* 1985;102:603–9.

10. Talcott JA, Garnick MB, Stomper PC, Godleski JJ, Richie JP. Cavitary lung nodules associated with combination chemotherapy containing bleomycin. *J Urol* 1987;138:619–20.

62 Thymoma

Julia White and George Haasler

Complete resection is the key to long-term survival

CASE PRESENTATION

This patient is a 41-year-old black woman who presented to another hospital in the area with a 3-week history of persistent cough, dyspnea, headache, sore throat, myalgias, bilateral ptosis, and generalized weakness. A neurologic evaluation was performed and she was diagnosed as having myasthenia gravis (MG) based on a positive tensilon test and electromyographic (EMG) findings. Anti-acetylcholine receptor antibodies were markedly elevated. The patient was begun on mestinon 60 mg qid with an apparently good initial clinical response. However, 3 days after her admission she was transferred to the medical intensive care unit for management of a worsening respiratory status and started on prednisone 40 mg daily and antibiotics. Re-evaluation of the admission CXR demonstrated fullness in the anterior mediastinum (Fig. 62–1). A computed tomography (CT) scan of the thorax was performed, demonstrating an estimated 5- to 6-cm anterior mediastinal mass (Fig. 62–2). The patient was subsequently transferred to our institution for further management of her MG and presumed thymoma.

Upon transfer, the patient reported improvement in her respiratory symptoms and less ptosis after mestinon. There was no previous history of autoimmune disease. Her previous medical history was significant only for a herniated lumbar disk for which she had a laminectomy 3 months ago and had residual right leg weakness. Physical exam was remarkable for a slight esotropia of the right eye, bilateral ptosis, and upward gaze fatigue at 25 s. Facial muscles were diffusely weak, but symmetric. Muscle strength testing revealed the right lower extremity weakness. Lung exam revealed poor inspiratory effort but

was otherwise clear to auscultation. Pulse oximetry demonstrated 98% saturation on room air.

The cardiothoracic surgeons evaluated the patient for possible resection of the anterior mediastinal mass. Fluo-

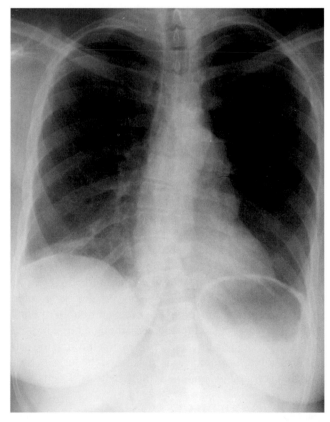

FIG. 62–1. PA view of the chest radiograph illustrates left-sided fullness in the mediastinum.

307

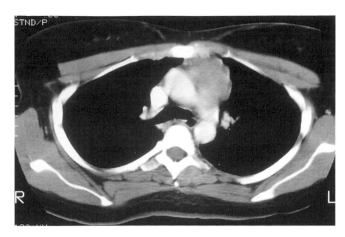

FIG. 62–2. CT scan section demonstrating large anterior mediastinal mass.

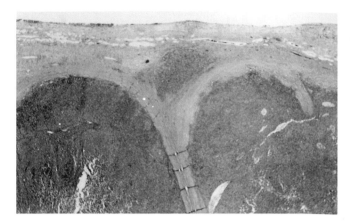

FIG. 62–3. Low magnification view of lymphocyte-predominant thymoma demonstrating thick fibrous capsule and intervening septa.

roscopy of the diaphragm was recommended because of the leftward position of the mass within the mediastinum to check the integrity of the left phrenic nerve. Observation of the diaphragm under fluoroscopy demonstrated paradoxical movement of the right hemidiaphragm and hypofunction of the left. An EMG revealed bilateral phrenic mononeuropathies, moderate on the right and severe on the left. In preparation for surgery, the patient underwent plasmapheresis twice and had her prednisone therapy weaned to 10 mg daily. Serial pulmonary function tests revealed a stable force vital capacity at approximately 2.0 L.

A transsternal thymectomy was performed without incident. At the time of surgery, the thymic mass was easily removed off most neck and mediastinal structures, except at the level of the left phrenic nerve. There, the tumor had encased the nerve and required significant sharp dissection to remove. Some tumor was left on the nerve over a 2-cm extent just anterior to the pulmonary hilum in the aortopulmonary window.

The patient had an uncomplicated postoperative course. She required mechanical ventilatory support and plasmapheresis in the first 24 hours. Three days after surgery she was transferred to a regular surgical bed and discharged to home on the eighth postoperative day.

On pathologic evaluation a 9.5 × 5.0 × 3.5 cm mass in greatest dimensions was appreciated grossly. Microscopically, sections of the tumor demonstrated a well delineated mass with a thick fibrous capsule and intervening fibrous septa (Fig. 62–3). The areas between the septa were extremely cellular and composed of an admixture of bland thymic epithelial cells interspersed among a large population of lymphocytes. Focal microinvasion through the capsule was noted. Immunostains confirmed the large cells as epithelial (Fig. 62–4) and the lymphocytes as T cells.

TUMOR BOARD DISCUSSION

Pathologist: Thymomas are tumors that originate from the epithelial component of the thymus. Review of this patient's pathology demonstrates classic findings of a predominantly lymphocytic type of thymoma. Thymoma can be classified histologically according to the predominant cell type as either lymphocytic, epithelial, or mixed. There is evidence that the predominantly epithelial tumors have a more aggressive course. However, the overwhelming prognostic factor for thymoma is evidence of invasion either macroscopically or microscopically.

Thoracic surgeon: This patient typifies many of the issues involved in the management of MG and thymoma. On review of the outside CT scan, it appeared that the mediastinal mass extended to the left in the region of the left phrenic nerve. Observing the diaphragm movement under fluoroscopy demonstrated that the right hemidiaphragm moved paradoxically and EMG confirmed bilateral mononeuropathies of the phrenic nerves. At the time of resection, invasion of the left phrenic nerve was evident. In view of the right phrenic nerve dysfunction, it was felt that resection of the left phrenic nerve would be unwise, potentially compromising her respiratory function further and removing any chance for some left-sided recovery, acknowledging the fact that this would result in a less than complete resection. Although unilateral involved phrenic nerve resection is feasible to cure a thymoma in the absence of MG and respiratory compromise, it is not wise if someone has significant respiratory difficulties already and there is still some function left in the affected nerve.

This patient did well perioperatively and her MG remained stable. Optimizing management of MG in the perioperative period is important for reducing morbidity and mortality. Patients with MG and thymoma generally have more difficulty with persistent myasthenic symptoms postoperatively than those without thymoma, with a poorer prognosis related independently to the effects of the MG. Conversely, the presence of MG has not been associated with poorer cancer control. Approximately 50% of patients with MG have thymoma, whereas only 10% to 20% of patients with thymoma have MG.

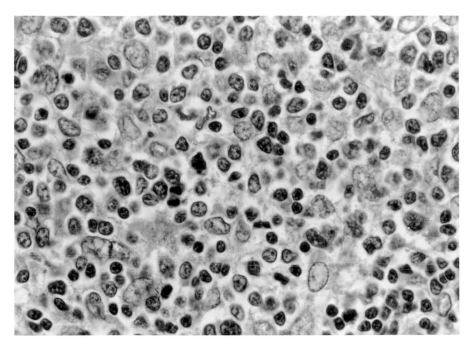

FIG. 62–4. High magnification view demonstrates the characteristic large epithelial cells interspersed among the lymphocytes.

Radiation oncologist: One of the more commonly applied staging systems is by Masoaka. Briefly, stage I is a completely encapsulated mass without microscopic evidence of invasion. Stage II is slightly invasive with either macroscopic invasion into the surrounding fat or mediastinal pleura or microscopic invasion into the capsule. Stage III is a more prominent invasion into neighboring organs such as pericardium, great vessels, or lung. Stage IV is subdivided into pericardial or pleural dissemination and lymphogenous or hematogenous metastases. This patient fits best into stage II.

Completely resected stage I patients have a risk of local recurrence of less than 2% to 3% and in general do not benefit from postoperative mediastinal irradiation. For stage II patients the mediastinal recurrence rate after resection alone varies from approximately 20% 45% in various reports. In the case of a subtotal resection, the risk for recurrent mediastinal disease is probably greater than 50%. Stage III and IV patients are at even higher risk of mediastinal recurrence after complete resection and more frequently have subtotal resections. For patients with stage II or greater disease, postoperative mediastinal irradiation is indicated even when complete resection has been achieved.

Irradiation of the mediastinum requires careful attention to the dose delivered to surrounding critical structures to minimize pneumonitis and avoid pericarditis or myelitis as late-occurring complications. In this patient's case, CT scan–based three-dimensional treatment planning has been used to design the treatment volumes and field arrangements. The plan is to deliver 40 Gy at 1.8 Gy per day to the entire mediastinum. The initial field is inclusive of T2 through T8 vertebral body levels. Inferiorly, the field covers the cardiac silhouette with adjacent pleura and more cephalad narrows to cover the superior mediastinum. A field size reduction will be made and the original tumor volume with a 2-cm margin will then be taken to 50.4 Gy with the same fractionation. A final field size reduction will be performed and the small area of gross residual disease with a 1-cm margin will boosted to a cumulative total dose of 59.4 Gy.

A CT scan was performed 6 weeks after surgery before initiation of irradiation. Five-millimeter cuts through the superior and anterior mediastinum failed to demonstrate any evidence of residual mass. A pleural-based density seen in the left lung base was felt to represent atelectasis because there was significant evidence of atelectactic changes in the lung bases bilaterally.

Medical oncologist: Cisplatin-based combination chemotherapy has been used for advanced, unresectable, or metastatic invasive thymoma. A small intergroup trial has evaluated the response rate in previously untreated patients. At this time, there is no role for systemic therapy in the management of this patient and it would be reserved for consideration in the treatment of local or distant recurrence.

REFERENCES

1. Masaoka A, Monden Y, Nakahara K, et al. Follow up study of thymoma with special reference to their clinical stages. *Cancer* 1981;48:2485–92.
2. Blumberg D, Port JL, Weksler B, et al. Thymoma: A multivariate analysis of factors predicting survival. *Soc Thorac Surg* 1995; 60:908–14.
3. Monden Y, Nakahara K, Iioka S, et al. Recurrence of thymoma: Clinicopathological features, therapy, and prognosis. *Ann Thorac Surg* 1985;39:165–9.

4. Kirschner PA. Reoperation for thymoma: Report of 23 cases. *Ann Thorac Surg* 1990;49:550–5.

5. Maggi G, Casadio C, Cavallo A, Cianci R, Molinatti M, Ruffini E. Thymoma: Results of 241 operated cases. *Ann Thorac Surg* 1991;51:152–6.

6. Wilkins EW, Grillo HC, Scannell JG, Moncure AC, Mathisen DJ. Role of staging in prognosis and management of thymoma. *Ann Thorac Surg* 1991;51:888–92.

7. Nakahara K, Ohno K, Hashimoto J, et al. Thymoma: Results with complete resection and adjuvant postoperative irradiation in 141 consecutive patients. *J Thorac Cardiovasc Surg* 1988;95:1041–7.

8. Lewis JE, Wick MR, Scheithauer BW, Bernatz PE, Taylor WF. Thymoma: A clinicopathologic review. *Cancer* 1987;60:2727–43.

9. Shamji F, Pearson FG, Todd TRJ, Ginsberg RJ, Lives R, Cooper JD. Results of surgical treatment for thymoma. *J Thorac Cardiovasc Surg* 1984;87:43–7.

10. Curran WJ, Kornstein MJ, Brooks JJ, Turrisi AT III. Invasive thymoma: The role of mediastinal irradiation following complete or incomplete surgical resection. *J Clin Oncol* 1988;6:1722–7.

11. Haniuda M, Morimoto M, Nishimura H, Kobayashi O, Yamada T, Iida F. Adjuvant radiotherapy after complete resection of thymoma. *Ann Thorac Surg* 1992;54:311–15.

12. Rea F, Sartori F, Loy M, et al. Chemotherapy and operation for invasive thymoma. *J Thorac Cardiovasc Surg* 1993;106:543–9.

COMMENTARY by Michael Burt

Thymomas are relatively uncommon tumors that are derived from the epithelial cells of the thymus. Although there are multiple histologic classification schemes, one accepted classification divides thymomas into five entities: (1) spindle cell, (2) predominantly lymphocytic, (3) mixed lymphoepithelial, (4) thymic carcinoma, and (5) predominantly epithelial thymoma. In the staging of thymomas, most series utilize the Masaoka staging system (1): stage I defined as encapsulated thymomas; stage II defined as microscopic capsular invasion or invasion into surrounding mediastinal fat or pleura; stage III defined as invasion into mediastinal structures; stage IVa defined as metastases confined to the thoracic cavity; and stage IVb defined as distant hematogenous metastases.

Patients with thymoma may have associated autoimmune disorders. In a recent report of 118 patients with thymoma, 10% had myasthenia gravis, 3% had hypogammaglobulinemia, 3% had red cell aplasia, 3% had systemic lupus erythematosus, 1% had positive antinuclear antibody, and 1% had limbic encephalitis (2). In this series and others, the presence of an autoimmune disorder did not have an impact on survival.

Resection remains the mainstay of therapy for patients with thymoma. The primary goal at operation is complete resection, as incomplete resection translates into decreased survival. In our series of 118 patients, there were 86 complete resections (73%), 18 incomplete resections (15%), and 14 biopsies (12%) (2). Pathologic staging demonstrated 21% of patients were stage I, 35% were stage II, 36% were stage III, and 9% were stage IVa. The overall survival was 77% at 5 years and 55% at 10 years.

When analyzing factors that would predict recurrence, only stage of disease is an independent predictor of recurrence (2-4).

In our series, a multivariate analysis of factors predicting survival demonstrated that stage, tumor size, histology, and complete resection were significant and independent predictors of survival (2). These factors have also been shown to affect survival in other reported series (5–9).

Although postoperative radiation therapy has evolved to be standard of care in patients after complete or incomplete resection of stage II, III, and IVa malignant thymoma (10,11), data from prospective, controlled clinical trials are sparse.

With the high recurrence rates for stage II, III, and IVa thymomas, (associated with a decreased survival) attention has been focused on preoperative multidrug chemotherapy. Data from one recent study demonstrated an overall response of 100% in 16 patients with stage III and IVa thymoma treated with doxorubicin, cyclophosphamide, vincristine, and carboplatin (12). The 3-year survival after resection was 70%. These data are encouraging but require confirmation in larger controlled clinical trials.

Table 62-1. *Resectability, recurrence, and survival by stage*

Stage	n	CR	PR	Bx	Recurrence (5y)	Survival 5y
I	25	100%			4%	95%
II	41	73%	10%	17%	21%	70%
III	43	56%	30%	14%	47%	50%
IVa	9	78%	11%	11%	80%	100%

Bx = biopsy; CR = complete resection; PR = partial resection

63

Malignant Pericardial Effusion

Kenneth B. Roberts and Bruce G. Haffty

*Early chemotherapy may be required despite other medical
complications*

CASE PRESENTATION

The patient was a 51-year-old woman who was well,
aside from her 25 pack-per-year smoking habit until mid-
December 1991, when she developed myalgia, cough,
nausea, vomiting, and chills. Before this time the patient
had been active; screening mammograms and a pap smear
had been negative just 2 months earlier. Hematemesis and
melenic stools subsequently occurred. The patient was
admitted to an outside hospital on December 21, 1991,
where upper endoscopy revealed erosive gastritis and
duodenitis consistent with effects from prior usage of
nonsteroidal anti-inflammatory agents. Ranitidine was
prescribed. Laboratory evaluation was otherwise remarkable only for renal insufficiency with blood urea nitrogen
and creatinine of 124 mg/dL and 4.4 mg/dL, respectively.
A chest radiograph showed bilateral, moderately sized
pleural effusions (Fig. 63–1). With progressive dyspnea
and acute respiratory failure requiring endotracheal intubation, a left chest tube thoracostomy yielded a large
amount of hemorrhagic fluid. Repeat chest radiograph
showed cardiomegaly. An echocardiogram showed a
large pericardial effusion with tamponade physiology. A
pericardiocentesis was performed with removal of 700 cc
of sanguinous fluid. The patient was then transferred to a
tertiary care medical center for further management on
December 23, 1991.

On initial evaluation, the patient was suspected to have
a viral or idiopathic pericarditis with effusion causing cardiac tamponade. Physical examination was remarkable
for an intubated woman in no distress with left chest tube
draining serosanguinous fluid. Vital signs were temperature 99.6°F, blood pressure 98/54, heart rate 104 and reg-

ular, respiratory rate 14. Head, eyes, ears, nose, and throat
were otherwise unremarkable. Neck was supple without
thyroidomegaly. There were a few small left posterior
cervical lymph nodes felt. The breasts were without
masses. The lungs had coarse rhonchi on the right on auscultation. The cardiac apex was enlarged and diffuse.
There was no right ventricular heave. On auscultation
there was normal S_1 and S_2, as well as an atrial gallop. No
murmurs or rubs were heard. Normal carotid impulse was
felt. Right atrial pressure was estimated at 8 cm with normal waveform. Abdomen was benign with normal bowel
sounds. There was no hepatosplenomegaly, masses, or
tenderness. Extremities were without edema and had normal peripheral pulses and perfusion. Neurologic exam
was without focal findings. Laboratory evaluation
showed white blood cells 12,700 per mm³ (differential of
5 bands, 86 segs, 5 lymph, 4 mono, and 3 nucleated rbc's)
Hgb 11.1 g/dL, platelets 175,000 per mm³, prothrombin
time 15.6 sec, PTT 27.9 sec, glucose 103 mg/dL, BUN
110 mg/dL, creatinine 2.8 mg/dL, Na 131 mEq/L, K 3.7
mEq/L, Cl 96 mEq/L, bicarbonate 22 mEq/L, Ca 7.7
mg/dL, bili 0.5 mg/dL, SGOT 370 U/L, SGPT 489 U/L,
alkaline phosphatase 102 U/L, CPK 482 U/L with 5.7%
MB fraction, negative ANA and rheumatoid factors, and
normal C_3 and C_4 antigens. Urinalysis showed nonspecific moderate pyuria and hematuria in the setting of bladder catheterization without evidence of casts, proteinuria,
or dysmorphic red cells. Repeat echocardiogram revealed
a small pericardial effusion without tamponade, global
left ventricular hypokinesis, and no significant valvular
abnormalities. Ejection fraction was estimated at 15%.
Electrocardiogram showed sinus rhythm and nonspecific
ST-T wave changes. A right thoracentesis yielded tran-

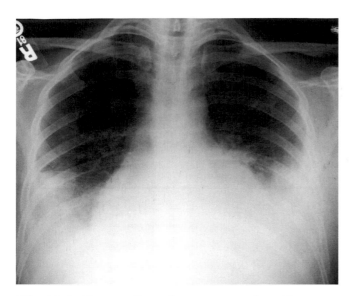

FIG. 63–1. Chest radiograph on presentation. There are bilateral pleural effusions seen in the bases of the lungs with pronounced cardiomegaly. The normal vascularity of the lung field excludes the possibility of congestive failure as a basis for the effusions.

sudative fluid with negative cytology, Gram stain, cultures, and LE prep. Left-sided pleural fluid obtained from the chest tube was also negative except for chemistries more compatible with an exudate. Cardiac hemodynamics by Swan-Ganz catheterization showed evidence of heart failure, which steadily improved over the next several days. With supportive care, limited low-dose dopamine infusion for the first 24 hours, and mild hydration, the patient's clinical status improved after several days, allowing her to be extubated and transferred out of the intensive care unit with removal of central lines and left chest tube. Azotemia and liver dysfunction secondary to transient ischemia gradually resolved. Repeat echocardiogram on December 26, 1991, showed improving left ventricular function (35% ejection fraction) and a small pericardial effusion. Later, a MUGA showed a 45% ejection fraction.

The etiology of the patient's acute illness finally became clear when the patient's pericardial fluid obtained at the outside hospital became available for cytologic analysis. Adenocarcinoma was diagnosed. A fine-needle aspirate of one of the small left posterior cervical nodes also showed adenocarcinoma. A computed tomography (CT) scan of the chest, abdomen, and pelvis showed thickened skin over the left breast, suspicious left axillary lymph nodes, multiple small wedge-shaped pulmonary nodules, pericardial and bilateral pleural effusions, and a left renal vein thrombus with collateral flow through the left gonadal vein. The patient was discharged from the hospital on January 3, 1992, in stable condition with a diagnosis of metastatic adenocarcinoma of unknown primary.

On follow-up with a medical oncologist on January 17, 1992, the patient complained of some new blurry vision with ophthalmologic and neurologic examinations showing no focal abnormalities. A magnetic resonance imaging (MRI) scan of the brain was scheduled. Repeat mammograms showed no suspicious lesions, although there was diffusely increased skin thickening over the left breast. Examination of the left breast now showed some subtle induration of the upper outer quadrant. In the meantime, hormone receptor assay on the pericardial fluid was reported as positive and weakly positive for estrogen and progesterone receptors, respectively. Bone scan was negative for metastases. With a presumption of breast cancer, tamoxifen was prescribed. On January 22, 1992, a surgeon performed a left breast punch biopsy, revealing invasive ductal carcinoma.

The patient's case was subsequently discussed at the multidisciplinary Breast Tumor Board. The initial difficulty in recognizing that the patient had a breast cancer primary was noted, but not felt to be unusual. Certainly, the initial problems with gastrointestinal bleeding and myalgias created some confusion. It was felt that malignancy would in retrospect have been a leading diagnostic possibility in a middle-aged women presenting with pericardial tamponade, with lung cancer also a high concern on a statistical basis. Records from the referring physician at the outside hospital were unclear as to whether any of the more classic signs and symptoms of tamponade were present (e.g., pulsus paradoxus, elevated venous pressures, low voltage on EKG, etc.). Clinically, events developed rapidly, with echocardiography critical in diagnosing the patient's underlying cardiovascular difficulties. Once diagnosed with cardiac tamponade, the proper therapeutic procedure—after initial resuscitation with intravenous fluids and, if needed, adrenergic agonists—was felt to be controversial with advocates for either pericardiocentesis or immediate subxyphoid pericardiotomy ("pericardial window" placement). This particular patient was felt to be at high risk for recurrent cardiac tamponade because a more definitive drainage procedure had not been performed. The patient was felt to be a candidate for systemic cytotoxic chemotherapy. It was unclear whether the patient would have a rapid enough response or that sufficient concentration of drugs would reach the pericardium to prevent further hemodynamic compromise. Although adriamycin-based regimens are the most active in metastatic breast cancer, another anthracycline mitoxantrone (along with cyclophosphamide and 5-fluorouracil; 5-FU) was selected, given its lower profile of cardiotoxicity.

Brain MRI showed multiple small metastatic lesions (Fig. 63–2). A Decadron taper was begun in light of a small degree of associated cerebral edema. Whole brain radiotherapy was initiated on January 28, 1992, 3,000 cGy in 10 fractions. The same day that radiotherapy was begun, the patient complained of increasing fatigue and

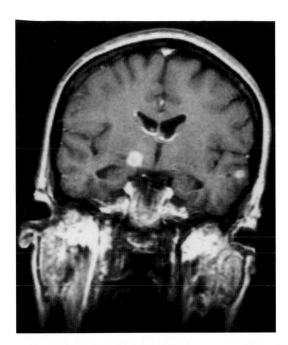

FIG. 63–2. MRI of brain showing multiple metastases. There are well-developed metastatic deposits in the left temporal lobe and in the region of the thalamus.

dyspnea on exertion. A chest radiograph suggested increasing pericardial and left pleural effusions. Another echocardiogram showed a large pericardial effusion, diastolic collapse of the right atrium, and normal left and right ventricular function. On January 30, 1992, the patient underwent an uncomplicated left thoracotomy and pericardial window. Inspection and palpation of the inferior surface of the pericardium showed extensive studding with tumor nodules and no areas of fluid loculation. Two days later, the patient received her first cycle of chemotherapy (cytoxan 500 mg/M^2, mitoxantrone 10 mg/M^2, and 5-FU 500 mg/M^2). Tamoxifen was continued. Several days thereafter, the patient resumed radiotherapy, had her chest tube removed, and was again discharged from the hospital in stable condition. Cranial irradiation was completed on February 14, 1992.

Two weeks later, when the patient presented for her second cycle of chemotherapy, she was again symptomatic with fatigue and dyspnea. Unfortunately, echocardiography again demonstrated reaccumulation of pericardial fluid with tamponade. Repeat CT scan of the chest (Fig. 63–3) showed massive enlargement of pericardial effusion with ill-defined borders between the heart and the fluid. Bilateral pleural effusions had increased as well. Otherwise, there was no evidence of other sites of rapidly progressive disease; left axillary adenopathy had slightly decreased and pulmonary nodules were not seen. A new 1.7-cm para-aortic node and a 2-cm left adrenal mass were described as well. On February 29, 1992, a subxyphoid pericardiotomy was performed with drainage of 800 cc of fluid and symptomatic improvement.

The case was again discussed at the Tumor Board. Treatment options discussed were (a) alternative chemotherapy, (b) bleomycin instillation within the pericardium, and (c) radiotherapy. Reliance on additional chemotherapy alone was not believed to be prudent because the patient had already failed a front-line regimen. It was thought that there was little evidence that bleomycin (or, alternatively, tetracycline) "sclerosis" of the pericardium would work, particularly because the penetration of drug into gross tumor nodules would be negligible. Radiotherapy was felt to be the best option given the desperate situation. It was commented that, historically, radioactive colloidal gold administered into the pericardial space might have been considered, but was no longer commercially available and would present a considerable radiation safety hazard. Theoretically, intrapericardial chromic phosphate-32, a beta emitter, could be considered but was without precedent in this situation and would have similar problems as bleomycin, in addition to radiation safety concerns. External beam radiotherapy was considered to make the most sense, recognizing that depending on dose and fractionation there would be some risk of late toxicity with pericardial and myocardial fibrosis. This realistically was a minor concern given the pressing need for effective palliation of the patient's recurring malignant pericardial effusion. Radiotherapy directed to the heart and mediastinum was begun on March 4, 1992, at 200 cGy per fraction with a planned total dose of 3,000 cGy.

Further complicating the patient's clinical course was a right lower extremity deep venous thrombosis. To avoid anticoagulation, an inferior vena cava filter was placed. Dyspnea in part due to progressive pleural effusions was managed with multiple therapeutic thoracenteses. With continued drainage through the pericardial tube, the effu-

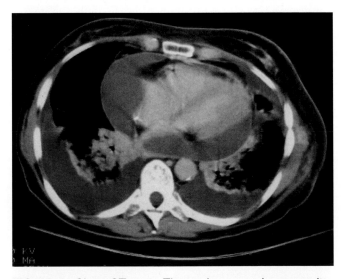

FIG. 63–3. Chest CT scan. The supine scan shows gravitation of the pleural fluid to the posterior gutters. The heart is essentially encased by the liquid. Some peripheral atelectasis of the lung is demonstrable posteriorly.

sion subsequently became superinfected with *Staphylococcus aureus*. Vancomycin was prescribed. A left lower extremity deep venous thrombosis occurred. With a ventilation/perfusion scan interpreted as high probability for embolic disease, heparin anticoagulation was reluctantly begun. The pericardial tube was finally removed on March 12, 1992, with resolution of purulent drainage. Radiotherapy continued to a total dose of 1,400 cGy and was discontinued on March 13, 1992. At that time, the patient had developed acute renal failure. The patient died on March 16, 1992.

COMMENTARY by Robert B. Livingston

In terms of the specific management of this patient's malignant pericardial effusion, the initial steps of pericardiocentesis, followed by subxiphoid pericardiotomy, appear reasonable and in keeping with currently accepted standard management (1). The failure of subxiphoid pericardiotomy to produce even short-term control of the effusion is distinctly unusual. I know of no evidence that the penetration of cytotoxic chemotherapy into the pericardium is compromised in patients with malignant effusion, and would agree with the initial use of systemic chemotherapy, as well as the subsequent reluctance to rely on further chemotherapy in view of apparent failure of the "first-line" regimen. However, there was disappearance of the "multiple wedge-shaped pulmonary nodules" described before chemotherapy, and some decrease in axillary adenopathy. Is it possible that tumor necrosis, associated with an increase in edema and associated lymphatic obstruction, accounted for the worsening of her pleural and pericardial effusions? Such a phenomenon is not inconceivable, and is one of the reasons why change in an effusion is not used as a major criterion for response (or progression) by medical oncologists. In this context, it would be helpful to know whether the cells removed on February 29 appeared necrotic, and whether there was an evident change in their proliferative activity (e.g., by flow cytometry or Ki-67 staining).

There is little experience with bleomycin instillation in the pericardium, although it may be superior to tetracycline as a sclerosant for pleural effusions (2). "Penetration of the drug into gross tumor nodules" would not be a consideration in the efficacy of a sclerosing agent, which are thought to act by producing an intense, localized inflammatory response, rather than through direct cytotoxicity. Although tetracycline has an extensive track record in the management of pericardial effusion, it is no longer commercially available (3). The related compound, doxycycline, is, however, available and would have merited consideration.

REFERENCES

1. Chan A, Rischin D, Clark CP, Woodruff RK. Subxiphoid partial pericardiectomy with or without sclerosant instillation in the treatment of symptomatic pericardial effusions in patients with malignancy. *Cancer* 1991;68:1021–5.
2. Ruckdeschel JC, Moores D, Lee JY, et al. Intrapleural therapy for malignant pleural effusions. A randomized comparison of bleomycin and tetracycline. *Chest* 1991;100:1528–35.
3. Davis S, Rambotti P, Grignani F. Intrapericardial tetracycline sclerosis in the treatment of malignant pericardial effusion: an analysis of thirty-three cases. *J Clin Oncol* 1984;6:631–6.

EDITORIAL BOARD COMMENTARY

It is easy for a physician to be deviated from the cancer problem by medical complications. Coping with the pericardial fluid in this case was not accompanied by an aggressive approach to the diagnosis and therapy of the cancer. The extensive evidence of disseminated cancer highly pointed to breast cancer (thickened skin of breast, axillary nodes). Tumor markers (CEA, CA-125, CA 15-3) might have given some evidence of malignancy. The clinical story is not consistent with a hormonally responsive tumor. Hormone receptor assay of pericardial fluid would be unproductive, even if possible. Tamoxifen as a hormonal therapy is not the treatment of choice. More than one course of aggressive chemotherapy early in the course of this disease would have been preferable, whereas radiotherapy would be of no help for such a disseminated cancer.

SECTION XV

Bone (Adult)

64

Chondrosarcoma of the Hemipelvis

Marvin M. Romsdahl

A technical challenge

CASE PRESENTATION

This 34-year-old man noted a mass in the left lower abdomen 3 months before referral. Although he was unable to discern any change in size during this period, his local physician thought it enlarged somewhat and attempted percutaneous biopsy with a Jamshidi needle. This biopsy being nondiagnostic, the patient submitted to a formal incisional biopsy, which revealed a proliferating cartilaginous tumor consistent with low-grade chondrosarcoma.

The patient had no prior history of surgery or past medical illnesses. Review of systems was within normal limits. The patient reported no change or alteration in bowel evacuation, urinary function, or sexual activity. He smoked one pack of cigarettes daily for the past 14 years and also drank beer daily. The patient's father had carcinoma of the colon and a maternal grandmother had carcinoma of the uterus.

Physical examination showed a 10 × 14 cm hard mass in the left iliac fossae described as rigid in location and fixed to the pelvis. A recent well-healing scar in the left lower quadrant extended diagonally in the direction of fibers of the external oblique muscle (Fig. 64–1). The abdomen above the mass was not tender, with no evidence of peritoneal irritation. Neurologic and vascular examination of the left lower extremity was normal, as well as elsewhere. Rectal sphincter tone was normal.

Initial abdomen and pelvis films showed a partially calcified mass attached on the left iliac bone, occupying much of the pelvis (Fig. 64–2). The excretory urogram revealed normal kidneys with no evidence of obstructive uropathy, although the left ureter was deviated medially because of the pelvic mass. Chest tomograms did not indicate metastases.

Further diagnostic evaluation at our institution included a computed tomography (CT) scan of the abdomen and pelvis, which indicated that the mass arose from the internal aspect of the ilium. It extended almost to the midline, appearing medial to the lateral extent of the transverse process of the fifth vertebral body and almost reaching the sacroiliac joint. The tumor extended into the pelvis in close proximity to the psoas muscle. (Fig. 64–3). The tissue slides of the original incisional biopsy were interpreted as grade I chondrosarcoma.

CONFERENCE PRESENTATION

The patient was presented to the Multidisciplinary Sarcoma Conference, at which wide surgical excision was recommended without prior radiotherapy or chemotherapy. Conference members did, however, raise the question as to whether a grade III chondrosarcoma component might be present in view of the large tumor size. A higher grade chondrosarcoma, especially a component of dedifferentiated chondrosarcoma, could serve to consider the merit of preoperative systemic therapy. The consensus was that the clinical, radiographic, and pathologic features favored a grade I and/or a grade II chondrosarcoma, thus supporting the decision for direct surgical intervention.

The conference participants agreed that the patient was a candidate for internal hemipelvectomy as opposed to formal hemipelvectomy with amputation. A question did arise as to whether the transection of the pelvis should be supra-acetabular or infra-acetabular. Conference members from the Department of Diagnostic Radiology offered that the relationship of the tumor to the acetabulum could be more accurately determined by 5-mm CT cuts at this level of the pelvis. Because transection of the pelvic bone above the

317

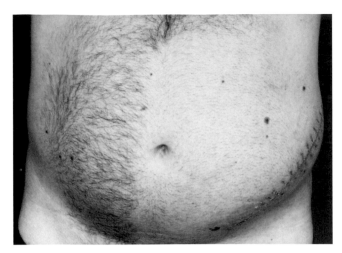

FIG. 64–1. Anterior view of lower abdomen after biopsy shows correctly placed incision to accommodate either standard or partial hemipelvectomy.

acetabulum allows for hip joint salvage, subsequent function is markedly better than with resection of the acetabulum and head of the femur. However, successfully oncologic management of the tumor should not be compromised to obtain this particular functional advantage. The surgical oncology team expressed concern that the size and location of the hard mass occupying a significant portion of pelvis space may preclude sufficient intraoperative definition of a safe margin above the acetabular ridge. In this setting, it is important not to risk transection or incision into the neoplasm, thereby increasing the risk of local recurrence and/or wound implantation of tumor cells.

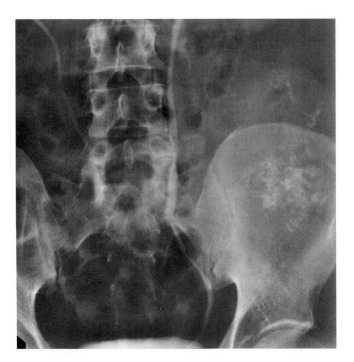

FIG. 64–2. Radiograph showing large tumor with calcium causing medical displacement of left ureter at inlet to pelvis.

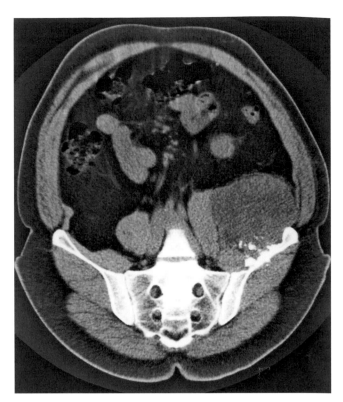

FIG. 64–3. CT scan demonstrates pelvic mass with destruction of ilium and compression of psoas muscle. The tumor extends medial to the superior aspect of the sacroiliac joint.

Surgical management consisted of left internal hemipelvectomy, transecting the femoral neck and the acetabulum in a manner to preserve integrity of the ischial and pubic bone components of this joint. The surgical incision "enveloped" the correctly placed incisional biopsy site, extending posterior adjacent to the wing of the ilium to gain exposure of the left sacral region. The posterior pelvic transection was performed to include the wing of the sacrum, medial to the sacroiliac joint, but lateral to the first and second sacral foramina (Fig. 64–4). This allowed complete removal of the iliac bone, minimizing the potential of tumor-positive surgical margins. The en bloc resection of the multilobulated 16 × 10 × 10 cm tumor showed focal involvement of the medullary cavity, extension into true soft tissue, and tumor-free margins at all bone and soft tissue surfaces (Fig. 64–5). Similarly, separate biopsies of the posterior sacral margin, inferior sacroiliac region, superior and anterior acetabulum margins, and synovial-covered connective tissue at the acetabulum showed no evidence of tumor. The wound was closed by suturing the posterior-based flap in two layers to the fascia of the anterior abdominal wall.

The patient sustained a small area of skin necrosis near the middle of the incision that healed with debridement and simple wound care. He rapidly became ambulatory with crutches, becoming able to transfer in and out of bed, and maneuver up and down stairs.

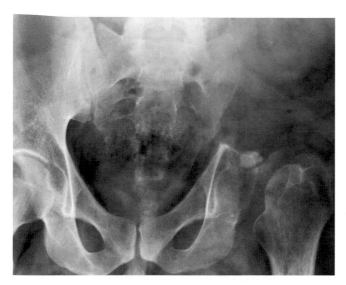

FIG. 64–4. Postoperative radiograph of pelvis shows relationship of transected femoral neck to remaining acetabulum and transection through wing of sacrum.

Routine follow-up at 6-month intervals failed to show evidence of recurrence. However, at 24 months after surgery, he developed progressive swelling of his operative region (Fig. 64–6). This was aggravated by his almost unrestricted activity as a farmer, including tractor driving, as well as substantial weight gain. Consequently, at 4 years post–internal hemipelvectomy, the patient had abdominal hernia repair utilizing Marlex and Dexon as a three-layer closure (Fig. 64–7). In the course of recover-

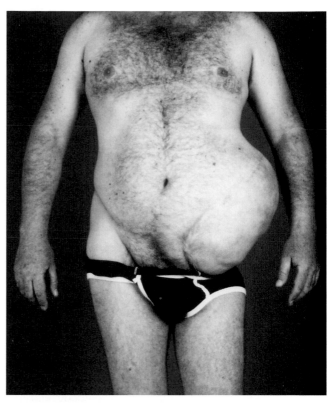

FIG. 64–6. Anterior view of patient shows large herniation of abdominal wall in surgical region.

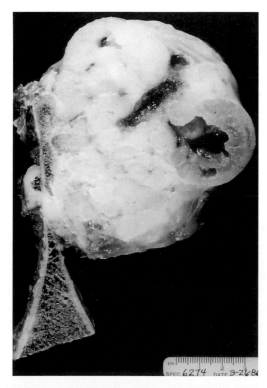

FIG. 64–5. The multilobulated cartilaginous tumor arises from the inner table of the ilium.

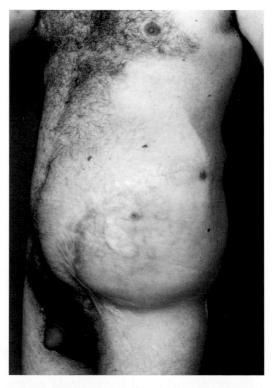

FIG. 64–7. Contour of operative region after repair of hernia, utilizing posterior flap for wound closure.

ing from this surgical procedure, the patient developed subsegmental atelectasis, interstitial changes, and pleural effusion. This problem, however, was successfully treated without long-term sequelae. He is now 7 years post-management of grade I chondrosarcoma of the ilium and free of evidence of recurrence.

REFERENCES

1. Evans HL, Ayala AG, Romsdahl MM. Prognostic factors in chondrosarcoma of bone: a clinicopathologic analysis with emphasis on histologic grading. *Cancer* 1977;40(2):818–30.
2. Romsdahl MM, Evans HL, Ayala AG. Surgical treatment of chondrosarcoma. In: *Current concepts in the management of primary bone and soft tumors.* The University of Texas System Cancer Center M. D. Anderson Hospital and Tumor Institute 21st Annual Clinical Conference on Cancer. Chicago, Yearbook Medical Publishers; 1977: 125–36.

COMMENTARY by John H. Healey

Dr. Romsdahl and colleagues expertly and successfully managed one of the most difficult oncologic problems, chondrosarcoma of the pelvis. The radiographic appearance is suggestive of chondrosarcoma, the most common malignant pelvic bone tumor. Diagnosis depends on biopsy. A CT-guided needle biopsy is frequently nondiagnostic in mineralized tumors, and may not be representative in heterogeneous tumors. Be it needle biopsy or open biopsy, it must be performed by the surgeon. Chondrosarcoma grows in a hypoxic environment, and can seed soft tissue. It is important to identify and tattoo the needle biopsy tract and excise it during resection. The biopsy must be planned as part of the extensive exposure necessary for internal hemipelvectomy. The most useful biopsy approach is typically along the iliac crest so that minimal amount of tissue need to be sacrificed on either side of the pelvis, maintaining sufficient tissue for closure after internal hemipelvectomy.

The grading of chondrosarcoma remains controversial. Most clinicians and pathologists consider three grades of chondrosarcoma reflecting metastatic potential. A special subset of dedifferentiated chondrosarcoma is also seen. Differential diagnosis in this case included an osteochondroma. Osteochondromas evolve into chondrosarcomas infrequently. But because the change appears to occur more often in the pelvis than the extremities, a high index of suspicion is needed for pelvic lesions. Even mild degrees of atypia should be sufficient to diagnose chondrosarcoma in the pelvis, whereas such changes would be innocuous in the distal extremities.

The value of biopsy is to specifically exclude the highest grade tumors for which chemotherapy may be considered and to rule out osteogenic sarcoma for which preoperative chemotherapy is established treatment. Whether or not preoperative chemotherapy should be given for high-grade chondrosarcomas is uncertain. Extremely poor patient survival is an important theoretic reason for seeking systemic therapy. Recent molecular biologic evidence suggests that virtually all high-grade chondrosarcomas overexpress a multidrug resistance gene. This correlates with a lack of histologic response to adriamycin and cisplatin given preoperatively in 20 patients from our institution. The potential to facilitate surgery by shrinking the tumor doesn't work because the extracellular matrix and calcified mass do not shrink even when tumor necrosis occurs. Finally, the patients are typically older adults and they are less tolerant of aggressive chemotherapy. Poor nutrition and wound healing are the common consequences, adding to the surgical morbidity.

Work-up includes chest CT scan, particularly if amputation is to be considered, and a whole-body bone scan to rule out multifocal disease, extrapulmonary metastases, and possible existence of multiple osteochondromatosis. Local diagnostic imaging includes CT scan with intravenous and oral contrast to properly identify intrapelvic structures. MRI including narrow T2-weighted cuts is very important to evaluate margins in the supra-acetabular area. Thallium scans have been misleading because they are often cold in all grades of chondrosarcoma.

Although local excision is the method to treat chondrosarcoma, this is just as true for a low-grade as a high-grade tumor. The surgical margin is essentially no different between a standard hemipelvectomy and a so-called internal hemipelvectomy. Preperitoneal fat and areolar tissue constitute the margin in each case. The decision to perform internal hemipelvectomy is often guided by the ability to preserve femoral and/or sciatic nerve function. The sciatic nerve in the area of the notch and lumbosacral plexus are particularly vulnerable in large medial tumors with intrapelvic extension. The femoral nerve may also be involved with tumor as it courses between the iliacus and psoas muscles. Extra-articular resection is strongly advised at the sacroiliac joint, as emphasized by the author. Although the tumor can course across ligamentous structures and traverse the joint, typically a good plane exists between the SI joint and the neural foramina. Similarly, an extra-articular resection of the hip is frequently necessary if the joint is contaminated. Careful imaging is important in this regard. Frequently, the resected segment of proximal femur is not specifically involved by tumor and it may be used as bone graft to help stabilize the pelvis or serve as a recipient bone for the socket and total hip replacement. Ligation of the internal iliac artery and vein are often required. Whenever possible, preservation of the gluteal vessels is recommended to retain vascularity to the flap. Plan the soft tissue and bone reconstruction. Whenever possible, the inferior epigastric artery and rectus abdominous muscle should be retained as a good source for soft tissue coverage. Pelvic resections are prone to develop serious bowel herniation and/incarceration. The smaller the defect, the more reconstruction of the pelvis and/or use of mesh should be considered. Skeletal reconstructive options include creating a flail limb with a girdlestone type hip resection, a total hip replacement, or hip fusion. The goals are to create a pain-free stable joint with suitable limb length to minimize energy expenditure during walking and maximize function. Femoral ischial arthrodesis is an excellent alternative if the acetabulum is resected (type II pelvic resection). Pelvic replacement with allograft or metal prosthesis may give spectacularly good results. Nevertheless, they are quite prone to infection because of the deficient soft tissue envelope. Fixation proximally to the sacrum remains a serious problem. When a solid post remains in the proximal ilium, a saddle prosthesis is an excellent and rapid reconstructive solution.

Careful follow-up is required for 10 years for chondrosarcoma. Its course is unpredictable. Despite the low-grade histology, metastatic potential is real in these cases. I would recommend examination and chest radiography every 3 months initially. Chest CT may be performed periodically as required. Imaging for potential local recurrence is quite difficult, particularly if there is a significant amount of orthopedic hardware in the reconstruction. Arteriography, although not perfect, seems to be the best mode at the present.

In conclusion, Dr. Romsdahl and his team are to be commended for their success with internal hemipelvectomy—the most challenging of musculoskeletal oncologic procedures.

65

Solitary Plasmacytoma

Robert Kyle

In contrast to rapidly lethal multiple myeloma, solitary plasmacytoma is an indolent form of the disease

CASE PRESENTATION

Case 1.

This 31-year-old white man noted a mass in his left cervical region in January 1988. This was treated with two courses of antibiotics without improvement. A biopsy on August 2, 1988, revealed a plasmacytoma (Fig. 65–1). Bone marrow examination, skeletal radiographs, and studies of the serum and urine were reported as negative. He received 50 cGy over 32 days from October 3, 1988, to November 4, 1988.

In December 1988, he developed pain in a right anterior rib while walking his dog. A needle biopsy of the right third rib revealed a plasmacytoma. He was given 40 cGy to the rib over a 4-week period, beginning March 20, 1989.

He was first seen at the Mayo Clinic on May 15, 1989. He said that he felt fine. He had noted some fatigue, but this was decreasing. He denied bone pain, weakness, recurrent infections, or bleeding. On physical examination he looked good. The blood pressure was 120/84. He was 75 inches in height and weighed 199 pounds. There was a healed incision in the left cervical area. The heart and lungs were negative. The liver and spleen were not palpable and there was no lymphadenopathy. Physical examination revealed grade 1 benign prostatic hypertrophy. There was no tenderness of his ribs or sinuses on palpation. The remainder of the physical examination was noncontributory.

The hemoglobin was 14.5 g/dL, hematocrit 41%, and erythrocytes 4.67×10^{12}/L. The leukocytes were 3.4×10^9/L with neutrophils 52%, lymphocytes 33%, monocytes 7%, eosinophils 7%, and basophils 1%. The

platelets were 197×10^9/L. The peripheral blood smear appeared normal. The calcium was 9.4 mg/dL, creatinine 1.2 mg/dL, uric acid 7.9 mg/dL, and alkaline phosphatase 134 U/L (nl 98–251 U/L). The lactate dehydrogenase was 77 U/L (nl 91–196 U/L). The serum β_2-macroglobulin value was 1.9 μg/mL (nl ≤2.7 μg/mL). Serum protein electrophoresis revealed no abnormalities. Immunoelectrophoresis and immunofixation showed no evidence of a monoclonal protein. The IgG was 1,240, IgA 183, and IgM 186 mg/dL. The routine urinalysis was negative for sugar and protein. Microscopic examination was negative. A 24-hour urine specimen contained 130 mg of protein. Electrophoresis showed no globulin band. Immunoelectrophoresis and immunofixation showed no evidence of a monoclonal protein. A metastatic bone survey including the humeri and femurs and localized views of the left anterior ribs revealed a lytic, expansile lesion in the anterior end of the right third rib. A chest radiograph showed no additional lesions. A bone marrow aspirate and biopsy showed no increase in plasma cells. The specimen for the bone marrow plasma cell labeling index contained insufficient plasma cells for the labeling index.

No treatment was advised. In September 1989, the patient had a bone marrow harvest of 1.4×10^{10} monoclonal cells at his home hospital in the event that high-dose chemotherapy/total body irradiation followed by bone marrow rescue would become necessary.

The patient returned to the Mayo Clinic for re-evaluation on September 12, 1990, November 5, 1991, and September 21, 1992. At his last visit he denied increased fatigue, bone pain, palpable masses, recurrent infections, or bleeding. His physical examination was unchanged.

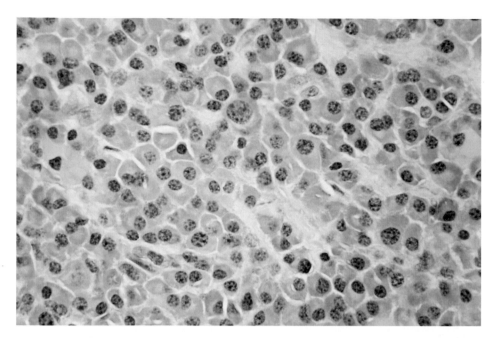

FIG. 65–1. Section of left cervical lymph node showing atypical plasma cells consistent with a solitary extramedullary plasmacytoma (H&E, ×640).

The hemoglobin was 15.0 g/dL, calcium 9.8 mg/dL, creatinine 1.2 mg/dL, and uric acid 7.9 mg/dL. Immunoelectrophoresis and immunofixation of the serum and urine showed no evidence of a monoclonal protein. A bone marrow aspirate and biopsy contained no evidence of a plasma cell proliferative disorder. The specimen for the plasma cell labeling index contained only polyclonal plasma cells. The peripheral blood labeling index of the cytoplasmic immunoglobulin-positive cells was 0.0%. No circulating plasma cells were detected. The chest radiograph and metastatic bone survey showed no change in the expansile lesion in the right third rib. No other lesions were seen. The β_2-microglobulin value was 1.2 μg/dL and C-reactive protein 0.15 mg/dL (nl <0.8 mg/dL).

He was advised to have his hemoglobin, calcium, creatinine, serum and urine evaluated at 4-month intervals. If any changes occur, he should have a metastatic bone survey and examination of the bone marrow and peripheral blood for the presence of plasma cells.

This patient is unusual in that he presented with an extramedullary plasmacytoma and shortly thereafter developed a solitary plasmacytoma of the rib. He has remained asymptomatic and without evidence of multiple myeloma for more than 4.5 years.

Case 2.

This 42-year-old white woman came to the Mayo Clinic on May 22, 1978, because of fluid retention, arthritic pains, recurrent sore throats, and a history of multiple allergies.

On physical examination, the blood pressure was 120/85. She was 67 inches in height and weighed 165 pounds. Physical examination revealed a carotid bruit. There was a short grade 2 systolic murmur on cardiac auscultation. The lungs were clear. The liver and spleen were not palpable and there was no lymphadenopathy. The remainder of the physical examination was noncontributory. The hemoglobin was 12.1 g/dL, erythrocytes $3,800,000 \times 10^{12}$/L, leukocytes $4,500 \times 10^9$/L with a normal differential, and platelets $280,000 \times 10^9$/L. The erythrocyte sedimentation rate was 32 mm/hr (Westergren). The calcium was 9.3 mg/dL, uric acid 5.4 mg/dL, and creatinine 0.8 mg/dL. Serum protein electrophoresis revealed no abnormalities. Immunoelectrophoresis revealed a probable small monoclonal IgA kappa protein. The quantitative immunoglobulins were as follows: IgG 1,278 mg/dL, IgA 422 mg/dL, and IgM 230 mg/dL. A skull film revealed a large lytic lesion involving the right mandible. Roentgenograms of the mandible confirmed the presence of a large lytic lesion (Fig. 65–2). A metastatic bone survey showed no other lytic lesions. A routine urinalysis contained no sugar or protein. Microscopic evaluation was negative. A 24-hour urine specimen contained no monoclonal protein.

Biopsy of the mandibular lesion revealed sheets of plasma cells consistent with a plasmacytoma (Fig. 65–3). A bone marrow aspirate and biopsy showed no evidence of myeloma. She received 40 Gy to the lesion from June 5–16, 1978. The monoclonal serum protein disappeared after radiation therapy.

Subsequent roentgenograms of the right mandible revealed inadequate healing of the lesion. On May 3,

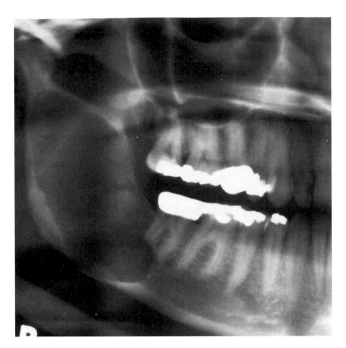

FIG. 65–2. Roentgenogram of right mandible showing a large lytic lesion.

1979, the mandible was re-explored and disclosed a small amount of granulation-like tissue within the cavity. This was debrided and histologic examination revealed a well differentiated plasmacytoma. Immunoperoxidase studies showed staining with only kappa antisera confirming the neoplastic nature of the process. Osteoradionecrosis occurred and required debridement and saucerization of

the right mandible on November 6, 1979. A right hemi-mandibulectomy was performed on December 11, 1979, and 6 months later mandibular reconstruction with rib and iliac crest grafts was attempted. This was unsuccessful. Reconstruction of the right mandible was attempted again on August 10, 1981.

A small monoclonal IgA kappa protein was again found in the serum on June 27, 1984. The serum IgA level was 328 mg/dL. On June 16, 1987, small lytic defects were seen in the clavicles and humeri. The hemoglobin was 12.2 g/dL, calcium 10.1 mg/dL, and creatinine 0.9 mg/dL. Immunoelectrophoresis and immunofixation of the serum revealed a small monoclonal IgA kappa protein. The quantitative immunoglobulins were as follows: IgG 1360 mg/dL, IgA 378 mg/dL, and IgM 159 mg/dL. A 24-hour urine specimen contained 104 mg of protein. No monoclonal protein was found with immunofixation. The lytic lesions increased slightly and on October 30, 1990, lytic lesions involved the calvarium, ribs, clavicles, humeri, and femurs. The hemoglobin was 12.0 g/dL, calcium 9.9 mg/dL, and creatinine 0.8 mg/dL. The IgA value was 390 mg/dL. A 24-hour urine specimen contained 35 mg of protein. Immunofixation showed no monoclonal protein. A bone marrow aspirate and biopsy on August 14, 1991, was nondiagnostic. The specimen for the labeling index contained 2% plasma cells. They appeared mature and stained with kappa antisera. The labeling index was 0.0%. She had no symptoms directly related to multiple myeloma, and no treatment was advised.

She was last seen on October 6, 1992. She denied increased fatigue, back pain, recurrent infections, or bleeding. Physical examination revealed no changes.

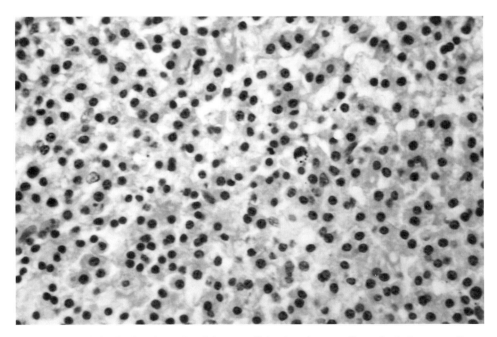

FIG. 65–3. Section of the lesion from the right mandible showing small atypical plasma cells consistent with a solitary plasmacytoma (H&E, × 640).

The hemoglobin was 12.6 g/dL, calcium 9.7 mg/dL, and creatinine 0.9 mg/dL. Immunoelectrophoresis and immunofixation revealed no change in the small monoclonal IgA kappa protein. The IgA value was 438 mg/dL. A 24-hour specimen contained 43 mg of protein. Immunofixation showed no evidence of a monoclonal light chain. A metastatic bone survey showed no change in the lytic lesions. She was advised to continue without chemotherapy.

The diagnosis of plasmacytoma was a serendipitous discovery from a skull film that was ordered because of a carotid bruit. In contrast to most patients, the plasmacytoma was not destroyed despite radiation, which produced radionecrosis. The residual plasmacytoma was removed by curettage. Six years after the recognition of the plasmacytoma, a small monoclonal IgA kappa protein recurred. Nine years after diagnosis, she developed multiple lytic bone lesions. However, the lesions did not progress and she has had no other evidence of multiple myeloma. Chemotherapy has been withheld, and she remains stable 14.5 years after recognition of a solitary plasmacytoma and more than 5 years after the discovery of lytic bone lesions. She will continue to be seen at 4- to 6-month intervals for appropriate laboratory and roentgenographic studies.

COMMENTARY by B.J. Kennedy

A 31-year-old man developed a neck mass and a rib lesion that were plasmacytomas. Each was given radiation therapy. Another expansile rib lesion has not been treated. Bone marrows were negative. After 4.5 years there is no evidence of progression of the disease.

The second case is that of a 42-year-old woman who had a mandibular plasmacytoma treated with radiation therapy. Nine years later she has multiple lytic bone lesions but no therapy has been given with survival of 14.5 years.

These cases illustrate the normal course of solitary plasmacytomas versus multiple myeloma. These solitary lesions usually occur in younger persons, are initially solitary lesions, have an absence of myeloma cells in the bone marrow, and lack anemia, hypercalcemia, or renal involvement (1–4). This rare phenomenon represents less than 10% of all plasma cell neoplasms (2). Local radiotherapy is used for relief of symptoms. Dissemination of the disease occurs in most of the patients with the eventual development of multiple myeloma. The general consensus is that solitary plasmacytoma of the bone and myelomatosis are the same disease process (4).

Because of the long duration of this phenomenon, intensive early chemotherapy has not been used, but surgery or radiation therapy are employed for symptomatic improvement. Observation and monitoring the long course of this disease appears to be the most efficacious method of management, as clearly demonstrated in the two cases.

REFERENCES

1. Batallo R, Sony J. Solitary myeloma: clinical and prognostic features of a review of 114 cases. *Cancer* 1980;48:845–50.
2. Knowling MA, Harwood AR, Bergsagel DE. Comparison of extramedullary plasmacytomas with solitary and multiple plasma cell tumors of the bone. *J Clin Oncol* 1983;1:255–62.
3. Dimopoulas MA, Goldstein J, Fuller L, et al. Curability of solitary bone plasmacytoma. *J Clin Oncol* 1992;10:587–90.
4. Chak LY, Cox RS, Bostwick DG, Hoppe RT. Solitary plasmacytomas of bone: treatment, progression, and survival. *J Clin Oncol* 1987;5:1811–15.

SECTION XVI

Soft Tissue Sarcoma (Adult)

66

Retroperitoneal Liposarcoma

Paul H. O'Brien, John S. Metcalf, and Stephen I. Schabel

Adjuvant therapy: yes or no?

CASE PRESENTATION

The patient was a 55-year-old woman who complained that over a period of 4 to 5 months she had noticed a fullness in her abdomen and vague discomfort in the lower right quadrant of her abdomen without alteration in bowel habit or genitourinary symptoms. On physical examination there was a palpable tender mass in the right abdomen, without guarding or rigidity. There were no signs of sepsis.

A double-contrast barium enema had been obtained by her primary physician, which was interpreted as showing some displacement of the right colon anteriorly and medially. The patient's stools were negative for blood. With this information, a computed tomography (CT) scan was ordered.

A CT axial image of the upper abdomen near the mid–left kidney shows a mixed water and fat density mass involving the retroperitoneum (Fig. 66–1A). The water density components of the mass measure about 20 Hounsfield units (cursor #1). Although the tumor seems relatively well encapsulated and is displacing adjacent bowel loops anteriorly on the right side, it has deeply invaded the paraspinal muscles and is extending to the neuroforamina on the right side.

The CT examination at the level of the midiliac wings reveals the extension of this same tumor into the pelvis (Fig. 66–1B). Although predominantly fatty in the pelvis, the tumor has septae of water density and again is deeply infiltrating the perirectal and peri-iliac soft tissues. From an imaging standpoint, this tumor has components of both mature fat and less mature water density tissue. It is infiltrating along tissue planes.

A CT scan of the chest was accomplished and showed no abnormalities or potential metastatic sites.

The preoperative diagnosis was retroperitoneal sarcoma, or less likely lymphoma. The patient underwent an exploratory laparotomy through a midline incision. After reflection of the right colon, the tumor was visualized and a longitudinal incisional biopsy accomplished, as the possibility of lymphoma was considered.

The tumor did not have extensive involvement with the mesocolon. It did seem to be located very posteriorly in the retroperitoneal space in close proximity to the aorta. It was yellowish white, medium density, with an irregular serrated border. Clinically, the assumption was liposarcoma based on its gross appearance and subsequent frozen section. Frozen section was not diagnostic but compatible with liposarcoma.

Because of the posterior extension, it was not felt to be resectable with a definitive margin. Tumor was removed, and the volume of tumor removed was estimated to be 95% of the total. Metallic clips were placed where the tumor was felt to be unresectable. Histologic sections of this large soft tissue mass showed a proliferation of fairly uniform neoplastic cells characterized by indistinct cytoplasmic boundaries and relatively small and uniform nuclei set in a myxomatous background. The tumor was well vascularized, with numerous small branching blood vessels coursing throughout (Fig. 66–2). On higher magnification, some of the nuclei of the neoplastic cells appeared indented by cytoplasmic vacuoles, with the cells having the configuration of lipoblasts (Fig. 66–3). Histochemical staining showed the myxoid staining matrix to be rich in hyaluronic acid. Sometimes, neutral fat can be identified within the tissue as well. The ultimate perma-

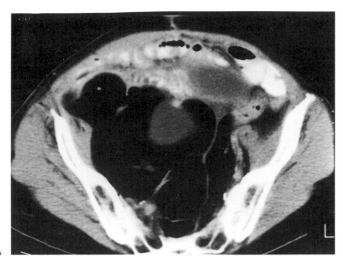
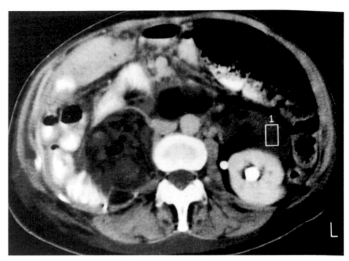

A   B

FIG. 66–1. CT scans of the abdomen and pelvis. **A:** Section through the upper abdomen at the level of the kidneys shows a mixed water and fat density mass in the retroperitoneum. **B:** Section at the level of the midiliac wings showing extension into the pelvis of the predominantly fatty mass. There is extensive infiltration of the perirectal and peri-iliac soft tissues.

nent histology on the resected tumor was a low-grade myxoid liposarcoma. The patient was treated with 5,000 cGy. The patient has been followed and is doing fairly well 4 years post-treatment. To the best of our information our patient remains without progressive disease.

COMMENTARY by Walter Lawrence, Jr.

Soft tissue sarcomas (STS) comprise only about 1% to 2% of all malignant neoplasms in adults and STS arising in the retroperitoneal area represent only 10% to 20% of STS (12.3% in the large pattern of care survey of the American College of Surgeons [1]. Approximately one third of all malignant neoplasms arising in the retroperitoneum prove to be primary lymphoma—a significant consideration in a patient such as this, because management of this condition relies heavily on nonresectional treatment whereas treatment of retroperitoneal STS is primarily operative.

Retroperitoneal STS represent both a diagnostic and therapeutic dilemma because of their "silent" growth, the large size they can reach before being detected, and their prognosis when compared with STS of more accessible sites (1–5). Five-year survival is approximately 50%

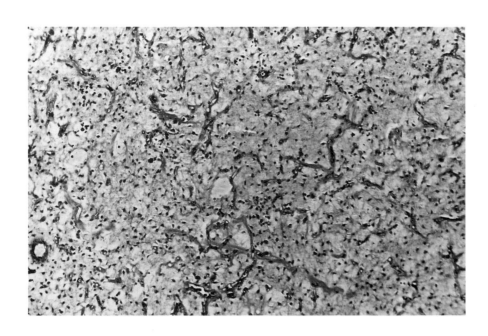

FIG. 66–2. Histologic specimen showing a well-vascularized tumor with numerous small branching blood vessels throughout.

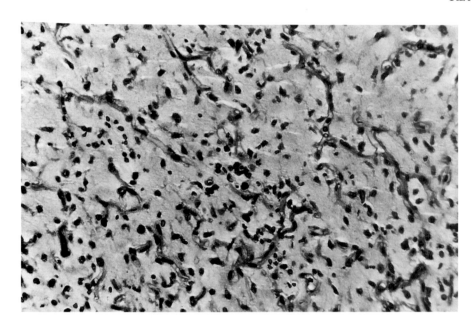

FIG. 66–3. Histologic speciment showing some of the nuclei of the neoplastic cells, which appear to be indented by cytoplasmic vacuoles.

when all gross disease is resected whereas more than 70% of patients with STS of the extremities survive at 5 years if there were no distant metastases at initial presentation and all gross disease was resected.

The most frequent histologic varieties of retroperitoneal STS in most studies are liposarcoma and leiomyosarcoma with malignant fibrous histiocytoma (MFH) rapidly becoming a major histology in more recent years (MFH was described as an entity only in 1961). The most favorable histologic variety in this location is liposarcoma because it is often well differentiated and associated with longer survival than other types as well as often being amenable to re-resection despite local recurrences.

The patient described presented with nonspecific symptoms of fullness and a vague discomfort, as well as a palpable abdominal mass, a rather typical clinical presentation for retroperitoneal STS. Diagnostic workup in this clinical situation often begins with "imaging" procedures, if there are no bowel or genitourinary symptoms, but the lower abdominal mass in this case prompted a barium enema, a not unreasonable initial test because right colon cancers are often palpable despite absence of obstructive symptoms. The histopathology in this case (myxoid liposarcoma) is one of the two most frequent types and might well have been suspected from the findings on this abdominal CT examination. Magnetic resonance imaging (MRI) is now considered preferable to CT for evaluation of many STS (particularly the extremities), but CT is still preferred for trunk sites because of motion artifacts associated with MRI. Whereas clinical examination is often a better guide to the extent of disease in patients with STS of the extremities, CT is invaluable for accurate assessment of lesions of the retroperitoneum (6) (as well as for later assessment of the lungs).

Despite the CT findings in this patient, lymphoma was considered a possible diagnosis before operation. Although an operative biopsy was planned to clarify this, another consideration would have been preoperative fine-needle or core-needle biopsy under CT guidance, an approach that would simplify the conduct of a subsequent operation. It would either enhance or eliminate the lymphoma diagnostic possibility. A second preoperative consideration in this case might have been preparation for possible application of brachytherapy with afterloading catheters at the time of operation because a narrow margin or incomplete resection might have been predicted in this patient from the CT. Adjuvant radiation by brachytherapy has not been shown to be superior to external beam radiotherapy for more accessible sites. However, radiation therapy by external beam generally has been unsuccessful in achieving local disease control in the retroperitoneum when gross disease remains after operation. In our own series there was no evidence of survival benefit from external beam radiotherapy in patients in whom gross disease remained after attempted resection (5).

No consideration of adjuvant chemotherapy was mentioned in this case presentation. This was for a good reason, because no clinical trials thus far have demonstrated a survival benefit from such therapy (7). Continued trials of this approach are necessary before adjuvant chemotherapy programs this approach can be established as "standard."

What is the outlook for this patient now that 4 years have elapsed since the primary treatment? In collected series there was 61% local treatment failure despite gross resection of retroperitoneal STS and a number of individual institutional reports have even higher rates of local treatment failure. Overall survival at 5 years after gross resection is usually 50% despite this because some retroperitoneal STS are low-grade, nonmetastasizing, and amenable to re-resection. The risk for ultimate local treatment failure in this patient is still considerable despite the 4-year interval so periodic follow-up physical examination and CT is appropriate.

REFERENCES

1. Lawrence W Jr, Donegan WL, Natarajan N, et al. Adult soft tissue sarcomas (a pattern of care survey of the American College of Surgeons). *Ann Surg* 1987;205:349–59.

2. Cody HS III, Turnbull AD, Fortner JG, Hajdu SI. The continuing challenge of retroperitoneal sarcomas. *Cancer* 1981;47:2147–52.

3. Moore SV, Aldrete JS. Primary retroperitoneal sarcomas: the role of surgical treatment. *Am J Surg* 1981;142:358–61.

4. Storm FK, Eilber FR, Mirra J, Morton DL. Retroperitoneal sarcomas: a reappraisal of treatment. *J Surg Oncol* 1981;17:1–7.

5. McGrath PC, Neifeld JP, Lawrence W Jr, et al. Improved survival following complete excision of retroperitoneal sarcomas. *Ann Surg* 1984;200:200–4.

6. Neifeld JP, Walsh JW, Lawrence W Jr. Computed tomography in the management of soft tissue tumors. *Surg Gynecol Obstet* 1982;155:535–40.

7. Lawrence W Jr, Neifeld JP. Soft tissue sarcomas. *Curr Probl Surg* 1989;26(11):755–827.

67

Extremity Soft Tissue Sarcoma

J. Milburn Jessup and Glenn D. Steele, Jr.

*A case of resection and microscopically positive margins
for functional limb preservation*

CASE PRESENTATION

R.L. is a 48-year-old Caucasian man who noticed pain in his left posterior thigh approximately 2 months before presentation. He did not have any other complaints and did not initially notice a mass in his thigh. However, as the dull, aching pain increased, he began to feel a mass on the posterolateral aspect of his left thigh. There were no radicular pains or any swelling of the lower extremity. The patient did not have any decrease in appetite, weight loss, or other significant past history. The patient was seen by his referring physician who obtained a magnetic resonance image (MRI), which revealed a 10 × 13 × 8 cm lesion in the posterior compartment of the left buttock. The mass arose in the head of the left biceps femoris muscle at the inferior aspect of the gluteus maximus muscle (Fig. 67–1B) and extended distally, involving the body of the left biceps femoris muscle. The sciatic nerve appeared to be on the edge of the tumor but not encompassed by it (Fig. 67–2).

On physical examination, the pertinent findings were restricted to the left thigh. The patient had a 10-cm, smooth, semimobile mass that was in the posterolateral left thigh and had as its superior aspect the gluteus maximus muscle. There was no pain on palpation. There were palpable dorsalis pedis, posterior tibial, and popliteal pulses below the mass. There was no evidence of altered sensation or joint position sense in the limb. The patient displayed good motor strength of all muscle groups of the thigh and lower leg. A computed tomography (CT) scan of the chest did not reveal any pulmonary metastases.

The patient's thigh was explored through a posterior thigh incision under general anesthesia. A core biopsy was obtained that on frozen section suggested the tumor was a malignant mesenchymal tumor without further classification. The lesion was then excised, along with removal of the left biceps femoris muscle from origin to insertion. A portion of the left gluteus maximus was removed because it was adherent to the mass. The left sciatic nerve was preserved, although it was clear that the tumor abutted the sciatic nerve. The skin was approximated with closed suction drains. The patient recovered uneventfully.

The final pathology revealed that the tumor was 12 × 9 × 8.5 cm in greatest dimensions. The tumor had a heterogeneous yellow-tan surface with scattered areas of necrosis, hemorrhage, and degeneration. On histologic and electron microscopic section, the tumor was diagnosed as a moderately to poorly differentiated, predominantly myxoid type of liposarcoma but with areas of focal round cell involvement (Figs. 67–3, 67–4). There were also foci of degeneration, necrosis, and blood vessel invasion. The area of the sciatic nerve was identified and showed a microscopic positive margin. The final AJCC pathologic stage was IIB (G2 T2 N0 M0).

At the Tumor Board discussion there was consideration of the best mode of limb preservation in this situation. The consensus opinion was that the sciatic nerve should be preserved and that postoperative radiotherapy to prevent local recurrence of this grade II liposarcoma was appropriate. Because this is not a high-grade lesion and active institutional or cooperative group protocols for this stage of soft tissue sarcoma are not available, it is not considered appropriate to give adjuvant chemotherapy to this patient. The discussion also centered on the possibility of preoperative radiotherapy or chemotherapy. The patient comes from a

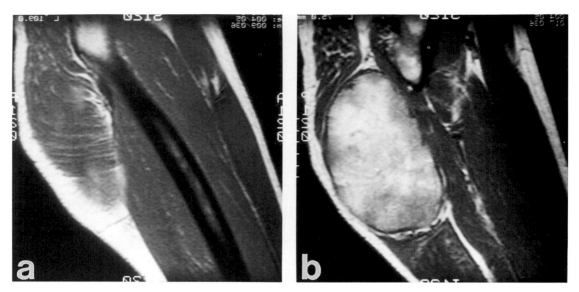

FIG. 67–1. MRI of proximal thigh soft tissue sarcoma, MRI scan, sagittal section. Tumor arises in head of biceps femoris muscle, inferior to gluteus maximus muscle. The gluteus maximus and biceps femoris are seen in the midplane of the femur (**A**) and then through the middle of the tumor (**B**). Note the tumor displaces the overlying gluteus maximus superiorly.

rural area in which access to such medical care is limited. The University of Texas M.D. Anderson Cancer Center series reported by Barkley et al. (1) suggests that there may be some benefit to preoperative radiotherapy for high-grade sarcomas. However, because this is an intermediate-grade sarcoma, it is not clear that such an approach is warranted without prospective trials. Similarly, the data with

neoadjuvant chemotherapy has not yet been proven in a prospective trial to be superior to excision and postoperative radiation. The recent experience from Memorial Sloan-Kettering (2) suggests that even if the patient has a local failure in the thigh, salvage may still be possible with further surgery, perhaps without loss of limb.

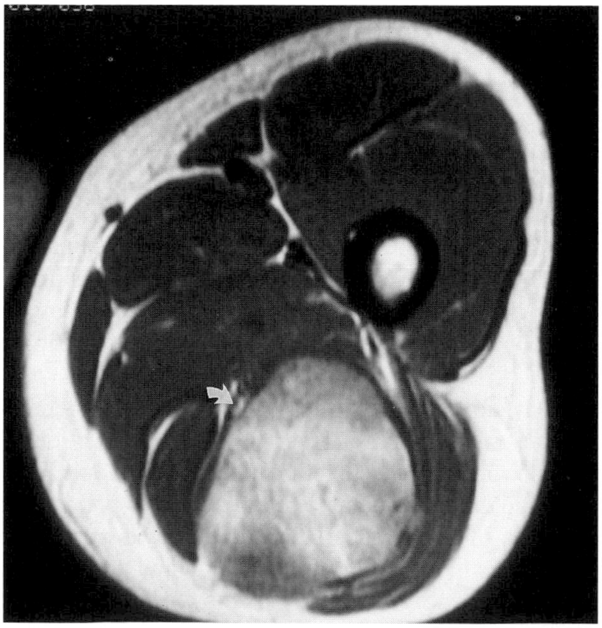

REFERENCES

1. Barkley HT Jr, Martin RG, Romsdahl MM, et al. Treatment of soft tissue sarcomas by preoperative irradiation and conservative surgical resection. *Int J Radiat Oncol Biol Phys* 1988;14:693–9.
2. Williard WC, Hajdu SI, Casper ES, Brennan MF. Comparison of amputation with limb-sparing operations for adult soft tissue sarcoma of the extremity. *Ann Surg* 1992;215:269–75.

COMMENTARY by Marvin M. Romsdahl

Management of this patient by the two modalities of surgery and radiotherapy is appropriate in view of our knowledge of the clinical behavior of this neoplasm.

The differential diagnosis of a large, expansive mass presenting in the thigh would include low-, intermediate-, or high-grade liposarcoma as well as a spectrum of other histologic types of sarcoma. It may have been feasible to establish preoperatively that this lesion was an intermediate- or high-grade sarcoma by either percutaneous fine-needle aspiration or core biopsy, thus allowing one to determine if radiotherapy could contribute to achieving local control. A low-grade tumor identified by this means would probably exclude a potential role for adjunctive radiotherapy. One aspect of preoperative diagnosis is that

FIG. 67–2. Transverse section of MRI scan through midportion of tumor. The relationship to the sciatic nerve is outlined *(arrow)* and the nerve is displaced but not encircled by tumor.

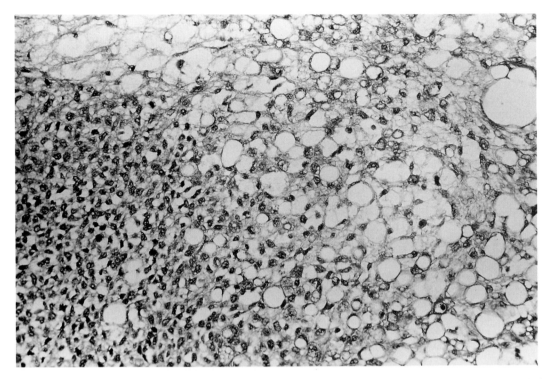

FIG. 67–3. Histologic section of the tumor demonstrating its pleomorphic features with a round cell infiltrate *(bottom left)* and lipid-filled adipocytes *(upper right)* (H&E, ×100).

it would allow a choice of preoperative versus postoperative radiotherapy.

Generally, when postoperative therapy is employed, it is considered appropriate to irradiate the entire surgical field to encompass neoplastic cells potentially contaminating surgically disturbed tissues. Preoperative irradiation of a field that extends well beyond the mass may still be smaller than one delivered postoperatively if one accepts that the entire surgically disturbed field should be irradiated. A smaller radiotherapy field should result in less long-term disability without compromising the prospects for local tumor control. Should a high-grade

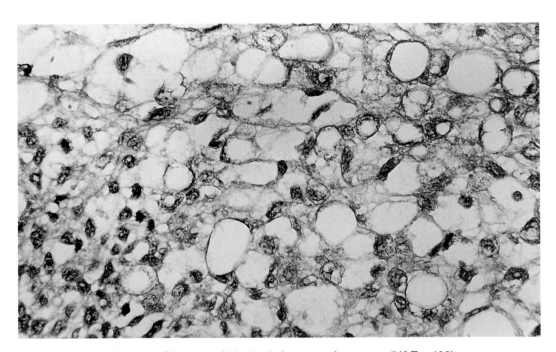

FIG. 67–4. Close-up of histologic features of sarcoma (H&E, ×400).

tumor be identified, a preoperative diagnosis may also allow the clinician to consider neoadjuvant chemotherapy to address promptly potential metastatic disease not identifiable by current means.

Radical surgery, as with muscle or compartment resection from origin to insertion, may often obviate the need for adjunctive radiotherapy. However, in this patient, the proximity of tumor to the sciatic nerve and the gluteus maximus muscle strongly suggested the employment of radiotherapy with limb salvage as the goal. This would have been the case for either an intermediate- or high-grade malignancy. Consequently, resection of the entire biceps femoris muscle here may not have contributed oncologically, yet necessitating extension of the radiation field distally in the thigh in order to encompass the surgical field.

It is our experience that local recurrence of intermediate-grade sarcomas can frequently be treated surgically with limb preservation and should be so considered in treatment planning.

REFERENCES

1. Fletcher GH. *Textbook of radiotherapy,* 3rd ed. Philadelphia: Lea & Febiger; 1980:219–24.
2. Lindberg RD. Soft tissue sarcoma. In: *Textbook of radiotherapy,* 3rd ed, Fletcher GH, ed. Philadelphia: Lea & Febiger; 1980:922–42.

EDITORIAL BOARD COMMENTARY

The present case and the discussion highlight some of the controversies in the management of such lesions. As the consultant correctly pointed out, it was difficult to understand a resection from the ischial tuberosity to below the knee for a lesion in the biceps femoris when the margin was indeed the sciatic nerve. One would argue for a lesser caudad cephalad resection when the margin is the sciatic nerve. There would be little debate that this patient should receive adjunctive radiation therapy, which has been shown to be of benefit in a prospective randomized trial.

Melanoma

68 Invasive Melanoma of the Midback

Hilliard Seigler

Adjuvant therapy?

CASE PRESENTATION

F.H., a 39-year-old Caucasian man, was referred to a plastic surgeon by his family physician for an enlarging pigmented lesion of his upper midback (Fig. 68–1). Excisional biopsy revealed that this was a Clark's level IV nodular melanoma with a Breslow thickness of 3.95 mm. Preoperative studies before completing the surgical procedure for the primary lesion should include a thorough history and physical examination. Diagnostic studies should include blood counts as well as liver function studies. A PA and lateral chest radiograph should also be completed to rule out metastatic disease to the lungs.

This patient completed a preoperative evaluation, which included normal blood counts, normal liver function studies, a normal radionuclide scan of the liver, and a PA and lateral chest radiograph that revealed no evidence of metastatic disease. After this, the plastic surgeon excised the lesion with 2-cm margins and closed the wound primarily. The slide material was forwarded to a tertiary care university medical center. Histopathologic review documented a Clark's level IV invasion with a Breslow thickness of 3.68 mm; 18 mitoses/mm^2 were documented and there was no ulceration of the lesion noted (Fig. 68–2). The patient was then referred to the medical center. He was evaluated by the melanoma study group, which includes a surgical oncologist, medical oncologist, and radiation oncologist.

The history revealed no significant past medical history. The patient was unaware of the lesion. He denied scaling, itching, bleeding, or trauma to the area. The patient also denied headaches, visual disturbance, bone pain, changes in appetite or weight, melena, abdominal symptomatology, and neurologic symptomatology. Phys-ical examination revealed that this man was fair skinned, with blue eyes and red hair. His physical appearance indicated excessive sunlight exposure to the trunk. There was no evidence of abnormality at the primary excision site. Nothing could be palpated to suggest intransit disease and there was absence of additional suspicious cutaneous pigmented lesions. Complete physical examination was unremarkable for neurologic, chest, or abdominal abnormalities. The patient had completely normal blood counts and liver function studies. The chest radiograph was clear.

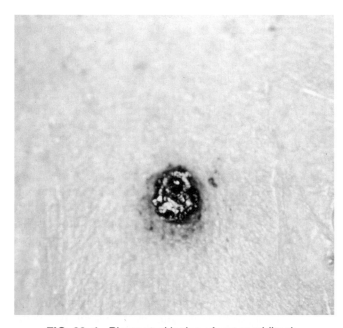

FIG. 68–1. Pigmented lesion of upper midback.

339

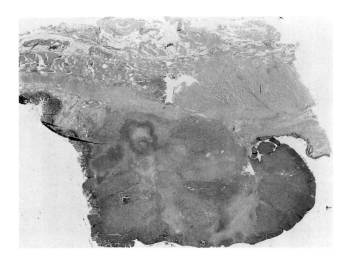

FIG. 68–2. Histopathologic photograph—Clark's level IV with a Breslow thickness of 3.68 mm.

At this point, a therapeutic strategy was discussed by the group. The relevant topics in this case included (a) the adequacy of the biopsy, (b) the histopathologic features of the primary lesion, (c) surgical margins around the excision of the primary lesion, (d) evaluation of the first order lymph nodes, (e) the possibility of distant disease, (f) adjuvant therapy, and (g) a plan for clinical follow-up.

Biopsy of pigmented cutaneous lesions should be entertained when irregular surfaces, irregular borders, changes in pigmentation, and ulceration are noted. The biopsy specimen should include the most advanced area of involvement and must include the entire skin thickness and a portion of subcutaneous fat. This type of biopsy will provide adequate material for the pathologist to determine microstaging information, including the level of invasion and tumor thickness. In this case, the excisional biopsy was adequate and did provide the pathologist with sufficient tissue to determine the Clark's level and Breslow's thickness of the primary lesion.

There is a general consensus of opinion that 2 cm of normal tissue around a primary cutaneous melanoma is adequate for local control. Surgical excision with these measurements will permit primary wound closure on most body sites. Truncal melanomas can almost always be closed by primary intention. In this case it was determined that 2-cm margins had been included and there was a well-healed wound without evidence of local abnormalities. Nothing could be palpated to suggest intransit disease and there were no additional suspicious cutaneous pigmented lesions.

Deeply invasive cutaneous melanomas can be associated with metastatic disease to regional lymph nodes. In this case the primary lesion was the upper midback. This represents an ambiguous site in terms of lymphatic drainage. Lymph node basins to both axillae and both

supraclavicular fossae are at risk. Lymphoscintigraphy could be carried out and lymph node drainage from this primary site could be determined using this technique. Unfortunately, elective lymph node dissection has not been associated with a statistically significant therapeutic benefit. In this case it was not deemed necessary to complete lymphoscintigraphy or elective lymph node dissection. All nodal basins were free from significant adenopathy by physical examination. A decision was made to follow the lymph node basins expectantly.

Distant disease secondary to metastatic melanoma is usually signaled by abnormalities determined by history, physical examination, blood counts, or blood chemistries. Specific bone pain should be evaluated by bone scan and radiography to document architectural changes. Neurologic signs or symptoms should be evaluated by magnetic resonance imaging (MRI) scans as well as by complete assessment of cerebral spinal fluid. Chest and abdominal abnormalities are best evaluated by computed tomography (CT). In this case there was nothing to suggest distant disease and scans were deemed not necessary.

The group believed that this young Celtic man had a high-risk nodular melanoma involving the midback. It was deemed that the patient was free from evidence of existing disease and should be considered for adjuvant therapy because of the significant risk of future disease dictated by the histopathologic features of his primary lesion. The group believed that a level IV primary with a Breslow's thickness of 3.68 mm associated with a high mitotic index was predictive of future recurrent problems in approximately 40% to 50% of patients studied. Adjuvant irradiation and adjuvant chemotherapy were discussed and it was deemed to be inadvisable and without therapeutic merit for this patient. Prior reported series have failed to show any therapeutic benefit of adjuvant radiation and chemotherapy. Hormonal therapy as a single agent has also been shown to be ineffective for patients with melanoma. The melanoma board felt that the patient was appropriate for an adjuvant-specific active immunotherapy protocol. Patients with high-risk stage I and stage II disease who have been rendered free from all measurable disease are considered for adjuvant immunotherapy. Recent studies have failed to show benefit for patients receiving nonspecific active immunization. Patients who are immunized specifically and actively against melanoma itself are currently being studied in an active immunization protocol. The patient was included in this trial and received four monthly vaccinations with approximately 2.5×10^7 x-irradiated melanoma cells with each immunization.

The patient was seen monthly for the first 6 months and quarterly for 2 years. After this, follow-up visits were semiannually for an additional 2 years and annual thereafter. At each clinical visit, the patient underwent complete history and physical examination. During the first 2 years he was subjected to quarterly blood counts and liver function studies and semiannual chest radiographs. After 2 years the chest radiographs were performed on an annual basis. Without history, signs, and symptoms, diagnostic scans are not deemed to be indicated or cost effective. If, however, the patient demonstrates findings relating to a specific organ system, diagnostic scans are appropriate and should be completed before surgical procedures for distant metastatic disease. This patient has been followed up for more than 3 years and, at present, he is free from evidence of recurrent disease.

COMMENTARY by Michael A. Warso

This case report is presented in an extremely logical fashion. I would emphasize the point made at the outset about routine workup. Routine liver scans, bone scans, and CT scans have not been shown to be effective measures for detecting occult metastases in patients with clinically localized melanoma (1,2).

The issue of surgical margins and the adequacy of excision has been the subject of recent investigation. The WHO trial (3) of 703 patients directly looked at the question of adequate margins in patients with thin (<2 mm) primary cutaneous melanoma. They found no significant increase in local recurrence with excision margins of 1 versus 3 cm, although four patients with melanomas of 1 to 2 mm and a 1-cm margin did develop local recurrence. Other reports from the Sydney Melanoma Unit directly suggest that resection margins of 2 to 3 cm may be adequate for melanomas greater than 3 mm in thickness (4). Balch et al. (5) recently investigated the difference in local control between 2- and 4-cm margins in localized melanoma from 1 to 4 mm in thickness. They too found that the extent of excision margin between 2 and 4 cm did not affect the outcome. This patient's excision margin of 2 cm would require no further treatment.

A cutaneous melanoma 3.95 mm thick and Clark's level IV also has a high chance of developing regional lymph node metastases (6,7). Retrospective studies have suggested that elective node dissection leads to improved survival in patients with intermediate thickness melanoma (8,9). However, the two prospective randomized trials that have been done failed to show any benefit of elective dissection (10,11). These studies are currently being repeated because of the positive results of the retrospective trials and methodologic problems with the prospective trials. At this point, though, after discussing the issues with the patient, a decision to follow the regional lymph nodes would be appropriate.

As stated, the decision as to which nodes are at highest risk would best be made by lymphoscintigraphy in those cutaneous melanomas that arise in areas of ambiguous drainage, including the midline of the torso, the area around the T10 dermatome, and the areas over the clavicle and edge of the trapezius. Ideally, this test should be performed before any surgical intervention to avoid altering drainage patterns. For a lesion in the upper midback, the most likely drainage would be to the axillary lymph nodes, and these areas should receive the most diligent observation.

Current data on adjuvant immunotherapy are scant, to say the least. Thus, no definitive statements can be made as to the relevance or lack thereof of presumed adjuvant immunotherapy. It appears this was a trial and such deserves to be pursued.

REFERENCES

1. Iscoe N, Kersey P, Gapski J, et al. Predictive value of staging investigation in patients with clinical stage I malignant melanoma. *Plast Reconstruct Surg* 1987;80:233–9.
2. Aranha G, Simmons R, Gunnarsson A, Grage T, McKhann C. The value of preoperative screening procedures in stage I and II malignant melanoma. *J Surg Oncol* 1979;11:1–6.
3. Veronesi U, Cascinelli N, Adamus J, et al. Thin stage I primary cutaneous malignant melanoma: comparison of excision with margins of 1 or 3 cm. *N Engl J Med* 1988;318:1159–62.
4. Ames F, Balch C, Reintgen D. Local recurrences and their management. In: *Cutaneous melanoma*, 2nd ed, Balch C, Houghton A, Milton G, Sober A, Soong S-J, eds. Philadelphia: JB Lippincott; 1992:287–94.
5. Balch C, Urist M, Karakousis C, et al. Efficacy of 2-cm surgical margins for intermediate-thickness melanomas (1 to 4 mm): results of a multi-institutional randomized surgical trial. *Ann Surg* 1993;218:262–9.
6. Das Gupta T. Results of treatment of 269 patients with primary cutaneous melanoma: a five-year prospective study. *Ann Surg* 1977;186:201–9.
7. Balch C, Murad T, Soong S-J, et al. Tumor thickness as a guide to surgical management of clinical stage I melanoma patients. *Cancer* 1979;43:883–8.
8. McCarthy W, Shaw H, Milton G. Efficacy of elective lymph nodes dissection in 2,347 patients with clinical stage I malignant melanoma. *Surg Gynecol Obstet* 1985;161:575–80.
9. Reintgen D, Cox E, McCarty K, et al. Efficacy of elective lymph node dissection in patients with intermediate thickness primary melanoma. *Ann Surg* 1983;198:379–85.
10. Veronesi U, Adamus J, Bandiera D, et al. Inefficacy of immediate node dissection in stage I melanoma of the limbs. *N Engl J Med* 1977;297:627–30.
11. Sim F, Taylor W, Pritchard D, Soule E. Lymphadenectomy in the management of stage I malignant melanoma: a prospective randomized study. *Mayo Clin Proc* 1986;61:697–705.

69 Upper Extremity Melanoma

J. Ralph Broadwater

How wide should the excision be and should the sentinel axillary node be biopsied?

CASE PRESENTATION

The patient is a 34-year-old woman who was referred by her dermatologist. She had a new mole on the inner aspect of her right arm that had increased in size over the last year. The dermatologist performed an excisional biopsy with a narrow margin. Results of this biopsy reveal her to have a nodular melanoma, Breslow thickness 3 mm.

She denies any history of weight loss, anorexia, bowel complaints, new pain, or change in her mental status. She denies any bleeding or ulceration in the mole. She does not have a family history of melanoma. She denies previous skin biopsies.

Physical examination reveals her to be a healthy woman. She has no obvious skin changes secondary to sun exposure. On the inner aspect of her right arm there is a healing biopsy incision approximately 2 cm in length. Sutures are in place, and there is no evidence of infection. There is no epitrochlear, axillary, or supraclavicular adenopathy. Examination of her body reveals no other worrisome lesions. Abdominal examination reveals no palpable organomegaly. A chest roentgenogram was performed for staging and was negative. A complete blood count was normal and liver functions, including an LDH, were unremarkable.

TUMOR BOARD DISCUSSION

Our pathologists agree that this an intermediate thickness melanoma that measures 3 mm in depth (Fig. 69–1). There is no indication of systemic spread. Her preoperative stage after initial biopsy is T3 N0 M0, AJCC stage IIA.

Important points in the patient history and physical exam to be noted are that she has had no previous biopsies or lesions excised. She has a negative family history of melanoma. On physical examination, she has no evidence of spread.

This patient's staging was completed with a chest radiograph, which was negative, and routine blood work to evaluate any spread to the liver. Some physicians would order more sophisticated testing such as a computed tomography (CT) scan of the liver, chest, or head, or bone scan. Without specific symptoms, the yield of these tests does not warrant their expense, and risks a false-positive test that would require further diagnostic evaluation. The initial biopsy by the dermatologist was appropriate; the mole was completely excised so that a full-thickness biopsy could be evaluated by the pathologist. This is critical because surgical decisions are based on the tumor thickness. A shave biopsy is inadequate.

Some surgeons would perform cutaneous lymphoscintigraphy in this patient to define the nodal basins at risk for subsequent spread of her melanoma (1). This was not performed in this patient because we do not routinely perform elective lymph node dissection as it is an unproven treatment. The location of the patient's primary lesion is not in an area of ambiguous drainage. Subsequent physical examination should carefully evaluate this patient for recurrence in the local region, the axillae, and supraclavicular regions.

This patient should be treated with additional surgery to excise the previous biopsy site. Initial analysis of the

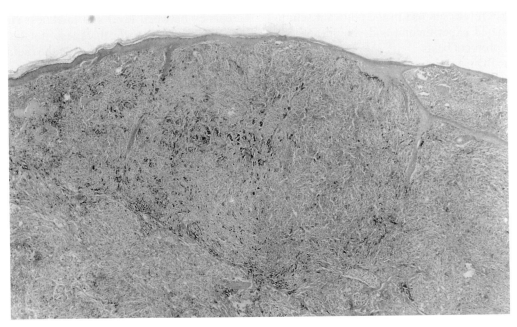

FIG. 69–1. Pathology indicates a 3.0 mm nodular melanoma.

Intergroup trial indicates that a 2-cm margin is adequate for patients who have an intermediate-thickness melanoma (2). It is recommended that this patient have a re-excision with a 2-cm margin. This should allow primary closure. The procedure can be done as an outpatient under local anesthesia.

We do not recommend elective lymph node dissection. Two randomized studies have not indicated a benefit in dissecting the lymph nodes prophylactically (3,4). This is in contrast to a multivariate analysis by Balch et al., which indicated a survival benefit of performing elective lymph node dissection in patients with intermediate-thickness melanoma (5). A recent randomized control study by several groups (Intergroup study) has been completed, but the data have not been analyzed because it is not mature. The results of this study will determine future treatment recommendations regarding elective lymph node dissection. At this time, it is not our recommendation that patients have elective lymph node dissection.

An appealing alternative to elective lymph node dissection is the use of intraoperative lymphatic mapping recently described by Morton et al. (6). This new procedure involves injecting a blue dye near the primary lesion. At the time of re-excision of the primary melanoma or excision of the melanoma, the lymph node draining basin is explored. A sentinel lymph node takes up the dye first. This node is excised. If this node is negative (not involved by tumor), subsequent lymph node dissection is not necessary because almost all patients are node negative. This procedure has the benefit of performing a lymph node dissection only on patients who have a positive sentinel

lymph node. This allows one to avoid the morbidity of lymph node dissection in patients who are node negative.

This procedure requires cutaneous lymphoscintigraphy to identify the areas of lymph node drainage that are at risk, and has a moderate learning curve to identify the sentinel lymph node.

This patient had a wide local excision as an outpatient with a 2-cm margin. Final pathology revealed her to have no residual tumor in the excision specimen.

This patient is at moderate risk for subsequent recurrence to her lymph nodes and other distant sites. The multivariate analysis of Balch et al. has determined that tumor thickness is the primary risk factor determining prognosis (7). Although this patient has several secondary factors that are favorable (she is female and has an extremity lesion that was not ulcerated), 10-year survival is approximately 60% and her risk of regional or systemic recurrence within the next 5 years is 35% to 60%. For this reason, she should be considered for adjuvant treatment.

There is no proven adjuvant treatment for melanoma that has been shown to improve patient survival. This patient is eligible for an adjuvant protocol at our institution. The study, SWOG 9035, would randomize her to receive melacine vaccine, an allogenic melanoma oncolysate, or observation. In this study, patients may receive a melanoma oncolysate as a vaccination. There is no role for adjuvant radiation therapy in this patient.

It should be said that a few centers in our country would consider this patient for prophylactic or elective isolation limb perfusion. Although isolation limb perfusion has been shown to be helpful in patients who have intransit disease of the extremities, its use in the adjuvant setting should be considered experimental and should be done only on a formal protocol basis.

A review of the PDQ data base for treatment options for stage IIA melanoma can provide several other potential adjuvant protocols that might be offered to this patient.

There are no firm guidelines for optimal follow-up of patients who have melanoma. Our routine policy in patients who have an intermediate-thickness melanoma are to examine them every 3 months for the first 2 years. We would perform a history and physical examination with careful attention to the primary site, the dermal lymphatics, axillae, and supraclavicular region. We would not perform routine laboratory or radiologic testing except annually. Without specific symptoms or abnormalities in routine testing, we would order only a chest radiograph, complete blood count, and routine liver functions, including an LDH. Subsequent follow-up would be every 6 months if the patient has not developed any recurrent disease.

REFERENCES

1. Lamki LM, Haynie TP, Balch CM, et al. The contribution of Tc-99m sulfur colloid lymphoscintigraphy to the surgical management of primary truncal melanoma of intermediate thickness. *J Nucl Med* 1988;29:554.
2. Singletary SE. Melanoma margins (meeting abstract). In *Advances in the biology and clinical management of melanoma*. November 20–23, 1991, Houston, TX; 15.
3. Sim FH, Taylor WF, Pritchard DJ, et al. Lymphadenectomy in the management of stage I melanoma: a prospective randomized study. *Mayo Clin Proc* 1986;61:697.
4. Veronesi U, Adamus J, Bandiera DC, et al. Inefficacy of immediate node dissection in stage I melanoma of the limbs. *N Engl J Med* 1977;297:627.
5. Balch CM, Soong SJ, Milton GW, et al. A comparison of prognostic factors and surgical results in 1,786 patients treated with localized (stage I) melanoma treated in Alabama, USA, and New South Wales, Australia. *Ann Surg* 1982;196:677.
6. Morton DL, Wen DR, Wong JH, et al. Technical details of intraoperative lymphatic mapping of early stage melanoma. *Arch Surg* 1992;127(4):392–9.
7. Balch CM, Soong SJ, Murad TM, Ingals AL, Maddox WA. A multifactorial analysis of melanoma:II. Prognostic factors in patients with stage I (localized) melanoma. *Surgery* 1979;86:343.

COMMENTARY by Charles M. Balch

I basically agree with the management approach described by Dr. Broadwater. The following salient comments are appropriate: The microstaging criteria (level and thickness) are in congruence, making this a stage II melanoma. In other circumstances where there is a discrepancy between level and thickness (i.e., level 4, 1.2-mm thickness), then the thickness, not the level, should be used for staging (in this example the melanoma would be a stage I) because thickness is a more accurate predictor of outcome.

The diagnostic workup should be modest, as described by Dr. Broadwater. There are no indications for CT scan, MRI, or bone scans unless there are symptoms to suggest metastatic disease.

Margins of excision should be 2 cm for intermediate-thickness lesions as described. Flaps should be mobilized and the defect closed primarily with a subcuticular suture. Drains usually are not necessary.

Elective lymph node dissection is optional. In my opinion, I would consider this for such a patient based on the retrospective publications. The Intergroup melanoma randomized surgical trial still does not have results to report about this issue. Keep in mind that the morbidity of an axillary dissection in such a patient should be minimal. I agree with the approach of using intraoperative lymphatic mapping, although this is still an investigational procedure.

There is no role for adjuvant treatment, such as limb perfusion, radiation therapy, or adjuvant therapy. Eligible patients should be entered into prospective clinical trials.

Follow-up as described by Dr. Broadwater is appropriate, although slightly more intensive than we would use. The most frequent sign of metastasis would be the regional lymph nodes. The most common sites of distant disease (in order of frequency) are skin and subcutaneous tissue, distant lymph nodes, lung, liver, and bone. Patients are at risk for developing a second melanoma and should have an annual skin examination on a long-term basis.

EDITORIAL BOARD COMMENTARY

A recently reported multi-institutional prospective surgical trial identified a subgroup of patients who had significant benefit in overall survival with elective lymph node dissection as initial management. The greatest benefit occurred to individuals younger than 60 with intermediate-thickness melanomas, especially those whose tumors were 1 to 2 mm thick (1).

REFERENCES

1. Balch CM, Soong SJ, Bartolucci AA, et al. Efficacy of an elective regional lymph node dissection of 1 to 4 mm thick melanomas for patients 60 years of age and younger. *Ann Surg* 1996;224:255–266.

70

Malignant Melanoma of the Distal Lower Extremity with Satellitosis and a Clinically Positive Inguinal Lymph Node

Daniel G. Coit

This constellation of findings requires wide excision, split-thickness skin graft, and inguinal node dissection

CASE PRESENTATION

B.H. is a 47-year-old Caucasian man referred for management of a recently biopsied melanoma of his left lateral calf.

He initially noted a gray scab on the left lateral calf 16 months before this admission. This was felt to represent a benign seborrheic keratosis at a routine dermatology screening clinic, and no biopsy was performed. Twelve months before admission, the patient underwent local excision of a number of benign skin lesions, as well as a basal cell carcinoma of his upper arm. Six months before admission, the patient required a re-excision of a local recurrence of the basal cell carcinoma. At that time, he underwent excision of the lesion on his leg. No pathology examination was performed on the latter specimen. Two months before admission, the patient noted the appearance of several dark nodules in the region of the biopsy site on the left lower leg. Repeat biopsy of this revealed malignant melanoma. These lesions appeared to represent histologic satellites, with no in situ component seen.

The patient underwent a complete history and physical examination. Screening blood work, including complete blood count and liver chemistry, were within normal limits. Chest radiography, as well as computed tomography

(CT) scan of the chest, abdomen, and pelvis were all completely normal.

The patient was initially confronted with a number of different therapeutic options, ranging from surgical excision alone to surgical excision with regional lymph node dissection, with or without associated adjuvant hyperthermic isolation limb perfusion or high-dose systemic chemotherapy.

Physical examination at the time of referral revealed a healthy-appearing man in no acute distress. Abnormal findings were confined to the local exam. There was a 0.4-cm nodular pigmented lesion on the left lateral calf. Immediately proximal to this were two small 0.2-cm satellite lesions and two small punch biopsy sites. There was no visible or palpable intransit disease. In the left groin, there was a soft, distinct, 1.5-cm lymph node palpable high in the femoral triangle. This was clearly asymmetric when compared with the right side. No other pigmented lesions were noted in the left lower extremity.

This patient was staged clinically as a T4 N1 M0, AJCC clinical stage III. At a minimum, he was felt to require wide excision of the primary site. The exact margin of excision for a melanoma of unknown thickness presenting with localized satellitosis is unknown. Recent histopathologic reviews have suggested the frequency of micro-

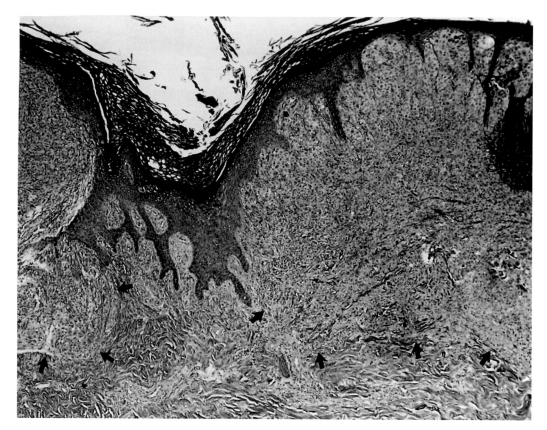

FIG. 70–1. Histologic specimen showing two nodules of melanoma in dermis *(black arrows)*, with no in situ component.

scopic satellitosis within 5.0 cm of the primary to be on the order of 30%. It would appear that a minimum acceptable margin in this setting would be 5.0 cm, if only to achieve local control. The impact of local control on ultimate survival is unproven.

With regard to management of the regional nodes, the patient was felt to have an asymmetric physical examination. Under those circumstances, therapeutic superficial inguinofemoral lymphadenectomy was advised. Deep pelvic lymphadenectomy would be considered in the presence of multiple positive superficial nodes, or a positive bridging or Cloquet's lymph node between the superficial inguinofemoral and deeper ilio-obturator nodal groups.

With regard to the issue of adjuvant regional hyperthermic isolation limb perfusion, many conflicting claims have been made relative to its efficacy, virtually all based on retrospective trials. Only one prospective trial has suggested a benefit to the use of adjuvant limb perfusion using phenylalanine mustard. This has yet to be confirmed by a large ongoing cooperative group study. Clearly, without participation in such an ongoing trial, adjuvant hyperthermic isolation limb perfusion cannot be considered standard therapy, and should not be routinely recommended.

With regard to adjuvant systemic therapy, either immunotherapy or chemotherapy, such use outside of an investigational trial should be discouraged. Eligibility for any such postoperative adjuvant trial would clearly be determined by the ultimate pathologic staging, after which a realistic estimate of recurrence risk could be made.

The patient underwent wide excision with split-thickness skin grafting of the primary site. At the same time, he underwent complete radical inguinofemoral lymphadenectomy. Frozen section examination of Cloquet's node was negative; deep pelvic node dissection was not performed.

Pathology revealed several foci of malignant melanoma in skin. No definite in situ changes were noted (Fig. 70–1). The thickest tumor nodule measured 1.6 mm in thickness. All lymph nodes were negative.

The patient's subsequent management was discussed at length in a multidisciplinary tumor board. Given his pathologic stage, T4 N0 M0 of a presumed extremity melanoma, he was felt to have an estimated 30% risk of systemic recurrence. Under these circumstances, he was not eligible for any ongoing adjuvant trials. A program of close expectant observation was advised.

The patient currently remains free of disease 15 months after lymphadenectomy.

COMMENTARY by Tapas K. Das Gupta

Under usual circumstances, in the presence of a localized cutaneous melanoma, the addition of CT scanning to the staging workup does not yield information that would result in a change in the patient's clinical stage (1,2). However, this man's initial risk is uncertain because the presumed primary was never examined pathologically. In addition, because of local recurrence with satellites, he is at a higher risk of systemic disease. In this case, therefore, it would be appropriate to proceed with a more extensive workup.

From the presentation it appears as though the patient was considered to have a clinically positive inguinal lymph node. On this basis, he was advised to have a therapeutic lymph node dissection. Presumably, the CT scan of the pelvis was done to evaluate the iliac nodes, but it should not be forgotten that a pelvic exam would also be beneficial in these circumstances.

Although the exact margin necessary for local control is unknown, the presence of satellites would necessitate wide excision. The decision to proceed with a lymph node dissection based on a suggestive physical exam shows good clinical judgment. As stated in the case presentation, the addition of an iliac dissection without multiple positive superficial lymph nodes has not been shown to confer any survival advantage, although it may give important prognostic information (3,4). The presence of positive iliac nodes portends a high risk of systemic disease. If positive iliac nodes are present, however, a portion of those patients can be salvaged with long-term survival by performing an iliac dissection (5,6). The possibility of survival benefit does mandate an evaluation of the iliac nodes, which in this case was performed by examining Cloquet's node.

REFERENCES

1. Iscoe N, Kersey P, Gapski J, et al. Predictive value of staging investigation in patients with clinical stage I malignant melanoma. *Plast Reconstruct Surg* 1987;80:233–39.
2. Aranha G, Simmons R, Gunnarsson A, et al. The value of preoperative screening procedures in stage I and II malignant melanoma. *J Surg Oncol* 1979;11:1–6.
3. Singletary S, Shallenberger R, Guinee V. Surgical management of groin nodal metastases from primary melanoma of the lower extremity. *Surg Gynecol Obstet* 1992;174:195–200.
4. Coit D, Brennan M. Extent of lymph node dissection in melanoma of the trunk or lower extremity. *Arch Surg* 1989;124:162–6.
5. Karakousis C, Emrich L, Rao U. Groin dissection in malignant melanoma. *Am J Surg* 1986;152:491–5.
6. Finck S, Giuliano A, Mann B, Morton D. Results of ilioinguinal dissection for stage II melanoma. *Ann Surg* 1982;196:180–6.

71 Melanoma of the Ethmoid Sinus

Andrew M. Trotti, Douglas Klotch, Ronald DeConti,
and Ken Schroer

*Mucosal melanoma: a poor prognosis tumor. An aggressive
head and neck–neurosurgical team combined with
postoperative irradiation offers the best approach for tumor
control and occasional cure.*

CASE PRESENTATION

P.B. is a 74-year-old man hospitalized for coronary artery bypass surgery in December 1992. Postoperatively he developed progressive symptoms consistent with sinusitis progressing to right orbital cellulitis. A computed tomography (CT) scan of the paranasal sinuses revealed opacification of the left maxillary sinus, left ethmoid sinus, and sphenoid sinus (Fig. 71–1). Examination revealed polypoid masses in the left nasal cavity, and he underwent exploration for presumed polyp disease. A 3 × 1 × 1 cm aggregate of tissue was removed on nasal polypectomy. Microscopic evaluation revealed large-cell undifferentiated malignancy. A panel of immunoperoxidase-labeled antibodies for cytokeratin, vimentin, epithelial membrane antigen, S100, HMB45, actin, and leukocyte common antigen were evaluated. Only the vimentin and HMB45 stains were positive. This biopsy was thought to be compatible with malignant melanoma.

Additional workup included CT scan of the neck that revealed no adenopathy. A CT scan of the chest and abdomen to include the liver was also performed. This showed only a right pleural effusion consistent with congestive heart failure related to the recent coronary artery bypass surgery. There was no evidence of lung or liver metastases. Magnetic resonance imaging (MRI) of the paranasal sinuses revealed apparent involvement of the medial orbital wall and sphenoid sinus (Fig. 71–2). The patient was felt to have a localized mucosal melanoma of

the left ethmoid sinus with extension to the nasal cavity. There was possible invasion of the sphenoid and maxillary sinuses.

He was then seen preoperatively by neurosurgery and radiation oncology, and a joint recommendation was made for a wide local excision using a craniofacial approach and postoperative radiotherapy.

He underwent en bloc resection of the ethmoid sinus via a craniofacial approach including the cribriform plate, nasal septum, floor of the orbit, and left maxillectomy. There was no invasion of the orbit noted during surgery. Reconstruction was performed with a temporalis fascia for dura, paracranial flap to seal the floor of the nose, and a split calvarial graft to reconstruct the orbital floor. His postoperative recovery was uneventful and without complications.

Examination of the surgical specimen revealed a large, pigmented, lobulated mass involving the ethmoid sinus, sphenoid sinus, nasal cavity, and maxillary sinus. The aggregate size of the mass was approximately 4.5 × 3 × 1.7 cm. Intraoperative frozen sections were used to assess margins. A microscopic focus of melanoma was seen in the floor of the medial orbit. Additional sections were taken showing no further malignancy. A maxillary prosthesis (obturator) was fashioned by the dental oncologist. Postoperative radiotherapy was recommended to enhance local control.

He received 5,480 cGy over 6 weeks to the primary site encompassing the ethmoid, sphenoid, and maxillary

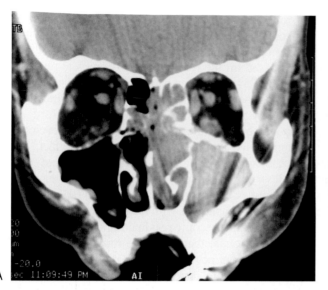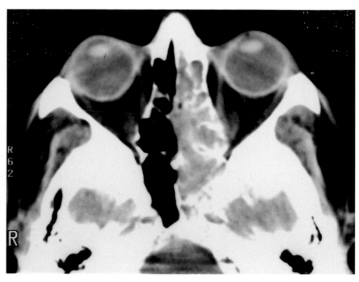

FIG. 71–1. A: Coronal CT scan of paranasal sinuses showing tumor involvement of ethmoid sinus, nasal cavity, and left maxillary sinus. Bone destruction is evident in the ethmoid cells and upper septum. **B:** Axial CT scan through orbits showing ethmoid sinus tumor encroaching on orbit and bony expansion.

sinuses including the entire nasal cavity. We generally prefer to deliver 6,000 to 6,600 cGy in the postoperative setting, but the tolerance of adjacent normal tissues can be limiting. Dose to the optic chiasm was limited to 4,500 cGy. The maximum dose to the ipsilateral optic nerve was 5,800 cGy because of a small hot spot in that region. He tolerated treatment well, with only modest irritation of the nasal cavity and fatigue.

He was last seen 2 years after completing postoperative radiotherapy and was without evidence of disease. He has occasional epiphora of the left eye but good vision bilaterally without diplopia. A maxillary prosthesis covers his hard palate defect, and the patient has full speech and

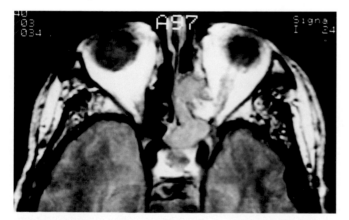

FIG. 71–2. Axial MRI through orbits showing ethmoid sinus tumor encroaching on orbit and invading sphenoid sinus.

swallowing function. Cosmesis was excellent, with only mild asymmetry of the eyes.

TUMOR BOARD DISCUSSION

Dr. Schroer: The histologic sections of the tumor demonstrate an anaplastic neoplasm composed of large cells with pleomorphic irregular vesicular nuclei, prominent nucleoli, and abundant clear cytoplasm (Figs. 71–3, 71–4). The mitotic rate is very high (about 10/HPF), and many of the mitoses are abnormal. The differential diagnosis of a large-cell anaplastic neoplasm includes undifferentiated carcinoma, high-grade lymphoma, and malignant melanoma. Immunostains with immunoperoxidase-labeled antibodies for cytokeratin, vimentin, epithelial membrane antigen, S100 protein, HMB45, actin, and LCA showed only positive staining with vimentin and HMB45. These results essentially exclude the diagnosis of carcinoma and malignant lymphoma and are quite typical for malignant melanoma arising in the nasal cavity. HMB45 is a highly melanoma-specific antibody, as only rare carcinomas have been reported to show staining. Up to 90% of melanomas will stain with either HMB45 or S100, and thus the sensitivity for diagnosis is increased with the use of both stains. Based on these results, the tumor was diagnosed as malignant melanoma of the ethmoid cavity.

Dr. Trotti: Mucosal melanoma has a reputation for local recurrence and distant disease. The 5-year survival is in the 10% to 20% range with less than 5% of patients surviving 10 years. There are scattered reports using radiotherapy in

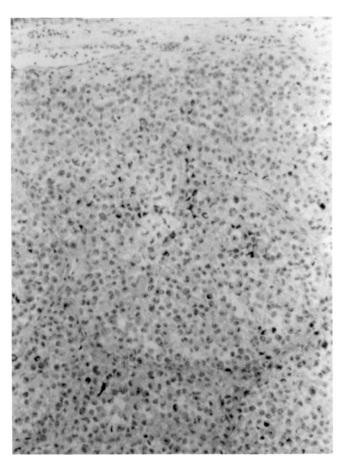

FIG. 71–3. Low power (×100) photomicrograph showing ethmoid mucosa with underlying malignant melanoma.

the postoperative setting, but very few institutions have used it routinely as an adjuvant to surgery. The rationale for delivering postoperative radiotherapy for mucosal melanoma is based on the relatively high complete response rate (50% to 75%) seen for patients with unresectable or recurrent disease. Long-term control has been achieved in approximately 50% of complete responders.

Melanoma, both cutaneous and mucosal, has developed a reputation for being "radioresistant." In fact, the responses to radiotherapy are quite variable and on average may be less than a typical carcinoma. However, many lesions are quite sensitive and responsive to radiotherapy. Results are better in patients with low-volume gross disease or patients with microscopic residual tumor after surgery.

Using the rationale that complete resection of the primary tumor and routine postoperative radiotherapy to sterilize any microscopic residual would result in the best chances for local regional control, we offered the patient an aggressive, potentially curative approach. Recognizing that the long-term outcome is generally bleak, the ability to obtain local control would still be of benefit from a standpoint of morbidity and enhanced disease-free interval.

Dr. Klotch: We chose to use a combined craniofacial approach on this case because of involvement of the ethmoid sinus and disease potentially invading the cribriform plate. Through the use of frozen section margin evaluation we were able to obtain negative margins and perform an en bloc resection. The assistance of our neurosurgical colleagues was crucial. We had a preoperative plan of resection, possible orbital preservation, and postoperative radio-

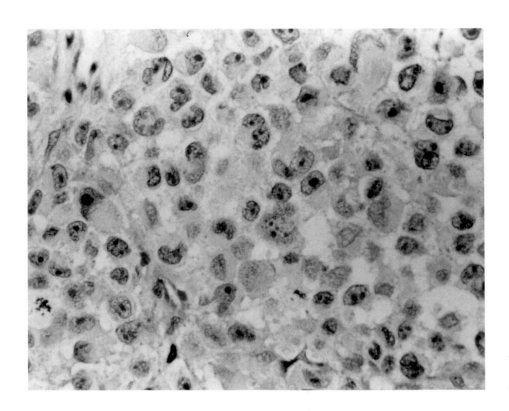

FIG. 71–4. High power (×400) photomicrograph showing marked pleomorphism with numerous mitoses and no apparent pigment.

therapy from the outset. Because the long-term survival of these patients is limited, we thought it best to try to preserve the orbit and enhance quality of life. We were willing to use an orbit-sparing approach because there is no convincing evidence that more aggressive surgery results in better local control or survival. The highest risk of disease recurrence in our opinion will be distant. Because the natural history of melanoma is highly unpredictable, he may go many years before developing distant disease.

We chose not to perform elective lymphadenectomy for several reasons. First, elective dissection in cutaneous melanoma has been controversial, with only a subset of patients appearing to benefit. Second, there are conflicting reports regarding the risk of nodal failure in mucosal melanoma. In general, cancers of the paranasal sinuses uncommonly spread to the neck. Considering the unpredictability of patterns of failure, we did not think additional surgery would impact survival.

Dr. DeConti: The adjuvant use of chemotherapy in melanoma, both cutaneous and mucosal, remains investigational. The response rate from combination chemotherapy is in the 20% to 40% range, with less than 10% obtaining complete responses. Considering this modest level of activity, we did not think it would be beneficial for this patient to have adjuvant chemotherapy. Recently high-dose interferon has been shown to delay or reduce recurrence rates and improve survival in patients with cutaneous melanoma (1). It is completely unstudied for the much rarer mucosal melanomas.

REFERENCES

1. Kirkwood JM, Strawderman MH, Ernstoff MS, et al. Interferon Alfa-2b adjuvant therapy of high-risk resected cutaneous melanoma. *J Clin Oncol* 1996;14:7–17.

COMMENTARY by Elliot W. Strong

Mucosal melanoma is a rare disease, representing approximately 2% of all melanomas (1) and 8% of melanomas of the head and neck (2). Nasal cavity and paranasal sinus melanomas comprise 3.5% of all sinonasal tract neoplasia (3,4). Within the sinonasal tract, melanoma most commonly involves the anterior nasal cavity on the septum, and then the middle or inferior turbinates. The maxillary antrum is the most commonly involved paranasal sinus (5). Mucosal melanoma is a disease of middle age with no specific sex predilection and of unknown etiology. Japanese are significantly more commonly afflicted than Caucasians (5). Most reported series (2–4,6–8) describe small numbers of patients with mucosal melanoma of varied extent and subjected to various treatment regimens from which statistically valid conclusions cannot usually be drawn.

The authors have described their investigation and treatment of an elderly man with melanoma of the ethmoid sinus. Often the primary lesion is so large that its precise site of origin cannot be identified with certainty. This patient typified the usual presentation with a short history of nonspecific complaints and a large primary tumor.

The extent of the clinical investigation is adequate. The true extent of the tumor is not fully described or illustrated. Was there bone destruction? Was opacification of the maxillary and sphenoid sinuses the result of tumor involvement or secondary to obstruction? An MRI scan with T_2-weighted images, especially when the diagnosis of melanoma was established, may have provided more precise information on the differentiation of tumor from infection/sinus obstruction. Such information may have been of critical importance in assessing surgical resectability, especially in the sphenoid sinus. Although CT gives better bone detail, MRI will provide more precise delineation of tumor versus infection (9). Such information is important in treatment planning, especially in predicting whether resection may be curative or palliative.

The importance of an accurate histologic diagnosis has been appropriately emphasized. Histologic examination should search for melanin, present in more than two thirds of melanomas, and premelanosomes (5). Not all melanomas are pigmented and melanin may be produced by other tumors of neural crest origin (5,10). The antibodies against melanoma-associated antigens (MAA-ab) recognize different antigens on human melanoma cells but no MAA-ab has been proven to have absolute specificity for melanoma (10); thus, the importance of a series of immunohistochemistry and monoclonal antibody panels in establishing the pathologic diagnosis (10).

Adequate wide surgical resection of mucosal melanoma is the accepted treatment of choice (2–4,6–8). Stern and Guillamondegui (8) report that in their experience those patients whose initial treatment was surgical resection alone had a statistically significant better 5-year survival rate than those whose treatment was multidisciplinary. This probably reflects a more favorable initial presentation. The role of palliative (incomplete) resection of mucosal melanoma cannot be ascertained from the reported reviews available. The importance of intraoperative frozen section analysis is uncertain because these primary tumors may be multifocal (5); in one report, almost all specimens demonstrated intralesional blood vessel and/or lymphatic permeations (3). Reconstruction of the orbital floor was appropriately performed to support the preserved globe. Because the occult incidence of regional lymph node metastases from nasal/paranasal sinus melanoma is low (3–6,10), no elective neck dissection was performed.

The rationale of postoperative radiation therapy has been well discussed (3,4,7,8,11). Its use in the primary setting for palliation is well accepted, but its curative potential is limited. Its best utility may be in the presence of close surgical margins for eradication of microscopic residual tumor, as illustrated in this case. Harwood and Cummings (11) reported complete remission after radiation therapy in 72% of 24 patients with mucosal melanoma, of whom 11 were free of disease for 9 to 54 months. Large fraction size, equal to or greater than 400 Gy, was employed. It is probably appropriate to treat all but the smallest, easily resected mucosal melanoma with adequate postoperative radiation. Ideal total dose and fraction size are still uncertain. The morbidity of radical radiotherapy to the preserved orbital contents, especially when the orbital floor has not been reconstructed, has been documented (12). In this series, only 17% of patients whose unreconstructed orbit was fully irradiated (for squamous carcinoma) retained significant function in the irradiated eye and in addition suffered local recurrence in 44%, leading the authors to plead for orbital exenteration in this clinical setting (12).

The use of other adjuvant therapy for mucosal melanoma is less clear. The authors justifiably concluded that adjuvant chemotherapy with its morbidity and low response rate was unjustified. Immunotherapy and biologic response modifiers remain experimental and should not be employed outside a research protocol, usually in the setting of recurrent disease.

This patient has done very well to date. Local recurrence is common, often in more than 50% of patients, usually occurring within the first postoperative year (7). However, melanoma is unpredictable and may have a long history with significant failures beyond the first 5 years, and even after 10 years (4,5,8). Most failures will include local/regional as well as distant failure at the time of death. Prognostic factors are uncertain with age, sex, site of origin, histology, and presence of regional nodal metastases apparently playing little role (3–8). Measurement of microscopic depth of infiltration, although difficult to standardize because of the absence of anatomical landmarks comparable to the papillary and reticular dermis of the skin, can be made on adequate tissue sections (5) and may be prognostically significant (3). The occult nature of the early lesion, the occasional difficulty with diagnosis, and the generally advanced stage of the melanoma when treated all contribute to the overall poor prognosis. The unpredictable nature of this disease with its occasional long natural history should encourage appropriate treatment, recognizing that in most patients such treatment will only be palliative.

REFERENCES

1. Milton GW. Melanoma of the nose and mouth. In: *Malignant melanoma of the skin and mucous membranes,* Milton GW, ed. Edinburgh: Churchill Livingston, 1977:157–64.
2. Conley J, Hamaker RC. Melanoma of the head and neck. *Laryngoscope* 1976;87:760–4.
3. Shah JP, Huvos AG, Strong EW. Mucosal melanomas of the head and neck. *Am J Surg* 1977;134;551–5.
4. Snow GB, van der Esch EP, van Slooten EA. Mucosal melanomas of the head and neck. *Head Neck Surg* 1978;1:24–30.
5. Batsakis JG, Regeji JA, Solomon AR, Rice DH. The pathology of head and neck tumors: mucosal melanomas, part 13. *Head Neck Surg* 1982;4:404–18.
6. Harrison DFN. Malignant melanoma of the nasal cavity. *Proc Roy Soc Med* 1968;61:12–8.
7. Hoyt DJ, Jordan T, Fisher SR. Mucosal melanoma of the head and neck. *Arch Otolaryngol Head Neck Surg* 1989;115:1096–9.
8. Stern SJ, Guillamondegui OM. Mucosal melanoma of the head and neck. *Head Neck* 1991;13:22–7.
9. Som PM, Shapiro MD, Biller HF, et al. Sinonasal tumors and inflammatory tissues: differentiation with MR imaging. *Radiology* 1988;167:803–8.
10. Henzen-Logmans SC, Meijer CJLM, Ruiter DJ, et al. Diagnostic applications of panels of antibodies in mucosal melanomas of the head and neck. *Cancer* 1988;61:702–11.
11. Harwood AR, Cummings BJ. Radiotherapy for mucosal melanomas. *Int J Radiat Oncol Biol Phys* 1982;8:1121–6.
12. Stern SJ, Goepfert H, Clayman G, et al. Orbital presentation in maxillectomy. *Otolaryngol Head Neck Surg* 1993;109:111–5.

72

Subungual Melanoma

Michael J. Edwards

*Level of amputation, prophylactic lymph node dissection
and regional isolation perfusion must be addressed in
treatment planning*

CASE PRESENTATION

History

A 54-year-old white man had an asymptomatic pigmented lesion for several months under the base of his right thumbnail. There was no history of previous thumb trauma. The patient did not complain of any symptoms consistent with systemic metastasis.

Physical Examination

Skin inspection of a healthy white man showed no other suspicious-appearing lesions, including the absence of any pigmented lesions of the right upper extremity suspicious for intransit melanoma. Examination of axillary, cervical, epitrochlear, inguinal, and supraclavicular lymph nodes showed no evidence of adenopathy. The patient had no evidence of hepatosplenomegaly, and guaiac stool test was negative. The neurologic examination was within normal limits. Examination of the right thumb showed an asymmetrical pigmented lesion with an irregular border (measuring 6 mm in greatest diameter) under the base of the right thumbnail. There was no gross evidence of nail destruction or ulceration.

Diagnostic and Staging Evaluation

A biopsy was performed by removing the thumbnail and excising a representative section of the pigmented lesion from the periphery to the center. Results of the biopsy con-

firmed a 2.3 mm, Clark's level IV, subungual melanoma extending to all margins (stage pT3a). The remainder of the staging evaluation was completed by the physical examination which showed no evidence of intransit disease or lymphadenopathy (N0) and anteroposterior and posterolateral chest radiographs and liver function tests, including alkaline phosphatase to screen for bone metastasis, which were all within normal limits (M0).

TUMOR BOARD DISCUSSION

Subungual melanoma is a rare subtype of melanoma, occurring in about 2% of cases. Unique clinical characteristics at presentation include a predominant occurrence in men, an increased frequency of lesions of the great toe or thumb, and an increased rate of occurrence in the 6th or 7th decade of life. This subtype usually has a more advanced stage at presentation, with an associated poorer prognosis, than other subtypes of melanoma. The general consensus is that a delay in diagnosis, caused by a misdiagnosis of subungual hematoma, is related to the advanced stage at presentation and the associated poor prognosis.

Staging should be accomplished by a thorough history and physical examination, supplemented with baseline chest radiographs and liver function tests. Extensive testing, using various scans and ultrasound techniques, are not indicated in the absence of suggestive symptoms or signs of metastasis. Extensive testing subjects the patient to risks inherent to a particular study as well as to risks associated with further interventions required to resolve false-positive results.

With regard to treatment, the role of radiation therapy and systemic chemotherapy in the treatment of localized subungual, or other subtypes of melanoma, is minimal. Effective therapy requires wide local surgical excision with digital amputation. Points of controversy include the extent of amputation and the role of adjuvant regional lymphadenectomy and isolated chemotherapeutic limb perfusion.

Treatment

The patient underwent thumb amputation at the metacarpophalangeal joint, axillary lymphadenectomy, and isolated chemotherapeutic limb perfusion with nitrogen mustard and actinomycin D. Results of pathologic examination of the amputated specimen identified a Clark's level IV subungual melanoma (3.9 mm thickness). There was no histologic evidence of ulceration, nail destruction, or bone invasion (Fig. 72–1), and no evidence of regional metastasis in the axillary lymph nodes (pT3b N0 M0, stage II).

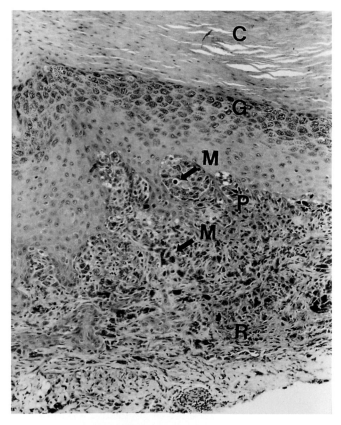

FIG. 72–1. Photomicrograph of subungual melanoma. The area marked **(C)** is the stratum corneum, **(G)** is the stratum germinativum, **(P)** is the papillary dermis, **(R)** is the reticular dermis, and **(M)** points to the melanoma. (H&E ×200).

Screening for Disease Recurrence

The patient was screened for symptoms and signs of recurrence every 2 months for the first year, every 3 months for the second year, every 4 months for the third year, and every 6 months for the fourth and fifth year. The screening history was directed toward symptoms suggestive of distant metastasis, while the screening physical examination concentrated on the primary site, the involved limb, and all lymph node-bearing regions for evidence of local recurrence, intransit disease, and suspicious lymphadenopathy. The skin of the patient also was inspected for the development of new primary melanomas. Chest radiographs were obtained annually to screen for pulmonary metastasis. Routine serum liver function tests and computed tomographic scans were not used. No evidence of recurrence or subsequent primary melanomas were seen after 6 years of follow-up.

COMMENTARY by Carl M. Sutherland

The presentation of any case of melanoma sparks controversy at any Tumor Board. This controversy is sometimes extremely heated. The presentation of a case of subungual melanoma particularly sparks controversy because of the limited number of cases available, making hard data difficult to obtain, and of the wide range of treatment options available with considerable difference in magnitude between them. Although the presentation of this patient does not document heated discussion at the original tumor board presentation, I would be surprised if that did not happen.

Management of the Primary

Most subungual melanomas are thick with a poor prognosis, and many have been present for a long time before the correct diagnosis is made. Apparently, the rate of nonmalignant lesions of the nail beds is sufficiently high and that of malignant lesions sufficiently low that both lay public and physicians are not inclined to think of subungual melanoma. Because of the aggressiveness of these tumors, adequate local excision needs to be done for local control, which usually results in amputation. At least two thirds of all subungual melanomas will occur in the major digit of the affected limb because at least one third of all subungual melanomas occur in the thumb and at least one third occur in the great toe (1,2). Amputation of the most distal joint possible is advantageous because major functional as well as cosmetic differences exist between proximal versus distal amputation of the major digit. It has been my practice to perform the most distal amputation possible. In 31 patients with subungual melanoma treated by the Surgical Oncology Group at Tulane University, local recurrence has not been a problem with treatment by perfusion and usually distal interphalangeal amputation. In addition, a recent study of 100 patients with subungual melanomas found no difference in survival rates of patients with local/proximal interphalangeal joint amputation, compared to those having a more proximal amputation (2). Therefore, until data are available that document improvement in local control, survival, or both, with more proximal amputation, I will continue to advocate distal amputations for tumors confined to the nail bed. I would not have performed the metacarpophalangeal joint amputation done in this case.

Management of the Nodes

A review of the history, theory, and current clinical trials of prophylactic node dissection (PND) for melanoma, in general, is beyond the scope of this discussion but was recently done elsewhere and was summarized in a previous Tumor Board presentation discussion (3,4). Since that summary, one of the major groups that advocated PND on the basis of a previous retrospective review of their findings has presented the findings of a new retrospective analysis of their data and conclude the new study does not support a survival benefit of PND (5). Therefore, until new data are presented with survival benefits of PND, I will rarely advise or perform PND for clinical node-negative malignant melanoma.

In addition to the general data on PND, regional perfusion for clinical stage I melanoma has been known to reduce the incidence of nodal failure (6). These data have recently been supported with findings from the EORTC/WHO/North America Perfusion Group Study of 13.9% nodal failure rate in the perfused group versus 21.9% in the non-perfused group (7). Because the morbidity rate of PND is significant and failure rate is low in nodes of perfused patients, I do not believe PND should be performed in patients being perfused with nodes that are clinically negative.

Regional Isolation Perfusion

The question of whether Regional Isolation Perfusion (RIP) is beneficial for patients with clinical stage I melanoma has been heatedly debated. Fortunately, good data are beginning to appear from the EORTC/WHO/North American Perfusion Group Study in which patients with malignant melanomas, at least 1.5 mm thick, were randomized to receive a wide local excision with or without an RIP (7). To date, there has been no difference in survival rate, but a significant difference does exist in disease-free survival rate. The type of first regional progression was significantly higher in patients without RIP compared to those with RIP. The rates of lymph nodes metastases, intransit metastases, and local recurrences were 13.5%, 1.5%, and 2%, respectively, in patients treated with RIP, compared with 21.9%, 6%, and 3.3%, respectively, in the control group without RIP. Unfortunately, the number of subungual cases will probably not be sufficient in this protocol to analyze differences in this specific subtype of melanoma. Patients with subungual melanoma treated without perfusion do have significant local, intransit, and nodal metastases (2). Because a regional perfusion will decrease those failures, it should at least be considered for patients with a poor prognosis.

Systemic Therapy

No discussion occurred regarding adjuvant systemic therapy. Although none has been found to be beneficial, the poor prognoses of most patients are such that I attempt to put them in randomized prospective trials of adjuvant therapy and would have attempted to do so in this case.

REFERENCES

1. Muchmore JH, Krementz ET, Reed RJ, et al. Melanoma of the hand and foot (volar and subungual melanoma). In: *Cutaneous Melanoma*, Balch CM, Houghton AN, Milton GW, et al., eds. Philadelphia: JB Lippincott, 1992:302.
2. Park KGM, Blessing K, Kernohan NM, et al. Surgical aspects of subungual malignant melanoma. *Ann Surg* 1992;216(6):692–5.
3. Sutherland CM, Mather FJ. Prophylactic lymph node dissection for malignant melanoma: what to do while we wait. *J Surg Oncol* 1992;51(1):1–4.
4. Sutherland CM, Extensive Hutchinson's melanotic freckle of the face. Commentary. Submitted for publication to the Tumor Board: Cancer Diagnosis and Treatment.
5. Ingivar C, Coates A, Petersen-Schaefer K, et al. Role of elective lymph node dissection in primary malignant melanoma 1.5 mm or thicker of the trunk and limbs without clinical node metastases. *Melanoma Res* 1993;3(1):103 (abstr).
6. Sugarbaker EV, McBride CM. Survival and regional disease control after isolation-perfusion for invasive Stage I melanoma of the extremities. *Cancer* 1976;37:188–98.
7. Lejeune FJ, et al. A randomized trial on prophylactic isolation perfusion for Stage I high-risk (i.e., 1.5 mm thickness) malignant melanoma of the limbs: an interim report. *Melanoma Res* 1993;3(1):95 (abstr).

73

Extensive Hutchinson's Melanotic Freckle of the Face

F. Kristian Storm

Give it enough time and a biologically significant invasive melanoma may develop

CASE PRESENTATION

H.S. is a 74-year-old Caucasian farmer with a 20-year history of a lightly colored homogeneous tan, flat lesion of his right malar eminence, estimated to be 4 cm in greatest dimension, clinically consistent with a lentigo maligna (Hutchinson's freckle). Over the past several months this lesion has developed a slightly raised, centrally located, irregular area of deep pigmentation (Fig. 73-1). The patient states the area has never bled or become ulcerated. The entire area of pigmentation was excised by the referring physician, and the patient was referred to the university for additional therapy if warranted.

The patient is pain-free and has no weight loss or fatigue. He is of northern German extraction. His red-headed blue-eyed granddaughter was treated for melanoma of the chest wall 2 years ago and is disease-free. He does not recall other family history of cancer and no family member is known to have multiple irregular moles.

Six years ago H.S. underwent a mitral valve annular reconstruction for regurgitation, and was placed on two aspirin a day for 5 years. Six months ago he had a transient ischemic episode, manifested by some flattening of his left facial contour. He had an extensive carotid artery workup at that time, which revealed a normal carotid ultrasound and normal brain computed tomography (CT) scan. He has chronic atrial fibrillation; however, a transesophageal cardiac echo and ultrasound failed to reveal any clot within the atrium. His thallium scan was only mildly abnormal, with 78% predicted. He was placed on

coumadin, 5 mg on day 1, 2.5 mg on days 2–3, then repeat. He is also on lanoxin, 0.125 mg daily, as well as calan SR, 180 mg, for mild hypertension. He is allergic to penicillin (urticaria) and clinoril (hyperactivity).

The patient is a well-developed, well-nourished, hardy, elderly, fair-skinned, blue-eyed gentleman in no distress. There is a well healed 4- to 5-cm vertical incision over the right malar eminence. There is no evidence of residual pigmentation, satellitosis, or intransit metastasis and no other suspicious skin lesions. No parotid, cervical, axillary, or inguinal adenopathy is noted. Examination of the heart revealed an irregularly irregular rhythm and a grade II regurgitation murmur. There were no other physical findings.

A review of the outside pathology slides was consistent with a lentigo maligna melanoma, level IV, 2.2-mm depth of invasion (Fig. 73-2). The complete blood count, SMA12, and CXR were all normal.

The patient was presented to the Surgical Oncology Tumor Conference. Members suggested additional diagnostic tests for occult metastatic disease, including CT scans of the brain, lung, and liver, as well as a bone scan. Treatment options included observation only versus re-excision of the primary site with wider margins, with or without a regional lymphadenectomy of radical or modified radical type.

No additional diagnostic tests were performed.

After 1-week withdrawal of anticoagulant, the patient underwent wide re-excision of his excisional biopsy site with 2-cm radial margins of normal skin, and incontinuity

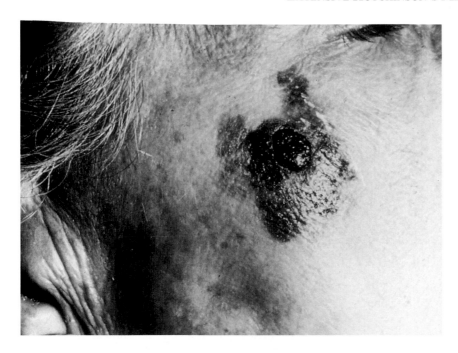

FIG. 73–1. Lentigo maligna melanoma, right cheek.

superficial parotidectomy and modified neck dissection. The wound was closed primarily with advancement flaps.

The final pathology report showed a wide excision specimen without evidence of residual melanoma; 0/4 parotid and 0/14 neck nodes containing metastatic melanoma were reported.

There were no treatment-related complications and the patient was discharged from the hospital on postoperative day 4.

SELECTED READINGS

1. Storm FK, Eilber FR, Sparks FC, Morton DL. A prospective study of parotid lymph node metastases in head and neck cancer. *Am J Surg* 1977;134:115–9.
2. Storm FK, Mahvi DM. Management of primary melanoma. In: *Malignant melanoma,* Das Gupta TK, Lejeune FJ, Chandhuri PK, eds. New York: McGraw-Hill; 1994;193–203.

COMMENTARY by Carl Sutherland

The Surgical Oncology Tumor Conference discussed several treatment options offered, including observation only versus re-excision of the primary site with wider margins, with or without a regional lymphadenectomy of radical or modified-radical type.

Unfortunately, there is not enough information provided by pathology to discuss fully the management of the primary site of this specific lesion. The photograph provided appears to be a typical vertical growth-phase melanoma in the middle of a lentigo maligna. As the lentigo maligna should not be invasive, it poses minimal, if any, risk of local recurrence. The dimensions are not given, but it is possible that the original excision of all the pigmented area may have attained a 2-cm margin around the invasive component of the melanoma. If so, I would have elected to do no further therapy on the primary because excision of this magnitude usually results in substantial cosmetic deformity, or in this case substantial additional surgery in generating flaps to cover the defect. Almost all these patients are elderly and usually with multiple other diseases. I favor keeping operative therapy to the minimum.

Although surgical resection is viewed as the standard of care in treatment of such lesions, and I would have favored surgery as the treatment of the primary in this case, it should not be forgotten that alternate methods of treatment of the primary exists. Again, most of these patients are in the older age ranges and frequently have concomitant cardiovascular disease and other diseases that put them at substantial risk for general anesthesia and surgery. As the risk for complications increase, consideration of the alternative increases. Radiation therapy has been used in Europe for decades for such lesions and more recently in Canada with apparently very good control rates (1).

Also, particularly in patients with higher risk for general anesthesia and surgery, it is possible that the magnitude of the excision can be greatly reduced by the use of topical 5-FU to control the lentigo maligna portion of the lesion, leaving only the invasive component that needs control with a surgical excision that might then be possible under local anesthesia (2).

Also controversial is whether or not a prophylactic lymph node dissection (PND) should be done for such cases. A full review of the history, theory, and current clinical trials of PND for malignant melanoma is beyond

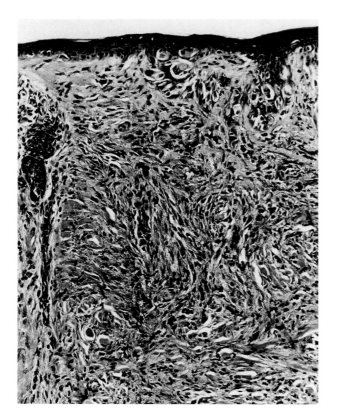

FIG. 73–2. Lentigo maligna melanoma (H&E, ×400).

the scope of this discussion, but has been done elsewhere recently (3). Briefly, PND in this century has been primarily based on the Hunterions lectures of Hanley of February 25 and February 27, 1907. Prospective trials of PND in both melanoma and breast cancer have not documented survival benefits from such therapy. Until clear-cut evidence is presented that will contradict these findings, I generally have not advised or performed PND for clinical stage I malignant melanoma in general and probably would not have advised so in this case.

To complicate this case additionally is the matter of prognosis of lentigo maligna melanoma. The available evidence indicates that patients who develop lentigo maligna melanoma in a pre-existing lentigo have a better prognosis than other types of melanoma, even when matched for tumor thickness (4). Therefore, even if one is an advocate of PND for primary malignant melanoma, it is not clear to me at what level of invasion or thickness lentigo maligna melanoma becomes at high enough risk for development of lymph node metastases to warrant PND.

This patient was not offered adjuvant systemic therapy, which is consistent with the standard of care. On the other hand, if I had thought the patient was at high enough risk for development of regional lymph nodes to warrant PND, I would have favored entry into one of the prospective systemic adjuvant therapy trials available.

REFERENCES

1. Harwood AR. Conventional fractionated radiotherapy for 51 patients with lentigo maligna and lentigo maligna melanoma. *Int J Radiat Oncol Biol Phys* 1982;9:1019.
2. Litwin MS, Krementz ET, Mansell PW, et al. Topical chemotherapy of lentigo maligna with 5-fluorouracil. *Cancer* 1975;35:721–33.
3. Sutherland CM, Mather FJ. Prophylactic lymph node dissection for malignant melanoma: what to do while we wait. *J Surg Oncol* 1992; 51(1):1–4.
4. Balch CM, Soong Seng-jaw, Shaw HM, et al. An analysis of prognostic factors in 8,500 patients with cutaneous melanoma. In: *Cutaneous melanoma*, Balch CM, Houghton AN, Milton GW, Sober AJ, Soong, Seng-jaw, eds. Philadelphia: JB Lippincott; 1991;2:165–99.

74

Hyperthermic Extremity Perfusion in the Management of Multiple Intransit Metastases of Malignant Melanoma

A. Benedict Cosimi and Robert W. Carey

Is there a role for intralesional therapy as well?

CASE PRESENTATION

A 74-year-old woman underwent removal of a 1.9-mm level IV melanoma from the anterior aspect of the left ankle in 1983. Six years later she developed two 3-mm nodules adjacent to the surgical site. At this time she had extensive staging and no distant metastases were found. Wide excision of the recurrent nodules was done, and she remained well for 1 year. Two new lesions appeared regionally, which were 4 mm in depth. These were also excised.

The patient was referred to the Massachusetts General Hospital. Multiple blue-black and gray-blue lesions, measuring 1 to 3 mm in diameter, were present on the leg (Fig. 74–1). Restaging included chest and abdominal computed tomography (CT) scans, which were negative for metastatic disease. Laboratory tests were normal. Therapeutic options considered by the Tumor Board were wide excision and skin grafting versus regional perfusion.

She underwent left lower extremity isolated perfusion with L-phenylalanine mustard (Fig. 74–2) and left inguinal lymph node dissection. A total of 80 mg of L-phenylalanine mustard was delivered through the perfusion pump. The total perfusion time was 1 hour. The patient's course was complicated by a drop in hematocrit to 18.8, for which she received two units of packed cells.

After completion of the perfusion, lymph node dissection was completed. Pathology review showed no evidence of metastasis to the regional nodes.

Figure 74–3 shows the appearance of the extremity 1 year after completion of perfusion. Complete remission of the extremity metastasis has persisted 4 years from regional perfusion of the extremity.

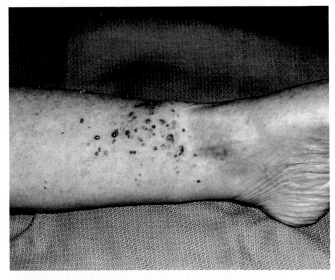

FIG. 74–1. Lower extremity showing numerous intransit melanoma metastases at time of extremity perfusion.

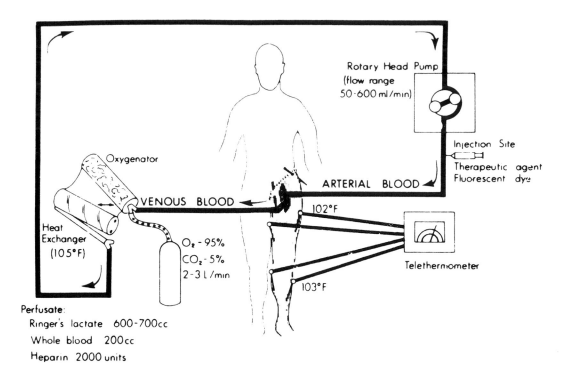

FIG. 74–2. Flow diagram for isolated hyperthermic regional chemotherapy of lower limb melanoma. The common femoral or external iliac artery and vein are surgically cannulated at the inguinal ligament. A tourniquet is held around the root of the limb by Steinmann pins inserted at the iliac crest and pubic ramus. The limb is perfused and oxygenated with warmed heparinized blood by the arterial and venous cannulas to a heart-lung machine circuit. Thermistor probes continuously monitor the subcutaneous temperature during the perfusion procedure. Once the limb temperature has stabilized at 39 to 40°C (102 to 104°F), fluorescent dye is added to the circuit to confirm there is no significant leakage from the isolated limb into the systemic circulation. The chemotherapeutic agent (e.g., L-phenylalanine mustard or cisplatin) is then added and perfusion continued for approximately 1 hour. The perfusion is terminated by washing out the extremity with Ringer's lactate solution. The cannulas and tourniquet are then removed and the vessels are repaired, thereby returning the limb to the systemic circulation.

COMMENTARY by Donald L. Morton and Richard Essner

More than 30 years ago Creech and associates (1) devised the technique of isolated limb perfusion to improve the efficacy of chemotherapy for patients with melanoma limited to a single extremity. This case presentation describes the successful use of hyperthermic isolated limb perfusion with L-phenylalanine (melphalan) to treat multiple intransit melanoma metastases on the lower leg of an elderly woman.

Extremity perfusion delivers high-dose chemotherapy with a reduced risk of systemic toxicity. Heating the chemotherapeutic agent theoretically increases its uptake by tumor tissue. Although the efficacy of hyperthermic extremity perfusion in primary or metastatic melanoma has not been proved by randomized trial, several retrospective studies demonstrate response rates as high as 40% to 60% (2). Krementz and associates (2,3) reported a 5-year survival rate of 59% in patients undergoing limb perfusion for recurrences within 3 cm of the primary lesion; however, survival dropped to 29% when satellite

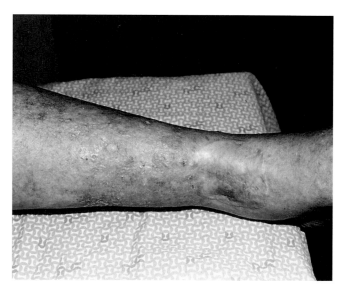

FIG. 74–3. Lower extremity condition 1 year after hyperthermic perfusion illustrating complete regression of intransit metastases. Post-treatment photographs demonstrate the impressive capacity of extremity perfusion to bring about regression of multiple cutaneous intransit metastases.

lesions were more than 3 cm from the primary. Other investigators have demonstrated 5-year survival rates of 58% (4) and 67% (5) for melanoma patients receiving limb perfusion to treat intransit metastases.

Stehlin and associates (6) reported a 43% rate of 5-year survival in melanoma patients undergoing adjuvant regional lymphadenectomy and perfusion for AJCC stage III disease. Ghussen and co-workers (5) demonstrated a significant ($p<0.01$) improvement in disease-free survival of melanoma patients undergoing adjuvant hyperthermic limb perfusion immediately after wide excision and regional node dissection. Ghussen's group (5,7) undertook a prospective randomized trial of hyperthermic limb perfusion in melanoma, but their highly favorable results (recurrence rate 7.5% with perfusion vs. 39% without perfusion) were biased by the predominance of women and low-risk lesions in the perfusion arm of the study. Also, the recurrence rate in the control arm of their study was much higher than that reported by other melanoma centers.

Melphalan is the chemotherapeutic agent most commonly used for isolated limb perfusion. Dacarbazine (DTIC), cisplatin, nitrogen mustard, and thiotepa, alone or in combination, are less effective than melphalan (8). However, recent phase II trials show that a combination of high-dose tumor necrosis factor, gamma-interferon, and melphalan may be more effective than melphalan alone (9,10).

Balanced against the potential efficacy of extremity perfusion is its frequent complication of fever (2). Patients may also experience transient or persistent edema, nerve dysfunction, lymph fistula, pain, or venous/arterial thrombosis, which in some cases can lead to limb amputation. Most importantly, inadequate isolation of the extremity can cause hypotension or shock, fatal leukopenia or thrombocytopenia (2,3,8,11,12).

In summary, there is no standard treatment for multiple intransit melanoma metastases to an extremity. Hyperthermic limb perfusion has been successful in some patients, as it was in the case reported here by Drs. Cosimi and Carey. Without nodal metastases, the addition of groin dissection to perfusion, as described in their case, has not been shown to improve survival and may increase the risk of postoperative complications. Surgical resection or nonsurgical modalities such as intralesional immunotherapy with bacille Calmette-Guerin (13), local radiation, monoclonal antibodies, melanoma vaccines, or systemic chemotherapy are some alternative methods to manage these patients.

Figure 74–4 outlines our protocol for managing patients with intransit melanoma metastases (14). We ini-

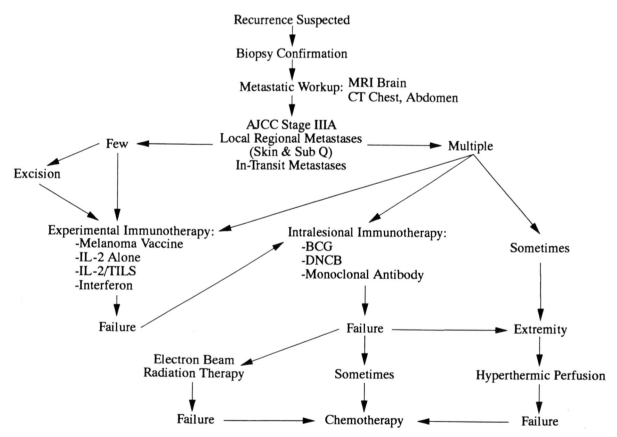

FIG. 74–4. Management of intransit melanoma metastases. (From Morton DL, et al. Malignant melanoma. In: *Cancer Medicine, Third Edition*, Holland JF, et al (eds). Philadelphia: Lea & Febiger, 1993, 1793–1824. Used by permission.)

tiate therapy with less toxic modalities such as resection (if there are only a few intransit lesions), intralesional BCG (13) or intralesional monoclonal antibodies (15), or active immunotherapy with melanoma vaccine (16). Surgical resection, intralesional immunotherapy, and local electron beam radiation are often successful initial therapies, and we tend to reserve perfusion for patients who do not respond to these simpler local therapies (17). We have found that intransit melanoma metastases can be controlled by delayed hyperthermic perfusion in most patients who fail intralesional therapy (18).

REFERENCES

1. Creech O, Krementz ET, Ryan RF. Chemotherapy of cancer: regional perfusion utilizing an extracorporal circuit. *Ann Surg* 1958;148:616–32.
2. Krementz ET, Ryan RF, Muchmore JH, et al. Hyperthermic regional perfusion for melanoma of the limbs. In: *Cutaneous melanoma,* 2nd ed, Balch CM, Houghton AN, Milton GW, Sober AJ, Soong SJ, eds. Philadelphia: JB Lippincott; 1992:403–26.
3. Krementz ET, Ryan RF. Chemotherapy of melanoma of the extremities by perfusion. Fourteen years clinical experience. *Ann Surg* 1972; 175:900–14.
4. Hartley JW, Fletcher WS. Improved survival of patients with stage II melanoma of the extremity using hyperthermic isolation perfusion with L-phenylalanine mustard. *J Surg Oncol* 1987;36:170–4.
5. Ghussen F, Kruger I, Smalley RU, Groth W. Hyperthermic perfusion with chemotherapy and melanoma of the extremities. *World J Surg* 1989;13:598–602.
6. Stehlin JS Jr, Giovanella BC, Delpolyi PD, et al. Results of hyperthermic perfusion for melanoma of the extremities. *Surg Gynecol Obstet* 1975;140:339–48.
7. Ghussen F, Kruger I, Groth W, Stutzer H. The role of hyperthermic cytostatic perfusion in the treatment of extremity melanoma. *Cancer* 1988;61:654–9.
8. Thompson JF, Gianoutsos MP. Isolated limb perfusion for melanoma: effectiveness and toxicity of cisplatin compared with that of melphalan and other drugs. *World J Surg* 1992;16:227–33.
9. Lienard D, Lejeune FJ, Ewalenko P. In transit metastases of malignant melanoma treated by high dose rTNF-α in combination with interferon-γ and melphalan in isolation perfusion. *World J Surg* 1992;16:234–40.
10. Lejeune F, Lienard D, Eggermont A, et al. Administration of high-dose tumor necrosis factor alpha by isolation perfusion of the limbs. Rationale and results. *Jx. Infusional Chemotherapy* 1995;5:73–81.
11. Hoekstra HJ, Koops HS, deVries LGE, et al. Toxicity of hyperthermic isolated limb perfusion with cisplatin for recurrent melanoma of the lower extremity after previous perfusion treatment. *Cancer* 1993;72:1224–9.
12. Thom AK, Alexander HR, Andrich MP, et al. Cytokine levels and systemic toxicity in patients undergoing isolated limb perfusion with high-dose tumor necrosis factor, interferon gamma, and melphalan. *J Clin Oncol* 1995;13:264–273.
13. Morton DL, Eilber FR, Holmes EC, et al. BCG immunotherapy of malignant melanoma: summary of a seven-year experience. *Ann Surg* 1974;180:635–43.
14. Morton DL, Wong JH, Kirkwood JM, Parker RG. Malignant melanoma. In: *Cancer medicine,* 3rd ed, Holland JF, Frei E, Bast RC Jr, et al., eds. Philadelphia: Lea & Febiger; 1993:1793–1824.
15. Irie RF, Morton DL. Regression of cutaneous metastatic melanoma by intralesional injection with human monoclonal antibody to ganglioside GD2. *Proc Natl Acad Sci USA* 1986;83:8694–8.
16. Morton DL, Foshag LJ, Hoon DSB, et al. Prolongation of survival in metastatic melanoma after active specific immunotherapy with a new polyvalent melanoma vaccine. *Ann Surg* 1992;216:463–82.
17. Storm FK, Sparks FC, Morton DL. Treatment for melanoma of the lower extremity with intralesional injection of bacille Calmette Guerin and hyperthermic perfusion. *Surg Gynecol Obstet* 1979;149:17–21.
18. Wong JH, Cagle LA, Kopald KH, et al. Natural history and selective management of in transit melanoma. *J Surg Oncol* 1990;44:146–50.

75

Extensive Metastatic Melanoma in the Axilla

Robert M. Barone

Unresectable disease converted to resectable disease with neoadjuvant chemotherapy

CASE PRESENTATION

This 38-year-old Caucasian man presented with a right axillary mass. He saw his family practitioner at the time, who treated him with antibiotics with improvement in the pain, as well as the size of the mass. After this, he had similar episodes of lymphadenitis on three other occasions, which again responded to antibiotics. Nine months later, the patient sustained a puncture wound to the right pectoral region that caused marked swelling of his right axillary lymph nodes. He was placed again on antibiotics with improvement in the swelling. However, over the ensuing months, the patient began to complain of increasing swelling in the right axilla, as well as increasing pain in his right shoulder and arm, especially with use. He was referred to a general surgeon, and at that time physical exam revealed a mass, measuring 4.5 cm in dimension, involving the right axillary fossa, as well as involvement of the skin of the axilla. An incisional biopsy was performed, which demonstrated amelanotic melanoma (Figs. 75–1, 75–2). Once the diagnosis was made, the patient volunteered that 2 to 3 years before his present illness, he had noticed a mole on his anterior chest wall that had become crusted and subsequently became covered with an eschar and spontaneously fell off. Because of the extensive amount of tumor that was noted in the axilla at the time of the incisional biopsy, as well as the fact that he also had infraclavicular lymphadenopathy, he was referred to a surgical oncologist, in late September 1992 for consideration of a forequarter amputation to remove the mass of disease presumed to involve the right axillary, infraclavicular, and brachial plexus regions.

The patient's main complaint at that time was excruciating pain and swelling in his right arm, axillary region, and shoulder with inability to use the right arm because of pain. The patient denied weight loss, headaches, or bone pain.

His physical examination was essentially negative except for a 4.5-cm mass involving the right axillary fossa fixed to overlying skin with several smaller lymph nodes palpated in the right infraclavicular area. There was no supraclavicular lymphadenopathy. There was no left axillary or left cervical lymphadenopathy. Examination of the abdomen revealed no evidence of organomegaly or masses. Skin examination revealed no evidence of a primary lesion. Neurologic exam revealed some muscle atrophy of the right arm but neurologic function was intact.

Metastatic workup was performed and included a computed tomography (CT) scan of the chest and abdomen. The CT scan of the chest revealed no evidence of metastatic disease to the lungs. Examination of the right axillary region revealed several nodular masses, measuring from 2 cm in diameter up to 3.2 cm in diameter with several smaller 1-cm nodular densities noted along the chest wall and pectoralis muscles in the infraclavicular regions (Figs. 75–3, A and B). There was no mediastinal lymphadenopathy. The CT scan of the abdomen was negative. A magnetic resonance image (MRI) of the brain also was negative. Blood chemistries also were within normal limits. The patient was clinically staged as TX N1 M0, stage III.

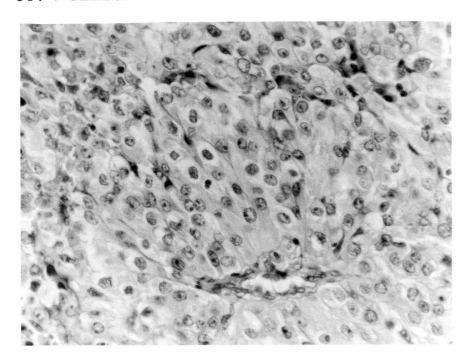

FIG. 75–1. Metastatic malignant melanoma involving axillary lymph node. Large cell malignant neoplasm with prominent nucleoli.

The patient was presented to the Tumor Board at Sharp Memorial Hospital for therapeutic considerations. The consensus of the Tumor Board was that surgical removal of all gross metastatic disease in the axilla should be performed first before considering some type of adjuvant therapy. However, it was the opinion of the surgical oncologist that, based on the physical examination and the CT scan results, it would be difficult to encompass all gross disease because the tumor burden in the axilla was bulky and probably would extend to, or beyond, the surgical margin, based on the amount of disease in the infraclavicular region and skin involvement. Several medical oncologists felt that the patient should be treated preoperatively with the McClay regimen, which consists of tamoxifen together with dacarbazine, carmustine, and cisplatin in the hopes of decreasing the bulk of the disease. This regimen has resulted in response rates of 50% in patients with metastatic disease (1). One should give a single course to assess the response. If the disease responds after one course, two or more courses are given,

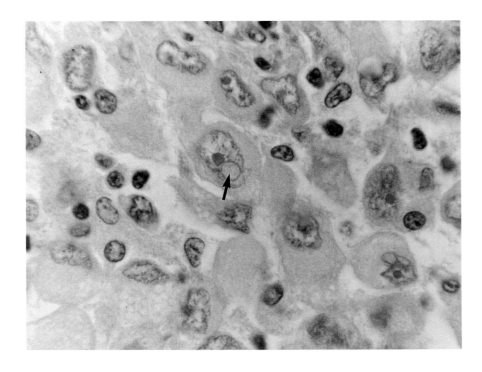

FIG. 75–2. High magnification: malignant neoplasm with macronucleoli and intranuclear cytoplasmic inclusions *(arrow)* characteristic of malignant melanoma.

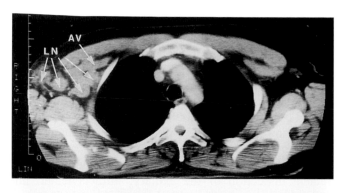

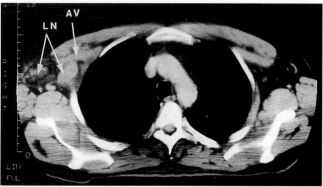

FIGS. 75–3, A and B: CT scans of the chest demonstrates multiple axillary lymph nodes *(LN)* in close proximity to axillary vein *(AV)*.

followed by surgery. After surgery, the radiation oncologist recommended radiation therapy to the axilla, chest wall, and supraclavicular area.

The patient received his first course of DTIC, platinum, BCNU, and tamoxifen with immediate improvement in his pain, as well as edema, and marked decrease in the size of the lymph nodes in the axilla and infraclavicular region. The patient then received a second course of this regimen a month later, again with continued reduction in the tumor volume in his axilla. One month later, the patient underwent an extended radical right axillary lymphadenectomy with infraclavicular and supraclavicular lymph node dissection, brachial plexus dissection, and axillary vein and artery dissection with partial resection of the axillary vein because a portion of one node was attached to the axillary vein.

Pathologic examination revealed metastatic melanoma involving 35 of 48 axillary lymph nodes. Supraclavicular lymph nodes were negative for metastatic tumor. The patient was still considered to be pathological stage III. Postoperatively, the patient made an uneventful recovery.

The patient was then referred for radiation therapy at the end of January 1993. It was the radiation therapist's opinion that because he responded well to the combination chemotherapy preoperatively, one of the drugs, cisplatin, should be used in conjunction with radiation for

radiosensitization. He was therefore given cisplatin with the initiation of radiation. The patient received a second course of platinum chemotherapy 1 month later and completed his radiation in 2 weeks. The patient received a total of 5,040 cGy to the right axilla, chest wall, and supraclavicular areas with AP/PA portals.

After completion of his radiation, the patient was again presented to the Sharp Memorial Hospital Tumor Board for consideration of further adjuvant therapy. It was pointed out that almost all the published phase III studies of adjuvant therapy for melanoma have shown no improvement in survival. However, a series of new studies suggest that the advent of recombinant DNA-produced cytokines and chemically defined antigens may have some effect in an adjuvant setting.

It was the feeling of the Board that adjuvant therapy be offered to this patient in a study setting. One could consider the ECOG Randomized Study, using interferon alpha-2B (2). Another study that could be considered would be that of Morton et al. (3) at John Wayne Cancer Center in Santa Monica, California, using allogeneic irradiated cell lines and BCG, with or without indomethacin. Other studies using allogeneic tumor cell vaccines are available through the Southwest Oncology Group (4) and the New York University Cancer Center (5).

The patient declined further adjuvant therapy. Physical examination, histochemical studies, and chest radiography performed 6 months after surgery were negative.

REFERENCES

1. McClay EF, Mastrangelo MJ, Sprandio JD, et al. Importance of tamoxifen to a cisplatin-containing regimen in the treatment of metastatic melanoma. *Cancer* 1989;63:1292–5.
2. Kirkwood JM, Ernstoff MS. Interferons—clinical applications: cutaneous melanoma. In: *Biologic therapy of cancer,* DeVita Jr VT, Hellman S, Rosenberg SA, eds. Philadelphia: JB Lippincott; 1991:311–33.
3. Morton DL, Foshag LJ, Hoon DS, et al. Prolongation of survival in metastatic melanoma after active specific immunotherapy with a new polyvalent melanoma vaccine. *Ann Surg* 1992;216:463–82.
4. Mitchell MS, Harrel W, Kan-Mitchell J, Deans R. The immunologic basis of active specific immunotherapy for human melanoma. *Prog Immunol* 1993;8.
5. Bystryn JC, Oratz R, Roses D, Harris M, Henn M, Lew R. Relationship between immune response to melanoma vaccine immunization and clinical outcome in stage II malignant melanoma. *Cancer* 1969: 5:1157–64.

COMMENTARY by Constantine P. Karakousis

This is a case of an apparently spontaneous regression of a cutaneous melanoma of the right anterior chest wall that was not diagnosed and was barely noticed by the patient. He presented 2 to 3 years later with right axillary adenopathy. This was treated with antibiotics with improvement, and periodic exacerbations were treated also with antibiotics when an incisional biopsy by a surgeon revealed amelanotic melanoma.

It is not surprising that, given no history of prior malignancy, the primary physician initially assumed the diagnosis of lymphadenitis and treated the patient with antibiotics. However, there are sufficient differences in the history, physical findings, and symptoms between reactive, inflammatory lymphadenopathy and malignant adenopathy, which, although by no means totally reliable, often permit the differential diagnosis.

Inflammatory nodal swellings usually have an antecedent course, that is, prior trauma or inflammation in the anatomic region drained by the particular nodal basin. There may be other signs or symptoms of an infection, such as tenderness, redness in the involved area, and fever. The white blood count usually reveals leukocytosis. Inflammatory swellings usually have a short history of development.

Malignant adenopathy is characterized by a more subtle onset. The history of development may have been long, but the patient may have noticed it just a few days before. These nodal swellings are usually painless and lack the concomitant signs and symptoms of inflammation. A primary tumor site may be evident in the anatomic region drained by this nodal basin.

On physical examination, inflammatory nodes usually retain their fusiform shape, are rather flat, soft, and may be tender on palpation. Nodes enlarged by a malignant process are usually spherical, firm, and not tender to palpation.

When the presumptive diagnosis of inflammation is made, antibiotics are prescribed. After 2 to 4 weeks, if the nodes have not returned to normal size, needle aspiration for cytology (also for culture and sensitivities if the diagnosis of inflammation is still entertained) should be done. If this is not diagnostic, an open biopsy should be performed. In malignant lymphadenopathy, although some improvement in size or symptoms may occur with antibiotic therapy, the nodal status does not return to normal as in inflammatory adenopathies.

By the time of presentation to the present group, the patient had extensive disease in the axilla and supraclavicular fossa, thought to require a forequarter amputation for its surgical extirpation.

The patient was started on a four-drug protocol. Marked objective and subjective improvement was noted after the first course and a second course was given, followed by extended radical axillary and supraclavicular node dissection.

There is no question that the correct approach was chosen in this patient with neoadjuvant chemotherapy because it was determined that the tumor could not be resected except by forequarter amputation. For cases of intermediate surgical difficulty, when the disease can be resected with limb preservation, the use of neoadjuvant chemotherapy is questionable. Malignant melanoma is still considered to be a chemoresistant tumor, and the likelihood is greater than 50% that the disease will be more extensive after one or two courses of chemotherapy. The cautious attitude espoused by Dr. Barone and the rest of multidisciplinary team, of evaluating the patient 3 to 4 weeks after the first course and before a second course would be advised, should be commended as opposed to prescribing two courses from the beginning and evaluation after the second course.

The correct surgical procedure was performed, that is, radical dissection of the axillary, infraclavicular, and supraclavicular nodes. We have followed the same approach for extensive disease in this area (1). For patients with massive disease extending under the clavicle, claviculectomy with en bloc resection of the supraclavicular, infraclavicular, and axillary nodes is tolerated well and provides the necessary exposure for complete extirpation of the disease (2). There should be no hesitation to resect a portion of the axillary vein when involved by the tumor with ligation of the two ends, because this does not cause in itself swelling of the arm and is followed by occasional long-term survival (1). Because of the frequent microscopic or gross involvement of the supra-axillary lymph nodes when there is extensive disease in the axilla, we mobilize the supra-axillary fat pad and nodes en bloc with the axillary nodes and do so even for the elective procedure, exposing routinely the brachial plexus (3).

Postoperative adjuvant radiation to the axillary region after resection of extensive nodal disease makes theoretical sense. It is by no means required often, but there is supportive evidence in the literature that the local control rate, at least, is thus increased (4).

It is true that there is no adjuvant therapy of proven efficacy at the present. Therefore, out of the context of a prospective randomized study, the patient may as well be simply observed.

In conclusion, the presented case, despite the regrettable but understandable delay in the diagnosis, was subsequently treated optimally. This patient obviously needs close follow-up particularly in the first two years, because most patients bound to relapse after therapeutic lymphadenectomy do so in the first 2 years.

REFERENCES

1. Karakousis CP, Goumas W, Rao U, Driscoll DL. Axillary node dissection in malignant melanoma. *Am J Surg* 1991;16:2:202–7.
2. Karakousis CP, Gupta BK, Zografos GC. Claviculectomy for the exposure and en bloc resection of adjacent tumors. *Am J Surg* 1992;164:63–7.
3. Karakousis CP, Rao U. Axillary node dissection in malignant melanoma. *Surg Gynecol Obstet* 1981;152:506–9.
4. Ang KK, Byers RM, Peters LJ, et al. Regional radiotherapy as adjuvant treatment for head and neck malignant melanoma. *Arch Otolaryngol Head Neck Surg* 1990;116:169

SECTION XVIII

Breast

76

T2 N0 M0 Cancer of the Right Breast

William G. Kraybill and Jeffrey F. Moley

Is young age a contraindication to breast conservation?

CASE PRESENTATION

The patient is a 39-year-old Caucasian woman who identified a mass in her right breast while performing breast self-examination. This was evaluated with mammography in her community, where it was estimated that this was a 1.5-cm lesion in the lateral aspect of the right breast. The lesion was described as being spiculated and calcified. Examination of the left breast revealed no evidence of mass or calcifications. This patient underwent needle localization on January 29, 1990, at an outside hospital (Fig. 76–1). Specimen radiograph revealed the presence of the mass within the specimen and confirmed removal of the mass identified on mammography. Pathologic examination revealed an infiltrating ductal carcinoma with an intraductal component of the comedo type (Fig. 76–2). On review of the outside pathology at this institution, it was the impression that the lesion had been incompletely excised, although the margins had not been inked. The patient's outside physician recommended a mastectomy to the patient. She was referred to Barnes Hospital for definitive surgery. Estrogen and progesterone receptors revealed an estrogen receptor level of 55 Fmol/MCP and a progesterone receptor value of 39 Fmol/MCP. Histologic staining confirmed the tumor to be ER positive and progesterone positive (Figs. 76–2A,C, F,G). By history she was otherwise healthy. She had a previous cholecystectomy and bilateral ligation of her fallopian tubes. There was a family history of fibrocystic change, but the patient denied any family history of breast cancer. She denied any history of hypertension, diabetes, or pulmonary disease. The patient smoked one pack of cigarettes per day. She denied any headaches, dizziness, or bone pain. She was gravida II para II with two healthy children.

On physical examination, she was found to be a well-developed slightly obese Caucasian woman. There was no adenopathy present in the neck, supraclavicular, or axillary regions. The breast examination was remarkable for a healing right circumareolar incision within an area of ecchymosis in the right upper outer quadrant and a firm mass presumably secondary to healing at the breast biopsy site. The left breast was without masses or discharge. Abdominal examination was not remarkable. There were no masses, nor was the liver palpated. The extremities were well perfused and otherwise normal. The patient had had a recent pelvic and rectal examination by her gynecologist.

In summary, this is a 39-year-old premenopausal woman with what was initially thought to be a T1 N0 M0 carcinoma. Physical examination after biopsy revealed the mass to be 2.5 cm. Presumably, this was secondary to healing at the biopsy site. Pathologic review revealed an invasive adenocarcinoma of the breast with about a 10% intraductal component of the comedo type. Because the margins had not been inked, no comment could be made concerning the adequacy of margins. Of note, this lesion was felt to be a high-grade tumor.

This case was presented to the breast conference at Barnes Hospital. On the basis of mammographic findings, history, physical exam, and pathology presented, it was felt that she was potentially a candidate for either modified radical mastectomy or breast conservation therapy with postoperative radiation therapy. The option of modified radical mastectomy with immediate reconstruction was also considered. Of note, the operating surgeon's

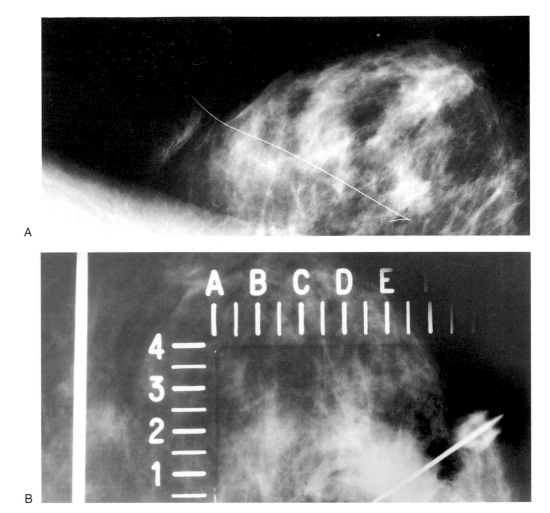

FIG. 76–1. A: Needle localization mammogram of the right breast, mediolateral position. The tip of the localization wire lies immediately behind a spiculated mass. **B:** Craniocaudal projection. Localization markers are in place, and the tip of the marker needle lies just posterior to the intramammary mass

feeling was that this patient, because of her age, would probably benefit most from having a mastectomy. Because of the presence of a high-grade breast cancer in a premenopausal woman, it was the recommendation of medical oncology that she be treated with adjuvant chemotherapy. After completion of chemotherapy, it was recommended that she receive tamoxifen.

These options were presented to the patient. She chose to have a modified radical mastectomy with immediate reconstruction. It was decided in consultation with plastic surgery as well as in discussions with the patient to perform a free TRAM flap reconstruction of the right breast using microvascular technique. On February 11, 1992, the patient underwent a right modified radical mastectomy with immediate breast reconstruction using a free TRAM flap. Immediately postoperatively, she did well. Her drains demonstrated decreasing drainage throughout her hospital stay and were discontinued by the seventh post-operative day. She did have mild duskiness of the mastectomy flaps with several areas of mild epidermolysis. At

the time of her discharge on the eighth postoperative day, her drains had been removed and her wounds were healing well with the exception of a small area of epidermolysis on the superior and inferior mastectomy flaps. These were stable.

Pathologic evaluation of the resected specimen demonstrated residual invasive ductal carcinoma. There was microscopic evidence of involvement of the intramammary lymphatics. The margins were free of tumor. Microcalcifications were present. Immunoperoxidase stains for estrogen and progesterone receptors were positive. There was no evidence of malignancy in 11 of 11 lower axillary nodes and in 9 of 9 upper axillary lymph nodes. The gross description of the lesion demonstrated it to measure 2.5 × 1.4 × 1.8 cm in greatest dimension. On the basis of this and previously excised tissue, this was staged as a T2 N0 M0 estrogen receptor–positive, progesterone receptor–positive adenocarcinoma of the breast.

Despite the recommendations by medical oncology, this patient refused to take adjuvant chemotherapy. She

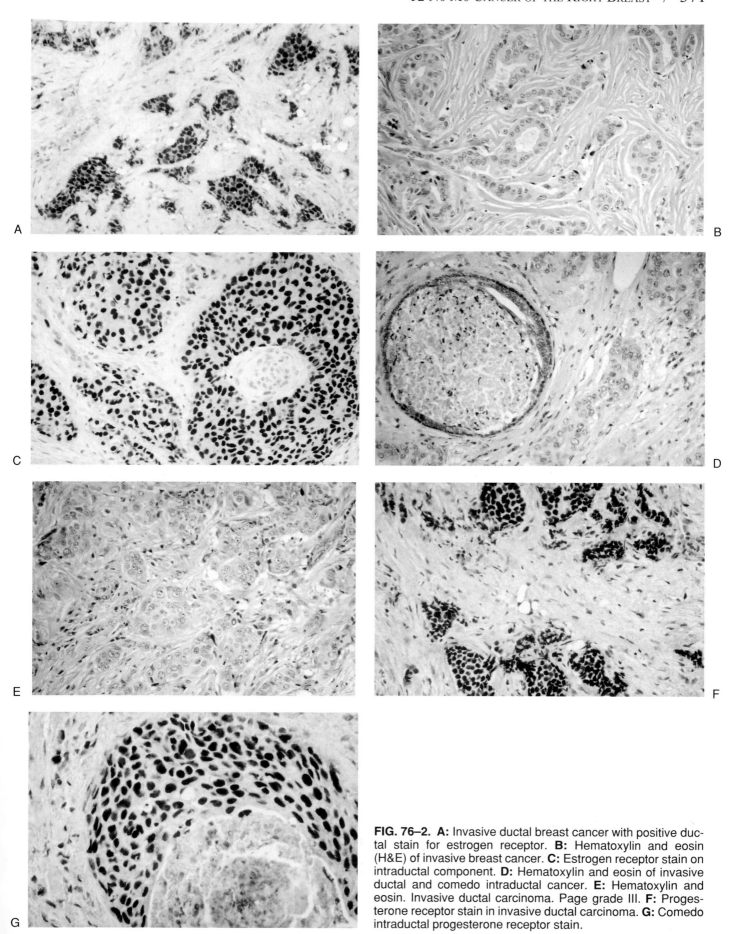

FIG. 76–2. A: Invasive ductal breast cancer with positive ductal stain for estrogen receptor. **B:** Hematoxylin and eosin (H&E) of invasive breast cancer. **C:** Estrogen receptor stain on intraductal component. **D:** Hematoxylin and eosin of invasive ductal and comedo intraductal cancer. **E:** Hematoxylin and eosin. Invasive ductal carcinoma. Page grade III. **F:** Progesterone receptor stain in invasive ductal carcinoma. **G:** Comedo intraductal progesterone receptor stain.

did agree to taking tamoxifen and continues on that medication at this time. Four months after her mastectomy and immediate reconstruction, her flap had healed well. She continued to do well until approximately 18 months after her surgery, when she began to experience some anxiety attacks. This consisted of her losing her temper with her family and occasionally with children in her capacity as a teacher. Arrangements were made for the patient to seek psychiatric consultation.

COMMENTARY by Robert T. Osteen

The patient is a young woman with a T1 breast cancer that ultimately turned out to be T2 on the basis of pathologic examination. The tumor was estrogen and progesterone receptor–positive but high-grade. Axillary lymph nodes were negative, but intramammary lymphatic metastases were seen.

This case offers multiple alternatives for management. First, it is not clear why a palpable mass discovered by the patient required a needle localized biopsy, which is usually used for nonpalpable, mammographically detected lesions.

The mammographic characteristics of the mass were such that cancer was a likely diagnosis. In addition to two-view mammograms, magnification views are helpful before the biopsy to assess the extent of disease, particularly when breast conservation is being considered.

When, as in this case, the diagnosis of cancer is likely, a one-stage biopsy and treatment would have been an appropriate consideration (1). Needle aspiration cytology, core needle biopsy of a palpable lesion, or stereotactically directed core needle biopsy for nonpalpable lesions can establish the diagnosis and the options for therapy, including a one-stage procedure. The only disadvantage of attempting a breast-conserving, one-stage procedure is the small number of patients who have either extensive invasive lobular carcinoma or ductal carcinoma in situ not detected by mammogram and extending far beyond the palpable margins of the tumor. The use of magnification views improves the rate of detection of extensive ductal carcinoma in situ, but does not eliminate the need for re-excision in some patients to obtain better margins (2).

As in this case, the failure to apply ink to the biopsy specimen inevitably raises a question regarding the adequacy of the initial excision. The inability to assess margins may compel a re-excision and compromise the cosmetic results. The amount of tissue to excise and the adequacy of margins are controversial (3–5). If permanent pathology shows that the tumor is a pure invasive ductal carcinoma with little or no ductal carcinoma in situ, excision may have been adequate, even if there is focal microscopic margin involvement (5).

This patient's pathology is described as being an infiltrating ductal carcinoma with a comedo type intraductal component. The amount of ductal carcinoma in situ (DCIS) and its relation to the margins must be included in considerations of breast conservation. With adequate margins, a small amount of DCIS does not predict an increased local recurrence rate. However, a large amount of DCIS is associated with a significant in-breast recurrence rate unless generous tumor-free margins are obtained (6,7).

Judging by her mammogram, the size of the tumor in relation to the size of this patient's breast would have allowed a satisfactory cosmetic result from breast conservation, even if a limited re-excision were thought to be necessary.

The decision to do a mastectomy was apparently based on the patient's age. Several studies have reported a higher risk of in-breast recurrence in young patients after breast-conserving surgery and radiation (8). The definition of young age has varied, but the problem appears to be of greatest concern in women under the age of 35 years who also tend to have significant amounts of ductal carcinoma in situ. It has been argued that even in that young age group with an increased risk of in-breast recurrence, the risk of dying from metastatic breast cancer is similar to mastectomy and that breast-conserving surgery is still a viable option.

The Tumor Board's recommendation to treat a T1 N0 M0 ER+ tumor with cytotoxic chemotherapy is debatable. Apparently, the pathologist's interpretation of the tumor as high grade (translated by the Tumor Board as undifferentiated) was the basis for this decision (9). Flow cytometry might have supported that decision (10). Because the mastectomy specimen showed that the tumor was 2½ cm in diameter (T2) with intramammary lymphatic invasion, the case for chemotherapy in a node-negative patient was strengthened (11). The usefulness of tamoxifen in premenopausal, node-negative patients is also debatable (12).

One can only wonder whether the anxiety attacks experienced by this patient may have been related to her hormonal changes and speculate on the relative effectiveness of cessation of the tamoxifen versus psychiatric intervention (13).

REFERENCES

1. Fisher B. Reappraisal of breast biopsy prompted by the use of lumpectomy. *JAMA* 1985;253:3585–8.
2. Healey EA, Osteen RT, Schnitt SJ, et al. Can the clinical and mammographic findings at presentation predict the presence of an extensive intraductal component in early stage breast cancer? *Int J Radiat Oncol Biol Phys* 1989;17:1217–21.
3. Harris JR, Connolly JL, Schnitt SJ, et al. The use of pathologic features in selecting the extent of surgical resection necessary for breast cancer patient treated by primary radiation therapy. *Ann Surg* 1984;201:164–9.
4. Wazar DE, DiPetrillo T, Schmidt-Ullrich R, et al. Factors influencing outcome and complication risk after conservative surgery and radiotherapy for early-stage breast carcinoma. *J Clin Oncol* 1992;10:356–63.

5. Vicini FA, Eberlein TF, Connolly JL, et al. The optimal extent of resection for patients with Stages I or II breast cancer treated with conservative surgery and radiotherapy. *Ann Surg* 1991;214:200–5.

6. Holland R, Connolly JL, Gelman R, et al. The presence of an extensive intraductal component following a limited excision correlates with prominent residual disease in the remaining breast. *J Clin Oncol* 1990;8:113–8.

7. Zafrani B, Vielh P, Fourquet A, et al. Conservative treatment of early breast cancer: prognostic value of ductal in-situ component and other pathological variable in local control and survival. *Eur J Cancer Clin Oncol* 1989;25:1645–50.

8. Kurtz JM, Jacquemier J, Almaric R, et al. Why are local recurrences after breast-conserving therapy more frequent in younger patients? *J Clin Oncol* 1990;8:591–8.

9. Fisher ER, Redmond L, Fisher B, et al. Pathologic findings from the National Surgical Adjuvant Breast and Bowel Projects (NSABP). *Cancer* 1990;65:2121–8.

10. Clark GM, Mathiew M-C, Owens MA, et al. Prognostic significance of S-phase fraction in good-risk, node-negative cancer patients. *J Clin Oncol* 1992;10:428–32.

11. Mansour EG, Gray R, Shatila A, et al. Efficacy of adjuvant chemotherapy in high-risk, node-negative breast cancer. *N Engl J Med* 1989;320:485–90.

12. Early Breast Cancer Trialists' Collaborative Group. Effects of adjuvant tamoxifen and of cytotoxic therapy in mortality in early breast cancer: an overview of 61 randomized trials among 28,896 women. *N Engl J Med* 1988;319:1681–92.

13. Jones S, Cathcart C, Pumroy S, et al. Frequency, severity and management of tamoxifen-induced depression in women with node-negative breast cancer. *Proc ASCO* 1993;12:78.

EDITORIAL BOARD COMMENTARY

Many surgeons categorically deny an opportunity for breast conservation in young women. This is based on the observation that young age is a risk factor for local recurrence after breast conservation. Although this remains a controversial issue, the balance of evidence now favors the hypothesis that local recurrence in young patients is more a function of the biology of the disease than the surgical procedure chosen.

77

T1c N0 M0, Stage I, ER Negative Breast Cancer

Ann McCunniff

Why tamoxifen and how long?

CASE PRESENTATION

A 44-year-old black premenopausal woman felt a lump in the lower aspect of the right breast. Her obstetric history was gravida 4, para 2, aborta 2. Mammography revealed an area of density in the inferior outer quadrant of the right breast. Fine-needle aspiration was not diagnostic. The patient underwent excisional biopsy, and pathologic results revealed a moderately differentiated infiltrating ductal carcinoma measuring 1.5 cm in greatest diameter. No vascular invasion was seen. Margins were free of tumor. Axillary dissection revealed 16 nodes, all of which were negative. Flow cytometry showed that the tumor was estrogen-receptor negative but highly progesterone-receptor positive (112 fmol/mg). The tumor was also found to be diploid and had an S phase of only 1%. The estrogen receptors were rechecked by means of an exchange method and were confirmed to be negative (Table 77–1).

The patient has no significant medical history. She does have a history of light-to-moderate smoking. Family history is significant in that her mother had breast cancer 15 years earlier and underwent modified radical mastectomy. Her disease has not recurred.

TUMOR BOARD DISCUSSION

The two options for local treatment of this patient's breast cancer were (a) modified radical mastectomy or (b) lumpectomy and axillary node dissection followed by radiation therapy to the intact breast. There were several factors to consider in deciding whether this patient was a candidate for conservation of the breast. Her breasts were moderate in size, and as the lesion was small (1.5 cm), cosmesis after excision was very good. No high-risk factors for recurrence in the breast, positive margins, or

TABLE 77-1. *Factors influencing choice of treatment*

Factor	Favorable	Unfavorable	
Estrogen receptor (fmol/mg of protein)		Standard 0 Exchange 0	(Procedure is biochemical)
Progesterone receptor (fmol/mg of protein)	112		Favorable is <10 units or positive staining by ICA
Cathepsin D (pmol/mg of protein)	29.5		Favorable is <40 units and unfavorable >62 units
Ploidy (DNA content/cell)	Diploid 1.00		
DNA synthesis (by flow cytometry) G 1/0 % = 98 S % = 1 G$_L$M % = 1			

374

extensive intraductal component were present. She had no connective-tissue disease that might result in poor cosmesis, and she agreed to come for therapy for approximately 6 weeks and after that to return regularly for follow-up. In this patient, local recurrence in the treated breast is expected to be approximately 10% (1). The patient therefore received 5,040 cGy in 28 fractions to the intact breast, followed by an electron boost of 1,000 cGy in 5 fractions to the lumpectomy site.

The second issue to consider in the treatment of this patient is the role of systemic therapy. There is evidence now from prospective, randomized studies that adjuvant systemic therapy significantly increases disease-free survival (DFS) in patients with negative axillary nodes. Some believe, however, that not all patients should be treated (2–5). In discussing further therapy for this patient, several prognostic features were examined to determine what, if any, further treatment was necessary.

The two factors of primary concern were the patient's age and estrogen-receptor status. In the above-mentioned trials, adjuvant chemotherapy resulted in a significant increase in DFS in estrogen-receptor–negative patients. Interestingly, though, these studies showed this benefit regardless of the patient's age.

However, other prognostic factors such as size of the tumor, progesterone-receptor level, proliferative rate, and ploidy, as well as cathepsin D level, were all in the favorable range.

Tumor size was evaluated in a large series of patients with negative axillary nodes by the Surveillance, Epidemiology, and End Results (SEER) Program of the National Cancer Institute, Bethesda, Maryland. They found that tumor size was related to recurrence and in lesions 1.0 to 1.9 cm, axillary nodes negative, relative 5-year survival was approximately 90% (6).

Using DNA flow-cytometric measurement on 345 patients, Clark et al. found that ploidy and S-phase fraction were important predictors of DFS and overall survival in axillary node–negative patients (7). They found that the probability of DFS at 5 years was approximately 90% in patients with diploid tumors with low S-phase fraction. Also, Sigurdsson et al., in a multivariate analysis of 250 patients with node-negative disease, found that S-phase fraction was an independent prognostic factor, followed by tumor size and progesterone receptor level (8). Results from the Danish Breast Cancer Cooperative Group have also shown that progesterone-receptor status may be as important as estrogen-receptor status in predicting outcome (9).

Although the use of cathepsin D level has not yet been proven an important prognostic factor, studies have shown correlation with outcome. Tandon et al. examined cathepsin D levels in patients with negative axillary nodes and found that the values were predictive of outcome, especially in patients with aneuploid tumors (10).

Certainly, some would recommend chemotherapy for this patient because of her premenopausal status, tumor size (>1.0 cm), and negative estrogen-receptor status. However, because the lesion was 1.5 cm in size and all other factors were favorable, it was decided that the benefits of cytotoxic chemotherapy would not likely be outweighed by its cost and potential toxicity. However, the question of hormonal treatment in this patient was then raised.

The Nolvadex Adjuvant Trial Organization study, as well as an earlier study done by the Scottish Breast Cancer Trials Committee, showed benefit with adjuvant tamoxifen, regardless of menopausal status or estrogen-receptor status in node-negative patients (11,12). Also, the possibility of reducing the patient's risk of developing contralateral breast cancer was also discussed (4,13,14).

The patient's medical oncologist then discussed these issues with the patient, after which the patient began receiving tamoxifen citrate, 20 mg twice daily, and was to continue close follow-up with her medical and radiation oncologists.

REFERENCES

1. Fisher B, Redmond C, Poisson R, et al. Eight year results of a randomized clinical trial comparing total mastectomy and lumpectomy with or without irradiation in the treatment of breast cancer. *N Engl J Med* 1989;320:822–8.
2. Fisher B, Redmond C, Dimitno N, et al. A randomized trial evaluating sequential methotrexate and fluorouracil in the treatment of patients with node negative breast cancer who have estrogen receptor negative tumor. *N Engl J Med* 1989;320:473–8.
3. Zambetti M, Bonadonna G, Valagussa P. CMF for node-negative and estrogen receptor negative breast cancer. *J Natl Cancer Monogr* 1992;11:77–83.
4. Fisher B, Costantino J, Redmond C, et al. A randomized clinical trial evaluating tamoxifen in the treatment of patients with node-negative breast cancer who have estrogen-receptor positive tumors. *N Engl J Med* 1989;320:479–84.
5. Mandor EG, Eudey L, Shatila AH. Efficacy of adjuvant chemotherapy in high-risk node negative breast cancer. *N Engl J Med* 1989;320:485–90.
6. Carter CL, Allen C, Hena DE. Relation of tumor site, lymph node status, and survival in 24, 74- breast cancer cases. *Cancer* 1989;63:181–7.
7. Clark GM, Dressler LG, Owens MA, Pounds B, Oldaher T, McGuire WL. Prediction of relapse or survival in patients with node-negative breast cancer by DNA flow cytometry. *N Engl J Med* 1989;320:627–33.
8. Sigurdsson H, Baldetoys B, Borg A, et al. Indicators of prognosis in node-negative breast cancer. *N Engl J Med* 1990;322:1045–53.
9. Thorpe SM, Rose C, Rasmussen BB, et al. Prognostic value of steroid hormone receptors: multivariate analysis at systemically untreated patients with node negative primary breast cancer. *Cancer Res* 1987;47:6126–33.
10. Tandon AK, Clark GM, Clamnes GC, et al. Cathepsin D and prognosis in breast cancer. *N Engl J Med* 1990;322:297–302.
11. Baum M. Nolvadex Adjuvant Trial Organization: controlled trial of tamoxifen as single adjuvant agent in management of early breast cancer; analysis at eight years. *Br J Cancer* 57:608–11.
12. Breast Cancer Trials Committee, Scottish Cancer Trial Office (MRC), Edinburgh. Adjuvant tamoxifen in the management of operable breast cancer: The Scottish Trial. *Lancet* July 25, 1987.
13. Early Breast Cancer Trialists' Collaborative Group. Systemic treatment of early breast cancer by hormonal, cytotoxic, or immune therapy. *Lancet* 1992;339:1–15, 71–85.

14. Early Breast Cancer Trialists' Collaborative Group. Systemic treatment of early breast cancer by hormonal, cytotoxic, or immune therapy: 133 randomized trials involving 31,000 recurrences and 24,000 deaths among 75,000 women. *Lancet* 1992;39(8785):71–85.

COMMENTARY by Alexander J. Walt

The surgical management of this patient and subsequent breast radiation follows the mainstream approach to a T1 N0 M0 lesion and does not warrant elaboration. The subsequent decisions do.

The administration of adjuvant chemotherapy for node-positive premenopausal patients has been well accepted since Bonadonna's pioneering work 15 to 20 years ago. In 1989, extension of this concept to the patient with a node-negative axilla followed the alert issued by the National Cancer Institute when a prospective study suggested that adjuvant chemotherapy provided an approximately 25% benefit in this specific group. By extrapolation, of patients with node-negative lesions less than 1.5 cm in whom the disease-free survival is about 90% at 5 years, only 25% of the 10% destined to have metastatic disease will be helped. Stated differently, about 97 of 100 patients in the group will receive chemotherapy unnecessarily. The quest has therefore been to identify the two or three patients who may benefit from adjuvant chemotherapy. An extensive array of prognostic indicators has been studied in an attempt to predict which patients might benefit (1). Preliminary and often conflicting reports have suggested that measurement of c-erb B2, p53 expression, the extent of angiogenesis, and other factors may by of value in assessing the degree of aggressiveness of individual tumors and thus encourage vigorous prophylactic therapeutic measures when appropriate. To this point, the efficacy of these and other laboratory tests in the node-negative patient has been disappointing. Regrettably, these measurements have added little to meticulous cytologic examination of the primary lesion by an experienced pathologist.

The patient under consideration, whose tumor had all the hallmarks of an excellent prognosis, was an ideal candidate for breast conservation. The finding of estrogen-negative/progesterone-positive receptors, carefully rechecked, is found in about 4% of patients. When the PGR is positive, the ER negativity seems not to influence prognosis adversely to any substantial degree. In practice, the hormone receptor status is more accurately predictive of potential response of subsequent metastases to estrogen deprivation rather than to prognosis for ultimate survival.

Nevertheless, many oncologists would recommend adjuvant chemotherapy in a patient with the findings of this case and, indeed, prescribe adjuvant chemotherapy in virtually all infiltrating cancers (1.2 cm is perhaps the most widely recommended dividing line between adjuvant chemotherapy and observation). Others would feel that no further treatment is warranted in this case. Still others, more commonly in Europe than in the United States, favor a middle course, as was selected here, by administering tamoxifen on the grounds that tamoxifen, like CMF, has been shown to have a beneficial effect in reducing recurrence in premenopausal patients, albeit to a somewhat lesser degree. Tamoxifen has the advantage of avoiding the morbidity of chemotherapy, which extends over a period of approximately 6 months, but has potential side effects of its own (2–4). Of the serious hazards ascribed to tamoxifen, endometrial carcinoma is the most threatening. Patients need to be clearly instructed in the potential side effects of the drug and, more particularly, in the importance of reporting, without delay, any vaginal bleeding. Many controversies remain. Should regular transvaginal ultrasonography be performed to assess endometrial thickness? (There are few if any data to support this approach.) Should endometrial biopsy by done annually? (This is not at present mandatory in the absence of symptoms.) What should the dose of tamoxifen be? (The administration of 20 mg b.i.d. as prescribed in this particular case seems excessive and may increase the hazard to the patient. 20 mg daily is as effective and is safer. Furthermore, the tradition of prescribing the tamoxifen into divided doses seems unnecessary, considering the half-life of the drug.) For how long should tamoxifen be given? (The optimal length remains disputed. Although many patients have received tamoxifen longer than 10 years and many from 5 to 10 years, there is a serious question as to whether extension beyond 5 years is beneficial because the complications from tamoxifen increase with the length of administration. In light of present knowledge, it would be hard to justify administering tamoxifen for longer than 5 years in this patient, and there are some who feel that 2 years is sufficient. Well-planned studies are underway and rational guidelines should be available within a few years.)

REFERENCES

1. Johnson H Jr, Masood S, Belluco C, et al, Prognostic factors in node-negative breast cancer. *Arch Surg* 1992;127:1386–91.
2. Cohen I, Rosen DJD, Shapira J, et al. Endometrial changes with tamoxifen: comparison between tamoxifen-treated and untreated asymptomatic, post-menopausal breast cancer patients. *Gynecol Oncol* 1994;52:185–90.
3. Fisher B, Costantino JP, Redmond CK, et al. Endometrial cancer in tamoxifen-treated breast cancer patients: findings from the National Surgical Adjuvant Breast and Bowel Project (NSABP) B-14. *J Natl Cancer Inst* 1994;86:527–37.
4. van Leeuwen FE, Benraadt J, Coebergh JWW, et al. Risk of endometrial cancer after tamoxifen treatment of breast cancer. *Lancet* 1994; 343:448–52.

EDITORIAL BOARD COMMENTARY

It is now widely accepted that adjuvant tamoxifen administered beyond 5 years offers no advantage.

78

A Postmenopausal, ER-Negative Woman with T1cN1M0 Infiltrating Ductal Carcinoma of the Breast

Homer H. Russ

Is adjuvant chemotherapy really indicated in a postmenopausal woman?

CASE PRESENTATION

Moderator: *Homer H. Russ (Radiation Oncologist)*
Our first case, to be presented by Dr. Mercier, may seem straightforward on the surface, but it does illustrate well, I think, some of the difficult choices our patients may be required to make.

Dr. Richart J. Mercier (Medical Oncologist): B.D. is a 67-year-old retired secretary from Northern Wisconsin, 100 miles away, who self-referred herself for management of a right breast carcinoma. She had seen her primary healthcare physician several times because of her concern about abnormalities she thought she detected in her breast. Mammography one year earlier had been called normal, but a change was found on a current study, which lead to an excisional biopsy in the upper central part of her right breast.

At age 53, she had undergone total abdominal hysterectomy with removal of the tubes and ovaries for benign disease. For about one year after that, she took replacement hormones. There was no family history of breast or any other cancer. She was known to have a large multinodular goiter but was not on any thyroid hormone therapy. She quit smoking cigarettes 10 years ago and drinks a little wine occasionally and a couple of cups of coffee daily.

Other than the easily palpable goiter and the ecchymotic biopsy site on the right breast, there were no significant abnormalities found on physical examination.

We asked Dr. Hoehn to see her.

Dr. James L. Hoehn (Surgical Oncologist): Radiology's review of the outside mammogram described an area of increased density with stellate edges and slight skin thickening, located immediately beneath the surface of the skin in the upper portion of the right breast with radiographic characteristics very suggestive of malignant disease (Fig. 78–1).

The tissue removed at home consisted of a 4-cm piece of yellow lobulated fat and white rubbery mammary tissue containing a poorly circumscribed hard gritty area approximately 1.5 cm in greatest dimension. A portion of that was submitted for estrogen and progesterone receptor levels. Permanent sections confirmed the frozen-section diagnosis of infiltrating ductal carcinoma, intermediate nuclear grade, but no vascular invasion was noted. There was a moderate lymphocytic reaction to the tumor, and considerable epithelial proliferation was seen, some representing intraductal carcinoma, some probably atypical epithelial hyperplasia, some cancerization of lobules, and some lobular hyperplasia as well. The slides were reviewed by the Pathology Department here, and those observations were confirmed.

We discussed the situation in depth with the patient, and she also spent considerable time talking with the oncology nurse clinician. The alternatives of conservation surgery, mastectomy, and reconstruction were out-

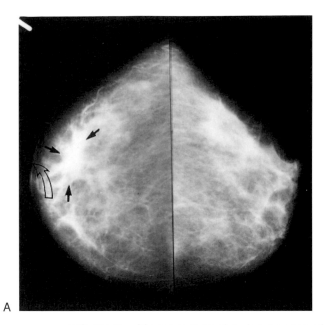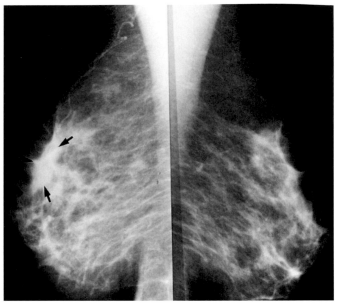

A B

FIG. 78–1. Mammograms showing an area of increased density with stellate edges (closed arrows) and slight skin thickening (open curved area) suggestive of malignant disease. **A:** Cephalocaudad projection; **B:** Mediolateral oblique projection.

lined to her. She indicated that she was interested in the mastectomy approach without immediate reconstruction.

A bone scan showed increased uptake in one rib. She remembered some trauma there, and plain films did show what was interpreted to be a healing fracture with no sign of malignancy.

Dr. Mercier: The various options for management of her breast cancer were presented to the patient several times. I discussed with her possible participation in the Eastern Cooperative Oncology Group study 4188 comparing FAC versus FAC plus tamoxifen versus tamoxifen alone. I indicated that I thought she would be an excellent candidate for this study and should strongly consider participating. At that time, hormone receptor status was still pending.

Dr. Hoehn: We went through the multiple options again, as I was a little concerned about her rapidity in making a decision. She was also seen again by the Oncology Nurse. She opted for mastectomy and lymph node removal only and did not wish reconstruction at the same time but seemed relieved that it was possible at some later date. The risks of arm swelling and numbness, blood transfusion reaction, hepatitis, AIDS, and other risks of exposure to blood products were discussed. I believed that she was well informed, and we scheduled her for operation the next morning.

A right modified radical mastectomy was the surgical procedure that was done. We chose a standard horizontally oriented approach, elevating flaps circumferentially ellipsing the nipple, areola, and biopsy site. In addition to removing the breast, we completely dissected the axilla, preserving the major vessels and nerves. The lateral bor-

der of dissection was the latissimus dorsi muscle. Blood loss was estimated at about 300 cc, and none was replaced. The apex of the axillary dissection was labeled with a long suture, the 12 o'clock radian of the skin ellipse was labeled with a clip, and the pathologist was asked to submit tumor from both the primary site and nodal sites if present for hormone receptors.

Dr. Mercier: About one week later, we saw the patient postoperatively. She was doing well without immediate complications. The pathology report indicated no evidence of residual tumor in the breast, but one of the 14 lymph nodes removed was affected by tumor. The studies done for hormone receptors, both on the primary tumor removed at home and on the lymph node found involved here were negative for hormone receptors, making her ineligible for randomization on the ECOG study we had discussed. She did agree to our idea of receiving adjuvant chemotherapy in the form of FAC as it would have been given on the study. Her EKG was normal, and there was no history or evidence of any heart disease. We scheduled her to be seen in the outpatient chemotherapy clinic the following week.

Kathy Tarcon: I gave the patient the booklet "Chemotherapy and You," to read. We discussed potential side effects, such as alopecia, mucositis, hemorrhagic cystitis, diarrhea, low blood counts, and so on. She was instructed to drink two quarts of water per day for three days, and have blood counts done at home in 10 days. A 23-gauge butterfly needle was inserted into a small left wrist vein and 10 mg of dexamethasone given over 10 minutes. She took 10 mg of Torecan and 50 mg of Benadryl by mouth. She was chewing ice chips for oral hypotherapy as we started giving 72 mg of Adriamycin intravenously. A combination of 725 mg of 5-FU and 725 mg of Cytoxan with 250 cc of normal saline solution was infused. Then, the butterfly needle was removed.

Dr. Mercier: The adjuvant chemotherapy went fairly well overall, but after the third cycle, there was significant nausea and vomiting, requiring a brief hospitalization at home for intravenous hydration and antiemetics. Subsequently, we added Ativan and a scopolamine patch to the antiemetics she had been getting. Also, because of moderate leukopenias, we found that we had to increase the interval between cycles from three weeks to four. The lowest white cell count was 1,300, and the lowest platelet count was 186,000, coming after the last cycle. Altogether, she received 300 mg/m^2 of the Adriamycin.

A chest roentgenography done at the time of her last cycle showed a patchy infiltrate in the right middle lobe that was new and did not appear to be metastatic disease. She was not symptomatic from this, but we did empirically put her on Ciprofloxacin, 500 mg twice a day for 10 days. One month later, her chest roentgenogram showed normal findings.

Dr. Hoehn: Dr. Mercier and I have seen the patient periodically since the completion of her adjuvant chemotherapy. The pectoral area is free of local or regional recurrence, and the axillae and supraclavicular areas are normal. As scheduled, she had a mammogram of her remaining breast at home. All roentgenograms and tests have remained normal. She did agree to be fitted with a breast prosthesis, which she does use. She seems happy and content with the way things have gone.

Dr. Mercier: Our plan is to see her at six-month interval for five years. Thereafter, we may continue to see her on an annual basis, while she sees her primary healthcare physicians at home for continuing surveillance of other health care needs.

Dr. Russ: Next summer will mark five years of disease-free follow-up for this patient. The results seem to speak for themselves. Do you think if she had lived closer to a major center she might have been interested in an alternative approach such as partial mastectomy followed by breast radiation?

Dr. Hoehn: Who can say? Certainly, we have seen more and more women of all ages showing interest in breast preservation, as attested to by the large numbers we have been able to enter into the NSABP studies. At the time this woman first came to us, there was no radiation facility in her community. It would have been a hard thing for her to do. Now, for the last year or so, there is a nice facility there that does provide this service, and a number of women who live in that area have chosen the approach of breast preservation surgery followed by radiation.

Dr. Russ: This woman had a number of hard choices to make. She chose to go with mastectomy and axillary dissection followed by adjuvant chemotherapy. She did not choose breast reconstruction or conservation surgery fol-

lowed by radiation. At this point, it appears that she has made good decisions and is happy with the way things are turning out.

COMMENTARY by Kirby I. Bland

This 67-year-old female patient was admitted with a T1c N1 M0 infiltrating carcinoma of intermediate grade and 1.5-cm transverse diameter. A right modified radical mastectomy was selected by the patient as the surgical procedure of choice, despite presentation of the alternative for conservation surgery and the necessity of postoperative irradiation. Of interest, the patient did not elect to have reconstructive surgery with myocutaneous flaps or with subpectoral saline implants. The latter choice is not surprising, due to her age.

In this circumstance, the surgeon selected the Patey axillary node dissection, in that all three levels were removed. The specimen was tagged as to the highest level of the nodes removed; no comment was made by the pathologist relative to the level of identification of the one of 14 nodes that was involved by tumor. Although this was an intermediate nuclear grade lesion without vascular invasion, tumor receptor analysis confirmed that the cancer was negative for hormone receptors (ER/PR receptors). The latter criteria made her ineligible for randomization on ECOG studies; thus, she was treated off-study with FAC adjuvant chemotherapy, following determination of her cardiac and pulmonary status.

The total duration of chemotherapy (in months) was not specifically stated; however, the patient received a total dose of 300 mg/m^2 of Adriamycin. Despite a recent interval in which there was concern about the possibility of metastatic disease, the chest roentgenogram cleared following antibiotic therapy; it was also evident that she did not have metastatic disease. The report does not document computed tomography on the chest to conclusively determine metastatic pulmonary disease or the planned interval for doing bone scans to determine if interval symptoms appeared, especially in light of her recent rib fracture. She has been followed up for five years and has been free of disease (NED) with regard to her physical exam, routine chest roentgenography, and liver function tests and has remained asymptomatic.

One would be remiss not to point out that a strong decision on the part of the medical oncologist and the surgeon to offer total mastectomy to this patient has to do with the modalities necessary to complete conservation surgery. The necessity for use of radiation to the intact breast after segmental mastectomy obviated this therapeutic approach, as this patient lived a considerable distance from a radiation therapy facility. I would agree that modified radical mastectomy is an appropriate approach if the patient is not desirous of breast preservation or, further, if logistic reasons dictate that this is not a proper choice. The decision to perform a complete axillary dissection (Level I–III, Patey dissection) is, in my view, not essential in this patient. No statistical differences have been confirmed in prospective studies that evaluate the Auchincloss-Madden axillary dissection (Levels I/II sampling) with modified radical mastectomy versus Patey axillary dissection (Levels I–III). Further, if one desires breast preservation, sampling of 10 nodes (minimum) is highly recommended for invasive tumors, especially since total breast irradiation, including portions of the axilla, is standard. However, should disease be palpated at Level II or Level III, it is advisable to complete the Patey dissection in these presentations to enhance local–regional control. Despite these considerations for conservative approaches, the patient has had an excellent result with both local–regional and, to this point, systemic control.

The decision by the medical oncologist to randomize her to ECOG studies was an excellent choice some five years ago. In addition, she has received a superior regimen for management of systemic disease in an adjuvant setting. The duration of therapy is not explicitly reported in this case, and the patient did not receive the maximum allowable dose of Adriamycin (450 mg/m^2). Therapy beyond six months is not essential; this has now been confirmed in European and North American studies. I would also agree that interval follow-up, as described by Dr. Mercier, at six-month interval for five years, and then on an annual basis thereafter, is proper. Preferentially, the operating surgeon and the medical oncologist should have input as to the findings at follow-up, but at least one physician knowledgeable in the biology of breast disease should be responsible for her care. Communication should also exist between the surgeon and the oncologist relative to subsequent findings in follow-up.

The question will arise as to the importance of tamoxifen in the adjuvant setting for an individual who is estrogen-receptor and progesterone-receptor negative. Unequivocally, tamoxifen has a major role in the ER-positive setting, but its role is less clear in the circumstance presented in this 67-year-old patient. Many medical oncologists encourage the use of this antiestrogen steroid in the ER-negative patient, because breast cancer is a heterogeneous neoplasm that is a mixture of both ER-positive and ER-negative cells, and the salutary benefit in both positive and negative tumors is evolving. In contrast, should there be any evidence of potential side effects that may discourage its use (e.g., thrombosis, venous stasis), withholding tamoxifen therapy would be considered the proper decision.

Finally, this patient with this stage IIA carcinoma of the breast by AJCC-TNM staging has an excellent prognosis, as manifested by her NED status at five years. Relapse of an additional 15% to 20% of this population of patients would be expected in the next five years, thus mandating the essentials of annual follow-up and restaging. Symptoms of pulmonary or osseous disease should be promptly evaluated using chest roentgenography, computed tomography of the chest, and bone scan imaging. In addition, routine CBC and hepatic function tests are indicated. Unfortunately, sensitive biomarkers indicative of early recurrence of breast cancer are not available in this patient population.

EDITORIAL BOARD COMMENTARY

Most individual trials have failed to demonstrate a beneficial effect from polychemotherapy for node-positive breast cancer in postmenopausal patients. The first choice of therapy in this patient group is tamoxifen if hormone receptor values are positive; however, in this case they were negative. If one accepts the validity of meta-analysis, a small reduction in mortality was demonstrated in patients receiving polychemotherapy. NSABP B-16 demonstrated a significant reduction in recurrence mortality with the use of doxorubicin and cyclophosphamide. In addition to tamoxifen, age, per se, should not represent a contraindication to systemic cytotoxic chemotherapy.

79

Postmenopausal Stage IIA Breast Cancer with Extracapsular Nodal Invasion and Positive Hormone Receptors

Richard G. Caldwell

Should postoperative radiation therapy in this breast-conserved patient be confined to the breast or include the axillary and supraclavicular area?

CASE PRESENTATION

Dr. Caldwell: This is a case of a 65-year-old white diabetic, hypertensive woman, who presented with a mass in the upper aspect of her right breast. A recent mammogram confirmed the presence of this lesion. The patient's significant history revealed that her menarche was at the age of 14, first child at 20, no nipple discharge or trauma, and her menopause was uncomplicated at age 45.

Examination of the right breast revealed a 1.5-cm mass in the upper outer quadrant that was firm with irregular edges. No other palpable abnormalities were found in either breast, and the axilla was negative for adenopathy.

Dr. Michael Siegfried: The mammograms (both mediolateral and craniocaudad views) reveal an irregular mass in the upper outer aspect of the right breast with stranding of tissue away from the mass. There are no calcifications in the immediate vicinity of the mass. I would conclude that this is a spiculated mass, highly suspicious for cancer (Figs. 79–1, 79–2, and 79–3).

Biopsy followed on an outpatient basis under local anesthesia with sedation.

Dr. Henry Carson: Within the tissue received, there was a 1.5-cm grayish–tan firm mass with an infiltrating margin. Microscopically, this revealed an infiltrating ductal carcinoma with dense desmoplastic reaction. The tumor cells formed tubules and nests of cells. This tumor was classified as a moderately well-differentiated adenocarcinoma, according to the Bloom-Richardson Grading System. On further review of the specimen, frank intraductal carcinoma (DCIS) as well as atypical ductal hyperplasia were noted. The DCIS is of the cribriform type and was found in the tumor mass. The components represented approximately 5% of the bulk tumor. Lymphatics were not involved (Figs. 79–4, 79–5, and 79–6).

Estrogen and progesterone receptors were strongly positive by the cytosol method. Flow cytometry revealed one tetraploid peak and an S phase of 5%. The later finding suggests a moderately poor prognosis.

Dr. Caldwell: Knowing the history and the pathologic findings, our next concern is the recommendations for the appropriate surgical treatment. It will be remembered that there are no significant calcifications seen on the mammogram, and the margins of the specimen were clear of tumor.

Dr. Bruce Stoehr: With the given history and the tumor parameters described by pathologic study, I think this patient is either a candidate for modified radical mastectomy or breast conservation followed by irradiation. The

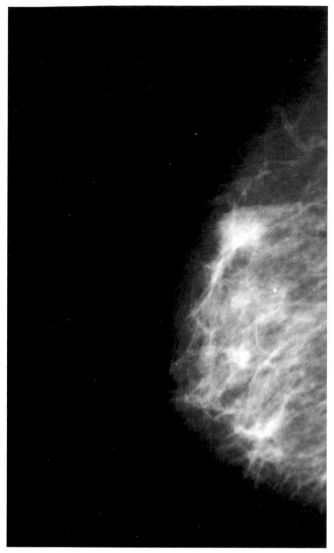

FIG. 79–1. Mammogram of the right breast in the mediolateral projection. There is a spiculated density in the upper outer quadrant.

main criteria that I would look at in terms of recommending therapy would first be the size of the tumor. This tumor was less than 2 cm. The second concern would be that of the DCIS, which represented 5% of the bulk tumor. I think that the risk of recurrence, if breast-conserving therapy is chosen, is in the neighborhood of 3% to 5%. It should be remembered, however, that if recurrence does take place, there is approximately a 40% chance that the recurrence will be in the form of infiltrating ductal carcinoma.

Because the chance of recurrence is low and the tumor size is small, I would discuss both options with the patient and I could support either.

Dr. Caldwell: If after breast conservation there is local recurrence, what percentage of these woman will have systemic disease?

Dr. Leonard Kosova: The probability of recurrence after adequate excision and regional therapy was known before Fisher's NSABP BO6 study. At least 85% of these patients will have demonstrable systemic disease or will have occult disease that becomes clinically manifest within a two-year period.

Dr. Jacob Bitran: I believe that we need to clarify local recurrence. I believe that patients treated with modified radical mastectomy and who develop local recurrence (as described by Dr. Kosova) are a subgroup, which after treatment with the radiation, chest wall resection, and/or chemotherapy, have a 10% to 15% chance of being disease free after 5 years.

On the other hand, in the NSABP BO6 studies, patients who received lumpectomy and axillary resection had a 23% recurrence rate. These patients, after salvage modified radical mastectomy, showed no difference in their survival curves when compared to the initial group.

Dr. Christopher Rose: Salvage rate for those patients whose disease do recur certainly is good; but, 50% of these patients will still have infiltrating disease. Local recurrence certainly is higher in tumors with a DCIS component when compared to infiltrating tumors alone. This patient's DCIS component was 5% of the bulk tumor.

Dr. Caldwell: Dr. Peckler, after hearing the details of this patient's presentation, what would be your surgical recommendations for treatment?

Dr. Scott Peckler: Because the DCIS component is 5% and the surgical margins of the excised specimen were free of additional tumor, I would do only an axillary dissection, to be followed by irradiation therapy.

Dr. Caldwell: Dr. Carson, would you describe the findings on the tissue removed from the breast as well as the axilla?

Dr. Henry Carson: Tissue removed from the breast revealed only ductal hyperplasia. Two of ten lymph nodes removed from the axilla revealed metastatic carcinoma in the lymphoid follicles. One of these metastatic nodes had capsular invasion with perinodal infiltration.

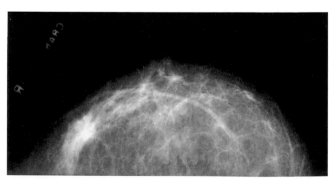

FIG. 79–2. Cephalocaudad projection of the right breast showing the mass in the periphery of the outer quadrant.

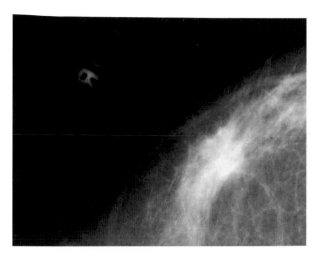

FIG. 79–3. Magnified cephalocaudad view demonstrating the details of the stellate lesion. The borders are not sharply defined with strands of tissue leading into the surrounding parenchyma. No significant calcium deposits are present. The findings are suggestive of a malignant lesion.

Dr. Caldwell: Dr. Rose, as treating medical oncologist, would you please describe your choice of adjuvant therapy?

Dr. Christopher Rose: Because this patient is 65 years of age, postmenopausal for many years, strongly positive for ER and PR receptors with a flow cytometry which is equivocal in terms of prognosis, I feel quite comfortable in treating this patient with hormonal manipulation.

Dr. Caldwell: Is extra nodal disease a marker for recurrence?

Dr. Rose: Yes.

Dr. Caldwell: Dr. Klein, would you please comment on the use of chemotherapy in this patient?

Dr. Leonard Klein: With the use of adjuvant chemotherapy, one tries to access the risk of recurrent disease. The interpretation of reports that study the use of chemotherapy in the postmenopausal patient has spawned controversy. It is clear, however, that adjuvant hormonal therapy has a clear benefit in the strongly positive ER patient. The question remains: How much benefit do the patients get, and can it be improved with the addition of chemotherapy? A number of studies indicate that patients with positive nodes or negative ER receptors may, in fact, have improved outcomes.

Dr. Kosova: I think I would try to separate a few of the issues. If this woman is predominantly ER-PR receptor negative, I think that this patient should be considered for adjuvant chemotherapy. Other factors, such as the patient's physiologic age and comorbidity, must be included in that decision, however. Because this patient is ER-PR receptor positive, tamoxifen is the first line of treatment. The addition of chemotherapy to this regimen may be beneficial, but the interpretation of the literature is unclear.

Dr. Bitran: First, let me consider recurrence. If indeed this patient was not treated with adjuvant therapy, there is a greater than 67% chance that she would recur within 10 years with two nodes positive. In addition, there has never been a study that showed a beneficial effect with chemotherapy alone in the postmenopausal woman without the use of Adriamycin-based therapy; this is to include the CMFVP trial that was SWOG-based.

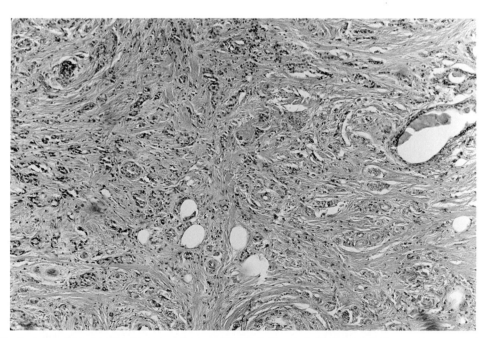

FIG. 79–4. Infiltrating ductal adenocarcinoma of breast. Tumor cells form tubules and nests, or infiltrate individually. Note marked desmoplastic reaction (H & E, original magnification × 100).

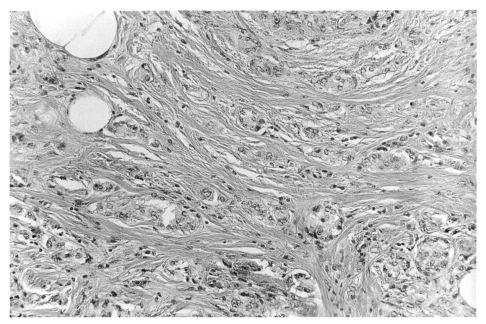

FIG. 79–5. Detail of Figure 4. Note high nuclear-to-cytoplasmic ratio, irregular nuclear membranes, prominent nucleoli, and occasional binucleation. Also note paucity of mitotic figures (overall, fewer than ten per ten high-power fields) (H & E, original magnification × 100).

If we used tamoxifen alone in the postmenopausal woman with high levels of estrogen and progesterone receptors, there is a benefit because there is a reduction in the rate of recurrence by approximately 20% in a 10-year period, reducing the recurrence level from 67% to 55%.

This benefit was also demonstrated with a regimen of Adriamycin-based chemotherapy and tamoxifen. Benefit was seen in the first 5 years of the trial, but not seen at 10 years, by virtue of the fact that these women died of comorbid disease.

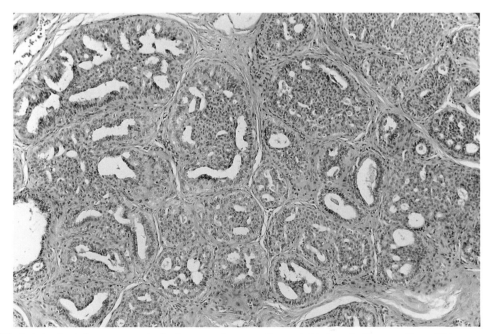

FIG. 79–6. Intraductal component of adenocarcinoma of breast. Note cribriform pattern. This component was within the main tumor, and accounted for less than 5% of the mass (H & E, original magnification × 100).

In this patient, if she was otherwise healthy, I would give an Adriamycin-based regime with tamoxifen. Because we are talking about an unhealthy obese patient with comorbid disease, I feel that the best treatment is tamoxifen.

Dr. Caldwell: Dr. Moran, in addition to adjuvant therapy, irradiation to the involved breast to control recurrent disease is necessary. Would you please comment on the irradiation given to this patient?

Dr. Moran: Postsurgically, this patient was given irradiation to the involved breast, the axilla, and supraclavicular region. Most authorities believe that the axilla should be irradiated if there are greater than four nodes positive or there is capsular penetration with perinodal involvement. However, Jay Harris has published a series of 1,000 patients where the supraclavicular region was treated if positive nodes were found in the axilla. With irradiation and chemotherapy, they found that there was a higher incidence of brachioplexopathy. At present, we are not irradiating the supraclavicular region for there is a 1% risk of recurrence and 6% chance of developing neuropathy. This complication may well be enhanced by the fact that this patient has insulin-dependent diabetes.

Dr. Rose: In this patient's case, the decision as related to adjuvant therapy was an easy one. The patient presented with comorbid disease, was 65-years old, and was strongly positive ER-PR receptors. Tamoxifen was therefore the choice.

Dr. Kosova: I cannot support using an Adriamycin-based regimen, because this would increase this patient's rate of survival by only approximately 5%. This 5% improvement of survival rate would be countered by at least a 5% chance of developing Adriamycin cardiomyopathy.

Dr. Bitran: Reviewing the figures, one starts out with a 67% chance of recurrence within 10 years. This could be reduced by using a regimen of tamoxifen and Adriamycin. It should be noted that there is a 20% improvement in survival at 10 years with tamoxifen, and a 5% increase in survival with Adriamycin. It is, therefore, obvious that the additional 5% use of Adriamycin is not indicated.

Dr. Klein: It should be remembered that any improvement in survival rate will be important to that patient. Decisions for therapy cannot be made unilaterally, but must be made with the understanding and knowledge of the patient.

COMMENTARY by William Wood

The choice of local therapy is discussed with the comment that any local recurrence has "a 40% chance that [it] . . . will be in the form of infiltrating ductal carcinoma." Extensive intraductal carcinoma is defined as DCIS in more than 25% of the primary tumor and in the surrounding ducts. That finding has been shown by Recht et al. (1) to identify a group of patients prone to more diffuse presentations of the primary tumor, and it has been further delineated by Holland et al. (2). Such patients exhibit local failure roughly equally divided between invasive and in situ disease. With only 5% DCIS, this patient does not have extensive intraductal component; any recurrence would be almost certainly infiltrating ductal carcinoma, either residual, or in later years, a new primary. The issue of systemic disease in women who fail locally after either mastectomy or breast-conservation therapy can be confusing. After mastectomy, nearly all local failures represent aggressive, disseminated disease, and about 85% to 90% will demonstrate systemic disease shortly after the local failure, as stated in the discussion. After breast-conservation therapy, these same women will fail locally; but, in addition, there will be new primary breast cancers arising in the conserved breast and areas of uncontrolled local disease in the breast becoming manifest. Neither of these can occur following mastectomy, and either can provide a focus for secondary metastasis and increased risk. Although it seems likely that this could occur, the finding of no significant difference in survival between mastectomy and breast-conservation therapy in the six randomized trials in the literature shows that any such occurrence is too rare to significantly affect survival.

Adjuvant tamoxifen therapy for a 65-year-old woman with two involved lymph nodes and strongly positive expression of ER and PR is the right choice. Two years is superior to shorter periods in the overview analysis by Peto, and cooperative group studies suggest but do not establish that 5 years may be better still. For a woman with one to three involved lymph nodes, the percent treatment failure at 10 years is 47% without adjuvant therapy (3), a little better than suggested in the discussion. It is this failure rate that is reduced by 29% in annual odds of events by tamoxifen in women 60 to 69 years of age (4). Nothing else produces benefit of this magnitude in this group of women. It is clear that there is an additional increment of survival benefit from the addition of combination chemotherapy to tamoxifen in postmenopausal women as gleaned from meta-analysis. Such incremental benefit is small and needs to be weighed against its cost to the patient in toxicity and inconvenience. With comorbid conditions described in this patient, I would not disagree with the discussants in not advocating its addition to tamoxifen alone.

Radiation is clearly indicated to control local, subclinical disease. At a minimum, this must encompass the entire breast. Whether a boost is of additional benefit in control has not been clarified in terms of the extent of the surgical margin achieved, the size of the primary, grade of the primary, and possible use of adjuvant chemotherapy. Until this is fully clarified, a boost is sometimes added if the margin is close. In this case, the margins of the excision were not stated but the re-excision ("segmental mastectomy" or "lumpectomy") contained no identifiable tumor, and I would not opt for a boost. The irradiation of the regional nodal areas is also controversial. Some make a case for axillary irradiation when a certain number of lymph nodes are involved—many if ten nodes are involved, some if only four nodes are involved. This patient had extracapsular extension of the nodal metastasis, and that is a widely accepted indication for irradiation of the axilla to reduce axillary failure. The virtue of supraclavicular irradiation is lost on me as the morbidity seems to render the slight putative benefit moot. I agree with the discussion provided on this point.

Were the patient an otherwise healthy 65-year-old woman, I would think it important to discuss the potential small but real benefit of adding combination chemotherapy (e.g., Adriamycin-cytoxan) versus the cost in alopecia, morbid symptoms, and the small risk of cardiomyopathy or profound marrow suppression. If I were she, I suspect I would still opt for tamoxifen alone.

REFERENCES

1. Recht A, Connolly JC, Schnitt SJ, et al. The effect of young age on tumor recurrence in the treated breast after conservative surgery and radiotherapy. *Int J Radiat Oncol Biol Phys* 1988;14:3–10.
2. Holland R, Connolly J, Gelman R, et al. The presence of an extensive intraductal component following a limited excision correlates with prominent residual disease in the remainder of the breast. *J Clin Oncol* 1990;3:113–118.
3. Fisher ER. Prognostic and therapeutic significance of pathological features of breast cancer. *NCI Monograph* 1986;1:29–34.
4. Early Breast Cancer Trialists' Collaborative Group: Systemic treatment of early breast cancer by hormonal, cytotoxic, or immune therapy. *Lancet* 1992;339:1–14,71–85.

EDITORIAL BOARD COMMENTARY

There is clear-cut evidence that radiation therapy for a case such as this is essential for local control in the patient undergoing breast-conserving surgery. Studies have demonstrated in mastectomy patients that chest wall and axillary radiation are beneficial to patients with extracapsular nodal disease. In the patient with a conserved breast, radiation therapy to the breast encompasses the chest wall and is extended to the axilla in cases of capsular penetration of nodes. It is difficult to justify supraclavicular radiation in this patient.

80

Adjuvant Systemic Chemotherapy and Hormonal Therapy for Postmenopausal, ER-Negative, Stage IIB Breast Cancer

Douglas E. Merkel

Tamoxifen alone for ER-negative, node-positive,
postmenopausal women?

CASE PRESENTATION

H.P. is a 67-year-old woman with a remote history of a left breast carcinoma who discovered a lump in her right breast. She was not in the habit of breast self-examination, and her last normal mammogram was in 1991. At presentation, a 2-cm hard, freely moveable mass was noted in the upper outer quadrant of the right breast. Mammography revealed a new irregular mass in the upper outer quadrant containing a few punctate microcalcifications. Aspiration cytology was consistent with adenocarcinoma, possibly colloid carcinoma, and she underwent modified radical mastectomy.

The specimen weighted 296 grams and consisted of a breast with intact pre-pectoral fascia, overlying skin, and level I, II, and III lymph nodes. Sectioning revealed dense, sclerotic, tan-white breast parenchyma dissecting amongst lobulated, yellow adipose tissue. A $2.0 \times 2.0 \times 1.5$-cm firm mass was noted; and after frozen section demonstrated infiltrating ductal carcinoma, a portion of this mass was reserved for flow cytometry and immunocytochemical receptor assays. On microscopic examination, this carcinoma exhibited a biphasic histology. One pattern consisted of conventional high-grade invasive ductal carcinoma with cords and nests of pleomorphic ductal cells infiltrating a desmoplastic stroma (Fig. 80–1). Nuclei were large and vesicular with dispersed chromatin and prominent nucleoli. This pattern was juxtaposed to and merged imperceptibly with a pattern composed of lobular aggregates of malignant cells dispersed in a chondromyxoid matrix suggestive of cartilagenous differentiation (Fig. 80–2). Invasion of lymphatic vascular spaces was noted, and 3 of 20 axillary lymph nodes contained metastases.

Neither estrogen receptor nor progesterone receptor proteins could be detected immunocytochemically. Flow cytometric DNA analysis demonstrated aneuploidy with a DNA index of 1.60 (Fig. 80–3). The S-phase fraction of the aneuploid component was elevated at 20.1%.

Risk profile included a previous carcinoma of the left breast 23 years ago, which reportedly did not involve any axillary lymph nodes. This was treated by radical mastectomy and adjuvant Cobalt therapy to the left chest wall. There has not been any recurrence. Family history is negative for breast cancer. She does not recall the age of menarche, but underwent menopause at the time of a hysterectomy in her forties. There was no exposure to exogenous estrogens. She completed the first of two full-term pregnancies at 23 years of age. Past medical history includes an episode of pancreatitis, complicated by pneumonia several years ago. She has a long-standing seizure disorder that is well-controlled by phenytoin, and hypothyroidism treated with synthroid. She smokes >1/2 a pack of cigarettes daily and has done so for 50 years. Currently, she enjoys a couple of beers each day.

On physical examination, this is an older-appearing woman in no acute distress. There are no palpable cervi-

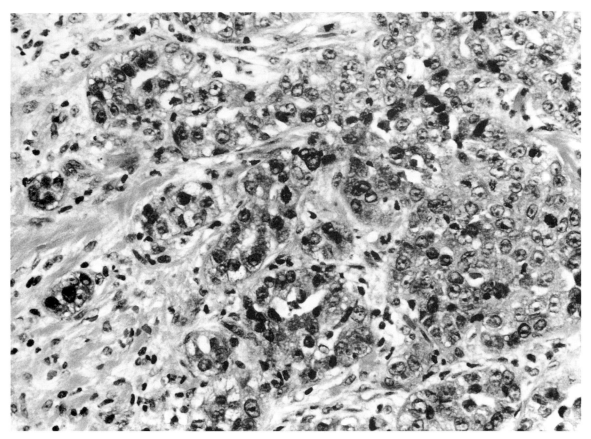

FIG. 80–1. A microscopic field demonstrating infiltrating ductal carcinoma, NOS, with grade 3 nuclear and architectural features.

cal, supraclavicular, or left axillary lymph nodes. The teeth are in reasonable repair. The lungs are clear to percussion and auscultation. The spine was nontender. The right mastectomy scar is healing nicely. The left mastectomy scar is free of nodularity. There is no edema present in either arm. On cardiac exam, there is an S1, S2, a midsystolic murmur along the left sternal border, and occasional premature beats. No gallup is audible. The liver edge is not palpable, and there are no abdominal masses, or evidence of ascites. Ankles are free of edema.

TUMOR BOARD DISCUSSION

To summarize, this was a 67-year-old woman with a metaplastic T1c carcinoma involving three axillary lymph nodes. Although the presence of three involved lymph nodes suggests approximately a 45% risk for recurrence over the next 5 years, the adverse biologic features of this tumor-negative receptor assays, elevated S-phase fraction, and perhaps metaplasia suggest that her actual risk is somewhat higher. Thus, systemic adjuvant therapy was clearly indicated. The choice of adjuvant therapy becomes somewhat problematic, however.

Although neither estrogen nor progesterone receptor proteins could be detected and would not be expected in a high-grade metaplastic carcinoma, tamoxifen might still provide some benefit to this 67-year-old woman. The overview analysis demonstrated a 16% reduction in recurrence and mortality rates among postmenopausal, estrogen-receptor negative women who were randomized to receive tamoxifen. Certainly, some of this observed effect could have been due to the misclassification of women with false negative estrogen receptor assays in older studies lacking adequate laboratory standardization or quality control measures. On the other hand, the improvement in prognosis seen for these patients could be a real effect, related to the recently observed decrease in circulating levels of insulinlike growth factor produced by tamoxifen in postmenopausal women.

Considering only those women aged 60 to 69, the overview analysis was able to demonstrate a 20% relative reduction in risk of recurrence and a 10% reduction in mortality rates for those patients randomized to polychemotherapy. Relatively few individual trials have demonstrated a reduction in recurrence or mortality rates associated with the use of adjuvant cytotoxic chemotherapy for postmenopausal, node-positive women. CMF (cyclophosphamide, methotrexate, fluorouracil)-based programs, in particular, seem not to reduce recurrence rates beyond that reduction already achieved with tamox-

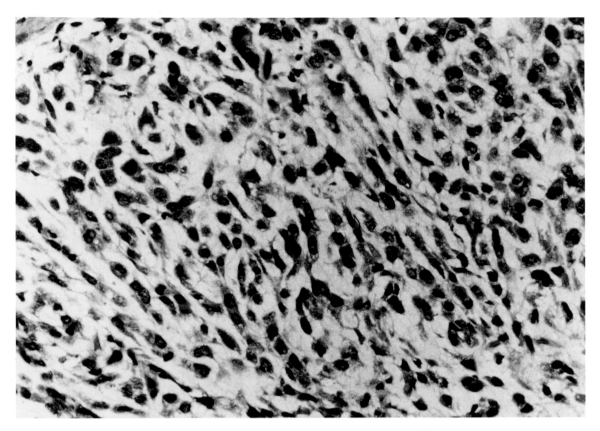

FIG. 80–2. A microscopic field showing chrondomyxoid differentiation.

ifen. Perhaps, the most promising phase III data comes from the NSABP B-16 trial, which enrolled 1,267 postmenopausal, node-positive patients. At 5 years, a highly significant reduction in recurrence and mortality rates were achieved by the addition of doxorubicin and cyclophosphamide to tamoxifen.

On this basis, a combination of doxorubicin and cyclophosphamide, administered every 3 weeks for four cycles, together with oral tamoxifen for 5 years was recommended to this patient. A particular concern with this patient was the potential for cardiac toxicity. Although this complication was reported for only 1% of the patients on the B-16 trial, this patient has risk factors for pre-existing cardiac damage: a long smoking history, prior radiotherapy to the left chest wall, and ongoing over-consumption of alcohol. Work done at our institution using a murine model of doxorubicin-induced cardiomyopathy has demonstrated synergistic toxicity with simultaneous exposure to ethanol (G.Y. Locker, personal communication). Before initiation of chemotherapy, a MUGA scan was obtained and showed normal left ventricular wall motion and an ejection fraction of 67%.

The last concern before treatment related to secure vascular access in a patient with bilateral axillary node dissection. As the chemotherapy program would be completed in 64 days, temporary placement of a Groshon catheter was recommended.

The patient underwent the recommended program of adjuvant therapy with generally good tolerance. Alopecia was complete, as expected, and grade 2 stomatitis was also encountered. There were no infectious complications, nor any symptoms suggestive of congestive heart failure. She will be followed up by physical examination, chemistry profile, and blood counts every 3 months for the first 3 years after diagnosis, and every 4 months thereafter. Chest radiography and bone scanning will be followed up on a yearly basis.

COMMENTARY by Paul P. Carbone

The patient described is a 67-year-old woman who presented with a T1 N1 M0 ER negative cancer, 23 years after a breast cancer in the opposite breast was treated with a mastectomy and postoperative radiation. In the pathologic assessment, three lymph nodes were involved. The tumor was said to have an undifferentiated component with an increased aneuploid segment and a high S phase. The patient has been a long-term smoker and consumed alcohol regularly. She was treated with Adriamycin and Cytoxan for four cycles and tamoxifen for five years.

Several aspects of this patient's history need comment. The first of these relates to the value of cytometry flow

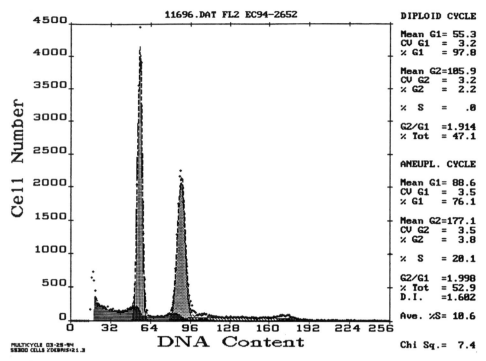

FIG. 80–3. The DNA histogram, revealing aneuploidy with a DNA index of 1.60. The S-phase fraction of the aneuploid component was elevated at 20.1, suggesting a worsening prognosis.

measurements such as S phase and aneuploidy. In this patient, we know that the tumor was high grade, three lymph nodes were involved, and that the tumor was ER negative. These would be compelling enough to suggest a poor prognosis and the need for chemotherapy. Measurement of the S phase in my opinion adds little information although presumably adding to the costs. The other piece of clinical information that influences outcome and therapy was size. In her case, size did not impact on the choice of therapy. In our environment, when concern for medical costs is high, are we justified in ordering tests that do not influence therapy? I do not think that even if the ploidy was normal and the S phase low that the treatment decision would be different. Based on most current approaches to management of patients with early breast cancer, the measurement of aneuploidy or S phase rarely impacts on therapy. The clinical situation where it might is when the tumor is small (<1.0 cm), the lymph nodes are found not to contain tumor cells and the ER is not obtainable. Even in that situation some centers do not treat the patient (1). Other parameters such as Her-2-neu and tumor necrosis although suggestive by some retrospective studies as descriminating in outcome have not been shown to be effected by therapy in well-designed prospective studies.

It is worthwhile to discuss briefly the option to undergo a mastectomy rather than elect a tumorectomy. We were not told whether the patient was informed about that option. In many states this is a requirement. The physical findings as described would have made this an appropriate alternative. Of interest, our studies in Wisconsin have indicated that older women are less likely to have referrals to oncologists and more likely to have all their treatment given in small hospitals (fewer than 100 beds) (2). Decision making needs to be informed and open. I like to make sure that the patient is seen by a radiation oncologist as well as a surgeon, preferably at the same clinic visit. In this patient, a needle-aspirate biopsy was done that indicated the diagnosis way before any major surgical procedure was done. A discussion of surgical options would have been appropriate.

Another aspect of the case that needs comment is the choice of chemotherapy or tamoxifen in a postmenopausal woman. Most individual studies using chemotherapy alone rarely show benefit in postmenopausal women. However, some individual trials do and the overview in 1992 showed a benefit. It is an option that women need to hear about. Dr. Merkel does point out that tamoxifen alone is also a reasonable choice. My policy has been to discuss the options with each woman with the pros and cons of each therapy. Many patients want to make the choice and they should not be made to feel uncomfortable if they decide to take tamoxifen alone rather than undergo chemotherapy. Others when told about the benefits of a combined approach elect to undergo both (3).

The next point I would like to discuss is the use of chemotherapy in the older patient. Many studies have shown that older patients defined as over 65 years are less likely to receive appropriate therapy when the effects of associated medical problems are factored out. The reasons for this are not clear but are given as fear of excessive toxicity, lack of effectiveness, and relative slower growing tumors in the elderly. Our own studies in ECOG have shown no such age effect in patients that are in relatively good physiologic condition (4). My axiom has been that physiologic age rather than chronologic age is the discriminating factor. Older people do have some increase in hematologic toxicity but this is confined to selective drugs that seem to require renal clearance or some biliary excretion. There was no evidence that most other toxicities are age-related. As a result, I manage most older patients with cancer that require chemotherapy with standard dosages of drugs, modifying some such as methotrexate and the vinca alkaloids. The fact that this patient had left chest wall radiation made the physicians appropriately sensitive to the potential synergy of adriamycin and radiation on the heart. Dr. Merkel also raises the issue of alcohol as a potential additive toxicity factor of drug therapy with the anthracyclines on the heart.

Finally, this patient was to be followed up with a battery of tests and routine visits. This practice is standard although evidence to support such routines as improving outcome is lacking. One however can avoid the routine measurements of tumor markers such as CEA as having impact on earlier disease detection or influencing therapeutic outcome. They clearly do not help.

REFERENCES

1. Fisher B, Gunduz N, Costantino J, et al. DNA flow cytometric analysis of primary operable breast cancer. Relation of ploidy and S-phase fraction to outcome of patients in NSABP B-04. *Cancer* 1991;68:1465–75.
2. Newcomb PA and Carbone PP. Cancer treatment and age: patient perspectives. *J Natl Cancer Inst* 1993;85(19):1580–4.
3. Early Breast Cancer Trialists Collaborative Group. Systemic treatment of early breast cancer by hormonal, cytotoxic, or immune therapy. *Lancet* 1992;339:1–85.
4. Begg CB and Carbone PP. Clinical trials and drug toxicity in the elderly: the experience of the Eastern Cooperative Oncology Group. *Cancer* 1983;52:1986–92.

EDITORIAL BOARD COMMENTARY

A small percentage of patients with postmenopausal node-positive ER-negative tumors will benefit from tamoxifen alone. The combination of Adriamycin-based polychemotherapy and tamoxifen increases benefits slightly; and in this patient with a high S phase fraction, a metaplastic tumor and three positive nodes, the option of Adriamycin-based chemotherapy and tamoxifen should be thoroughly discussed with the patient as it was in this case. Some oncologists would begin treatment with tamoxifen after the chemotherapy is given, based on animal studies suggesting that with concomitant use tamoxifen may interfere with the effectiveness of cytotoxic chemotherapies.

In follow-up, just as the CEA is of little value, bone scans are not necessary unless the patient has bone pain.

81

Locally Advanced Breast Cancer Requiring Neoadjuvant Chemotherapy

Monica Morrow and Wendy Recant

The importance for the surgeon to recognize unresectability
for N2 disease

CASE PRESENTATION

The patient is a 37-year-old gravida five, para five woman; age 19 at first birth; no prior history of breast disease; and a negative family history of breast carcinoma. The patient is premenopausal and takes no medications. She was in good health until 1 year prior to presentation when she first noted a left breast mass. The mass increased in size over the last 12 months, and finally caused the patient to seek medical attention. She denies weight loss, bone pain, increased fatigue, or other systemic symptoms.

On physical examination, fullness of the upper outer quadrant of the left breast was evident with the arms raised. There were no skin or nipple changes. Examination of the right breast, axilla, and supraclavicular areas was normal. In the left breast a hard, irregular 7 cm × 8 cm mass was present occupying the upper half of the breast. The mass was not fixed to the chest wall or the skin. A mass of matted, fixed nodes measuring 4 cm was palpable in the left axilla. There was no supraclavicular adenopathy. The tumor was clinically staged as T3N2, stage III, and the diagnosis of carcinoma was confirmed by aspiration cytology. Bilateral mammography confirmed the presence of a large left breast mass and dense axillary nodes consistent with metastatic disease (Fig. 81–1). No abnormalities were noted in the right breast. A metastatic workup consisting of screening chemistries, chest roentgenogram and bone scan was within normal limits.

This case was discussed at tumor board and felt to be unresectable on the basis of the matted axillary nodes.

There was agreement that this patient should be treated initially with chemotherapy in an effort to 1) shrink the primary tumor and the axillary nodes, rendering the local disease technically resectable and 2) to reduce the very high risk of distant relapse. It was elected to begin treatment with cyclophosphamide, doxorubicin and 5-fluorouracil (CAF) with a plan to deliver four cycles and then reevaluate the patient for resectability.

The patient tolerated chemotherapy well, with alopecia being the only significant treatment-related side effect. At reevaluation on day 28 of the fourth cycle of chemotherapy, complete resolution of the axillary mass was noted. A 2-cm area of firmness was present at 12 o'clock in the left breast, and the remainder of the left breast mass had resolved. A repeat mammogram was obtained that showed only some stellate architectural distortion at 12 o'clock and mild skin thickening (Fig. 81–2). A repeat metastatic workup was negative. The patient was believed to have had a clinical complete remission, and was re-presented to the tumor board for discussion of local therapy. Considerable debate ensued over whether this patient was now an appropriate candidate for lumpectomy, axillary dissection, and radiotherapy. It was noted that clinical response often correlates poorly with the amount of residual tumor in mastectomy specimens. In addition, it is unclear whether tumor regression is a uniform process or occurs in a spotty fashion, making the entire upper half of the breast at risk for viable residual tumor. However, because of the impressive clinical response, and the fact that local fail-

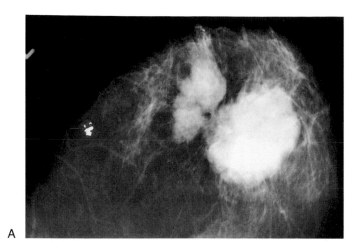

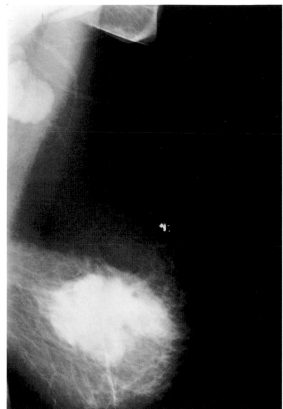

FIG. 81–1. A: Craniocaudal view of the left breast demonstrating the large, spiculated tumor mass. An incidental calcified fibroadenoma is seen in the lateral breast. **B**: Lateral mammogram demonstrating the primary tumor mass and enlarged, dense axillary lymph nodes highly suspicious for metastatic disease.

ure in the breast will have no impact on this patient's survival, it was decided to proceed with a lumpectomy of the palpable thickened area and axillary dissection. It was explained to the patient that if extensive viable residual tumor was found in the lumpectomy specimen, a mastectomy would be necessary.

The lumpectomy specimen measured 6.0 × 6.0 × 2.0 cm. No gross tumor was identifiable. Microscopic sections revealed marked stromal fibrosis (Fig. 81–3), non-proliferative fibrocystic disease and no evidence of residual tumor. Thirteen axillary nodes were identified, and none contained tumor. In three nodes, areas of fibrosis and low cellularity thought to represent areas of tumor regression were noted (Fig. 81–4). The patient's postoperative course was uncomplicated. She began radiotherapy 2 weeks postoperatively and received 4,600 Gy to the whole breast with a 1,400 Gy boost to the lumpectomy site. After the completion of radiotherapy, two additional cycles of CAF were administered. The patient remains free of disease 9 months after the completion of therapy.

COMMENTARY by Paul P. Carbone and Jordan Berlin

In evaluating the case presented, the major issues in the treatment of locally advanced breast cancer are reviewed.

The issues relate to the use of initial or neoadjuvant chemotherapy prior to local therapy and how this affects survival and disease control. Another controversy is utilizing breast-conserving surgery and radiation (XRT) for "local" therapy of locally advanced breast cancer.

Locally advanced breast cancer is encompassed in the current AJCC stage III (1). Stage III is divided into stage IIIA, defined as tumor greater than 5 cm, possibly adherent to underlying muscle or with ipsilateral matted or fixed axillary nodes; and stage IIIB which contains inflammatory breast cancer as well as tumor extending to the chest wall or involvement of ipsilateral periclavicular nodes.

Recently, clinicians have been approaching stage III breast cancers with a combined modality approach. Pilot studies reviewed by Dorr et al. favored improved prognosis for stage III patients treated with chemotherapy when compared with retrospective reviews of patients treated with local therapy only (2). In a retrospective study by the M.D. Anderson Cancer Center, Hortobagyi et al. evaluated combined modality therapy in stage III patients. Five-year survival rates were 84% for stage IIIA patients, and 35% for stage IIIB patients (3). This was in contrast to 5-year survival rates of 30% to 45% and 10% to 28% for stages IIIA and IIIB, respectively, cited from previous reports. In addition, Pierce et al. reported a prospective study of combined modality therapy in stage III breast cancer demonstrating that this strategy can produce excellent local–regional control rate (4). In his editorial based

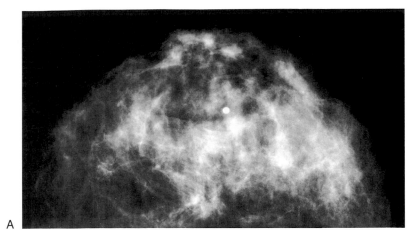

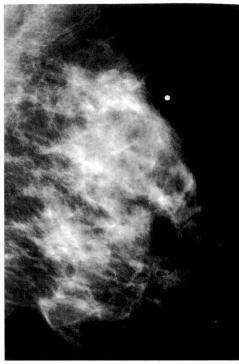

FIG. 81–2. **A**: Craniocaudal and **B**: lateral mammograms taken after four cycles of chemotherapy demonstrate resolution of the large breast mass and axillary nodes. The marker was placed on the area of residual firmness.

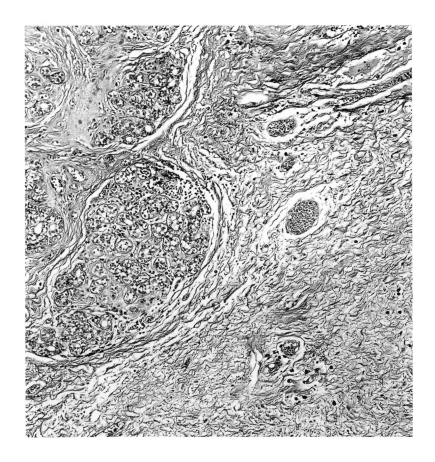

FIG. 81–3. High-power photomicrograph demonstrating residual breast tissue (top right) and hylanized scar. No tumor is seen.

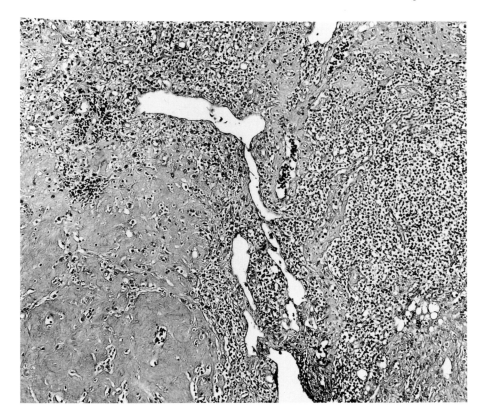

FIG. 81–4. High-.power photomicrograph of a lymph node demonstrating lymphoid tissue (right) and hylanized scar (left) at the site of apparent tumor regression.

on the aforementioned publication, Hortobagyi discusses that the study by Pierce et al., as well as other studies, demonstrate that neoadjuvant chemotherapy has a role in reducing inoperable malignancies to operable disease, as was the case for the patient presented here (5). Although data provide some evidence for a role of combined modality therapy in stage III breast cancer, randomized protocols are needed to provide definitive data.

Once this patient was found to have a remission (CR) following neoadjuvant chemotherapy, the next phase of her therapy was local control. Treatment options included surgery alone, XRT alone, or the two combined. In addition, surgical options included mastectomy or breast-conserving surgery.

The use of both surgery and XRT in stage III breast cancer has been studied. In a retrospective analysis by the M.D. Anderson Cancer Center, the combination of mastectomy and XRT resulted in an actuarial local–regional control rate of 82% at 10 years (6). Another retrospective analysis by Graham et al. demonstrated that their patients treated with mastectomy and XRT had significantly improved local–regional control rates when compared with those patients treated with XRT alone (7).

When evaluated in a randomized trial, chemotherapy and XRT resulted in similar local control rates compared with chemotherapy and surgery (8). Therefore, the efficacy issue of combining XRT and surgery compared with either therapy alone is still not settled.

The role of breast-conserving surgery in earlier stage (stages I and II) breast cancer has been established (9). However, far less is known with regards to locally advanced disease. The premise in this case that local failure does not affect survival appears to be a sound one. In treated stage III breast cancer, the majority of patients with recurring disease have distant metastases with or without local–regional recurrence (3,4,6,7). Bonadonna et al. have shown that neoadjuvant chemotherapy, indeed, does make it possible to perform breast-conserving surgery in patients with bulky disease (10). Again, further evaluation, preferably in randomized studies, may establish more firmly the role of breast-conserving surgery in patients with response to neo-adjuvant chemotherapy, such as in the case presented.

From the data presented, it can be concluded that the choice of combined modality treatment for this patient is supported by the literature and may improve her chances at long-term survival. In addition, breast-conserving surgery with postoperative XRT is a feasible option and should not impact negatively on her survival.

REFERENCES

1. American Joint Committee on Cancer. In: *Manual for staging of cancer,* Beahrs OH, Henson DE, Hutter RVP, and Kennedy BJ, eds. Philadelphia: J.B. Lippincott; 1992:149–54.
2. Dorr FA, Bader J, Friedman MA. Locally advanced breast cancer cur-

rent status and future directions. *Int J Radiation Oncology Biol Phys* 1989;16:775–84.

3. Hortobagyi GN, Ames FC, Buzdar AU, et al. Management of stage III primary breast cancer with primary chemotherapy, surgery and radiation treatment. *Cancer* 1988;62:2505–16.

4. Pierce LJ, Lippman M, Ben-Baruch N, et al. The effect of systemic therapy on local–regional control in locally advanced breast cancer. *Int J Radiat Oncol Biol Phys* 1992;23:946–60.

5. Hortobagyi GN. Local control for locally advanced breast cancer: many opinions, few facts. *Int J Radiat Oncol Biol Phys* 1992;23:1085–6.

6. Strom EA, McNeese MD, Fletcher GH, Romsdahl MA, Montague ED, Oswald MJ. Results of mastectomy and postoperative irradiation in the management of locoregionally advanced carcinoma of the breast. *Int J Radiat Oncol Biol Phys* 1991;21:319–23.

7. Graham MV, Perez CA, Kuske RR, et al. Locally advanced (noninflammatory) carcinoma of the breast: results and comparison of various treatment modalities. *Int J Radiat Oncol Biol Phys* 1991;21:311–8.

8. Perloff M, Lesnick GJ, Korzun A, et al. Combination chemotherapy with mastectomy or radiotherapy for stage III breast carcinoma: a cancer and leukemia group B study. *J Clin Oncol* 1988;6(2):261–9.

9. Fisher B, Redmond C, Poisson R, et al. Eight-year results of a randomized clinical trial comparing total mastectomy and lumpectomy with or without irradiation in the treatment of breast cancer. *N Engl J Med* 1989;320:822–8.

10. Bonadonna G, Veronesi U, Brambilla C, et al. Primary chemotherapy to avoid mastectomy in tumors with diameters of three centimeters or more. *J Natl Cancer Inst* 1990;82(10):1539–45.

EDITORIAL BOARD COMMENTARY

This case illustrates the importance of understanding the surgical implications of matted axillary lymph nodes in treatment planning. The general surgeon must understand that matted axillary nodes (N2) cannot technically be completely removed, and that preoperative chemotherapy will usually convert the patient to a resectable status. Most patients will subsequently undergo a mastectomy, but this case illustrates the feasibility of a breast-conserving approach, which may be more broadly applied if supported by mature data.

82

T3 N1 M0 Stage IIIA Breast Cancer

Robert M. Quinlan

Is mastectomy as an initial approach contraindicated in stage III patients?

CASE PRESENTATION

C.M. is a 44-year-old woman who presented to the office with a several month history of an enlarging right breast mass. The patient had no other complaints. She continued to menstruate and was on no medications. She had no known allergies and no family history of breast cancer. The first of three full-term pregnancies began at age 24. She gave no history of exogenous hormone intake. Her physical exam was essentially within normal limits with the exception of a 6-cm rock-hard mass involving the upper outer quadrant of the right breast (Fig. 82–1A,B). There was mild skin retraction but no dimpling or peau d'orange. There were one or two easily movable nodes measuring more than 1 cm in the right axilla. All masses were easily movable over the underlying chest wall and under the overlying skin. There was no evidence of a contralateral left breast mass or other adenopathy. There was no hepatomegaly. The patient's chest radiograph showed no evidence of metastatic disease. Her liver function tests, including bilirubin and alkaline phosphatase, were within normal limits. Her hematocrit was 34% and her hemoglobin 11.2 gm/dL. Her albumin was 3.8 gm/dL with a normal of 3.9 to 5.0. The patient underwent a needle biopsy of the right breast mass, which was positive for adenocarcinoma, and immunoperoxidase staining for estrogen receptor showed the tumor to be focally positive but negative for progesterone receptor.

After a discussion at our tumor conference, it was decided to proceed with neoadjuvant chemotherapy and reevaluate the clinical response after two cycles. The patient understood that perhaps we would go to four or five cycles of chemotherapy before maximum response

was noted. The chemotherapy chosen was Cytoxan, Adriamycin, and 5-FU. This chemotherapy regimen was to be a 28-day cycle with Cytoxan, Adriamycin, and 5-FU being given on day 1 in the dose of 600 mg/M^2, 60 mg/M^2, and 600 mg/M^2 respectively. The 5-FU at 600 mg/M^2 was to be repeated on day 8, and then the entire cycle repeated beginning on day 28. The patient was not given tamoxifen at this time. Following two cycles of chemotherapy, there was a dramatic response; however, the third cycle of therapy was given. Because of the timing of the surgery, she also received a fourth cycle, and was taken to the operating room 4 months following her initial presentation. She underwent a right total mastectomy, axillary node dissection, and synchronous prosthetic implant. Findings were consistent with infiltrating duct cell carcinoma of the breast with residual lymphatic invasion and metastases to 12 of 17 axillary lymph nodes. The residual tumor was close to the deep resection margin. There was no gross tumor seen on the fresh specimen but found only on permanent pathology. One lymph node was grossly involved with tumor. After the operation, participants at our Tumor Board Conference discussed various options for treatment, including continuation with an additional five cycles of Cytoxan, Adriamycin, and 5-FU, or switching to Cytoxan, methotrexate, 5-FU, vincristine, and platinum for an additional five cycles. There was a discussion of possibly considering bone marrow transplantation at that time; however, because of the neoadjuvant chemotherapy, she was not a candidate for protocols in our area. She completed an additional five cycles of Cytoxan, Adriamycin, and 5-FU approximately 10 months following her initial diagnosis, and then underwent 5,000 Gy in 25 fractions to the right chest wall, including the prosthesis

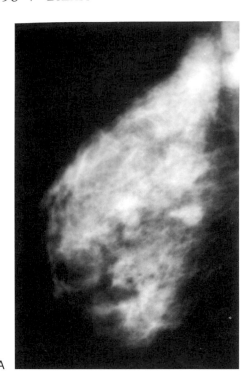

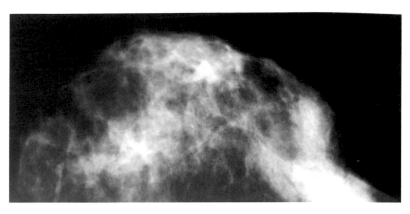

FIG. 82–1. Mammograms showing carcinoma of the upper outer quadrant of the right breast. **A**: Mediolateral view of the breast showing a dense tumor mass in the right upper breast. An enlarged lymph node is seen immediately behind the major tumor mass. **B**: An exaggerated cephalocaudal view of the right breast showing tumor involving the upper outer quadrant and axillary tail.

and internal mammary nodes as one setting through a tangential field. A separate field included the supraclavicular nodal area angled away from the spinal cord. All the patient's therapy was completed at approximately 1 year from her diagnosis. Tamoxifen was begun at the completion of standard chemotherapy.

At 2 years from diagnosis she was free of recurrent disease, although the prosthesis was removed because of a painful chest wall. Two and half years following her diagnosis, she developed mid-back pain and repeat bone scan revealed possible involvement of a vertebrae at T-10 or T-11 (Fig. 82–2A). A computed tomography scan of this area confirmed probable metastatic disease (Fig. 82–2B) and discussion at Tumor Board Conference conferred on essentially either bone marrow transplantation or changing her tamoxifen to Megace. She was also offered a course of radiotherapy to the thoracic spine. The patient chose to receive the radiotherapy and to be switched to Megace, with which she is currently being treated.

COMMENTARY by Craig Henderson

The management of this patient conforms to standard practice in the United States in the 1990s, and the options considered at each decision point are similar to those that might be discussed at tumor boards across the country. Most clinicians would treat stage III breast cancer with primary (or neoadjuvant) chemotherapy. Regimens that include doxorubicin are most frequently employed. After four to six cycles of chemotherapy, local treatment con-

sisting of mastectomy and radiotherapy are administered. Finally, most American physicians would administer further chemotherapy after the completion of local treatment. Because of the perception that these patients have a universally poor outlook, various types of investigational treatment, such as bone marrow transplant or, in this case, platinum therapy, are often used. From the case presentation, it seems likely that this cancer was technically operable at presentation, and thus, the mastectomy could have been performed first.

Although patients with locally advanced or stage III breast cancer are thought to have a poor prognosis, this is in actuality a very heterogenous group. In fact, very few studies are limited only to patients with stage IIIA, stage IIIB (technically inoperable), or inflammatory breast cancer. In a study from the Joint Center for Radiotherapy and Dana-Farber Cancer Institute, the 5-year survival of a group of stage III breast cancer patients treated with limited surgery and radiotherapy was 38% (1). In a nonrandomized comparison, the 5-year survival of patients in this series to receive both radiotherapy and chemotherapy was 51%.

The relative importance of mastectomy and radiotherapy in the management of locally advanced breast cancer was addressed in a randomized trial conducted by the Cancer and Leukemia Group B (CALGB). In this study, all patients were initially treated with three courses of a chemotherapy regimen that included doxorubicin. At that point they were randomized to receive either mastectomy followed by further chemotherapy, or radiotherapy with-

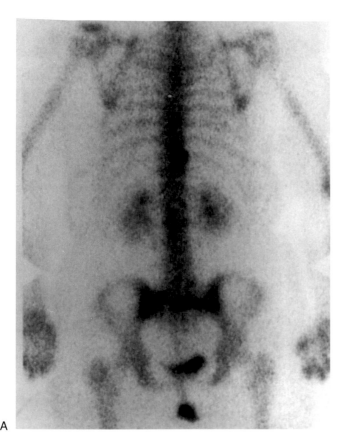

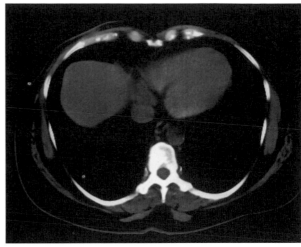

FIG. 82–2. Metastases involving the thoracic spine. **A**: radionuclide scan showing increased uptake in the right lateral aspect of T-10. **B**: CT scan of the lower chest and upper abdomen showing invasion of the body of T-10 on the right by tumor.

out mastectomy followed by further chemotherapy (2). There was no difference in the overall disease-free survival of patients in the two arms of this study. Local recurrence was the first site of relapse in 55% of the patients randomized to radiotherapy and only 42% of the patients randomized to mastectomy ($p = 0.43$). While it is reasonable to assume that local control will be improved by the use of both mastectomy and radiotherapy, there are no data from randomized controlled trials demonstrating an improved survival from the use of both forms of local treatment for stage IIIA breast cancer.

Since the use of adjuvant chemotherapy or endocrine therapy has been shown to prolong the lives of patients with early breast cancer (3) it seems plausible that systemic therapy given either before or after local treatment of stage III disease will prolong survival as well. Three randomized trials have been conducted to address this issue (4–6). Only the trial from Finland—in which stage III patients were randomized to radiotherapy alone, chemotherapy alone, or a combination of chemotherapy and radiotherapy—demonstrated a survival advantage from a combination of radiation and chemotherapy (4). In the trial conducted by the EORTC, 363 postmenopausal women were randomized to receive radiotherapy alone or radiotherapy plus hormone therapy, radiotherapy plus chemotherapy, or radiotherapy plus both hormone and chemotherapy. No survival advantage was seen from the

systemic treatment of these mostly postmenopausal and inoperable stage III women, but there was a prolongation of disease-free survival and improved local control with the addition of both hormone and chemotherapy (6). Taken together, the results from the overview of all adjuvant therapy trials (many of which included patients with stage IIIA disease) and the studies of adjuvant treatment in patients with locally advanced (operable and inoperable) breast cancer, suggest that the addition of systemic treatment (chemotherapy for premenopausal women, tamoxifen for postmenopausal) to local therapy will improve local control (or at least delay the time to the appearance of a local recurrence) and have a modest impact on the survival of these patients.

There are two potential advantages for using neoadjuvant chemotherapy (i.e., chemotherapy before local treatment) of stage IIIA breast cancer: it may reduce the need for mastectomy, allowing additional patients to be treated with lumpectomy and radiation, and it may prolong patient survival. In a recently published study, 196 pre- and postmenopausal women with T-2 and T-3 lesions between 3 cm and 7 cm in size were randomized to receive either two cycles of the combination doxorubicin, cyclophosphamide, 5-fluorouracil (ACF) followed by local treatment with radiation and/or surgery and four more months of chemotherapy or initial radiotherapy and/or surgery followed by six courses of ACF (7). The two courses of preoperative ACF resulted in either a partial or complete response for 45% of the patients; a complete response was seen in 13%. In this study, fewer patients required surgery if neoadjuvant chemotherapy was given before radiation, but there was no significant disease-free or overall survival difference for the patients receiving neoadjuvant chemotherapy. These investigators have recently completed a second study in which 414 premenopausal women with tumors measuring between 3 cm and 7 cm were randomized to receive either four courses of chemotherapy followed by radiation and surgery or local treatment followed by the adjuvant chemotherapy, but no results are available (8). The available data suggest that preoperative chemotherapy may improve local control or increase the number of patients who may receive breast conserving surgery, but a longer follow-up will be needed from studies such as this to confirm these preliminary observations. There is as yet no evidence from controlled trials that neoadjuvant chemotherapy will prolong survival.

Because of the perception that patients with stage III breast cancer have a poor prognosis, it is tempting to use very high dose chemotherapy and autologous bone marrow transplant (9). Many uncontrolled trials suggest that this approach may improve the response rate in patients with metastatic breast cancer or prolong the time to recurrence in patients with early breast cancer (10). However, these studies have not yet demonstrated that this strategy will prolong life, and there is certainly no evidence that patients who cannot be cured with more conventional therapy will be cured by high-dose chemotherapy and bone marrow transplant.

In summary, studies of stage III patients have demonstrated that many of these patients will have a 5-year survival in excess of 50% if treated with a combination of chemotherapy and radiation (11,12). The precise role of neoadjuvant chemotherapy, the importance of mastectomy, and the ideal sequence of treatment to maximize survival have not been demonstrated in properly controlled trials.

REFERENCES

1. Sheldon T, et al. Primary radiation therapy for locally advanced breast cancer. *Cancer* 1987;60:1219–25.
2. Perloff M, et al. Combination chemotherapy with mastectomy or radiotherapy for stage III breast carcinoma: A cancer and leukemia group B study. *J Clin Oncol* 1988;6:261–9.
3. Early Breast Cancer Trialists' Collaborative Group. Systemic treatment of early breast cancer by hormonal, cytotoxic, or immune therapy: 133 randomised trials involving 31,000 recurrences and 24,000 deaths among 75,000 women. *Lancet* 1992;339:1–15,71–85.
4. Grohn P, et al. Adjuvant postoperative radiotherapy, chemotherapy, and immunotherapy in stage III breast cancer. *Cancer* 1984;54:670–4.
5. Schaake-Koning C, et al. Adjuvant chemo- and hormonal therapy in locally advanced breast cancer: A randomized clinical study. *Int J Radiat Oncol Biol Phys* 1985;11:1759–63.
6. Rubens RD, et al. Locally advanced breast cancer: The contribution of cytotoxic and endocrine treatment to radiotherapy. An EORTC Breast Cancer Co-operative Group Trial (10792). *Eur J Cancer Clin Oncol* 1989;25:667–78.
7. Scholl SM, et al. Neoadjuvant chemotherapy in operable breast cancer. *Eur J Cancer* 1991;27(17):1668–71.
8. Scholl SM, et al. Neoadjuvant vs. adjuvant chemotherapy in operable breast cancer: a controlled trial. *Breast Cancer Res Treat* 1991;19(2):162.
9. Henderson IC. Window of opportunity. *J Natl Cancer Inst* 1991;83:894–6.
10. Peters WP, et al. High-dose chemotherapy and autologous bone marrow support as consolidation after standard-dose adjuvant therapy for high-risk primary breast cancer. *J Clin Oncol* 1993;11:1132–43.
11. Sheldon T, et al. Primary radiation therapy for locally advanced breast cancer. *Cancer* 1987;60:1219–25.
12. Frank JL, et al. Stage III breast cancer: is neoadjuvant chemotherapy always necessary? *J Surg Oncol* 1992;49:220–5.

EDITORIAL BOARD COMMENTARY

As Dr. Henderson points out, this patient is technically resectable. There appears to be no local control or survival benefit lost with this approach. The disadvantage of initial mastectomy is that breast-conserving surgery would be eliminated as an option, but most would perform mastectomy because of lack of mature data supporting the breast-conserving approach for locally advanced tumors. Continued research in this area may allow us to extend our indications for breast-conserving surgery.

83

Inflammatory Breast Cancer

Frederick L. Greene and Douglas Dorsay

A poor-prognosis tumor mandating multimodality therapy

CASE PRESENTATION

Mrs. G.C., a 39-year-old African-American woman, was referred to the Breast Clinic at the University of South Carolina Department of Surgery after being evaluated in a rural South Carolina physician's office with findings consistent with inflammatory carcinoma of the right breast. The patient had noted change in her right breast during the 3 months prior to this admission. She sought medical care and a biopsy was performed at an outlying hospital. The patient's history was significant for asthma, during a 20-year period, for which she is taking Theo-Dur, 300 mg p.o., b.i.d., and Proventil. She has a history of mild hypertension, which is currently being controlled medically. The patient does not smoke or ingest alcohol.

On physical examination, the patient was a moderately obese lady in no acute distress. Examination of the head and neck was entirely unremarkable. There was no evidence of any adenopathy in the cervical or supraclavicular areas. The chest was remarkable for an indurated right breast with erythema of the breast, extending to the axillary area. There were several firm nodes in the right axilla. The left breast showed minimal nodularity. There was no evidence of any adenopathy in the left axillary area. The abdomen was unremarkable. Pelvic examination showed a normal cervix and vaginal area. Rectal examination was unremarkable. Neurological examination was normal.

TUMOR BOARD DISCUSSION

During the Tumor Board discussion, the Medical Oncology group discussed plans for chemotherapy to achieve local control prior to using external beam irradiation or surgical debulking. The Surgical Service recommended that a venous access device be placed to facilitate chemotherapy. It was recommended that a mammogram be performed of the left breast to assure that there were no suspicious lesions that would require early biopsy and local treatment. The pathological specimen from the outside hospital was reviewed and found to be consistent with inflammatory carcinoma (Figs. 83–1 and 83–2). The patient was staged as a T4 N3 M0 tumor. The Medical Oncology group recommended that the patient receive combined chemotherapy utilizing 5-FU, Adriamycin, and Cytoxan. This was instituted as an outpatient therapy.

Tumor Board Discussion (3 Months Follow-up)

The patient completed three cycles of chemotherapy, using 5-FU, Adriamycin, and Cytoxan, and had undergone marked reduction in the size of the tumor. On physical examination, a palpable tumor in the right breast measured 7 cm to 8 cm with fixed nodes palpable in the axilla. On that visit, she was also noted having a swollen right cheek, and intra-oral examination showed an obvious abscess of a right upper molar tooth. She was referred to the dental unit for extraction or incision and drainage of her gingival abscess.

Tumor Board Discussion (4 Months After Initial Presentation)

Discussion at Tumor Board dealt with the marked reduction in the amount of obvious tumor in the right breast with the successful application of multidrug

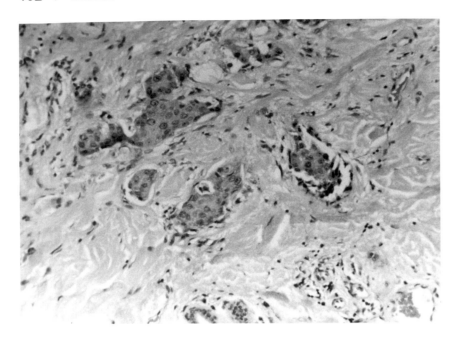

FIG. 83–1. Multiple dilated lymphatics with "plugs" of tumor cells. Endothelial lining cells are recognizable. (Hematoxylin and eosin stain ×250.)

chemotherapy. A discussion centered on the importance of utilizing external beam radiation at this point, or achieving local control with surgical debulking in the form of mastectomy and axillary clearance. It was the feeling of the Surgical Oncology service that this would be the best time to perform mastectomy prior to the radiation effects caused by external beam therapy. In light of this, the patient was scheduled for a right modified radical mastectomy, and underwent this procedure 4 and 1/2 months after initial presentation. The pathology specimen showed a lesion 20 cm in diameter. The nipple was replaced by an irregular mass with erosion of the skin's surface. Biopsy at the time of the mastectomy was utilized to send tissue for estrogen receptor and flow cytometric examination. The microscopic sections showed scattered foci of residual ductal carcinoma (Fig. 83–3). There was no evidence of any lymphangitic or intravascular involvement. The deep margin of the resection was negative for neoplasm. It was believed that the gross and microscopic changes in the breast may be secondary to chemotherapy effect on the

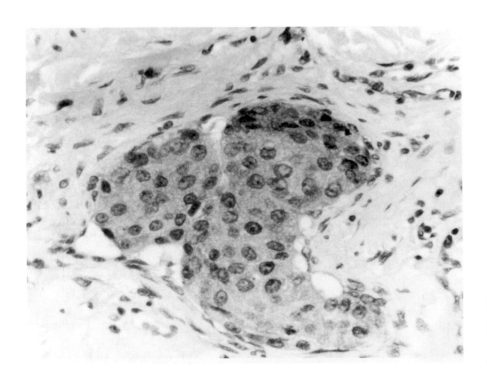

FIG. 83–2. Expanded lymphatic vessel containing a cluster of malignant epithelial cells. Note the recognizable endothelial cells at the periphery. (Hematoxylin and eosin stain ×500.)

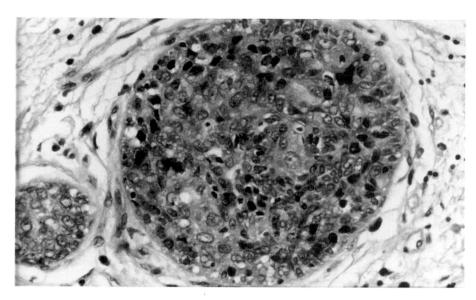

FIG. 83–3. In situ mammary (ductal) carcinoma. Note slight "retraction artifact" with separation of cell clusters from surrounding stroma. No evidence of stromal invasion at this site. (Hematoxylin and eosin stain ×500.)

neoplasm, since no radiation had been used. The pathologist at Tumor Board questioned the initial diagnosis of "inflammatory carcinoma" because of the dramatic reduction in tumor secondary to chemotherapy alone.

Tumor Board Discussion (5 Months After Initial Presentation)

The patient had now undergone an additional cycle of 5-FU, Adriamycin, and Cytoxan, after the completion of a right modified radical mastectomy. Estrogen receptor findings showed negative ER and an aneuploid tumor on flow cytometry. The S-phase fraction was greater than 10%. The radiation oncologist recommended that the patient now be considered for a course of radiation to the right chest wall that would encompass the supraclavicular area and the internal mammary chain. A repeat chest radiograph was viewed during this Tumor Board discussion and showed a left pleural effusion (Fig. 83–4). Although no mass lesions were noted in the pulmonary parenchyma, a concern was voiced regarding the possibility of pleural metastases from the right breast lesion. Laboratory data were all within normal limits. A follow-up left mammogram showed several benign-appearing soft tissue masses but no evidence of any abnormal calcifications or suspicious lesions. Following this Tumor Board conference, a bone scan was performed, which was found to be within normal limits. The patient was referred to the Radiation Oncology service.

Six months after initial presentation, the patient was begun on external beam radiation. The supraclavicular and axillary apex areas were treated with anterior fields, using 18 MV X-rays with 2 cm of bolus across the entire field.

This area received 55.8 Gy in 31 treatments. A posterior axillary field was used to boost the dose by giving 8 Gy in four treatments, calculated at an 8-cm depth with 18 MV X-rays. The chest wall was treated with 6 MV electrons for an initial dose of 50.4 Gy in 28 treatments. The surgical incision was given an additional 12 Gy in six treatments for a

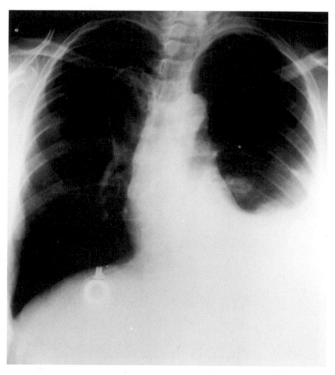

FIG. 83–4. Chest radiography performed 4 months after presentation showing left pleural effusion and satisfactory position of venous access device.

total of 62.4 Gy. The internal mammary chain was treated with 12 MV electrons to a dose of 50.4 Gy in 28 treatments. The upper half of the field was then boosted for an additional 5.4 Gy in three treatments. Radiation therapy extended for a 6-week period, and following completion of radiation, the patient was re-presented to the Tumor Board.

Tumor Board Presentation (9 Months After Initial Presentation)

The patient had undergone her sixth cycle of 5-FU, Adriamycin, and Cytoxan with current plans to have a full 12 cycles. The patient was tolerating her chemotherapy well but was concerned about continued alopecia. Her Karnofsky index was excellent. Her weight was stable and she was taking a satisfactory diet, and she had returned to full employment. She had moderate hyperpigmentation from her irradiated areas with a small amount of desquamation of the skin of the anterior chest wall.

Tumor Board (28 Months Following Initial Presentation)

The patient had completed chemotherapy. She had undergone a replacement of the Port-A-Cath, 18 months

following original placement of the device because of an infected pocket. She voiced hope that the venous access device would be removed at some future date. A repeat left mammogram showed multiple size nodules in the left breast, unchanged from the previous study (Fig. 83–5). These were interpreted as being consistent with degenerating fibroadenomas. Breast examination was unremarkable. Follow-up chest radiograph showed residual left pleural effusion, but no evidence of any parenchymal masses. Laboratory data, including liver function studies, were entirely normal.

The patient continues to do well without evidence of recurrence, 36 months after initial presentation and discussion at Tumor Board.

COMMENTARY by Deborah K. Armstrong and Martin D. Abeloff

This case describes the clinical course of a 39-year-old woman who presented with a 3-month history of changes in her right breast. Initial examination revealed clinical characteristics of inflammatory breast cancer and a biopsy showed tumor embolization to lymphatic vessels. Her initial treatment consisted of systemic chemotherapy with an Adriamycin-containing regimen, resulting in marked tumor regression. This was followed by modified radical

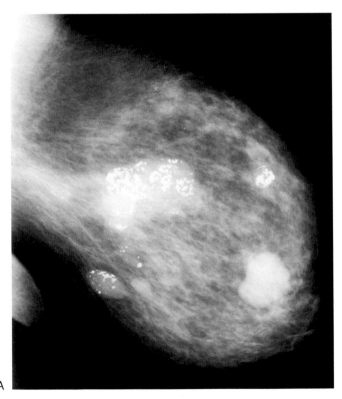
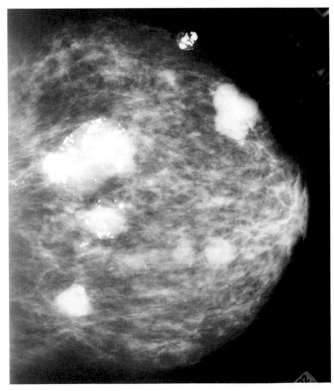

FIG. 83–5. A. Lateral view of left breast on mammography showing multiple lesions throughout breast with coarse calcifications interpreted as being degenerating fibroadenomas. **B** Craniocaudal view of left breast showing multiple degenerating fibroadenomas.

mastectomy, radiation therapy and further chemotherapy. The patient's course was complicated by a persistent idiopathic pleural effusion, but she remains without documented evidence of recurrence 3 years after her initial presentation.

The diagnosis of inflammatory breast cancer carries with it a particularly dismal prognosis. Local disease control is seldom obtained with mastectomy or radiotherapy alone, and most patients will die of distant metastatic disease within 2 years of diagnosis. These characteristics suggest that women with inflammatory breast cancer have systemic disease at presentation, and thus, require early intensive systemic therapy. Fortunately, the use of chemotherapy for women with inflammatory breast cancer has improved both local control and survival (1).

Inflammatory breast cancer is defined by its clinical features, which consist of erythema accompanied by heat, edema with characteristics of peau d'orange, and induration, usually involving at least one third of the breast. The breast is enlarged and tender, and the area of induration may end with a palpable ridge; however, a frank mass is frequently not appreciated. Although these characteristics are believed to arise from dermal lymphatic invasion by tumor emboli, this pathologic finding, while confirmatory, is not required for the diagnosis of inflammatory breast cancer (2). The initial pathologic findings from the case presentation clearly shows tumor embolization to lymphatic vessels. It does not appear that these are dermal lymphatic vessels, and thus, this finding does not provide confirmatory pathologic evidence for inflammatory breast cancer. Since the diagnosis is made on clinical grounds, however, there is no diagnostic difficulty.

The aggressive nature of inflammatory breast cancer is verified by the finding that greater than 25% of patients present with distant metastatic disease and 75% to 100% have regional nodal involvement (1). Although it is essential to treat inflammatory breast cancer as a systemic disease, the presence of overt metastatic disease has important therapeutic and prognostic significance. At the Johns Hopkins Oncology Center, women who present with inflammatory breast cancer are evaluated with radiographic studies of the chest, abdomen, and bone as part of their initial staging. The staging designation for the patient presented is T4, N3, M0. According to the 1989 edition of the *American Joint Committee on Cancer Staging* (3), N3 denotes metastases to ipsilateral internal mammary lymph nodes. We are, however, given no information to document this designation. In the absence of documented ipsilateral internal mammary lymph node involvement, the presence of fixed ipsilateral axillary lymph nodes would be designated N2, and the presence of "several firm nodes" would be designated N1 if these nodes were mobile.

In the case presented here, the dramatic reduction in tumor at pathologic examination of the mastectomy specimen prompted the Tumor Board pathologist to question the initial diagnosis of inflammatory carcinoma; however, it has clearly been shown that the use of preoperative induction chemotherapy for women with inflammatory breast cancer results in objective clinical responses (1). In a pilot study from our institution, we used a 16-week dose-intense chemotherapy regimen as induction therapy in women with inoperable, locally advanced breast cancer. Although 84% of these women had inflammatory breast cancer, a clinical response was noted in all study patients; 37% had a complete response, 63% had a partial response. All of these women were rendered operable, and 29% had no microscopic evidence of disease in the breast at mastectomy (4). It is thus not surprising to see the marked clinical and pathologic responses noted in this case.

As documented by the case presented, treatment strategies that use induction chemotherapy may have the dual benefits of rendering patients more responsive to local therapy as well as eradicating micrometastatic disease. After systemic therapy, improved local control can be obtained by surgery or radiation therapy. Because local–regional failure is still a significant problem, utilization of both modalities may be warranted (5) particularly if residual disease is documented at mastectomy. Although a number of studies have examined the effect of sequence of radiation therapy and surgery, there has been no consistently observed sequencing benefit on either local or distant relapse rates (1). Thus, in the case under discussion, the combined modality treatment approach using induction chemotherapy followed by modified radical mastectomy and subsequent radiation therapy is entirely appropriate.

The appearance of a pleural effusion in the patient under discussion appropriately raised concern over the possibility of pleural metastases. A diagnostic thoracentesis would have provided important information regarding the possible etiologies of this patient's pleural effusion. Repeated thoracenteses are frequently necessary to establish a diagnosis of metastatic breast cancer and are warranted in the case under question because of the importance of documenting metastatic disease. Fortunately, the patient is now almost 3 years from the initial appearance of this effusion without any documented evidence of metastatic disease thus far.

The need for maintenance chemotherapy following induction chemotherapy and local treatment of inflammatory breast cancer has not been well studied in recent randomized clinical trials. Most current clinical trials in inflammatory breast cancer use maintenance chemotherapy after combined modality therapy, based on the efficacy of such therapy in resectable breast cancer. It is thus appropriate for the patient presented to have received further chemotherapy after mastectomy and radiation therapy.

The mammogram included as part of the patient's follow-up care points out the need for continued evaluation of remaining breast tissue in women with a history of breast cancer. It is important to note, however, that there is no known association of breast fibroadenoma(s) with breast cancer. Because there are specific mammographic findings in inflammatory breast cancer, it would have been helpful to see the original mammogram at presentation of inflammatory breast cancer, if one was obtained.

In summary, this patient presented with typical clinical findings of inflammatory breast cancer and was appropriately treated with induction chemotherapy followed by local therapy with mastectomy and radiation therapy and subsequent maintenance chemotherapy. Our recommendations are that a patient such as this should additionally have a thorough metastatic evaluation at the time of presentation and that the appearance during treatment of a new pleural effusion warrants an aggressive search for the etiology.

REFERENCES

1. Waldman S, Toonkel LM, Davila, E. Inflammatory breast cancer. In: *High-risk breast cancer*, Ragaz J, Ariel IM, eds. Berlin: Springer-Verlag; 1991:319–33.

2. Parker LM, Boyages J, Eberlien TJ. Inflammatory carcinoma of the breast. In: *Breast diseases,* 2nd ed., Harris JR, Hellman S, Henderson IC, Kinne DW, eds. Philadelphia. J.B. Lippincott; 1991:775–82.

3. Harris JR. Staging of breast carcinoma. In: *Breast diseases,* 2nd ed., Harris JR, Hellman S, Henderson IC, Kinne DW, eds. Philadelphia. J.B. Lippincott; 1991:327–32.

4. Armstrong DK, Beveridge RA, Donehower RC, et al. Sixteen week dose intense chemotherapy for inoperable, locally advanced breast cancer (LABC). *Breast Cancer Res Treat* 1991;19:160.

5. Swain SM. Selection of therapy for Stage III breast cancer. *Surg Clin North Am* 1990;70:1061–80.

EDITORIAL BOARD COMMENTARY

The sequence of therapy for inflammatory carcinoma most commonly involves induction chemotherapy followed by mastectomy and radiation therapy for local control, followed by maintenance chemotherapy for a variable period of time. These patients are technically inoperable at the time of presentation. With modern induction chemotherapy they may become resectable, and while the absolute improvement in survival for this disease has not been dramatically improved, the quality of life has.

84

Paget's Disease of the Nipple

Morton C. Wilhelm

Don't treat eczema of the nipple with salves—biopsy it

CASE PRESENTATION

HISTORY

A 68-year-old woman with a 6-month history of drippings of the right nipple and nodularity of nipple was seen. There had been a slight bloody tinge on the right side for 2 months.

On examination, the contour of the breast was normal. The right nipple was slight irregular, with erosion of the central and outer aspects. There was no mass effect in the nipple or the breast. The left nipple was enlarged with a nodule in the central portion. There was no erosion and no mass was felt in the underlying breast. Both axillae were negative.

Mammography revealed dense glandular breasts with vascular calcifications and calcifications of fat necrosis. There were occasional punctate calcifications on the left with round morphology on magnification. The right breast revealed extensive irregular casting type microcalcifications in the upper inner quadrant at 2 o'clock. (Figs. 84–1A and 84–1B) These were deep in the breast and separate from the nipple. No subareolar calcifications were observed. The right breast findings were categorized as highly suspicious for ductal carcinoma in situ, most likely comedo type.

The patient was taken to the operating room, and under local anesthesia, bilateral nipple biopsies were performed.

The pathologic findings revealed a benign nipple adenoma on the left side and Paget's disease of the right nipple (Figure 84–2A). On low magnification, Paget's cells infiltrated the surface squamous epithelium, which in some places was attenuated and had overlying crusts. High-magnification views (Figure 84–2B) showed Paget's cells inter-

mixed both singly and in groups with the squamous epithelium of the nipple. The Paget's cells were characterized as large with clear cytoplasm, large nuclei, and prominent nucleoli. Immunohistochemical studies express low molecular weight keratins common in Paget's cells.

TUMOR BOARD DISCUSSION

No further treatment was indicated for this patient for the left nipple adenoma. For the right breast, the stage was TisN0N0—stage 0. In view of the extensive suspicious microcalcifications in the right breast separated from the Paget's disease of the nipple, it was believed that a total mastectomy would be required to remove involved areas. Excision of the microcalcifications as a separate procedure was not thought technically feasible. Level I axillary dissection was recommended in view of possible microinvasive cancer. Subsequently, the patient underwent total mastectomy, with residual Paget's disease in the nipple, which did not extend into the breast. There was extensive ductal carcinoma in situ of the comedo, solid cribriform types in the upper inner quadrant of the breast. There was no evidence of invasion. The level I lymph nodes were negative for tumor. Final pathologic stages was TisN0N0—stage 0.

The patient had an uneventful recovery. No further treatment was recommended. A follow-up mammography in the left breast in 6 months to assess stability of the nonsuspicious calcifications was recommended.

COMMENTARY by Kirby I. Bland

This 48-year-old Caucasian woman presented with encrustation and drippings of the right nipple, which had

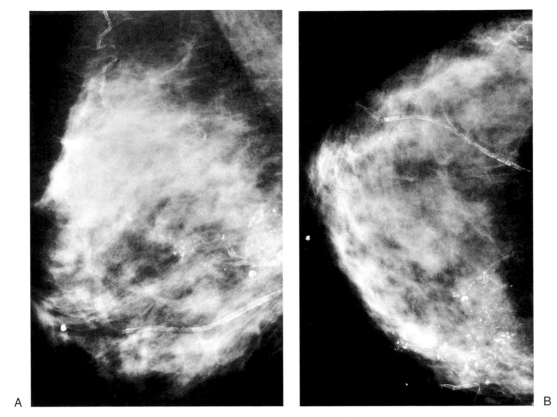

FIG. 84–1. **A**: Right mediolateral view. **B**: Right craniocaudal view.

slight irregularity and erosion of the central and outer aspect of the areola. Physical exam disclosed no mass effects in the nipple or the breast. The clinical presentation is typically that for one of the most important malignancies of the skin of the breast—Paget's disease. The mammogram of this individual has important implications for subsequent therapy. The right breast (Fig.84–1A,B) identifies irregular casting-type microcalcifications, which were extensive in the upper inner quadrant of the right breast at two o'clock. Of concern are calcifications that are separate from the subareolar breast; thus, are suspicious for a remote *second* primary of the right breast. No further therapy of the left breast or nipple was necessary because biopsy confirmed "benign nipple adenoma."

DISCUSSION

Essentially, all cases of mammary Paget's disease have an underlying ductal adenocarcinoma, which may be in situ or invasive. Paget's disease of the nipple may be regarded as an extension of subareolar ductal carcinoma in situ (DCIS) to the nipple epithelial surface (1). Thus, the associated disease within the breast may be extensive and invasive. Between 5% and 10% of individuals with Paget's disease have DCIS confined to the nipple (2,3).

The cells of mammary Paget's disease are believed to originate in adenocarcinomas of the lactiferous ducts, and subsequently ascend to involve the epidermis. However, only rarely does adenocarcinoma in situ of the nipple, areola, or skin of the breast arise within underlying ductal carcinoma. Many pathologists contend that carcinoma will invariably be discovered if searched for exhaustively. Approximately one fifth of patients with Paget's disease present with a nipple lesion *without* a palpable breast mass (4). Dabski and Stoll noted that approximately one half of cases present as a nipple lesion with a palpable mass at the first examination; 10.2% present as a palpable breast tumor with Paget's disease identified only on microscopic examination (4). This patient presented with the typical gross lesion of the nipple–areola with encrustation, weeping, and associated ulceration. Often the adjacent skin has a persistent eczematous dermatitis with erythema, scaling, oozing, and crusting. On occasion, a purulent or bloody discharge may be observed. Photomicrographs of the right nipple (Fig. 84–2A,B) identify at low- and high-magnification typical Paget's cells intermixed both singly and in groups with squamous epithelium of the nipple. These are typically large pale-staining cells within the epidermis, generally above the basement membrane (Figure 84–2B). Paget's cells have a large nucleus and abundant cytoplasm with basal epidermal cells that are flattened between Paget

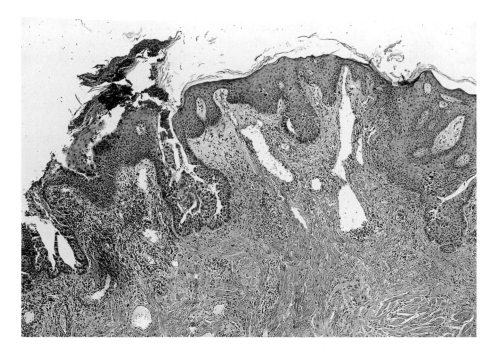

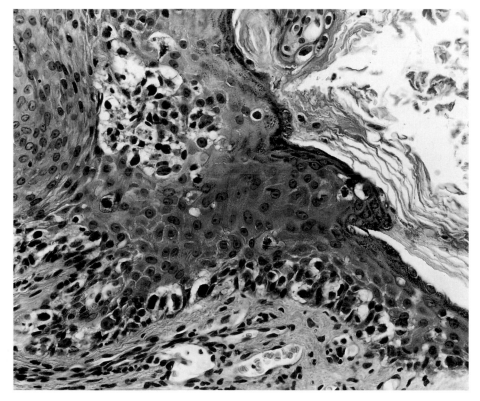

FIG. 84–2. A: At low magnification, Paget's cells have infiltrated the surface squamous epithelium, which in some places is attenuated and has an overlying crust. **B**: At high magnification, Paget's cells are intermixed both singly and in groups with the squamous epithelium of the nipple.

cells and epidermis. These cells are PAS-positive and diastases-resistant and may be positive for carcinoembryonic antigen (CEA) by immunoperoxidase techniques. This lesion may be identified within large ducts beneath the nipple and may arise within a background of other chronic skin lesions. The clinicians involved in the management of this patient proceeded appropriately with biopsy of the nonhealing skin lesion. Other skin abnormalities may be associated with carcinoma of the breast. Four variants of

cutaneous metastasis are observed to disseminate via lymphatics: *inflammatory carcinoma, nodular carcinoma, telangiectatic carcinoma,* and *carcinoma-en-cuirasse.*

Discussion of Patient Management

The patient was clinical stage Tis N0 M0-stage 0. In my view, the case was appropriately managed with total mastectomy, as segmental mastectomy with planned postoperative radiation would not allow proper therapy of the upper inner quadrant microcalcifications, which were mammographically suspicious for carcinoma. Further, extensive excision of large volumes of breast, especially inner quadrant lesions, leave cosmetically deforming defects. For the individual in whom complete resection of the central breast with clear margins is essential to diminish local–regional recurrence, a biopsy of an inner quadrant lesion would create a deformed breast and, in great probability, would not have allowed complete resection of the extensive volume of microcalcifications. The appropriate option exercised by the surgeon was that of total mastectomy with en bloc resection of level I lymphatics. With resection of the tail of Spence, the en bloc resection of level I nodal group is inclusive of the external mammary, subscapular, and lateral axillary groups. Ideally, flap development is accomplished via modified Orr (oblique) incision that adequately incorporates the nipple–areola complex with microscopically free margins about the Paget's lesion.

Final pathologic findings confirmed residual Paget's disease in the nipple without extension into the deep breast parenchyma. Of note was the finding of extensive DCIS of comedo, solid and cribriform types in the upper inner quadrant of the breast. No evidence of invasion was found. All recovered lymph nodes in level I were negative. As no adverse pathologic data were evident to suggest microinvasion or positive margins of the resection specimen, there is no indication for postoperative irradiation to the skin flaps, chest wall, or peripheral lymphatics.

Follow-up

Four- to 6-month follow-up is advisable. Further, left mammogram at 6 months will be completed to evaluate changes of nonsuspicious calcifications evident in breast parenchyma. Total mastectomy has abrogated the necessity of repeated mammographic and clinical follow-up of an intact breast and the potential necessity for biopsies of the extensive microcalcifications.

For many decades, mastectomy has been advocated as the appropriate therapy of DCIS for the perceived hazards of multicentricity, and the subsequent risk for progression of an in situ lesion to an invasive variant. Bloodgood originally viewed DCIS as a "pure comedo tumor" and as being essentially benign (5,6). Lewis and Geschickter (7) noted excellent results for mastectomy, although simple excision of the tumor in their series produced a 75% recurrence rate within 4 years. These authors attributed this finding to the inability to reliably ascertain the "malignant potential" of the lesion (distinction of invasive from DCIS variants; the former were apparently included in this patient population). Godwin

(8) recommended Halsted radical mastectomy for DCIS because of the difficulties of identifying areas of microinvasion as well as the concern that DCIS is a rapidly growing and aggressive lesion. The recent trial of the NSABP (B-17) confirmed the value of postoperative radiation to the intact breast to reduce local–regional recurrence for the patient with localized disease and in whom breast size is amenable to conservation surgery (9). However, investigators (10–17) have long recognized that simple (total) mastectomy is appropriate therapy of DCIS. Total mastectomy, thus, will cure virtually all patients who have pathologically identifiable DCIS and currently represents the gold standard of therapy. Ipsilateral mastectomy has generally been considered adequate, as the overall incidence of contralateral occult disease appears to be similar to that for invasive disease. Axillary dissection is *not* recommended for "pure" DCIS unless associated microinvasion is evident (18). Only 1% to 2% of patients with DCIS will have nodal metastases; the only potential benefit from any level of axillary dissection is to insure the completeness of the mastectomy rather than to improve the reliability of pathological staging (19). However, the minimal morbidity of low-axillary dissection (level I) en bloc with the axillary tail and the small probability of identifying *unexpected* invasive disease make this a reasonable alternative to the total mastectomy. Various series (10,11,17,20–23) confirm a recurrence rate of 3%, and a survival rate of approximately 98% for DCIS treated with total mastectomy. This survival is expected with the patient who presents with combination Paget's disease and DCIS in a remote quadrant.

REFERENCES

1. Page DL, Anderson TJ, Rogers LW. Carcinoma in situ (CIS). In: *Diagnostic histopathology of the breast.* Page DL, Anderson TJ. Edinburgh: Churchill Livingstone; 1988:157.
2. Chaudary MA, Millis RR, Lane EB, Miller NA. Paget's disease of the nipple: A ten year review including clinical, pathological, and immunohistochemical findings. *Breast Cancer Res Treat* 1986;8:139–46.
3. Lagios MD, Westdahl PR, Rose MR, Concannon S. Paget's disease of the nipple: Alternative management in cases without or with minimal extent of underlying breast carcinoma. *Cancer* 1984;54:545–51.
4. Dabski K, Stoll HL. Paget's disease of the breast presenting as a cutaneous horn. *J Surg Oncol* 1985;29:237–9.
5. Bloodgood JC. Borderline breast tumors. *Ann Surg* 1931;93:235–49.
6. Bloodgood JC. Comedo carcinoma (or comedo-adenoma) of the female breast. *Arch Surg* 1921;3:445–542.
7. Lewis D, Geschickter CF. Comedo carcinoma of the breast. *Arch Surg* 1938;36:225–44.
8. Godwin JT. Chronology of lobular carcinoma of the breast: Report of a case. *Cancer* 1952;5:229–66.
9. Fisher B, Costantino J, Redmond C, et al. Lumpectomy compared with lumpectomy and radiation therapy for the treatment of intraductal breast cancer. *New Engl J Med* 1993;328(22):1581–1586.
10. Ackerman LV, Katzenstein AL. The concept of minimal breast cancer and the pathologist's role in the diagnosis of "early carcinoma." *Cancer* 1977;29:2755–63.
11. Ashikari R, Hajdu SI, Robbins GF. Intraductal carcinoma of the breast (1960–1969). *Cancer* 1971;28:1182–87.
12. Brown PW, Silverman J, Owens E, et al. Intraductal "noninfiltrating" carcinoma of the breast. *Arch Surg* 1976;111:1063–7.

13. Millis RR, Thynne GSJ. In situ intraduct carcinoma of the breast: A long term follow-up study. *Br J Surg* 1975;63:957–62.
14. Rosen PP, Braun DW, Kinne DE. The clinical significance of preinvasive breast carcinoma. *Cancer* 1980;46:919–25.
15. Rosen PP, Senie RT, Schottenfeld D, et al. Noninvasive breast carcinoma: Frequency of unsuspected invasion and implications for treatment. *Ann Surg* 1979;189:377–82.
16. Schuh ME, Nemoto T, Penetrante RB, et al. Intraductal carcinoma: Analysis of presentation, pathologic findings, and outcome of disease. *Arch Surg* 1986;121:1303–7.
17. Schwartz GF, Patchefsky AS, Feig SA, et al. Clinically occult breast cancer: Multicentricity and implications for treatment. *Ann Surg* 1980; 191:8–12.
18. Von Rueden DG, Wilson RE. Intraductal carcinoma of the breast. *Surg Gynecol Obstet* 1984;158:105–11.
19. Silverstein MJ, Rosser RJ, Gierson ED, et al. Axillary lymph node dissection for intraductal breast carcinoma—Is it indicated? *Cancer* 1987;59:1819–24.
20. Carter D, Smith RL. Carcinoma in situ of the breast. *Cancer* 1977;40:1189–93.
21. Fisher ER, Sass R, Fisher B, et al: Pathological findings from the National Surgical Adjuvant Breast Project (protocol 6), I. Intraductal carcinoma (DCIS). *Cancer* 1986;57:197–208.
22. Lagios MD, Westdahl PR, Margolin FR, et al. Duct carcinoma in situ: Relationship of extent of noninvasive disease to the frequency of occult invasion, multicentricity, lymph node metastases and short-term treatment failures. *Cancer* 1982;50:1309–14.
23. Sunshine JA, Moseley HS, Fletcher WS, et al. Breast carcinoma in situ: A retrospective review of 112 cases with a minimum of 10 year follow-up. *Am J Surg* 1985;150:44–51.

EDITORIAL BOARD COMMENTARY

Delay in the diagnosis of Paget's disease is common, and often exceeds the 6-month delay in this case. Any weeping, crusted eczematous type lesion of the nipple–areola complex should be promptly biopsied to rule out Paget's disease.

The treatment chosen in this patient with central disease as well as upper inner quadrant ductal carcinoma in situ was appropriate. Had the disease been confined to the nipple, consideration could be given to a breast-conserving approach with resection of the nipple–areola complex and surrounding breast tissue, no lymph node dissection unless invasion were identified and postoperative radiation therapy. Both the patient and surgeon need to thoroughly discuss and understand the compromise in cosmetic outcome with loss of the nipple.

85

DCIS with Cancerization of the Lobules

Robert R. Kuske, Gunnar Cederbom, Gist Farr, and John Bolton

Breast-conserving surgery or mastectomy for extensive DCIS?

HISTORY AND PHYSICAL EXAMINATION

C.L. is a 53-year-old asymptomatic woman who had had a routine screening mammography at another hospital. Based on mammographic findings, a biopsy was recommended. She sought a second opinion at our Multidisciplinary Breast Oncology Clinic.

She has been in excellent health with no medical illnesses. Her risk factors for breast cancer include a family history positive for postmenopausal breast cancer in a paternal aunt. She has taken no exogenous hormones or oral contraceptives. She is gravida 3, para 2, abortion 1, with her first pregnancy at age 24, menarche age 13, last menstrual period in 1986 prior to a hysterectomy without oophorectomy. Over the past year she has had some hot flashes, but she reports that a vaginal smear by her gynecologist revealed that she is premenopausal. She is a special education teacher living in central Louisiana with her husband, who is a lawyer.

Examination revealed a healthy-appearing, cooperative Caucasian woman. There was no supraclavicular or axillary adenopathy. The breasts were full and symmetric in size and shape, with no skin discoloration or dimpling. There were no palpable breast masses, even with special attention to the upper outer quadrant of the right breast. The rest of the examination was unremarkable.

DIAGNOSTIC EVALUATION

Interpretation of outside mammography films by our radiologist revealed scattered fibroglandular elements of rather high density mixed with fatty involuted regions (Fig. 85–1A). There is no suspicious mass in either breast. There is a series of clustered calcifications within the upper outer quadrant of the right breast starting approximately 1.6 cm from the nipple and extending to a distance of approximately 8 cm from the nipple, encompassing an entire lobe (Fig. 85–1B). The total area containing microcalcifications is 6.5 × 1.5 cm. The calcifications are pleomorphic, some have a "casting" appearance. The clusters are essentially in 3 separate groups located 2–2.5 cm apart, and are suspicious for malignancy. Needle-directed biopsy is suggested.

FIRST DISCUSSION AT TUMOR BOARD

Surgeon: I agree with the radiologist that this lesion certainly warrants a biopsy. My concern is that excision of the entire mammographic abnormality may require an extensive resection of the upper outer quadrant of her breast. If this were an invasive cancer, which it is unlikely to be, it would clinically be a T3 lesion.

Radiologist: I can needle-localize the proximal and distal extents of the microcalcifications. That may allow you to excise the whole lesion.

Surgeon: What if this lesion proves to be benign? An excision of that volume of breast tissue may deform her breast, and if the results are benign, it may be preferable to sample some of these microcalcifications to confirm malignancy.

Radiologist: These microcalcifications are quite suspicious for comedo carcinoma . . . I would be surprised if this turned out to be benign.

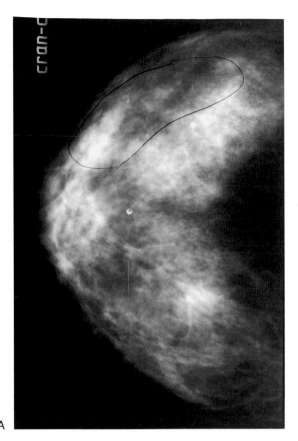
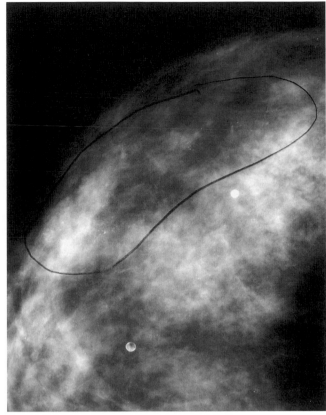

A

B

FIG. 85–1. A: Initial craniocaudal mammogram. Microcalcifications are seen in the large area laterally. **B:** Closeup of microcalcifications. Multiple clusters of pleomorphic calcifications.

Radiation Oncologist: This woman has relatively large breasts. The cosmesis can be surprisingly favorable when there is ample breast tissue, even in lesions of this size. I think an excisional biopsy should be performed. If this proves to be purely DCIS, she may be a candidate for the NSABP protocol B-24.

Medical Oncologist: I agree with that approach. The NSABP protocol permits enrolling patients even if there are microscopically positive surgical margins, or even in the presence of microcalcifications left within the breast.

TREATMENT

The radiologist placed two needle-localizing wires in the upper outer quadrant of the right breast, bracketing the sizeable area of microcalcifications (Fig. 85–2). The guide wires were approximately 6 cm apart, extending from close to the nipple in a radial fashion to the upper outer quadrant. Therefore, a radial incision was used, and a generous core of tissue incorporating the tips of both guide wires was excised. In the area underneath the nipple, a small amount of cheesy material suggesting comedo necrosis was noted, but there was no palpable mass.

Specimen radiography confirmed the presence of the vast majority of calcifications within the specimen, although the radiologist was not sure all of them had been removed (Fig. 85–3).

PATHOLOGY RESULTS

There are multifocal areas of comedo and apocrine-like DCIS seen. The tumor involves lobules by extension. There is no evidence of infiltrating carcinoma. The tumor is cut across by the superior margin resection line and the tumor is directly against the posterior and anterior margins. Other margins contain tumor within 1 mm of the inked margin.

SECOND PRESENTATION AT TUMOR BOARD

Surgeon: The pathologic stage is now Tis NX M0. Her breast is still cosmetically acceptable, but we have multiply positive surgical margins which I believe require a re-excision. She may be better treated by mastectomy if more surgery deforms her breast. The only randomized study in the literature, NSABP protocol B-17, demonstrated a three-

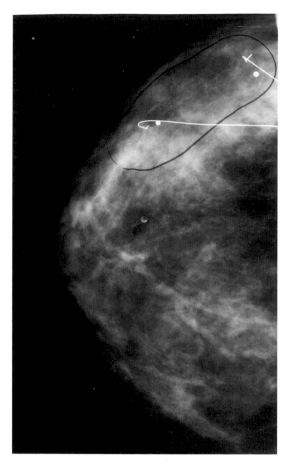

FIG. 85–2. Craniocaudal view after needle localization. Two wires were inserted in the area marked for the first biopsy.

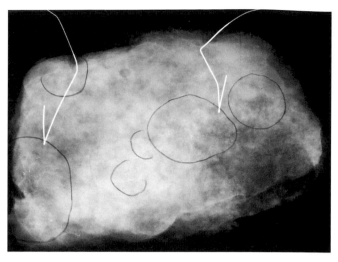

FIG. 85–3. Specimen radiogram from first excisional biopsy.

fold reduction in the risk of an invasive recurrence when lumpectomy is followed by radiation therapy, but we still do not know if and when a mastectomy is preferred.

Medical Oncologist: The NSABP protocol B-24 does not require complete excision of the lesion, and she can be entered right now. The entire breast is irradiated, and she will receive either tamoxifen or placebo on this protocol.

Radiation Oncologist: At our institution, we have elected to present this protocol only to women who have had a complete excision of the lesion as judged by a post-tylectomy mammogram demonstrating the absence of any remaining suspicious calcifications and re-excision with negative surgical margins. Considering this young woman's desire for breast preservation, and the good cosmetic outcome thus far, there is no reason why we should not attempt a re-excision to achieve these goals. What is the clinical significance of the pathologic finding of "lobular extension?"

Pathologist: Intraductal carcinomas can travel linearly down the duct. The malignant cells can spread in both directions, towards the nipple and peripherally into the terminal duct-lobular unit. As far as I know, with respect to treatment, there are no implications (Fig. 85–4).

Surgeon: I agree with our radiation oncologist that a post-tylectomy mammogram is indicated. Can any remaining microcalcifications be needle-localized again to direct the extent of my re-excision?

Radiologist: Any remaining microcalcifications can be needle-localized facilitating removal of the entire initial biopsy cavity along with the wire guides.

Surgeon: I hope that all this can be performed with an acceptable cosmetic result.

SECOND DIAGNOSTIC EVALUATION

The post-tylectomy mammogram revealed suspicious microcalcifications remaining beneath the nipple (Fig. 85–5A and Fig. 85–5B).

SECOND TREATMENT

A re-excision of the right upper outer quadrant removed a specimen measuring 8 × 6.5 × 3 cm, containing a 3.5 cm biopsy cavity. The specimen radiogram confirms removal of the remaining calcifications (Fig. 85–6).

The pathology report revealed ductal carcinoma in situ in two of the sections directly beneath the nipple, but not in any other areas of specimen. The carcinoma does not extend to any inked surgical margin.

A post-re-excision mammogram revealed complete excision of all microcalcifications.

THIRD PRESENTATION AT TUMOR BOARD

Surgeon: I now feel comfortable with this patient entering onto the NSABP protocol B- 24, if she desires. The only remaining potential carcinoma now is subclinical disease of a multicentric nature which radiotherapy will hopefully eradicate.

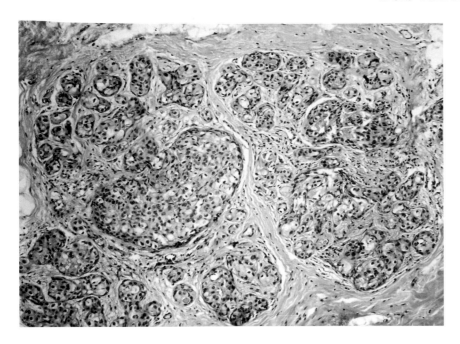

FIG. 85–4. Multifocal areas of comedo and apocrine-like DCIS are seen with involvement of the lobules by extension.

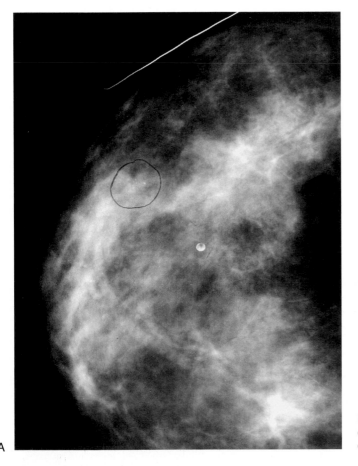

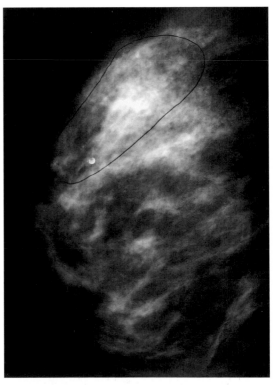

FIG. 85–5. A: Post-tylectomy mammogram. Calcifications remain anterior, close to the nipple. **B:** Needle localization of remaining calcifications.

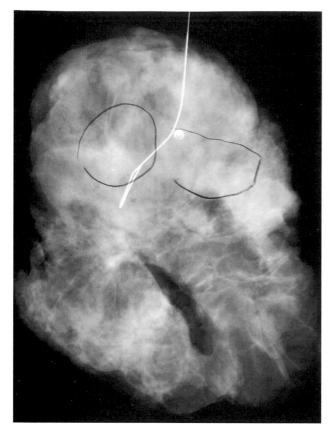

FIG. 85–6. Specimen radiogram after second excision, showing removal of microcalcifications.

Radiation Oncologist: I agree, this patient has already consented to the protocol. It is interesting that her cosmetic outcome remains favorable following excision and re-excision of a 6.5 cm mammographic lesion.

THIRD TREATMENT

The patient received pills which were either tamoxifen 10 mg or placebo to be taken twice daily. She started taking these pills at the start of breast irradiation. She received 50 Gy in 25 fractions to the right intact breast using medial and lateral tangential ports covering all mammary tissue. This was followed by a one week boost electron to the tylectomy site, measuring 7.5 × 11 cm because of the size of her excision. The boost also included the entire nipple. The boost dose was 10 Gy in 5 fractions utilizing 9 MeV electrons.

STATUS OF PATIENT

The patient has just been seen 4 months following the completion of breast irradiation, and 6 months from her diagnosis. Her first post-treatment mammogram revealed a large 9 × 4 cm seroma in the upper outer quadrant of the

right breast, with no microcalcifications. A mild lymphedema pattern consistent with her recent radiotherapy was noted (Fig. 85–7). The corrective result was excellent (Fig. 85–8).

The patient will be seen every 3 months for the first year, every 4 months for the second year, and every 6 months thereafter. Yearly bilateral mammography will be performed from the date of her first post-treatment mammographic evaluation. She will continue her tamoxifen/placebo for a duration of 5 years per the stipulations of the NSABP program.

COMMENTARY by Jay Harris

This case illustrates the careful mammographic and histologic evaluation and close cooperation and communication between specialists that is necessary when dealing with patients given the diagnosis of DCIS. DCIS is a breast lesion associated with the subsequent development of an ipsilateral invasive breast cancer. There has been a large increase in the incidence of the lesion over the last decade, due in large part to the more widespread use of

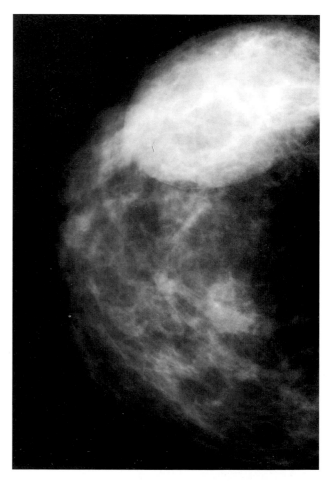

FIG. 85–7. Post-treatment mammogram.

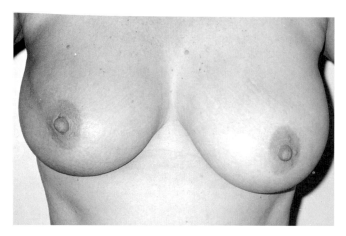

FIG. 85–8. Post-treatment photograph of the patient.

screening mammography. There is, however, uncertainty regarding the diagnostic criteria for the lesion and how frequently it will progress to invasive cancer. The comedo subtype of DCIS has a more malignant appearance histologically and appears to be associated with a greater risk of subsequent invasive cancer than the other subtypes of DCIS. As seen in this case, it is not uncommon for DCIS to involve a large portion of the breast (typically in a segmental pattern). Mastectomy is associated with a "cure" rate in the range of 99%, but is likely to represent overtreatment for many patients. Many women with DCIS prefer to have breast-conserving treatment if this can be shown to be reasonably "safe." As demonstrated in this case, for patients being considered for breast-conserving treatment, careful mammographic and histologic evaluation is critical to determine the extent of the lesion and the adequacy of the resection. Careful mammographic evaluation is very useful in assessing the full extent of the lesion and, on occasion, the presence of multicentric involvement. In particular, magnification views of the site of the lesion and the area extending toward the subareolar region are recommended to assess the full extent of the microcalcifications. A radiograph of the specimen and a post-excision mammogram are both mandatory to assess the adequacy of the resection. The pathologic evaluation of the resected breast specimen should include a description of the extent of the lesion within the specimen, the relationship between any calcifications observed microscopically and the lesion, and the proximity, presence, and extent of involvement in relation to the inked margin.

The risk of recurrence following breast-conserving treatment is higher than that for mastectomy (in the range of 10% to 20% percent at 10 years) and approximately one half of such recurrences contain invasive cancer. (It is anticipated that the risk of local recurrence will be decreased by the use of careful mammographic and histologic evaluation as described above.) A comparison of retrospective studies suggests that breast irradiation

decreases the rate of recurrence by about 50% to 70%. The 5-year results of the NSABP trial in patients with DCIS testing the utility of RT confirms this finding. However, in this trial, the size of the lesions is poorly described, and additional follow-up is required; it is uncertain which patients require mastectomy and which are adequately treated with breast-conserving surgery alone. For instance, it is not now known if the recurrence rate is higher than average for a patient with an extensive, but localized case of comedo-DCIS managed by breast-conserving therapy, as described here. A recent NSABP trial tests the value of tamoxifen in patients with DCIS treated with irradiation. This trial allowed entry for patients with involved margins and/or residual microcalcifications on mammography. Until the results of this trial are available, it is my view that, outside of a clinical trial, standard practice is to require negative margins of resection and removal of all suspicious microcalcifications seen on mammography.

How are we to judge the results from the available studies and interpret them for patients? One endpoint to judge the results of treatment is the risk of a recurrence, either DCIS or invasive, in the treated breast. It can now be questioned whether treatment with excision is a reasonable option of patients with the comedo subtype. For many patients and clinicians, the 25 percent recurrence rate seen in the Lagios experience and the 43 percent recurrence rate in the Schwartz experience may be too high. The use of excision alone for small areas of noncomedo DCIS, on the other hand, appears attractive based on this endpoint. This is particularly true for patients with *very* small non-comedo lesions, some of which may be difficult to distinguish from atypical ductal hyperplasia. Another and probably more relevant endpoint is the risk of an invasive cancer in the treated breast. In considering this endpoint, it may be useful to put this issue into a broader perspective. Breast cancer is a common disease in industrial societies. In the US, about 2% of women aged 50 will develop an invasive breast cancer over the following decade. In women with risk factors for the development of breast cancer, this risk is even higher. Among patients given the diagnosis of lobular carcinoma in situ, the risk of an invasive breast cancer is about 10% to 15% over 10 years. For all of the preceding groups of patients, it is now uncommon to recommend prophylactic mastectomy. Among the patients with DCIS treated with breast conserving treatment, the risk of an invasive cancer is about 5% to 10% over 10 years. When viewed from this perspective, the use of breast-conserving treatment appears reasonable. A further endpoint that is relevant for many patients is the risk of losing their breast. At this time, it is not certain what percent of patients with a limited area of DCIS treated by breast conserving treatment will require a mastectomy in the event of a recurrence. This issue is of particular relevance in patients with a relatively small breast where further excision (in the event of a recurrence) will not be feasible. In such patients, the use of irradiation may be important simply to minimize the risk of mastectomy. Finally, the endpoint of greatest relevance is the risk of dying of the breast cancer. At this time, it is not certain whether invasive cancers that follow conservative treatment for a mammographically-detected DCIS have a more favorable (or less favorable) outcome. Many more patient-years of follow-up will be required to address this critical question.

DCIS represents both a challenge and an opportunity for the 1990s. The identification of biological markers for progression to invasive breast cancer would greatly improve the management of patients with DCIS. Given the importance of breast conservation for many women, it is important to develop rules for the successful use of breast-conserving treatment. Long-term studies are needed to define the mortality risk associated with breast-conserving treatment. Finally, it may be useful to consider patients with DCIS as "high risk" and thus candidates for trials testing the value of prevention (e.g., with tamoxifen, as done by the NSABP).

REFERENCES

1. Fisher B, Constantino J, Redmond C, et al. Lumpectomy compared with lumpectomy and radiation therapy for treatment of intraductal breast cancer. N Engl J Med 1993; 328:1581–6.
2. Morrow M, Schnitt SJ, and Harris JR. Ductal Carcinoma In Situ. In: *Disease of the Breast*, Harris JR, Lippman ME, Morrow M, and Hellman S, eds. Philadelphia: Lippincott-Raven, 1996.

86

Incidental Finding of Lobular Carcinoma In Situ of the Breast with Duct Involvement in a Biopsy Done for Mammographic Microcalcification

Jonathan F. Lara, Robert V.P. Hutter, and Richard A. Michaelson

A combination of DCIS and LCIS: a challenge for patient communication and treatment

CASE PRESENTATION

Clinical History: This 41-year-old asymptomatic woman was referred for further evaluation of a lesion, discovered by mammography, in the upper outer quadrant of the right breast. The patient's past medical history was unremarkable, and she had no known increased risk factors. She has had two normal spontaneous vaginal deliveries and no family history of cancer. She is a nonsmoker and drinks socially. Her physical examination was completely within normal limits. Because of the mammographic findings, needle localization with directed excisional biopsy of the retroareolar region of the right breast was done.

Radiology (Dr. Kalisher): A cluster of fine microcalcifications was localized (Fig. 86–1). The remaining breast parenchyma consisted of dense fibroglandular tissue.

Pathology (Dr. Lara): A single segment of fibrofatty mammary tissue with localizing needle in place weighing 18.5 g and measuring 4.2 × 4.0 × 2.2 cm was received for intraoperative consultation. The tissue was gritty and firm. A frozen section of the area was prepared and interpreted as intraductal carcinoma, cribriform, and solid type with extension into terminal ducts and lobules. In subsequent paraffin sections (Fig. 86–2A) there was evidence of a florid proliferation of in situ carcinoma, involving mainly the lobular units with retrograde extension into terminal ducts and evident pagetoid foci (Fig. 86–2B). Other sections disclosed a dichotomous growth pattern, some ductules with typical features of lobular carcinoma in situ, others with a pattern more consistent with ductal carcinoma in situ (Fig. 86–2C). In another area, there was cribriform architecture (Fig. 86–2D). The specimen was replete with microcalcifications. There was no evidence of invasion. The inked surgical margins were involved by lobular carcinoma in situ. Our final diagnosis was predominantly in situ lobular carcinoma with focal extension into terminal ducts and displaying features of ductal carcinoma in situ.

DISCUSSION

The case presented was that of a young woman with diffuse changes of lobular carcinoma in situ with focal evidence of retrograde extension into ducts showing a pattern of ductal carcinoma in situ. The questions to be addressed are what is the nature of this entity, and what do we have to offer this patient and future patients with similar disease in terms of initial therapy, adjuvant therapy and follow-up?

419

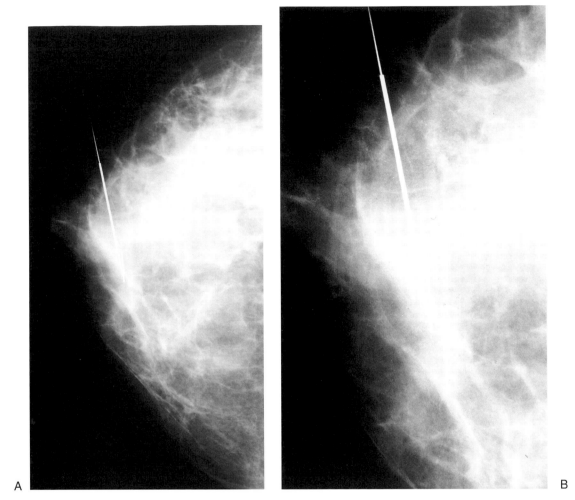

FIG. 86–1. A: Cephalocaudal mammogram with a localization wire in place. **B:** Magnification view of **A**. There is no mass component; the radiographic diagnosis was made on the basis of fine calcium deposits. The hook wire indicates the optimum biopsy site.

The discussion was initiated by the pathologist, who explained the microscopic anatomy of the breast. He pointed out that the excretory pathway of the mammary gland starts from the terminal ductule of the lobular unit, which is surrounded by an intralobular stromal complex. The terminal ductules extend to the intralobular terminal duct, which becomes the extralobular terminal duct. The terminal ducts extend into small ducts, major ducts, and lactiferous sinus, and finally out to the nipple–areola complex. At any point in this continuum of epithelial-lined spaces, there is a proliferation of epithelium. It has been pointed out that proliferations with ductal patterns (i.e., cribriform, solid, and micropapillary) often occur within "inflated" terminal ductules of the lobular units and occasionally within terminal ducts. It is therefore not a specific cell of origin that determines the type of epithelial proliferation, but the morphologic pattern and pathway of growth undertaken.

The radiologist pointed out that lobular carcinoma in situ is usually a serendipitous finding with a high degree of multifocality and bilaterality. It is more common in dense breasts and usually the microcalcifications are not within the lobular carcinoma in situ, as they are in this case. He also pointed out that patients with lobular carcinoma in situ had a 20% to 30% risk of developing an invasive carcinoma within the next 15 to 20 years, and that often the invasive lesion was of ductal histology rather than lobular.

Based on the pathologic findings, it is apparent that the patient has a florid proliferation involving lobules and terminal ducts with histologic patterns satisfying criteria for both lobular and ductal carcinoma in situ. The next question of how to proceed with treatment was then raised.

A breast surgeon felt that in this situation he would disregard the lobular component and concentrate on the ductal component. However, due to the size of the lesion, as well as the presence of tumor at the biopsied margin,

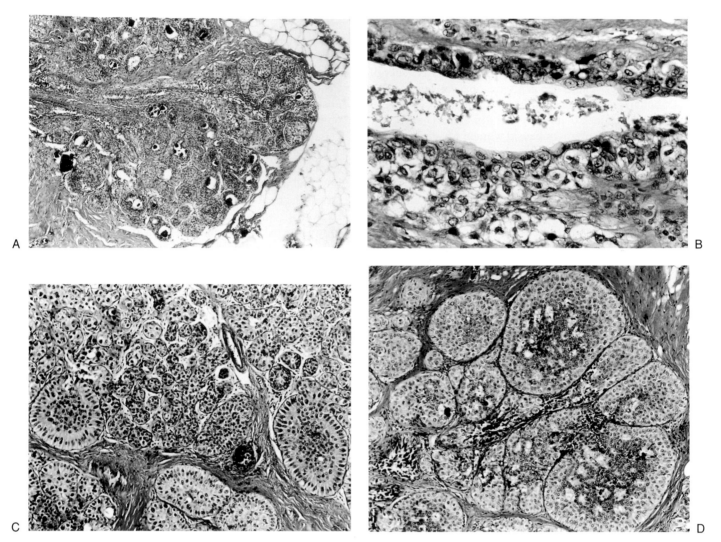

Fig. 86–2. A–D: Lobular carcinoma in situ with terminal duct extension.

he felt that a simple mastectomy would be in order rather than a breast-sparing procedure. He did not think that an axillary dissection was necessary because the percentage of positive nodes in ductal carcinoma in situ is less than 1%, which is virtually unheard of in lobular carcinoma in situ. Also, the ductal component was of the cribriform type as opposed to the comedo type. He did not feel it was necessary to do a contralateral biopsy as the likelihood of finding an occult invasive cancer would be remote, and the findings of lobular carcinoma in situ would not warrant treatment.

Another surgeon commented that lobular carcinoma in situ is a marker for a neoplastic condition and that ductal carcinoma in situ is a pre-invasive malignant process.

Radiation oncology was asked about the role of adjuvant radiation therapy for this patient. They believed that if the patient would be offered a lumpectomy, then certainly adjuvant radiation therapy would be recommended based on the recently published B17 study of the NSABP, although the data of short-term and long-term benefits are still uncertain. If mastectomy is the chosen therapy, there would be no need for adjuvant radiation.

The medical oncologist raised several important issues. First, the choice of lumpectomy versus mastectomy. Mastectomy has always been the gold standard. Most of the long-term studies available, however, are small and retrospective. The need for negative surgical margins with lumpectomy was also addressed. It was believed that most investigators support the need for negative surgical margins although the B24 protocol from the NSABP—which randomized patients with ductal carcinoma in situ, treated with lumpectomy and radiation, to tamoxifen or placebo—allows for positive margins.

He also raised the question of the role of tamoxifen not only for ductal carcinoma in situ but for lobular carcinoma in situ. Would it be of benefit to this patient? Would it reduce the risk of a second primary breast cancer? Can the risk to benefit ratio be justified in this young patient?

Finally, what is the significance of this patient's malady to her female offspring or siblings? There was general agreement that because she is premenopausal, her daughters would likely have a significantly higher risk of developing breast cancer than the general public. The role of mammography in premenopausal women was briefly discussed. It was felt that while the benefit of screening mammography in women under 50 is not accepted by all investigators, women under 50 with associated risk factors will probably benefit from screening.

In summary, the consensus was that a total mastectomy should be recommended and that there was no need for an axillary dissection or adjuvant radiation or hormonal therapy. Her prognosis is excellent, although the patient should be closely watched in view of her increased risk of a contralateral cancer. A mirror image biopsy was not considered to be necessary. A final comment was made that perhaps in the near future identification of the BRCA-1 gene may be available for testing. However, the identification of a carrier along with the social and ethical ramifications associated with such a finding have to be addressed. No further questions were raised and the Tumor Board meeting was adjourned.

COMMENTARY by Robert T. Osteen

This case exemplifies the uncertainties and frustrations that result from mammographic screening and our current state of knowledge regarding in situ carcinoma. The patient, a 41-year-old woman, had a needle localized biopsy of an area of microcalcifications found on a screening mammogram. The pathologic appearance was a mixture of ductal carcinoma in situ (DCIS) and lobular carcinoma in situ (LCIS). The microcalcifications were diffusely spread throughout the specimen and appeared to be associated with the in situ carcinoma. The growth patterns and histologic appearances of DCIS and LCIS can merge, making distinctions between the two difficult and perhaps meaningless (1,2).

Since the work of Haagensen et al., the natural history of lobular carcinoma in situ has been relatively well understood (3). It is considered a marker lesion that is usually discovered accidentally in a biopsy performed for some other reason. It predicts a risk of cancer in either breast of about 20% to 30% over a long period of time. The fact that LCIS is not detected mammographically means that the entity Haagensen described is the one we are dealing with today. Unlike LCIS, the natural history of DCIS is unclear. The ability to identify small areas of nonpalpable DCIS by microcalcifications on a screening mammogram has defined a new clinical entity. Before screening mammography DCIS was identified as a palpable lesion, usually with comedo necrosis, which had a sig-

nificant risk of turning into an invasive cancer if not treated by mastectomy. This new mammographically discovered entity usually has a lower proliferative thrust, probably has a longer premalignant phase, and has been treated so effectively that its natural history remains obscure (4,5). Faced with such a problem, the clinician's obligation is to treat the more dangerous component of the pathology.

The options for therapy are well discussed by the Tumor Board. The risk of axillary nodal metastases is low, and axillary nodal dissection is not justified regardless of the treatment of the breast (6). Although the risk of microinvasion is related to the extent of ductal carcinoma in situ, the risk of lymph node metastases remains low (7). Furthermore, in this situation, it is not clear that a given amount of tissue with this pathology would have the same risk for microinvasion as the same volume of pure DCIS.

The choice of local therapy, lumpectomy or mastectomy, is often related to the volume of breast tissue believed to be involved, the size of the breast, and the location within the breast. These factors bear on the potential for achieving the goals of minimizing the risk of recurrence in the breast while preserving a satisfactory cosmetic outcome.

The volume of DCIS may be difficult to determine. The mammographic microcalcifications by which it is commonly identified often define only a portion of the disease and not its extent. In this patient, the area of mammographic microcalcification is not given and does not reproduce well in the photograph. The biopsy specimen was $4.2 \times 2.0 \times 2.2$ cm, and this specimen was said to be "replete with microcalcifications." One must assume that additional DCIS, perhaps a substantial amount, remained in the breast after the diagnostic biopsy since no specimen radiograph or postexcision mammogram is included.

The needle localization film shows the needle in the subareolar position. DCIS tends to track toward the nipple. Pagetoid-type progression was seen in the specimen. The surgeon had to consider the major ducts of the nipple to be at risk.

A role for radiation therapy in patients who have a lumpectomy has been suggested by the NSABP-B17 protocol and others (8,9). Radiation therapy appears to decrease the risk of recurrence by about one half. The precise indications for radiation therapy and the need for radiation therapy in all circumstances remains debatable. The safety of substituting radiation therapy for negative surgical margins is unknown and will not be resolved by the NSABP-B24 protocol. Similarly, the possibility of reduction of local recurrence by use of tamoxifen is unproven, and the use of tamoxifen for that purpose is best confined to experimental protocols.

The declaration of negative margins is subject to limitations. Because of potential multifocality, narrow, negative margins should be viewed with skepticism (10). No uniform definition of negative margins exists, but the band of normal tissue surrounding any identifiable focus of DCIS should be wider than the band of normal tissue that would permit a case of invasive carcinoma to be declared as having negative margins. Wide excisions may interfere with a satisfactory cosmetic result. When all of these factors are considered in this case, the choice for mastectomy appears to be a good one.

The Tumor Board raised several interesting questions regarding the risk for other family members. Although the risk for first-degree relatives appears to be increased by having breast cancer at a premenopausal age, the risk associated with premenopausal DCIS is unknown. The relationship between family risk and histologic subtype has not been thoroughly investigated; however, a relationship between family history and LCIS has been suggested (11,12). The safest course is to screen family members as if they are at higher risk.

REFERENCES

1. Kerner H, Lichtig C. Lobular cancerization: incidence and differential diagnosis with lobular carcinoma in situ of breast. *Histopathology* 1986;10:621–9.
2. Ottesen LL, Graversen HP, Blicher-Toft M, et al. Lobular carcinoma in situ of the female breast. Short-term results of a prospective nationwide study. *Am J Surg Pathol* 1993;17:14–21.
3. Haagensen CD, Lane N, Lattes R, Bodian C. Lobular neoplasia (so-called lobular carcinoma in situ) of the breast. *Cancer* 1978;42:737–69.
4. Meyer JS. Cell kinetics of histologic variants of in situ breast carcinoma. *Breast Cancer Res Treat* 1986;7:171–80.
5. Lagios MD, Margolin FR, Westdahl PR, Rose MR. Mammographically detected duct carcinoma in situ. Frequency of local recurrence following tyelectomy and prognostic effect of nuclear grade on local recurrence. *Cancer* 1989;63:618–24.
6. Silverstein MH, Gierson ED, Colburn WJ, et al. Axillary lymphadenectomy for intraductal carcinoma of the breast. *Surg Gynecol Obstet* 1991; 172:211–14.
7. Silverstein MH, Gierson ED, Waisman JR, et al. Axillary lymph node dissection for T1a breast carcinoma. Is is indicated? *Cancer* 1994;73: 664–7.
8. Fisher B, Costantino J, Redmond C, et al. Lumpectomy compared with lumpectomy and radiation therapy for the treatment of intraductal breast cancer. *New Engl J Med* 1993;328:1581–6.
9. Solin LJ, Recht A, Fourquet A, et al. Ten-year results of breast conserving surgery and definitive irradiation for intraductal carcinoma (ductal carcinoma in situ) of the breast. *Cancer* 1991;68:2337–44.
10. Holland R, Veling SHJ, Mravunac M, Hendricks JHCL. Histologic multifocality of Tis, T1-2 breast carcinomas. Implications for clinical trials of breast conserving surgery. *Cancer* 1985;56:979–90.
11. Rosen PP, Lesser ML, Senie RT, Kinne DW. Epidemiology of breast carcinoma III. Relationship of family history to tumor type. *Cancer* 1982;50:171–9.
12. Claus EB, Risch N, Thompson WD, Carter D. Relationship between breast histopathology and family history of breast cancer. *Cancer* 1993;71:147–53.

87

Tubular Carcinoma of the Breast

Scott M. Noel and John F. Foley

Less aggressive treatment for an excellent prognosis tumor?

CASE PRESENTATION

This 46-year-old white woman requested that her primary physician see her regarding a newly discovered breast mass. The patient had been known to have fibrocystic changes in the breast for more than 10 years. Ten months before the above problem, she had routine screening mammography. The mammograms showed dense tissues with multiple lobulated areas (Fig. 87–1). After consulting with the surgeon, ultrasound examination of the breasts showed the nodules were cystic and no further study was deemed necessary.

At this time, examination of her breasts demonstrated a 1- to 2-cm firm mass in the upper inner quadrant of her left breast. A mammogram confirmed the presence of the mass (Fig. 87–1A,B), which had developed in the 10-month interval since her last study. An ultrasound of the mass showed a complex cyst (Fig. 87–2).

The patient had had a hysterectomy without removal of her ovaries 14 years previously. She is nulliparous. There is one aunt who has had breast cancer. Past medical history includes subtotal thyroidectomy for benign disease with subsequent hypothyroidism and trigeminal neuralgia associated with significant depression requiring psychiatric care.

Laboratory studies included a hemoglobin level of 11.8 g/dL and a normal white blood cell count, chemistry profile, and chest roentgenogram.

After presenting the case at the Tumor Board, it was the opinion of the board that the nodule should be surgically removed with adequate margins. The patient requested only the "lumpectomy" with a decision on further surgery after final pathologic examination.

The excisional biopsy specimen consisted of a portion of breast tissue that was 3.5 cm in greatest dimension. In addition to focal fibrosis and cystic change, the cut surfaces exhibited an ill-defined, infiltrative mass with dimensions of $1.4 \times 1.2 \times 0.9$ cm. This mass was very firm, white, and had a gritty consistency. The cryostat impression was deferred to permanent sections, which demonstrated invasive adenocarcinoma. The invasive component consisted of well-formed, oval to round glands with open lumina infiltrating dense fibrous stroma (Fig. 87–3). Many of the glands were partially compressed by the dense fibrosis and appeared curved and angulated ("comma shaped") (Fig. 87– 4). A single row of uniform neoplastic epithelial cells lined each space. The tumor cells displayed low-grade nuclear features and abundant cytoplasmic projections (apical snouts) extending from the luminal surface (Figs. 87–5 and 6). The initial biopsy specimen also demonstrated fibrocystic changes characterized by varying degrees of ductal hyperplasia and papillomatosis and multifocal ductal carcinoma in-situ.

On presentation to the Tumor Board, there was considerable discussion on further management of this unusual case. Tubular carcinomas generally have a good prognosis with only one in 10 having axillary metastases. As less than 10% have been treated with simple mastectomy or excisional treatment, there was insufficient data to make firm recommendations to the patient. However, because excision and radiation therapy is acceptable in invasive carcinomas and equal to modified radical mastectomy in results, it was believed by the Board that this could be offered to the patient. After discussion with her surgeon, oncologist, and primary physician, the patient decided on

424

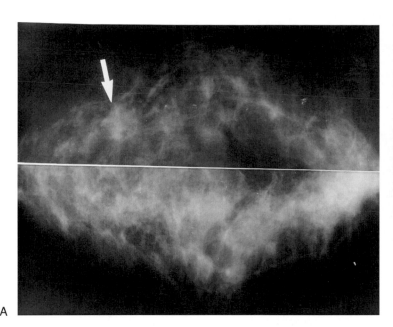
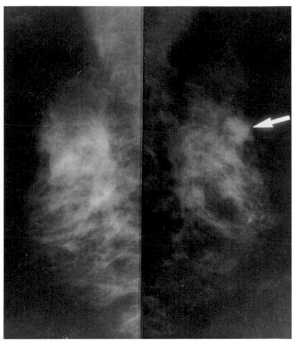

A   B

Fig. 87–1. Craniocaudal **(A)** and mediolateral oblique **(B)** mammograms of the left breast. Baseline mammogram on left and study before surgery. Arrows indicate a spiculated mass on the presurgical films. The images are mounted back-to-back for comparative purposes. The mass may have been present on the baseline study but was not reported.

a modified radical mastectomy with immediate reconstruction.

She had the definitive surgery 4 days after her excisional biopsy. A pathologic study disclosed residual ductal carcinoma *in situ* and invasive tubular and ductal adenocarcinoma with deep surgical margins free of tumor. There was infiltrating nontubular ductal carcinoma in only one area, whereas there were extensive areas of tubular carcinoma. Twenty-two lymph nodes were free of metastatic carcinoma. The tumor was T1 N0 M0, stage I. Indirect immunoperoxidase stain of the initial tumor was done for antibodies to human estrogen and progesterone receptor. There was weak staining with estrogen receptor whereas there was intense staining for progesterone staining.

The patient had immediate breast reconstruction with a Becker implant/expander underneath the pectoralis minor muscle and had a smooth convalescence.

Adjuvant therapy with cytoxan, methotrexate, and flourouracil was offered to the patient with the clear understanding that it would help only a minority of such patients as they have a good prognosis without further therapy. Nevertheless, the patient decided to receive adjuvant therapy and received her program without difficulties. The radiation therapist believed that local radiation therapy was not indicated and that tamoxifen was not offered to her after the chemotherapy.

Ten months after her surgery, a suspicious 2-cm nodule was noted in the patient's right breast. She decided to have a simple mastectomy and not endure further biop-

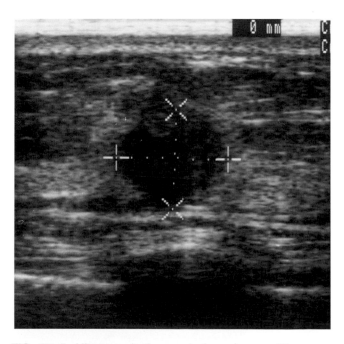

FIG. 87–2. Ultrasound of mass before surgery. There are some features consistent with a complex cyst, but a solid tumor could not be excluded.

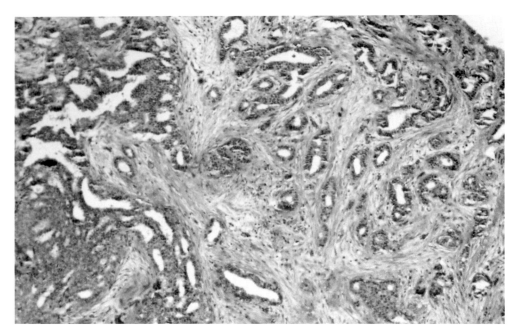

FIG. 87–3. Tubular carcinoma. The infiltrating tumor consists of round to oval glands with open lumina. Also note the ductal hyperplasia and papillomatosis at the left (Hematoxylin and eosin; ×40).

sies. The breast showed only fibrocystic disease with focal ductal hyperplasia and two fibroadenomas. No non-invasive or invasive tubular carcinoma was found. One could speculate that the chemotherapy may have elimi-nated them. The patient remains well 3 years after initial surgery.

COMMENTARY by Blake Cady

This patient referred by Drs. Noel and Foley brings up several interesting points. This is a 46-year-old woman who had a 1.4 cm tubular carcinoma with negative nodes and was treated with mastectomy, reconstruction, and

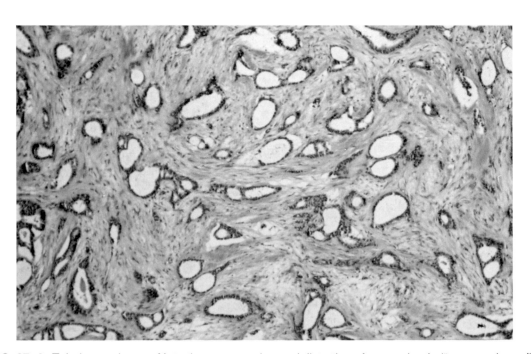

FIG. 87–4. Tubular carcinoma. Note the compression and distortion of some glands ("comma shaped") (Hematoxylin and eosin; ×40).

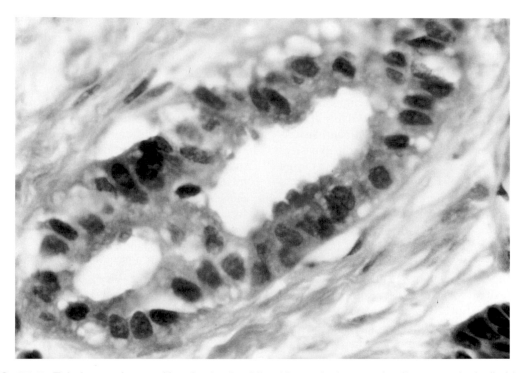

FIG. 87–5. Tubular carcinoma. Neoplastic gland lined by a single row of uniform, cytologically bland cells (Hematoxylin and eosin; ×400).

adjuvant chemotherapy. Ten months later, the patient elected to have a contralateral mastectomy even though she had no biopsy of a small palpable mass and had only fibrocystic changes on pathology of the opposite breast. That mastectomy of the opposite side presumably was accompanied by immediate reconstruction just as her original mastectomy had been.

This case is most interesting because it illustrates many contemporary issues about breast cancer and, in particular, brings forth issues that need to be addressed about very

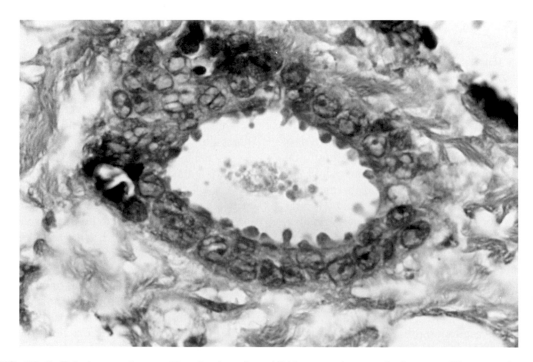

FIG. 87–6. Tubular carcinoma. Neoplastic cells exhibiting prominent apical snouts (Hematoxylin and eosin; ×400).

small or very low grade breast cancers that are increasingly found with mammographic screening. For instance, almost 10% of mammographically discovered cancers 1 cm or less in diameter (T1A T1B) are of tubular histology. Such tubular cancers have an exceedingly good prognosis.

It would be the hope that increasingly common recognition of very small breast cancers might lead to still more conservative modifications of current treatment. Just as radical mastectomy gave way to modified radical mastectomy as breast cancers decreased in size and extent during the 1950s and 1960s and just as mastectomy gave way to local excision and radiation therapy with still smaller cancers in more recent times, so we can expect lumpectomy, axillary dissection, and radiation therapy to give way to still more conservative options as the size of breast cancers continues to decrease under the impact of extensive screening programs in this country. In the SEER data ending in 1988, 13% of all invasive breast cancers were less than 1 cm in diameter. Such very small cancers may continue to increase (as a proportion of breast cancer) because more women have screening mammography and adhere to screening guidelines.

This patient had a normal screening mammography 10 months before she palpated a mass. At the time of the palpated mass, another mammogram was obtained and the mass was seen. Obviously, the presence of a palpable suspicious mass demands biopsy even though a mammogram might show nothing. An ultrasound of the mass supposedly showed a "complex cyst". Whether the lesion that was called a "complex cyst" was actually the cancer or not is uncertain but breast cancers do not generally present with any cystic component. Cancers appearing in cysts are quite rare so that the usual echographic finding of a true cystic lesion generally eliminates the possibility of a cancer. It was unnecessary to obtain the echogram of a palpable mass that was to be aspirated at least and removed by biopsy eventually.

At the described presentation of a mass, no needle aspiration or aspiration cytology was done. Masses in 40-year-old women are frequently found to be cysts and can be diagnosed without ultrasonography by the insertion of a needle into the palpable mass. Needle aspiration in the office is a far cheaper, and more reliable, and more rapid in diagnosis of a cyst than is ultrasound. This saves time and money and relieves the patient immediately when the cyst disappears. A benign diagnosis of cyst is certain if fluid is obtained and the mass disappears; but if the mass is solid or does not disappear with insertion of the needle, then cellular material can be withdrawn by aspiration and submitted for cytology examination. At least 75% of cancers that have a needle aspiration can be diagnosed with this simple technique. In the office, I personally perform an immediate needle aspiration of any mass that appears in a woman's breast because this is the most cost-efficient, rapid, and accurate way of separating palpable cysts from other lesions and making a cytologic diagnosis of

cancer. Every surgeon who deals with women having breast lumps should insert a needle in every palpable breast mass in the office on the first visit. Cytologic study will usually provide a diagnosis of cancer if that is the diagnosis and sometimes can even eliminate the need for open biopsy if the woman wishes to proceed directly with mastectomy. This might apply particularly to elderly women but only infrequently to women in the their 40s.

The patient had a hysterectomy at the age of 32, but the ovaries were left in place. That is certainly appropriate treatment for a young woman requiring hysterectomy but the surgeon should know why the hysterectomy was performed. Whether it was done for carcinoma in-situ, invasive carcinoma of the cervix, or for a benign condition is helpful in understanding the woman's general situation upon presentation with breast complaints. There was one aunt who has had breast cancer; however, the aunt's age is not given. Premenopausal first-degree relatives communicate significant increase in risk of breast cancer to patients (risk ratios of 3 to 6); however, second degree relatives (aunts, grandmothers) have an unknown risk communication. Postmenopausal first-degree relatives communicate a far lower risk of cancer (risk ratio of only 1 to 3).

The presentation then stated that the patient requested only the lumpectomy with the decision for further surgery after final pathologic examination. It should be standard in 1993 for the surgeons and physicians to insist on only a lumpectomy/biopsy performed under local anesthesia as the first step; the patient should be relieved of the anxiety and fear that the surgeon would even consider immediate mastectomy. In this age of sophisticated treatment of breast cancer, it is critical to obtain thorough pathologic information before mastectomy, lumpectomy, axillary dissection or *any* further treatment. It is inappropriate to do one-step biopsy and mastectomy or biopsy/lumpectomy and axillary dissection because sophisticated therapeutic decisions require detailed understanding of the final pathology report, not just the frozen section, in contemporary breast cancer management.

This mass was firm, white, and gritty with a maximum gross dimension of 1.4 cm. typical of a carcinoma. The excisional biopsy specimen was 3.5 cm in greatest dimension for a mass described as 1 to 2 cm in diameter; therefore, she had the equivalent of a satisfactory lumpectomy with a 1-cm margin around the tumor apparently. Cryostat impression was deferred to permanent sections indicating that the pathologist had difficulty in making a diagnosis of cancer quite characteristic of tubular carcinomas. The histologic feature of the invasive carcinoma was typical of a tubular type. In addition, the biopsy revealed ductal hyperplasia and multifocal ductal carcinoma in-situ (DCIS), both commonly accompanying the tubular pattern. It is unclear what the extent of the DCIS was and whether it fulfilled the requirements of an extensive intraductal component (EIC positive). One prime reason for separately analyzing the final pathology in detail before proceeding with discussions regarding surgery for breast cancer is the diagnosis of an extensive intraductal component defined by at least 25% of the invasive tumor consisting of DCIS and moderate or marked amount of DCIS in surrounding tissues (both components of the in-situ carcinoma have to be present to be labelled as EIC positive) and the histologic analysis of tissue margins. Patients that are EIC-positive or -negative may both be highly suitable for lumpectomy, but in EIC-negative cases, the lumpectomy surgical margins do not have to be pathologically negative. However, for EIC-positive cases, the margins of the lumpectomy should be pathologically negative to achieve a relatively low recurrence rate and thus re-excisions may be required.

There is ample data for any Tumor Board in the United States today to make recommendations to patients and physicians that because survival results are absolutely equivalent when comparing lumpectomy with mastectomy in any type of breast cancer, these two options are available and should be presented to the patient. This is particularly true with small invasive carcinomas with or without extensive intraductal component. In addition, there are ample data regarding the biology of tubular carcinoma and the unusually good prognosis, particularly when it is a pure tubular carcinoma or where there is only a small (<10%) proportion of other features such as ductal carcinoma, as was true in this case. Because of their particularly low rate of recurrence and metastases, tubular carcinomas are uniquely suitable to lumpectomy and breast preservation, particularly when the carcinoma is small.

It is wise to separate the two components of failure of breast cancer management: local recurrence in the retained breast and distant metastatic disease. Although survival rate is exactly the same comparing lumpectomy and mastectomy, local recurrence rates may be quite different. In EIC-positive cases, local recurrences in the retained breast after conservative surgery may be as high as 40% or more, particularly if the final lumpectomy margins are positive. While that may not deter some patients who are particularly anxious to keep their breast, (since this still leaves a 60% chance to keep their breast) other patients might choose mastectomy in such a situation because of concern about vigilance for the in-breast recurrence. It is difficult and requires time and discussion to explain to patients the difference between local in-breast recurrence, which has no impact on survival, and distant metastases, which clearly governs survival. However it is critical to explain these aspects of biology in order to get the best informed decision by the patients. Patients may well be willing to accept a significant risk of local recurrence, particularly if they know that in-breast recurrence does not interfere with their survival expectations.

The final pathology of the mastectomy specimen disclosed residual ductal carcinoma in-situ but does not describe how much residual disease was present. Was this disease that would have been encompassed with a re-

excision of the original lesion if the patient had been fully desirous of keeping her breast? The pathology was noted to show only "one area with infiltrating non-tubular ductal carcinoma whereas there are extensive areas of tubular carcinoma" (i.e., < 10% non-tubular). The data in the literature regarding the excellent outcome from treatment of tubular carcinoma is based on a definition that includes the vast majority of the pathology being tubular, not that every single slide of the tumor shows the tubular pattern. Thus this patient had a tubular carcinoma and that diagnosis is not changed by a few slides showing features of invasive ductal carcinoma. It is not known how much residual tumor there was volumetrically but the disease-free survival of a 1.4 cm tubular carcinoma, even if there is some residual ductal carcinoma in-situ and invasive disease is extremely good. Small tubular carcinomas have an extremely good prognosis with probably at least a 95% survival. It is noted that the 22 lymph nodes were free of metastatic carcinoma in the axillary dissection that accompanied the mastectomy. The likelihood of a lymph node metastases in tubular carcinoma is extremely low, probably not more than 5% in a tubular carcinoma of 1.4 cm in maximum diameter. Whether such a low risk of an axillary lymph node metastasis justifies an axillary dissection is a question to be decided; however, the benefit/risk ration is extremely low.

The patient had a breast reconstruction with a silicone implant under the pectoralis muscle, with a smooth convalescence. It should be pointed out that there are no scientific data whatsoever that indicate any major health penalty or impairment of cure from breast cancer or induced illness from the use of silicone implants for breast reconstruction. The wide publicity about the dangers of breast reconstruction with implants at the hearings in Washington was completely without any scientific foundation. The rulings of that panel and of the FDA Commissioner were not based on science but on political expediency. Therefore, breast reconstruction can be offered to every person undergoing mastectomy. This is a reasonable way to restore the breast mound and shape with minimal risk and inconvenience if mastectomy is required or requested.

After surgery, the patient was offered cytoxan, methotrexate, and fluorouracil therapy (CMF). This is astonishing given the fact that the patient had a 1.4-cm tubular carcinoma with negative nodes. Those pathologic findings meant she had at least a 95% disease free survival expectation at 5 years; indeed, survival might well be higher than that.

Proportional reduction in recurrence by the use of adjuvant chemotherapy is at most 25% to 30%. Thus, the maximum increase in disease-free state such a patient could achieve would be only 1% or 2% (i.e., 30% of 5%). This means that for every 100 patients like this woman in such an extremely low-risk situation who are given CMF adjuvant chemotherapy 98% to 99% of patients would be treated unnecessarily. Adjuvant chemotherapy was clearly not designed to improve an already superb result but should be offered to patients who have a poor prognosis. Clearly, a patient with a small tubular carcinoma should be told that she does not need adjuvant chemotherapy because the gains would be so small compared with the price paid in terms of morbidity and expense.

The Tumor Board also indicated that the radiation therapist believed that radiation therapy was not indicated and tamoxifen was not offered to her after the chemotherapy. I might ask why even consider radiation therapy after mastectomy? There is ample data to indicate that post-mastectomy radiation therapy does not change the survival rate whatsoever and therefore there should be few if any indications for it, particularly in this case when the cancer was so small and of such low grade.

Lastly, the other issue brought up by this case is that 10 months later, the patient had a palpable nodule in the opposite breast and elected to have mastectomy apparently for prophylaxis although no biopsy was performed to indicate whether she had a cancer or any high-risk ductal changes. It is my experience that most women in their mid 40s have a great desire to keep at least one natural breast; and as long as it is explained to them that with a careful mammographic screening program and with a risk of a cancer developing in the opposite breast of no greater than 1% per year, most are quite happy to keep their breast and undergo surveillance rather than have a "prophylactic" mastectomy. Certainly prophylactic mastectomy may be very important when women are at extremely high risk, as when multiple family members have premenopausal breast cancer. However, when data are presented indicating that women who are screened carefully by a mammographic screening program have less than a 10% risk of dying of any discovered cancer and thus the real risk to the patient's life of a cancer that arises in the opposite breast is on the order of 1% or 2% of ever dying of the cancer that might arise rather than the 25% or 30% risk of the cancer itself. Most patients choose to be observed carefully rather than to undergo prophylactic mastectomies when counselled with such data.

So many decisions in current breast cancer management involve value judgements regarding the acceptance of risk, such as the likelihood of response, the usefulness of adjuvant chemotherapy, the desire to preserve the breast, the likelihood of in-breast recurrence, etc., that the woman's values should be paramount in all the discussions regarding treatment. Perhaps, the major reason for an apparent wide variation of breast preservation rates across this country is the orientation and conviction of the surgeons counselling patients. Carefully balancing all aspects of management and patient attitudes is essential for modern breast cancer management. This particular patient exemplifies some of the possibilities of surgical and adjuvant therapy variations based on careful analysis of disease features such as small size and low-grade histology, Such variations need to be presented to patients because many of them are quite willing to accept modifications of therapy for the perceived gains of simplified surgery, and avoidance of radiation or chemotherapy when added benefits are marginal at best or insignificant.

88

Local Recurrence After Lumpectomy for a Patient with Extensive Intraductal Disease

Monica Morrow

An indication for mastectomy

CASE PRESENTATION

The patient is a 59-year-old white woman who underwent a routine screening mammogram that revealed a new area of microcalcifications in the right breast. The patient is gravida 4, para 4, age 29 at first birth. She has been surgically postmenopausal for 12 years, and takes Provera for 10 days each month. She has no prior history of breast disease. Her family history includes a mother who developed breast cancer at age 43. The patient has no complaints referable to her breasts and denies breast masses, nipple discharge, skin changes or axillary masses.

Physical examination revealed the breasts to be symmetric without skin or nipple changes. There were no palpable axillary or supraclavicular nodes. No nipple discharge could be expressed. No masses were palpable in either breast. Review of the mammograms revealed diffuse scattered calcifications throughout both breasts. However, in the medial portion of the left breast, one clustered area of calcification was noted. Spot compression views of the calcifications (Fig. 88–1) revealed them to be of moderately low suspicion for malignancy based on their appearance. However, review of the patient's previous mammogram of one year ago did not reveal the calcifications, so needle localization biopsy was undertaken.

Review of the pathology at tumor board revealed a 3.0 × 2.5 × 1.0 cm specimen with no gross abnormalities. Microscopically, infiltrating ductal carcinoma (0.8 cm)

with an associated intraductal component was present. The calcifications were associated with the intraductal tumor (Fig. 88–2). Tumor was noted to be present at the inked margins of resection.

Discussion in this case centered on the suitability of this patient for breast-conserving therapy. The presence of extensive intraductal carcinoma in the biopsy specimen was believed to increase the risk of local failure in the breast, but not to a prohibitive degree, if negative margins could be obtained by re-excision. No other suspicious lesions were noted on mammogram, and no other contraindications to breast preservation were present. The tumor was clinically staged as T1 N0 M0, stage I. Staging workup consisting of complete blood count, chemistry profile, and chest radiograph was obtained, and all studies were normal. Bone scan was not believed to be indicated due to the early stage of the tumor and the absence of symptoms.

The patient underwent re-excision lumpectomy and axillary dissection. A small amount of residual intraductal carcinoma was found in the lumpectomy specimen and none of the 12 axillary nodes contained metastases. Immunohistochemical staining for hormone receptors was negative. The patient was not believed to require adjuvant chemotherapy due to the small size of her primary tumor and the lack of nodal involvement. She began radiotherapy 2 weeks postoperatively, and received 4600 Gy to the whole breast and a 1,400-Gy boost to the tumor bed the following week. There was a small amount of

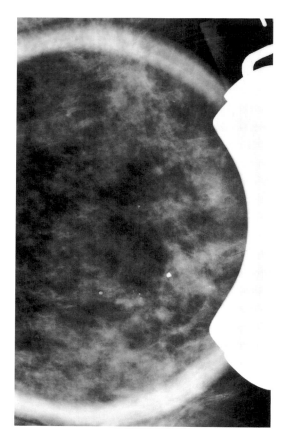

FIG. 88–1. Spot compression view of microcalcifications of the left breast, demonstrating a small number of indeterminate microcalcifications.

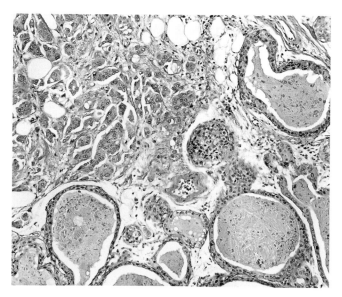

FIG. 88–2. High-power photomicrograph demonstrating infiltrating ductal carcinoma *(upper right)* and ductal carcinoma in situ of the comedo type *(lower half).*

moist skin desquamation during radiation, but no other complications were noted.

The patient was followed up at 3-month intervals and underwent a baseline post-treatment mammogram 3 months after completing radiotherapy. Mammograms of the treated breast were obtained at 6-month intervals, and mammograms of the contralateral breast were obtained annually. The patient's physical exams and mammograms remained normal for 26 months postoperatively. At that time a new group of calcifications with an ill-defined mass density was noted in the left breast adjacent to the previous biopsy site (Fig. 88–3). Needle localization biopsy was done (Fig. 88–4), which revealed a 2-cm area of infiltrating ductal carcinoma with associated ductal carcinoma in situ. A metastatic workup consisting of chest roentgenogram, bone scan, and screening chemistries was normal.

This case was re-discussed at tumor board for consideration of further management. The tumor was believed to represent a "true" local recurrence, since it occurred within the previous boost volume. Management of the patient by

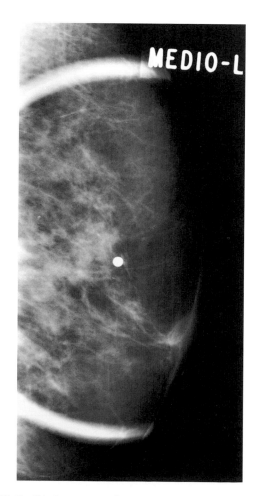

FIG. 88–3. Spot compression mammogram demonstrating ill-defined mass not seen on previous mammograms. The marker is on the lumpectomy scar.

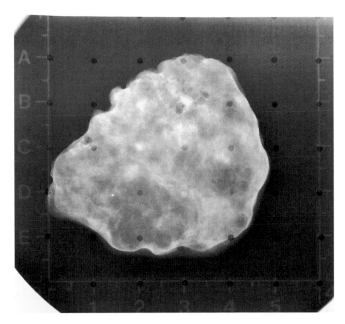

FIG. 88–4. Specimen mammogram demonstrating excision of the mass density. Calcifications not evident on the preoperative film are seen in the specimen.

re-excision alone was considered. Both the radiation oncologists and the surgeons believed that experience with this form of treatment was extremely limited, and that local failure rates with short-term follow-up are high. The risk of further local failure in this patient with such an approach was believed to be particularly high due to the finding of large amounts of intraductal carcinoma in all of the biopsy specimens. For these reasons, completion mastectomy was believed to be the procedure of choice. The patient was offered the option of immediate breast reconstruction at the time of mastectomy. Because of the prior radiation, the use of implants was believed to be contraindicated.

The patient opted for a TRAM flap reconstruction, and completion mastectomy with reconstruction was performed without incident. The pathology of the specimen revealed multifocal ductal carcinoma in situ in two of the four quadrants of the breast. The estrogen receptor content of the invasive tumor was 50 fm, the progesterone receptor 20 fm. The case was again discussed regarding the need for adjuvant therapy. There was agreement that local failure after breast-conserving therapy does not have a negative impact on prognosis. However, there is minimal data on the need for systemic chemo or hormonal therapy after local failure. Because this patient had positive hormone receptors, it was elected to treat her with tamoxifen. The medical oncologists believed that in addition to its systemic antitumor effects, tamoxifen would decrease the risk of second primary carcinoma in the opposite breast and stabilize bone density and lower blood cholesterol in this postmenopausal woman.

The patient remains free of disease 12 months after mastectomy. She will continue tamoxifen for 5 years.

COMMENTARY by Barbara Fowble

This case raises a number of issues including the clinical presentation of extensive intraductal component (EIC) positive tumors, the suitability of EIC-positive tumors for breast-conservation therapy, the appropriate follow-up procedure for patients undergoing conservative surgery and radiation, the detection of a breast tumor recurrence after breast-conservation therapy, and its treatment and prognosis.

The pathologic entity of an extensive intraductal component was first described by Schnitt et al. (25) and consists of the simultaneous presence of an intraductal carcinoma comprising 25% or more of the primary invasive ductal carcinoma and the presence of intraductal carcinoma in surrounding normal breast tissue. The definition also includes predominantly ductal carcinoma in situ in which there are focal areas of invasion, also termed *microinvasive ductal carcinoma*. Approximately 20% of women with early-stage breast cancer, undergoing conservative surgery and radiation for invasive ductal carcinoma, are found to have an extensive intraductal component (2,3,8,14,31). As in this case, the clinical presentation of EIC-positive tumors is most often one of mammographic microcalcifications without an associated mass (12). In general, EIC-positive tumors are more common in younger women (3,14). However, in this particular case, the patient is postmenopausal.

The pathologic extent of the disease in EIC-positive tumors may be significantly underestimated by the clinical and mammographic findings. Holland et al. (13), in a serial subgross and correlated mammographic examination of 217 mastectomy specimens, found that EIC-positive tumors were significantly more likely to have residual tumor and tumor at greater distances from the primary than EIC-negative tumors after an excisional biopsy. The residual tumor was predominantly noninvasive cancer. At a distance of 2 cm from the edge of the primary tumor, 59% of EIC-positive tumors had residual disease compared to 29% of EIC-negative tumors. At a distance of 6 cm from the edge of the primary tumor, 21% of EIC-positive tumors had residual carcinoma compared with 8% of EIC negative tumors. Schnitt et al. (26) reported that 88% of EIC-positive tumors were found to have a positive re-excision compared to 48% of EIC negative tumors. After re-excision, 60% of EIC-positive tumors continued to have a margin of resection that was positive compared with 31% of EIC negative tumors. Krishnan et al. (15) also reported a higher incidence of residual tumor at the time of re-excision for EIC-positive tumors.

The presence of an extensive intraductal component has been associated with an increased risk of breast recurrence in patients undergoing conservative surgery and radiation in several series (3,9,14,31). In these series, the risk ranges from 20% to 30% at 5 and 10 years. Based on these observations, some authors have suggested that the presence of an extensive intraductal component is a contraindication to conservative surgery and radiation. However, for the most part, in these early series, the assessment of resection margins was not standard. Recent information suggests that in patients with EIC-positive tumors in whom negative margins can be achieved, the risk of a breast recurrence is 10% or less. Fisher et al. (8) reported an 11% breast recurrence rate in EIC-positive tumors with negative margins of resection compared with 9% in EIC-positive tumors. The median follow-up was 8 years. Abner et al. (1) from the Joint Center for Radiotherapy reported a 0% crude incidence of breast recurrence in EIC-positive tumors with negative, close, or focally positive margins of resection. The crude incidence of breast recurrence increased markedly to 54% for EIC-positive tumors with more extensive margin involvement. The median follow-up was 75 months in this series. Bartelink et al. (2) also reported a 0% breast recurrence rate in EIC-positive tumors with negative margins of resection. Jacquemier et al. (14) and Kurtz et al. (18) reported that the presence of an extensive intraductal component was a predictor for breast recurrence only in premenopausal women and not in postmenopausal women. Therefore, in the present case, the finding of residual tumor at the time of re-excision was not unexpected, and the presence of an EIC-positive tumor with negative margins of resection would not have placed the patient at a significant risk for breast recurrence especially since she is postmenopausal. However, before initiation of radiation, a postbiopsy mammogram should have been obtained. If residual calcifications had been demonstrated, a second re-excision would have been indicated to remove all calcifications near the cluster. The presence of residual calcifications has been associated with a 100% breast recurrence rate in patients with ductal carcinoma in situ undergoing conservative surgery and radiation (20). In this particular case, a postbiopsy mammogram was not obtained and the baseline was obtained at 3 months after treatment.

An additional consideration was the presence of a positive family history and whether this impacts on breast recurrence in patients undergoing conservative surgery and radiation. A single report has addressed this issue and found no increased risk of breast recurrence in patients undergoing conservative surgery and radiation (19).

While the optimal frequency of mammographic follow-up for a patient who has undergone conservative surgery and radiation remains unknown, a policy of mammograms of the treated breast every 6 months can be questioned especially during the first year. The median interval to a breast recurrence is 3 to $3^{1}/_{2}$ years (10,11,23,24,30). Recurrences within the first year are rare (10,23). At the University of Pennsylvania, the initial post-treatment mammogram is obtained at 9–12 months (22). This interval allows for the resolution of radiation changes whose disappearance may also be delayed by chemotherapy. If the first follow-up mammogram reveals a linear or contracting scar or dystrophic calcifications, further studies are performed on a yearly basis unless subsequent clinical or mammographic findings warrant closer follow-up or biopsy. A nodular scar or ambiguous calcification merits a repeat study in 6 months. The presence of increasing nodularity or calcification requires a biopsy.

Approximately one third of all breast recurrences are detected by mammography alone (10,11,21,22,28), and the mammographic finding of microcalcifications associated with a mass is virtually always indicative of a recurrence (27,28) as in this patient. Eighty-five to 90% of patients with breast recurrences have an invasive histology (10,23). The majority of recurrences occur in the vicinity of the primary tumor (10,11,16,23). Approximately 80% of EIC-positive tumors recur in the vicinity of the original primary (3,14). Therefore, in this particular case, the appearance of the recurrence at 26 months is not unusual and it is in the most common location for EIC-positive tumors.

The standard treatment of a breast recurrence after conservative surgery and radiation has been mastectomy. Five-year survival after salvage mastectomy for an operable breast recurrence has ranged from 60% to 80% (4,10,16,23,29). The role of surgical procedures less than mastectomy in the treatment of an isolated breast recurrence has been evaluated by Kurtz et al. (17). Fifty patients with an isolated breast recurrence after conservative surgery and radiation underwent wide excision alone. The subsequent 5-year actuarial breast recurrence rate was 37%. The only group of patients in whom the subsequent risk of breast recurrence was under 10% was the group of patients in whom the disease-free interval exceeded 5 years. The incidence of recurrence was unrelated to the margins of resection or the use of supplemental radiotherapy. In an attempt to identify a subset of patients for whom wide excision alone may be appropriate treatment, pathologic findings from patients undergoing salvage mastectomy at the University of Pennsylvania were reviewed (10). At the time of salvage mastectomy, 13 of 31 patients whose initial biopsy for recurrence was excisional had no residual tumor as determined by random sections from quadrants separate from the recurrence and in multiple sections from the area of the recurrence. Detailed sectioning of the breast was not performed. No significant factors could be identified that would predict for patients who would have no residual tumor. Patients whose recurrence had an associated intraductal component were more likely to have residual tumor at the time of mastectomy. In the present case, residual ductal carcinoma in situ was identified in two of four quadrants, and mastectomy clearly was indicated. It is stated that because of the prior radiation, the use of implants was believed to be contraindicated. However, at the University of Pennsylvania, immediate reconstruction employing prosthetic implants has not resulted in significant complications (10).

The prognosis of a breast recurrence after conservative surgery and radiation is primarily related to the extent of the recurrence, the histology of the recurrence, and the time interval to the development of the recurrence. Patients whose recurrence is purely noninvasive have an improved prognosis (10,23). Patients with diffuse recurrences or axillary node involvement have a decreased survival (4,10,11,16,29). Breast recurrences appearing after 5 years have not had an adverse impact on overall survival (16). In the present case, favorable prognostic factors include the presence of a localized recurrence that was detected solely by mammography. However, the interval to recurrence of less than 5 years may result in a somewhat decreased survival when compared with patients without such a recurrence.

The role of tamoxifen after salvage mastectomy for an isolated breast recurrence is unknown. However, tamoxifen use has reduced the risk of ipsilateral breast recurrence in patients undergoing conservative surgery and radiation (7) and has decreased the risk of contralateral breast cancer (6). In the meta-analysis (5), tamoxifen provided an improvement in survival and disease-free survival in postmenopausal women.

In summary, the majority of breast recurrences after conservative surgery and radiation are operable and are associated with a 5-year survival of 60% to 80%, which is superior to that of a chest wall recurrence after mastectomy. The median interval to recurrence is approximately three years. The risk of a breast recurrence is not increased in EIC-positive tumors provided that negative margins of resection are achieved. Mastectomy offers optimal local control, especially for recurrences within 5 years. Recommendations for systemic therapy, either chemotherapy or tamoxifen, are based on the presence of adverse prognostic factors such as extensive involvement of the breast, dermal lymphatic or vascular lymphatic invasion, positive axillary nodes, and a short interval to recurrence.

REFERENCES

1. Abner A, Recht A, Connolly JL, et al. The relationship between positive microscopic margins of resection and the risk of local recurrence in patients treated with breast conserving therapy. *Int J Radiat Oncol Biol Phys* 1992;24:130.
2. Bartelink H, Border JH, van Dongen JA, Peterse JL. The impact of tumor size and histology on local control after breast-conserving therapy. *Radiother Oncol* 1988;11:297.
3. Boyages J, Recht A, Connolly J, et al. Early breast cancer: predictors of breast recurrence for patients treated with conservative surgery and radiation therapy. *Radiother and Oncol* 1990;19:29.
4. Clarke DH, Le MG, Sarrazin D, Lacombe M, et al. Analysis of local-regional relapse in patients with early breast cancers treated by excision and radiotherapy: experience of the Instituut Gustave-Roussy. *Int J Radiat Oncol Biol Phys* 1985;11:137.
5. Early Breast Cancer Trialists' Collaborative Group. Systemic treatment of early breast cancer by hormonal, cytotoxic or immune therapy. 133 randomized trials involving 31,000 recurrences and 24,000 deaths among 75,000 women. *Lancet* 1992;339:1–15;71–84.
6. Fisher B, Costantino J, Redmond C, et al. A randomized clinical trial evaluating tamoxifen in the treatment of patients with node-negative breast cancer who have estrogen receptor positive tumors. *N Engl J Med* 1989;320:479.
7. Fisher B, Wickerham DL, Deutsch M, et al. Breast tumor recurrence after lumpectomy with and without breast irradiation: an overview of recent NSABP findings. *Sem Surg Oncol* 1992;8:153–60.
8. Fisher ER, Anderson S, Redmond C, Fisher B. Ipsilateral breast tumor recurrence and survival following lumpectomy and irradiation: pathologic findings from NSABP protocol B06. *Sem Surg Oncol* 1992;8:161–2.
9. Fowble B, Solin LJ, Schultz DJ. Conservative surgery and radiation for early breast cancer. In: Fowble B, Goodman RL, et al. *Breast cancer treatment—a comprehensive guide to management.* St. Louis, C.V. Mosby; 1991.
10. Fowble B, Solin LJ, Schultz DJ, et al. Breast recurrence following conservative surgery and radiation: patterns of failure, prognosis and pathologic findings from mastectomy specimens with implications for treatment. *Int J Radiat Oncol Biol Phys* 1990;19:833.
11. Haffty BG, Fisher D, Rose M, et al. Prognostic factors for local recurrence in the conservatively treated breast cancer patient: a cautious interpretation of the data. *J Clin Oncol* 1991;9:997.
12. Healey EA, Osteen RT, Schnitt SJ, et al. Can the initial clinical and mammographic features predict the presence of an extensive intraductal component in early-stage breast cancer? *Int J Radiat Oncol Biol Phys* 1989;17:1217.
13. Holland R, Connolly J, Gelman R, et al. The presence of an extensive intraductal component following a limited excision correlates with prominent residual disease in the remainder of the breast. *J Clin Oncol* 1990;8:113.
14. Jacquemier J, Jurtz JM, Amalric R, et al. An assessment of extensive intraductal component as a risk factor for local recurrence after breast-conserving therapy. *Br J Cancer* 1990;61:873.
15. Krishnan L, Jewell WR, Krishnan EC, et al. Breast cancer with extensive intraductal component: treatment with immediate interstitial boost irradiation. *Radiology* 1992;183:273.
16. Kurtz JM, Almaric R, Brandone H, et al. Local recurrence after breast-conserving surgery and radiotherapy. Frequency, time course, and prognosis. *Cancer* 1989;63:1912.
17. Kurtz JM, Jacquemier J, Amalric R, et al. Is breast conservation after local recurrence feasible? *Eur J Cancer* 1991;27:240.
18. Kurtz JM, Jacquemier J, Amalric R, et al. Why are local recurrences after breast conserving therapy more frequent in young patients? *J Clin Oncol* 1990;8:591.
19. Kurtz JM, Spitalier JM, Brandone H, et al. Mammary recurrences in women younger than forty. *Int J Radiat Oncol Biol Phys* 1988;15:271.
20. McCormick B, Rosen PP, Kinne D, et al. Ductal carcinoma in situ of the breast. An analysis of local control after conservative surgery and radiotherapy. *Int J Radiat Oncol Biol Phys* 1991;21:289.
21. Orel SG, Fowble BL, Solin LJ, et al. Prognostic significance of method of detection of local recurrence after lumpectomy and irradiation for early stage breast cancer. *Radiology* 1993;188:189.
22. Orel SG, Troupin RH, Patterson EA, et al. Breast cancer recurrence after lumpectomy and irradiation. Role of mammography in detection. *Radiology* 1992;183:201.
23. Recht A, Schnitt SJ, Connolly JL, et al. Prognosis following local or regional recurrence after conservative surgery and radiotherapy for early stage breast carcinoma. *Int J Radiat Oncol Biol Phys* 1989;16:3.
24. Recht A, Silen W, Schnitt SJ, et al. Time course of local recurrence following conservative surgery and radiotherapy for early stage breast cancer. *Int J Radiat Oncol Biol Phys* 1988;15:255.
25. Schnitt SJ, Connolly JL, Harris JR, et al. Pathologic predictors of early local recurrence in stage I and II breast cancer treated by primary radiation therapy. *Cancer* 1984;53:1049.
26. Schnitt SJ, Connolly JL, Khettry U, et al. Pathologic findings on re-excision of the primary site in breast cancer patients considered for treatment by primary radiation therapy. *Cancer* 1987;9:675.
27. Solin LJ, Fowble BL, Schultz DJ, et al. The detection of local recurrence after definitive irradiation for early stage carcinoma of the breast. *Cancer* 1990;65:2497.
28. Stomper PC, Recht A, Berenberg AL, et al. Mammographic detection of recurrent cancer in the irradiated breast. *AJR* 1987;148:39.

29. Stotter A, Atkinson EN, Fairston BA, et al. Survival following local-regional recurrence after breast conservation therapy for cancer. *Ann Surg* 1990;212:166.
30. Veronesi U, Banfi A, Del Vecchio M, et al. Comparison of Halsted mastectomy with quadrantectomy, axillary dissection, and radiotherapy in early breast cancer: long-term results. *Eur J Cancer Clin Oncol* 1986;22:1085.
31. Zafrani B, Vielh P, Fourquet A, et al. Conservative treatment of early breast cancer: prognostic value of ductal in situ component and other pathologic variables on local control and survival. *Eur J Cancer Clin Oncol* 1989;25:1645.

EDITORIAL BOARD COMMENTARY

Breast-conserving surgery for invasive carcinoma with an extensive intraductal component in a background of other scattered mammographic calcifications should be done with caution. These scattered microcalcifications with benign radiographic criteria may take on a different meaning with a diagnosis of ductal carcinoma in situ.

89

Chest Wall Recurrence After Modified Radical Mastectomy for Stage I Disease

Marie E. Taylor

Ordinarily an ominous finding, but there were favorable factors in this patient.

CASE PRESENTATION

A 67-year-old white woman presents for treatment recommendations with a finding of left chest wall recurrence after modified radical mastectomy.

HISTORY OF PRESENT ILLNESS

The patient had been in excellent health when a routine mammogram demonstrated an approximate 2 cm lesion in the upper inner quadrant of the left breast. Examination at that time confirmed palpable changes in this region, without cervical, supraclavicular, or axillary adenopathy.

An excisional biopsy was completed. A $3.5 \times 3.0 \times 1.5$ cm specimen contained a $1.0 \times 0.3 \times 0.5$-cm firm, whitish gray area with ill-defined borders. Microscopically, this was consistent with an invasive ductal carcinoma, and foci of intraductal carcinoma were seen.

Routine staging studies were completed and these were within normal limits. The patient underwent a left modified radical mastectomy. Grossly, the breast was remarkable for a recent biopsy cavity in the upper inner quadrant, and in addition there was a firm area that measured 6.0×4.5 cm, which demonstrated irregular bands of grayish white fibrous-appearing tissue. This fibrous tissue extended to an area adjacent to the previous biopsy cavity. None of the observed lymph nodes appeared grossly abnormal.

Histologically, sections from the upper inner, lower inner, and lower outer quadrants demonstrated invasive ductal carcinoma, grade II/III (Fig. 89–1). The breast tissue was also remarkable for cystic change with fibrosis, hyperplasia, and sclerosing adenosis with mitosis. The resection margin and nipple were uninvolved. None of the 14 lymph nodes found contained metastatic disease. Estrogen receptor (ER) was 542 and progesterone receptor (PR) was 178. Flow cytometries were not reported.

The patient did not receive any adjuvant therapy and was followed with regular check-ups by her primary care physician and annual right mammography.

Four-and-one-half years later she noted a painless mass in the left mastectomy scar. On physical examination, a 3.0×2.5 cm mobile mass was noted in the middle of the scar. The overlying chest wall tissues had a puckered appearance. There were no skin changes, and there was no peripheral adenopathy. Mammography could be completed on the remaining chest wall tissues, and this confirmed a spiculated density deep to the scar. A fine-needle aspiration cytology was positive for ductal carcinoma.

Metastatic workup included chest roentgenography, complete chemistry profile and complete blood count, all of which were within normal limits. A bone scan was completed, which demonstrated multifocal uptake consistent with degenerative disease. There was increased activity in the anterior lateral aspect of the left proximal tibia, which correlated with plain radiographic findings consistent with a chronic process (Paget's disease) as well as in

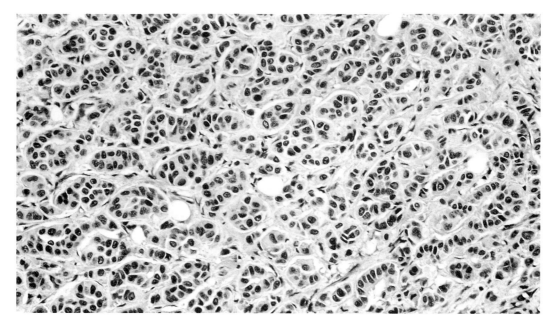

FIG. 89–1. Grade II/III invasive ductal carcinoma.

the right anterior seventh or eighth ribs, which correlated with old rib fractures.

The patient underwent an excisional biopsy. The oriented and inked specimen confirmed a 2.5 × 1.5 × 1.5 cm mass of firm, white and tan nodular tissue suspicious for malignancy. This tissue extended close to the deep surgical margin focally. Histologically, this lesion was compatible with an infiltrating ductal carcinoma, Pages grade II/III, and there was focal cancerization of lobules (Figs. 89–2 and 89–3). A single focus of ductal carcinoma in situ was present and consisted of cribriform and solid types. Areas of the invasive tumor component resembled infiltrating lobular carcinoma. In some areas the tumor demonstrated signet ring features; other areas showed the overall pattern of infiltrating ductal carcinoma. Individual tumor cells were present less than 0.1 mm from the inked

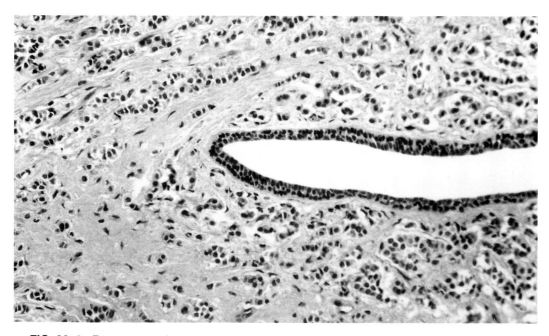

FIG. 89–2. Recurrence—large mammary duct surrounded by tumor (residual breast tissue).

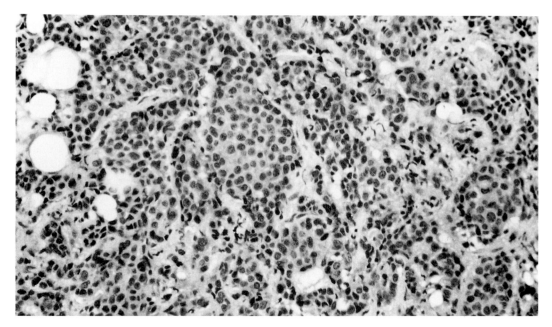

FIG. 89–3. Recurrence—grade III/III invasive ductal carcinoma.

deep surgical margin from the inferior medial aspect of the specimen. Lymph–vascular invasion was identified. Flow cytometry indicated that the tumor was diploid with an S-phase fraction of 4.4% and a DNA index of 1.0. ER was 346 and PR was 181.

It was recommended that the patient receive postoperative radiation therapy to the left chest wall and regional lymphatics as well as adjuvant tamoxifen therapy. Also notable was a past surgical history of hysterectomy for dysfunctional uterine bleeding.

Radiation treatments were completed over an elapsed time of 51 days. Treatment consisted of left chest wall medial and lateral tangents with inclusion of ipsilateral IMC for a total dose of 5,040 cGy at 180 cGy per fraction, 28 fractions over an elapsed time of 39 days. Because of a mid-bridge separation of 26 cm, treatments were given with 18-MV photons with 2-cm layer bolus applied daily. The entire left mastectomy scar and recurrent tumor site were additionally boosted 900 cGy for a total of 5,940 cGy. Treatments were given with 16 MV electrons utilizing 1-cm surface bolus and dose prescribed to 3.2 cm. The chest wall recurrent site received a final boost dose of 720 cGy for an overall dose of 6,660 cGy at that site. The left supraclavicular region was treated to a total dose of 4,500 cGy at 180 cGy per fraction, and the posterior left axilla was supplemented to a mid-plane dose of 5,000 cGy.

The patient tolerated her radiation therapy relatively well with the anticipated skin responses of dry desquamation and mild erythema. She eventually progressed to patches of moist desquamation in the left axilla, and these were treated with routine topical measures with good resolution.

POSTTHERAPY

Her course was notable for a 2 × 2 cm area of induration approximately 1–2 cm superior to the mastectomy incision at 4 months postirradiation. Clinically, this was not believed to be suspicious for recurrent cancer but was eventually excised and found to be fat necrosis. At approximately 7 months posttherapy, early telangiectasias were present in the region overlying boost portals, and at approximately 1 year posttherapy, mild left upper extremity lymphedema was noted throughout the extremity. There was no significant cosmetic or functional compromise from this mild lymphedema. She continues with tamoxifen at last evaluation, noting that previously observed hot flashes have now ceased. There is no evidence of disease, and her performance status is 100% at 1 year and 2 months postirradiation.

TUMOR BOARD DISCUSSION

This case presents several features of interest. One is that the recurrence pathology describes cancerization of lobules, with the implication that residual breast tissue was left postmastectomy. The patient also had an apparent clinically localized process, initially by mammography and physical examination, but pathologic analysis of the breast indicated diffuse infiltration in three of four breast quadrants. In spite of surgical margins, extensive tumor involvement of this nature would prompt recommendation for adjuvant local radiation therapy at the time of initial diagnosis in an effort to decrease the risk of local recurrence.

Recurrent chest wall carcinoma is treated with or without surgical debulking, depending on the tumor burden of the chest wall and assessment for operability. Without operation or with larger tumor volumes, higher doses of radiation are necessary. With smaller tumor volumes, the probability of local control on the chest wall area is greater. Tumor debulking with chemotherapy and/or hormonal manipulation may be of great value in reducing chest wall tumor burdens prior to initiation of radiation therapy in cases where operation is not feasible. The value of adjuvant tamoxifen in the setting of chest wall recurrence is uncertain, but was offered to optimize the probability of disease-free survival.

COMMENTARY by Barbara Fowble

The case presentation is that of a postmenopausal woman who underwent a modified radical mastectomy for a clinical T1 N0 M0 stage I invasive ductal carcinoma of the breast and 4½ years later developed a solitary chest wall recurrence measuring 3 cm in diameter, which is estrogen and progesterone receptor positive, and after excision is treated with radiation and tamoxifen. The issues for discussion include the incidence of local–regional recurrence after mastectomy for operable breast cancer, the sites of recurrence and the interval, the role of surgery and radiation for local–regional disease, optimal radiotherapy technique, the role of adjuvant systemic therapy, and prognostic factors for outcome after treatment.

The overall incidence of local–regional recurrence after radical or modified radical mastectomy for operable breast cancer is 10% to 15% and local–regional recurrences represent approximately one third of all first recurrences (6,10,18,19,23,38). The risk of a local–regional recurrence has been related to primary tumor size and the axillary nodal status. Patients with primary tumors greater than or equal to 5 cm and/or four or more positive axillary nodes are considered high-risk patients with a 25% to 30% incidence of local–regional recurrence after mastectomy with or without adjuvant chemotherapy (10,16,19,38). However, for primary tumors less than or equal to 2 cm (T1) and negative axillary nodes, the risk is less than 10% (10,16,40). The presence of diffuse multicentric disease at the time of mastectomy has not been associated with an increased risk of local–regional recurrence unless four or more axillary nodes are positive or the gross primary tumor size is greater than or equal to 5 cm (21); therefore, in this patient, the finding of microscopic involvement of all three quadrants of the breast despite the clinical appearance of localized disease, would not be expected to result in a higher risk of local–regional recurrence. An increased risk of local recurrence has also been associated with increasing tumor grade (16).

The most common site for a local–regional recurrence after mastectomy is the chest wall (1,2,4,8,9,12,14,34,

39). The majority of recurrences occur within the first two years after treatment (10,13,15,16,29,32–36,41). However, for initial clinical stage I disease, the mean interval to local–regional recurrence after mastectomy has been reported to be 6–7 years (3,22). Therefore, the 4½ year interval to recurrence in this patient is not unusual.

Treatment options for local–regional recurrence after mastectomy include surgery alone, surgery and radiation, or radiation alone. For recurrences that can be excised, surgery alone has resulted in a subsequent relapse rate in the initial site of recurrence of 45% to 73% (2–4,11,16). Wide excision followed by radiation has resulted in improved local–regional control when compared with radiation alone (1,3,16,34,37). Therefore, where appropriate, surgical excision should precede radiation. Optimal radiotherapy consists of treatment of the entire chest wall with a minimum dose of 5,000 cGy. The use of small fields to treat portions of the chest wall has resulted in subsequent recurrence rates of 18% to 43% (4,8,27,30,37). Elective treatment of uninvolved nodal sites is controversial. For patients with a chest wall recurrence, failure rates in the untreated supraclavicular region range from 16% to 20% (4,24). There is no evidence to suggest that for a chest wall recurrence elective treatment of the internal mammary nodes or the axilla results in improved regional control (4,24,34). Therefore, in this particular patient, treatment could have been limited to the chest wall and supraclavicular region. Several studies have suggested that doses above 5,000 cGy do not result in improved local control in completely excised recurrences (4,24,34). The additional radiation given to the areas of recurrence in this case may be warranted because of the close margin of resection. Overall long-term local–regional control rates in patients who have received adequate radiotherapy range from 50% to 70% (4,8,9,24,30,34,39).

The majority of patients who develop a local–regional recurrence after mastectomy subsequently develop distant metastasis (1,5,31). This observation has resulted in the frequent use of adjuvant systemic chemotherapy or tamoxifen. However, most studies have demonstrated no survival benefit from adjuvant chemotherapy when compared with radiation alone (14,26,28,31,39). Schwaibold et al. reported an improved overall and disease-free survival with the addition of adjuvant chemotherapy in patients whose local–regional recurrence was excised and treated with radiation (34). Two recent series have demonstrated a significant improvement in 5-year disease-free survival with the addition of tamoxifen (7,26). Halverson et al. reported a significant improvement in overall and disease-free survival and a significant decrease in distant metastasis in patients receiving tamoxifen and radiation (26). Tamoxifen, however, had no impact on local–regional control. In contrast, in a randomized trial reported by Borner et al., comparing radiation with tamoxifen and radiation for patients with local–regional recurrences after mastectomy that were estrogen receptor positive, ≤3 cm in size and less than or equal to three nodules, there was no impact on overall survival or distant metastasis with the addition of tamoxifen (7). However, there was a significant improvement in local–regional control, which translated into a significant improvement in disease-free survival. Schwaibold et al. reported an improved survival for tamoxifen only in patients whose local–regional recurrence could not be excised (34).

A number of factors have been reported to correlate with overall and disease-free survival after local–regional recurrence after mastectomy. These factors include the initial tumor size and pathologic nodal status, the initial estrogen receptor status, the disease-free interval, the size and extent of the recurrence, the number of sites involved, the ability to excise the recurrence, and ultimate local–regional control (20). The most important prognostic factors appear to be the initial tumor size and pathologic nodal status (2,3,8,10,15,30), the disease-free interval (≤2 years vs. ≥2 years) (1,2,5,12,14,15,25,30,34,36), and the extent of recurrence including the number of sites involved and size of the recurrence (4,14,17,25,28,30). The overall survival after a local–regional recurrence after mastectomy is 30% to 50% (1–3,12,14,25,30,31,34,39). However, a number of series have identified a favorable subgroup of patients whose 5-year survival is 60% to 70% with a disease-free survival of 50% to 60% (2,3,7,15,25,34). This group is characterized by the following factors: isolated chest wall recurrence less than 3 cm that is excised and is estrogen and progesterone receptor positive, disease-free interval greater than 2 years, and initial pathologic axillary nodal status that is negative. However, only 18% of all local–regional recurrences after mastectomy are in this favorable subgroup (25,34). The recurrence in this patient demonstrates a number of these favorable prognostic factors.

In summary, the case for discussion represents that of a postmenopausal woman with a clinical stage I breast cancer treated with mastectomy whose risk of local–regional recurrence would be expected to be low. Unfortunately, the patient developed a chest wall recurrence that was optimally treated with local excision, radiation, and tamoxifen. The recurrence was characterized by a number of favorable prognostic factors including: a single nodule in the chest wall that could be excised; positive estrogen and progesterone receptors and a relatively long disease-free interval. The prognosis in this particular patient, unlike the majority of local–regional recurrences after mastectomy, is not dismal, and the 5-year overall survival is 60% to 70%.

REFERENCES

1. Aberizk WJ, Silver B, Henderson IC, et al. The use of radiotherapy for treatment of isolated locoregional recurrence of breast carcinoma after mastectomy. *Cancer* 1986;58:1214–18.
2. Andry G, Suciu S, Vico P, et al. Locoreginal recurrences after 649 modified radical mastectomies: incidence and significance. *Eur J Surg Oncol* 1989;15:476–85.
3. Beck TM, Hart NE, Woodward DA, et al. Local or regionally recurrent carcinoma of the breast: results of therapy in 121 patients. *J Clin Oncol* 1983;1:400–5.
4. Bedwinek JM, Fineberg B, Lee J, et al. Analysis of failures after local treatment of isolated local regional recurrence of breast cancer. *Int J Radiat Oncol Biol Phys* 1981;7:581–5.
5. Bedwinek JM, Lee J, Fineberg B, et al. Prognostic indicators in patients with isolated local-regional recurrence of breast cancer. *Cancer* 1981;47:2232–5.
6. Bonadonna G, Valagussa P, Rossi A, et al. Ten-year experience with CMF-based adjuvant chemotherapy in resectable breast cancer. *Breast Cancer Res Treat* 1985;5:95.
7. Borner M, Bacchi M, Goldhirsch A, et al. First isolated locoregional recurrence following mastectomy for breast cancer: results of a phase III multicenter study comparing systemic treatment with observation after excision and radiation. *J Clin Oncol* 1994;12:2071–7.
8. Chen KKY, Montague ED, Oswald MJ. Results of irradiation in treatment of locoregional breast cancer recurrence. *Cancer* 1985;56:1269–73.
9. Chu FCH, Lin FJ, Kim JH, et al. Locally recurrent carcinoma of the breast: results of radiation therapy. *Cancer* 1976;37:2677–81.
10. Crowe JP, Gordon NH, Antunez AR, et al. Local-regional breast cancer recurrence following mastectomy. *Arch Surg* 1991;126:429–32.
11. Dahlstrom KK, Anderson AP, Andersen M, et al. Wide local excision of recurrent breast cancer in the thoracic wall. *Cancer* 1993;72:774–7.
12. Danoff BF, Coia LR, Cantor RI, et al. Locally recurrent breast carcinoma: the effect of adjuvant chemotherapy on prognosis. *Radiology* 1983;147:849–52.
13. Demaree EW. Local recurrence following surgery for cancer of the breast. *Ann Surg* 1951;134:863–8.
14. Deutsch M, Parsons JA, Mittal BB. Radiation therapy for local regional recurrent breast carcinoma. *Int J Radiat Oncol Biol Phys* 1986;12:2061–5.
15. Di Pietro S, Bertario L, Piva L. Prognosis and treatment of locoregional breast cancer recurrences: critical considerations on 120 cases. *Tumori* 1980;66:331–6.
16. Donegan WL, Perez-Mesa CM, Watson FR. A biostatistical study of locally recurrent breast carcinoma. *Surg Gynecol Obstet* 1966;122:529–40.
17. Fentiman IS, Mathews PN, Davison OW, et al. Survival following local skin recurrence after mastectomy. *Br J Surg* 1985;72:14–16.
18. Fisher B, Fisher ER, Redmond C. Ten-year results from the NSABP clinical trial evaluating the use of L-phenylalanine mustard (L-PAM) in the management of primary breast cancer. *J Clin Oncol* 1986;4:929–35.
19. Fowble B, Gray R, Gilcrist K, et al. Identification of a subgroup of patients with breast cancer and histologically positive nodes receiving adjuvant chemotherapy who may benefit from postoperative radiotherapy. *J Clin Oncol* 1988;6:1107–17.
20. Fowble B, Schwaibold F. Local-regional recurrence following definitive treatment for operable breast cancer. In: Fowble B, Goodman RL, Glick JH, Rosato EF, eds. *Breast cancer treatment: a comprehensive guide to management.* St. Louis: C.V. Mosby; 1991:373–402.
21. Fowble B, Yeh IT, Schultz DJ, et al. The role of mastectomy in patients with stage I-II breast cancer presenting with gross multifocal or multicentric disease or diffuse microcalcifications. *Int J Radiat Oncol Biol Phys* 1993;27:567–73.
22. Gilliand MD, Barton RM, Copeland EM. The implications of local recurrence of breast cancer as the first site of therapeutic failure. *Ann Surg* 1983;197:284–7.
23. Goldhirsch A, Gelber R. Adjuvant treatment for early breast cancer: the Ludwig Breast Cancer studies. *NCI Monogr* 1986;1:55.
24. Halverson KJ, Perez CA, Kuske RR, et al. Isolated local-regional recurrence of breast cancer following mastectomy: radiotherapeutic management. *Int J Radiat Oncol Biol Phys* 1991;19:851–7.
25. Halverson KJ, Perez CA, Kuske RR, et al. Survival following locoregional recurrence of breast cancer: univariate and multivariate analysis. *Int J Radiat Oncol Biol Phys* 1992;23:285–91.
26. Halverson KJ, Perez CA, Kuske RR, et al. Locoregional recurence of breast cancer: A retrospective comparison of irradiation alone versus irradiation and systemic therapy. *Am J Clin Oncol* 1992;12:177–85.

27. Jackson SM. Carcinoma of the breast–the significance of supraclavicular lymph node metastases. *Clin Radiol* 1966;17:107–112.

28. Janjan NA, McNeese MD, Buzdar AU, et al. Management of locoregional recurrence of breast cancer. *Cancer* 1986;58:1552–6.

29. Karabali-Dalomaga S, Souhami RL, O'Higgins NJ, et al. Natural history and prognosis of recurrent breast cancer. *Br Med J* 1978;2:730–4.

30. Mango L, Bignardi M, Micheletti E, et al. Analysis of prognostic factors in patients with isolated chest wall recurrence of breast cancer. 1987;60:240–4.

31. Mendenhall NP, Devine JW, Mendenhall WM, et al. Isolated localregional recurrence following mastecomy for adenocarcinoma of the breast treated with radiation therapy alone or combined with surgery and/or chemotherapy. *Radiother Oncol* 1988;12:177–85.

32. Oliver DR, Sugarbaker ED. The significance of skin recurrences following radical mastectomy. *Surg Gynecol Obstet* 1947;85:360–5.

33. Pawlias KT, Dockerty MB, Ellis FH. Late local recurrent carcinoma of the breast. *Ann Surg* 1958;148:192–6.

34. Schwaibold F, Fowble BL, Solin LJ, et al. The results of radiation therapy for isolated local-regional recurrence after mastectomy. *Int J Radiat Oncol Biol Phys* 1991;21:299–310.

35. Shimkin MB, Lucia EL, Low-Beer VA, et al. Recurrent cancer of the breast: analysis of frequency, distribution and mortality at the University of California Hospital, 1918 to 1947, inclusive. *Cancer* 1954;7:29–34.

36. Spratt JS. Locally recurrent cancer after radical mastectomy. *Cancer* 1967;20:1051–3.

37. Stadler B, Kogelnik D. Local control and outcome of patients irradiated for isolated chest wall recurrences of breast cancer. *Radiother Oncol* 1987;8:105–10.

38. Stefanik D, Goldberg R, Byrne P, et al. Local-regional failure in patients treated with adjuvant chemotherapy for breast cancer. *J Clin Oncol* 1985;3:660–5.

39. Toonkel LM, Fix I, Jacobson LH, et al. The significance of local recurrence of carcinoma of the breast. *Int J Radiat Oncol Biol Phys* 1983;9:33–9.

40. Valagussa P, Bonadonna G, Veronesi U. Patterns of relapse and survival following radical mastectomy: analysis of 716 consecutive patients. *Cancer* 1978;41:1170–8.

41. Zimmerman KW, Montague ED, Fletcher GH. Frequency, anatomical distribution and management of local recurrences after definitive therapy for breast cancer. *Cancer* 1966;19:67–72.

90 Axillary Metastasis with Occult Breast Primary

Kent C. Westbrook and Denise Greenwood

This 44-year-old woman presented with occult breast cancer and an axillary metastasis.

CASE PRESENTATION

This patient was a 44-year-old woman with a 3-year history of a lump in her left axilla that had increased in size in the 6 months immediately prior to presentation. She performed monthly breast self examinations, and denied any palpable masses. She had no family history of breast cancer. She denied weight loss, anorexia, change in bowel habits or fatigue. She denied a history of previous breast pathology or pigmented lesions of her trunk or extremities.

Problem Delineation

On physical exam, the patient had a 1 × 1.5 cm firm mass in the upper outer quadrant of the left breast or low in the axilla. As breast tissue often extends into the axilla, differentiation between the axilla or the tail of Spence can be difficult. The exam of the right breast and axilla was normal. Head and neck examination revealed no thyromegaly, and there was no evidence of trunk or upper extremity pigmented lesions.

DISCUSSION OF WORKUP, BIOPSY, AND DIAGNOSIS

A mammogram showed a 7-mm soft tissue nodule in the tail of the left breast (Fig. 90–1). There were no other mammographic abnormalities. The radiologists were not sure whether this was a lesion in the breast or in an axillary node. The lesion was very smooth and round and appeared benign. Cancer of the breast that presents as an axillary metastasis without a physical abnormality will have an abnormal mammogram in a small percentage (about 12%) of cases (1). An earlier paper indicated that mammograms may reveal abnormalities in a higher percentage of patients with tumors presenting simply as an axillary metastasis and no physical abnormality, possibly up to 50% (2).

To obtain a histologic diagnosis on this lesion, an excisional biopsy was performed. The specimen was described grossly as a well-encapsulated mass, 1.5 cm in greatest dimension. Upon sectioning, the tissue had a tannish-grey coloration and a relatively soft consistency. Microscopy revealed that the mass was a lymph node with metastatic adenocarcinoma (Fig. 90–2). Thus, a firm diagnosis of lymph node metastasis was dependent on biopsy and pathologic exam.

Once a diagnosis of metastatic adenocarcinoma was obtained, the next task was to identify a primary. In these instances, the most likely source is the breast, but other sites to consider are thyroid, lung, kidney, gastrointestinal tract, and melanoma (1–3). Physical examination, laboratory and radiologic studies ruled out these potential sites in this patient. Additionally, immunohistochemical stains for tumor markers were positive for estrogen and progesterone and strongly supported the diagnosis of occult breast cancer metastatic to the lymph node (4).

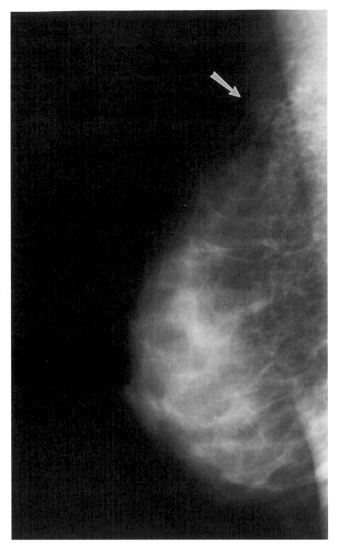

FIG. 90–1. Mediolateral oblique mammogram of the left breast showing a small, smoothly marginated mass in the axillary tail *(arrow).* Differentiation between a lymph node and a primary breast tissue tumor was not possible.

MANAGEMENT DECISIONS: LOCAL AND REGIONAL TREATMENT — TUMOR BOARD DISCUSSION

Cancer of the breast presenting as axillary metastasis without an obvious breast lesion occurs in 1% of all breast cancers. Authors are not always clear on the definition of *clinically occult.* This makes interpretation of the recommendations in the literature difficult. We define clinically occult as axillary metastasis without any physical abnormality. Mammograms for these patients may be abnormal or normal. The term *mammographically occult* is used to describe normal mammograms. The presence of an abnormal mammogram indicates that a breast biopsy of that area must be carried out.

Generally, the prognosis for these patients is equivalent to or better than stage IIB breast carcinoma. Surgical options are similar to those for patients with similar nodal stages and proven primaries (5–7). Current options for patients who present with metastasis in an axillary node, a negative breast exam and a negative mammogram are 1) modified radical mastectomy, 2) axillary node dissection with radiation therapy, or 3) axillary node dissection without radiation.

Traditionally, these patients were treated locally with radical mastectomy and later with modified radical mastectomy. As the management of early breast cancer has evolved to a more conservative approach, the options for this subset of patients have also become more conservative. Today, many surgeons believe that even the modified radical mastectomy may be excessive when a lesion cannot be seen or felt.

In a recent retrospective study from Memorial Sloan-Kettering, Baron et al. showed similar 5-year survival after mastectomy or breast preservation (77% and 65%, respectively) in patients with occult breast cancer (8). In another article comparing the survival of patients treated with mastectomy, axillary dissection and radiation therapy or axillary dissection with observation, Merson et al. concluded that there was no significant difference (5). However, study of their data results and survival curves indicate that treating the breast may be more effective than not doing so. Disease-free survival at 10 years was approximately 70% compared with 58%, which gave a *P* value of .06 (5). Additionally, since postoperative pathologic evaluation reveals carcinoma in more than two thirds of the breast specimens, we believe that simple observation of the breast may be inadequate (5–8).

The NSABP B-06 trial showed a decreased local recurrence rate in patients treated with partial mastectomy and radiation therapy when compared with those treated with surgery alone (9). We extrapolate that addition of radiation to the breast would decrease recurrence in women with clinically occult disease. Radiation of the axilla is considered only when there are four or more positive nodes or evidence of extranodal disease (10). This is usually not necessary because the majority of these patients does not have extensive nodal disease.

Our patient chose breast conservation. Axillary node dissection with resection of the tail of the breast was done. No cancer was identified in the portion of the breast removed, and 18 axillary nodes were negative for malignancy. Subsequently, she received 5,000 cGy to the entire remaining breast; however, her axilla was not irradiated.

Systemic Treatment

With regard to systemic adjuvant therapy, benefit has long been recognized when used to treat breast cancer patients with positive nodal disease. In a recent review,

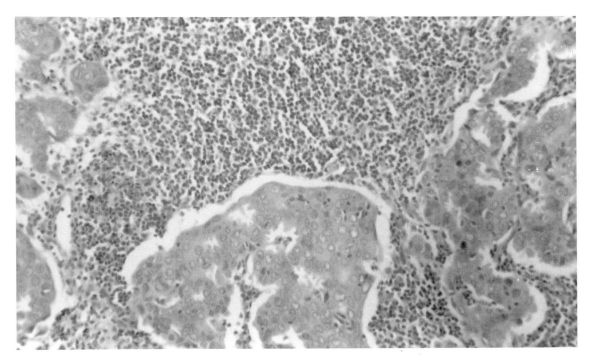

FIG. 90–2. Microscopic section of excised mass revealing lymphatic tissue with island of metastatic adenocarcinoma.

Patterson pointed out the limited data on adjuvant therapy in patients with occult primaries (10). In the previously mentioned article from the Milan group, they suggested that the addition of adjuvant therapy for these patients does not alter the survival curves, although the data from Baron et al.'s review concluded otherwise (5,8).

Our medical oncologists currently recommend multi-drug chemotherapy for these patients, as they do for most patients with early breast cancers and disease in the axilla. This patient received Cytoxan, 5-FU, and methotrexate. She was also placed on a 5-year course of tamoxifen because of her receptor status.

Follow-up

Routine follow-up consists of physical examination every 3 months and mammography of the involved breast every 6 months for 2 years following radiation. Mammography of the contralateral breast is done annually. In the absence of symptoms, we do not recommend routine chest roentgenography, laboratory tests, or bone scan.

Summary

This patient had an occult breast cancer that presented as an isolated axillary mass. She was treated with axillary node dissection and radiation to the breast. Additionally, she received multidrug chemotherapy and tamoxifen. After 7 years, she has not had evidence of recurrence.

The optimal treatment for this presentation remains controversial. Just as treatment for early-stage breast cancer is becoming more conservative, most oncologists believe that less-aggressive therapy may be equally efficacious in this subset of patients. We believe that the breast that is found to be negative by both mammogram and physical exam may be treated with radiation after node dissection. Some surgeons believe that strict follow-up after axillary dissection without radiation is a viable alternative, provided that a resection is performed if the tumor becomes evident. However, we continue to believe that all nodes should be removed and that the breast should receive radiation. Radiation to the axilla is seldom recommended in patients with clinically occult disease, because most do not have extensive nodal disease. Systemic adjuvant therapy is still routinely advocated and, again, based on known benefit to patients with proven disease, we are willing to extrapolate that benefit to these patients. Regardless of the management, there is a general consensus that the prognosis associated with this presentation is quite favorable.

REFERENCES

1. Ashihari R, Rosen PP, Urban JA, Senoo T. Breast cancer presenting as an axillary mass. *Ann Surg* 1976;183:415–7.
2. Westbrook KC, Gallager HS. Breast carcinoma presenting as an axillary mass. *Am J Surg* 1971;122(5):607–11.
3. Copeland E, McBride C. Axillary metastasis from unknown primary sites. *Ann Surg* 1973;178(1):25–7.

4. Bhatia SK, Saclarides TJ, Witt TR, Bonomi PD, Anderson KM, Economou SG. Hormone receptor studies in axillary metastases from occult breast cancers. *Cancer* 1987;59(6):1170–2.

5. Merson M, Andreola S, Galimberti V, et al. Breast carcinoma presenting as axillary metastases without evidence of a primary tumor. *Cancer* 1992;70(2):504–8.

6. van Ooijen B, Bontenbal M, Henzen-Logmans SC, Koper PC. Axillary nodal metastases from an occult primary consistent with breast carcinoma. *Br J Surg* 1993;80(10):1299–300.

7. Ellerbroek N, Holmes F, Singletary E, et al. Treatment of patients with isolated axillary nodal metastases from an occult primary carcinoma consistent with breast origin. *Cancer* 1990;66:1461–7.

8. Baron PL, Moore MP, Kinne DW, Candela FC, Osborne MP, Petrek JA. Occult breast cancer presenting with axillary metastases. *Arch Surg* 1990;125(2):210–5.

9. Fisher B, Redmond C, Poisson R, et al. Eight year results of the NSABP randomized clinical trial comparing total mastectomy and lumpectomy with or without radiation in the treatment of breast cancer. *N Engl J Med* 1989;320(13):822–8.

10. Patterson WB. Occult primary tumor with axillary metastases. In: Harris JR, Hellman S, Henderson IC, Kinne DW, eds. *Breast diseases.* Philadelphia: JB Lippincott; 1987:608–13.

COMMENTARY by David J. Winchester

This case demonstrates how the concept of breast preservation has grown to encompass many forms and presentations of cancer of the breast. As mentioned in the discussion, treatment of the unknown primary of the breast has evolved from a radical mastectomy to breast-preserving approaches, as described by Dr. Westbrook. Fewer than 1% of all cases of breast cancer present in this fashion, making the study of this entity difficult (1,2). Although there have been no randomized comparisons between the treatment approaches described, retrospective information from several studies suggest that risk of relapse and survival may be no different for patients treated with breast preservation (1,2).

As outlined, there are several definitions of occult breast cancer. All definitions include the presence of palpable axillary adenopathy as the presenting sign of disease. The initial diagnostic maneuver should be fine needle aspiration cytology to establish the diagnosis of cancer. If unsuccessful, an excisional lymph node biopsy is performed. Although metastatic carcinoma to the axilla is deemed carcinoma of the breast until proven otherwise, many other sources remain possibilities, and a careful evaluation should include consideration of thyroid carcinoma, melanoma, gastrointestinal adenocarcinoma, neuroblastoma, sarcoma, carcinoid, mesothelioma, choriocarcinoma, lymphoma, basal cell carcinoma, squamous carcinoma, and various lung cancers (3). Clinically occult cancers refer to nonpalpable but radiographically identifiable breast cancers with palpable axillary metastases. With the increased utilization and improvements in mammography, the diagnosis of this type of presentation has probably increased. Mammographically, occult tumors are neither palpated nor imaged mammographically. Unknown primaries of the breast are defined after an exhaustive evaluation, which should include a normal physical examination, mammogram, and ultrasound of the breast. Any abnormalities in the diagnostic evaluation of the breast should be excised with a low threshold, maintaining the possibility of identifying a less distinct invasive lobular carcinoma. If physical examination, mammography, and ultrasound are negative, no other diagnostic studies of the breast are indicated. As nuclear magnetic resonance (NMR) spectroscopy and positron emission tomography (PET) scanning technology improves, these and other imaging modalities may prove to be more sensitive in identifying microscopic primary disease. However, a thorough search fails to identify a primary tumor in as many as one third of mastectomy specimens (1).

In the treatment of this disease, several important concepts emerge. First, these patients all present with metastatic disease and thus display the propensity for distant failure. Therefore, systemic treatment decisions are as important as the locoregional management. Although no difference in the rates of overall regional control were demonstrated between axillary radiation and surgery in patients enrolled in NSABP-04 (4), most would prefer to perform an axillary lymphadenectomy for the added benefit of providing more complete staging information, which may help to define prognosis and guide therapeutic decisions. A complete histologic analysis of axillary contents should include hormonal receptor assays.

Treatment of the breast includes three options: observation, radiation, and mastectomy. As known from NSABP-06, radiation is effective in controlling microscopic disease within the breast (5). The choice of observation carries the risk of leaving an untreated primary in as many as 66% of patients (1), with the potential of continued metastatic behavior. Ellerbroek et al. examined the 5-year actuarial risk for the appearance of occult primaries of the breast and found that patients treated with observation alone had a 57% risk as compared with a 17% risk in patients treated with radiotherapy to the breast (2). Mastectomy remains a viable treatment option for patients not interested in undergoing a course of radiotherapy. Based on the available information, either breast irradiation or mastectomy appear to be the safest options for treatment of the breast.

Finally, systemic treatment should be emphasized, as in any breast cancer patient with nodal involvement. Although information directly addressing the role of adjuvant chemotherapy for these patients is limited, there is clear consensus regarding the use of systemic treatment for node-positive breast cancer (6,7). In our institution, the selection of therapy for patients with an occult primary of the breast depends upon the extent of lymph node involvement, age, and the functional status of the patient. Patients under the age of 70 usually receive poly-chemotherapy. Those older than 70 may be treated with either tamoxifen or chemotherapy depending upon their functional status.

In conclusion, the case presented represents an appropriately evaluated and treated patient presenting with an occult carcinoma of the breast. Although little information exists for this presentation, lessons learned from more common forms of breast cancer have helped to define a successful treatment approach that includes multimodality therapy and breast preservation.

REFERENCES

1. Baron PL, Moore MP, Kinne DW, et al. Occult breast cancer presenting with axillary metastases. *Arch Surg* 1990;125:210–5.
2. Ellerbroek N, Holmes F, Singletary E, et al. Treatment of patients with isolated axillary nodal metastases from an occult primary carcinoma consistent with breast origin. *Cancer* 1990;66:1461–7.
3. Altman E, Cadman E. An analysis of 1539 patients with cancer of unknown primary site. *Cancer* 1986;57:120–4.
4. Fisher B, Redmond C, Fisher ER, et al. Ten-year results of a randomized clinical trial comparing mastectomy and total mastectomy with or without radiation. *N Engl J Med* 1985;312:674–81.
5. Fisher B, Redmond C, Poisson R, et al. Eight-year results of the NSABP randomized clinical trial comparing total mastectomy and lumpectomy with or without radiation in the treatment of breast cancer. *N Engl J Med* 1989;320:822–8.
6. Consensus conference: Adjuvant chemotherapy for breast cancer. *JAMA* 1985;254:3461–3.
7. Glick JH, Gelber RD, Goldhirsch A, Senn HJ. Meeting highlights: Adjuvant therapy for primary breast cancer. *J Natl Cancer Inst* 1992;84(19):1479–85.

91

Small Breast Cancer with Eventual Osseous Metastasis

Alan A. Lewin and James G. Schwade

A metastatic tumor responsive to several regimens. Continuous therapy may be superior to intermittent therapy.

CASE PRESENTATION

Mrs. G.B. is a 32-year-old gravida 0, para 0, white woman, who noted a small hard mass in the upper outer aspect of her right breast while showering. Bilateral mammograms confirmed a 1-cm irregular mass in the upper outer aspect of the right breast. Fine-needle aspiration showed cellular evidence of carcinoma. Metastatic evaluation included a chest radiography, bone scan, CBC and chemistry profile, all of which were within normal limits. The patient denied a family history of breast cancer. Menarche commenced at age 13. Aside from an appendectomy in childhood, the past medical history was unremarkable. She denied a history of conjugated estrogen use.

After diagnosis, the patient was referred for consideration of further treatment. On initial evaluation, she was a moderately obese and in no acute distress. There was no palpable cervical, supraclavicular or axillary lymphadenopathy. The breasts were of moderate size and symmetrical. No dimpling of the skin was noted in either breast. On examination of the right breast, a 1-cm nodule was palpated in the upper outer quadrant. There was no evidence of skin or chest wall fixation. No other masses were noted in either breast. The remainder of the physical examination was unremarkable. The patient was clinically staged as having T1b N0 M0 carcinoma of the right breast. Her case was referred to the Tumor Board for discussion of appropriate local and systemic therapies.

TUMOR BOARD DISCUSSION

After evaluation, the surgical oncologist explained to the patient the local treatment alternatives, including modified radical mastectomy and conservative surgery and radiation therapy. He thought that she would be an excellent candidate for the latter. The patient had a strong wish to preserve her breast. Favorable factors for conservative surgery and radiation therapy included a small tumor mass in a moderate size breast, which could be easily excised without adverse cosmetic effect. No contraindications to conservation treatment, including multifocal disease or pre-existing collagen vascular disease, were noted. It was elected to withhold recommendations on adjuvant systemic therapy until a wide local excision of the primary lesion with margin control and right axillary lymph node dissection were performed.

Tumor Board (2-Week Follow-Up)

The patient underwent a needle localization and wide local excision of the primary right breast lesion and a right axillary lymph node dissection. The right breast specimen measured $2 \times 4.5 \times 2$ cm and contained within it a poorly circumscribed tumor measuring 7 mm in greatest dimension. The tumor was grossly 1 cm from the nearest resection margin. On microscopic evaluation, an infiltrating ductal carcinoma was seen (Fig. 91–1). The tumor cells had a high nuclear grade. Additional tissue was obtained from the superior, medial, deep, anterior, inferior, and lateral margins of resection. All margins were free of tumor. Three of eight level I axillary lymph nodes were positive for tumor. Twelve level II and III nodes were negative for tumor. The tumor was aneuploid with an S-phase fraction of 16%. The tumor was ER–PR negative. Poor prognostic factors in the patient included young age, three positive axillary lymph nodes as well as tumor aneuploidy, high S-phase fraction and receptor negativity. The medical oncologist recommended adjuvant chemotherapy, because this had been shown to improve both disease-free survival (First Milan Trial) and survival (Early Breast Cancer Trialists' Collaborative Group) in premenopausal patients with a similar nodal status. The medical oncologists debated the potential risks and benefits of entering the patient in a prospective clinical protocol comparing CMF and a doxorubicin-containing regimen. If the patient refused entrance into a protocol, standard CMF was recommended. The duration of therapy with CMF was then debated. Since the patient refused entrance into a prospective clinical trial, it was elected to treat her for 6 months with CMF. Chemotherapy and radiation were to be given concurrently. After three cycles of CMF, primary radiation would be given with Cytoxan and 5-fluorouracil; the methotrexate would be withheld until completion of radiation treatment. The need to avoid pregnancy during radiation therapy and chemotherapy and the potential for decreased fertility or infertility with chemotherapy were discussed with the patient. Because the tumor was receptor negative, it was felt that adjuvant tamoxifen would provide little benefit and so was not recommended. General follow-up guidelines were recommended for the patient, including a routine history and physical examina-tion, CBC, chemistry profile and tumor markers every 3 to 4 months for approximately 3 years following completion of therapy and base-line mammography at 6 months following conservative surgery.

Tumor Board (6-Month Follow-Up)

The patient completed six cycles of chemotherapy, as well as radiation therapy to the right breast, supraclavicular region, and axillary apex. Forty-five hundred cGy in 180 cGy fractions were given to the right breast and adjacent nodal drainage areas, followed by an electron boost of 1,600 cGy in eight fractions to the area of previous gross disease in the right breast. The total dose to the tumor bed in the right breast was 6,100 cGy. The patient tolerated both chemotherapy and radiation treatment well without significant ill effects. Cosmetic result remained excellent. In addition to medical oncology and radiation oncology follow-up, the patient was advised to participate in a breast cancer support group. At the time of her follow-up, history, physical examination and laboratory studies showed no evidence of active disease.

Tumor Board (3 Years After Initial Presentation)

The patient was seen by her medical oncologist, with a complaint of left hip pain. On physical examination, mild tenderness to palpation was noted in the region of the left acetabulum. Physical examination was otherwise unremarkable. Bone scan and plane films of the pelvis confirmed metastatic disease in the area of pain (Fig. 91–2). Chest roentgenogram and computed tomography (CT) scan of the abdomen showed no evidence of pulmonary or hepatic metastasis. CEA, CA15-3, and alkaline phosphatase were mildly elevated.

The Tumor Board discussed the use of local and systemic therapies. The radiation oncologist recommended palliative radiation therapy to the left acetabular area. It was thought reasonable to follow the patient's disease progression without further systemic treatment at this time if symptoms were relieved with radiation treatment, because there was an absence of indicator lesions to follow and the disease-free interval was long. It was also recommended that more-aggressive experimental approaches, including the use of high-dose chemotherapy with bone marrow transplantation be discussed with the patient. She elected to receive local radiation treatment alone, and experienced relief of pain.

Tumor Board (3½ Years After Initial Presentation)

The patient complained of progressive bone pain in multiple areas. Bone scan showed multiple areas of abnor-

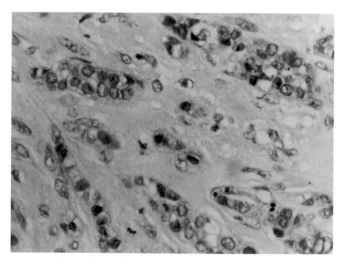

FIG. 91–1. Infiltrating ductal carcinoma (Hematoxylin and eosin stain ×200).

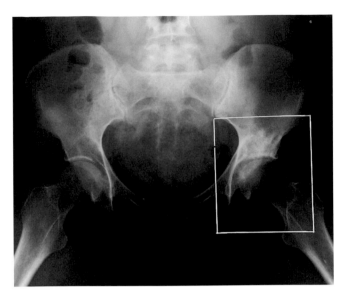

FIG. 91–2. AP view of the pelvis showing an irregular sclerotic lesion in the left acetabular area.

mal uptake consistent with progressive diffuse metastatic disease. CT scan of the chest and abdomen showed no evidence of parenchymal metastasis. The areas of most severe pain included the lower thoracic and mid-lumbar spine. The neurologic exam was within normal limits. The radiation oncologist recommended palliative radiation to the above-noted areas for pain relief. The medical oncologists discussed various treatment regimens, including re-treatment with CMF or CAF. The duration of treatment in a palliative situation was also discussed.

The patient received six cycles of CAF. She noted a transient increase in bone discomfort during the first six weeks of CAF treatment, but thereafter, noted relief of bone pain. On evaluation 6 months later at completion of CAF, the bone scan results remained unchanged.

Tumor Board (4½ Years After Initial Presentation)

Six months after completing CAF, the patient complained of mild nausea and a 5-lb weight loss over a 1 month period. On evaluation, the hepatic edge was now felt 1 cm below the right costal margin in the mid-clavicular line. No tenderness was noted. Increased levels of CEA and CA15-3 were seen, as well as elevation of alkaline phosphatase. A CT scan of the abdomen confirmed multiple metastatic deposits in the liver, as well as extensive metastatic disease throughout the dorsal and lumbar vertebra. Palliative treatment was discussed. The advantages and disadvantages of various treatment regimens were discussed in detail, including the use of high-dose chemotherapy with autologous marrow rescue, Taxol and other alternative third-line chemotherapeutic agents (cisplatinum, mitomycin-C, Velban, 5-FU, and leucovorin).

Tumor Board (4¾ Years Following Initial Presentation)

The patient elected to receive Taxol. After three cycles, a minor response was seen: The patient's hepatic metastases decreased in size. Aside from transient myalgia-arthralgia, the patient tolerated treatment well. Her appetite and sense of well-being are improved. CEA, CA15-3, and alkaline phosphatase have decreased. Treatment will continue.

COMMENTARY by Deborah K. Armstrong and Martin D. Abeloff

This case presentation unfortunately documents an all too frequent scenario of the progressive nature of metastatic breast cancer. Although small primary tumor size is a good prognostic sign (1), this patient had a number of poor prognostic factors, including lymph node metastases, negative hormone receptors, high nuclear grade, and elevated S-phase fraction. These poor prognostic factors might prompt consideration of the use of an anthracycline-containing adjuvant chemotherapy regimen for this patient. A number of trials in metastatic breast cancer have documented the efficacy of doxorubicin both as a single agent and in combination (2–4). The demonstrated activity of doxorubicin in advanced breast cancer has led to speculation that this drug may be beneficial in the adjuvant therapy of breast cancer, particularly node-positive breast cancer. Although data from the National Surgical Adjuvant Breast and Bowel Project (NSABP) suggest a benefit of including doxorubicin in the postoperative treatment of patients with stage II breast cancer, these regimens included the use of 2 years of melphalan, and are difficult to compare with CMF or CAF (5). Cooperative group trials comparing CAF and CMF have recently been completed; however, results of these studies are currently unavailable. Thus, the role of doxorubicin in the adjuvant therapy of breast cancer remains controversial (6).

This patient received concurrent chemotherapy and radiation therapy, including dose alterations of drugs received during radiation therapy. The ideal sequencing of radiation and chemotherapy after conservative surgery has not been established; however, simultaneous irradiation and full-dose CMF has been shown to produce inferior cosmetic results. In addition, patients receiving radiation therapy prior to chemotherapy have an increased incidence of lymphocytopenia (7). At the Johns Hopkins Oncology Center, we thus routinely recommend radiation therapy after completion of adjuvant chemotherapy.

Autopsy studies indicate that breast cancer is the epithelial malignancy with the greatest propensity to metastasize to bone (8). Bone is the most common site of first recurrence after primary therapy for breast cancer, either alone or in combination with other metastatic sites (9). Although studies have documented a greater propensity for ER-positive tumors to recur in bone, ER-negative tumors can clearly relapse in bone as illustrated by the case presentation (10,11). Evaluating the response of bony lesions to systemic therapy presents a particularly difficult problem. Re-ossification of lytic bone lesions may not be detectable by plain radiography for months, and osteoblastic metastases, frequently seen in breast cancer, are particularly difficult to follow by plain radiograph. Bone scintigraphy has the advantage of allowing for measurement of activity, with decreased activity indicating healing. A small percentage of patients responding to systemic treatment may have a temporary "flare" reaction on bone scan which can occasionally be associated with pain and may be difficult to distinguish from disease progression (12). This phenomenon rarely lasts more than six months after the initiation of therapy. The clinical flare described in this case and the unchanged bone scan after six cycles of CAF, suggest that the patient had, at best, a modest partial response to this regimen.

For patients who have a response to systemic chemotherapy for metastatic disease, the issue of duration of therapy inevitably arises. The physician and patient must carefully weigh the risk of further toxicity versus potential benefit of greater "tumor kill." Two separate randomized studies comparing intermittent with continuous therapy of metastatic breast cancer have demonstrated a longer time to progression for patients receiving continuous therapy (13,14). One of these studies additionally documented an improved response rate and enhanced "quality of life" measures for continuously treated patients (14). Although a number of studies have documented that responses can be durable off therapy and that patients who progress may be reinduced with the same regimen, continuing CAF therapy past six cycles might have been beneficial in this case if excessive toxicity was not encountered. The patient under discussion developed progressive bone disease as well as new liver metastases within 6 months of discontinuing CAF and has now had a minor response to three cycles of Taxol.

An important focus of treatment of women with bony metastases from breast cancer is prevention of associated morbid events. In this regard, pamidronate, a bisphosphonate inhibitor of bone resorption, has been shown to significantly decrease the occurrence of hypercalcemia, severe bone pain and overall complications in this patient group (15). Although pamidronate therapy did not impact on survival, the significant reduction in skeletal morbidity and improvement in quality of life remain important treatment goals. The patient discussed here might benefit from this type of supportive therapy, which can be given regardless of other systemic treatments.

In summary, for this woman with a small infiltrating ductal carcinoma of the breast with three involved lymph nodes, we would have considered the use of an Adriamycin-containing adjuvant chemotherapy regimen, and we would have continued treatment of metastatic disease until progression. Unfortunately, the patient has had only modest responses to treatment of metastatic disease with CAF and Taxol, and we would have limited expectations for response to further chemotherapy at this point. If available, investigational new drug therapy would be appropriate at the time of relapse.

REFERENCES

1. Rosen PP, Groshen S, Saigo PE, et al. A long-term follow-up study of survival in Stage I (T1 N0 M0) and Stage II (T1 N1 M0) breast carcinoma. *J Clin Oncol* 1989;7:355–66.
2. Taylor SG IV, Gelber R. Experience of the Eastern Cooperative Oncology Group with doxorubicin as a single agent in patients with previously untreated breast cancer. *Cancer Treat Rep* 1982;66: 1594–5.
3. Smalley RV, Carpenter J, Bartolucci A, et al. A comparison of cyclophosphamide, Adriamycin, 5-fluorouracil (CAF) and cyclophosphamide, methotrexate, 5-fluorouracil, vincristine, prednisone (CMFVP) in patients with metastatic breast cancer: a Southeastern Cancer Study Group project. *Cancer* 1977;40:625–32.
4. Tormey DC, Gelman R, Falkson G. Prospective evaluation of rotating chemotherapy in advanced breast cancer—An Eastern Cooperative Group trial. *Am J Clin Oncol* 1983;6:1–18.
5. Fisher B, Redmond C, Wickerham DL, et al. Doxorubicin-containing regimens for the treatment of stage II breast cancer: The National Surgical Adjuvant Breast and Bowel Project experience. *J Clin Oncol* 1989;7:572–82.
6. Davidson NE, Abeloff MD. Adjuvant chemotherapy of axillary lymph-node-positive breast cancer. In: Henderson IC, ed. *Adjuvant therapy of breast cancer*. Kluwer Academic Publishers; 1992.
7. Harris JR, Recht A. Conservative surgery and radiotherapy. In: Harris J, et al., eds. *Breast diseases*. Philadelphia: J.B. Lippincott; 1991.
8. Abrans HL, Spiro R, Goldstein N. Metastases in carcinoma. Analysis of 1000 autopsied cases. *Cancer* 1950;23:74–85.
9. Hayes DF, Kaplan WD. Evaluation of patients following primary therapy. In: Harris J, et al., eds. *Breast diseases*. Philadelphia: J.B. Lippincott; 1991.
10. Campbell FC, Blamey RW, Elston CW, et al. Oestrogen-receptor status and sites of metastasis in breast cancer. *Br J Cancer* 1981;44:456.
11. Wazi R, Chuang J-L, Drobyski W. Estrogen receptors and the pattern of relapse in breast cancer. *Arch Intern Med* 1984;144:2365.
12. Malawer MM, Delaney TF. Treatment of metastatic cancer to bone. In: DeVita VT Jr., et al., eds. *Cancer: principles and practice of oncology*. Philadelphia: J.B. Lippincott; 1993.
13. Muss HB, Case LD, Richards F, et al. Interrupted versus continuous chemotherapy in patients with metastatic breast cancer. *N Engl J Med* 1991;325:1342–8.
14. Coates A, Gebski V, Bishop JF, et al. Improving the quality of life during chemotherapy for advanced breast cancer. *N Engl J Med* 1987;317:1490–5.
15. van Holten-Verzantvoort ATM, Kroon HM, Cleton FJ, et al. Palliative pamidronatre treatment in patients with bone metastases from breast cancer. *J Clin Oncol* 1993;11:491–8.

92

T2 N1 M0 Breast Cancer, Second Trimester Pregnancy

Rache Simmons and John M. Daly

Breast cancer occurring during pregnancy

CASE PRESENTATION

A 36-year-old woman who was 17 weeks pregnant (G4,P2,Ab1) discovered a lump in her right breast. Physical examination revealed a 5-mm firm mobile breast mass, without skin changes and with no palpable axillary or supraclavicular lymphadenopathy. Physical examination 2 months previously showed no breast abnormality. The most recent mammograms, 6 months before this time, showed a density in the right breast that was stable and was not in the location of the palpable mass. Fine-needle aspiration of the nodule was performed and no fluid was obtained. The cytology of this aspirate was indeterminate. The patient underwent an excisional biopsy of the right breast mass, which revealed an infiltrating ductal carcinoma, 1.5 cm in diameter, that was poorly differentiated with focal medullary features. At that time the patient was scheduled for a modified radical mastectomy. This pathology revealed a residual focus of infiltrating ductal carcinoma, and axillary dissection confirmed 4 of 17 axillary lymph nodes positive for metastatic carcinoma.

When the patient was 25 weeks into her pregnancy, treatment plans discussed with her included induction of delivery at 28 weeks and subsequent initiation of chemotherapy, or immediate treatment with antineoplastic drugs. The patient was also to have the systemic workup for distant metastatic disease with bone scan, CXR, and hepatic ultrasound postpartum. The decision by the patient was to have a therapeutic abortion at 25 weeks.

TUMOR BOARD DISCUSSION

Pregnancy-associated breast cancer is not a common clinical presentation. Two to three percent of all breast cancers are pregnancy associated (1). One in 3,000 pregnancies is complicated by a diagnosis of breast cancer (2).

The treatment of pregnancy-associated breast cancer is complex, and is best undertaken with the consultation of a team whose members include the general surgeon, the medical oncologist, and the obstetrician. The approach is generally to be aggressive in treatment of the patient. Treatment of the patient should not be delayed in consideration of the pregnancy. If intensive therapy, including antineoplastic agents or radiation therapy, is recommended in the first trimester, the conservative approach would be to advise therapeutic abortion because of risk to the fetus. The options for treatment in the second and third trimester are more complicated. The treatment plan must also be individualized to the emotional, religious, and philosophical needs of the patient.

Any mass that persists or enlarges during pregnancy must be considered potentially malignant, and must be treated as such. All suspicious masses should have fine-needle aspiration (FNA) and cytology, or surgical biopsy. If the cytology is inconclusive, an excisional biopsy should be performed. During the pregnancy, surgery is the treatment modality with the least risk of fetal complications. A FNA or surgical biopsy under local anesthesia has almost no risk to the developing fetus (3).

The correct diagnosis is often delayed because of breast hypertrophy during pregnancy, making detection of a mass difficult (4). Because of this delay in diagnosis, pregnant women are significantly more likely to be diagnosed at a later stage than nonpregnant women (3,5). In pregnancy-associated breast cancer, 53% to 89% are axillary lymph node–positive at diagnosis (1,6). Pregnant women are 2.5 times as likely as nonpregnant controls to have metastatic disease at the time of diagnosis (5).

The routine metastatic evaluation for staging of a woman diagnosed with breast cancer would include a chest roentgenogram, hepatic ultrasound or computed tomography (CT) scan, and radionuclide bone scan. A chest roentgenogram, can be obtained with minimal risk to the fetus if abdominal shielding is done (7). Radionuclide bone scans and CT scans are contraindicated in pregnancy unless pregnancy termination is planned. Hepatic ultrasound is acceptable during pregnancy with no risk to the fetus.

The standard treatment of breast cancer diagnosed during pregnancy is a modified radical mastectomy. Unless the patient is within weeks of delivery, operative treatment should not be delayed for completion of the pregnancy (4). The risk of spontaneous abortion due to mastectomy is less than 1% (8).

Breast conservation, lumpectomy, and radiation therapy is not appropriate therapy during pregnancy because of radiation effects to the fetus (1,4,9). If a patient is within weeks of delivery (either spontaneous or induced), breast conservation can be considered with initiation of radiation therapy immediately postpartum.

After the first trimester, the weight of the gravid uterus on the aorta and vena cava in a supine position can cause vascular compromise to the fetus and the mother, so the patient should be placed slightly on her left side during the operative procedure. A knowledge of the changes in maternal physiology is important for the anesthesia and surgical teams, to assure the best postoperative outcome.

Radiation treatment is not recommended during pregnancy because of significant risk of fetal malformation. The effect of radiation treatment is related to dose, dose frequency, field size, and gestational age of the fetus. The risk to the fetus is highest at the time of organogenesis, during the second to eighth weeks (3). In the first 10 weeks of gestation, irradiation in therapeutic doses produces severe anomalies in 50% of fetuses; between 10 and 20 weeks less severe anomalies are noted, and after 20 weeks no severe anomalies are noted; however, it is common to see anemia and pigmentation changes in the infant. There is also evidence that in utero exposure to radiation in therapeutic ranges leads to a higher incidence of future neoplastic disease in the child/adult (10).

Most tumors diagnosed during pregnancy are estrogen-receptor and progesterone-receptor (ER/PR) negative (1,9). There is controversy surrounding whether breast cancers associated with pregnancy are truly negative, or if they are falsely negative because of high levels of circulating estrogens binding to all available ER sites (11). It is proposed that the hormonal stimulation of pregnancy should have no effect on the growth of the breast cancer in hormone-receptor–negative tumors. Indeed, elective or spontaneous termination of pregnancy has no effect on prognosis (1,5,9,11,12) (see Fig. 92–1), and there is also no effect on prognosis with elective oophorectomy (11). It is therefore appropriate to infer that the pregnancy-associated tumors are actually hormone-receptor negative (11). Termination of pregnancy is not routinely recommended,

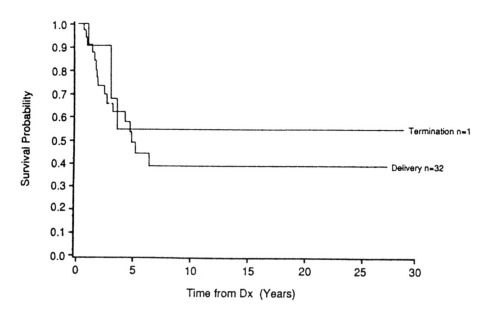

FIG. 92–1. Kaplan-Meier cause-specific survival curve for breast cancer comparing women who were delivered against those whose pregnancy was terminated (*p*=0.5, nonsignificant). (Adapted from ref. 15.)

TABLE 92-1. *Chemotherapeutic agents for treatment of breast cancer in pregnancy*

Fetal risk	Drug
Probably low	Doxorubicin
	Vincristine
Intermediate	Cyclophosphamide
High	Antimetabolites
	5-fluorouracil
	Methotrexate

Adapted from ref. 4.

unless chemotherapeutic drugs are to be given before the second trimester.

In women with stage II and III breast cancer, chemotherapy offers a significant survival advantage. There is, however, a risk of chemotherapy-induced fetal malformations, particularly in the first trimester during the time of organogenesis and rapid cell division. The probability of teratogenesis depends on the trimester of exposure, the drug dose, the duration of treatment, and the frequency of administration. There may be a synergistic teratogenic effect with combination drugs and sequential drugs, or sequential drug and radiation treatment (3). The rate of fetal malformation in the first trimester ranges from 12.7% (13) to 23% (8), compared with the second and third trimesters, which are significantly less, ranging from 0% (13–15) to 1.5% (3). If chemotherapy is indicated in the first trimester, then pregnancy should be terminated (1,6,9), unless the initiation of chemotherapy can be safely postponed until the second or third trimester. If a woman is at the point in her pregnancy when delivery is imminent or can be safely induced, chemotherapy should be postponed until postpartum. If a woman is in her second or third trimester and delivery is not possible, it is reasonable to initiate chemotherapy, with low risk to the fetus.

If chemotherapeutic drugs must be given during pregnancy, they should be chosen from those with the least teratogenic effects. The use of folic acid antagonists, such as methotrexate, is to be avoided if possible (14). If combination regimens can be avoided, it is ideal (14) (see Table 92-1).

The prognosis of pregnancy-associated breast cancer is no different at the same stage and age than that of women who are not pregnant (2,6,9). In a study by Zemlickis et al., in which women with breast cancer diagnosed during pregnancy were control matched with a group of nonpregnant women, the survival was no different between the two groups (5) (see Fig. 92–2). There was also no difference in survival in women diagnosed in the first, second, or third trimester (5) (see Fig. 92–3).

There is no evidence that suppression of lactation has any influence on prognosis. It is advisable to abstain from breast feeding if the patient is receiving chemotherapy.

There does not appear to be a difference in survival in women who choose to become pregnant subsequent to the diagnosis of breast cancer (1,12). In an age- and stage-matched study of subsequent breast cancer, the patients who became pregnant actually had a better 5-year survival rate than the controls, 72% and 50%, respectively (11). It is still considered a reasonable suggestion to delay any subsequent pregnancy to after the first few years, when recurrence is most likely.

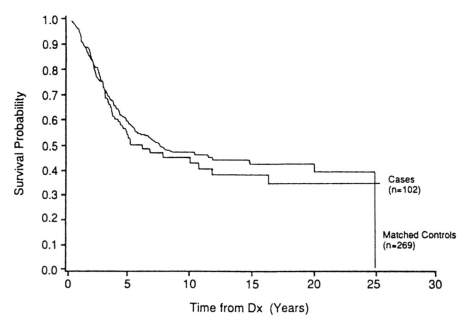

FIG. 92–2. Kaplan-Meier cause-specific survival curve for breast cancer comparing women who became pregnant against matched nonpregnant controls (*p*=0.6, nonsignificant). (Adapted from ref. 15.)

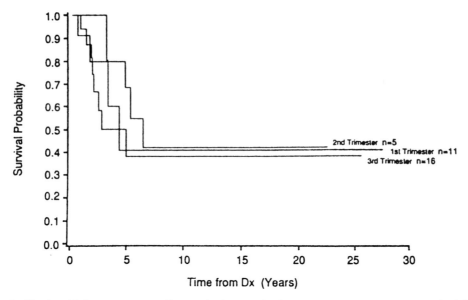

FIG. 92–3. Kaplan-Meier cause-specific survival curve for breast cancer comparing survival for pregnant women with diagnosis during first, second, and third trimesters ($p = 0.8$, nonsignificant). (Adapted from ref. 15.)

REFERENCES

1. Saunders CM, Baum M. Breast cancer and pregnancy: a review. *J Roy Soc Med* 1993;86:162–5.
2. Tobon H, Horowitz LF. Breast cancer during pregnancy. *Breast Dis* 1993;6:127–34.
3. Doll DC, Ringenberg QS, Yarbro JW. Management of cancer during pregnancy. *Arch Intern Med* 1988;148:2058–64.
4. van der Vange N, van Dongen JA. Breast cancer and pregnancy. *Eur J Surg Oncol* 1991;17:1–8.
5. Zemlickis D, Lishner M, Degendorfer P, et al. Maternal and fetal outcome after breast cancer in pregnancy. *Am J Obstet Gynecol* 1992;166:781–7.
6. Petrek JA, Dukoff R, Rogatko A. Prognosis of pregnancy-associated breast cancer. *Cancer* 1991;67:869–72.
7. Jones SE. Management of breast cancer in the pregnant patient. *Contemp Oncol* 1992;July/August:19–24.
8. Theriault RL, Hortobagyi GN. When breast cancer complicates pregnancy: what options are available? *Primary Care Cancer* 1989;February:27–32.
9. Petrek JA. Breast cancer and pregnancy. Incidence of pregnancy-associated breast cancer. In *Breast diseases*, Harris JR, Hellman S, Henderson IC, Kinne, DW, eds. Philadelphia: Lippincott; 1991:809–15.
10. Sweet DL, Jr Kinzie J. Consequences of radiotherapy and antineoplastic therapy for the fetus. *J Reprod Med* 1976;17:241–6.
11. Gallenberg MM, Loprinzi CL. Breast cancer and pregnancy. *Semin Oncol* 1989;16:369–76.
12. Nugent P, O'Connell TX. Breast cancer and pregnancy. *Arch Surg* 1985;120:1221–4.
13. Schapira DV, Chudley AE. Successful pregnancy following continuous treatment with combination chemotherapy before conception and throughout pregnancy. *Cancer* 1984;54:800–3.
14. Barber HRK. Fetal and neonatal effects of cytotoxic agents. *Obstet Gynecol* 1981;58:41S–7S.
15. Sokal JE, Lessmann EM. Effects of cancer chemotherapeutic agents on the human fetus. *JAMA* 1960;172:1765–71.

COMMENTARY by William L. Donegan

The patient is a young woman early in the second trimester of pregnancy who discovered a lump in her right breast. She is at the age when breast cancer is most likely to coincide with pregnancy. In the mid-30s the rising incidence of breast cancer coincides with a still fertile and reproductive population. Although lactating adenoma is the most frequent cause of a lump in the breast of a pregnant or lactating woman, it is important to realize that a palpable lump during pregnancy has the same chance of being malignant as does one in a nonpregnant woman of the same age. This woman's discovery of a mass as small as 5 mm suggests that she practices breast self-examination conscientiously. Her mammogram 6 months earlier is said to show a stable density in the right breast, indicating that she had earlier evaluations for problems with her breasts.

No mammogram was done on the occasion of this new finding; mammograms during pregnancy are unlikely to provide useful information because of the dense glandularity of the breasts and because they might needlessly expose the fetus to irradiation. An ultrasound examination could have determined whether the nodule was solid or cystic, but a fine-needle aspiration is more expedient and provides an opportunity to obtain a specimen for cytology when the nodule is solid. An indeterminate or negative cytology result is no reason for complacency in this situation and should not delay a biopsy for diagnosis.

The cancer that was found in this case was considerably larger than the palpable mass, an indication of the extent to which pregnancy can interfere with physical findings, and potentially with clinical staging. The tumor had focal medullary features, but this is of no consequence when it occurs in an invasive ductal carcinoma with poor differentiation. On histology alone, this tumor is likely to be ER negative, have a high S phase, and a poor prognosis. Although the tumor is relatively small and unlikely to have disseminated, staging is appropriate at this point to determine whether treatment will be for cure or for palliation. I would not choose a modified radical mastectomy for palliation. Staging should not risk radiation of the fetus unless the patient has symptoms that suggest dissemination, such as recent bone pain or headaches. In their absence, staging should be performed with a chest roentgenogram using proper shielding, serologic tests of liver function, and an ultrasound examination of the liver.

The pregnant patient with breast cancer in an early stage is potentially as curable as others, and treatment should not be compromised or delayed. It may entail some difficult choices, however, and the patient must thoroughly understand her options and the consequences of each. Decisions are best made after consultation with surgeon, radiation therapist, medical oncologist, and obstetrician/gynecologist. Certain guidelines are clear. Radiation therapy at any time during pregnancy can result in fetal damage or impairment and is to be avoided. Adjuvant chemotherapy also is avoided during the first trimester when organogenesis is taking place, but it can be given with relative safety during the second and third trimesters. Operations on the breast under local or general anesthesia do not jeopardize fetal development; the hazard is confined to a small risk of spontaneous abortion or premature labor. Experience is scant with tamoxifen, but animal studies suggest it can cause maldevelopment of fetuses and for this reason it is contraindicated. Because radiation therapy is a necessary component of breast conservation, breast-conserving therapy is not an option for the pregnant patient unless the pregnancy is terminated or unless she is near term and radiation can be given after delivery without entailing a delay. Unless these conditions are satisfied, modified radical mastectomy is the treatment of choice.

The presence of metastases in four axillary lymph nodes makes future recurrence highly likely and this patient is clearly a candidate for adjuvant chemotherapy. Nonpregnant patients with four or more involved nodes have an 86% chance of recurrence within the first 10 postoperative years. Adjuvant chemotherapy can reduce this by about 25% to 30%. As she is well into the second trimester of pregnancy, systemic therapy could begin as soon as healing is complete, avoiding methotrexate and other antifolates. A doxorubin/cytoxan combination would be a reasonable choice. The schedule should be designed to avoid a nadir around the time of delivery, and breast feeding should be avoided during chemotherapy because it can cause neutropenia in the infant. In this particular case, the patient's decision to have a therapeutic abortion at 25 weeks obviates further considerations relevant to the fetus. However, therapeutic abortion will not enhance chances for cure, nor does oophorectomy at the same time. Oophorectomy is an unproved adjuvant in this young age group either alone or in conjunction with chemotherapy. Oophorectomy is also not necessary to prevent future pregnancies, as they have shown no influence on the prospects for remaining disease free. It should be noted that spread of breast cancer to a fetus has not been documented.

SELECTED READINGS

1. Donegan WL. Breast cancer with pregnancy. In *Treatment of pre-cancerous lesions and early breast cancer*, Ariel IM, Cahan AC, eds. Philadelphia: Williams and Wilkins; 1993:214–22.
2. Wallack MK, Wolf JA, Bedwinck S, et al. Gestational carcinoma of the female breast. *Curr Probl Cancer* 1983;7(9):1–58.
3. Gallenberg MM, Loprinzi CL. Breast cancer and pregnancy. *Semin Oncol* 1989;16(5):369–76.
4. Early Breast Cancer Trialists' Collaborative Group. Systemic treatment of early breast cancer by hormonal, cytotoxic, or immune therapy. *Lancet* 1992;339:71–84.

SECTION XIX

Cervix

93 Stage IB Cancer of the Cervix

John P. Curtin

Radical hysterectomy or radiation therapy?

CASE PRESENTATION

The patient is a 43-year-old woman who is gravida 5, para 2; she has had three elective abortions. The patient went to a local Planned Parenthood Clinic in July 1992 for pregnancy testing. The patient's last menstrual period was approximately 10 weeks prior to admission. At the time of her initial evaluation, the pregnancy test was positive and a physical examination demonstrated an enlarged uterus consistent with a 10-week gestation. As part of her routine initial evaluation, cervical cytology was obtained.

The patient elected to undergo a termination of the pregnancy, which was performed without complications. On return to the Clinic, the patient was informed that the Pap smear obtained at the initial evaluation was abnormal, and it was recommended that the patient be seen for colposcopy.

The patient's past gynecologic history was unremarkable. She had normal menses and had not been using contraception recently. She had taken oral contraception pills for approximately 10 years between age 25 and 35. She had no history of previous abnormal cervical cytology. She had no history of any sexually transmitted diseases, and, specifically, no history of genital warts or human papilloma virus infection. Although her Pap smears were reported to be normal in the past, the patient had not had a cervical cytology specimen in over seven years.

The patient's review of systems were unremarkable. Specifically, she denied any unusual vaginal bleeding or discharge.

On presentation for initial evaluation, the patient's general physical examination was unremarkable. On pelvic examination, the external genitalia and vagina were normal. The cervix was paras and there were no gross abnor-malities noted. The Pap smear was repeated. There was no bleeding noted at the time of Pap smear.

Colposcopy was performed and was unsatisfactory. Although there was no gross lesion present, under colposcopic examination and after application of acetic acid, there was an area of thick white epithelium with atypical vessels present on the posterior lip of the cervix extending into the endocervical canal. Palpation with a cotton swab demonstrated an area of firmness corresponding to the area of abnormal epithelium noted at colposcopy. An endocervical curettage, as well as a cervical biopsy, were obtained. The Pap smear was consistent with invasive cancer (Fig. 93–1). Cervical biopsy demonstrated in situ and invasive squamous cell carcinoma extending deeply

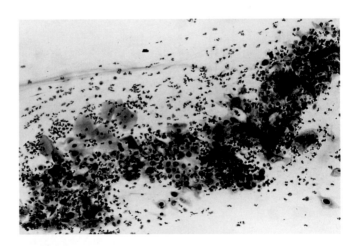

FIG. 93–1. Cervical smear: pleomorphic malignant cells from a squamous carcinoma are found in abundance. (Papanicolaou stain, original magnification × 400).

459

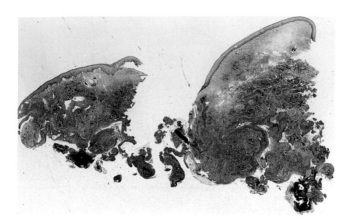

FIG. 93–2. Whole mounts of the pieces from a cervical biopsy showing squamous carcinoma in situ and infiltrating to the deep edges of the biopsy fragments (H&E stain).

into the stroma with a minimal depth of at least 3 mm (Figs. 93–2 and 93–3).

The patient was informed of the results of the biopsies, and her case was presented at the Tumor Board Conference. There was a consensus at the Conference that in a 43-year-old woman who is otherwise healthy and able to withstand an operation, that the recommended treatment for this presumed early stage cancer of the cervix (FIGO stage IA2/IB) would be radical hysterectomy. Should the patient not desire surgery, then a combination of whole pelvic irradiation plus intercavity radiation would probably be equally effective. The advantage of the surgery would be a more directed treatment approach, shortening

the treatment interval. It was also discussed that the complication rates are similar for the two treatment options. However, complications due to surgical treatment are often more amenable to repair.

The patient agreed to proceed with a recommended radical hysterectomy. At age 43, she was also counselled regarding the advisability of bilateral salpingo-oophorectomy at the time of radical hysterectomy. The patient opted to have a bilateral salpingo-oophorectomy at the same time as a radical hysterectomy and agreed to take estrogen replacement therapy postoperatively.

The patient underwent a preoperative evaluation, including chest roentgenography and intravenous pyelogram (IVP) and screening mammography. These radiographic studies were normal. The patient also donated one unit of autologous blood prior to surgery.

The patient was admitted to the hospital and under anesthesia, underwent exam, cystoscopy, and proctoscopy followed by exploratory laparotomy and a type III radical hysterectomy, bilateral salpingo-oophorectomy, bilateral pelvic lymphadenectomy, and paraaortic lymph node sampling. The pathology demonstrated residual invasive squamous cell carcinoma in the cervix minimally invasive to the middle third of the cervix (Fig. 93–4). There was no vascular space involvement, there was no parametrial involvement, and all lymph nodes were negative. The uterus, tubes, and ovaries were pathologically normal. Peritoneal cytology was also normal.

The patient recovered well and was discharged on the eighth postoperative day. Prior to discharge, her Jackson-Pratt drains were removed. She was discharged with a

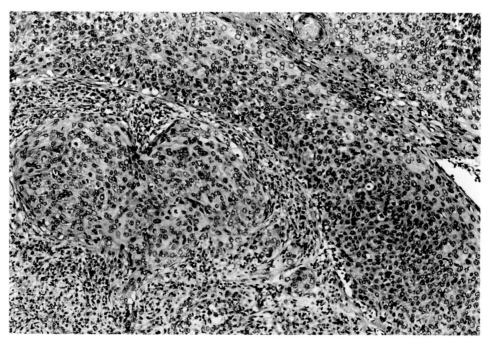

FIG. 93–3. Higher magnification of the biopsy fragment showing squamous carcinoma, in situ and infiltrating (H&E stain, original magnification × 200).

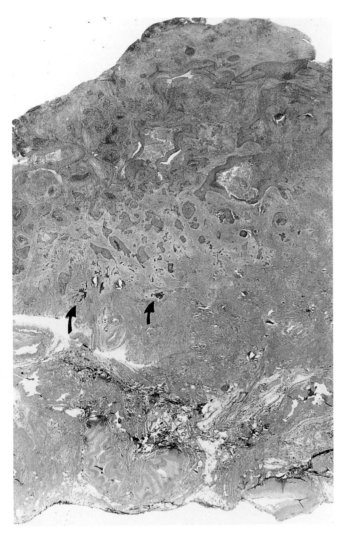

FIG. 93–4. Whole mount of the cervix from the hysterectomy specimen showing the deeply infiltrating squamous carcinoma; the deepest extent of infiltration is marked with arrows (H&E stain).

Foley catheter in place, which was removed 3 weeks later when she returned to the Clinic.

The patient has been followed up at 3-month intervals. Because of the minimal invasion and the lack of any risk factors, she was not offered adjuvant therapy. She was placed on hormonal replacement therapy via an estrogen patch. Her Pap smears done every 3 months have remained normal. A chest roentgenogram at 1 year was also normal.

COMMENTARY by Edward L. Trimble

Worldwide, cervical cancer remains the leading cause of cancer deaths among women (1). In the United States and other developed countries, however, widespread screening programs and the concomitant availability of treatment for preinvasive disease have decreased the incidence of cervical cancer dramatically (2). In 1994, it was estimated that 15,000 women in the United States would be diagnosed with cervical cancer and 4,600 would die of the disease (3).

In the United States, younger women are more likely to be screened for cervical cancer with Pap smears than older women. According to the 1992 National Health Interview Survey, 84% of women 30 to 39 years of age had a Pap smear within the last 3 years compared with 63% of women aged 60 to 69 years, and 46% of women older than 70 years (4). These percentages were stable between 1987 and 1992, despite efforts at health education. Women in their reproductive years visit healthcare providers who routinely screen with Pap smears more often than postmenopausal women. The younger women visit for contraception, for pregnancy, and for benign gynecologic disorders. In this case, the patient received her Pap smear as part of a routine physical examination at a Planned Parenthood Clinic. It should be noted, however, that the patient's previous Pap smear had been 7 years earlier.

The patient was 10 weeks pregnant when her Pap smear was done. Cervical cancer is rarely diagnosed in pregnancy. Boutselis reported 71 invasive tumors of the cervix in 95,000 deliveries (5). Survival rates for pregnant patients appear to be similar to those for nonpregnant patients (6). Had she still been pregnant at the time her cervical cancer was diagnosed, she and her physician would have needed to resolve the issue of her pregnancy and intercurrent cancer. In the first trimester, most gynecologic oncologists recommend definitive treatment of the cancer. In the third trimester, treatment may be delayed for 4 to 6 weeks, until the fetus is assured of intact survival outside the womb, at approximately 32 weeks gestation. Most oncologists would then advise cesarean delivery, followed by radical abdominal hysterectomy. One retrospective study found no adverse maternal outcome in pregnant women with stage IB cervical cancer attributable to delays in treatment of up to 17 weeks (7).

Stage IA cervical cancer can, in some cases, be safely managed with fertility-conserving surgery. Cervical cone biopsy, for example, has been shown to be adequate therapy for stage IA lesions with less than 3-mm invasion and no evidence of lymph–vascular space invasion (8). In this case, a cone biopsy would have been necessary to determine whether this patient's tumor was the appropriate stage for such conservative treatment.

Radiotherapy and radical hysterectomy have equal efficacy for stage I cervical cancer (9). Surgery, however, conveys less long-term toxicity than does radiotherapy. Radiation-associated toxicities include vaginal stenosis, chronic cystitis, proctitis, and sigmoid stricture (10).

The patient received appropriate counseling about the issue of bilateral oophorectomy at the time of her operation. Parker et al. recently published a retrospective study of 84 women who retained ovaries at the time of their radical hysterectomies (11). They experienced a 7% re-operation rate for ovarian pathology, and a 20% rate of early ovarian failure. These risks must be weighed against the need for continued estrogen-replacement therapy to ward off osteoporosis and heart disease, as well as to support the tissues of the bladder, urethra, and vagina.

Postoperative radiation therapy has not been shown, in prospective studies, to prolong survival in patients with cervical cancer. It can, however, decrease the chance of local recurrence. Identified risk factors for recurrence include status of the lymph nodes, the size of the tumor, involvement of paracervical tissues, the depth of invasion, and the presence or absence of lymph–vascular space invasion (12).

A majority of recurrences (80%) occur in the first 2 years after radical hysterectomy (13). The postoperative surveillance offered the patient is consistent with that provided by the majority of gynecologic oncologists (14). The optimal regimen for such surveillance has not yet been identified prospectively.

REFERENCES

1. International Federation of Obstetricians and Gynecologists. *FIGO 21st Annual Report*. London; 1991.

2. Bergstrom R, Adami HO, Gustafsson L, et al. Detection of preinvasive cancer. *J Natl Cancer Inst* 1993;85:1050.

3. Boring CC, Squires TS, Tong T, Montgomery S. Cancer statistics, 1994. *CA Cancer J Clin* 1994;44:7.

4. National Center for Health Statistics.

5. Boutselis JG. Intraepithelial carcinoma of the cervix associated with pregnancy. *Obstet Gynecol* 1972;40:557–66.

6. Creasman WT, Rutledge FN, Fletcher GH. Carcinoma of the cervix associated with pregnancy. *Obstet Gynecol* 1970;36:495.

7. Greer BE, Easterling TR, McLennan DA, et al. Fetal and maternal considerations in the management of stage IB cervical cancer during pregnancy. *Gynecol Oncol* 1989;34:61.

8. Lohe KJ: Early squamous cell carcinoma of the uterine cervix. I. Definition and histology. *Gynecol Oncol* 1978;6:10.

9. Pilleron JP, Durand JC, Lenoble JC. Carcinoma of the uterine cervix, stages I and II, treated by radiation and extensive surgery (1000 cases). *Cancer* 1972;29:593.

10. Perez CA: Uterine cervix. In: Perez CA, Brady LW, eds. *Principles and practice of radiation oncology*. 2nd ed. Philadelphia: J.B. Lippincott; 1992.

11. Parker M, Bosscher J, Barnhill D, et al. Ovarian management during radical hysterectomy in the premenopausal patient. *Obstet Gynecol* 1993;82:187.

12. Delgado G, Bundy B, Zaino R, et al. Prospective surgical–pathological study of disease-free interval in patients with stage IB squamous cell carcinoma of the cervix: a Gynecologic Oncology Group study. *Gynecol Oncol* 1990;38:352.

13. Krebs HB, Helmkamp BF, Sevin B-U, et al. Recurrent cancer of the cervix following radical hysterectomy and pelvic lymph node dissection. *Obstet Gynecol* 1982;59:442.

14. Barnhill D, O'Connor D, Farley J, et al. Clinical surveillance of gynecologic cancer patients. *Gynecol Oncol* 1992;346:275.

94 Stage IIB Cervical Cancer

Henry M. Keys

Increasing cost effectiveness in the pretreatment evaluation
of patients with cervical cancer

CASE PRESENTATION

The patient is a 54-year-old divorced woman, gravida 5, para 4, AB1, and postmenopausal since age 49. She has had postcoital spotting since several months ago and has developed first a clear, and subsequently yellowish discharge with some odor. She has had a sense of heaviness and dragging discomfort in her lower back for the past month. Her last pelvic exam and Pap smear was at the time of the birth of her last child, 22 years ago. She has had some increased urinary frequency and urgency without dysuria or hematuria. She has been slightly constipated.

She was seen by a family practitioner, who detected an obvious cervical abnormality and referred her to a gynecologist, who examined her and obtained an office biopsy. This was interpreted as showing squamous cell carcinoma without definite evidence of invasion. Because of this pathology report she was taken to the operating room, where a D&C was performed, followed by a LEEP procedure. Pathology of the D&C showed fragments of squamous cell carcinoma and benign endometrial tissue, while the LEEP tissue revealed invasive squamous cell carcinoma extending to the margins of resection (both deep and superior). The patient was referred to the Gynecology Oncology and Radiation Oncology Services at Albany Medical Center.

Her past medical history is unremarkable. She was 13 at first intercourse; became pregnant at age 16, which was terminated by abortion. She had several sexual partners prior to her marriage at age 20. Over the next 12 years, she had four spontaneous vaginal deliveries of her four children. She was divorced at age 40, and has a steady boyfriend at present. She has never had a mammogram. She has smoked $1^1/_2$ packs of cigarettes per day since age 15, and continues to smoke at the present time. She drinks alcohol occasionally and does not use drugs. She takes no medications on a regular basis. She works full time in her local hospital in the laundry department. She has no family history of gynecologic cancer. Her father died of lung cancer and her mother is alive with hypertension and adult onset diabetes. She has five siblings, all alive and well.

On initial examination, she was found to be a healthy appearing middle aged woman. She weighed 157 lbs. Blood pressure 140/80, with a regular pulse of 80. She had no palpable cervical or supraclavicular lymphadenopathy. The breasts were normal. No axillary masses were noted. Lungs were clear to auscultation and percussion except for a few coarse inspiratory wheezes. There was no ascites and the abdomen was benign. The liver and spleen were not enlarged. There was no inguinal adenopathy. The vulva and perineum were unremarkable. On speculum examination, the vagina was normal except for a moderately heavy yellow–green vaginal discharge. The cervix was largely replaced by a ragged appearing tumor mass measuring 3×5 cm. The cervical os was visible in the center of the cervix. On bimanual and recto-vaginal examination, there was a globular feeling cervical mass with extension into the mid-right parametrium, and a nodule measuring about 5 mm in size was felt in the left uterosacral ligament close to the cervix. There was no obvious extension anteriorly or posteriorly. There was a clear space felt along both pelvic sidewalls. There was no edema of either lower extremity. Stool was negative for occult blood.

The patient was scheduled for an abdominal/pelvic CT scan with intraluminal and intravenous contrast, and PA and lateral chest roentgenograms. The chest films were normal. The CT scan showed no ureteral obstruction. There were no enlarged lymph nodes in the pelvis or para-aortic areas. The cervix was enlarged, measuring $5 \times 3.5 \times 3$ cm. There appeared to be some nonspecific streaking in the pelvic soft tissues to the right of the cervical mass. This finding was suspicious for tumor extension into the right parametrium. The uterus was slightly enlarged with what appeared to be fluid collection in the endometrial cavity.

The tumor was staged FIGO stage IIB and presented for discussion of management.

PATHOLOGY

The outside slides were reviewed. Dr. Ambrose's diagnosis was moderately differentiated nonkeratinizing squamous cell carcinoma with invasion into the cervical stroma, and capillary–lymphatic space involvement extending to the deep and superior margins of the slides available for review. While there are fragments of squamous cell carcinoma in the endometrial curettings, these could be contaminants from the cervical neoplasm. The films were reviewed with Dr. Peters with the findings outlined above.

DISCUSSION OF MANAGEMENT

Diagnostic Evaluation

This patient initially did not have an intravenous pyelogram, barium enema, cystoscopy, or sigmoidoscopy. Lymphangiogram was not performed, and the patient was not examined under anesthesia for staging purposes. Surgical lymph node staging was not performed. In the past, some or all of these procedures would have been utilized to precisely stage the patient's cancer. However, in the absence of clinical suspicion, the yield from barium enema, cystoscopy, and sigmoidoscopy has been nearly zero. Intravenous pyelogram does yield some positive findings, but CT scan with IV contrast provides just as much urinary tract information while also visualizing the primary tumor, its pelvic extension, and identifying enlarged pelvic and para-aortic lymph nodes as well. Lymphangiography is the best imaging modality for lymph nodes, but it is infrequently performed today and, hence, few radiologists are proficient at performing or interpreting this procedure. Surgical extraperitoneal lymph node staging has been used in research settings to eliminate patients from protocol study who are found to have para-aortic lymph node involvement. However, the yield of positive para-aortic nodes in Gynecologic Oncology Group (GOG) studies has been dropping, making this expensive and morbid procedure of little practical use. The tremendous cost savings of this more selective and tailored diagnostic work up can be achieved while hastening the onset of therapy without detracting from the patient's opportunity for successful therapy.

Treatment Options

There are a variety of treatment programs which could be offered to this patient.

(a) Participation in the currently active GOG study (#120) for locally advanced cervical cancer. This is a three-pronged randomized trial in which all patients receive external and intracavitary radiation in conjunction with one of three concomitant chemotherapy programs; cisplatin and 5-FU, weekly cisplatin infusion, or cisplatin, 5-FU and hydroxyurea. This study requires surgically negative para-aortic lymph node sampling for the patient to be eligible for study entry. Our program has discontinued surgical evaluation of para-aortic lymph nodes as not cost effective nor is it in the patient's best interest, and thus we would not enter this patient into the GOG trial.

(b) Conventional external and intracavitary radiation will produce a long-term (5 year) disease-free survival of 65%–75% in a population of patients like the one under discussion. Our standard treatment program would involve approximately 4,000 cGy external radiation followed by two intracavitary applications to raise the central (point A) dose to at least 8,000 cGy, and pelvic sidewall boost to obtain a pelvic sidewall dose (point B) of 5,500 cGy minimum combined external and intracavitary dose.

(c) There is considerable interest in the international gynecologic oncology community in neoadjuvant chemotherapy programs for cervical cancer followed by surgery, radiation therapy, or both. The studies done to date have demonstrated high response rates with an uncertain effect on relapse rate or survival. As this approach has not demonstrated any survival benefit in head and neck cancers, where it has been studied for considerably longer, we would not consider this kind of treatment outside of a formal study setting.

(d) Concomitant weekly cisplatin and radiation therapy have been used in our program for several years, initially for patients with positive para-aortic lymph nodes, and has appeared to give better than expected complete remissions with a surprisingly high rate of unrelapsed patients. Because of their involved para-aortic nodes, this initial patient group was treated to extended pelvic and para-aortic fields with excellent patient tolerance. Cisplatin is given once a week during the patient's external radiation program at a dose of 1 mg/kg body weight, up to a maximum weekly cisplatin dose of 60 mg. We aim to achieve six weekly doses of cisplatin, and accomplish that in almost 80% of patients.

(e) Extended field pelvic and para-aortic external radiation was associated with improved survival in the Radiation Therapy Oncology Group (RTOG) study with 5-year follow-up data now available. There was a suggestion in the data that this program was more likely to benefit the earlier stages of cervical cancer, and that there was little, if any, benefit seen in the stage IIIB patients. Patients in the RTOG study did not have surgical staging of para-aortic nodes.

Synthesis

Based on the above background, we have embarked on a standard cervical cancer diagnostic work-up and treatment program, which will be offered to this patient. The initial work-up has already been described above. The treatment program combines standard pelvic external and intracavitary radiation with the addition of elective concomitant para-aortic lymph node irradiation and weekly cisplatin chemotherapy. For most patients, the para-aortic lymph nodes are treated through anterior and posterior extended pelvic and para-aortic fields to deliver a para-aortic lymph node dose of 150 cGy/day and continued to a total para-aortic dose of 4,500 cGy in 30 fractions over 6 weeks total time. The pelvis dose is boosted laterally to a daily pelvic dose of 180 cGy. After 3,960 cGy in 22 fractions and a good response, the treatment field is reduced to exclude the pelvic area and the para-aortic treatment completed. The patient will then undergo two intracavitary applications with 2 weeks between applications. The treatment would then be completed with pelvic sidewall boost treatment, if needed, to achieve a minimum dose of 5,500 cGy at point B. Stage IIIB patients, or stage IIB patients who have an unusually slow or poor response, would have their pelvic external treatment continued to 5,040 cGy in 28 treatments prior to undergoing a single intracavitary implant.

COMMENTARY by Carlos A. Perez

It is noteworthy that a patient with an obvious cervical abnormality would have a biopsy that showed no definite evidence of invasion. It is emphasized in textbooks that care must be exercised in obtaining biopsies of clinically apparent lesions in the cervix by taking multiple punch biopsies in the various quadrants of the cervix, obtaining them at the junction of normal tissue and tumor with enough depth in the stroma to assess the degree of invasion (20). If this principle had been followed, the LEEP procedure would not have been necessary, considering the other findings on pelvic examination. Also, multiple punch biopsies of the cervix could have been obtained at the time of examination under anesthesia. The depth of stromal invasion and the presence of capillary–lymphatic space involvement have been reported to be important prognostic factors in patients with operable cervical carcinoma (stages IB and IIA) (2). Stehman et al. (23) recently

reported that important prognostic factors that correlated with progression-free interval in 626 patients treated with radiation therapy for various stages of carcinoma of the cervix were patient age, performance status, tumor size, and pelvic and periaortic lymph node status. In addition to these factors, clinical stage and bilateral parametrial extension correlated with survival.

The FIGO staging system requires chest roentgenogram and intravenous pyelogram. In recent years, the IVP has been replaced by CT scan of the pelvis and abdomen with contrast material. However, there is no definite evidence that the CT scan is more accurate than pelvic examination in assessing pelvic tumor extent (15), although some authors (1,6) have reported 67% to 80% accuracy with CT scanning or MRI in staging of carcinoma of the cervix (compared with surgical findings). Hricak et al. (8) noted a correlation between findings on the CT scan and outcome in 66 patients with bulky stage IB or greater.

I concur with Dr. Keys's statement that surgical staging in these patients may not be warranted, considering the cost, risk, and relatively small impact on outcome. Nelson et al. (11) reported no significant impact on survival in patients staged surgically and treated with irradiation compared with a group treated without surgical staging.

Regarding therapeutic options, we believe that radiation therapy alone is the best treatment. Irradiation doses of 8,500–9,000 cGy to point A with a combination of external beam irradiation (delivered with high-energy photons) and two intracavitary insertions with standard applicators provide approximately 80% pelvic tumor control and 75% 5-year survival (18,19). The potential benefit of elective irradiation of the periaortic lymph nodes has been documented by RTOG protocol 79–20, in which 4,500 cGy was delivered to a group of these patients, and results were compared with those of a control group treated to the pelvis only (21). A recent update of the data (22) confirms better pelvic tumor control and 5-year disease-free survival (67%) compared with the control group (56%) (p=0.029). A similar study by the EORTC (5) failed to show benefit for elective periaortic lymph node irradiation. However, in that protocol, patients with stage IIIB disease were included; thus, the populations are not comparable.

With regard to use of neoadjuvant or adjuvant chemotherapy in advanced carcinoma of the uterine cervix, except for the reports by Park et al. (13,14), no other studies show any improvement in tumor control or survival in patients receiving chemotherapy and irradiation compared with definitive irradiation alone (17).

Several studies strongly suggest that higher doses of irradiation alone will correlate with improved pelvic tumor control (3,19). Also, we have reported that patients with pelvic tumor control have a lower incidence of distant metastasis and higher survival than those developing pelvic failure (4). Therefore, we deliver 8,500–9,000 cGy to point A (irradiation alone) for stage IB–IIA bulky tumors and stage IIB and III carcinoma of the cervix (16).

At our institution the external beam dose to the lateral pelvic wall with parametrial disease is 6,000 cGy, in addition to the intracavitary dose contribution. This is the treatment I recommend for this patient.

REFERENCES

1. Camilien L, Gordon D, Fruchter RG, Maiman M, Boyce JG. Predictive value of computerized tomography in the presurgical evaluation of primary carcinoma of the cervix. *Gynecol Oncol* 1988;30:209–15.
2. Delgado G, Bundy B, Zaino R, Seven B-U, Creasman WT, Major F. Prospective surgical-pathological study of disease-free interval in patients in stage IB squamous cell carcinoma of the cervix: A Gynecologic Oncology Group study. *Gynecol Oncol* 1990;38:352–7.
3. Eifel PJ, Thoms WW Jr., Smith TL, Morris M, Oswald MJ. The relationship between brachytherapy dose and outcome in patients with bulky endocervical tumors treated with radiation alone. *Int J Radiat Oncol Biol Phys* 1994;28:113–8.
4. Fagundes H, Perez CA, Grigsby PW, Lockett MA. Distant metastases after irradiation alone in carcinoma of the uterine cervix. *Int J Radiat Oncol Biol Phys* 1992;24:197–204.
5. Haie C, Pejovic MH, Gerbaulet A, Horiot JC, et al. Is prophylactic para-aortic irradiation worthwhile in the treatment of advanced cervical carcinoma? Results of a controlled clinical trial of the EORTC radiotherapy group. *Radiother Oncol* 1988;11:101–12.
6. Hricak H, Lacey CG, Sandles LG, Chang YCF, et al. Invasive cervical carcinoma: Comparison of MR imaging and surgical findings. *Radiology* 1988;166:623–31.
7. Hricak H, Phillips T. The influence of tumor size and morphology on the outcome of patients with FIGO stage IB squamous cell carcinoma of the uterine cervix (editorial). *Int J Radiat Oncol Biol Phys* 1994;29:201–3.
8. Hricak H, Quivey JM, Campos Z, Gildengorin V, et al. Carcinoma of the cervix: predictive value of clinical and magnetic resonance (MR) imaging assessment of prognostic factors. *Int J Radiat Oncol Biol Phys* 1993;27:791–801.
9. Kottmeier H-L. *Annual report on the results of treatment in gynecological cancer.* vol 18. Stockholm: International Federation of Gynecology and Obstetrics; 1982.
10. Leibel S, Bauer M, Wasserman T, Marcial V, et al. Radiotherapy with or without misonidazole for patients with stage IIIB or stage IVA squamous cell carcinoma of the uterine cervix: preliminary report of a Radiation Therapy Oncology Group randomized trial. *Int J Radiat Oncol Biol Phys* 1987;13:541–9.
11. Nelson JH, Boyce J, Macasaet M, Lu T, et al. Incidence, significance, and follow-up of para-aortic lymph node metastases in late invasive carcinoma of the cervix. *Am J Obstet Gynecol* 1977;128:336–40.
12. Overgaard J, Bentzen SM, Kolstad P, Kjoerstad K, et al. Misonidazole combined with radiotherapy in the treatment of carcinoma of the uterine cervix. *Int J Radiat Oncol Biol Phys* 1989;16:1069–72.
13. Park TK, Choi DH, Kim SN, Lee CH, et al. Role of induction chemotherapy in invasive cervical cancer. *Gynecol Oncol* 1991;41:107–12.
14. Park TK, Lee SK, Kim SN, Hwang TS, et al. Combined chemotherapy and radiation for bulky stages I–II cervical cancer: comparison of concurrent and sequential regimens. *Gynecol Oncol* 1993;50:196–201.
15. Parker LA, McPhail AH, Yankaskas BC, Mauro MA. Computed tomography in the evaluation of clinical stage IB carcinoma of the cervix. *Gynecol Oncol* 1990;37:332–4.
16. Perez CA. Uterine cervix. In: Perez CA, Brady LW, eds. *Principles and practice of radiation oncology.* 2nd ed. Philadelphia: JB Lippincott; 1992.
17. Perez CA, Grigsby PW. Adjuvant chemotherapy and irradiation in locally advanced squamous cell carcinoma of the uterine cervix. *PPGO Update* 1993;1(4):1–20.
18. Perez CA, Kao M-S. Radiation therapy alone or combined with surgery in the treatment of barrel-shaped carcinoma of the uterine cervix (stage IB, IIA, IIB). *Int J Radiat Oncol Biol Phys* 1985;11:1903–9.
19. Perez CA, Kuske RR, Camel HM, Galakatos AE, et al. Analysis of pelvic tumor control and impact on survival in carcinoma of the uterine cervix treated with radiation therapy alone. *Int J Radiat Oncol Biol Phys* 1988;14:613–21.
20. Perez CA, Kurman RJ, Stehman FB, Thigpen JT. Uterine cervix. In: Hoskins WJ, Perez CA, Young RC, eds. *Principles and practice of gynecologic oncology.* Philadelphia: JB Lippincott; 1992:591–662.
21. Rotman M, Choi K, Guze C, Marcial V, et al. Prophylactic irradiation of the para-aortic lymph node chain in stage IIB and bulky stage IB carcinoma of the cervix: initial treatment results of RTOG 7920. *Int J Radiat Oncol Biol Phys* 1990;19:513–21.
22. Rotman M, Pajak T, Choi K, Clery M. Prophylactic extend-field irradiation of para-aortic nodes in cervical stages IIB and bulky IB and IIA: 10-year results of RTOG 79-20. *JAMA* 1995;274:387–93.
23. Stehman FB, Bundy BN, DiSaia PJ, Keys HM, et al. Carcinoma of the cervix treated with radiation therapy. I. A multi-variate analysis of prognostic variables in the Gynecologic Oncology Group. *Cancer* 1991;67:2776–85.
24. Stehman FB, Bundy BN, Thomas G, Keys HM, et al. Hydroxyurea versus misonidazole with radiation in cervical carcinoma: long-term follow-up of a Gynecologic Oncology Group trial. *J Clin Oncol* 1993;11:1523–8.

95

36-Year-Old HIV-Positive Woman with Stage IIB Squamous Cell Carcinoma of the Cervix

Beth Erickson

The increasing challenge of HIV positivity in patients with gynecologic cancer

CASE PRESENTATION

A 36-year-old black woman was admitted with a 1-year history of daily vaginal bleeding in addition to her regular monthly menses. Approximately 1 month before admission, she noted the onset of left lower quadrant abdominal, groin, and left leg pain and the passage of vaginal blood clots. She was admitted to the emergency room, at which time gynecologic consultation was requested. A urine pregnancy test was performed, with negative results. Pelvic examination revealed a friable, bleeding cervix that was deviated to the left, obscuring visualization of the cervical os. There appeared to be visible and palpable involvement of the left lateral vaginal fornix with the cervix firm and nonmobile and the left parametria infiltrated and nodular. A biopsy was obtained, which revealed an invasive squamous cell carcinoma with no histologic evidence of human papilloma virus (HPV) (Fig. 95–1). Staging was initiated including a chest roentgenogram, which was normal except for some vague lucent areas within both humeral heads. A CT scan of the pelvis with contrast demonstrated an enlarged cervix that measured 4×5 cm in size. The cervix was contiguous with the left ureter with some stranding in the paracervical fat. No pelvic adenopathy was identified. A CT scan of the abdomen did not demonstrate hydronephrosis or retroperitoneal adenopathy and demonstrated a normal liver and spleen. Magnetic resonance imaging (MRI) of

the pelvis revealed a soft tissue mass involving the cervix and lower uterine segment and proximal anterior vaginal wall (Fig. 95–2). Laboratory analysis included a CBC with a hemoglobin of 8.7 and hematocrit of 27 with an MCV of 66, a white blood cell count of 9,000 with normal differential, and a platelet count of 400,000. Liver functions were normal as were the electrolytes with a creatinine of 0.9. Due to a history of IV drug abuse, an enzyme-linked immunoabsorbent assay (ELISA) for HIV was obtained and was found positive. The western blot technique reported viral bands P17, P24, P55, P31, P51, P66, GP41, GP120, and GP160. The total number of T-cells was $82/mm^3$ with $27/mm^3$ T helper and $54/mm^3$ T suppressor cells with a helper to suppressor ratio of 0.5. The absolute number of lymphocytes was $1,749/mm^3$, absolute T11 was $1,434/mm^3$, absolute T4 was $472/mm^3$, absolute T8 was $944/mm^3$, and the B4 population was 14%. The interpretation was that a decrease in helper T-cells and a slight increase in suppressor T-cells resulted in a decreased helper/suppressor ratio with a normal percentage of B-cells.

The patient's past history was significant for a remote history of HIV positivity without obvious progression to AIDS. The patient was gravida 4, para 4 with last menstrual period 1 week before admission. She had normal spontaneous vaginal deliveries in 1971, 1972, 1975, and a low transverse C-section in 1978 with tubal ligation. Menarche began at age 17 with 28-day cycles lasting 3 to

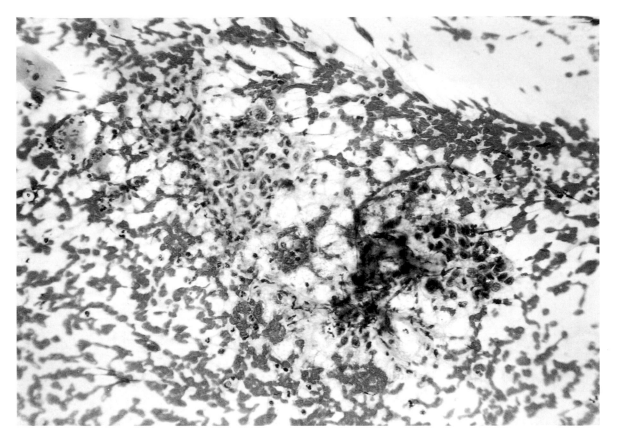

FIG. 95–1. Cervical biopsy. There is an invasive squamous cell carcinoma with no histologic evidence of human papilloma virus.

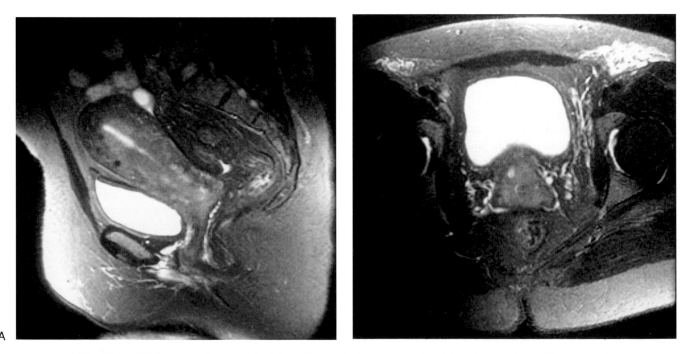

A

B

FIG. 95–2. MR images of the pelvis. There is a soft tissue mass involving the cervix and lower uterine segment with extension to the proximal anterior vagina. **A:** Sagittal cross section. **B:** Transverse section.

5 days. The onset of sexual intercourse was at age 14 with over 10 partners since that time. There was no previous history of an abnormal Pap smear. The patient did have a history of IV cocaine abuse and cigarette smoking. Family history was pertinent for a niece with cervical carcinoma and a sister with breast cancer.

An Infectious Disease consultation was obtained regarding therapeutic intervention for her HIV seropositivity, but the patient refused discussion of this topic and all further phlebotomy.

The patient was also referred to the Radiation Oncology Department after staging was completed and the patient confirmed as stage IIB. Definitive irradiation was recommended consisting of external beam irradiation followed by intracavitary or interstitial implantation. External radiation was initiated with AP/PA pelvic fields due to the very posterior nature of her disease and the possibility of involvement of the left uterosacral ligament. Twenty-two X-17 cm fields with custom blocking were designed, delivering 4,500 cGy in 25 fractions over the next 38 days with 18 MV photons. Her treatment course was significant for multiple treatment breaks due to poor patient compliance. At only 1,080 cGy, the patient began to complain of hourly urinary frequency and dysuria. A urine specimen was obtained, and no organisms were found on subsequent culture. Pyridium was implemented to decrease bladder irritability. Despite this, the patient continued to have marked dysuria and also developed pain with defecation. The patient's abdominal and groin pain persisted with pain radiating down the left leg. Lomotil was implemented as well as MS Contin and Tylenol with codeine. With further continuation of her bladder symptomology, at a dose of 2,880 cGy, another urinalysis was obtained revealing greater than 100 white blood cells per high-powered field, and 50 to 100 red blood cells with no bacteria. The colony count revealed greater than 100,000 gram negative bacilli, and the patient was begun on Bactrim. At a dose of 4,500 cGy the patient required hospitalization for severe bladder pain and frequency. A catheterized urine specimen revealed only 20 to 25 white blood cells per high-powered field with all cultures negative. The patient was again started on Bactrim DS. While hospitalized, an exam under anesthesia was performed, because the patient had refused pelvic examination in the office. The few pelvic exams that the patient had allowed during preceding irradiation demonstrated little change in the cervical and parametrial disease. The exam under anesthesia confirmed this with the cervix again noted to be retracted and deviated to the left. The os was palpably stenotic, and tumor was again noted to involve the left parametrium. Insertion of intracavitary applicators was attempted but the os was too stenotic to admit a uterine sound or dilators, and the procedure terminated. While hospitalized, the patient was seen by psychiatry because of suicidal claims and was diagnosed with a borderline personality disorder. She was discharged on Ditropan,

Bactrim, MS Contin, codeine, and ferrous-sulfate, and resumed external radiation. Consideration of further radiation included interstitial implementation versus external beam only. The patient was thought to be at high–risk for infection if interstitial implantation was performed, making definitive irradiation the treatment of choice. There was also concern over intraoperative needle puncture risk and employee exposure to the patient's body fluids during the implant. Subsequently, the patient was positioned prone on a belly board to displace the small bowel from the radiation field and lateral portals were simulated which were implemented, and through shrinking fields delivered 7,020 cGy to the cervix and paracervical tissues over 74 days. During treatment, the patient lost a total of 20 pounds. The patient was treated with vaginal suppositories for a vaginal trichomonas infection. She did complain of occasional left hip pain in a sciatic distribution. Little regression of tumor was noted at the conclusion of treatment.

At a 1-month follow-up visit, she again complained of continued hip pain in a sciatic distribution. Bimanual examination revealed some reduction in size of the cervix, which remained retracted. A Pap smear was obtained, which revealed only acute inflammation and atypia. At a 3-month follow-up visit, the patient continued to have left hip pain radiating into the left leg and groin without any complaints of vaginal bleeding or discharge. Pelvic examination revealed persistent thickening in the left parametria with bleeding noted at the time of the Pap smear. An MRI of the pelvis demonstrated no cervical mass with residual stranding in the paracervical tissues. The patient returned 6 months after radiation and had continued discharge from the vagina and persistent left hip pain. Pelvic exam revealed mild thickening of the cervix and paracervical tissues on the left; a Pap smear was positive for inflammatory changes. Restaging ensued including an MRI of the pelvis, which again confirmed the absence of a cervical mass and identified an 8-mm lymph node in the left common iliac chain. New abnormal signal intensity was seen in both pyriformis muscles in the region of the sciatic nerves, indicating granulation tissue, postradiation changes, or recurrent disease. A CT scan of the abdomen was negative and a CT scan of the chest showed normal bilateral axillary lymph nodes. Despite efforts to have the patient report to the Infectious Disease Department for intervention regarding her HIV seropositivity, the patient refused. Eleven months following completion of radiation, the patient returned for follow-up and now complained of bilateral leg pain and tingling and low back pain. The patient was referred to the Pain Clinic for evaluation because there did not appear to be any evidence of recurrent disease causing her symptomology. One year following treatment, the patient reported severe abdominal and left flank pain and was ultimately thought to be "drug seeking" in the emergency room on several occasions. It was suggested that she return to the Pain Clinic, but she was then lost to follow-up. Though the patient has failed to return to the Radiation Oncology Department for further follow-up, she remains alive, seemingly free of disease 4 years following definitive irradiation. She continues to refuse active intervention for her HIV positivity, but has not manifested further progression of AIDS during this same time frame.

TUMOR BOARD DISCUSSION

The Center for Disease Control (CDC) recently amended the AIDS surveillance case definition to include invasive cervical carcinoma among the conditions diagnostic of AIDS in women with HIV infection. Originally, this was not the case, despite the fact that Kaposi's sarcoma is considered diagnostic of AIDS (1). Cervical cancer may be the first sign of compromised immunity in these HIV-positive patients. Strong epidemiologic, serologic, and molecular evidence suggests that the occurrence of malignancies in AIDS patients may be related to coexistent or antecedent viral infection, which may be HPV in cervical carcinoma patients. Many women with HIV are co-infected with HPV. The incidence of cervical intraepithelial neoplasia (CIN) is increased in patients with HPV (2). The immune deficit induced by HIV infection may play a permissive role, allowing more rapid HPV proliferation, a facilitated conversion to CIN, or a more rapid emergence of invasive carcinoma once malignant transformation has occurred (2,3). It is probable that the immunodeficiency resulting from HIV infection allows an oncogenic virus to flourish and inhibit the body's natural immunologic defense mechanism that suppresses the development of neoplasia (4). There is also a suggestion that HIV-infected women with cervical carcinoma have a much more fulminate course than HIV-negative women. It has been demonstrated that malignancies do occur more frequently and in unusual patterns in patients who are HIV-positive, suggesting that significant immune deficits may occur in patients soon after infection with the virus, which may predispose to the initiation or progression of cancer (2). A more advanced stage of presentation, higher recurrence and death rates, and the shorter interval to recurrence and death in HIV patients has been documented (4). The T-cell status may impact on the rate of progression. There is some suggestion that when the T4 cell counts drop, there is rapid progression of disease. Cervical intraepithelial neoplasia is more common among HIV-infected patients with lower CD4+ T-lymphocyte counts or more advanced clinical stage of HIV disease (1, 5). Cervical HPV is more common among HIV patients with lower CD4+ T-lymphocyte counts (1, 6). CD4 status may also influence outcome: Patients with suboptimal immune responses in the series of Maiman et al. responded poorly to therapeutic intervention, whereas those with CD4 cell counts greater than $500/mm^3$ had more favorable courses (7). The mean T4:T8 ratio in HIV-positive patients in the series of Maiman et al. was 0.49 versus 1.86 in the HIV-negative patients (4). Cellular immunity indeed is depressed in the HIV-infected patient, and this has an impact on both their susceptibility to neoplasia and their response to standard treatment. Currently, strong recommendations are made regarding screening for cervical intraepithelial neoplasia and cervical carcinoma in HIV-positive patients, and early intervention with anti-AIDS drugs to enhance their chance of responding to standard therapy. When irradiated, there is some suggestion that mucosal reactions maybe more severe and at lower doses than typically expected (8).

Our patient confirmed several of these conclusions. Her very slow regression of disease during treatment may in fact infer that she was unable to immunologically defend herself against the malignancy and, once treated, had very slow clearance of tumor from her body. Our patient's T4:T8 ratio was 0.5 at presentation. Unfortunately, she refused all further testing to document her immune status and refused intervention with anti-AIDS drugs. Despite this, she remains free of disease 4 years following irradiation and has not been hospitalized for other HIV-related infections. She has not demonstrated the fulminant form of cervical carcinoma despite her low T4 counts. Her course of radiation was significant for marked dysuria, perhaps pointing to early and severe mucosa reactions, as has been seen in other patients treated for oral Kaposi's. Perhaps, one of the most difficult aspects of her management was her limited cooperation with treatment; this remains problematic in light of her HIV status.

REFERENCES

1. Northfelt DW. Cervical and anal neoplasia and HPV infection in persons with HIV infection. *Oncology* 1990;8:33–7.
2. Rellihan MA, Dooley DP, Burke TW, et al. Rapidly progressing cervical cancer in a patient with human immunodeficiency virus infection. *Gynecol Oncol* 1990;36:435–8.
3. Rogo KO, Kavoo-Linge. Human immunodeficiency virus seroprevalence among cervical cancer patients. *Gynecol Oncol* 1990;37:87–92.
4. Maiman M, Fruchter RG, Serur E, et al. Human immunodeficiency virus infection and cervical neoplasia. *Gynecol Oncol* 1990;38:377–82.
5. Schafer A, Friedmann W, Mielke M, et al. The increased frequency of cervical dysplasia-neoplasia in women infected with the human immunodeficiency virus is related to the degree of immunosuppression. *Am J Obstet Gynecol* 1991;164:593–9.
6. Conti M, Agarossi A, Parazzini F, et al. HPV, HIV infection, and risk of cervical intraepithelial neoplasia in former intravenous drug abusers. *Gynecol Oncol* 1993;49:344–8,
7. Maiman M, Fruchter RG, Guy L, et al. Human immunodeficiency virus infection and invasive cervical carcinoma. *Cancer* 1993;71:402–6.
8. Watkins EB, Findlay P, Gelmann E, et al. Enhanced mucosal reactions in AIDS patients receiving oropharyngeal irradiation. *Int J Radiat Oncol Biol Phys* 1987;13:1403–8.

COMMENTARY by Andrew K. Saltzman and Leo B. Twiggs

The patient under discussion presents with FIGO stage IIB squamous cell carcinoma of the uterine cervix, and is also seropositive for the human immunodeficiency virus (HIV). The presentation is interesting not only from the clinical management standpoint, but also as an illustration of the relationship between immunologic competence of the host and the development of cervical cancer.

A 36-year-old woman with a "remote" history of HIV seropositivity, along with other cervical cancer risk factors, early onset of sexual activity and multiple sexual partners, was admitted with a grossly visible cervical lesion. The history in regard to cervical cancer screening is unavailable. The patient was clinically staged, and primary radiotherapy was recommended.

As recommended by FIGO, staging of cervical cancer is clinical, and is based on inspection, palpation, cystoscopy, sigmoidoscopy, colposcopy, endocervical curettage, biopsies, and roentgenographic examination of the chest, kidneys, and skeleton, as necessary. Studies such as lymphangiograms, CT, MRI, laparoscopy and laparotomy, although often useful for patient management, are not used in clinical staging (1). The discrepancy between clinical and surgical staging ranges from 20%–48%, depending on the clinical stage (2). The primary rationale for surgical staging is its ability to identify patients who may benefit from extended field irradiation. Although the value of surgical staging remains controversial, management decisions based on the information gained results in a 2.5%–7% improvement in overall cure rate (2,3). Microscopically positive lymph nodes are not seen with the resolution of CT or MRI, and, importantly, it is this group of patients most likely to benefit from extended field radiotherapy. Other advantages of surgical staging include the removal of bulky lymph nodes, removal of diseased adnexae, and ovarian transposition. If surgical staging is not employed, then CT or MRI are both more accurate than clinical staging in advanced cervical cancer (4). In a recent comparison, MRI was superior to CT in differentiating stage IB from stage IIB in both the evaluation of parametrial extension and overall accuracy (5).

The patient had poor compliance with her external beam radiation therapy as evidenced by her missing many appointments. Under anesthesia, placement of the intrauterine tandem for brachytherapy was unsuccessful, and the procedure was terminated. Interstitial radiation implants were considered but avoided due to unfounded concerns over the risk of infection in the patient as well as exposure risks for the staff at placement. The omission of brachytherapy was unfortunate, as it has been shown that brachytherapy is integral to the radiotherapeutic management of cervical cancer (6). A recent study from the "Patterns of Care" data base showed that for patients with locally advanced cervical cancer, local pelvic control and survival was improved for those with "ideal" or "satisfactory" brachytherapy implants versus those with "unacceptable" insertions (7). Although the achievement of a technically adequate implant may be affected by tumor geometry and/or anatomic distortions due to the external radiation, avoidance of interstitial implants because of the aforementioned concerns is questionable. Maiman et al. (in the same reference cited in the Tumor Board discussion) stated "we believe surgery is safe in patients with relatively good immune function and should be used as indicated with standard surgical precautions" (8). In the 4 years since this patient was treated, our understanding of HIV and the use of universal precautions has increased; hopefully, patients are not being inadequately treated because of physician fear. This difficult patient should have the benefit of a multidisciplinary approach to her care with early intervention by social workers, clinical psychologists, and other skilled professionals who have experience in dealing with the psychosocial aspects of these two devastating diseases.

The relationship between cervical cancer and immunocompetence has implications beyond HIV infected patients. At initial evaluation, the patient had a CD4 count of $472/mm^3$, and a T-cell helper/suppressor (CD4/CD8) ratio of 0.5. She refused all subsequent immunologic testing. According to the "immuno-surveillance" theory, a defective cellular-mediated immune system is thought to allow potentially neoplastic cells to proliferate, leading to the development of cancer (9). The hallmark of HIV infection is a marked decrease in T-helper lymphocytes, resulting in a deficiency of cellular-mediated immunity. As pointed out by the case discussion, there is a growing body of literature detailing the relationship between HIV status and premalignant and malignant lesions of the cervix.

Three studies concerning the development of premalignant cervical lesions in HIV infected women, not mentioned in the case discussion, warrant comment. Vermund and colleagues investigated the interactions between HIV, HPV, and cervical cytologic abnormalities. They showed that women who were HIV seropositive and symptomatic were over three times more likely to be infected with HPV than those who were seropositive but asymptomatic. Furthermore, there was a clear association between viral presence and cervical lesions: Women with both viruses had a 58% rate of squamous intraepithelial lesions versus 18% for those with either virus, and 9% for uninfected women (10). Adachi and associates reported the findings of a longitudinal, prospective study of cervical cytology in HIV-seropositive women (11). Contrary to other reports, they found that cytologic findings reliably predicted the colposcopic and histologic findings, and they did not see a rapid progression of disease in their study population. Maiman et al. looked prospectively at the recurrence rate of cervical dysplasia in women who were treated at his clinic. Thirty-nine percent of HIV-seropositive women recurred, compared to 9% of the seronegative patients. In addition, when the first group was stratified according to their CD4 counts, those who were below 500/mm³ had a 45% incidence of recurrence versus 18% for those seropositive but with greater counts (12).

In the context of cervical cancer and immunocompetence, HIV infection may "simply" be an extreme example of the more general concept. In 1986, Carson et al. looked at twenty patients with multiple recurrent genital condylomata and neoplasias all with HPV–DNA demonstrated in the involved tissues. Compared to controls, patients had a statistically significant decrease in their CD4/CD8 ratio (13). The group from the National Cancer Institute in Naples, Italy divided patients with cervical neoplasia into three groups: CIN III, microinvasive cancer, and invasive cancer. They found that the CD8 cells were increased (and the CD4/CD8 ratio therefore decreased) in patients in the first two groups, versus both control women and those in the third group. They postulated that cellular-mediated immunity plays a role in the premalignant and early stages of cervical cancer (14). The relationship between host immunocompetence and viral infection, specifically HPV, needs more attention. Viral replication may have a local effect on immunocompetent cells, and such an effect may lead to the host developing incompetent systemic immunity.

Pillai and colleagues in India have investigated this area for a number of years. In one report they looked at 67 women with stages I–IV squamous cell carcinoma of the cervix. In contrast to the Italian findings, where the third group of patients (those with invasive cancer) had normal immune indices, they found derangements in the T-cell helper and suppressor populations in patients with *all* stages of cervical cancer, the imbalance being most prominent in the advanced stages (15). In a subsequent paper involving over 200 patients, they found five immunological variables that were consistently abnormal in all stages of cervical cancer, among which were the CD4 count and the CD4/CD8 ratio. They constructed an immunologic scoring system and purported to show that a patient's prognosis could be predicted, even before treatment (16).

As the Tumor Board discussion pointed out, the CDC has recently included invasive cervical carcinoma among those conditions diagnostic of AIDS in HIV-positive women. The management of these patients is challenging, and the interactions between viral status (HPV, HIV), immunocompetence (CD4 counts), and premalignant and malignant cervical disease deserve close scrutiny.

REFERENCES

1. Carcinoma of the cervix uteri. In: Pettersson F. ed. Annual report on the results of treatment in gynecological cancer. *Int J Gynecol Obstet* 1991;36(Suppl):27–31.
2. LaPolla JP, Schlaerth JB, Gaddis O, Morrow CP. Influence of surgical staging on the evaluation and treatment of patients with cervical carcinoma. *Gynecol Oncol* 1986;24:194–206.
3. Potish RA, Twiggs LB, Okagaki T, Prem KA, Adcock LL. Therapeutic implications of the natural history of advanced cervical cancer as defined by pretreatment surgical staging. *Cancer* 1985;56:956–60.
4. Walsh JW. Computed tomography of gynecologic neoplasms. *Radiol Clin North Am* 1992;30(4):817–30.
5. Kim SH, Choi BI, Lee HP, et al. Uterine cervical carcinoma: comparison of CT and MR findings. *Radiology* 1990;175:45.
6. Lanciano RM, Won M, Coia LR, Hanks GE. Pre-treatment and treatment factors associated with improved outcome in squamous cell carcinoma of the uterine cervix: a final report of the 1973 and 1978 patterns of care studies. *Int J Radiat Oncol Biol Phys* 1991;20:667–76.
7. Corn BW, Hanlon AL, Pajak TF, Owen J, Hanks GE. Technically accurate intracavitary insertions improve pelvic control and survival among patients with locally advanced carcinoma of the uterine cervix. *Gynecol Oncol* 1994;53:294–300.
8. Maiman M, Fruchter RG, Guy L, Cuthill S, et al. Human immunodeficiency virus infection and invasive cervical carcinoma. *Cancer* 1993;71(2):402–6.
9. Burnett FM. The concept of immunological surveillance. *Prog Exp Tumour Res* 1970;13:1–43.
10. Vermund SH, Kelley KF, Klein RS, et al. High–risk of human papillomavirus infection and cervical squamous intraepithelial lesions among women with symptomatic human immunodeficiency virus infection. *Am J Obstet Gynecol* 1991;165:392–400.
11. Adachi A, Fleming I, Burk RD, Ho GYF, Klein RS. Women with human immunodeficiency virus infection and abnormal Papanicolaou smears: a prospective study of colposcopy and clinical outcome. *Obstet Gynecol* 1993;81(3):372–7.
12. Maiman M, Fruchter RG, Serur E, Levine PA, et al. Recurrent cervical intraepithelial neoplasia in human immunodeficiency virus seropositive women. *Obstet Gynecol* 1993;82:170–4.
13. Carson LF, Twiggs LB, Fukushima M, Ostrow RS, et al. Human genital papilloma infections: an evaluation of immunologic competence in the genital neoplasia-papilloma syndrome. *Am J Obstet Gynecol* 1986;155:784–9.
14. Castello G, Esposito G, Stellato G, Dalla Mora L, et al. Immunological abnormalities in patients with cervical carcinoma. *Gynecol Oncol* 1986;25:61–4.
15. Balaram P, Pillai MR, Padmanabhan TK, Abraham T, et al. Immune function in malignant cervical neoplasia: a multi-parameter analysis. *Gynecol Oncol* 1988;31:409–23.
16. Pillai MR, Balaram P, Chidambaram S, Padmanabhan TK, Nair MK. Development of an immunological staging system to prognosticate disease course in malignant cervical neoplasia. *Gynecol Oncol* 1990;37:200–5.

SECTION XX

Uterus

96
Endometrial Carcinoma

John R. Lurain

The necessity for a tailored multidisciplinary approach to the treatment of endometrial carcinoma

CASE PRESENTATION

R.C. is a 74-year-old white woman, gravida 2, para 2, who presented to her gynecologist with a two-week history of light vaginal bleeding. She had been menopausal since 1977 and had been on hormone-replacement therapy since 1982. In 1989, she had some uterine bleeding, and an endometrial aspiration biopsy had revealed benign endometrial glandular fragments. Her hormone therapy had been changed to continuous conjugated estrogens 0.625 mg and medroxyprogesterone acetate 2.5 mg daily. She had not had any bleeding since then until recently. A pelvic ultrasound in 1990 had revealed a normal-sized uterus with normal endometrial stripe and no adnexal masses.

The patient's past medical history was significant for hypertension, currently being treated with lisinopril and hydrochlorothiazide; diverticulosis; and mild granulocytopenia of 20 years' duration. Review of systems was positive only for moderate urinary stress incontinence.

On physical examination, she was 61 inches tall, weighed 140 lbs, and her blood pressure was 150/80. Her head and neck examination was normal. There was no supraclavicular or cervical lymphadenopathy. Both breasts were without masses, and the axillae were negative. Her heart and lungs were clear. The abdomen was soft and nontender; there was an ill-defined left lower quadrant mass; the liver was of normal size; and there was no ascites. The vulva, vagina, and cervix appeared normal. The uterus was normal size and mobile. There were no adnexal masses on bimanual examination. Rectal examination, including stool for occult blood, was negative.

A Pap smear and endometrial aspiration biopsy were performed. The Pap smear was normal. The endometrial biopsy showed grade II adenocarcinoma. Preoperative testing including a chest roentgenogram, electrocardiogram, complete blood and platelet counts, serum chemistries, and urinalysis were within normal limits, except for a white blood count of 3,000.

The patient underwent exploratory laparotomy with total abdominal hysterectomy, bilateral salpingo-oophorectomy, pelvic and para-aortic lymph node biopsies, and a retropubic urethropexy, as well as peritoneal washings for cytologic examination. The left adnexa was found to be bound up in adhesions with a diverticular mass involving the sigmoid colon. The remainder of the peritoneal cavity including the liver, kidneys, stomach, large and small bowel, and peritoneal surfaces appeared and felt normal. The patient made an uneventful postoperative recovery, and was discharged from the hospital on the fifth postoperative day.

Pathologic examination of the uterus revealed a moderately differentiated (grade II) adenocarcinoma of the endometrium that involved almost the entire endometrial cavity but did not extend into the lower uterine segment or cervix (Fig. 96–1). The endometrial cancer invaded into the outer half of the myometrium (approximately two thirds of the myometrial thickness), but not to the uterine serosa (Fig. 96–2). There was one focus of lymphvascular space invasion within the myometrium (Fig. 96–3). All 15 lymph nodes were negative for tumor, as were both tubes and ovaries. Peritoneal washings from the right and left paracolic gutters and pelvis were cytologically negative.

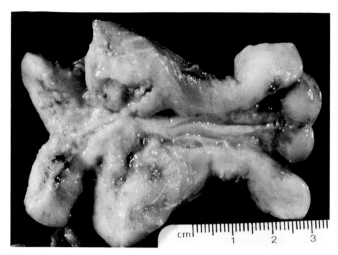

FIG. 96–1. Adenocarcinoma diffusely involving almost the entire endometrial cavity, but not the lower uterine segment or endocervix, and invading deeply into the myometrium.

Based on the surgical–pathologic findings, the patient was assessed as having stage IC, grade II endometrial cancer. Because of the deep myometrial invasion, as well as the size of the tumor and presence of lymph–vascular space invasion, the Tumor Board recommended postoperative pelvic radiotherapy, 4,500 cGy in 25 180-cGy fractions, followed by a vaginal boost of 1,500 cGy (total dose = 6,000 cGy to the vaginal apex). The patient toler-ated the radiotherapy with minimal gastrointestinal toxic-ity. She has remained well and without evidence of recur-rent disease.

DISCUSSION

Adenocarcinoma of the endometrium is the most common malignancy of the female genital tract. Approximately 33,000 cases are diagnosed annually in the United States, resulting in an estimated 5,500 deaths. Several risk factors for the development of endometrial carcinoma have been identified. Most of these involve unopposed estrogen due to increased estrogen, decreased progesterone, or a combination of these. Endogenous estrogen excess is associated with estrogenic ovarian tumors, such as granulosa cell tumors, polycystic ovarian disease, and other anovulatory states, which result in decreased progesterone production, and obesity where adrenallyderived androstenedione is converted to estrone in fat by aromatization. Estrogen therapy without progestins for gonadal dysgenesis and hypopituitarism or menopause also increases the risk for developing endometrial cancer. Other predisposing conditions may be diabetes mellitus, hypertension, hypothyroidism, infertility, endometrial hyperplasia, and the Lynch type II cancer family syndrome. This patient had hypertension but was not obese. She had been on menopausal estrogen replacement therapy, albeit in conjunction with a progestin.

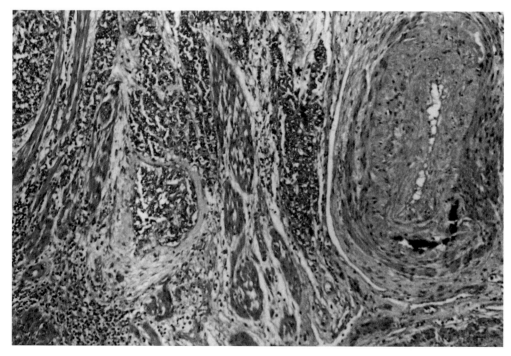

FIG. 96–2. Moderately differentiated endometrial adenocarcinoma with myometrial invasion (H&E stain, ×100).

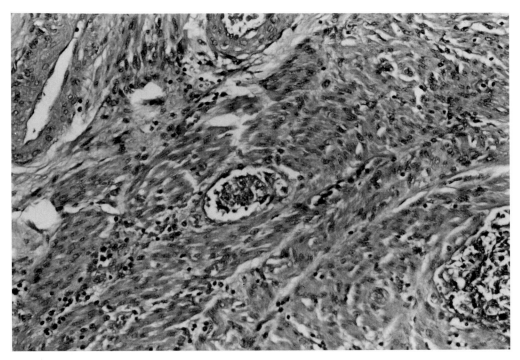

FIG. 96–3. Endometrial carcinoma with lymphvascular space invasion (H&E stain, ×100).

Usually, the only symptom of endometrial carcinoma is abnormal peri- or postmenopausal uterine bleeding, such as this patient had, but only 10%–20% of patients with this complaint have endometrial cancer. Only 1%–5% of cases of endometrial cancer are diagnosed while the patient is asymptomatic. This usually results from investigation of a Pap smear showing atypical or malignant glandular cells or discovery of cancer in a uterus removed for another gynecologic condition. Physical examination seldom reveals any evidence of endometrial carcinoma. Only 30%–50% of patients with endometrial cancer will have an abnormal Pap smear, making this an unreliable diagnostic test. Office endometrial aspiration biopsy is the accepted first step in evaluating abnormal uterine bleeding or whenever endometrial pathology is suspected. Hysteroscopy and dilation and curettage should be reserved for situations in which cervical stenosis or patient tolerance does not permit adequate office evaluation, bleeding recurs after a negative endometrial biopsy, or an inadequate specimen to explain the abnormal bleeding is obtained. Transvaginal ultrasound may be useful as an adjunct to endometrial biopsy for evaluating abnormal bleeding and selecting patients for additional testing. Patients receiving hormone-replacement therapy should undergo endometrial sampling prior to initiating therapy, possibly periodically (every 1 to 2 years during treatment, and if any unscheduled bleeding occurs).

In recognition that nearly all patients with endometrial carcinoma undergo surgery as the primary mode of therapy, and that preoperative clinical staging is incorrect up to 50% of the time, the International Federation of Gynecology and Obstetrics (FIGO) changed from clinical to surgical staging in 1988. Preoperative clinical evaluation is still important in planning for surgery and correlates well with prognosis. In approximately 75% of cases, there is no clinical evidence of extra-uterine disease on physical examination, and the only additional preoperative studies required are chest roentgenogram and routine serum chemistries. More extensive preoperative evaluation, such as computed tomography of the abdomen and pelvis, may be warranted for patients whose disease characteristics (e.g., poorly differentiated tumor) or physical examination findings (e.g., parametrial, vaginal, or cervical extension or adnexal masses) put them at greater risk for extra-pelvic metastases.

For most patients, exploratory laparotomy with total abdominal hysterectomy, bilateral salpingo-oophorectomy, pelvic and aortic lymph node biopsies, and peritoneal cytology should be the initial step in staging and treating endometrial cancer. Approximately 18% of patients with clinically early stage disease will have evidence of extra-uterine spread, including 12% with positive peritoneal cytology, 10% with pelvic and 8% with para-aortic node metastases, 7% with adnexal spread, and 3% with peritoneal implants. In addition, 20% will have outer one-half myometrial invasion, 8% will have occult extension to the cervix, and 7% will have lymphvascular space invasion (LVSI). The value of surgical–pathologic staging has been clearly demonstrated. The survival in patients with surgical stage I disease (tumor confined to the uterine corpus) and stage II disease (cervical involvement without extrauterine extension) is over 90%, whereas survival decreases to 75%–80% with stage IIIA disease (positive peritoneal cytology, uterine serosal involvement or adnexal metastasis), and to 45%–50% with stage IIIC (40% for aortic node and 60%–75% for pelvic node metastasis).

Several prognostic factors for endometrial cancer recurrence or survival have been identified. Increasing patient age has consistently been found to be associated with a greater risk of disease recurrence. Patients with endometrial cancer diagnosed before age 50 rarely die of disease, whereas the 5-year disease-free survival for patients over age 75 years is only 65%–70%. Histologic type and tumor grade, as well as depth of myometrial invasion have prognostic input, even in the absence of extra-uterine disease. Patients with grade III tumors are three to five times more likely to develop recurrence than are patients with grade I or II tumors (16%–36% versus 4%–10%). The histopathologic subtypes of adenosquamous, papillary and clear cell adenocarcinomas also carry an increased risk for recurrence. Increasing tumor anaplasia is highly associated with deep myometrial invasion. Recurrence develops in less than 10% of patients, with less than one-half myometrial invasion compared with approximately 30% in patients with greater than or equal to one-half myometrial invasion. Recurrence risk is approximately 17% for tumors exceeding 2 cm in size, 22% for positive peritoneal cytology, 25% for adnexal metastasis, 25% for pelvic lymph node metastasis, 35% for LSVI, and 60% for aortic lymph node metastasis. Other tumor factors that may have prognostic importance are steroid hormone receptor content and DNA ploidy.

Most women with early endometrial cancer can be cured by hysterectomy, with or without radiotherapy. Survival with hysterectomy is greater than with radiation alone by 15%–25%. Extending the operation to some form of radical hysterectomy does not seem to improve the results. In general, patients with disease clinically confined to the uterus are subjected to exploratory laparotomy as the initial step in the treatment program. This approach recognizes that most patients will not need adjuvant pelvic radiotherapy, that preoperative radiation can obscure important surgical–pathologic information, and that postoperative irradiation is as safe and effective as preoperative irradiation. Surgical–pathologic staging data, including peritoneal cytology and lymph node sampling, obtained concurrently with hysterectomy and bilateral salpingo-oophorectomy, will provide the basis for selection of postoperative adjuvant therapy. Extended surgical staging adds little morbidity. More recently, laparoscopically assisted vaginal hysterectomy and bilateral salpingo-oophorectomy with pelvic and aortic lymph node biopsies has been advanced as a surgical treatment option.

Postoperatively, patients can be divided into groups based on risk for recurrence and need for adjuvant therapy. Patients with small (less than 2 cm) grade I or II endometrioid tumors not involving the lower uterine segment or cervix, no or very superficial myometrial invasion, no LSVI and no extra-uterine spread are at low risk (less than 5%) for recurrence and require no further treatment. Patients with grade I or II tumors larger than 2 cm with less than one-half myometrial invasion and/or extension to the lower uterine segment and no evidence of extra-uterine disease have a 5%–10% risk of recurrence and should be treated with postoperative vaginal cuff irradiation (intravaginal brachytherapy or high-dose rate). Patients with grade III tumors or high-risk histologic subtypes, greater than or equal to one-half myometrial invasion, cervical involvement, adnexal metastasis, LVSI, or pelvic lymph node metastasis are at high risk for recurrence and are candidates for postoperative pelvic irradiation (4,500–5,000 cGy in 180 daily fractions). If aortic node metastases are present, in the absence of more widespread disease, extended field para-aortic radiation (4,500 cGy) is recommended. Adjuvant medical therapy with progestins or cytotoxic chemotherapy is not indicated.

When the cervix is clinically involved by tumor, whole pelvic radiation therapy, intracavitary brachytherapy, and adjunctive simple hysterectomy-bilateral salpingo-oophorectomy with selective para-aortic lymph node dissection is usually the treatment of choice. Patients with parametrial or vaginal extension (clinical stage III) are best treated with pelvic radiation therapy after a thorough metastatic work-up. When radiation therapy is completed, exploratory laparotomy is recommended for those patients whose disease seems to be resectable. Patients with an adnexal mass should, after proper evaluation, undergo primary surgery to determine the nature of the mass (inflammatory, benign, or malignant primary ovarian tumor, benign uterine tumor, metastatic endometrial cancer), to perform surgical–pathologic staging and to carry out tumor reductive surgery, including hysterectomy and adnexectomy. Patients with clinical or pathologic evidence of disseminated metastatic endometrial cancer are usually most suitable for systemic hormonal therapy or chemotherapy. Occasionally, hysterectomy or pelvic radiotherapy are indicated for local tumor control. Whole abdominal radiation may have a place for treatment of microscopic intra-abdominal disease found at surgery.

Follow-up of patients after treatment for endometrial cancer should consist of a history, physical examination including lymph node survey, breasts, abdominal and pelvic examinations, and vaginal cytology every 3 months during the first 2 years and every 6 months thereafter. Blood work including a complete blood count, serum chemistries, and possibly a CA-125, as well as a chest roentgenogram, should be obtained periodically. Other tests, such as CT scans and MRI, are not indicated unless the patients' symptoms warrant them. Estrogen-replacement therapy for women at low risk for recurrence does not seem to be contraindicated.

SUGGESTED READINGS

1. Boronow RC, Morrow CP, Creasman WT, et al. Surgical staging in endometrial cancer. Clinical-pathologic findings of a prospective study. *Obstet Gynecol* 1984;63:825–32.
2. DiSaia PJ, Creasman WT, Boronow RC, Blessing JA. Risk factors and recurrent patterns in stage I endometrial cancer. *Am J Obstet Gynecol* 1985;151:1009–15.
3. Lurain JR, Rice BL, Rademaker AW, et al. Prognostic factors associated with recurrence in clinical stage I adenocarcinoma of the endometrium. *Obstet Gynecol* 1991;78:63–9.
4. Morrow CP, Bundy BN, Kurman RJ, et al. Relationship between surgical-pathological risk factors and outcome in clinical stage I and II carcinoma of the endometrium. *Gynecol Oncol* 1991;40:55–65.

COMMENTARY by Perry W. Grigsby

Multiple prognostic factors have been identified for patients with endometrial carcinoma. Standard therapy for stage I disease has traditionally been surgery. The role of radiation therapy has been in an adjuvant setting, either preoperative or postoperative. Appropriate studies to test the effectiveness of irradiation have not been successfully performed.

When asked to evaluate patients postoperatively for consideration of irradiation, I require information concerning the surgery, the pathologic specimens, and the patient's performance status.

The patient in this case apparently tolerated surgery well but was found to have adhesions and a diverticular mass involving the sigmoid colon. Pathologic findings revealed grade II adenocarcinoma, 2/3 myometrial invasion, lymph vascular space invasion, no extra-uterine (pelvic) disease, negative pelvic and para-aortic lymph nodes, and negative peritoneal cytology. I will assume the patient has a performance status that is average for her age.

I would recommend postoperative external beam pelvic irradiation and an intracavitary implant for this patient, based on deep myometrial invasion and lymph vascular space involvement. There is no extra-pelvic disease and no consideration would be given for whole abdominal irradiation. Our standard treatment policy at the Mallinckrodt Institute of Radiology for a patient with these pathologic findings would be to deliver 2,000 cGy whole pelvis, 3,000 cGy split field, and a single low dose rate vaginal cuff implant with Fletcher-Suit colpostats (2 cm) for 6,500 cGy surface dose. I would modify this prescription for this patient. The external irradiation dose would be decreased to 2,000 cGy whole pelvis; and 2,500 cGy split field because of the previously described adhesions.

Rather than a single low-dose rate intracavitary implant (6,500 cGy surface dose), an alternative form of brachytherapy utilizing high dose rate brachytherapy can be performed (500 cGy at 0.5 cm depth, ×3 [total; 1,500], each procedure separated by 2 weeks).

Although not recommended by myself, an alternative school of thought for this patient is that since the pelvic and para-aortic lymph nodes are negative, then no postoperative irradiation should be administered. Since routine lymph node sampling is a relatively recent development for patients with endometrial carcinoma, long-term follow-up for a large group of patients with negative lymph nodes and who were not treated with irradiation is not available. This issue will need further review as data becomes available.

97

Carcinosarcoma of the Uterus, Clinical Stage I

Peyton T. Taylor, Jr., Willie A. Andersen, and Laurel W. Rice

A rare tumor of mesodermal origin, often treated with success locally but with a high propensity for metastases

CASE PRESENTATION

Gynecologic Oncologist: The patient is a 71-year-old woman, gravida 4, para 4, who presented to a local gynecologist with a 2-month history of light vaginal spotting and occasional bleeding. This was noticeable after voiding and as blood stains in her underclothing. She was otherwise healthy and without specific complaints on a review of systems.

On her initial examination her vulva, vagina, and cervix were normal to inspection and palpation. The uterus was small and of normal size. There were no adnexal or rectal abnormalities to palpation, and there was no palpable lymphadenopathy. Referral to a urologist was made because of the suspicion of hematuria, revealing a normal urinalysis, excretory urogram, and cystoscopic examination.

Two weeks later, she returned to her gynecologist after having experienced heavy vaginal bleeding. At that time, she was found to have blood flowing from the cervical os and the uterus was enlarged to three to four times normal size. Examination under anesthesia with dilatation and curettage was performed, significant only for an abundant amount of endometrial tissue. The referring pathologist described a carcinosarcoma with cartilaginous elements. The patient was then referred to our institution. The findings on pelvic examination were notable only for an enlarged uterus.

Surgical Pathology: The curettings contained a mixture of malignant glands and malignant stromal elements. We were in agreement with the diagnosis rendered by the referring pathologist of a malignant mixed Mesodermal tumor with heterologous elements. (Fig. 97–1).

Tumor Board Moderator: Do we have radiographic studies on this patient?

Radiologist: The plain chest radiogram and the previous excretory urogram were normal. The CT of the abdomen and pelvis revealed a gallstone, a benign liver cyst without evidence of hepatic metastasis, no para-aortic or pelvic lymphadenopathy, and no ascites. There is a midline pelvic mass consistent with an enlarged uterus filled with soft tissue and blood or fluid (Figs. 97–2 and 97–3).

Tumor Board Moderator: I would like to start the discussion of the patient's management by asking one of the gynecologic oncologists to give us an opinion.

Gynecologic Oncologist: This patient has what was formerly known as a malignant mixed mesodermal tumor of the uterus with heterologous elements. The term carcinosarcoma is now preferred by the International Society of Gynecologic Pathologists and the World Health Organization. All of these tumors are very aggressive with an extremely poor 5-year survival rate (1). The majority of patients with this disease relapse within 18 months of their original diagnosis and most commonly succumb with distant metastases.

The disease appears to be clinically confined to the uterus. I would advise exploration, formal surgical staging, and hysterectomy with bilateral salpingo-oophorectomy. I also advocate careful surgical staging to include omentectomy and selective pelvic and para-aortic lymphadenectomy at the time of hysterectomy.

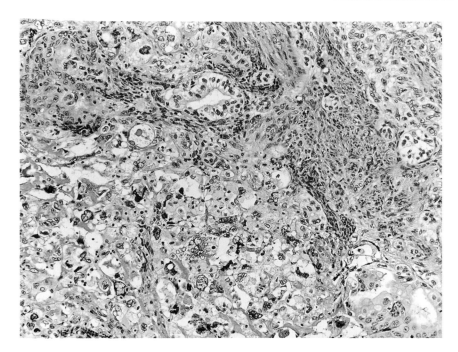

FIG. 97–1. Photomicrograph revealing malignant glands and diffuse pleomorphic malignant stomal cells (× 250).

Tumor Board Moderator: Does the size of the lesion, depth of invasion, or any of a number of histologic variants affect your recommendation? Would anyone comment on the need for postoperative treatment if the disease is surgical stage I.

Surgical Pathology: The histologic factors useful in predicting prognosis in other uterine sarcomas (degree of cytologic atypia, mitotic index, DNA ploidy, or nature of invasion) are not helpful in uterine carcinosarcomas. Several studies have noted that patients' tumors containing heterologous elements do worse than those with homologous elements (2). This has not been consistently found to

be the case (3). The presence of cartilage is likewise a feature of dubious prognostic significance (4).

Radiation Oncologist: If there is no evidence of extrauterine disease at the time of hysterectomy, postoperative whole pelvic radiation therapy should be considered to increase the probability of local control. Although the role of radiation therapy in tumors confined to the uterus is somewhat controversial, several authors have shown that supplemental pelvic radiation provides a higher rate of local control and, perhaps, improved survival (5). Preoperative therapy is, in general, associated with a slightly lower rate of complications than postoperative therapy;

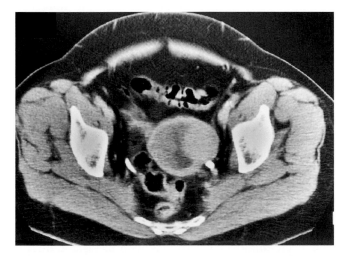

FIG. 97–2. Computed axial tomogram through the pelvis revealing uterine enlargement: The uterine cavity contains fluid and sessile soft tissue mass.

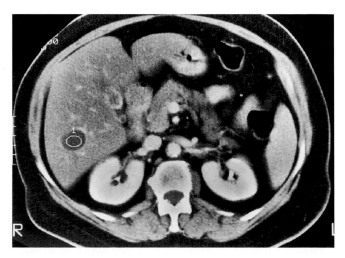

FIG. 97–3. Computed axial tomogram revealing no hepatic parenchymal metastases, no ascites, and a normal spleen and kidneys. There is a benign hepatic cyst.

for that reason, one can argue for preoperative whole pelvic radiation therapy.

Gynecologic Oncologist: I think the data regarding the beneficial effects of radiation therapy in this setting are conflicting and I specifically have reservations about preoperative radiation therapy. A large percentage of patients with disease clinically limited to the uterus have been reported to have extra-uterine disease at exploration (a higher surgical–pathologic stage) (6–8). In addition, a number of authors have shown no survival advantage in those series in which surgery has been combined with radiation as compared with series of patients treated by surgery alone (9–11).

I support Dr. W.A.'s recommendation for primary surgical staging. If the patient has *surgical* stage I disease, I would encourage her to participate in the adjuvant chemotherapy trial being conducted by the Gynecologic Oncology Group (GOG). The objective of that trial is to determine if 'prophylactic' postoperative chemotherapy will decrease the risk of relapse.

Tumor Board Moderator: What are the specifics of the current GOG trial?

Medical Oncologist: The current trial is a prospective nonrandomized trial designed to determine whether postoperative chemotherapy with ifosfamide/Mesna and platinum will decrease the rate of either local recurrence or distant metastases in patients with completely resected stage I or stage II disease. Patients are begun on therapy within 8 weeks of surgery and treated for 4 days every 3–4 weeks. Patients are not eligible for this study if they have received prior radiation or chemotherapy.

Gynecologic Oncologist: I know that some of you disagree with the value of radiation in these cases, but over the years I have found that my patients have higher rates of local control when I've used radiation adjunctively with surgery. I'm not impressed with the data supporting adjuvant chemotherapy trials, and because of this, I'll stick with my previous plan for combination radiation therapy and surgery.

SUBSEQUENT TUMOR BOARD MEETING

Tumor Board Moderator: May we please have an update on the patient with carcinosarcoma discussed by the Tumor Board a few months ago? Did she have any extra-uterine disease at exploration? Was any further therapy advised or given?

Gynecologic Oncologist: The patient received preoperative whole pelvic radiation through parallel opposed ports. She received 4,400 cGy in 22 fractions over 30 days. Except for occasional loose stools (controlled with antiperistaltics) and dysuria caused by a simple lower urinary tract infection (controlled with oral antibiotics) there were no complications of therapy. Exploration and hysterectomy were performed 3 weeks after completion of her radiation therapy.

I reviewed the specimen with the pathologist. There was a small focus of residual malignancy that invaded the muscle wall about 50%. The oviducts, ovaries, nodes, and omentum were negative.

We decided not to advise chemotherapy at this point, and plan to follow her regularly.

SUBSEQUENT TUMOR BOARD MEETING, 16 MONTHS LATER

Radiation Oncology: I would like to re-present the patient with carcinosarcoma discussed on two previous occasions. She gave a history of being well until August 1993 when she had a bout of transient bronchitis, which completely resolved with antibiotic therapy. Three weeks later she developed fever, exertional dyspnea, and cough. She was seen in the Emergency Department of the community hospital, where a chest radiogram revealed collapse of the right middle and lower lobes (Fig. 97–4). She underwent bronchoscopy, which revealed an endobronchial tumor that almost completely obstructed the right mainstem bronchus. A fine-needle aspiration and a biopsy were obtained, both of which confirmed a malignant lesion. The patient gave a history of smoking a pack of cigarettes a day for 40 years, but quit smoking almost 8 years ago.

Surgical Pathologist: We have both fine needle aspiration cytology and biopsy material on this patient. The first is a transbronchial aspirate on which the preliminary diagnosis rendered was positive for malignancy. The cells are those of a poorly differentiated malignant neoplasm (Fig. 97–5).

The biopsy sample was a 1-cc aggregate of hemorrhagic and necrotic-looking yellow-green/pink-tan tissue. We performed stains for vimentin, desmin, cytokeratin and epithelial membrane antigen (EMA) to help us classify the tumor. In addition, the biopsies were compared with the original tissue removed at dilation and curettage.

The tumor appeared to be biphasic. There were areas with malignant glandular structures as well as areas of undifferentiated malignancy. The latter areas were consistent with her original carcinosarcoma.

The carcinomatous areas stained for both cytokeratin and EMA, whereas the undifferentiated areas stained only with vimentin. The malignant cartilaginous areas were desmin positive in the original curettings and variably positive in the undifferentiated areas of the current biopsy.

Medical Oncologist: I saw this unfortunate woman in consultation. She is dyspneic at rest, coughing and hypoxemic. I did not advise chemotherapy at this point. Although there are a number of cytotoxic agents which have been employed in patients with metastatic uterine sarcomas, they very rarely produce rapid or complete regression of metastatic foci (12,13). The patient's needs are acute, and I concurred with the recommendation for

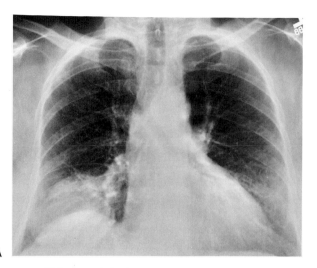 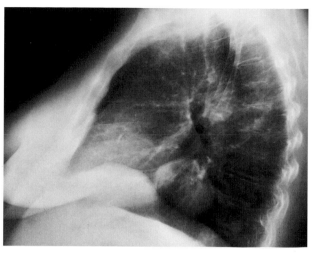

A   B

FIG. 97–4A,B. PA chest and lateral roentgenograms of the chest demonstrating a large, circular mass in right lower lobe.

palliative radiation therapy. Hopefully, this will promptly relieve or diminish the obstruction of the bronchus.

Gynecologic Oncologist: I saw the patient and found no evidence of local recurrence. I discussed her care in Radiation Oncology and with Gynecologic Oncology. We were in agreement with the recommendation for radiation therapy. This seems to offer the greatest possibility of a true palliative response.

Gynecologic Oncologist: I understand that the patient did not have pelvic recurrence felt on pelvic examination.

Since most patients with pulmonary metastasis also have occult metastatic disease elsewhere, I would get a CT of the head as well as the abdomen and pelvis. If she has multiple sites of metastasis I would advise we change the focus of therapy toward palliative and supportive (hospice) care after completion of radiation therapy. The commercially available chemotherapeutic agents, even ifosfamide and Platinum combinations, are woefully inactive in metastatic carcinosarcomas. I think they offer little help for this patient, especially given her current performance status.

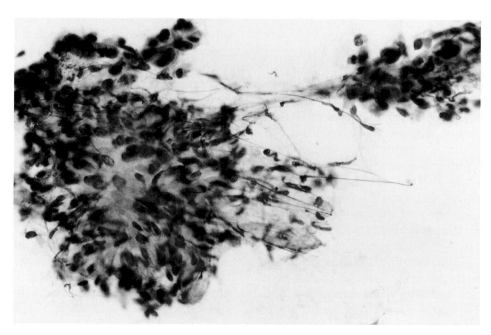

FIG. 97–5. Transbronchial fine needle aspiration cytology (× 250) showing malignant cells, some with glandular features; others have diffuse pleomorphic features.

REFERENCES

1. Ali S, Wells M. Mixed Mullerian tumors of the uterine corpus: a review. *Int J Gynecol Cancer* 1993;3:1–11.
2. Ober WC, Tovel HMM. Mesenchymal sarcomas of the uterus. *Am J Obstet Gynecol* 1959;77:246–68.
3. Nielson, et al. ibid.
4. Gallup DG, Gable DS, Talledo OE, Otken LB Jr. A clinical-pathologic study of mixed Mullerian tumors of the uterus over a 16 year period—The Medical College of Georgia experience. *Am J Obstet Gynecol* 1989;161:533–9.
5. Larson B, Silversward C, Nilsson B, Petterson F. Mixed Mullerian tumors of the uterus-prognostic: a clinical and histopathologic study. *Radiother Oncol* 1990;17:123–32.
6. Spanos WJ, Wharton JT, Gomez L, et al. Malignant mixed Mullerian tumors of the uterus. *Cancer* 1984;53:311–6.
7. Doss LL, Llorens AS, Henriques EM. Carcinosarcoma of the uterus: a 40 year experience from the State of Missouri. *Gynecol Oncol* 1984;18:43–53.
8. Major FJ, Blessing JA, Silverberg SG, et al. Prognostic factors in early-stage uterine sarcoma. *Cancer* 1993;71:1702–9.
9. Nielson et al. ibid.
10. Peters WA III, Kumar NB, Fleming WP, Morley GW. Prognostic features of sarcomas and mixed tumors of the endometrium. *Obstet Gynecol* 1984;63:550–6.
11. Hornback NB, Omura G, Major FJ. Observations on the use of adjuvant radiation therapy in patients with stage I and II uterine sarcoma. *Int J Radiat Oncol Biol Phy* 1986;12:2127–30.
12. Grosh WW, Jones HW III, Burnett LS, Greco FA. Malignant mixed mesodermal tumors of the uterus and ovary treated with cisplatin-based combination chemotherapy. *Gynecol Oncol* 1986;25:334–9.
13. Gershenson DM, Kavanagh JJ, Copeland LJ, et al. Cisplatin therapy for disseminated mixed mesodermal sarcoma of the uterus. *J Clin Oncol* 1987;5:618–21.

COMMENTARY by William T. Creasman

Unfortunately, this patient presentation follows an all too predictable course. Carcinosarcomas of the uterus historically have had a very dismal course almost irrespective of treatment and, unfortunately, even today, the exceptions to that statement are unusual.

Case History

This patient presented with the usual history of postmenopausal bleeding. Patients with a carcinosarcoma (CS) are usually postmenopausal, as are most women with uterine sarcomas of all types. Occasionally, one of these lesions may primarily appear as an endocervical polyp with a mass protruding through the cervix. This may lead to uterine cramping but is usually accompanied with bleeding. It is noted that when this patient was first seen with this history, her pelvic exam was apparently within normal limits. With this history, a sampling of the endometrial cavity is the first diagnostic test performed that can be done easily in the office. Why that was not done in this particular case is unclear. She continued to bleed and was seen 2 weeks later, at which time blood was seen at the cervical os and of interest was that her uterus was now three to four times normal size. An examination under anesthesia and dilatation and curettage was performed. Again, an endometrial biopsy should have been done first, because when intercavitary pathology is present, the ability of an endometrial biopsy to make the diagnosis is very high. This will therefore save the patient the time, expense, and morbidity from a general anesthetic. As with any malignancy, the extent of disease (stage) is the most important prognostic factor. Patients with sarcomas in general and CS specifically have a high incidence of extra uterine disease, even though clinical and laboratory data would suggest disease is limited to the uterus. In a large surgical staging study by the GOG, those patients with a CS had an incidence of lymph node metastases of 20% versus only 4% for leiomyosarcoma. This is about twice the incidence of lymph node metastases in patients with endometrial cancer thought to be confined to the uterus. Intraperitoneal metastasis is not uncommon, with distant disease being found quite frequently. An autopsy study of 73 primary uterine sarcoma patients showed that essentially all sites are vulnerable for disease, including the peritoneal cavity, lungs, lymph nodes, bone, and liver parenchyma. The hematologic spread for this disease entity is well known.

The work-up for these patients is essentially the same as for an individual who might have the other types of corpus cancer (endometrial cancer). Obviously a chest roentgenogram to identify occult disease is appropriate. How beneficial a CT scan is in this patient remains debatable. A large study evaluating its use has not been done. It is assumed that it may be beneficial in identifying occult disease. Metastases to the lymph nodes from corpus cancer is usually microscopic; very seldom are clinically enlarged lymph nodes appreciated in this disease. As a result, the CT scan will probably not identify lymphadenopathy.

The management of corpus cancer has changed dramatically over the last several years. Prior to that time, preoperative radiation in one form or another was the usual adjuvant treatment, followed by a total abdominal hysterectomy and bilateral salpingo-oophorectomy. The data generated by the GOG and other groups identified a significant number of patients who were thought to have intrauterine disease but had extra-uterine metastasis. This finding has therefore eliminated preoperative radiation in most patients. This applies to sarcomas of the uterus also. In 1988, FIGO changed the staging for corpus cancer from a clinical to a surgically staged disease. As a result, I think most today would proceed initially to surgical staging at which time lymph node involvement would be ascertained as well as a thorough exploration of the abdominal cavity along with a total abdominal hysterectomy and bilateral salpingo-oophorectomy. Depending upon the extent of disease determined through surgical staging, subsequent therapy could then be addressed. Since prognosis for this disease entity is guarded even with early stage disease, adjuvant therapy has been evaluated. It would appear that external irradiation postoperatively does give local control; however, it does not prevent distant metastasis and produces essentially no change in survival. Since metastatic disease is probably hematogenous spread in most instances, different chemotherapeutic agents have been tested in an attempt to decrease the recurrence rate. In a prospective randomized study by the GOG, doxorubicin was used as an adjunct in patients with stage I and II sarcomas in which all gross disease was removed. In 156 evaluable patients, no statistically significant difference in progression free interval or survival was found between those receiving doxorubicin and the patients not treated. In small phase II studies, it has been suggested that cisplatin and adriamycin as an adjuvant may be of benefit in these early staged patients. Ongoing studies with ifosfamide, Mesna, and platinum may identify an effective regimen.

In patients with recurrent disease, effective chemotherapy has been limited. Reports in the literature have suggested that various combinations have shown some response with a handful of complete responders. Median survival for the complete responders is in the neighborhood of 2 to 5 years. Those with a partial response or nonresponders have a very short life expectancy. Ifosfamide and Mesna have shown activity in phase II studies. The GOG currently has a phase III study comparing ifosfamide and Mesna with and without cisplatin in patients with advanced or recurrent carcinosarcomas. Until more active drugs in sarcoma are identified, this disease entity will remain dismal.

SUGGESTED READINGS

1. Silverberg SG, Major FJ, Blessing JA, et al. Carcinosarcomas of the uterus: a Gynecological Group Pathology Study of 200 cases. *Intl J Gynecol Pathol* 1990;9:9–19.
2. Rose PG, Piver MS, Tsukada Y, Lau T. Patterns of metastases in uterine sarcoma: an autopsy study. *Cancer* 1989;63:935–8.
3. Peters WA, Rivkin SE, Smith MR, Tesh DE. Cisplatin and Adriamycin combination chemotherapy for uterine stromal sarcoma and mixed mesodermal tumors. *Gyn Oncol* 1989;34:323–7.

98

Stage I Uterine Cancer with Positive Peritoneal Washings

John L. Lewis, Jr.

What causes a positive peritoneal cytology and what should one do about it?

CASE PRESENTATION

The patient is a 52-year-old woman (gravida 3, para 2, elective abortion 1) referred for treatment because a dilatation and curettage 1 week earlier had shown a well-differentiated adenocarcinoma of the endometrium. She had undergone spontaneous menopause at age 49 and did not receive hormonal replacement. Before menopause, her menstruation had been regular. Although she said that she had had intermittent vaginal staining off and on for 18 months and had seen a gynecologist at regular intervals during that time, no diagnostic procedure was carried out until she bled daily for a month.

Her medical history indicated evidence for mitral valve prolapse, chronic obstructive pulmonary disease (45 pack-per-year smoking history), allergy to sulfa, and migraine headaches. She had not been obese, hypertensive, or diabetic. However, several members of her family had malignancies that are associated with an increased likelihood of her developing an endometrial cancer: three paternal aunts had breast cancer (one also had endometrial cancer); two uncles had colon cancer; and two of her maternal grandmother's sisters had breast cancer.

Her physical exam and vital signs were within normal limits. Pelvic exam revealed a small, mobile uterus and no adnexal masses. A medical consultant recommended antibiotic coverage for her mitral valve prolapse, pre- and postoperative use of low-dose heparin, and the use of a nebulizer and incentive spirometer. Her preoperative chest roentgenogram, EKG, blood tests, and urinalysis were all normal. An intravenous pyelogram was normal except for a 5-mm left renal calculus. Proctoscopy the evening before surgery was normal. She was presented to our equivalent of a Tumor Board preoperatively. It was recommended that she have an endocervical curettage and frozen section at the beginning of anesthesia because the outside dilatation and curettage (D&C) slides had shown no endocervical tissue in the slide-labelled endocervical curettage.

At the time of exam and D&C, the uterus was only 5 cm in depth, was freely movable, and no adnexal or pelvic wall masses were palpable. On frozen section exam there was no abnormal tissue in the endocervix. At laparotomy, all abdominal and pelvic structures were normal except for the unsuspected finding of approximately 20 mL of serosanguinous fluid in the cul-de-sac. (It should be noted that hysteroscopy was not carried out at the time of the D&C, so this could not account for this finding.)

A total abdominal hysterectomy and bilateral salpingo-oophorectomy were carried out uneventfully. The uterus was bisected and on gross inspection there was no evidence of significant myometrial invasion. However, because of the unexpected finding of ascites, normal-appearing lymph nodes were removed from each pelvic side wall. The procedure was "sampling" and not a formal node dissection. The para-aortic space was opened but no palpable nodes were felt and none were removed.

The patient's postoperative course was unremarkable. The pathology demonstrated a well differentiated adenocarcinoma that was limited to the fundus and showed no myometrial invasion (Figs. 98–1 and 98–2). The cervix,

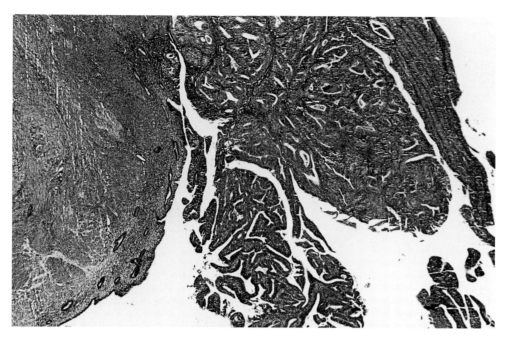

FIG. 98–1. Exophytic growth pattern of the FIGO grade 1 endometrial adenocarcinoma with a tubulovillous pattern confined to the endometrium (H&E stain, original magnification × 40).

fallopian tubes, ovaries, and pelvic nodes were all normal. The ascitic fluid was reported as "positive for malignant cells—adenocarcinoma." (Fig. 98–3).

At the next Tumor Board, this patient's case was of great interest. Few clinicians could remember a similar case in which a well-differentiated adenocarcinoma showing no myometrial penetration and no spread to the adnexal or intraperitoneal structures had been associated with positive cytology. (In fact, a review of our records indicates that there has been no other patient meeting these criteria in the 7½ years since she was cared for.) It was decided to administer Megace at a dose of 40 mg

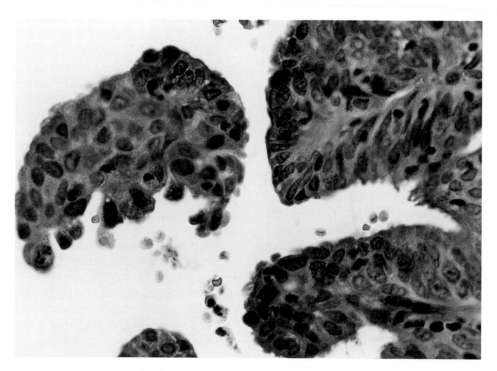

FIG. 98–2. Higher magnification of the surface of the papillary fronds (H&E stain, original magnification × 200).

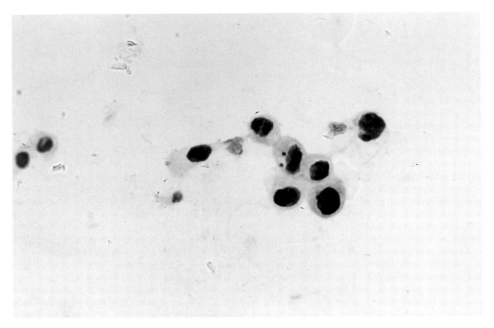

FIG. 98–3. The malignant cells in a cul-de-sac fluid showing pleomorphism and having nuclei with prominent nucleoli (Papanicolaou stain; original magnification × 400).

b.i.d. for a minimum of 2 years. This was recommended on the basis of the likelihood that a well-differentiated adenocarcinoma would be receptor positive. No receptor studies were done. Vaginal brachytherapy is usually recommended for all of our patients with endometrial adenocarcinoma, but it was not used in this patient because of the lack of myometrial invasion.

The patient has remained free of disease for eight years.

COMMENTARY by William T. Creasman

Endometrial carcinoma is the most frequently seen pelvic gynecological malignancy. It is usually seen in the postmenopausal patient; however, about 25% of patients will be premenopausal. Postmenopausal bleeding is the most common symptom, which usually leads to sampling of the endometrium and ultimately the diagnosis. Irregular bleeding during the menopause has, in many situations, been ignored, suggesting that the bleeding is due to the menopause. Bleeding during this time interval should be lighter and lighter and further and further apart. This patient, although only 52 years of age, had apparently been amenorrheic for about 18 months prior to her year and a half of intermittent vaginal staining. She was not taking hormone-replacement therapy, which may have accounted for her postmenopausal bleeding. The reason she was not evaluated earlier is unknown.

Before 1988, when FIGO changed the staging for endometrial cancer from a clinical to a surgical stage clas-

sification, an adequate evaluation of the endocervical canal was an important preoperative test. If cancer is present in the endocervical specimen, by definition, the patient was classified as stage II. Considerable overstaging was noted by several authors as "contamination" from the endometrial cavity, which made an endocervical biopsy "positive" and upstaged as many as 50% of patients who were classified with stage II disease. In many instances this led to an overtreatment of the disease process. With the negative ECC the authors preceded with standard treatment for a grade I, stage 1 cancer, i.e., total abdominal hysterectomy and bilateral salpingo-oophorectomy.

At the time of operation, many surgeons routinely obtained peritoneal cytology in all patients with endometrial cancer. In this particular patient, approximately 20 cc of serosanguinous fluid was present in the cul-de-sac. This was removed for cytology. It is not unusual to see fluid in the cul-de-sac at the time of surgery. It has been suggested that up to 100 cc could be considered normal. On the other hand, there are times when it appears that there is no fluid in the cul-de-sac. The question asked many times is whether or not malignant cells in the cytology could have been caused by manipulation of the uterus, i.e., D&C before surgery. To date this is unanswerable. A prior D&C (several days or weeks) before abdominal surgery apparently has no impact on the finding of positive peritoneal cytology, but it may have in this case. It is generally accepted that the passage of malignant cells from the uterus into the peritoneal cavity is most likely via patent fallopian tubes; however, instances have been reported in which positive peritoneal cytology is present in patients who have had a previous tubal ligation (1). The uterine lymphatics may play a role here.

The real question of this case is what, if any, significance the positive peritoneal cytology may be and does it affect further management? The literature on this subject is mixed. Most investigators have noted that positive cytology is an independent risk factor for advanced disease (i.e., lymph nodes, etc.) (2). Others have suggested that the positive findings do not predict recurrence or poor survival (3,4), while others have shown that it is a poor prognostic factor (5). Various postsurgical managements have been suggested. For many years we have used intraperitoneal ^{32}P, with a significant improvement in survival of these patients (6). Other investigators have used progestins, whole abdominal radiation, or no further treatment (7).

The authors note that this patient was unique in their experience in that she had a grade 1 lesion with no myometrial invasion but positive peritoneal cytology. Over the years we have seen several patients like the one presented. Initially, as we were gaining experience with this situation, no treatment was given and patients recurred very rapidly with extensive intra-abdominal disease. These patients obviously influenced our assessment of this parameter, and as a result, we began to actively treat this patient. The use of progestins is interesting, particularly in light of the rationale the authors used for its use. Our early experience with receptors in endometrial cancer identified a small number with positive cytology. At that time we were using progestins as a possible reasonable therapy. In all patients treated with progestins who had positive cytology and positive receptors, none recurred. In all patients with negative receptors, all recurred and died. Certainly in this patient, the chances of having positive receptors is very high, and the use of progestins may have been therapeutic.

REFERENCES

1. Creasman WT, Lukeman J. Role of the fallopian tube in dissemination of malignant cells in corpus cancer. *Cancer* 1972;29:456–7.
2. Sutton GP, Geisler HE, Stehman FB, Young PC, Kimes TM, Ehrlich CE. Features associated with survival and disease-free survival in early endometrial cancer. *Am J Obstet Gynecol* 1989;160:1385–93.
3. Kennedy AW, Peterson GL, Becker SN, Nunez C, Webster KD. Experience with pelvic washings in stage I and II endometrial carcinoma. *Gynecol Oncol* 1987;28:50–60.
4. Lurain JR, Rumsey NK, Schink JC, Wallemark CB, Chmiel JS. Prognostic significance of positive peritoneal cytology in clinical stage I adenocarcinoma of the endometrium. *Obstet Gynecol* 1989;74(2):175–9.
5. Turner DA, Gershenson DM, Atkinson N, Seige N, Wharton AT. The prognostic significance of peritoneal cytology for stage I endometrial cancer. *Obstet Gynecol* 1989;74(5):775–80.
6. Creasman WT, DiSaia PJ, Blessing J, Wilkinson RH, Johnston W, Weed JC. Prognostic significance of peritoneal cytology in patients with endometrial cancer and preliminary data concerning therapy with intraperitoneal radiopharmaceuticals. *Am J Obstet Gynecol* 1981;141:921–9.
7. Piver MS. Progesterone therapy for malignant peritoneal cytology surgical stage I endometrial adenocarcinoma. *Semin Oncol* 1988;15(2):50–2.

99

Stage IIA Carcinoma of the Endometrium

William J. Hoskins

The potential relationship between adjuvant tamoxifen therapy for breast cancer and endometrial carcinoma

CASE PRESENTATION

J.B. is a 65-year-old Caucasian woman who became menopausal at age 52. She described menarche at age 15 with regular menstrual periods and an uneventful menopause.

The patient had never taken estrogen replacement therapy although she had taken oral contraceptives for 6 years. The patient had four pregnancies, all resulting in normal vaginal deliveries. The patient had taken tamoxifen 10 mg twice daily since 1988, when she had been diagnosed with breast cancer. In July 1992 the patient experienced vaginal spotting for 2 weeks; in August 1992 she had a single episode of heavy vaginal bleeding. She consulted a gynecologist, who performed a fractional dilatation and curettage. He also performed three cervical biopsies. The pathologic review of this material revealed poorly differentiated (grade 3) adenocarcinoma of the endometrium. The endocervical curettings and the cervical biopsies revealed chronic endocervicitis. The patient was referred to Memorial Sloan-Kettering Cancer Center for therapy.

Past medical history revealed that the patient had been diagnosed with infiltrating ductal carcinoma of the breast, stage I (T1c, N0) in 1988. The carcinoma had been diagnosed by routine mammography, was 1.5 cm in diameter, and had been treated by lumpectomy and axillary dissection followed by irradiation. Estrogen receptors were positive and the patient had taken tamoxifen, as stated above, since completing radiation. A recent evaluation for metastatic breast cancer was negative. A mammogram was reported to have been normal in January, 1992. She had been diagnosed with hypertension in 1982 and took Tenormin 50 mg daily with good control of her blood pressure. She reported occasional episodes of asthma secondary to "allergies." She reported a tonsillectomy as a child. The remainder of her past medical history was negative.

Review of systems was entirely negative except for occasional leg cramps and the vaginal bleeding described in the present illness.

On physical examination the patient was 158 cm in height, weighed 76 kg, and her blood pressure was 150/80 mm Hg. The general physical examination was normal except for the lumpectomy scar in the upper outer quadrant of the left breast and the scar from the left axillary dissection. Her abdomen was moderately obese with no scars. On pelvic examination, the external genitalia were normal as was the vagina. The cervix had been recently biopsied, but was otherwise normal. The uterus was enlarged to twice normal size (10 cm in length), and was slightly globular. The uterus was mobile and the parametria were normal. No adnexal masses were palpable. Rectal examination confirmed the vaginal examination; there were no intrinsic abnormalities of the rectum, and the stool guaiac was negative.

The preliminary diagnosis was endometrial adenocarcinoma, probable stage I.

A chest roentgenogram, CT scan of the abdomen and pelvis (with double contrast), and routine laboratory studies (CBC, liver function studies, BUN, creatinine and PT, PTT) were conducted. The patient was scheduled for cystoscopy, proctoscopy, total abdominal hysterectomy, and para-aortic nodal sampling pending presentation at the Gynecology Service Tumor Board.

On September 18, 1992, the patient was presented at the Gynecology Service Tumor Board. There were 22 individuals present, including five gynecologic oncologists, two medical oncologists, two radiation oncologists, one pathologist, and 12 residents and fellows from gynecology, medical oncology, and radiation oncology.

Review of the outside pathology slides were interpreted as endometrioid endometrial adenocarcinoma, FIGO grade 3 (nuclear grade 3) in the endometrial curettings. The endocervical curettings and cervical biopsies were read as showing chronic cervicitis. The chest roentgenogram and CT scan of the abdomen and pelvis showed an enlarged uterus with no parametrial abnormality. There was no adenopathy in the pelvis or para-aortic lymph nodes. The attending gynecologist outlined his plan for therapy: cystoscopy, proctoscopy, total abdominal hysterectomy, and para-aortic node biopsy. He stated he would not routinely perform pelvic nodal sampling because the decision to treat the pelvis with irradiation is based on tumor grade and depth of invasion. He pointed out that there are no data available to show that patients with negative node sampling but who have other high–risk factors (depth of invasion and grade) do not benefit from irradiation. The radiation oncologist stated that because the tumor is grade 3, he would recommend whole pelvis irradiation as well as vaginal brachytherapy if there was any myometrial invasion. He stated that he would use whole pelvis irradiation for grade 1 or grade 2 tumors only if there was either myometrial invasion of greater than 50% or if the cervix was involved, but that for grade 3 tumors he would recommend whole pelvis irradiation for any degree of myometrial invasion. He concurred with the gynecologist's plan to perform only para-aortic nodal sampling, pointing out the increased risk of complications in patients who have extensive pelvic dissection followed by pelvic irradiation. The medical oncologist stated there was no evidence of any benefit for preoperative chemotherapy or hormonal therapy. He also stated that a recent case control study from Sweden (Fornander, T, et al, Lancet, Jan 21, 1989) had shown a 6% risk of endometrial cancer in women taking a higher dose (20 mg b.i.d.) of tamoxifen for 5 years. The gynecologist pointed out that a review of the literature shows over 40 reported cases of endometrial cancer in women taking tamoxifen, and that the reported cases were a mixture of histologic grades.

On September 21, 1992, the patient underwent cystoscopy (negative), proctoscopy (negative to 22 cm), total abdominal hysterectomy, left and right para-aortic nodal sampling, and left pelvic lymph node biopsy. Findings at surgery included a negative upper abdomen, normal-appearing para-aortic lymph nodes, and a single 2-cm, enlarged, left external iliac lymph node. The uterus was enlarged to twice normal size, but there was no evidence of any tumor spread outside the uterus. The estimated blood loss was 400 cc, and there were no intraoperative complications. There were no postoperative complications and the patient was discharged on the fifth postoperative day.

On October 2, 1992, the patient was again presented in the Gynecology Service Tumor Board. Attendance was essentially the same as listed above. Review of the pathology surgery revealed endometrioid adenocarcinoma of the endometrium, FIGO grade 3 (>50% solid growth), nuclear grade 2–3. Myometrial invasion was less than 50% (10 mm where the maximal myometrial thickness was 29 mm). Endocervical invasion was present in the mucosa only. There was no vascular invasion and the parametria and vaginal margins were negative. Leiomyomata were present. The fallopian tubes and ovaries were negative. The left and right para-aortic lymph nodes (11 nodes) were negative for tumor. Four left external iliac lymph nodes were negative. The pathologic findings are illustrated in Figures 99–1 through 99–4. Based on the findings at surgery and the pathology report, the patient was FIGO stage IIA. The radiation oncologist recommended whole-pelvis irradiation, 4,500 cGy, followed by intravaginal irradiation with high dose rate brachytherapy to 2,100 cGY. The medical oncologist stated he did not recommend any postoperative chemotherapy or hormonal therapy for the endometrial carcinoma but would recommend that the patient continue her tamoxifen therapy for her breast cancer. A discussion followed as to the benefit of removing enlarged pelvic lymph nodes when irradiation to the pelvis was planned. The consensus of the group was that enlarged lymph nodes should be removed because the irradiation dose usually administered (4,500 cGy) was probably effective for microscopic disease but not for gross disease.

From October 26, 1992, through December 2, 1992, the patient received 4,500 cGy of irradiation in 25 fractions, using a four field technique and a 15-MV linear accelerator. She tolerated the treatment well except for lower abdominal cramping and loose stools. The loose stools were treated with Lomotil as needed. On December 18 and 31, 1992, and January 8, 1993, the patient received three treatments of 700 cGy each to the vagina using a Gamma-med high-dose-rate applicator.

The patient was seen by the gynecologic oncologist in the office on February 18, 1993, for a follow-up examination. The examination was normal. A Pap smear was not performed because the patient had only recently completed her radiotherapy. The follow-up plan outlined for the patient was examination every 3 months for 2 years, and examinations every 6 months for an additional 3 years. After 5 years, examination at yearly intervals was recommended. Pap smears would be performed at each

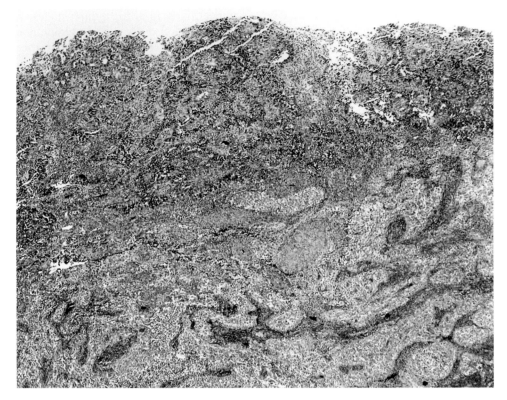

FIG. 99–1. Endometrial adenocarcinoma, FIGO grade 3, infiltrating into the myometrium. The depth of infiltration was 10 mm in an area where the myometrium measured 29 mm (H&E stain, × 40).

examination and chest roentgenograms were recommended every 6 months for 2 years and every year thereafter. A CT scan of the abdomen and pelvis was recommended at 1 year and 2 years following completion of therapy.

COMMENTARY by Philip J. DiSaia

This case brings to life many interesting facets in diagnosis and therapy of endometrial carcinoma. The patient was taking the so-called "anti-estrogen" tamoxifen for approximately 4 years prior to the diagnosis of a grade 3 adenocarcinoma of the endometrium. Several publications of the past few years have suggested that the incidence of endometrial adenocarcinoma is increased in patients taking tamoxifen. A convincing study (1) from Sweden reported a significant elevation of endometrial cancer incidence among tamoxifen-treated women who had previously undergone mastectomy for breast cancer. After an interval of 3 to 4 years, the increase in the incidence of endometrial cancer reached an overall relative risk of 6.4-fold. However, the dose used in this study was 40 mg/day, as opposed to the 20 mg/day taken by the patient in this report. In point of fact, my experience has

been that most of the patients who develop endometrial carcinoma on tamoxifen have well-differentiated lesions similar to those patients who developed endometrial lesions on unopposed estrogen.

A preliminary diagnosis of adenocarcinoma of the endometrium grade 3, stage 1 was made for this patient, and therapy was planned at the Tumor Board. Cystoscopy and proctoscopy were carried out. Our institution has abandoned the practice of cystoscopy and proctoscopy in clinical stage I lesions because of the low yield and seemingly unjustifiable expense. Upon review of the hysterectomy specimen, mucosal involvement of the endocervix with the neoplasm was detected despite the fact that the patient had endocervical curettings and cervical biopsies that showed only chronic cervicitis. With the new FIGO staging system (surgical criteria), the patient was eventually staged as stage IIA. A pelvic lymphadenectomy was not conducted but periaortic sampling yielded 11 negative nodes. Based on the fact that myometrial invasion existed to the junction of the inner and middle thirds of the myometrium, postoperative radiation therapy was recommended.

Most clinicians have interpreted the FIGO staging changes issued in October, 1988, (2) to require pelvic lymphadenectomy for staging, especially in high-grade

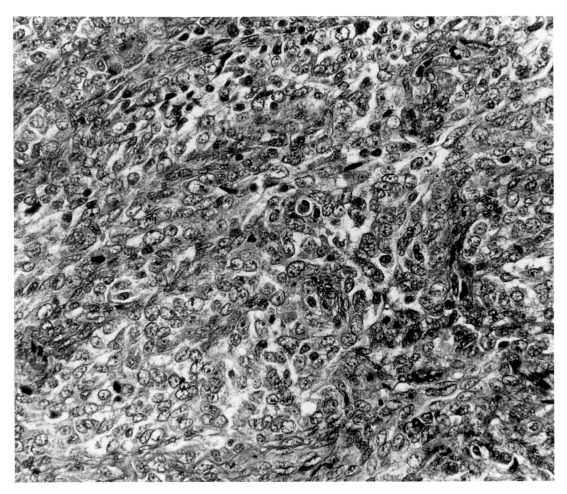

FIG. 99–2. High magnification of the tumor cells shows oval nuclei with prominent nucleoli. The cells are arranged in sheets with areas of spindling (H&E stain, × 400).

lesions. In this case, it was chosen not to do a pelvic lymphadenectomy, presumably on the basis that the patient needed pelvic irradiation anyway. This brings up some very interesting issues. Can we assume that pelvic radiation will sterilize all positive nodes, if they exist? Can we expect a better result if pelvic irradiation is given following removal of positive nodes ("debulking")? The answers to many of these questions are obscure, but I believe we cannot assume that irradiation therapy will sterilize all positive nodes. One could argue that a patient with pelvic nodes is incurable, but we have several reports showing a 40% survival in patients with documented positive nodes. Most of these patients have received pelvic irradiation, so we are left with the basic question of whether radiation is as effective as lymphadenectomy followed by irradiation. Creasman et al. (3) showed that 75% of patients with grade 3 lesions failed distally, even when the malignancy was confined to the uterus, and raised the question as to whether radiation therapy to the pelvis is of any value for these patients.

Multiple adjuvant studies utilizing various hormone regimens, and in a few instances chemotherapy, have been unsuccessful in improving the outcome for this group of patients. A search is desperately needed for new and effective methods of providing systemic therapy to the high-risk group of patients with endometrial carcinoma. Endometrial adenocarcinoma is currently the most common of all gynecological malignancies, and the high-risk group seems to be well defined. Additional information comes from a very interesting recent report by Podratz et al. (4), which showed that the deoxyribonucleic acid index provided an excellent stratification of aneuploid tumors and a multivariate analysis identified the proliferative index as the most cogent, independent prognostic factor for all endometrial cancers. Increased recurrence, or decreased survival rates were correlated with aneuploidy and increasing percent of S-phase fraction, DNA index, and proliferative index. Further confirmation of this report may eclipse the standard methods of analyzing histopathologic factors for identifying high-risk patients.

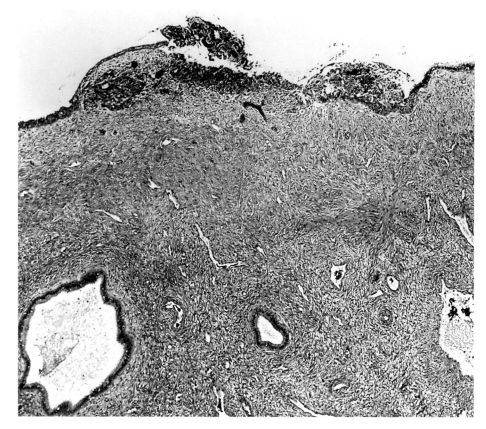

FIG. 99–3. Low-power photomicrograph shows the focal, limited area in the endocervical mucosa involved by the carcinoma (H&E stain, × 100).

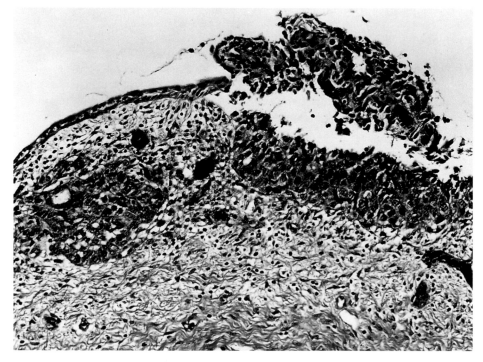

FIG. 99–4. High magnification shows that the cytology is similar to the endometrial primary (H&E stain, × 200).

REFERENCES

1. Fornander T, Cedermark B, Mattsson A. Adjuvant tamoxifen in early breast cancer: occurrence of new primary cancers. *Lancet* 1989; 1:117–20.
2. International Federation of Gynecology and Obstetrics. Annual report on the results of treatment in gynecological cancer. *Int J Gynecol Obstet* 1989;28:189–90.
3. Creasman WT, Morrow CP, Bundy L. Surgical pathological spread patterns of endometrial cancer. *Cancer* 1987;60:2035.
4. Podratz KC, Wilson TO, Gaffey TA, Cha SS, Katzman, JA. Deoxyribonucleic acid analysis facilitates the pretreatment identification of high-risk endometrial cancer patients. *Am J Obstet Gynecol* 1993;168:1206–13.

100 Choriocarcinoma with Pulmonary and Brain Metastases

Walter B. Jones

Choriocarcinoma: A rare malignant neoplasm that can masquerade as a common cancer

CASE PRESENTATION

The patient is a 39-year-old woman with a history of infertility who was unsuccessfully treated with clomiphene citrate in 1981. She underwent a laparoscopy in 1983 and was found to have endometriosis for which she received danazol therapy over a 9-month period. Two months after discontinuing this therapy she became pregnant and delivered at term a normally developed male infant in December, 1983. She breast fed the infant until July, 1984, during which time she had normal menses. She then developed irregular menstrual cycles until March, 1985 when she began to have severe headaches. This was followed by a visual disturbance in April, 1985, for which she was evaluated by a neurologist. Computer axial tomography of the brain revealed a large enhancing tumor in the left occipital lobe (Fig. 100–1). Chest roentgenogram showed a 5.5-cm soft tissue mass in the posterior segment of the right upper lobe consistent with bronchiogenic carcinoma (Fig. 100–2). On April 14, 1985, she underwent left occipital craniotomy with total excision of a large hemorrhagic tumor mass. Pathological evaluation of the specimen revealed a metastatic poorly differentiated large cell carcinoma, mucin negative, consistent with lung primary. Transbronchial biopsy of the lung lesion was interpreted as showing poorly differentiated carcinoma of large cell type similar to the tumor removed from the brain. She was initially treated with approximately 3,000 Gy of whole-brain radiotherapy. Serum tumor markers revealed a human chorionic gonadotrophin

(hCG) concentration of 1,882 mIU/ml (normal value, 5 mIU/mL).

She was admitted to the Memorial Sloan-Kettering Cancer Center on May 8, 1985, where review of histopathologic slides prepared elsewhere were interpreted as showing a metastatic anaplastic tumor consistent with choriocarcinoma with positive staining for hCG. Initial serum hCG concentration was 260 ng/mL (normal value, <2 ng/mL). She was begun on combination chemotherapy consisting of methotrexate, actinomycin D, and chlorambucil. She improved clinically with a decrease in serum hCG concentration and received two additional courses of therapy. However, hCG levels began to rise in June, 1985, and for this reason in July, 1985, she underwent right upper lobectomy of the lung containing choriocarcinoma (Fig. 100–3). Following surgery, she received four courses of etoposide and cisplatin and achieved normal hCG levels in October, 1985. Treatment was discontinued after a final abbreviated course of this therapy because of ototoxicity. The patient has remained clinically and hormonally free of disease since 1985. Her response to treatment measured in the subunit assay for hCG is shown in Figure 100–4.

This case demonstrates that metastatic choriocarcinoma to the brain may occur in the absence of gynecologic complaints and should alert physicians to the fact that any woman of childbearing age who presents with symptoms of intracerebral hemorrhage, increased intracranial pressure, or a primary brain tumor, should be evaluated for metastatic choriocarcinoma. In this situation, a

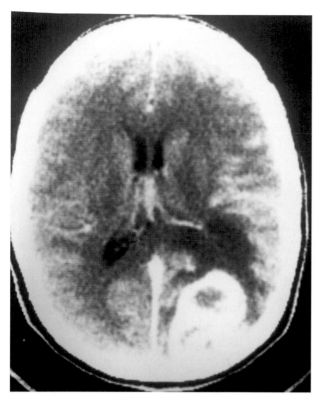

FIG. 100–1. Large enhancing tumor in the left occipital lobe on CAT scan of brain.

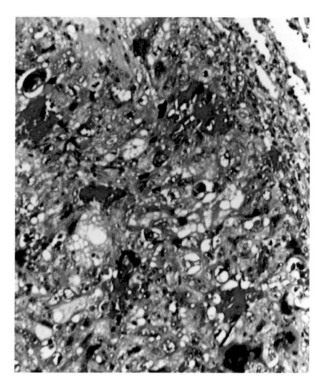

FIG. 100–3. Histologic section of lung metastasis of choriocarcinoma.

routine pregnancy test is usually positive; and in this case, the evaluation could have saved the patient an unnecessary craniotomy.

Intracerebral metastases occur in as many as 20% of patients with gestational choriocarcinoma and are poten-

tially lethal. Whereas intrathecal prophylaxis with chemotherapy reduces the incidence of central nervous system disease, an average of no more than 50% of patients survive once tumor in this location is diagnosed. Chemotherapy alone can cure tumors in the brain, but most authorities recommend combination chemotherapy with simultaneous whole-brain irradiation. The role of craniotomy is unclear,

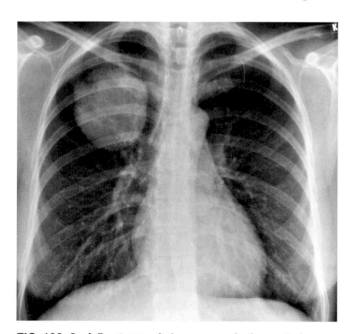

FIG. 100–2. A 5 × 6 cm soft tissue mass in the posterior segment of the right upper lobe consistent with bronchogenic carcinoma.

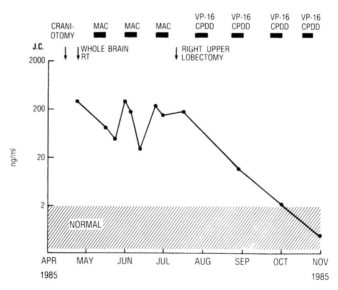

FIG. 100–4. Hormonal response to treatment of metastatic choriocarcinoma.

but the operation appears to be of minimal value in patients with resistant systemic disease and in patients with tumor in multiple areas of the brain. Moreover, craniotomy may cause severe morbidity. Nevertheless, it may be of therapeutic value in an occasional patient who has a stationary solitary focus of persisting tumor after metastases elsewhere have regressed clinically. Craniotomy may also be lifesaving in the patient who is deteriorating from intracerebral hemorrhage or hematoma formation.

The integration of surgery into the management of patients with a metastatic choriocarcinoma, in this case thoracotomy, can play a major role in the patient's curability. Indications for thoracotomy are as follows:

1. The patient must be a good surgical risk.
2. The primary malignancy must have been controlled (the uterus has already been removed or is free of disease on CAT scan or MRI, and there is no evidence of metastatic disease elsewhere in the pelvic cavity).
3. There is no evidence of metastatic disease elsewhere in the body.
4. Roentgenography shows pulmonary metastasis is limited to one lung.
5. The urinary hCG is below 1,000 mIU per mL.

The operation should be carried out on the third day of a 5-day course of single-agent chemotherapy. If the patient is to receive methotrexate, the dose is 0.3 mg per kg of body weight. This amount represents approximately 80% of the dose used when the drug is given alone. Wedge resection is the surgical procedure of choice so as to preserve as much normal pulmonary tissue as possible. On gross examination, these resected tumors appear as dark, hemorrhagic, well-defined masses. Histologic studies frequently show a disorderly growth of a few trophoblastic cells scattered in areas of hemorrhagic necrosis. Such findings suggest that chemotherapy failure may be accounted for by an ineffective concentration of drug reaching some of the cells.

Successful surgical extirpation of all residual tumor should result in the hCG levels returning to normal within 4 to 10 days after the operation. Depending on the hCG level prior to thoracotomy, one or two additional courses of chemotherapy should be given after normal values are achieved in an attempt to eliminate any residual trophoblastic cells that may be present but secreting insufficient hCG to be detected with current assay techniques. Excellent results from thoracotomy can be expected in properly selected patients, as demonstrated in a collected series of 55 patients, in which an average of 69% (range 55%–87%) entered complete and sustained remission after the operation.

SUGGESTED READINGS

1. Chaganti RSK, Koduru PRK, Chakraborty R, Jones WB. Genetic origin of trophoblastic choriocarcinoma. *Cancer Res* 1990;50:6330–3.
2. Jones WB, Lewis JL Jr. Integration of surgery and other techniques in the management of trophoblastic malignancy. *Obstet Gynecol Clin North Am* 1988;15:565–76.
3. Tomoda Y, Aril Y, Kaseki S, et al. Surgical indications for resection in pulmonary metastasis of choriocarcinoma. *Cancer* 1980;46:2723–30.
4. Jones WB, Wagner-Reiss KM, Lewis JL Jr. Intracerebral choriocarcinoma. *Gynecol Oncol* 1990;38:234–43.
5. Rustin GJS, Newlands EE, Begent RHJ, Dent J, Bagshawe KD. Weekly alternating etoposide, methotrexate, and actinomycin/vincristine and cyclophosphamide chemotherapy for the treatment of CNS metastases of choriocarcinoma. *J Clin Oncol* 1989;7:900–3.

COMMENTARY by Hyman B. Muss

The patient described in this report depicts the life-threatening end of the spectrum of trophoblastic malignancy. Her presentation, although not common, was not atypical, and underscores the variable natural history of choriocarcinoma. Although this patient lacked major gynecologic symptoms, the rarity of bronchogenic carcinoma in a 39-year-old woman who did not smoke should have alerted the clinician to consider other primary sites as the origin for this patient's tumor. A complete physical examination including a carefully done pelvic examination may have suggested a primary source earlier in this patient's course. Moreover, the patient's presentation illustrates the limitations of the surgical pathology review as the keystone for a conclusive diagnosis. Only the serum hCG concentration provided the major clue necessary for making the correct diagnosis. Because metastatic choriocarcinoma represents one of the potentially curable human solid tumors, a serum or urine hCG determination should be performed in any premenopausal patient who presents with a metastatic malignancy unless the primary site is obvious. In addition, immunohistochemical staining of either the cranial or pulmonary lesion for hCG would have suggested the correct diagnosis earlier in the patient's course.

Choriocarcinoma remains among the most exquisitely sensitive human tumors to cytotoxic chemotherapy (1). Those with early stage disease (stage I, confined to uterus; stage II, outside the uterus but limited to genital structures; and stage III, pulmonary metastases) have cure rates ranging from 80%–100% after treatment with single agent chemotherapy, with cure rates approaching 100% with tumor confined to the uterus. Methotrexate, dactinomycin, fluorouracil, and etoposide are equally effective in early stage, low-risk patients, but methotrexate appears to have the least toxicity (2). The patient reported had stage IV disease and, more importantly, had brain metastases, a poor prognostic feature. Several investigators have pointed out the limitations of standard anatomical staging, and other classifications that more accurately define the risk of treatment failure have been developed. Clinical characteristics indicative of poor prognosis include long duration (>4 months) since last pregnancy, pretreatment serum hCG level, >40,000 mIU/mL, prior chemotherapy, antecedent-term pregnancy, or liver or brain metastases. Tumor size and number of metastatic lesions also appear to be important (3). Patients with "high-risk" features should be considered for initial combination chemotherapy treatment including methotrexate, dactinomycin, and chlorambucil or cyclophosphamide ("MAC"), or newer and probably more effective combination regimens that contain etoposide and cisplatin. Durable remissions have been reported in 60%–80% of high-risk patients treated with MAC chemotherapy.

An essential ingredient in the treatment of all patients with metastatic choriocarcinoma is meticulous follow-up during treatment with assessment of serum beta-hCG (hCG) levels before each treatment course and periodic assessment of metastatic sites (if present). The hCG determination remains a key factor in the diagnosis, prognostication, and treatment monitoring for patients with trophoblastic disease (4). In this patient, combination chemotherapy with MAC failed to result in normalization of hCG levels and mandated a change in therapy. The use of etoposide and cisplatin, two of the most effective agents for the treatment of choriocarcinoma and other related germ cell malignancies, resulted in normalization of the hCG level and probable cure. After completion of chemotherapy, hCG levels should be measured at two-week intervals for the first several months, then at least monthly for one year, and then every six months. Most relapses occur in the first 12 months but late relapses have been reported in a small percentage of patients.

The role of surgery in the management of patients with metastatic choriocarcinoma is well presented by Dr. Jones. Surgery should be reserved for patients who have metastatic lesions resulting in rapid clinical deterioration, or those with residual radiographic abnormalities after chemotherapy and persistent hCG elevation. For patients who achieve normalization of hCG levels after several courses of chemotherapy, residual radiographic abnormalities frequently represent residual necrotic or fibrotic tissue without residual malignancy, and some experts suggest that surgical resection is unnecessary in this group. Patients with persistent elevation of hCG will almost always have residual tumor, and the decision to proceed with surgery as opposed to changing the chemotherapy regimen will depend on previous treatment and the site(s) and extent of organ involvement. Whole-brain irradiation is frequently recommended for patients with CNS metastases, although its contribution to current, more effective, chemotherapy treatment programs is unclear. Likewise, some have advocated the use of low-dose hepatic irradiation for patients with liver metastases to decrease the risk of catastrophic hemorrhage associated with these lesions. Radiation therapy in both these situations has been associated with only minimal toxicity.

The patient described in this report illustrates many of the clinical problems associated with the diagnosis and treatment of metastatic trophoblastic disease. Multimodality therapy, including surgery, irradiation, and chemotherapy, is frequently necessary for the management of patients with metastatic trophoblastic disease, and such treatment should be administered by gynecologic, radiation, and medical oncologists familiar with the treatment of this highly aggressive, but usually curable cancer.

REFERENCES

1. Soper JT, Hammond CR, Lewis JL, Jr. Gestational trophoblastic disease. In: Hoskins WJ, Perez CA, Young RC, eds. *Principles and practice of gynecologic oncology.* Philadelphia: J.B. Lippincott; 1992:795–825.
2. Kohorn EI. Single-agent chemotherapy for non-metastatic gestational trophoblastic neoplasia: perspectives for the 21st century after three decades of use. *J Reprod Med* 1991;36:49–55.
3. DuBeshter B. High-risk factors in metastatic gestational trophoblastic neoplasia. *J Reprod Med* 1991;36:9–13.
4. Bagshawe KD. Choriocarcinoma. *Rev Oncol* 1992;5:99–106.

SECTION XXI

Ovary

101 Stage IIIB Ovarian Cancer

Stephen C. Rubin

*If ovarian carcinoma is suspected preoperatively, informed
consent might avoid two operations*

CASE PRESENTATION

D.M. is a 29-year-old nulligravid woman who presented to her local gynecologist in September, 1991, for a routine gynecologic examination. She had been on oral contraceptives for approximately 2 years. Pelvic examination revealed bilateral adnexal masses of approximately 6 to 7 cm on the right and 5 cm on the left. The uterus was normal in size, and there was no cul de sac nodularity. The general physical examination was unremarkable. Her past medical history was noncontributory. There was no family history of cancer.

Computed tomography (CT) of the pelvis and abdomen obtained locally was reported as showing bilateral complex adnexal masses (Fig. 101–1). There was no ascites, and no evidence of disease elsewhere in the abdomen. Serum CA-125 was reported as 55 µ/mL (nl 0–35). The patient was taken to the operating room at her local community hospital. Laparoscopy revealed bilateral ovarian enlargement with surface excrescences seen on both ovaries. The omentum was noted to be adherent to the uterus and left adnexal region. On inspection of the upper abdomen, the liver surface and both hemidiaphragms appeared free of tumor. Because of the suspicion of malignancy, laparotomy was performed through a low midline incision. Washings were taken from the pelvis on entering the abdomen. Because the patient had not given consent for complete surgery, only right salpingo-oophorectomy and partial omentectomy were performed. The pathology report indicated serous cystadenocarcinoma involving the right ovary, with metastases to the omentum of less than 2 cm in size. Washings were positive for malignant cells.

The patient was referred for further management 2 weeks later. Physical examination at that time was remarkable for a left adnexal mass. On discussion of the management options with the patient and her family, she indicated that she would like to preserve the option of childbearing but not at the expense of compromising her cancer treatment. On review, her histologic material was reported as showing papillary serous cystadenocarcinoma, grade 1, involving the right ovary, fallopian tube, and omentum. Washings were confirmed to be positive for malignant cells. The case was presented to the Multidisciplinary Treatment Planning Conference. Because complete staging and cytoreduction had not been performed at the initial operation, and because of the likelihood of tumor being present in the left ovary, re-exploration was recommended. A preoperative barium enema was normal.

The patient was taken to the operating room and pelvic examination under anesthesia revealed a 5-cm left adnexal mass. Proctoscopy and cystoscopy were normal. Fractional dilatation and curettage of the uterus was performed, with the curettings reported as benign on frozen section. Abdominal exploration was performed through a midline incision. A 6-cm mass involving the left ovary had the gross appearance of carcinoma. Left salpingo-oophorectomy was performed, with frozen section confirming cancer. Exploration of the diaphragm, upper abdomen, liver, spleen, stomach, kidneys, intestines, and retroperitoneal regions was normal. The residual omentum was removed, as was the uterus. The pathology report indicated a well differentiated papillary serous cystadenocarcinoma involving the left ovary (Fig. 101–2). There were additional foci of carci-

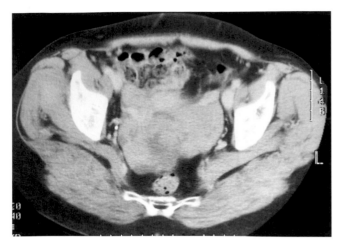

FIG. 101-1. CT showing bilateral complex adnexal masses.

noma in the omental tissue. The patient was staged as a stage IIIB adenocarcinoma of the ovary, with no gross residual disease. Her postoperative course was unremarkable. She was begun on estrogen replacement therapy on the fourth postoperative day.

After definitive surgery, the patient was re-presented to the treatment planning conference. Because of her youth, general good health, and low tumor burden, it was felt that she was a good candidate for protocol chemotherapy involving two courses of high-dose intravenous cyclophosphamide (1,000 mg/M²) and cisplatin (200 mg/M²)

followed by re-exploration, intraperitoneal catheter placement, and a subsequent four courses of intraperitoneal carboplatin (200 mg/m²) and etoposide (100 mg/m²), with interleukin 3 used for hematologic support. After discussion of the treatment options, the patient gave her informed consent for protocol entry.

She began her first treatment on the ninth postoperative day. One month later, just before her second chemotherapy cycle, her CA-125 was 14. She required a brief hospitalization for antibiotic treatment of nadir fever after her second cycle. As per protocol, she underwent re-exploration of January 7, 1992. There was no gross evidence of tumor found. Cytologic washings were obtained from the pelvis, both paracolic gutters, and the undersurfaces of both hemidiaphragms. Biopsies were taken from multiple areas, including the stumps of both infundibulopelvic ligaments, the pelvic cul de sac and the bladder peritoneum, the left and right paracolic gutters, the diaphragms, and a number of areas of filmy intestinal adhesions. Bilateral pelvic and aortic lymph node sampling was also performed. An intraperitoneal catheter and subcutaneous port were placed. All cytologic and histologic specimens were negative for tumor. The patient's postoperative recovery was uneventful.

The patient was treated with a subsequent four courses of intraperitoneal carboplatin and etoposide, which she tolerated well. Because the previous exploration had revealed no tumor, exploration at the completion of chemotherapy was not recommended. Her intraperitoneal port was removed under local anesthesia after her last

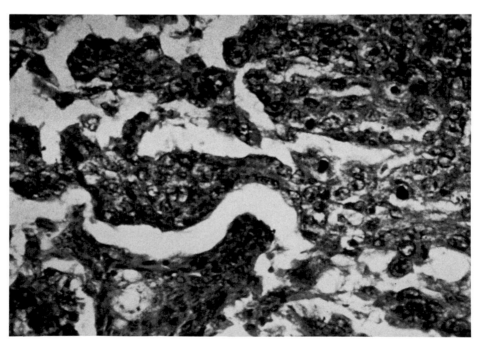

FIG. 101-2. Histologic section from the left ovary section showing well differentiated papillary serous cystadenocarcinoma (original H&E, × 100).

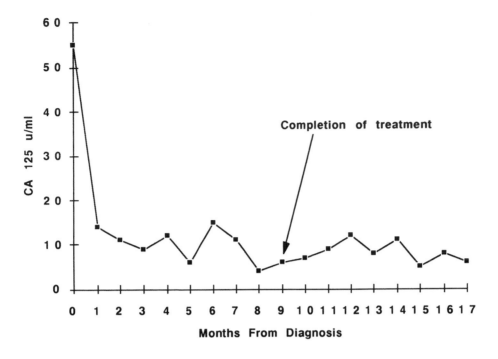

FIG. 101–3. Serum CA-125 levels from diagnosis to last follow-up (nl 0–35 æ/mL).

treatment. She has since been followed with examinations every 2 months and CA-125 determinations every month. She remains clinically free of disease, with her CA-125 in the normal range (Fig. 101–3).

COMMENTARY by William J. Hoskins

Although the finding of a malignant epithelial cancer in a 29-year-old woman is unusual, it is by no means a rare occurrence. The incidence of epithelial ovarian cancer in the 25- to 34-year age group is 3 per 100,000, as compared with 40/100,000 in women aged 55 to 64 years. The maximum incidence in the United States is 50/100,000 in women aged 65 to 84 years. Despite the relative infrequency of a diagnosis of cancer, the findings of bilateral complex ovarian masses and an elevation of the serum CA-125 must be considered suspicious for cancer. Although a variety of factors can cause a false-positive CA-125 (e.g., endometriosis, menses, hepatic disease, and leiomyomata uteri), the combination of bilateral complex ovarian masses and an elevated serum CA-125 must be considered ovarian cancer until proved otherwise. Additional tests that would be indicated in this patient would be a beta human gonadotropin level and an alpha-fetoprotein level. These tests may be elevated in a patient with a malignant germ cell tumor of the ovary. Malignant germ cell tumors usually occur in women under the age of 35 years.

The use of laparoscopy in this patient is reasonable to rule out endometriosis, which could explain the bilateral complex ovarian masses and the elevated serum CA-125 level. Considerable skill and experience with the laparoscope, however, is required to manage masses of this size without rupture of the masses inside the abdominal cavity. Once the diagnosis of an obvious cancer is made by diagnostic laparoscopy, the patient should be managed by a gynecologic oncologist in a facility with the availability of frozen section pathologic analysis.

The appropriate management of this patient would have been frozen section analysis of both ovarian masses and the omental nodule. With intraoperative confirmation of the diagnosis of advanced ovarian cancer, the appropriate surgical procedure would have been total abdominal hysterectomy, bilateral salpingo-oophorectomy, omentectomy, and a full surgical staging procedure, including sampling of pelvic and para-aortic lymph nodes. In this patient, an inadequate procedure led to the need for a second operation to complete the surgical therapy. Although one can and should be conservative in ovarian cancers of low grade confined to one ovary, this patient had obvious advanced disease.

This patient was treated postoperatively on an experimental protocol using high-dose chemotherapy with cisplatin and cyclophosphamide. Because of the poor survival of patients with advanced epithelial ovarian cancer [5-year survival of 21% according to the National Cancer Institute's Surveillance, Epidemiology and End Results

(SEER) Program], such patients should be encouraged to participate in prospective clinical trials. Standard chemotherapy at the time of this patient's diagnosis would have been five or six courses of chemotherapy with cisplatin (or carboplatin) and cyclophosphamide. Currently, the standard therapy would be five or six courses of chemotherapy with cisplatin (or carboplatin) and Taxol. The Gynecologic Oncology Group has demonstrated improved survival in patients with advanced ovarian cancer using a combination chemotherapy regimen containing Taxol.

SELECTED READINGS

1. Curtin JP. Diagnosis and staging of epithelial cancer. In: *Cancer of the ovary*, Markman M, Hoskins WJ, eds. New York: Raven Press; 1993:153–62.
2. Ozols RF, Rubin SC, Dembo AJ, Robboy S. Epithelial ovarian cancer. In: *Principles and practice of gynecologic oncology*, Hoskins WJ, Perez CA, Young RC, eds. Philadelphia: JB Lippincott Co; 1992:731–81.
3. McGuire WP, Hoskins WJ, Brady MF, et al., for the Gynecologic Oncology Group, Buffalo NY. A phase III trial comparing cisplatin/cytoxan and cisplatin/Taxol in advanced ovarian cancer. *Proc ASCO*, abstract #808, 1993.

102

Ovarian Serous Borderline Tumors with Peritoneal Implants

J. Taylor Wharton

The dilemma of low malignant potential tumors

CASE PRESENTATION

The patient is a 41-year-old woman who saw her gynecologist for an annual examination. She had been on oral contraceptives for the last 18 years without any problems. She works with her husband on their horse and cattle ranch and teaches school. Pelvic exam revealed an irregular pelvic mass, and an ultrasound showed a 12-cm complex cystic mass involving the left ovary. The patient was asymptomatic and had not experienced weight gain, a change in abdominal girth, or changes in bowel function. She had noted a decrease in bladder capacity that she attributed to the aging process.

There were no significant prior medical or surgical illnesses. She had one normal spontaneous vaginal delivery 18 years ago. She takes no medications except for oral contraceptives (for last 18 years). She drinks occasionally and has never used tobacco. Her mother died at age 35, and a sister died at age 40, both of breast cancer.

Pertinent physical findings were on abdominal and pelvic examination. There was a lower abdominal, firm, irregular, nontender mass extending to the level of the umbilicus. No ascites was detected. On bimanual pelvic exam, the cervix was displaced laterally and the uterus was confluent with an anterior 15 × 20 cm irregular firm mass. Rectovaginal examination confirmed the high anterior position of this mass, and the cul-de-sac was free.

The patient had a chemistry profile, electrolyte battery, hematology survey, coagulation studies, alpha fetoprotein, beta HCG, and CA-125. These studies were normal except for a CA-125 of 284 units/mL (normal range

0–35). Diagnostic imaging studies included a chest roentgenogram, single contrast barium enema, screening mammogram, and intravenous pyelogram. The barium enema showed a large pelvic mass displacing the midsigmoid posteriolaterally and to the right (Fig. 102–1). The intravenous pyelogram revealed a large pelvic mass compressing the superior aspect of the bladder, and normal kidneys and ureters (Fig. 102–2). The chest x-ray and mammograms were normal. Since the patient was on oral contraceptives and had a normal Pap smear and no irregular bleeding, cervical and endometrial biopsies were not performed. A CT scan of the abdomen and pelvis was not indicated.

The operative findings revealed an 8 × 10 cm irregular left ovary and an 8.5 × 3.5 cm right ovary covered by loops of small bowel and omentum. Both ovaries contained numerous external papillary excrescences (Fig. 102–3), and the left ovary was densely adherent to the sigmoid colon. A separate 2.5 cm implant was on the peritoneal surface of the cul-de-sac. No implants were discovered in the upper abdomen. Pelvic and abdominal washings were taken for cytological analysis. The patient had a total abdominal hysterectomy and bilateral salpingo-oophorectomy. A 22 × 15 cm segment of the omentum was removed. The cul-de-sac nodule was excised. Multiple biopsies were taken from selected abdominal peritoneal surfaces. Pelvic and aortic lymph nodes were removed. Biopsies were taken from suspicious areas on the serosal surface of the small bowel. Enlarged mesenteric lymph nodes were removed. All visible tumor was removed and suspicious sites biopsied.

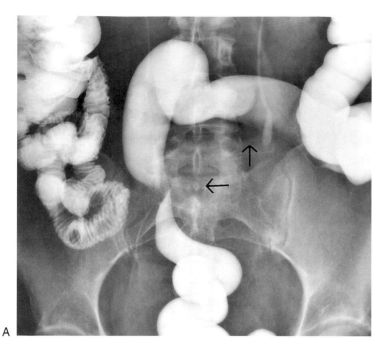

A

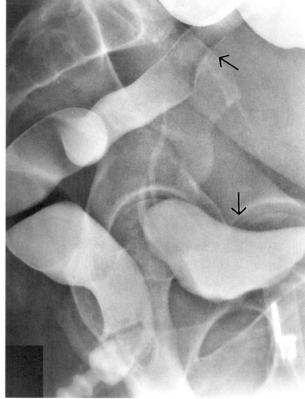

B

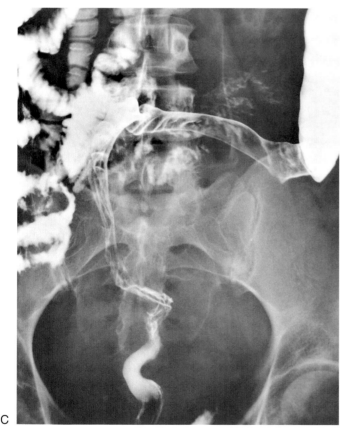

C

FIG. 102–1. Pelvic mass with displacement of the colon. **A:** The sigmoid colon is displaced to the right and superiorly by a soft tissue mass arising from the pelvis *(arrows).* **B:** The proximal sigmoid is displaced posteriorly against the first sacral segment, and the bladder is indented from above by the soft tissue mass *(arrows).* **C:** The postevacuation film confirms the colonic displacement and shows some interference with evacuation of the proximal colon.

The pathology report revealed a papillary serous tumor of low malignant potential (Fig. 102–4) with multiple foci of microinvasion (Fig. 102–5) involving the right and left ovaries. The cul-de-sac nodule showed a noninvasive implant of serous tumor of low malignant potential. The pelvic and abdominal washings showed numerous papil-

lary groups with psammoma bodies consistent with serous tumor of low-grade malignant potential. The lymph nodes were negative for tumor, and the suspicious serosal and mesenteric areas showed fat necrosis and fibrosis. The omentum and peritoneal biopsies from the upper abdomen showed no tumor. The tumor involved

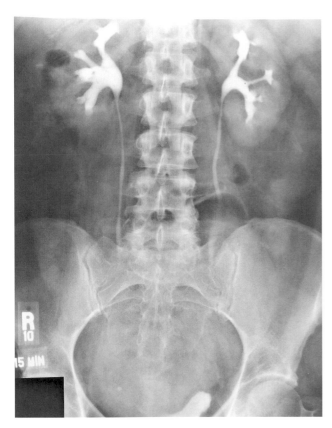

FIG. 102–2. Intravenous pyelogram. The upper tracts are normal, but a soft tissue mass indents the bladder from above.

both ovaries and extended to the pelvis, and the peritoneal washings contained malignant cells. The extent of disease was consistent with a FIGO stage IIC (TNM category T2c) papillary serous tumor of low malignant potential. The enlarged ovaries extended above the true pelvis, and the complex mass was adherent to the omentum and loops of small bowel; however, no microscopic disease was found above the true pelvis.

The patient experienced no postoperative problems, and bowel function resumed on the fifth postoperative day. She was discharged on the seventh postoperative day. A repeat CA-125 at the time of discharge was 80.4 units/mL.

The case was presented at the Gynecologic Oncology weekly tumor conference for a therapy decision. Members present were gynecologic oncologists, radiation oncologists, pathologists, residents, fellows, and clinical nurse specialists. Presentation to the board was initiated with a definition of the neoplasm being discussed. The category of borderline tumors of common epithelial origin represents a histologic subgroup of malignant carcinomas with a good prognosis. The World Health Organization defines serous borderline tumors as serous neoplasms that show epithelial proliferation greater than that seen in serous cystadenomas, as evidenced by cellu-

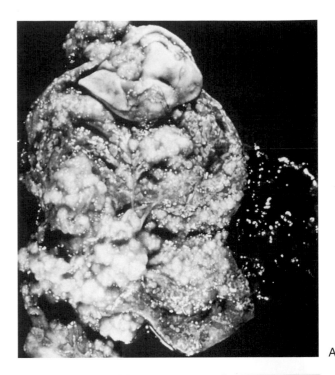

A

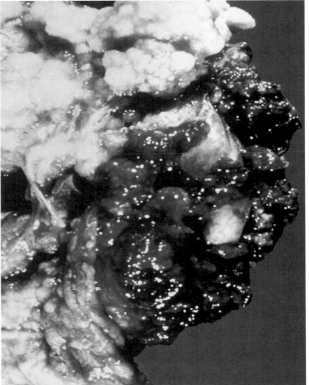

B

FIG. 102–3. Gross or surgical specimen. **A:** Low magnification. **B:** Higher magnification.

lar stratification, cytologic atypicality, and epithelial tufting, but which exhibit no evidence of "destructive stromal" invasion. Significant or destructive stromal invasion was not observed in either ovary. There were several areas of microinvasion.

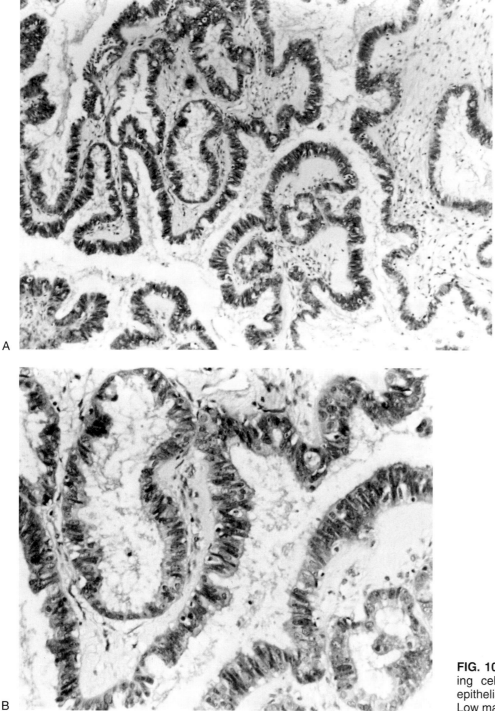

A

B

FIG. 102–4. Serous borderline tumor showing cellular stratification, cytologic atypia, epithelial tufting, and no stromal invasion. **A:** Low magnification. **B:** Higher magnification.

The majority of patients with serous borderline tumors with extra-ovarian spread usually have metastatic implants that are small and resectable. The patient being discussed is in this category. The cul-de-sac implant was easily removed. Positive peritoneal cytology was not considered important in the therapy planning for patients with serous borderline tumors. This patient had the ovaries and all visible implants removed.

This aspect of the case was considered pertinent because patients with no visible residual remaining after surgery rarely experience tumor progression. The histologic features of the implants received considerable discussion. Histologic review of the 2.5-cm implant in the cul-de-sac and the microscopic foci found in pelvic peritoneum biopsies showed no invasion, and only mild cytologic atypia was observed.

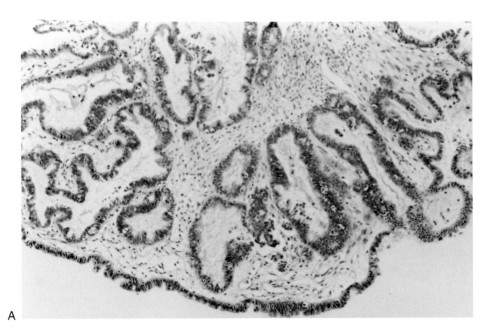

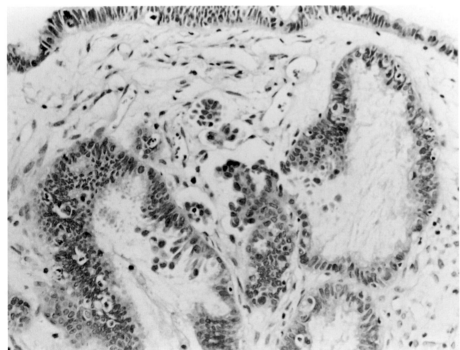

FIG. 102–5. Serous borderline tumor showing foci of microinvasion. **A:** Low magnification. **B:** Higher magnification.

There was a consensus reached by the disciplines present at the meeting. Patients with serous tumors of low malignant potential with extra-ovarian implants completely resected do not require postoperative chemotherapy or radiation therapy.

The patient was seen 4 weeks after surgery and pelvic examination was normal for a patient receiving TAH and BSO. A repeat CA-125 was 7.3 units/mL. The patient will have a pelvic examination and CA-125 performed every 3 months for the first year, every 4 months during the second year, and then every 6 months from the second to the fifth year.

Evaluations have continued as recommended, and the patient has not developed evidence of tumor progression. The CA-125 levels have remained normal. The patient is 24 months following surgery.

COMMENTARY by L. Stewart Massad

Low malignant potential (LMP) tumors of the ovary are uncommon but troubling management problems for treating physicians. Often, these are termed "borderline" tumors because their histologic features are intermediate between those of benign cystadenomas and malignant cancers of the ovary. Recurrences are rare and often present years after initial diagnosis. As indicated in the case report, adjuvant therapy is of uncertain benefit.

LMP tumors of the ovary were first described by Taylor in 1929 and are defined by the World Health Organization as having "some, but not all, of the morphologic features of malignancy," including stratification, apparently detached clusters of cells, mitotic activity, and nuclear atypia without obvious invasion of the adjacent stroma (1). Diagnosis requires that at least one slide should be examined for every centimeter of greatest tumor diameter. The number of slides examined in this case is not noted but should have been at least 10 for the left ovary, 8 for the right. Less intensive evaluation risks underdiagnosis of an invasive cancer for which chemotherapy may be lifesaving.

This patient presents several interesting features. She developed an ovarian neoplasm while on oral contraceptives, despite their protective effects against ovarian cancer (2). No association between oral contraceptives and LMP tumors has been demonstrated. Initial symptoms were vague, as are those of most ovarian neoplasms. The significant family history of breast cancer suggests a genetic etiology, but LMP tumors, unlike invasive ovarian cancers, have not been convincingly linked to family syndromes. The elevated CA-125 level was suggestive of ovarian neoplasm, but LMP tumors may present with a normal level of CA-125, and the degree of elevation of CA-125 cannot be used reliably to distinguish LMP tumors from frank ovarian carcinomas. Elevation of CA-125 in a patient with an LMP tumor suggests extra-ovarian disease, as seen in this case (3). The case report notes that "a CT scan... was not indicated." Although such a scan may provide information that cannot be obtained by other noninvasive modalities, the finding of a complex pelvic mass in a woman with a markedly elevated CA-125 level is suspicious for malignancy, and laparotomy by a surgeon capable of performing staging and debulking procedures was the indicated next step.

Controversy exists about the importance of formal staging procedures, especially since some series have reported good long-term survival after conservative surgery (6,7). Nevertheless, intraoperative decisions on appropriate staging procedures are based on frozen section. Since diagnosis of an LMP tumor is one of exclusion, patients with a diagnosis of LMP tumor at frozen section should be considered to have invasive cancer and staged accordingly. The only exception to this may be the patient who preoperatively decides to limit procedures to preserve fertility with the understanding that reoperation for formal staging may be required, especially since some series have reported good long-term survival after conservative surgery (6,7).

Recurrence and death are rare among patients with LMP tumors. Estimates of these endpoints are limited by short follow-up times in many series, but in an extensive literature review, the incidence of recurrence of persistent disease was 2.1% for stage I tumors, 7.1% for stage II tumors, and 14.4% for stage III/IV tumors, while death from tumor occurred in 1.9% of stage I tumors, 5.9% of stage II tumors, and 21.0% of stage III/IV tumors, findings corroborated by more recent single-institution studies (5,8,9). Patients who have no residual disease at the conclusion of initial surgery, like the one presented here, have the best prognosis.

The value of adjuvant chemotherapy for ovarian LMP tumors has been studied. A randomized trial of limited power found no benefit to adjuvant treatment of patients with stage I LMP tumors (10). Some suggest that chemotherapy may benefit patients with more advanced disease (11). However, review of a series of patients with stage III tumors failed to show disease regression after being treated erroneously under a protocol for invasive ovarian cancer by members of the Gynecologic Oncology Group (GOG) (12). Use of oral alkylating agents as treatment for LMP tumors of the ovary has been associated with the development of fatal leukemias and should probably be avoided (13). Better understanding of the value of adjuvant treatment for women with LMP tumors should follow the publication of results from an ongoing GOG study of this issue.

The borderline between LMP tumors and invasive cancers is a broad one. The pathologists who reviewed this case found a tumor with many of the proliferative features of LMP tumors in association with multiple foci of stromal invasion but no evidence of "destructive" invasion. Cases of this type are even more rare than usual LMP tumors, and their behavior is even less well defined. In the absence of clear data, a decision not to administer adjuvant chemotherapy must be made in consultation with the patient after assessing the potential toxicity of chemotherapy.

Appropriate follow-up for patients with ovarian LMP tumors in complete remission should consist of frequent physical examination, including pelvic examination, and CA-125 levels. Recurrences have been identified as late as 24 years after initial diagnosis, so the 24 months of disease-free survival noted here, though encouraging, is not definitive. The value of routine screening for recurrences via imaging is dubious, although new symptoms and physical findings should be pursued aggressively. LMP tumors have been linked to synchronous and metachronous second primaries, especially of the breast, endometrium, and colon; therefore, surveillance with mammography and sigmoidoscopy are likely to be beneficial (5). Surgery with complete resection appears to be the best modality for diagnosis and treatment of recurrent tumor, especially since recurrences may be invasive and aggressive (14).

REFERENCES

1. Serov SF, Scully RE, Sobin LH, eds. Histological typing of ovarian tumors. World Health Organization (WHO), Geneva, 1973.
2. Gross TP, Schlesselman JJ. The estimated effect of oral contraceptive use on the cumulative risk of epithelial ovarian cancer. *Obstet Gynecol* 1994;83:419–24.
3. Rice LW, Lage JM, Berkowitz RS, Goodman A, Muto MG, et al. Preoperative serum CA-125 levels in borderline tumors of the ovary. *Gynecol Oncol* 1992;46:226–9.
4. Leake JF, Rader JS, Woodruff JD, Rosenshein NB. Retroperitoneal lymphatic involvement with epithelial ovarian tumors of low malignant potential. *Gynecol Oncol* 1991;42:124–30.
5. Massad LS, Hunter VJ, Szpak CA, Clark-Pearson DL, Creasman WT. Epithelial ovarian tumors of low malignant potential. *Obstet Gynecol* 1991;78:1027–32.
6. Tazelaar HD, Bostwick DG, Ballon SC, Hendrickson MR, Kempson RL. Conservative treatment of borderline ovarian tumors. *Obstet Gynecol* 1985;66:417–22.
7. Lim-Tan SK, Cajigas HE, Scully RE. Ovarian cystectomy for serous borderline tumors: a follow-up study of 35 cases. *Obstet Gynecol* 1988;72:775–81.
8. Leake JF, Currie JL, Rosenshein NB, Woodruff JD. Long-term follow-up of serous ovarian tumors of low malignant potential. *Gynecol Oncol* 1992;47:150–8.
9. Kaern J, Trope CG, Abeler VM. A retrospective study of 370 borderline tumors of the ovary treated at the Norwegian Radium Hospital from 1970 to 1982. *Cancer* 1993;71:1810–20.
10. Creasman WT, Park R, Norris H, DiSaia PJ, et al. Stage I borderline ovarian tumors. *Obstet Gynecol* 1982;59:93–6.
11. Fort MG, Pierce VK, Saigo PE, Hoskins WJ, Lewis JL. Evidence for the efficacy of adjuvant therapy in epithelial ovarian tumors of low malignant potential. *Gynecol Oncol* 1989;32:269–72.
12. Sutton GP, Bundy BN, Omura GA, Yordan EL, et al. Stage III ovarian tumors of low malignant potential treated with cisplatin combination therapy (a Gynecologic Oncology Group study). *Gynecol Oncol* 1991;41:230–3.
13. O'Quinn AG, Hannigan EV. Epithelial ovarian neoplasms of low malignant potential. *Gynecol Oncol* 1985;21:177–85.
14. Bostwick DG, Tazelaar HD, Ballon SC, Hendrickson MR, Kempson RL. Ovarian epithelial tumors of borderline malignancy. *Cancer* 1986;58:2052–65.

EDITORIAL BOARD COMMENTARY

A decrease in bladder capacity or urgency of urination are early signs of ovarian cancer.

103

Stage III Ovarian Carcinoma with Positive Peritoneal Cytology at Second-Look Laparotomy

Hervy E. Averette and Michael Rodriguez, with Michael M. Method and Bernd-Uwe Sevin

Do we know how to manage patients with second-line chemotherapy?

CASE PRESENTATION

L.H. is a 24-year-old nulligravid woman who presented to her primary gynecologist with the chief complaint of dysmenorrhea and abdominal bloating beginning in January, 1994. Initial work-up was performed by her primary physician, who referred her to the University of Miami Sylvester Comprehensive Cancer Center for treatment. Past medical and surgical history was unremarkable, but a history of colon cancer was present in the maternal grandmother. The patient had been taking oral contraceptives for 1 year, and there was no history of alcohol, tobacco, or drug abuse. On physical exam she was a well developed Caucasian woman with a large, 18-cm abdominal-pelvic mass. Cul de sac nodularity was noted on rectovaginal exam. The remainder of the exam was unremarkable. Blood work included an elevated CA-125 of 731 (nl 0–35), a normal AFP of 0.9 (nl 0–15), CEA of 2.0 (nl 0–3), Hcg of less than 5. Computed tomography (CT scan) of the abdomen and pelvis demonstrated a large abdominal-pelvic mass most likely originating from the pelvis, with omental caking and ascites (Fig. 103–1). Individual gynecologic organs were obscured by the complexity and size of the mass. Ultrasound supported the diagnosis of an ovarian neoplasm by identifying bilateral adnexal masses and ascites, but a normal uterus.

On March 28, 1994, L.H. underwent surgical exploration at the University of Miami Hospital. A midline incision was used for exploration. Upon entry into the abdomen, 1.5 L of ascites was encountered and was sent for cytologic analysis. Bilateral ovarian masses were identified measuring $6 \times 7 \times 7$ cm (right) and $8 \times 10 \times 12$ cm (left). In addition, tumor involved the uterus and cul de sac. Palpation and visual inspection of the upper abdomen revealed gross tumor nodules greater than 2 cm within the omentum. The right and left paracolic peritoneal gutters also had large plaques of tumor involvement greater than 2 cm. The liver, spleen, and diaphragm were normal, and no enlarged lymph nodes were palpated retroperitoneally. The operation included tumor debulking, abdominal hysterectomy, bilateral salpingo-oophorectomy, appendectomy, para-aortic and pelvic lymph node sampling, and placement of an intraperitoneal port-a-cath. Peritoneal stripping was performed in the cul de sac and abdominal gutters to leave the patient with no visible residual disease at the end of the procedure. Tissue from the ovarian carcinoma was sent for *in vitro* chemosensitivity testing with the adenosine triphosphate cell viability assay (ATP-CVA). This *in vitro* assay tests standard chemotherapeutic drugs alone and in combination at five concentrations to assess an individual patient's tumor sensitivity to chemotherapeutic agents (1,2). Results indicated the

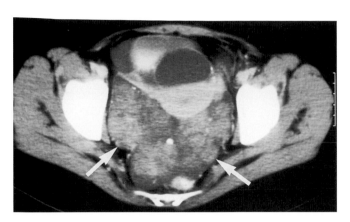

FIG. 103–1. CT of pelvis shows a large complex soft tissue mass.

tumor to be sensitive to both the combination of cisplatin/paclitaxel and cisplatin/cyclophosphamide. Pathology results showed a well differentiated papillary serous cystadenocarcinoma with metastases to the abdominal gutters and the omentum (Fig. 103–2). Two lymph nodes were positive, one from each external iliac nodal area. The final surgical stage was stage IIIC based on disease more than 2 cm in the upper abdomen as well as positive lymph nodes. Postoperatively, she recovered without complication and was discharged on the sixth day.

Gynecologic Oncology Group (GOG) protocol #114 for patients with optimally cytoreduced stage IIIC ovarian carcinoma that compares standard-dose intravenous cisplatin/paclitaxel to high-dose intravenous carboplatin followed by intravenous paclitaxel and intraperitoneal cis-

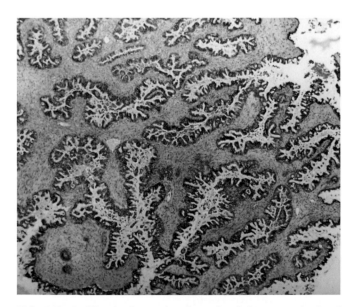

FIG. 103–2. Histologic section from the right ovary obtained at the initial debulking procedure showing well differentiated papillary serous cystadenocarcinoma.

platin was offered as adjuvant chemotherapy. The patient declined protocol and was subsequently treated with intravenous paclitaxel (135 mg/m^2) and cisplatin (75 mg/m^2). Postoperatively, the CA-125 declined rapidly into the normal range and was 18 by the beginning of the second treatment. An interim CT scan was taken after the third course of chemotherapy and was normal. She completed six courses of chemotherapy with tolerable toxicities including complete alopecia, moderate neutropenia, and thrombocytopenia between treatments, and mild peripheral neuropathy after the fifth treatment. No toxicity was severe enough to cause treatment delay.

At completion of six treatments of chemotherapy, the CA-125 was 12, and a repeat CT scan and physical exam showed no evidence of disease. Therefore, by definition she had a complete clinical response to the chemotherapy. As part of an institutional protocol, a radioimmunoscintigraphic scan (Oncoscint CR/OV) was performed and was positive for persistent disease (Fig. 103–3). Diffuse uptake of radiolabeled antibodies was noted within the posterior pelvis, along the right external iliac blood vessels, and in the area of the inguinal lymph nodes. This pattern, in our experience, has been consistent with small (<0.5 cm) residual or microscopic disease. The patient elected to undergo surgical re-exploration (second-look laparotomy) for definitive assessment of disease status, which was performed on August 29, 1994. Peritoneal washings were obtained in several regions of the pelvis and abdomen.

There was no sign of gross residual tumor. A thin layer of fibrotic material (1–2 mm) covering the bowel and many of the peritoneal surfaces was noted. Several biopsies of this material were taken and analyzed by frozen section, which revealed only fibrosis. The remaining omentum, peritoneal, para-aortic, and pelvic lymph node biopsies were performed. Postoperative recovery was uneventful, and the patient was discharged on day 4. Peritoneal cytology showed cells histologically identical to her primary papillary serous cystadenocarcinoma. One peritoneal cul de sac biopsy demonstrated one microscopic focus of serous adenocarcinoma in dense fibrous tissue. An addition 34 biopsies performed were negative for persistent carcinoma. Therefore, the patient had shown a complete clinical response, yet surgically only a partial response to previous chemotherapy.

The patient was presented at the University of Miami Sylvester Comprehensive Cancer Center multidisciplinary tumor board to discuss the next step in her treatment. Each option will be listed and elaborated on in this review.

Intraperitoneal (IP) Chemotherapy/Radiocolloid Therapy

Many studies have been performed looking at intraperitoneal chemotherapy. Its major role is in patients with microscopic or small volume disease (1–3 mm) after

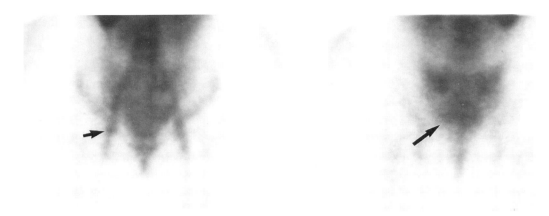

FIG. 103–3. Anterior and posterior views of a radioimmunoscintigraphy (Oncoscint) study showing increased uptake of radiolabeled antibodies in the pelvis and the right lower quadrant overlying the external ileal vessels and in the inguinal area.

laparotomy. Studies have shown that high concentrations of chemotherapy can be delivered to the peritoneal cavity via the IP route. This is especially true for paclitaxel, which has been shown to deliver as high as 1,000-fold higher plasma peak concentration (PPC) of drug to the peritoneal cavity via the IP route versus the intravenous route (3). Intraperitoneal paclitaxel may be appropriate consolidation therapy for this patient.

Radioactive phosphorous (32-P) has been used for the treatment of ovarian cancer since the 1950s. With the advent of effective systemic chemotherapy, its role has become more restricted. The feasibility, efficacy, and toxicity have been elucidated in several retrospective studies evaluating 32-P after adjuvant chemotherapy in early stage ovarian carcinoma. The efficacy is less well established for advanced stages. Currently, the GOG is conducting a randomized prospective trial in stage IIIC ovarian cancer patients with negative second-look laparotomies. Patients are being randomized to receive 32-P or no further treatment. The findings of this investigation are pending. Because of uncertain benefits from this mode of consolidation treatment in this high-risk group for recurrence, IP 32-P is not appropriate treatment in this setting until a randomized prospective trial is performed evaluating patients with microscopic residual disease at second-look laparotomy.

Whole Abdominal Radiation

Even though whole abdominal radiation (WAR) was the treatment of choice for residual disease after surgery for ovarian carcinoma for many years, no prospective randomized trial has been performed comparing cisplatin-based chemotherapy to WAR. This is true for primary disease as well as persistent disease after chemotherapy. Most of the literature on the subject is retrospective and is based on ovarian cancer patients who were primarily treated with

WAR (4). Potential complications of WAR in this setting are substantial. Fistula formation or small bowel obstruction can be catastrophic and are increased in patients with prior multiple surgical explorations and higher doses (pelvis > 4,500, abdomen > 2,250–2,500 Gy) of radiation therapy. Radiotherapy at this point in treatment would make future surgical options limited or impossible if bulky recurrence occurred at a later date. In addition, future chemotherapy tolerance is reduced secondary to compromise to the bone marrow from radiation. Because of the uncertain benefit of WAR, with its potential complications, it is not the first treatment of choice in this setting.

Standard High-Dose Chemotherapy/High-Dose Chemotherapy with Stem Cell Rescue

High-dose chemotherapy may be appropriate in this setting because the patient appeared to respond to primary chemotherapy. In addition, her young age and outstanding performance status would make her a good candidate for an intense high-dose regimen with granulocyte-colony stimulating factor (G-CSF) support. The use of marrow-toxic doses of chemotherapy with stem cell rescue is more controversial in this setting. Phase II studies have been performed showing short-term responses in heavily pretreated patients with ovarian carcinoma, but because of high costs and uncertain benefits, high-dose regimens with stem cell rescue should be reserved for investigative protocol settings.

Individualized Chemotherapy Based on *In Vitro* Chemosensitivity Testing

The adenosine triphosphate cell viability assay (ATP-CVA) has been shown to correlate well with clinical response to chemotherapy in preliminary studies (5). The assay is currently being evaluated by the GOG in a large prospective multi-institutional study in the treatment of primary ovarian carcinoma. We have found this assay to be a great value to assess patients with persistent or recurrent ovarian carcinoma. Statistical analysis with the median effect principle showed a supra-additive relationship between cisplatin and cyclophosphamide based on the *in vitro* assay. This patient's initial tumor showed greatest sensitivity to the combination of cisplatin and cyclophosphamide.

After discussion of the treatment options, the patient favored high-dose combination of carboplatin (cisplatin analog) and cyclophosphamide with G-CSF support.

REFERENCES

1. Sevin BU, Averette HE, Donato DM, Penalver MA. Chemosensitivity testing in ovarian cancer. *Cancer* 1994;71:1613.
2. Kochli OR, Sevin BU, Haller U, eds. *Chemosensitivity testing in gynecologic malignancies and breast cancer.* Basel: Karger; 1994.
3. Markman M, Rowensky E, Hakes T, et al. Phase I trial of intraperitoneal taxol: a Gynecologic Oncology Group Study. *J Clin Oncology* 1992;10:1485–91.
4. Thomas GM, Dembo AJ. Integrating radiation therapy into the management of ovarian cancer. *Cancer* 1993;71(suppl):1710.
5. Gerhardt RT, Perras JP, Sevin BU, et al. Characterization of in vitro chemosensitivity of perioperative human malignancies by ATP chemosensitivity analysis. *Am J Obstet Gynecol* 1991;165:2245–55.

COMMENTARY by Daniel H. Shevrin

Typically, ovarian cancer (OC) is a disease of older age. Presentation in a very young woman, such as the patient in this case, may be due to genetic factors (1). An ovarian neoplasm arising in a young woman may be a germ cell tumor, and alpha-fetoprotein and human chorionic gonadotropin levels should be measured. This patient's presentation was otherwise quite typical of advanced OC.

Patients with advanced OC should undergo cytoreductive surgery followed by six cycles of platinum-based chemotherapy (2). This patient had successful cytoreductive surgery, with no visible disease at the end of the procedure. The presence of positive external iliac lymph nodes and disease more than 2 cm in the upper abdomen made her stage IIIC. Pathology showed a well differentiated papillary serous cystadenocarcinoma. This patient was then treated with paclitaxel and cisplatin. Although the two-drug regimens of carboplatinum or cisplatin and cytoxan remain the standard treatments after cytoreductive surgery, the combination of paclitaxel and cisplatin has been shown to have significant activity as first-line therapy in poor prognosis disease (3). This regimen will likely become the new standard for first-line therapy in advanced OC.

After achieving a clinical complete remission, the patient underwent surgical re-exploration, or second-look laparotomy (SLL). The value of SLL has been questioned in recent years (4). Although SLL provides the most accurate assessment of residual disease and, therefore, an objective measure of response to therapy, a favorable impact on survival has never been proven (5). This is presumably due to the lack of effectiveness of second-line therapies that are used on the basis of the information gained by SLL. Clearly, SLL has a role in selecting patients for experimental second-line therapies. In this patient, after optimal debulking with no visible disease and six cycles of paclitaxel/cisplatin, SLL showed evidence of persistent microscopic cancer.

The primary question is whether any second-line therapy can be curative or, at least, prolong survival in this patient. If such therapies are not available, then treatment must be considered palliative, and experimental therapies should be considered. There are various therapies that are currently being employed in patients with persistent OC seen at surgical reexploration.

Whole abdominal radiation (WAR): WAR has been studied in patients with residual disease. Fuks et al. reported that 19 of 25 patients failed after WAR, and the actuarial 5-year disease-free survival was only 17% (6). Others have reported similar high relapse rates (7). There is no evidence that WAR given in this setting improves survival, and it cannot be recommended.

Standard high-dose chemotherapy: Retrospective data by Levin suggest that outcome in advanced OC is directly correlated with the intensity with which therapy is administered (8). Unfortunately, no prospective trial has shown any improvement in survival with high-dose therapy. The GOG prospectively evaluated cisplatin/cytoxan at two intensity levels but failed to show a survival advantage (9). A prospective randomized study by the Milan group using higher intensity cisplatin showed a similar response rate to standard therapy (10). High-dose carboplatinum has been studied in refractory OC. A high response rate was observed, but it was limited to patients showing prior objective responses to cisplatin (11). The overall median survival was only 12 months. The patient presented in this case had persistent disease after paclitaxel/cisplatin therapy. Despite the *in vitro* assay that showed the tumor to be sensitive to this combination, the presence of cancer after six cycles of treatment signifies clinical resistance to these drugs. It is therefore unlikely that carboplatinum given at a high dose will result in a significant response in this patient, and even more unlikely that this approach will prolong her survival.

Intraperitoneal (IP) therapy: IP therapy has the potential for the greatest dose intensity to the peritoneal surface. It is clear from multiple phase II studies that IP therapy results in frequent pathologically complete responses when used as salvage therapy in microscopic disease, and it may have a favorable impact on survival (12). Patients with minimal residual disease at SLL have a highly variable long-term survival with either salvage therapy or no therapy (13). Therefore, the true impact on survival of IP therapy awaits results of prospective randomized trials. Finally, prospective trials of IP therapy in optimally cytoreduced stage III patients are ongoing. It is unlikely that IP therapy will be pursued as second-line therapy if benefit is not demonstrated in this "good prognosis" group.

High-dose chemotherapy with autologous bone marrow transplantation (ABMT): High-dose chemotherapy with ABMT may be applicable in the management of refractory OC. Unfortunately, few adequate trials have been performed. Most studies, which have looked at heavily pretreated patients, have reported high response rates, but favorable impact on survival has not been proved (14). Stiff et al. reported a high response rate (6 out of 11 CRs), but 2-year progression-free survival for these responders was only 18% (15). Several European centers have evaluated high-dose chemotherapy with ABMT in patients with persistent disease after SLL (16). These studies also report high response rates, but follow-up is too short to make any firm conclusions on survival.

In conclusion, there is no evidence that second-line therapy in this patient will result in prolongation of survival or cure. Therefore, given the patient's young age, participation in an NIH-approved trial of high-dose chemotherapy with ABMT would seem appropriate. If this was not possible, treatment with IP chemotherapy, preferably in a clinical trial, would be a reasonable approach. This case underscores the many controversies and uncertainties surrounding the management of patients with stage III OC with persistent disease at SLL.

REFERENCES

1. Lynch HT, Lynch JF. Hereditary Ovarian Cancer. *Hematol/Oncol Clin North Am* 1992;6:783–811.
2. Heintz AP. Surgery in advanced ovarian carcinoma: is there proof to show the benefit? *Eur J Surg Oncol* 1988;14:91–9.
3. McGuire WP, Hoskins WJ, Brady MF, et al. A phase III trial comparing cisplatin/cytoxan and cisplatin/taxol in advanced ovarian cancer. *Proceed ASCO* 1993;12:255, #808.
4. Ho AG, Beller U, Speyer JL, et al. A reassessment of the role of second-look laparotomy in advanced ovarian cancer. *J Clin Oncol* 1987;5:1316–21.
5. Young RC. A second look at second-look laparotomy. *J Clin Oncol* 1987;5:1311–37.
6. Fuks Z, Rizel S, Biran S. Chemotherapeutic and surgical induction of pathologic complete remission and whole abdominal irradiation for consolidation does not enhance the cure of stage III ovarian cancer. *J Clin Oncol* 1988;6:509–16.
7. Bolis G, Zanaboni F, Vanoli P, et al. The impact of whole-abdomen radiotherapy on survival in advanced ovarian cancer patients with minimal residual disease after chemotherapy. *Gynecol Oncol* 1990;39:150–4.
8. Levin L, Hryniuk WM. Dose intensity analysis of chemotherapy regimens in ovarian cancer. *J Clin Oncol* 1987;5:756–67.
9. McGuire WP, Hoskins WJ, Brady MS, et al. A phase II study of dose intense versus standard dose cisplatin and cytoxan in advanced ovarian cancer. *Proc Int Gynecol Cancer Soc* 1991;3:35.
10. Pecorelli S, Marsoni S, Belloni C, et al. Controlled clinical trial of two different dose-intensity induction regimens in advanced ovarian cancer patients. *Proc Int Gynecol Cancer Soc* 1991;3:215.
11. Reed E, Janik J, Bookman MA, et al. High-dose carboplatinum and recombinant granulocyte macrophage colony-stimulating factor in advanced-stage recurrent ovarian cancer. *J Clin Oncol* 1993;11:2118–26.
12. McClay EF, Howell SB. Intraperitoneal therapy in the management of patients with ovarian cancer. *Hematol/Oncol Clin North Am* 1992;6:915–26.
13. Copeland LJ, Gershenson DM, Wharton JT, et al. Microscopic disease at second-look laparotomy in advanced ovarian cancer. *Cancer* 1985;55:472–8.
14. Schilder RJ. High-dose chemotherapy with autologous hematopoietic cell support in gynecologic malignancies. In: *Principles and practice of gynecologic oncology updates,* Hoskins, Perez, Young, eds. 1992;1:1–14.
15. Stiff PJ, McKenzie RS, Alberts DS, et al. Phase I clinical and pharmacokinetic study of high-dose mitoxantrone combined with carboplatin, cyclophosphamide, and autologous bone marrow rescue: high response rate for refractory ovarian carcinoma. *J Clin Oncol* 1994;12:176–83.
16. Viens P, Maraninchi D, Legros M, et al. High-dose melphalan and autologous marrow rescue in advanced epithelial ovarian carcinomas: a retrospective analysis of 35 patients treated in France. *Bone Marrow Transplant* 1990;5:227–33.

EDITORIAL BOARD COMMENTARY

This patient should also be closely followed up for breast cancer in view of the family history.

104

Stage IA Carcinoma of the Ovary Incidentally Discovered at Surgery

John P. Curtin

Early detection can be a winner

CASE PRESENTATION

The patient is a 37-year-old Caucasian married woman who is gravida 4, para 2, elective abortions 2, who presented to her gynecologist for a routine examination in January, 1992. At that time she was noted to have a slightly prominent right adnexa noted on pelvic exam. An ultrasound was obtained, which showed a small right ovarian cyst. A repeat ultrasound 6 weeks later did not demonstrate the presence of this cyst. The patient returned to her gynecologist in May, 1992, where again the right adnexa was prominent on examination. An ultrasound obtained on May 6, 1992, demonstrated a normal left ovary and uterus. The right ovary was filled with a 4.4 × 4.0 cm thickened walled bilocular cyst with minimal debris. A repeat ultrasound on July 8, 1992, demonstrated again a right ovarian cyst, bilocular with debris 4.1 × 3.1 cm. A CA-125 on May 26, 1992, was 24 æ/mL (nl <35 æ/mL) and a repeat CA-125 on June 24, 1992, was 27 æ/mL.

The patient did not complain of any other symptoms and specifically denied abdominal bloating, change in bowel habits or urinary tract function. Her medical history is significant for a history of mitral valve prolapse with occasional arrhythmias. She is otherwise in good health and is not a smoker and does not drink.

The patient's family history is significant in that her mother was diagnosed with a breast cancer at age 38 and died of metastatic breast cancer at age 41. The patient's maternal grandmother is alive and well. There is no other family history of breast and/or ovarian cancer.

The general physical examination was unremarkable. On pelvic examination the cervix and uterus were normal.

The uterus was mobile and the left adnexa were normal. On rectovaginal examination the right ovary was slightly enlarged, approximately 4 to 5 cm, smooth, and mobile.

The ultrasounds were reviewed by another radiologist. The consulting radiologist was concerned that there was a possibility of some internal papillations and raised the suspicion that this right ovarian mass could be a malignancy.

The patient was counseled concerning the various treatment options available at this time. The options presented were either to proceed directly to laparotomy with either an ovarian cystectomy or oophorectomy, depending on findings at the time of surgery. The second option would be to pursue a laparoscopy and attempt cystectomy or oophorectomy through the laparoscope. The patient stated that she had completed her child-bearing plans but was worried that if she underwent a bilateral salpingo-oophorectomy that this would require estrogen replacement therapy. She expressed a concern that because of her family history of breast cancer she would like to avoid estrogen replacement therapy, if possible.

After multiple consultations, the patient opted to be treated by an infertility expert because it was his thought that this mass most likely represented endometriosis. On August 5, 1992, the patient underwent laparoscopy. The description of the ovary was that it was enlarged with no external excrescences or papillations. The surgeon then proceeded to open the cyst using a carbon dioxide laser. Immediately upon opening the cyst, there was chocolate brown fluid that was released, and there was evidence of papillary neoplasia present within the cyst. A biopsy of these papillations was obtained and sent for frozen section. The biopsy returned probable papillary serous adenocarcinoma of the ovary. The laparoscope was removed, and through a small Pfannenstiel incision the surgeon performed a right salpingo-oophorectomy and an omental biopsy. There was no obvious spread of tumor beyond the right ovary.

The pathology review demonstrated a papillary serous adenocarcinoma of the ovary confined to the ovary. The fallopian tube was negative. The omental biopsy was also negative. The grade of the tumor was interpreted as a moderately differentiated tumor (Figs. 104–1, 104–2).

The patient then returned for further consultation. Her case was presented at the Gynecologic Treatment Planning Conference. The various options discussed were to proceed to a second surgery immediately with left salpingo-oophorectomy, total abdominal hysterectomy, and complete surgical staging for ovarian carcinoma. The other option was to proceed with chemotherapy because it was the opinion of the medical oncologists that, regardless of the findings of another surgery, at this time the patient would require a course of platinum-based chemotherapy because of the grade of the tumor as well as because it was ruptured before removal.

It was decided to offer the patient a course of five cycles of cisplatin and cyclophosphamide given at 4-week intervals. The patient agreed to this, and tolerated the course of chemotherapy without significant toxicity. Postchemotherapy, the serum CA-125 remained normal. A screening mammogram was negative, as was a colonoscopy. Approximately 6 weeks after completion of her

chemotherapy, the patient underwent an exploratory laparotomy through a low transverse Mallard incision. Because of the patient's small size and thinness, there was easy access to the upper abdomen. A left salpingo-oophorectomy and total abdominal hysterectomy were performed. An infracolic omentectomy was also performed. Multiple biopsies were obtained, including pelvic and periaortic lymph nodes, and these all returned negative for residual tumor.

The patient recovered well from her second surgery and, after counseling with her physician who follows her for breast disease, opted for estrogen replacement via the estrogen patch.

COMMENTARY by J. Taylor Wharton

This 37-year-old woman had a surgically unstaged papillary serous carcinoma arising from the right ovary. A right adnexal mass was suspected in January, 1992, and the surgery was done in August, 1992. There was little if any change in the size of the mass during this interval. Endometriosis was suspected. The tumor was inspected at laparoscopy, and the surface of the involved ovary was smooth. The enlarged ovary was then incised through the laparoscope and biopsied. The frozen-section diagnosis of cancer prompted an abdominal incision, and a right salpingo-oophorectomy and omental biopsy were performed. No spread beyond the ovary was observed. The

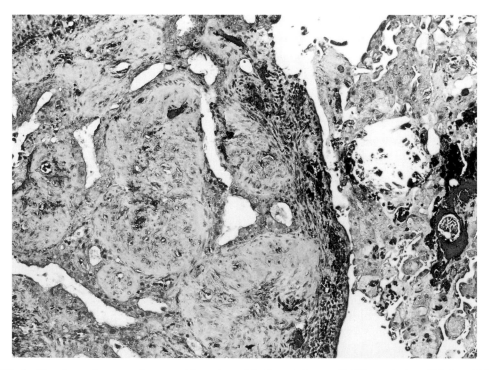

FIG. 104–1. Ovarian adenocarcinoma with endometrioid and clear cell differentiation (H&E, × 100 original magnification).

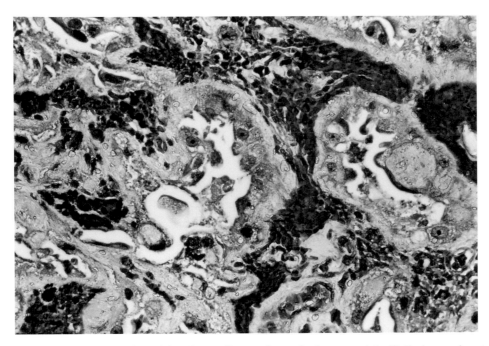

FIG. 104–2. Higher magnification of the clear cell area shows the large nuclei with their prominent nucleoli (H&E, × 400 original magnification).

pathologist stated that the tumor was moderately differentiated, which I will interpret as a histologically grade 2 cancer. The assigned FIGO stage was IA, or TNM category T1a. That stage was assigned because the operation performed did not give the necessary information for surgical staging.

The gynecologic oncologist has two therapy options. The first is to perform a laparotomy, remove the uterus and remaining tube and ovary, obtain peritoneal washings for cytology, biopsy the pelvic and aortic lymph nodes, biopsy selected peritoneal sites, obtain additional omentum, inspect the surface of the right diaphragm, and biopsy any suspicious areas. If upon this pathologic staging the lesion remains FIGO stage IA and histologic grade 2, or well or moderately differentiated, it is an acceptable option to give no further therapy. The literature supports the position that pathologically staged patients with stage IA, grade 2 lesions rarely develop recurrent disease. In contrast, patients with stage IA lesions that are histologically grade 3 or undifferentiated have a much worse prognosis, and chemotherapy has not improved survival in most studies.

The second option in the patient described is to give the patient chemotherapy. The more important reason for giving chemotherapy is inadequate staging information. It is well known that patients with suspected stage IA cancer are frequently up-staged when a comprehensive staging procedure is performed. The histologic grade in this case

or the intra-abdominal spillage of the cyst contents are less compelling reasons to give chemotherapy. If this second option were to be selected, we would give the patient carboplatin (300 mg/m^2) plus cyclophosphamide (400–600 mg/m^2) intravenously every 28 days for six courses. A laparotomy would be performed 6 weeks after completion of chemotherapy and would involve total abdominal hysterectomy and salpingo-oophorectomy plus the necessary biopsies to complete the staging procedure. The patient's therapy would be complete if all the biopsies and the remaining ovary, as well as peritoneal cytology, were negative. I concur with the therapy program completed by this patient's physicians.

SELECTED READINGS

1. Monga M, Carmichael JA, Shelley WE, et al. Surgery without adjuvant chemotherapy for early epithelial ovarian carcinoma after comprehensive surgical staging. *Gynecol Oncol* 1991;43:195–7.
2. Rubin SC, Wong GY, Curtin JP, Barakat RR, Hakes TB, Hoskins WJ. Platinum-based chemotherapy of high-risk stage I epithelial ovarian cancer following comprehensive surgical staging. *Obstet Gynecol* 1993;82:143–7.

EDITORIAL BOARD COMMENTARY

The ovarian cyst should have been removed entirely and not opened with a laser.

SECTION XXII

Prostate

105

A 67-Year-Old Man with T1c, Gleason's Grade 2 + 2 Prostate Cancer

William R. Fair

*PSA screening was particularly important in this patient
with a strong family history of prostate cancer*

CASE PRESENTATION

J.R., a 67-year-old Caucasian man, had a routine physical examination in November, 1991. The examination found him to be in overall excellent condition with the exception of an elevated prostate-specific antigen (PSA) of 6.7 ng/mL. A digital rectal examination revealed a minimally enlarged prostate consistent with the patient's age, but no discrete irregularities or prostatic nodules were palpated. The patient denied any significant urinary symptoms except nocturia once nightly, and a slight thinning of the urinary stream over a period of several years. His family history was significant in that his father died of prostatic cancer at age 86 and his 72-year-old brother had external beam radiation therapy for clinically localized prostate cancer at age 64. His brother was recently noted to have a rising PSA. A bone scan revealed multiple areas of increased uptake in the thoracic and lumbar spine consistent with metastatic disease. Similar osteoblastic lesions on the 5th, 7th, 9th, and 10th ribs were seen on bone scan and confirmed with rib films.

Based on the elevated PSA, his family physician had him return in 1 month for a repeat evaluation, including a digital rectal examination and PSA before the physical exam. On rectal examination, the prostate again was felt to be free of nodules, but a repeat PSA was 5.9 ng/mL when measured by the Hybritech method.

At this time, he was referred to Memorial Sloan-Kettering Cancer Center (MSKCC) for evaluation and possible biopsy. At our initial examination, we again confirmed a slightly enlarged but normal-feeling prostate to palpation, but with his family history and in the presence of two documented elevated PSA examinations, a transrectal ultrasound (TRUS) and bilateral needle biopsy of the prostate were performed after the patient had been administered prophylactic ciprofloxacin and a cleansing Fleet's enema. The overall prostatic volume measured 23.6 cm^3. There were small stippled calcifications found in both the right and left lobes, but most significantly, a small hypoechoic area was noted in the midline of the peripheral lobe, extending somewhat more into the left lobe than the right lobe (Fig. 105–1). Using the biopsy gun, sextent biopsies were done from six areas of the prostate as well as a direct biopsy of the hypoechoic area. The biopsy from the hypoechoic area, as well as ultrasound-directed biopsies from the two of the three sextent biopsies of the left lobe and one of the three from the right lobe, were positive for a well differentiated (Gleason 2 + 2) adenocarcinoma of the prostate.

At the time of the prostatic needle biopsy, a third PSA value was again elevated at 6.2 ng/mL and a serum acid phosphatase was in the normal range at 0.2 Sigma units (normal = 0 - 0.6 Sigma units). An extent of disease work-up consisting of a chest radiograph, bone scan, and magnetic resonance image (MRI) of the abdomen and pelvis

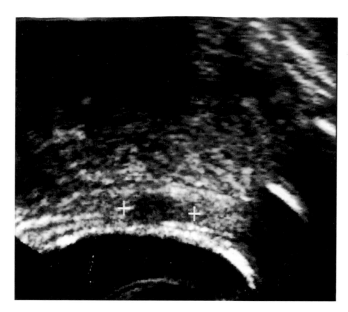

Fig. 105–1. Transrectal ultrasound of the prostate showing mid-line hypoechoic lesion in the peripheral zone.

were negative for metastatic disease. Although a patient with a well differentiated carcinoma of the prostate and a PSA below 10 would not routinely be subjected to an imaging study of the abdominal or pelvic nodes such as an MRI or computed tomography (CT) scan, in this case the MRI was ordered by the family physician with the full concurrence of the patient, who wanted to "be absolutely sure" that there were no suspicious pelvic nodes. Thus, the clinical stage of the patient was stage T1c NX M0.

The patient was again seen in our outpatient offices of the Urology Service at MSKCC for a full discussion of treatment options available. The patient expressed interest in the potential of "watchful waiting" with no immediate therapy; this approach was discussed in some detail, relying heavily on the Memorial experience in this area. The patient was told that although it is true that many patients will die *with* their disease rather than *of* their disease, this is most true in men over the age of 70, and in all cases followed with "watchful waiting" or "expectant management," tumor progression was noted, even if localized lesions did not progress to metastatic disease during the follow-up period. The option of radical prostatectomy with a bilateral pelvic lymph node dissection was also discussed in detail with the patient and his wife. At his request, an appointment was made for him to be evaluated by the Radiation Oncology Department. The final recommendation to the patient was that he had an apparently localized lesion with a low Gleason grade and that definitive therapy with either a radical prostatectomy or radiation therapy would be appropriate given his age, excellent physical condition, overall life expectancy of greater than 10 years, and his family history. When seen by the radiation therapist, he was offered the option of external beam

radiation using a three-dimensional conformal therapy technique, or interstitial implantation of [125]iodine pellets.

The patient considered the recommendations he had been given, and finally opted for a radical retropubic prostatectomy. Major factors influencing his decision were primarily his age, his overall excellent general physical condition, and his own conviction that psychologically he would prefer to know for sure the nodal status and the pathologic stage of the lesion. In addition, he expressed concern about the possibility of positive biopsies persisting after radiation therapy, and the fact that his brother had received radiation therapy only to develop metastatic disease subsequently. In March, 1992, the patient had a bilateral pelvic lymph node dissection for normal-appearing pelvic lymph nodes (frozen sections on the nodes were not done). He also had an uneventful radical retropubic prostatectomy with a bilateral nerve-sparing technique. The final pathologic stage revealed an organ-confined adenocarcinoma of the prostate that was read as moderately differentiated in both lobes: on the right Gleason 3 + 2 and on the left 3 + 3. No capsular penetration was noted, and the urethral and bladder neck margins were negative for tumor, as were the seminal vesicles and lymph nodes. He was reassured that despite the poor correlation between clinical and pathologic staging in prostate cancer and the high degree of clinical understaging that exists, it was indeed encouraging that his tumor was found to be totally organ confined within the prostatic capsule.

Postoperatively, the patient did very well. After his catheter removal 3 weeks after the surgery, he was able to stop and start his urinary stream without difficulty and experienced only stress incontinence, for which he wore a pad that required changing two to three times a day. By the end of the third month he was completely dry and has remained totally continent. After regaining his continence, the patient expressed a desire to consider some aid to potency, and he was started on the use of the vacuum erection device between the third and fourth month postoperatively. This worked satisfactorily, and by the seventh month, he was experiencing semi-erections on his own that progressed to full erections by December, 1992, at which time he stopped using the vacuum device.

His subsequent course has been uneventful. His PSA remains undetectable and the rectal examination reveals an empty prostatic fossa. Given the favorable pathology stage (pT2 N0 M0) and his subsequent course, he has been encouraged that he has a high probability of total cure of his cancer. He has enrolled his own two sons, aged 33 and 37, in our genetic epidemiology counseling service to address their own concerns about the future risk of prostate cancer.

COMMENTARY by William J. Catalona

This patient is an excellent example of the value of routine serum PSA testing in the early detection of prostate cancer; PSA testing probably saved his life. Currently, more than 80% of patients I see for treatment of prostate cancer had their cancer detected because of an elevated serum PSA concentration.

I agree completely with the management of this patient. His tumor was called stage T1c; however, according to the TNM classification, because the tumor was visible on ultrasonography, technically it would be classified as stage II.

This case was probably selected for presentation to raise discussion about the role of watchful waiting in a man approaching age 70 who has a nonpalpable, low-grade tumor. There are some who would recommend watchful waiting; however, I do not believe that we can identify with a high degree of accuracy men whose tumors are latent.

Epstein et al., in one of the most complete analyses of this issue in patients with T1c disease, developed criteria that took into account the Gleason grade, PSA density, and the extent of cancer on the biopsy specimens (1). They achieved 90% accuracy in identifying tumors that appeared to be clinically important (as defined by the histologic findings in the radical prostatectomy specimen) and about 70% accuracy in identifying tumors that appeared to be clinically unimportant. Thus, even if Epstein's criteria had predicted that Dr. Fair's patient's tumor was latent (which they would not, because the presence of cancer in four cores, including both lobes of the prostate, and the PSA density of 0.28 would be considered unfavorable parameters), there would be a 30% chance of being mistaken. In this case, the tumor was upgraded from Gleason 4 to Gleason 6 on the radical prostatectomy specimen. Thus, there is a substantial risk that in many men, watchful waiting may delay treatment until it is too late.

All available evidence indicates that prostate cancer progresses in a high percentage of men managed with watchful waiting. A recent study from Sweden also demonstrated substantial prostate cancer death rates in younger men managed with watchful waiting (2). The patient was aged 67 and healthy and therefore is likely to have 13 years or more in which to get into trouble from his prostate cancer. Moreover, his PSA value of 6.7 ng/mL also suggests that if he were treated immediately, there would be a 70% to 75% chance that his tumor would be organ-confined and curable (the corollary is that there is a 25%–30% chance that it has already spread). In fact, the

final pathology report showed that this tumor was worse than expected, and it is possible that a significant delay might have changed the ultimate outcome.

This case also illustrates the familial features of prostate cancer. The patient had two primary relatives with prostate cancer, which would increase his risk of having prostate cancer fivefold. It was appropriate to advise genetic counseling for his sons. Their risk of developing prostate cancer may be as high as 50%, and they may develop it at an earlier age. Although there are no data that bear directly on this issue, I would counsel them to begin screening with annual PSA testing and rectal examinations beginning at age 40.

The patient's father died of prostate cancer and his brother has a rising PSA and distant metastases after radiation therapy. Although there are no data to suggest that because his relatives had aggressive tumors, his tumor also will behave aggressively, I would certainly be concerned that this may be the case.

This case also shows the importance of performing systematic biopsies in men with PSA concentrations in the 4 to 10 ng/mL range despite the absence of symptoms and normal findings on rectal examination. In our studies, the chances of finding cancer in this setting are about 20%. His PSA density (0.28) also strongly suggests the need for biopsy. Finally, the hypoechoic lesion on ultrasonography is yet another strong indication.

I agree that the likelihood of metastases is low in men with PSA concentrations less than 10 ng/mL. Thus, the usual metastatic work-up such as bone scan, acid phosphatase concentration, and abdominal-pelvic MRI or CT scans are not necessary. These studies should be performed in patients with poorly differentiated tumors, because histologically documented bone metastases have been reported in some patients with PSA levels less than 10 ng/mL.

Overall, Dr. Fair's patient had an excellent outcome, being rendered tumor free while preserving potency and urinary continence.

REFERENCES

1. Epstein JI, Walsh PC, Carmichael M, Brendler CB. Pathologic and clinical findings to predict tumor extent of nonpalpable (stage T1c) prostate cancer. *JAMA* 1994;271:368–74.
2. Aus G, Hugosson J, Norlen L. Risk of dying of prostate cancer in different stages, grades and age at diagnosis. *J Urol* 1994;151:278A.

106

A 68-Year-Old Man With a Low PSA and a T2A (B1) Gleason's Grade 2 + 2 Prostate Carcinoma

Joseph P. Imperato

Radical prostatectomy versus radiotherapy in a patient with significant comorbid conditions

CASE PRESENTATION

Dr. Imperato: The patient, A.G., is a 68-year-old man who presented on a routine physical exam with an abnormal prostate exam. At that time, a prostate-specific antigen (PSA) was drawn and found to be 4.1; subsequently, on January 8, 1992, he underwent an ultrasound-guided needle biopsy. The pathology was read out as a Gleason's 2+2 adenocarcinoma of the prostate. At this point, the issue was raised as to what the different alternatives for management were. Let us start by looking at the pathology first, and then the radiologic evaluation.

Dr. Janes: We had one needle biopsy, and on microscopic exam I would call it a Gleason 2+2 (Fig. 106–1).

Dr. Imperato: The patient underwent a routine metastatic evaluation, which included a bone scan and a CT scan of the abdomen and pelvis.

Dr. Goodman: A CT scan was done of the abdomen and pelvis. The liver and retroperitoneum were negative for evidence of metastatic disease. The prostate is seen here; there are a few calcifications that are not uncommon. Prostatic calcifications are not indicative of malignant disease. The periprostatic planes are intact, and the fat planes around the prostate are distinct. There is a little deformity on the floor of the bladder, which is not unusual with benign prostatic enlargement.

Dr. Imperato: The patient's past medical history is most significant for two myocardial infarctions in the past, and he had a demand pacemaker in place. The patient has no other illnesses. There is no family history of any malignancy. The patient used to work as a lithographer. On exam, he had no peripheral lymph adenopathy. His abdomen was soft and nontender without organomegaly. His prostate exam was remarkable only for a 1.5-cm nodule in the right lower lobe of the gland. Based on my exam and the staging studies, I staged his disease as a stage II adenocarcinoma of the prostate. At this point, the issue is how to best manage this patient.

Dr. Janson: This T2 situation is probably the classic dilemma in urology. In other stages of the disease it is much easier to decide what to do. The options in most of these men is treating with radical prostatectomy, radiation therapy, or potentially even observation only. This is especially true in men who are significantly older or if their life expectancy is limited due to comorbid disease.

Dr. Cochran: What would be the major surgical option for this gentleman?

Dr. Janson: In this man I would not consider a radical prostatectomy under any circumstances.

Dr. Cochran: Is that because of his underlying cardiac disease?

Dr. Janson: He's had two myocardial infarctions, he has a pacemaker, he has a 2+2 Gleason's that is fairly nonaggressive, and he's 68 years of age. My choice in this situation is radiation, and the only question I would have

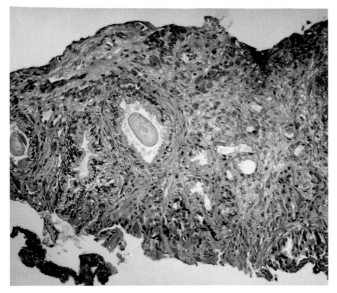 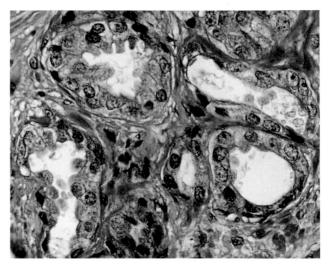

FIG. 106–1. A: Low-power view showing small neoplastic glands infiltrating the stroma between larger benign glands. **B:** Higher magnification view of neoplastic glands with enlarged nuclei and prominent nucleoli.

is whether or not he would have any benefit from a staging pelvic lymphadenectomy.

Dr. Cochran: In your experience, what has been the risk of doing a staging pelvic lymphadenectomy?

Dr. Janson: Historically, the risks of a staging pelvic lymphadenectomy have been primarily lymphocele and wound infection delaying treatment by a period of several weeks. But now that we're draining these people for 48 hours I have not seen any significant lymphoceles or wound infection.

Dr. Cochran: What's the incidence of upstaging such a patient with lymphadenectomy?

Dr. Janson: It depends upon the Gleason's scale and the clinical exam. In this situation with a Gleason's 2+2 and a tiny little nodule, the odds of having positive nodes are very low.

Dr. Imperato: I would agree. I think in this gentleman the risk of having positive nodes would certainly be less than 10%, probably about 5%. At that point you start coming into an adverse risk/benefit ratio. On the other hand, if you had a Gleason 9 or 10 or a PSA that was markedly elevated, then the likelihood of positive nodes may justify the surgery.

Dr. Ganshirt: How about laparoscopic staging?

Dr. Janson: I'm fairly familiar with the procedure and have been involved with a number of those procedures. My bias has been to choose laparotomy that takes 30 minutes over the option of doing something that may take several hours, and you get about 60% to 70% of the nodes that you would get on an open staging pelvic lymphadenectomy. The complication rate is also significantly higher with injury to bowel and ureter. I think a pelvic laparoscopic lymphadenectomy is the procedure of choice when

on CT scan you can see a node you're pretty sure has metastatic disease and you're going in to a specific target.

Dr. Imperato: One additional side benefit of the staging laparotomy is that you can clip the prostate gland. For patients who subsequently undergo radiation therapy, having the clips outline the circumference of the gland allows us to use a field that minimizes the volume of normal tissue irradiated. That's something you can't do as easily with the laparoscope.

Dr. Janes: Have you found the DNA ploidy analysis useful in predicting the stage?

Dr. Janson: Not at this time. In the urologic literature, ploidy studies are more useful as predictors of the risk of metastatic disease, but I haven't been using it at this time.

Dr. Cochran: Ken, would you review what the risks are for radical prostatectomy in terms of complications?

Dr. Janson: The basic risk of radical prostatectomy would be the high potential of impotence. We have, over the last few years, used a nerve-sparing procedure that can preserve potency.

Dr. Cochran: What about incontinence?

Dr. Janson: Incontinence had been a problem in the past. However, now that we do more anatomic operations, I haven't seen incontinence as a major problem. The biggest technical hassle can be bladder neck strictures, but this is only a problem for a few months, not long-term.

Dr. Cochran: Dr. Imperato, what happened to this patient?

Dr. Imperato: Due to the patient's medical history, he was referred for radiation therapy. His Gleason grade and stage made the likelihood of his having pelvic lymph nodes extremely low and, therefore, I treated this patient to the prostate only with an arc wedge technique on our 10-MV linear accelerator. He was given 6,660 rads over $7\frac{1}{2}$ weeks, which he tolerated well. He had the usual side effects of urinary frequency and burning toward the end of treatment and some mild diarrhea which was controlled with Lomotil. Both resolved within 2 weeks of treatment. The two major risks we are concerned about are permanent proctitis, which occurs less than 5% of the time; and permanent cystitis, which occurs less than 1% of the time. Impotence can also occur—the incidence is about 50% over 5 years; however, in patients treated with smaller fields the incidence may be less. Follow-up in these patients is accomplished with the digital rectal exam and PSA.

The patient was scheduled for his routine 6-week follow-up after completing radiation; however, on a routine visit to his internist for an unrelated reason, he had an arrhythmia in the office and died, despite attempts at resuscitation.

Obviously, in retrospect, this is one of those cases where observation would have been a real consideration. It points out how difficult these cases can be since you have a number of alternatives ranging from very radical to palliative. In patients with severe comorbid disease who are at risk of dying within the near future, simple observation or treatment with hormones is certainly to be considered; however, our selection criteria are not perfect. In the future, other tests, such as ploidy analysis, may allow us to further define our population so that we will better know who needs treatment and who can be observed.

COMMENTARY by Jeffrey M. Ignatoff

Few areas of urologic oncology have generated more controversy than the management of localized prostatic carcinoma. Case A.G. illustrates a frequent dilemma facing clinicians who manage this malignancy. Decisions such as how—or even whether—to treat stage T2 carcinoma should be predicated on an understanding of the variable natural history of this disease, one which is common in a patient population subject to mortality from frequent comorbid conditions. Delayed therapy, therefore, may be an appropriate alternative for some patients. Johansson et al. found a relative 5- and 10-year survival of 98.8% and 92.7%, respectively, for patients with lower-grade localized prostatic carcinoma treated by observation and delayed hormonal therapy, and/or transurethral resection when symptomatic (1). Patients of younger age, however, and particularly those with higher-grade tumors, are at greater risk to develop distant metastases and experience the morbidity of local tumor extension.

When a decision is made to treat aggressively localized prostatic carcinoma with curative intent, considerable controversy exists as to the respective roles of radical prostatectomy and radiation therapy. Current treatment recommendations are generally based on uncontrolled retrospective data and individual practitioner experience and training. The only randomized prospective trial comparing radical prostatectomy and radiation therapy demonstrated a shorter interval to recurrence or metastasis in the radiation treated group (2). A number of methodologic criticisms, however, have been raised to question the validity of this conclusion (3). It seems unlikely that a prospective controlled study will be completed in the near future to answer this question.

Failing this answer, several clinical observations can serve as a basis for rational decision making in the selection of surgery or radiation therapy for patients in whom curative efforts are deemed appropriate. The NIH consensus panel on prostate cancer concluded in 1987 that radical prostatectomy and radiation therapy have equivalent 10-year survival rates for patients with localized prostate cancer; there was not sufficient data to carry this observation to 15 years—a pertinent interval for younger or healthier patients with prostate cancer (4). Furthermore, a number of reported series have demonstrated a high rate of tumor persistence on rebiopsy—generally over 50%—in patients undergoing radiation therapy with curative intent (5). Individuals presenting with stage T2A tumors have been classically described as ideal candidates for radical prostatectomy. Ninety percent of these patients will have pathologically confined carcinoma, and less than 10% will have lymphatic metastasis. Radical prostatectomy has produced a disease-specific 15-year survival rate of about 85% (6).

The preceding factors have directed, for many clinicians, an approach wherein patients having an actuarial survival in excess of 10 to 15 years are optimally treated by radical prostatectomy. Radiation therapy deserves serious consideration in situations where curative therapy is appropriate, but anticipated actuarial survival is less than 10 to 15 years due to age or comorbid conditions.

The setting in this case is a clear illustration of a clinically confined prostatic malignancy in an individual with significant coronary disease. The findings of a T2A lesion, a low histologic grade, and virtually normal PSA, all argue against the likelihood of metastasis, as do the results of skeletal and CT scans. This author, in fact, has stopped using CT scans as a metastatic staging modality in low-probability settings, although the CT scan can be very useful as a localization study in patients for whom radiation therapy is planned. Further, some have argued that isotope bone scanning is not necessary in many patients with lower-grade tumors and PSA levels less than 10 ng (7); however, it remains my practice to obtain a baseline bone scan in virtually all prostate cancer staging evaluations.

With respect to the decision to omit pelvic lymph node staging, I fully concur that, given all the clinical findings of this case, the probability of lymph node metastasis is well under 10%, and justifies omitting lymphadenectomy. My preference in some surgical candidates, in fact, is to proceed to radical perineal prostatectomy without pelvic node staging in the face of organ-confined tumors of Gleason grade 6 or less, and PSA levels under 10 ng.

In the case presented, my approach would have been identical to that undertaken, and the alternative of serial observation alone would have been discussed as well. One could not foresee the unfortunate early demise of this patient shortly after therapy; however, this emphasizes the very reason why enthusiasm for aggressive therapy must be tempered in the face of competing causes of mortality. Whether or not A.G. would have elected curative therapy, it was appropriate not to seriously consider surgical extirpation as an option in this setting.

REFERENCES

1. Johansson JE, Andersson SO, Krusemo U, Adami H, Bergstrom R, Kraaz W. Natural history of localized prostatic cancer. *Lancet* 1989;I: 799–803.
2. Paulson DR. Randomized series of treatment with surgery versus radiation for prostate adenocarcinoma. *J Urol* 1979;7:127–31.
3. Hanks GE. External beam radiation therapy for clinically localized prostate cancer: Patterns of care studies in the United States. *NCI Monogr* 1988;7:75–85.
4. Grayhack JJ. The management of clinically localized prostate cancer: National Institute of Health Consensus Development Conference. *J Urol* 1987;138:1369–75.
5. Kabalin JN, Hodge KK, McNeal JE, Freiha F, Stamey T. Identification of residual cancer in the prostate following radiation therapy: role of transrectal ultrasound-guided biopsy and prostate specific antigen. *J Urol* 1989;142:326–31.
6. Lepor H, Kimball AW, Walsh PC. Cause specific actuarial survival analysis: a useful method for reporting survival data in men with clinically localized carcinoma of the prostate. *J Urol* 1989;141:82–4.
7. Oesterling JE, Martin S, Bergstralh E, Lowe FC. The use of prostate specific antigen in staging patients with newly diagnosed prostate cancer. *JAMA* 1993;269:57–60.

107

Cancer of the Prostate - T2b, Gleason's Grade 3 + 3, PSA of 14

James W. Keller and Lawrence W. Davis

*The impact of radical prostatectomy or radiation therapy
on potency*

CASE PRESENTATION

The patient is a 55-year-old man with a long-standing history of prostatic hypertrophy. He had a syncopal episode in 1985 with bradycardia which required hospital admission for suspected cardiac arrhythmia; no cause was found. However, his prostate was noted to be enlarged and he underwent a biopsy which was benign. In 1987 another biopsy was performed and again interpreted as benign. He was seen by another urologist recently who noted an enlarged prostate with a nodule about 1 cm in size in the midline. Repeat biopsy this time was interpreted as adenocarcinoma, Gleason 6/10. Bone scan was negative as was CT scan of the abdomen and pelvis. Currently the patient experiences nocturia twice per night, but a good urinary stream. Sexual function was intact.

Past Medical History:

Surgery: Appendectomy - Age 12
Removal of benign growth from ear, 1978
Medical: Evaluation for hoarseness by ENT in the recent past revealed a white patch on the anterior portion of left vocal cord; evaluation to be completed.
Medication: None
Allergies: None known
Family History: Father died of colon cancer at age 48. Brother died of cancer, unknown site.
Review of Systems: Patient smokes 2-3 packs of cigarettes per day. There is a history of hypertension, but the patient takes no medication.

Physical Examination: Weight 240 pounds, BP 170/110, P 80, regular. He was noticeably hoarse. Indirect laryngoscopy was unremarkable except for edematous cords.

Breath sounds were decreased. DRE revealed a gland approximately 4 cm in transverse diameter with a 1 cm nodule at the apex of the gland. Because of his size, the base of the gland and seminal vesicles could not be evaluated adequately.

Staging: Review of recent chest x-ray was negative and CT of the abdomen/pelvis did not reveal any adenopathy or capsular extension. Transrectal ultrasound confirmed a hypoechoic area at the apex of the gland measuring 1.5 cm in greatest diameter. There was no suspicion of involvement of the seminal vesicles with either the CT scan or ultrasound. PSA was 14. PAP was 2.6. CBC and SMA-12 were normal.

The patient was considered to have disease confined to the prostate but occupying both lobes and therefore stage B2 or T2b.

There was discussion regarding the treatment options which included surgery (radical retropubic prostatectomy) or radiation. Since the patient's PSA was >10 it was noted that he had approximately a 25% chance of disease not being localized; with a Gleason score of 6/10 he had a 15%-25% chance of lymph node spread. Generally patients with stage B2 disease have a higher incidence of unfavorable features at the time of surgical resection, namely lymph node spread, positive surgical margins, capsular penetration, or seminal vesicle invasion. However, it was stressed that within stage B2 there exists a spectrum of disease activity in the midline, but into both lobes, and this could be more favorable than disease that infiltrated both lobes extensively. Because of this, some of the urologists believed he could still be a good surgical candidate, but they would proceed with laporascopic pelvic lymph node sampling prior to any final recommendation.

Radiation was strongly favored by the patient with the belief that he would have a higher chance of retaining sexual activity. It was conceded that normally patients with stage B2 disease may have a lower chance for sexual activity since a thorough dissection bilaterally is necessary, but this might not be the case for this patient. The radiation oncologists were divided on whether they would treat the pelvic nodes with the prostate or just the prostate alone. There was some discussion about the use of adjuvant hormonal therapy, namely LHRH agonist + antiandrogen, before, during, and after the radiation. It was believed that the final information on the impact of this strategy on overall survival versus sequential radiation followed by hormonal therapy at the time of relapse was not available.

The patient elected to proceed with radiation.

TREATMENT:

The patient was treated to a large pelvic field using a 4 field box technique which included the prostate, seminal vesicles, obturator, and iliac nodes to a dose of 4500 cGy in 180 cGy fractions. The field was then reduced to include only the prostate gland with a 2 cm margin to a dose of 2200 cGy in 200 cGy fractions. The final dose to the prostate was 6700 cGy in 36 fractions over 51 days.

The patient tolerated the treatment well with only mild diarrhea, which was well controlled with Lomotil. At the completion of therapy the gland was flatter and softer; the nodule was smaller but still present.

When seen in follow-up at one month he was doing well. In the interim he was seen by his internist and started on medication for his hypertension. He was also seen in ENT consultation and biopsy of the vocal cords did not reveal any malignancy. His PSA was 6.7. Sexual function was still intact.

At 8 months his PSA was 2.1 and he was doing well. The prostate was flat without nodularity.

COMMENTARY by W. Bedford Waters

The case presented is a 55-year-old male with newly diagnosed prostate cancer. The patient had two previous negative prostate needle biopsies for cancer. The digital rectal examination (DRE) was positive for a 1 cm nodule at the apex. The prostate specific antigen (PSA) was 14. Transrectal ultrasound (TRUS) revealed a hypoechoic area that corresponded to the nodule felt on DRE. The

metastatic workup was negative. The options of radical prostatectomy and external beam radiation were offered to the patient as treatment alternatives. The patient elected to proceed with radiation therapy, primarily because of his concerns of maintaining potency. The patient received 6700 cGy with minimal complications. At 8 months after therapy the PSA was 2.1, the prostate was flat without nodularity, and potency was maintained.

It is estimated that 165,000 new cases of prostate cancer will be diagnosed in 1993 with 35,000 deaths. The early detection of prostate cancer while it is still organ confined is receiving increasing emphasis. The American Cancer Society and The American Urological Association now recommend that men over the age of 50 undergo a DRE and PSA on an annual basis to improve the early detection of prostate cancer. The early detection program should begin at age 40 if there is a family history of prostate cancer or if the person is African-American because of the higher incidence in these two populations. There is a lot of controversy about the use of PSA in the early detection of prostate cancer. Much of this controversy is due to the lack of any randomized, prospective studies demonstrating a reduction in disease-specific mortality as a result of prostate cancer screening using any method. While screening studies employing DRE, PSA, and TRUS have in some cases demonstrated an increased detection of localized tumors and improved survival (1–7), this does not necessarily guarantee a reduction in cancer deaths. Reasons for this include several potential errors such as lead and length time bias (8), which can occur in uncontrolled trials leading to incorrect conclusions. The upper age limit for routine screening or early detection has not been established, however, there is increasing evidence that the disease specific survival for patients with untreated low stage, low grade prostate cancer is excellent at 10 years.(9,10) Therefore, in most cases, screening and treatment of patients with clinically organ confined disease, should be limited to patients with at least a 10-year life expectancy (11).

The PSA level may be useful in determining the need for additional diagnostic studies, i.e. bone scans, CT, or surgical staging of the pelvic lymph nodes, and it may impact on the choice of treatment . Oesterling et al.(12) reported that only 3 of 561 (0.5%) patients with newly diagnosed prostate cancer and a PSA less than 10.0 ng/mL had positive bone scans for metastatic disease, with one additional patient having an indeterminate scan. In addition, none of 467 men with a PSA level less than 8.0 ng/mL had an abnormal bone scan. Based on these results, the authors recommend that those patients with newly diagnosed prostate cancer, no skeletal symptoms, and a PSA level of 10.0 ng/mL or less not undergo a staging bone scan. This would lead to a significant savings to the health care system. PSA has been used to predict nodal status and to evaluate the risk of local extracapsular extension into the periprostatic tissues (13–21). There is considerable overlap among groups which reduces the predictive value for individual patients. These reports suggest that the combination of PSA, tumor grade, and tumor stage may be very helpful in predicting the presence of metastatic disease to the pelvic lymph nodes and to help counsel patients considering radical prostatectomy regarding the relative risk of extracapsular disease spread, positive surgical margins, and the resultant need for further postoperative adjuvant therapy such as external radiation or hormonal therapy.

The most appropriate treatment for the patient with clinically localized prostate cancer continues to be hotly debated. Thus far, no published randomized trial has proven the efficacy of no therapy versus surgery, radiation therapy, or hormonal therapy in equivalent patient populations. However, if the patient has a ten-year life expectancy and is under 70 years of age, then external beam radiation therapy or radical prostatectomy is offered to the patient. Other than age, results of treatment which affect quality of life must be considered. The patient for whom sexual potency or fertility are extremely important and are unlikely to be preserved may be better served by other therapies. The technique of radical prostatectomy has been modified by Walsh and others (22). This has resulted in less blood loss, improved continence, and preservation of sexual potency in many patients. Radical prostatectomy appears to provide the most effective local control of prostate cancer due to the recent proven high persistence of tumor after radiation therapy. The risk of local failure following external beam radiation therapy increases with increasing tumor stage and length of followup. Up to 12% of patients with T1b (A2); 29% of T2 (B), and 35% of patients with T3 will have clinical evidence of regrowth from 5 to 15 years following radiation therapy (23–34). However, the results with radiation therapy in patients having early tumors compare favorably with the early outcome results of the John Hopkins surgical series when adjusted for tumor stage and the absence of surgically-proven pelvic lymph nodal metastases (35). The significance of postradiation PSA values is less clear compared with patients after radical prostatectomy. It is uncommon for PSA levels to become undetectable, and rising PSA levels after radiation therapy generally indicate the presence of disease progression that is often metastatic (17, 36–38). The treatment of organ confined prostate cancer is controversial and continues to evolve as more clinical and pathological data are analyzed.

REFERENCES

1. Gerber GS. Prostate specific antigen. *Principles and Practice of Oncology Updates* 1993;7(10):1–8.
2. Catalona WJ, Smith DS, Ratliff TL, et al. Measurement of prostate specific antigen in serum as a screening test for prostate cancer. *New Engl J Med* 1991;324:1156.
3. Dalton, DL. Elevated serum prostate-specific antigen due to acute bacterial prostatitis, *Urology* 1989;33:465.
4. Yuan, JJJ, Coplen DE, Petros JA, et al. Effects of rectal examination, prostatic massage, ultrasonography, and needle biopsy on serum prostate specific antigen levels. *J Urol* 1992;147:810.
5. Gilbertson VA. Cancer of the prostate gland. Results of early diagnosis and therapy undertaken for cure of the disease. *JAMA* 1976;215:81.
6. Jenson CB, Shahon DB, Wangensteen OH. Evaluation of annual examinations in the detection of cancer. Special reference to cancer of the gastrointestinal tract, prostate, breast and female reproductive tract. *JAMA* 1960;174:1783.
7. Cooner WH, Mosley BR, Rutherford CL, Jr., et al. Prostate cancer detection in a clinical urological practice by ultrasonography, digital rectal examination and prostate-specific antigen. *J Urol* 1990;143:1146.
8. Love RR, Camilli AE. The value of screening. *Cancer* 1981;48:489.
9. Johansson JE, Adami HO, Anderson SW, et al. High 10-year survival rate in patients with early, untreated prostatic cancer. *JAMA* 1992;267:2191.
10. Chodak GW, Thisted R, Gerber GS, et al. Multi-variate analysis of outcome following observation/delayed therapy of clinically localized prostate cancer. *J Urol* 1993;149:396A.
11. Walsh PC. Why make an early diagnosis of prostate cancer. *J Urol* 1992;147:853.
12. Oesterling JE, Martin SK, Bergstralh EJ, Lowe FC. The use of prostate specific antigen in staging patients with newly diagnosed prostate cancer. *JAMA* 1993;269:57.
13. Stamey TA, Kabalin JN. Prostate specific antigen in the diagnosis and treatment of adenocarcinoma of the prostate. I. Untreated patients. *J Urol* 1989;141:1070.
14. Stamey TA, Kabalin JN, McNeal JE, et al. Prostate-specific antigen in the diagnosis and treatment of adenocarcinoma of the prostate. II. Radical prostatectomy-treated patients. *J Urol* 1989;141:1076.
15. Gerber GS, Rukstalis DB, Chodak GW. Correlation of prostate-specific antigen and tumor grade with nodal status in men with clinically localized prostate cancer. *J Urol* 1993;149:448A.
16. Lange PH, Ercole CJ, Lightner DJ, et al. The value of serum prostate-specific antigen determinations before and after radical prostatectomy. *J Urol* 1989;141:873.
17. Hudson MA, Bahnson RR. Catalona WJ. Clinical use of prostate-specific antigen in patients with prostate cancer. *J Urol* 1989;142:1011.
18. Partin AW, Carter HB, Chan DW, et al. Prostate-specific antigen in the staging of localized prostate cancer: Influence of tumor differentiation, tumor volume, and benign hyperplasia. *J Urol* 1990;143:747.
19. Oesterling JE, Chan DW, Epstein JL, et al. Prostate-specific antigen in the preoperative and postoperative evaluation of localized prostatic cancer treated with radical prostatectomy. *J Urol* 1988;139:766.
20. Kleer E, Larson-Keller JJ, Zincke H, Oesterling JE. Ability of preoperative serum prostate-specific antigen value to predict pathological stage and DNA ploidy. *Urology* 1993;41:207.
21. Rukstalis DB, Bales GB, Gerber GS, Chodak GW. Radical perineal prostatectomy as monotherapy for localized prostatic cancer. *J Urol* 1993;149:380A.
22. Walsh PC. Radical prostatectomy, preservation of sexual function, cancer control. *Urol Clinic No Amer* 1987;14:663.
23. Bagshaw MA, Cox RS, Ray GR. Status of radiation treatment of prostate cancer at Stanford University. *Nat Cancer Inst Monogr* 1988;7:47–60.
24. Hanks GE, Diamond JJ, Krall JM, et al. A ten year followup of 682 patients treated for prostate cancer with radiation therapy in the United States. *Int J Radiat Oncol Biol Phys* 1987;13:499–505.
25. Personal communication, Dr. James D. Cox, Chairman, RTOG from patients not receiving any elective endocrine therapy on protocol 75–6 and 77–6.
26. Perez CA, Pilepich MV, Garcia D et al. Definitive radiation therapy in carcinoma of the prostate localized to the pelvis: experience at the Mallinckrodt Institute of Radiology. *Nat Cancer Inst Monog* 1988;7:85–94.
27. Kuban DA, El-Mahdi AM, Schellhammer PF. 1-125 interstitial implantation for prostate cancer: what have we learned 10 years later? *Cancer* 1989;63:2415.
28. Kaplan ID, Prestige BR, Bagshaw MA, et al. The importance of local

control in the treatment of prostatic cancer. *J Urol* March 1992 (in press).

29. Zagars GK, Von Eschenbach AC, Johnson DE, et al. The role of radiation therapy in stages A2 and B carcinoma of the prostate. *Int J Radiat Oncol Biol Phys* 1988;14:701–9.

30. Shipley WU, Prout GR Jr., Coachman NM, et al. Radiation therapy for localized prostatic carcinoma: the experience at the Massachusetts General Hospital (1973-1981). *NCSI Monogr* 1988;7:67–74.

31. Hanks GE, Asbell SO, Krall JM et al. Outcome for lymph node dissection negative T-lb, T-2 (A-2, B) prostate cancer treated with external beam radiation therapy in RTOG 77-06. *Int J Radiat Oncol Biol Phys* (in press).

32. Zagars GK, Von Eschenbach AC, Johnson DE, et al. Stage C adenocarcinoma of the prostate. An analysis of 551 patients treated with external beam radiation. *Cancer* 1987;60:1489–99.

33. Zagars GK, Johnson DE, Von Eschenbach AC, et al. Adjuvant estrogen following radiation therapy for stage C adenocarcinoma of the prostate: Long term results of a prospective randomized study. *Int J Radiat Oncol Biol Phys* 1988;14:1085–91.

34. Dugan TC, Verhey LJ, Shipley WU, et al. Post-irradiation biopsy of the prostate in stage T3 prostatic cancer: correlation with original histologic grade and with current PSA values. *Int J Radiat Oncol Biol Phys* 1990;19(1):198–9.

35. Morton RA, Steiner MS, Walsh PC. Cancer control following anatomical radical prostatectomy: Interim report. *J Urol* 1991;145:1197–200.

36. Stamey TA, Kabalin JN, Ferrari M. Prostate-specific antigen in the diagnosis and treatment of adenocarcinoma of the prostate, III. Radiation treated patients. *J Urol* 1989;141:1084.

37. Kaplan ID, Cox RS, Bagshaw MA. Prostate-specific antigen after external beam radiotherapy for prostatic cancer: Follow-up. *J Urol* 1993;149:519.

38. Kaplan ID, Prestidge BR, Cox RS, Bagshaw MA. Prostate specific antigen after irradiation for prostatic carcinoma. *J Urol* 1990;144:1172.

108

Prostate Cancer: Radical Prostatectomy for B1 Disease Management?

Seymour H. Levitt and G. Philip Engeler

Risk assessment for persistent disease following radical prostatectomy and the evolving role of adjuvant radiotherapy

CASE PRESENTATION

R.R. is a 65-year-old white man who had a normal physical exam in January, 1989. He was approaching retirement and made contact with an internist in Florida in March of the same year, and another physical exam was performed. On digital rectal exam, a suspicious area in the left lobe of the prostate was discovered. A prostate specific antigen (PSA) was performed demonstrating an elevated value of 10 (normal 0–3.9). He returned to Minneapolis, Minnesota, and examination confirmed the previous findings. A transrectal prostatic ultrasound (Fig. 108–1) demonstrated on the left side of the prostate in the peripheral zone an area of decreased echogenicity. This was most prominent at the levels of the base and mid-gland. Seminal vesicles appeared normal. The suspicious area was biopsied and revealed adenocarcinoma, Gleason grade III-IV (Fig. 108–2). Additional evaluation included a bone scan that showed a small area of increased uptake in the left hip, thought likely secondary to degenerative changes; a chest roentgenogram that showed mild increase in pulmonary vasculature and slightly enlarged cardiac silhouette; and an EKG that showed left axis deviation and normal sinus rhythm. Review of systems revealed no history of bone pain, bladder outlet obstructive symptoms, dysuria, or hematuria. Past medical history was remarkable for an appendectomy 9 years ago, bilateral pulmonary infiltrates status postbiopsy with diagnosis of interstitial pneumoni-

tis, and a history of podagra. His medications were allopurinol, an aspirin a day, and a daily multivitamin. A family history of a brother with laryngeal carcinoma was noted. The patient was a practicing lawyer in the Twin Cities, married with three healthy sons.

His clinical stage was B1 (T2 N0 M0) adenocarcinoma of the prostate, and a decision for treatment with radical

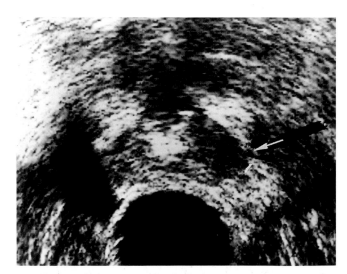

FIG. 108–1. Transrectal ultrasound; arrow demonstrates hypoechoic area in the left peripheral zone of the prostate, suspicious for malignancy.

536

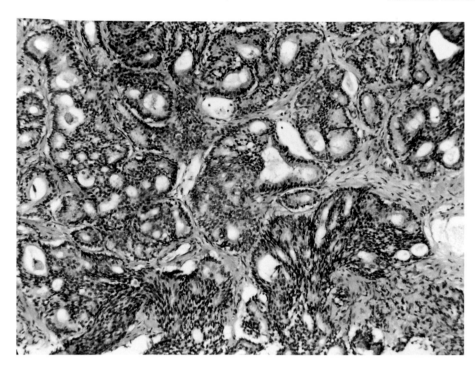

FIG. 108–2. Photomicrograph of biopsy specimen showing extensive infiltration of prostate gland by malignant glandular proliferation. (Hematoxylin and eosin × 120).

prostatectomy was made. On April 6, 1989, a radical prostatectomy and pelvic lymph node dissection were performed without circumstance. The pathologic specimen (Fig. 108–3) revealed Gleason's grade III-IV adenocarcinoma involving the left inferior posterior, left inferior posterior lateral, superior anterior, and left superior posterior lateral portions of the gland. The tumor extended into the periprostatic adipose tissue in the left superior posterior lateral aspect of the gland, and extended to the resection margins designated left inferior posterior, left inferior posterior lateral, and left superior posterior lateral. The seminal vesicles, bladder neck, and sections of 21 pelvic lymph nodes contained no evidence of tumor.

Postoperatively the patient did well, though he developed nocturia once or twice nightly and became impotent. A postoperative PSA, measured June 5, 1989, was 0.2. Despite the low PSA, a number of factors led to the decision to offer external beam radiation therapy, including high-grade, deep-lobe involvement and positive margins. His exam at the time (July 3, 1989) of radiation oncology consultation revealed no evidence of any gross residual disease on digital rectal exam. Review of systems showed that the patient was having nocturia once or twice nightly and impotence. A CT scan of the abdomen and pelvis (Fig. 108–4) obtained July 5, 1989, showed postoperative changes in the pelvis, no evidence of lymphadenopathy in the pelvic or para-aortic nodes, and some residual prostatic tissue at the gland apex. Soft tissue planes were preserved around the rectum with no evidence of tumor invasion.

The patient received external beam radiation to the prostate bed and pelvic nodes using a 19 × 17 cm field size,

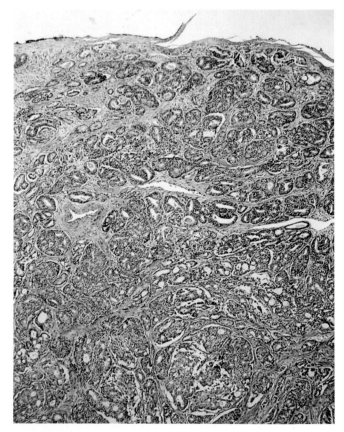

FIG. 108–3. Photomicrograph of prostatectomy specimen showing tumor extension to the inked resection margin. (Hematoxylstin and eosin × 48).

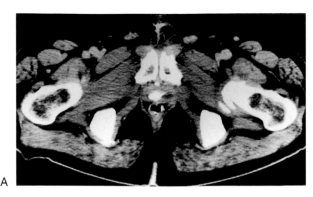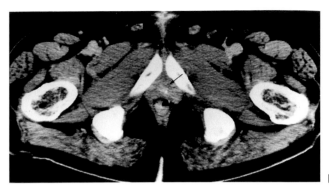

FIG. 108–4. A,B: Computed tomography scans at level of base of prostatic bed showing some residual soft tissue signal consistent with residual prostatic tissue *(arrow)*.

anterior posterior fields, and 18 MV. A total of 4,500 cGy was delivered to this field. A boost field was delivered to the prostate bed with anterior, right and left lateral fields for an additional 1,620 cGy, for a total dose to the prostate bed of 6,120 cGy. The radiation was delivered between July 6 and August 23, 1989. Radiation therapy was well tolerated except for mild diarrhea and a small patch of wet skin desquamation in the gluteal area. Both side effects were well managed with conservative measures and resolved shortly after treatments were completed.

The patient has been followed routinely and has done well. His impotence was addressed initially with a external vacuum suction device, but he was unhappy with the results. In June, 1992, he underwent placement of a Diaflex penile prosthesis.

He was doing well at his most recent date of follow-up in July, 1994. His PSA was at 0.2; digital rectal exam showed an empty prostatic vault; and his prosthesis was functioning well.

COMMENTARY by Paul H. Lange

By 1989 standards, this case was handled well and reflects established care of the time. Today, however, it would probably be handled somewhat differently, both pre- and posttherapy.

Before therapy, today six-sector core biopsies of the prostate would be obtained in order to get a better idea of tumor volume and its status on the other side. These factors are important to consider particularly if a nerve-sparing radical prostatectomy is contemplated. I have no argument with the performance of the radical prostatectomy. Of course, primary radiotherapy also was an option and the choice between the two has been, and still is, very controversial. We still do not have a randomized study that everyone will accept. Currently, the best way to compare the results of these two therapies is using multiple preoperative risk factors, with PSA being the most important, and 5-year posttherapy PSA results as the best surrogate

endpoint. We have fairly mature data for radical prostatectomy using these parameters, but we do not yet have reliable data for primary radiotherapy. What data are available for comparison suggests to me that radical prostatectomy is better at producing a 5-year PSA "negative" result, though admittedly the outcomes currently seem close enough to claim both therapies equally effective. However, one prevailing advantage of radical prostatectomy is that effective adjuvant radiotherapy is possible; and, of course, was done in this case.

Parenthetically, I do not believe that a "watch and wait" approach for this patient would have been acceptable to most experts, either before or after the diagnosis. This man has a life expectancy of more than 15 years, and it would appear that the DRE and biopsy results suggest that the tumor was of a volume considered to be potentially lethal (i.e., >1 cm), and finally, the preoperative PSA value is of a level that portends serious disease.

The radical prostatectomy appears to have gone well. I presume that a nerve-sparing approach was not done. This is significant because nerve-sparing surgery does increase the possibility that the positive margins are iatrogenic. I also presume that the lymphadenectomy was "modified"; that is, lymphatic tissue lateral to the external iliac artery was preserved. This is important because if adjuvant radiotherapy is given, leg edema is much less if a modified lymphadenectomy is performed. The major question in this case today is what is the best management for a patient after radical prostatectomy who presumably has positive margins. This issue is complicated and involves two major factors: Are the margins truly positive, and if so, what is the best therapy?

There are many different methods for determining pathologically from the radical prostatectomy specimen the extent of disease and consequently, the chances of persistent disease; but there is still no consensus on the definitions. Yet a consensus will soon evolve: (1) because pathologists are slowly beginning to agree on parameters (e.g., volume, grade, margins) and on the methods of measuring them; and, (2) 5-year postoperative PSA values are a very good surrogate endpoint for persistent disease after radical prostatectomy because the hazard rate after 5 years for patients with undetectable PSAs is almost negligible.

What can be said today is that involvement of the pelvic lymph nodes is almost a sure sign of persistent (usually systemic) disease; involvement of the seminal vesicles has a greater than 75% chance of portending persistent disease; however, the extent of seminal vesicle involvement is an important although still poorly defined factor. Positive margins are of course important but still a "mixed bag" because approximately 50% of men with positive margins seem to be cured, and this is most true if the margins involve primarily the prostate apex. The importance of tumor volume as an independent prognostic variable for persistent disease is controversial. Thus, until the positive margin and tumor margin controversies are settled, I believe one must individualize postoperative risk assessment, usually after careful discussion with a pathologist.

So, what should the therapy be in cases where the postradical prostatectomy is said to have pathologic risk factors for persistent disease? Of course, the choices are expectant management, androgen ablation therapy, or adjuvant radiotherapy. Androgen ablation therapy is not curative. It is also uncertain whether its application is better "early" or only after the onset of symptoms; I believe early therapy does improve the quality and probably quantity of life, if potency is not an issue for the patient. Today this question is somewhat moot because few patients are willing to "watch" their PSA continually rise without intervention. Adjuvant radiotherapy is well tolerated if a modified lymphadenectomy was done, the patient is continent, the incision is well healed, and there is no identified or impending bladder neck contracture. However, the question is whether adjuvant radiotherapy is effective.

There are many experts, particularly in the urologic community, who are disillusioned with the therapeutic results of adjuvant radiotherapy. The reasons can be summarized as follows:

1. All the adjuvant radiotherapy series are uncontrolled. What good data does exist taken together suggests that as a group adjuvant radiotherapy decreases local recurrence but does not affect cancer survival. The SWOG/ECOG randomized study of adjuvant therapy is many years from completion. Until the study is completed, posttherapy PSA levels are the best parameters we have to elucidate the effects of adjuvant radiotherapy. Postoperative PSA levels should be undetectable if all prostate tissue, either malignant or benign, has been removed. In 1989, a PSA level of 0.2 ng/mL was considered "undetectable." However, today using more sensitive assays, a level greater than 0.1 usually means persistent disease, although a rising level is a better indicator.

2. Almost all persistent disease after radical prostatectomy is portended by rising PSA levels. If the PSA level is clearly elevated and/or rising after radical prostatectomy, approximately 30%–50% will have prostate cancer detected on a biopsy of the prostatic fossa. Usually this occurs despite an "unimpressive" DRE. In about 20% of cases, these biopsies are only positive after the second or third biopsy of the fossa. Rarely do the biopsies consistently reveal only BPH, presumably because a "button" of normal prostate was left behind at the apex by the surgeon (the CT scan in this case shows a persistent apex, which is a curious finding that could possibly be validated by cystoscopy). Thus, the somewhat surprising postoperative biopsy results might be used to argue in favor of "early" adjuvant radiotherapy, but they also jeopardize the "old" local adjuvant therapy results: Indeed, more than 25% of patients who receive adjuvant radiotherapy and have elevated PSA levels subsequently have prostatic fossa biopsies that are positive even though the DREs remain "unimpressive."

3. In patients who have decreased PSA levels and have adjuvant radiotherapy, the PSA levels decrease dramatically in most (about 80%) and to undetectable levels in about 50%. However, this PSA suppression is not durable; less than 20% of patients overall have "durable" undetectable PSA levels. These facts of course could either mean that the disease has already extended beyond the radiation ports or, more likely, that in many cases the disease is primarily or completely localized, but radiotherapy as currently given is ineffective. These aforementioned facts have led some urologists to abandon adjuvant radiotherapy altogether or to give it only if the postoperative PSA levels are unequivocally elevated.

4. Recently, additional facts about postoperative PSA have come to light. For example, if the postoperative PSA levels do not decrease to undetectable levels, systemic disease is usually soon discovered. Also, in these patients, adjuvant radiotherapy rarely results in a permanent PSA suppression. If the PSA does initially descend to undetectable levels but then rises, if the doubling time is "slow" (e.g., >10 months), the disease seems usually to be local only, whereas if the doubling time is "fast" (<3 months), the disease is usually systemic.

In light of these facts (and until more is known), I believe the physician can formulate a management plan for the postoperative radical prostatectomy at risk who otherwise has a good surgical result. If the postoperative PSA levels do not become undetectable (the half-life of PSA is about 3 days), adjuvant radiotherapy is not usually indicated and I would recommend androgen ablation therapy, unless potency is an overriding issue. If the PSA levels are initially undetectable, I would wait until a PSA rise occurs, unless the pathology results and/or the surgeon's intraoperative knowledge strongly suggests a high likelihood of persistent disease, in which case, adjuvant radiotherapy would be my choice. If a "watch and wait" approach is chosen, if the PSA does become detectable and rises slowly (and especially if it begins to rise after the first year), I would recommend adjuvant radiotherapy without a biopsy of the prostatic fossa because the disease in this case is usually local, and prostatic fossa biopsies are initially falsely positive about 20% of the time. However, if the PSA level rises early and/or faster, I would probably recommend a prostatic fossa biopsy and adjuvant radiotherapy only if the biopsy were positive. Adjuvant radiotherapy in patients with positive lymph nodes, and probably in most with positive seminal vesicles, seems of little value.

In brief, I agree with the management of this case; I assume that the PSA levels were in fact undetectable but that the patient had unequivocal signs of persistent disease pathologically (e.g., large volume, multiple positive margins into the fat, significant grade of disease). If the risk assessment was somewhat uncertain, waiting for a PSA to rise is also acceptable. I believe the excellent outcome that resulted would have occurred by either approach.

Finally, I believe that in several years one will almost certainly write a different commentary. First, I think the available evidence suggests that the apparent ineffectiveness of adjuvant radiotherapy is, in part, due to insufficient dosimetry and not from pre-existing systemic disease. Better machines and technique(s) will yield better results. Also, the randomized studies will probably reveal important information upon which to build. Also, further information about pathology and postoperative PSA results, possibly with the addition of ultrasensitive PSA assays and the application of more sophisticated stratification techniques (neural network computer approaches), will help clarify patient subgroups. Finally, new biological approaches may even further sub-stratify the postradical prostatectomy man. The approaches might include radioimmunoscintigraphy, which promises to identify the occult sites of metastasis in patients with positive PSA levels and also reverse transcriptase PCR techniques, which now can detect circulating cancer cells with great sensitivity and promises to identify those PSA-positive patients who have systemic disease.

REFERENCES

1. Takayama TK, Lange PH. Radiation therapy for local recurrence of prostate cancer after radical prostatectomy. *Urol Clin North Am* 1994;21(4):687–700.
2. Kahn D, Williams RD, Seldin DW, et al. Radioimmunoscintigraphy with 111-indium labeled CYT-356 for the detection of occult prostate cancer recurrence. *J Urol* 1994;152(5):1490–5.
3. Wood DP Jr., Banks ER, Humphreys S, et al. Identification of bone marrow micrometastases in patients with prostate cancer. *Cancer* 1994;74(9):2533–40.
4. Katz AE, Olsson CA, Raffo AJ, Cama C, et al. Molecular staging of prostate cancer with the use of an enhanced reverse transcriptase–PCR assay. *Urology* 1994;43(6):765–75.

109

T2c, M1b Carcinoma of the Prostate

James M. Holland

*Androgen deprivation therapy is beneficial for patients with
hormonally sensitive prostate cancer*

CASE PRESENTATION

A 63-year-old Caucasian man developed acute urinary
retention after approximately 1 month of increasing frequency, nocturia, and slowing of his stream. He was taking
no drugs having an anticholinergic or adrenergic effect. His
father died of prostatic carcinoma at age 70. A kidney stone
had been removed in 1963. Chronic osteomyelitis of his
right ankle, present since childhood, was well controlled.
No bone pain was present at diagnosis.

Pertinent physical findings were limited to his prostate,
which was about twice enlarged, the right lobe being somewhat larger and firmer with no palpable induration of the
seminal vesicles or beyond the capsule. There was no palpable supraclavicular adenopathy or bony tenderness.

Abnormal staging evaluation findings were PSA 136
and 141 (nl 0–4) and prostatic acid phosphatase 2.2 (nl
0–0.8).

Transurethral resection of his prostate allowed resumption of normal voiding. The pathologic diagnosis was
poorly differentiated adenocarcinoma (Gleason grade 5 +
4 = 9) diffusely infiltrating the specimens (Figs. 109–1,
109–2).

Bone scans (Tc99m) revealed a small focus of
increased uptake in the left ischium (Fig. 109–3) and in
the right ankle. Bone radiographs of the pelvis were originally interpreted as normal, but correlation with the bone
scan revealed a corresponding small area of slightly
increased density and smudged trabecular pattern consistent with an osteoblastic metastasis (arrows, Fig. 109–4).
Because of the subtle changes, a magnetic resonance
(MRI) abdominal scan was done that showed abnormal
signal intensity in that area (arrows, Fig. 109–5). No other

areas of bony metastases were seen, nor was there abdominal or pelvic lymphadenopathy. The ankle uptake was
due to osteomyelitis.

The patient was presented to our multidisciplinary Uro-
oncology Board for discussion of treatment alternatives.
Pathology, nuclear medicine, and radiology consultants
agreed with the interpretation of the above studies. There
was unanimous agreement that androgen deprivation
therapy was indicated for this aggressive prostatic carcinoma grade 3–4 (poorly differentiated Gleason 5 + 4),
staged T2c (involves both lobes) and M1b (bone metastases), or stage D-2 by the previous method.

The choice of androgen deprivation therapy lay between castration or luteinizing hormone–releasing hormone (LHRH)-agonist treatment with preliminary flutamide administration to block the initial androgen flare.
The medical oncologist discussed the equal efficacies of
these treatments over the long term. In this patient, who
has minimal bone metastases, continued administration of
flutamide with LHRH-agonists appears to confer a somewhat longer term of remission to this subset of patients.
He acknowledged that the data in support of this finding
are relatively weak and wished to offer the patient entry
into a randomized clinical trial comparing orchiectomy
with or without flutamide. The patient was given a full
explanation of the options for management, including
delaying hormonal treatment until there was a complication requiring it. This option was discouraged because of
concern that a complication difficult to reverse would
occur, such as ureteral obstruction or spinal cord compression. He declined castration or randomization into a
clinical trial. Therefore, flutamide 250 mg every 8 hours
was begun, and 10 days later Zoladex pellet implantation

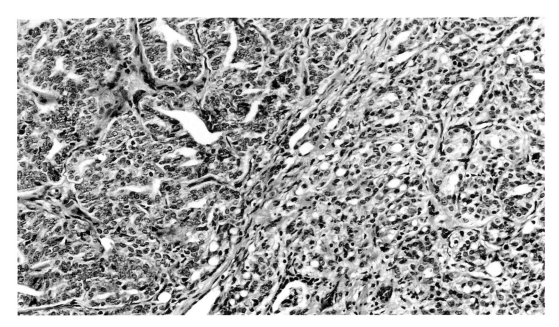

FIG. 109–1. Photomicrograph of grade 4 and 5 adenocarcinoma of prostate gland side by side. Grade 4 shows fused glands; grade 5 shows rudimentary glands with ragged infiltration and some signet ring cells (H&E, formalin fixed, × 50).

was given. He will continue to take flutamide along with monthly Zoladex implants. He chose to observe a vegetarian diet and began taking beta carotene.

Three weeks after the first Zoladex implants, his PSA had fallen to 13. Side effects of treatment included mild looseness of his stools, a common effect of flutamide, and hot "flashes" that are a common effect of LHRH agonists.

When evaluated 2 months after beginning flutamide and Zoladex, he felt well and had no voiding symptoms. His prostate now felt normal in size and consistency without nodules or induration. The PSA was 0.4 and prostatic acid phosphatase 0.3. Pelvic bone radiograph showed less density of the osteoblastic metastasis than was noted before treatment.

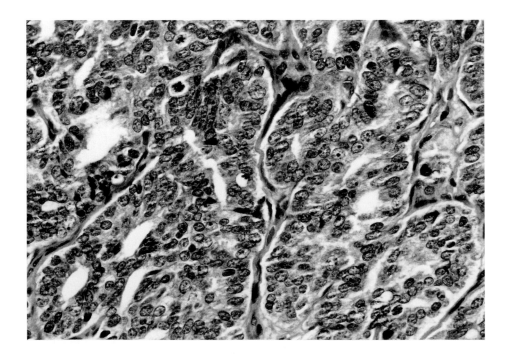

FIG. 109–2. Photomicrograph of the grade 4 adenocarcinoma of the prostate with fused glands and prominent nucleoli. (H&E, formalin fixed, × 100).

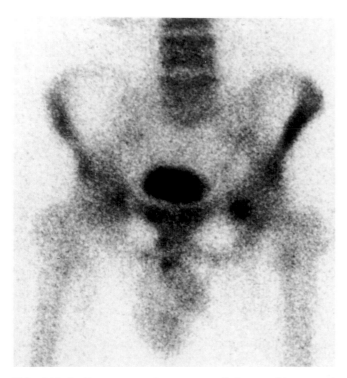

FIG. 109–3. Bone scan shows a small focus of increased uptake medial to the left acetabulum in the ischium.

He will receive subcutaneous Zoladex every 4 weeks and have a digital rectal exam and PSA every 3 months. A repeat bone scan will be done if the digital rectal exam or PSA become abnormal or other bone pain develops.

Salient issues illustrated by this patient include:

1. Rapid increase in outlet obstructive symptoms should alert the clinician of the greater risk of prostate cancer being present.
2. The positive family history of prostate cancer (patient's father) increases the patient's risk of developing it approximately threefold.

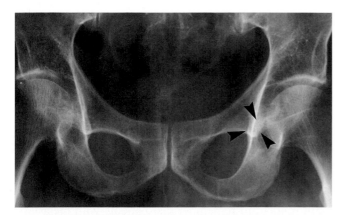

FIG. 109–4. Bone radiograph of the pelvis shows a poorly defined osteoblastic lesion (*arrows*) corresponding to the bone scan finding noted in the left ischium. Smudging of the trabecular pattern and indistinct margination suggest a neoplastic cause.

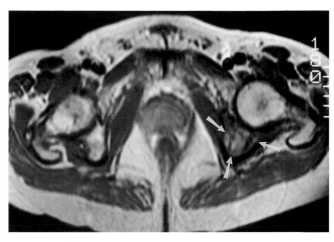

FIG. 109–5. MRI scan traverse section through the lower pelvis shows expansion of the posterior aspect of the left ischium and an abnormal signal intensity consistent with an osseus metastasis at the site of increased uptake on the bone scan.

3. The aggressiveness of poorly differentiated prostate cancer is shown by the spread to bone despite apparent confinement to the prostate by digital rectal exam.
4. Very subtle osteoblastic or osteolytic bony metastases are better appreciated by radionuclide bone scan (Tc99m). The MRI of bone to confirm the bony abnormality is rarely necessary but helped confirm to the patient that radical prostatectomy or radiotherapy to the prostate would be of no value. MRI scans should not be used on a routine basis.
5. Healing of bony metastases often is accompanied by an increased osteoblastic appearance, but this was not apparent in this patient 2 months after beginning androgen ablation.
6. Upon androgen deprivation treatment, prompt and rapid normalization of PSA and PAP levels to nearly undetectable levels often predicts a longer period of regression than in an incomplete or delayed response.
7. The true role of long-term flutamide administration requires recruiting patients into randomized studies comparing castration (or LHRH agonists) with or without flutamide.

COMMENTARY by Robert C. Flanigan

This well-presented case represents an all too common finding of disseminated prostate cancer at the time of the patient's initial diagnosis. Although this is less common today in the era of PSA than it was previously, it still remains true that many patients with prostate cancer present with advanced disease. This particular patient has a family history of prostatic cancer, which should alert the physician to an increased likelihood of cancer of approximately two- to fourfold. If a patient has two first-degree relatives with prostate cancer, the increased risk is approximately 5- to 10-fold (1).

This patient's cancer also illustrates an important concept regarding rectal examination in the diagnosis of prostate cancer. No palpable nodule was reported at the initial digital rectal exam, but rather an asymmetry of the gland with a firmer texture was noted. It is important for physicians to have a high index suspicion when doing rectal examinations and to consider any abnormality, including asymmetry or change in texture, as abnormal, not relying only on the presence of a nodule to suggest the diagnosis of prostate cancer.

This specific patient's markedly high PSA (136 nq/mL) suggests the probability of extension of the cancer beyond the prostate and should alert the clinician to the possibility of bony metastasis. Clearly, a PSA of this level necessitates the performance of a bone scan, particularly in a patient with high-grade malignancy, as was demonstrated in this man. An even more disturbing finding was an elevation in the PAP. If this determination is done by an enzymatic technique, it is the opinion of most individuals that this suggests the significant likelihood of disseminated disease, thereby making the patient stage D0 (American staging system). A patient with elevation of enzymatic acid phosphatase is like to have disseminated disease, even without a positive bone scan or imaging study of the pelvic lymph nodes (CT or MRI). In only 10% of cases are such patients found to have organ-confined disease. In contrast, they usually display a rapidly progressive course to demonstrable distant metastasis in most cases within the next 2 years (2). It is our practice, therefore, not to suggest the use of local therapy only (including radical prostatectomy or radiation therapy) in these individuals but rather to concentrate on hormonal treatment (with addition of radiation therapy to control the primary tumor in some patients).

This case also demonstrates the usefulness of bone scanning with correlative radiographs, and in some situations MRI, to confirm bony abnormalities suggestive of metastatic disease. Although there is no unanimous consensus among urologic oncologists regarding the necessity of bone scanning and CT scanning (or MRI) of the abdomen and pelvic areas for detecting lymphadenopathy, there is a general feeling that patients with PSAs greater than 50 ng/mL, bulky palpable disease in the prostate, or aggressive histologic disease (as was illustrated in this patient) with a Gleason sum of greater than or equal to 7 portends a high likelihood of metastasis, particularly lymphatic metastasis, and therefore indicates the need for evaluation of the bones and lymph nodes.

The treatment of this patient was clearly appropriate in the sense that his physicians concluded that androgen ablation was the appropriate therapy for his metastatic disease (M+). Although there still remains some controversy regarding the most prudent way to achieve androgen deprivation, it is increasingly clear in the literature, I believe, that a combination of standard therapy designed to block the production of androgens from the testicles with an antiandrogen to block the impact of adrenal androgen at the cellular

level is the most prudent treatment plan, particularly for a patient like this one who appears to be of good performance status and displays minimal bone metastasis. Castration or LHRH agonist therapy can both successfully eliminate the production of the testicular androgens, which account for approximately 95% of the serum androgen level. On the other hand, the adrenal androgens can be concentrated by the prostate cancer cell. The addition of the antiandrogen flutamide was selected in this patient. It is a receptor blocker that blocks the effect on circulating androgens at the cellular level. Large cooperative trials have been completed that suggest that combined (or total) androgen suppression (using castration or LHRH agonist therapy combined with an antiandrogen) results in an improved survival of patients with metastatic disease. In a large Intergroup trial completed in the United States, there was an overall 7-month increased survival in patients with metastatic prostate cancer treated with LHRH agonist plus flutamide as compared with patients who received LHRH agonist plus placebo (3). More important, as was suggested by the presenters of this case, in patients with good performance status and minimal bony disease, the survival advantage exceeded 20 months. Similar findings have recently been reported in a large European Cooperative Oncology Treatment Consortium (EORTC) study that described nearly identical survival advantages and also suggested that good-risk patients had a more significantly increased survival than did the entire population of metastatic patients as a whole (4). Even more important, the study suggested that the quality of life of patients treated with LHRH agonist plus antiandrogen therapy exceeded that seen in patients treated with orchiectomy plus placebo. The case presenters, however, correctly conclude that additional research must be completed. The current United States Intergroup study evaluating orchiectomy with and without flutamide is the last critical step in the overall evaluation of combined maximal androgen deprivation versus standard hormonal therapy.

Finally, the fact that this patient showed an excellent biochemical (PSA) response during his androgen deprivation therapy (his PSA dropped to normal levels within 2 months) suggests that this patient will have a more prolonged response to hormonal manipulation than a patient in whom this decrease in PSA does not occur. If and when PSA elevation should occur in this patient, it may be prudent to stop flutamide therapy in that recent reports of flutamide withdrawal have suggested that approximately 25% of patients seeming to progress with PSA elevation while being treated with combination hormonal therapy stopping the flutamide result in a decrease in their PSA and improvement of their clinical picture.

Despite advances in maximum androgen deprivation, it is still prudent to remember that patients with metastatic (M+) disease have an overall survival of only approximately 30 months. Once androgen insensitivity has developed, life expectancy of patients averages 6 months. To date, no reliably successful agents have been identified for use in the setting of androgen unresponsiveness, although current research with a variety of agents continues.

REFERENCES

1. Steinberg GD, Carter BS, Beaty TH, Childs B, Walch PC. Family history and the risk of prostatic cancer. *Prostate* 1990;17:337.

2. Bruce A, Mahan D, Sullivan L, et al. The significance of prostatic acid phosphatase in adenocarcinoma of the prostate. *J Urol* 1981;125(1): 357.

3. Crawford ED, Eisenbeyer MA, Investigators INT-0036. A Controlled Trial of Leuprolide with and without Flutamide in prostate cancer *N Engl J Med* 1990;321:428–32.

4. Denis LJ, Careiro de Moura JL, Bono A, et al. Goserelin acetate and flutamide versus bilateral orchiectomy: a Phase III EORTC Trial (30853). *Urology* 1993;42:119–130.

110

Advanced Prostate Carcinoma and Flutamide Withdrawal Response

Maria Theodoulou and Howard Scher

Flutamide withdrawal as a treatment strategy for advanced metastatic hormone refractory prostate cancer

CASE PRESENTATION

S.W. is a 55-year-old man who presented in 1987 with symptoms of dysuria, increased frequency of urination, and low back pain. Computed tomography (CT) scan revealed a mixed blastic and lytic lesion in the lumbar spine. Physical examination was remarkable for firmness on the right side of his prostate. Percutaneous needle biopsy of the prostate revealed adenocarcinoma Gleason score 8 (4 + 4). Serum prostatic acid phosphatase (PAP) was 33.5 IU/l and testosterone 1,259 ng/dl. Extent of disease work-up was significant for a lesion at L2 vertebral body with associated soft tissue mass. The patient was treated with combined androgen blockade with leuprolide (Lupron) and flutamide (Eulexin). He improved with decreased symptoms and a nadir PAP of less than 1.5 IU/l.

In May, 1990, patient relapsed with increased PAP to 9.89 IU/l. Prostate-specific antigen (PSA) was 8.5 ng/dl, serum testosterone was at castrate levels. Chemotherapy was started with cyclophosphamide (Cytoxan) single agent. Leuprolide and flutamide were continued. By September, 1990, the patient's back pain increased with associated right leg weakness. Repeat bone scan showed increased uptake at L2; PSA was increased to 23.7 ng/dl, PAP 29.57 IU/l. Myelogram showed slight epidural disease at T12 through L3. Spinal fluid contained a high total protein content (3,000 mg/dl). The patient was treated with steroids and external beam radiation therapy, to a total dose of 3,250 cGy; symptomatic improvement resulted.

The patient progressed biochemically with PSA peaking to 96 ng/dl. He was treated with various combinations of chemotherapy, including 5-FU/mitomycin/doxorubicin (Adriamycin), cisplatin-containing regimens, and estramustine (Emcyt)/vinblastine (Velban). Androgen ablation was continued with leuprolide and flutamide throughout the various treatment regimens. PSA plateaued at 18 to 20 ng/dl. Back and leg pain returned in early 1992, and an MRI of the spine showed progression of epidural disease in the lumbar spine. In February of that same year, the patient underwent a multilevel lumbar laminectomy with relief of radicular leg pain.

In July, 1992, an MRI of the lumbosacral spine showed a large soft tissue mass extending from the L3–4 level on the right causing significant compression on the dural sac and entering the spinal canal. Radicular pain and right leg weakness returned, limiting ambulation. The patient was referred to Memorial Sloan-Kettering Cancer for further evaluation and treatment options.

On admission at Memorial Sloan-Kettering Cancer Center in August, 1992, the patient had been on flutamide and leuprolide for more than 5 years, and estramustine and vinblastine for 1 year. Physical examination was significant for restricted flexion at the hip on the right, with motor strength of the right lower extremity 1 out of 5. There was decreased sensation along the anterior right thigh and anterior tibial region. PSA measured 19.5 ng/mL. Review of the bone scan confirmed multiple bony lesions; MRI confirmed epidural disease (Fig. 110–1).

The patient was evaluated by our Neurosurgery Service and the Genitourinary Oncology Service. Neurosurgery examined the patient and reviewed both the scans and the MRI with the question of potential surgical management of documented epidural progression in a radiation portal. It was felt that surgical intervention was not warranted at this time, although there was a recognized risk of further compression and compromise of function. If further pro-

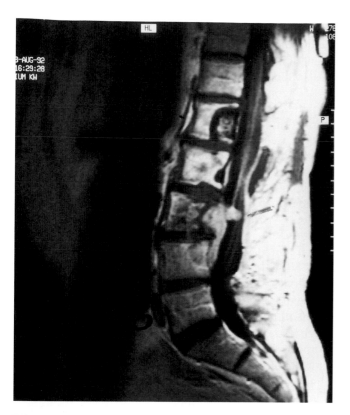

FIG. 110–1. An MR image of the patient with a lumbar epidural mass that had progressed despite combined androgen blockade with flutamide, chemotherapy, radiation therapy, and surgery.

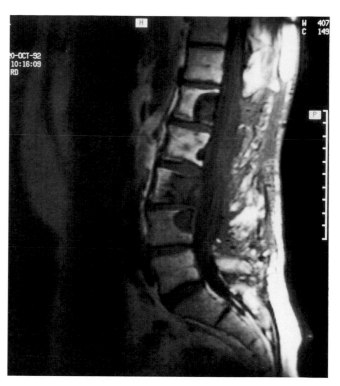

FIG. 110–2. MRI of the lumbar spine 8 weeks after flutamide was discontinued; note the regression of the epidural mass. No other therapeutic interventions were performed.

gression was documented clinically, then a surgical procedure would be contemplated, specifically with insertion of rods through a posterior approach. Radiation oncology was consulted to review the radiation portals. Pathology reviewed the submitted slides of the primary prostate biopsy, confirming the diagnosis of adenocarcinoma. Medical oncology discontinued estramustine, vinblastine, and flutamide (the latter was known to have agonistic action) (1), maintaining him on leuprolide only. The patient was asked to return in 2 weeks for re-evaluation with a new MRI. A back brace was recommended.

On return visit, the patient reported improvement in his symptoms, with marked decrease in his pain. MRI of the spine and plain films were without change. Physical examination showed improved sensory exam of the right lower extremity, as well as increased strength when compared to the exam 2 weeks prior. PSA had decreased to 4.9 ng/mL. It was decided to follow the patient's biochemical markers and clinical picture, without intervention, as he had improved. Two weeks later, the patient's PSA decreased to 1.5 ng/mL. He was able to walk on a treadmill for 15 minutes.

The patient was seen 1 month later. A new MRI of the spine showed partial response of the epidural mass in the lumbar spine (Fig. 110–2). PSA measured 1.2 ng/dl. His

back pain was nearly completely resolved. This was consistent with flutamide withdrawal response (2).

MRI of the spine repeated 6 months after flutamide withdrawal shows complete response of the epidural mass (Fig. 110–3). The patient continues to be followed, 13 months after flutamide withdrawal, on leuprolide maintenance alone. He is asymptomatic with normal exercise tolerance.

REFERENCES

1. Kelly WK, Scher HI. Prostate specific antigen decline after antiandrogen withdrawal. *J Urol* 1993;149:607–9.
2. Scher HI, Kelley WK. Flutamide withdrawal syndrome: its impact on clinical trials in hormone-refractory prostate cancer. *J Clin Oncol* 1993;11:1566–72.

COMMENTARY by Donald L. Trump

Drs. Theodoulou and Scher describe an all-too-common problem—widely disseminated prostate cancer. Prostate cancer is diagnosed in 320,000 men each year and accounts for 42,000 deaths annually. All too often patients are first diagnosed with widely disseminated disease as was the case in the gentlemen presented by Drs. Theodoulou and Scher. The case presented has some unique features: The serum PSA level was relatively low (8.5 ng per dl) at a time when symptomatic disease was

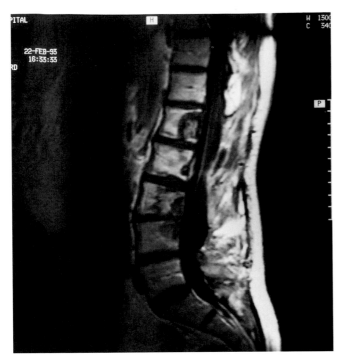

FIG. 110–3. MRI of the lumbar spine 23 weeks after flutamide withdrawal; note the continued response.

developing, and bone and prostate disease was evident. There is a rough, albeit imperfect, correlation between tumor burden and PSA value. One should keep in mind that when the apparent tumor volume and plasma PSA are discordant, consideration of an alternative histology or even diagnosis should be entertained. Small cell carcinomas arising in the prostate, or large duct carcinomas of the prostate, may be associated with extensive disease and low PSA. We have recently seen patients in this setting who turned out to have non-Hodgkin's lymphoma or transitional cell carcinoma arising in the bladder who presented in such a fashion. Another unusual feature of this case is the suggestion that this man possessed both lytic and blastic disease. Prostate cancers characteristically cause blastic bone lesions; mixed morphology bone disease is unusual. Finally, throughout the course of this patient's illness, his metastatic disease was predominantly situated in the lower lumbar spine and associated soft tissue. Again, this is unusual. The primary use for mentioning unusual features is to remind the reader that at some point atypical features in a clinical presentation should stimulate consideration of alternative diagnosis.

Primary Management of Metastatic Prostate Cancer

The patient presented was treated initially with luteinizing hormone releasing hormone (LHRH) agonist therapy and the antiandrogen, flutamide. Considerable data exists that support the superiority of combined hormone therapy

("total androgen deprivation") as the initial approach to advanced prostate cancer (2,3). It has been argued that the extent of improvement in time to treatment failure and survival, which occurs when an antiandrogen is added to an LHRH agonist, is small; it is nonetheless significant. The magnitude of the survival advantage with total androgen deprivation is comparable to the survival advantage seen with the use of tamoxifen for adjuvant therapy of stage I or II postmenopausal breast cancer. The mechanism whereby total androgen deprivation is superior to LHRH analogue alone remains uncertain. The leading hypothesis is that antagonism of both adrenal and testicular androgens is necessary to maximally deprive endocrine-sensitive cells of androgen stimulation. An additional variable that must be considered is the potentially unfavorable implications of the surge in plasma testosterone that occurs in the first 10–14 days following initiation of LHRH agonist therapy. Although LHRH agonists reduce gonadotropins with continuous therapy, there is an initial LH and FSH surge, which leads to rise in plasma testosterone. The role of total androgen deprivation in combination with orchiectomy is somewhat less clear-cut. Superiority in this setting would argue that the utility of total androgen deprivation is linked to antagonism of testicular and adrenal androgens rather than antagonism of the initial testosterone surge. A large multi-institutional trial in the United States has completed and analysis is awaited. A recent European study supports the superiority of antiandrogen plus orchiectomy, compared with orchiectomy alone (4).

Chemotherapy in Advanced Prostate Cancer

The patient described in this report received a number of cytotoxic drug therapies. Although all clinicians appreciate the pressures and needs that many patients and their families feel to "do something," there is little or no evidence to support the use of most of the agents that this patient received. Cyclophosphamide, 5-FU, mitomycin C, and doxorubicin- and cisplatin-based regimens have very small objective response rates and no documented impact on survival (5). Considerable enthusiasm has recently been generated by the apparent high response rate (40%–60%) seen with the use of estramustine and vinblastine (6). Whether this regimen will have an impact on survival is unclear. A strong case can be made for the treatment of patients, such as described in this report, with new agents on well-designed protocols rather than the serial utilization of a variety of essentially useless chemotherapeutic agents.

Flutamide Withdrawal Response

The authors of this report leave the impression that the flutamide response was well recognized at the time that they were managing the patient described. The recognition of the flutamide-withdrawal response is quite recent.

Dr. Scher and his group were among the very first to recognize it and conducted the most careful analysis of this phenomena. Flutamide-withdrawal response is a real phenomena, occurring in perhaps 25% of men with prostate cancer progressing on flutamide therapy (7). Those patients most likely to experience flutamide-withdrawal response are those who have been on flutamide for more than 12 months. The physiologic explanation for flutamide-withdrawal response is still elusive. There are in vitro data that show that a least one subline of the human prostate cancer cell line LNCaP is stimulated by flutamide treatment (8). Mutated androgen receptors have been characterized in this line (9). A reasonable hypothesis to explain the flutamide-withdrawal response is that long-term therapy with flutamide permits the selection of tumor cells with a mutated androgen receptor. Growth advantage is conferred on these cells by the application of flutamide, which in the situation of a mutated receptor, results in a growth stimulatory signal. Selection of this population of cells leads to overgrowth of this phenotype. With cessation of flutamide regression of these "flutamide-dependent" cells occurs in perhaps 25% of cases.

When to Treat

The case presented by Dr. Scher dramatically illustrates an important principle in the care of the patient with advanced hormone refractory prostate cancer: simply because one *can* provide active therapy it is not necessarily true that active therapy should be provided. This case illustrates the futility of sequential application of essentially ineffective cytotoxic regimens. It also illustrates that occasionally not giving therapy or withdrawing active therapy can be the best course to follow. Androgen deprivation is the only effective systemic therapy for prostate cancer. Considerable excitement surrounds the recent results of the estramustine-vinblastine and astramustine-etoposide combination, as well as the new putative growth factor antagonist, suramin (10). Studies demonstrating that either of these two systemic therapies affect survival or dependably improve the quality of survival are now underway. Flutamide withdrawal should be remembered as an important

maneuver. It may help some patients and does no harm to any patient. Given this very short list of active treatment strategies for hormone refractory prostate cancer, a strong case can be made for the judicious use of radiation therapy and generous application of analgesics in men with bone pain. Rather than applying any of the large number of readily available agents, which are ineffective, individuals with advanced hormone refractory prostate cancer should be entered on clinical trials, which will attempt to define agents with activity in this very important disease.

REFERENCES

1. Oesterling JE, Martin SK, Bergstralh EJ, Lowe FC. The use of prostate-specific antigen in staging patients with newly diagnosed prostate cancer. *JAMA* 1993;269:57–60.
2. Crawford ED, Eisenberger MA, McLeod DG, Spaulding JT, Benson R, Dorr FA, Blumenstein BA, David MA, Goodman PJ. A controlled trial of leuprolide with and without flutamide in prostatic carcinoma. *N Engl J Med* 1989;321:419.
3. Denis L, Smith P, deMoura C, Newling D, Bono A, Keuppens K, Mahler C, Robinson M, Sylvester R, DePauw M, Vermeylen K, Ongena P, and members of the EORTC GU Group. Total androgen ablation: European experience. *Urol Clin North Am* 1991;18:65.
4. Janknegt RA, Abbou CC, Bartoletti R, Bernstein-Hahn L, Bracken B, Brisset JM, Calais Da Silva F, Chisholm G, Crawford ED, Debruyne FMJ, Dijkman GD, Frick J, Goedhals L, Knonagel H, Vennerg PM. Orchiectomy and nilutamide or placebo as treatment of metastatic prostatic cancer in a multinational double-blind randomized trial. *J Urol* 1993;149:77–83.
5. Eisenberger MA. Chemotherapy for prostate carcinoma. *NCI Monogr* 1988;7:151.
6. Hudes GR, Greenberg R, Krigel RL, Fox S, Scher R, Litwin S, Watts P, Speicher L, Tew K, Comis R. Phase II study of estramustine and vinblastine, two microtubule inhibitors, in hormone-refractory prostate cancer. *J Clin Oncol* 1992;10:1754–61.
7. Scher HI, Kelly WK. Flutamide withdrawal syndrome: its impact on clinical trials in hormone-refractory prostate cancer. *J Clin Oncol* 1993;11:1566–72.
8. Wilding G, Chen M, Gelmann EP. Aberrant response in vitro of hormone-responsive prostate cancer cells to antiandrogens. *Prostate* 1989;14:103–14.
9. Veldscholte J, Ris-Stalpers C, Kuiper GGJM, et al. A mutation in the ligand binding domain of the androgen receptor of human LNCaP cells affects steroid binding characteristics and response to anti-androgens. *Biochem Biophys Res Commun* 1990;173:534–43.
10. Eisenberger MA, Reyno LM, Jodrell DI, Sinibaldi VJ, Tkaczuk KH, Sridhara R, Zuhowski EG, Lowitt MH, Jacobs SC, Egorin MJ. Suramin, an active drug for prostate cancer: interim observations in a phase I trial. *J Natl Cancer Inst* 1993;85:611–21.

SECTION XXIII

Testis

111

A 28-year-Old Man, Treated with Antibiotics for a Testicular Mass, Found to Have Stage II Embryonal Carcinoma and Positive Nodes

Gregory Warren and Stephen D. Williams

A compliant patient makes a difference in the method of treatment

CASE PRESENTATION

A 28-year-old Caucasian man noted swelling and some tenderness in his right testis. After a brief delay, he saw his family physician, who diagnosed "epididymitis" and treated the patient with scrotal support and antibiotics. The tenderness improved but the swelling persisted, and later increased somewhat. Two months later, he again saw his physician, who recommended urology consultation. The urologist noted a mass in the parenchyma of the right testis that did not transilluminate. Testicular ultrasound confirmed the findings noted on exam. On further questioning, the patient gave a history of an undescended left testis. He had undergone orchiopexy at age 10. General physical examination was otherwise unremarkable.

A β–subunit human chorionic gonadotropin (HCG) and a-fetoprotein (AFP) were obtained. The patient was scheduled for right radical inguinal orchiectomy, which was accomplished without event. Grossly, there appeared to be a malignant neoplasm involving the right testis. On microscopic exam, the tumor was a pure embryonal carcinoma (Fig.111–1). No vascular invasion was noted. Subsequent to the orchiectomy, the HCG was reported to be normal, and the AFP 74 (normal < 5 ng/mL). Radiographic staging included a chest CT scan, which was normal, and an abdominal CT scan, which showed borderline enlarged nodes in the draining zone of the right testis.

TUMOR BOARD DISCUSSION

The patient has nonseminomatous testicular cancer (Table 111–1). The clinical presentation is quite typical for such a condition. Even now, these tumors are frequently initially misdiagnosed as epididymitis. A brief trial of antibiotics may be reasonable, but in the absence of dramatic clinical improvement, further evaluation is warranted. Ultrasound confirmed the nature of the tumor and the orchiectomy confirmed the diagnosis and initiated therapy. The procedure must be done by the inguinal route, as scrotal violation complicates subsequent management. Tumor markers are important but are not particularly useful in the diagnosis of a scrotal mass, because they are ordinarily normal in patients with seminoma and frequently normal in patients with early stage nonseminomatous testis cancer. Of interest, on careful questioning: the patient did have a history of an undescended testis. These patients are at higher risk of testis cancer, both in the ipsilateral and contralateral testis.

In patients with true clinical stage I disease (Table 111–2), options for management include surveillance or

553

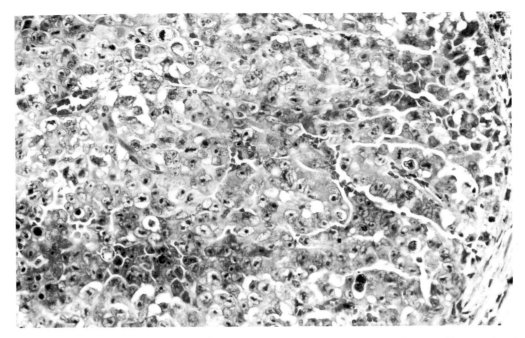

FIG. 111–1. A microscopic view shows a mostly solid pattern of embryonal carcinoma with occasional slit-like spaces. The nuclei are large and vesicular with macro-nucleoli; cytoplasmic borders are not distinct.

retroperitoneal lymphadenectomy (RPLND). The main advantage of the former approach is that it avoids surgery. Historically, observation also had the potential to avoid the major disadvantage of RPLND, which was disruption of the autonomics that control ejaculation with resultant infertility. More recently, however, an RPLND can be done effectively with preservation of these nerves and ejaculatory capability. The advantages of this so-called nerve-sparing RPLND are that it provides precise surgical staging, allows the rational use of adjuvant chemotherapy; cures many patients with nodal involvement; and avoids the necessity of chemotherapy (now the biggest threat to fertility) in some.

The situation is somewhat different for this patient. He does not have true stage I disease in that his abdominal CT scan is equivocal (a not uncommon finding). Further, his AFP was not normal although it may yet normalize with time after orchiectomy. Given these considerations, it was recommended that the patient undergo RPLND, to which he agreed.

Second Presentation

Prior to RPLND, his AFP had fallen to 14, with a rate of decline nearly consistent with the known half-time of AFP (about 5 days). The surgical procedure was accomplished without difficulty. Although there was no gross nodal involvement, the final pathology report noted involvement

of three lymph nodes, with tumor identical to that noted in his testis. His postoperative course was uneventful and a subsequent determination of AFP was normal.

Discussion

The patient has pathologic stage II testis cancer. Before 1980s, the "standard" management of patients with completely resected stage II testis cancer was postoperative adjuvant chemotherapy in an effort to prevent relapse, which was deemed unacceptable. However, in the 1970s and early 80s, it was recognized that cisplatin-based chemotherapy would permanently eradicate tumor in 70%–80% of patients with more advanced stage II or stage III disease. Further, the cure rate of patients with very small volume metastatic testis cancer was 95% or greater. The documentation of the high level of effectiveness in the treatment of metastatic disease mandated a reassessment of the management of patients with completely resected stage II tumors. Pilot data confirmed that brief cisplatin-based chemotherapy would prevent relapse in patients with resected stage II disease. However, an alternative management strategy would be to observe such patients carefully after RPLND. Those destined to be cured by surgery alone would avoid chemotherapy, with its potential acute and chronic adverse effects. On the other hand, with close follow-up, patients destined to recur would have their relapse

TABLE 111–1. *Pathology*

Seminoma
Nonseminoma
  Embryonal
  Teratoma
  Endodermal sinus
  Choriocarcinoma
  Mixed tumors

detected at a time when it is of small volume with a resultant high cure rate with chemotherapy. These two approaches were compared in an international randomized trial. About 50% of approximately 100 observed patients recurred versus only one of a similar number of patients who received adjuvant chemotherapy. However, nearly all relapsing patients were treated successfully, and the overall cure rate on both arms was identical and nearly 100%. In this particular patient, the risk of relapse is somewhat less because of the fact that the nodal involvement was microscopic only. It is thus reasonable to offer compliant patients the option of either immediate adjuvant treatment or deferral until the development of metastatic disease. Risk of relapse is highest in the first year after RPLND, and very rare after two years. It must be emphasized that follow-up must be meticulous in observed patients. Patients should have a chest radiograph, markers (HCG and AFP), and brief exam monthly for 1 year and every other month for the second year. Relapse may be detected by any one of those means.

It was decided, given this patient's high level of motivation and desire to avoid chemotherapy, that he would not receive adjuvant treatment but rather be followed monthly for one year and every other month for the second.

Third Presentation

The patient remained well after his RPLND. However, 5 months after the surgery, in routine follow-up, he was noted to have an AFP of 42. A repeat value was 53. He was without symptoms and his physical exam, including chest roentgenogram, was normal. However, a chest CT scan showed two new pulmonary nodules that were sev-

TABLE 111–2. Staging

Stage I	Tumor confined to testis
Stage II	Involvement of testis plus retroperitoneal nodes
Stage III	Supra-diaphragmatic or visceral involvement

eral millimeters in size. Abdominal CT scan showed postoperative changes but was otherwise normal.

Discussion

This patient has clearly suffered a recurrence of his tumor. In this clinical situation, a rising marker confirmed with another determination is diagnostic. The development of new abnormalities on chest CT scan further confirms, but really is not necessary to establish, the diagnosis. Further, no diagnostic biopsy is needed.

There is no one totally satisfactory prognostic factor system for patients with recurrent or metastatic testis cancer. Systems in use consider tumor bulk, degree of marker elevation, and number of sites of metastases. However, by whatever system is used, this patient has favorable prognosis disease because of only modest marker elevation and limited bulk and extent of metastatic disease. Chemotherapy should be initiated promptly because these patients occasionally progress very rapidly. Patients such as this one with "minimal" disease have about a 90%–95% chance of long-term survival, whereas only about 60% of patients with "advanced" tumor will remain continuously free of disease.

The most widely used chemotherapy regimen for patients with disseminated testis cancer is cisplatin and etoposide with or without bleomycin (BEP or EP; Table 111–3). In good prognosis patients, the Southeastern Cancer Study Group (SECSG) compared four courses of BEP with three courses of the identical regimen. Complete remission rates (97% and 98%) and long-term disease-free survival (91% and 92%) were identical. Investigators at Memorial Sloan-Kettering Cancer Center compared their four-drug VAB-6 regimen with four courses of cisplatin plus etoposide (EP). Complete remission rates and survival were identical and similar to the SECSG trial. The two-drug regimen was less toxic. A recent trial of the Eastern Cooperative Oncology Group (ECOG) compared three courses of BEP with the same regimen without bleomycin. The trial was terminated prior to completion of planned accrual because of an unexpectedly high failure rate on the arm that did not include bleomycin. In the BEP arm, 16% of patients experienced an unfavorable event (persistent or recurrent cancer or death) versus 31% on the arm that did not contain bleomycin. There were no episodes of serious pulmonary toxicity and only one drug-related death, which occurred on the BEP arm. A recently completed Memorial Hospital/Southwest Oncology Group (SWOG) study compared four courses of cisplatin plus etoposide with four courses of carboplatin plus etoposide. The cisplatin arm proved to be the superior regimen.

In summary, reasonable treatment options for patients with favorable prognosis tumor are three courses of BEP or four courses of EP. Considering the low risk of serious pulmonary toxicity seen in the ECOG trial, the dose-related potential of leukemogenesis from etoposide (see below), and general unpleasantness of chemotherapy, most individuals use three courses of BEP, as was selected for this patient. It is not appropriate to substitute carboplatin for cisplatin.

Modern antiemetics and other supportive care aspects have now made this form of chemotherapy relatively well tolerated. However, treatment must be given on schedule, in appropriate doses, to be optimally effective. Chemotherapy courses should almost never be delayed. Cisplatin dose is not altered. Etoposide dose previously was reduced 25% for previously irradiated patients and those with an intervening episode of neutropenic fever. However, with the availability of hematopoietic growth factors, it seems most appropriate to maintain dose and administer one of these for subsequent courses. Bleomycin is immediately discontinued for clinical or radiographic signs of pulmonary fibrosis. Subtle clinical findings that should warrant discontinuation of bleomycin include basilar rales or a lag or diminished expansion of a hemithorax.

An important consideration in these patients is potential late effects of treatment. There have been some important recent developments in this area. There have been anecdotal reports that have suggested that cisplatin-based chemotherapy may be associated with an increased risk of cardiovascular disease. A recent study investigated the likelihood of these events in patients entered several years previously on the Testicular Cancer Intergroup Study. This study registered and observed patients with pathologic stage I tumors; some ultimately relapsed and required chemotherapy. Patients with stage II tumors randomly received either two courses of adjuvant chemotherapy or were observed. Relapsing patients received four courses of therapy. Thus, a defined patient population received either no chemotherapy or two or four courses of chemotherapy. There were no differences seen in the incidence of the development of cardiovascular disease or hypertension. The only differences were the frequencies of distal extremity paresthesia or Raynaud's phenomenon, which were more likely to be present in patients who received more chemotherapy.

Another concern is the recent discovery that etoposide is associated with the late development of a distinctive type of leukemia. However, this event appears to be dose-related and very rare in patients who receive less than a total dose of etoposide of 2,000 mg/M^2. This total dose should not be exceeded in testis cancer patients, unless warranted by extenuating circumstances.

TABLE 111–3. *BEP*

Cisplatin	20 mg/M^2	days 1–5
Etoposide	100 mg/M^2	days 1–5
Bleomycin	30 units	weekly

Three to four courses given at 3-week intervals.

The impact of chemotherapy on fertility is less than originally thought. In the short term, all patients will have profound oligospermia or azoospermia. Many patients recover to a substantial degree after 2 to 3 years. Some patients will have longstanding chemotherapy-induced oligospermia or azoospermia. However, many, if not most, will resume normal or nearly normal spermatogenesis, and a significant number have fathered children.

As noted above, this patient was treated with three courses of BEP. Acute toxicity of treatment was fairly modest, with reversible alopecia and nausea and vomiting controlled reasonably well with the newer antiemetic agents available. He recovered quickly from the acute sequelae and is well without evidence of disease 3 years after treatment.

COMMENTARY by B.J. Kennedy

This case illustrates the need for patients with testicular cancers to be managed by oncologists experienced in this disease. The decision-making process involves options in the selection of therapy. Fortunately, the outcome was favorable. This disease continues to be a learning process.

The patient's swollen testis was initially treated with antibiotics—a common practice. If such is done, it is mandatory that the patient be seen no more than 2 weeks later to assure that the inflammatory process has subsided. If not, more vigorous diagnosis is required. This patient had a 2-month delay, which almost doubles his chance of having a stage II disease (1).

The patient had microscopic tumor in two retroperitoneal lymph nodes. Although the risk of recurrence is less than with more bulky nodes, it still is present. The process of observation instead of adjuvant chemotherapy has become popular. As stated in the discussion, however, "nearly all relapsing patients were treated successfully and the overall cure rate was nearly 100%," but not 100%, which might occur with adjuvant chemotherapy (2). The option of offering patients immediate adjuvant treatment or deferral until the development of metastatic disease is one that should be offered only to *compliant* patients, and the rigid follow-up must be meticulously done; otherwise, the failure to do so can be catastrophic.

Five months later, this patient has recurrent disease with distant metastases in the lungs. His lifestyle is again interrupted because of the need for chemotherapy. This is one of the disadvantages of the observation policy. Under the circumstances, chemotherapy must be initiated promptly. In patients in whom the disease has become more than "minimal," as stated, only about 60% of the patients remain free of disease.

The trend of some investigations to decrease the amount of therapy or to delete agents is of concern in view of the fact that failures have occurred. The continuing investigations emphasize that carboplatin cannot replace cisplatin

(3); patients receiving etoposide should be informed of the risk of acute leukemia, even if it is of very low occurrence (4); and they need to be cognizant of the phenomenon of vascular spasm (5). Fortunately, this patient was a compliant one, and hence, is potentially cured. All patients with testicular cancer do not fit in this category.

Staging of testicular cancer is being further matured. The method still retains the three stages, but the prognostic values of the AFP, HCG, and LDH will be incorporated in the revised staging systems to help distinguish between low-risk and high-risk patients. The 1997 *AJCC Manual for Staging of Cancer* will have this revised system incorporating prognostic factors into the anatomic system.

REFERENCES

1. Bosl GJ, Vogelzang NJ, Goldman A, Fraley EE, Lange PH, Levitt SH, Kennedy, BJ. Impact of delay in diagnosis on clinical stage of testicular cancer. *Lancet* 1981;2:970–3.
2. Kennedy BJ, Torkelson JL, Fraley EE. Adjuvant chemotherapy for stage II non-seminomatous germ cell cancer of the testis. *Cancer* 1991;73:1485–9.
3. Bosl GJ, Bajorin DF. Etoposide plus carboplatin or cisplatin in good-risk patients with germ cell tumors: a randomized comparison. *Sem Oncol* 1994;21(Suppl 12):61–4.
4. Bokemeyer C, Hans-Joachim S. Treatment of testicular cancer and the development of secondary malignancies. *J Clin Oncol* 1985;13: 283–92.
5. Vogelzang NJ, Bosl GJ, Johnson S, Kennedy BJ. Raymond's phenomenon: a common toxicity after combination chemotherapy for testicular cancer. *Ann Intern Med* 1981;95:288–92.

112

Nonseminomatous Germ Cell Malignancy

Louis F. Diehl and Raymond B. Weiss

*A complete regression is when all evidence of the cancer
has been removed*

CASE PRESENTATION

A 23-year-old white man presented with a scrotal mass, left back pain, and hemoptysis. He was well until 4 months before evaluation when he first noticed a nontender, left scrotal mass. Six weeks before evaluation he complained of pain in the right flank area. On the day prior to admission, he had several episodes of hemoptysis. Because of the hemoptysis, he sought medical attention. His past medical history was negative, including no history of cryptorchidism. Medical evaluation demonstrated a 4-cm, firm, nontender left scrotal mass. The remainder of the examination was normal with special attention to the right testis, inguinal lymph nodal areas, abdominal examination for masses, and the supraclavicular lymph nodes.

Initial laboratory evaluation demonstrated a normal complete blood count, normal serum chemistries except an LDH of 875 U/L (normal <175). His β–HCG was 247,439 mIU/mL (normal <5) and his AFP was 471 ng/mL (normal <15). A posteroanterior chest radiograph demonstrated multiple bilateral pulmonary nodules, ranging in size from 1 to 3 cm (Fig. 112–1). Computed tomogram of the chest confirmed the chest nodules. Computed tomogram of the abdomen and pelvis demonstrated peripancreatic lymphadenopathy as well as periaortic lymph

Acknowledgement:

The Tumor Board acknowledges the following participants: Dr. Edgar Colon, Department of Radiology, Walter Reed Army Medical Center, for interpretation of the radiographs and the computed tomograms.

nodes with the largest being 5 × 6 cm. Pulmonary function testing included a forced vital capacity, forced vital capacity in 1 second, and a carbon monoxide diffusion capacity.

The day after admission he had a left radical orchiectomy. Pathologic evaluation of the testicular mass revealed predominately embryonal cell carcinoma with elements of yolk sac carcinoma. Tumor did not invade the capsule. The distal spermatic cord was free of malignancy.

On the fourth day after admission, with the pathology confirmed as a nonseminomatous germ cell tumor (NSGCT), he was started on PEB (cisplatin, etoposide, bleomycin) chemotherapy given every 3 weeks for four cycles. He tolerated the chemotherapy well.

After the fourth cycle of chemotherapy, he had a re-evaluation of the sites of malignancy. The symptoms of flank pain and hemoptysis had resolved. The physical examination was normal. The laboratory studies were normal except for chemotherapy-induced anemia. The LDH was normal at 123 U/L. The β-HCG was 34 mIU/mL and the alpha-fetoprotein (AFP) was 6.1 ng/mL 91 days after the radical orchiectomy and 64 days after the beginning of chemotherapy. The chest radiograph and chest CT showed multiple small pulmonary nodules with all nodules being smaller than initially. The abdominal and pelvic CT was normal except that the largest periaortic mass was now reduced to 3 × 3 cm. He was observed off therapy for an additional 52 days when his β-HCG was 4.4 mIU/mL and his AFP was less than 5.0 ng/mL. Computed tomograms of the chest showed nodules in the right lung (Fig. 112–2) and left lung (Fig. 112–3). After treatment, the left periaortic lymph node, although

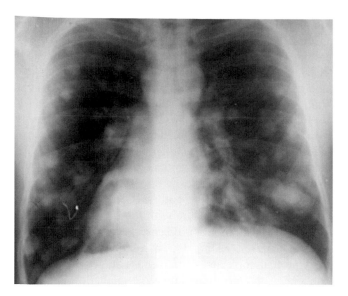

FIG. 112–1. Pretreatment chest radiograph demonstrating more than 40 pulmonary nodules.

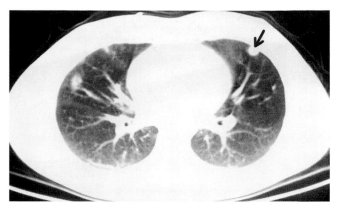

FIG. 112–3. Posttreatment CT of the lung showing the residual left lung nodule against the chest wall *(arrow).*

DISCUSSION

It is expected that approximately 6,600 patients will continue to be diagnosed with testicular cancer each year (1). This translates into a 0.2% life time risk for white men or an incidence of 3.7 cases per 100,000 white men (2). The peak incidence is between 20 and 40 years of age. Testicular cancer is exceedingly rare in blacks for unknown reasons.

Although rare, NSGCT malignancies deserve very special study because the careful application of advances in serum tumor markers, diagnostic radiology, surgical techniques, and the principles of combination chemotherapy have taken one of the most rapidly fatal cancers and turned it into a disease that can be cured in 90% of patients. This discussion of the treatment of a patient with advanced NSGCT examines these concepts from five perspectives: presentation, initial evaluation

decreased from the pretreatment size (Fig. 112–4) was still present (Fig. 112–5).

Because of the masses that persisted on abdominal CT, he had a left retroperitoneal lymph node dissection. Pathologic evaluation documented only fibrosis and necrosis. Four weeks later he had a right thoracotomy in which the largest of the two lung masses was removed. Pathology again showed only necrosis and fibrosis. It was decided to follow up the left lung nodule.

With 3.5 years of observation, he has remained without symptoms. The physical examination has remained normal. Serum β-HCG and AFP remain normal. Chest radiographs have remained normal with an unchanging nodule in the left lung. Abdominal computed tomograms remained normal.

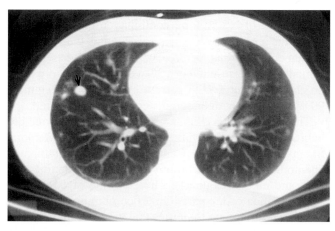

FIG. 112–2. Posttreatment CT of the lung showing the residual right lung nodule *(arrow).*

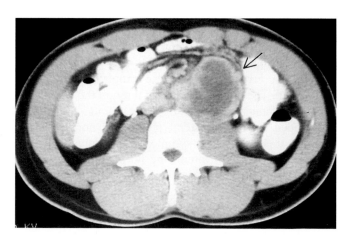

FIG. 112–4. Pretreatment abdominal CT demonstrating the largest of the periaortic lymph nodes. The enlarged lymph node *(arrow)* is ipsilateral to the testicular cancer *(both on the left)* and is necrotic.

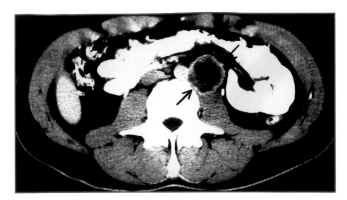

FIG. 112–5. Posttreatment abdominal CT demonstrating that the periaortic, necrotic lymph node is smaller but still present. Because of this finding, a left retroperitoneal lymph node dissection was performed. Pathologically, the mass contained only necrotic and fibrotic tissue.

and treatment, initial chemotherapy, evaluation post-chemotherapy with serum markers, and the approach to residual masses.

PRESENTATION

The central concept in understanding the presentation of NSGCT is to understand the method of spread. After originating in the testis, metastases occur through the lymphatics and through the blood (3). Lymphatic spread generally follows the spermatic vessels to spread to the ipsilateral periaortic lymph nodes. The right testis drains into the periaortic lymph nodes around T-12, and the left testis drains to the periaortic lymph nodes just below the renal hilum. From there, spread via the thoracic duct may lead to supraclavicular lymph node involvement. Hematogenous spread is usually to the lungs but may lead to liver involvement. If the scrotum is violated, the inguinal lymph nodes (which drain the scrotum) may be involved.

Against this background, our patient presented with a left scrotal malignancy that spread to the periaortic lymph nodes. The involvement of these lymph nodes led to the flank pain. The tumor also spread through the blood to the most common site of hematogenous spread—the lung. He developed multiple bilateral pulmonary nodules, which caused the presenting symptom—hemoptysis. β-HCG mimics the action of luteinizing hormone (LH) and may lead to gynecomastia, which was not present.

Initial Evaluation and Treatment

Patients who present with a testicular mass require two separate sets of diagnostic studies. The first set is the study of the anatomic sites to which the tumors can metastasize. These studies consist of the chest radiograph as an initial screening study, the chest CT for more detail of the chest, the abdominal CT to assess the periaortic lymph nodes, and the pelvic CT to assess the low periaortic and iliac lymph nodes. These studies documented multiple pulmonary nodules (Fig. 112–1) along with periaortic lymph nodes (Fig. 112–4) and a peripancreatic mass. They provided the pretreatment baseline against which tumor regression and eventual resolution is measured. The second set of studies is the serum tumor markers. These studies, the β-HCG and AFP, are virtually diagnostic in this setting, correlate with the bulk of disease, and can be used to monitor disease resolution. The lactic dehydrogenase (LDH) is an ubiquitous intracellular enzyme that correlates with disease stage in a variety of cancers. Although the simplistic explanation is that this intracellular enzyme is released in increasing quantities with increasing bulk of tumor, data are emerging that LDH is produced in response to as yet unknown mechanisms and correlates well with the bulk of disease. Thus, the initial evaluation consisted of an examination of the sites of spread by physical examination (testis, inguinal lymph nodes if appropriate, and supraclavicular lymph nodes); CTs of the chest, abdomen, and pelvis; the LDH; and serum tumor markers of β-HCG and AFP.

Although this patient's disease had spread beyond the testis, radical orchiectomy still played a critical therapeutic role. It was clear from the outset that this patient would need chemotherapy. Like the blood-brain barrier, there exists a blood-testis barrier that would keep the testis "protected" from the chemotherapy. This protection afforded by the blood-testis barrier, together with the fact that chemotherapy is least effective against bulk sites of disease, dictate that the testicular mass needs to be removed through a radical orchiectomy for both diagnostic and therapeutic purposes.

Initial Chemotherapy

The cure of NSGCT by combination chemotherapy is one of the great success stories of medicine. It needs only to be remembered that before chemotherapy, disseminated testicular cancer resulted in a 30-week median survival and no chance of cure. With current chemotherapy regimens, 90% of patients with disseminated NSGCT are cured.

The story of this dramatic success and the principles behind it are worth detailing. Investigators at Memorial Sloan-Kettering Cancer Center reported on combination chemotherapy with dactinomycin, L-phenylalanine mustard, and methotrexate (4). The cure rate of 10% in this disease validated the paradigm of combining active drugs with nonoverlapping toxicities that would lead to the cure of many other malignancies. Other drugs were being found to be active in NSGCT, with bleomycin and vinblastine among the most active. Investigators at the M.D. Anderson Hospital, using the principle of combining drugs without overlapping toxicities, combined the pulmonary toxic agent bleomycin and the myelosuppressive agent vinblastine. This bleomycin–vinblastine combination resulted in a 60% response rate and a 25% durable complete response rate (5). But it was the discovery of the activity of cisplatin that completely eclipsed the early therapeutic successes. In a study of 11 heavily treated, advanced stage patients with NSGCT, single-agent cisplatin caused 6 partial responses and 3 complete responses in 11 patients (6). Because the toxicity of cisplatin was mostly renal, the paradigm of using combinations of active drugs with nonoverlapping toxicities was applied again by adding cisplatin to the bleomycin–vinblastine regimen. At Memorial Sloan-Kettering Cancer Center, the cisplatin–vinblastine–bleomycin regimen was incorporated into the dactinomycin–chlorambucil regimen that Li had developed there (7). At Indiana, Einhorn added the newly found cisplatin to vinblastine and bleomycin to form the PVB regimen. The cure of disseminated NSGCT of 60% of the patients with these regimens again validated the concept of combinations of active drugs with nonoverlapping toxicities.

Two events have occurred that have led to the development of a standard regimen. The finding that etoposide was a very active agent in relapsed patients led to the substitution of etoposide into the PVB regimen for the neurotoxic drug vinblastine, thus creating the PEB regimen. The Southeastern Cancer Study Group compared the PEB regimen with the PVB regimen with overall survival of 78% versus 66%, respectively (not significantly different) but with the elimination of the neuromuscular toxicity of vinblastine (8). PEB was less toxic with equal or better survival. The second event was an analysis of the toxicity in a study in which either VAB-3 or PVB could be used as adjuvant chemotherapy for stage II. This study by Weiss et al. demonstrated that the VAB-6 regimen is slightly more nephrotoxic, and the PVB regimen is slightly more myelotoxic (9). The combination of PEB being less toxic than PVB, and PVB about equally toxic with VAB-6 (PEB < PVB = VAB-6), have made PEB the standard chemotherapy regimen for advanced-stage NSGCT.

This patient clearly had disseminated disease. His radical orchiectomy had removed the site of disease that would be protected (blood-testis barrier) from chemotherapy. A body of information was available to select a curative chemotherapy regimen. The most active drugs, best combinations, doses, schedules, and routes had been well studied. Based on a slightly higher response rate and less toxicity, the PEB regimen was selected. Although three cycles may be adequate with minimal tumor burden, a standard four cycles were given to this patient.

Evaluation Postchemotherapy: Serum Marker Studies

In order to interpret the β–HCG and AFP in this patient, a understanding of the serum half-life of these markers is critical. β-HCG is a hormone, normally produced by trophoblastic tissue, that is composed of α and β chains. Although the alpha subunit is distinct from the pituitary hormone LH, the β subunit has marked homology with LH. In germ cell tumors, HCG is produced by the syncytiotrophoblastic cells. It is found in 100% of choriocarcinomas, 50% of embryonal cell subtypes, and in 5%–10% of seminomas. It normally has a serum half-life of 30 to 36 hours. When the source of β-HCG is completely removed (a tumor confined to the testis removed by a radical orchiectomy), the serum $T^{1/2}$ is 30 hours. However, when the NSGCT producing the β-HCG is disseminated and is killed by chemotherapy, there is an initial burst of β-HCG into the serum that raises the β-HCG. This initial surge of β-HCG into the serum may represent up to a 500% increase in the level of β-HCG as the starting point. When this higher level is taken into consideration, the actual calculated half-life of β-HCG can be as long as 96 hours (10). It is critically important to remember that β-HCG values are rarely measured in the time after starting chemotherapy, so this initial surge in β-HCG level is not often seen. However, it does enter into the calculation of the half-life of β-HCG. Thus, the β-HCG initially rises for 1 to 5 days, then decreases with a $T^{1/2}$ of 30 to 36 hours but possibly as long as 96 hours. A measurable β-HCG (beyond the time it should have been cleared from the serum) virtually documents the presence of residual disease.

Alpha-fetoprotein is a single chain 7,000 MW embryonic protein that declines to nearly undetectable levels by 1 year of age. In the fetus, it is produced by the yolk sac, the liver, and the GI tract. In the adult, cancers of these organs can give elevated levels of AFP. It is produced by yolk sac, pure embryonal, and teratocarcinomas, but not by pure choriocarcinomas, and definitely not by seminomas. It has a $T^{1/2}$ of 5 to 7 days, but in starting chemotherapy there is a surge of AFP into the serum, just as there is a surge of β-HCG discussed above. This surge, unmeasured and unnoted, makes the AFP calculated $T^{1/2}$ after starting chemotherapy appear closer to 7.5 days. This long half-life for AFP means that when the initial AFP is high, the AFP will be elevated for prolonged periods of time. An example of this is seen in Figure 112–6. As can be seen, 64 days after starting therapy, the AFP is still markedly elevated. However, the $T^{1/2}$ is 5 days, and the level of residual AFP falls on the $T^{1/2}$ plot, indicating that this residual AFP represents slow clearance of a protein with a long half-life and not new production (and hence, residual NSGCT) of AFP. Although the AFP remained elevated for several months after chemotherapy, the tumor was completely responding.

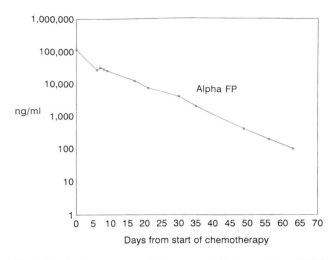

FIG. 112–6. An example of the rate of decline of the AFP in a patient with a yolk sac testicular malignancy. The initial AFP was 114,770 ng/mL. Note that the rate of decline is linear when plotted on a log scale.

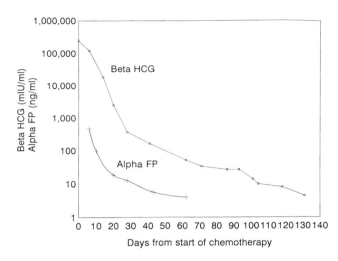

FIG. 112–7. A graph of the β–HCG and AFP for this patient. The most critical elements are the continued decline and the length of time it can take very high levels of β-HCG to return to normal.

After appropriate chemotherapy, there were two problems in this patient: the residual masses and the β-HCG-elevation. Correctly interpreting the β-HCG is of critical importance. If the β-HCG elevation represents slow clearance from the serum of a very high initial amount, the residual masses will then require surgical removal. If, on the other hand, the β-HCG is inappropriately high for the time from starting chemotherapy, the patient has residual malignancy and salvage chemotherapy would be the correct choice. The clinical decision hinges on the correct interpretation of the half-life of the β-HCG. The β-HCG values for this patient are plotted in Figure 112–7. Using simple arithmetic, there are 14 half-lives between the value of 247,439 on day 1 of chemotherapy, and the β-HCG value of 34 mIU/mL on day 64 postchemotherapy. This makes the $T^{1}/_{2}$ = 4.5 days—too long for simple serum clearance but within the range for clearance after chemotherapy. The second consideration in deciding whether the β-HCG is persistently elevated from slow clearance or residual malignancy, is whether the measurement of β-HCG is continuing to decrease with an constant $T^{1}/_{2}$. A review of the plotted data in Figure 112–7 indicates that for our patient, the $T^{1}/_{2}$ is constant; again supporting the fact that the β-HCG and AFP are not inappropriately elevated. The question now becomes what do you do with residual masses after the treatment for NSGCT?

Evaluation Postchemotherapy: Residual Masses

In treating NSGCT there are a number of possible outcomes. There could be necrosis or scarring (fibrosis) in the masses. There might be teratoma (the benign tumor of teratocarcinoma) or residual malignancy. The clinical question: How do you treat residual masses after the treat-ment of NSGCT? When residual masses are resected, there is general agreement that 40% will be necrotic/fibrotic, 40% will be teratoma, and 20% will have residual germ cell tumor (11). The survival of those with necrosis/fibrosis is 85%; those with teratoma is 90%, and those with residual germ cell malignancy is 50% (11). Moreover, if there is teratoma present, there are important reasons to resect the teratoma: it can grow locally; disease-free survival is dependent on the completeness of resection; malignant transformation can occur in 14%; late recurrences of teratoma occur in 19%; and, recurrent NSGCT occurs in 19% (11). Just as important, these percentages apply whether the mass is in the abdomen or the chest (12).

After four cycles of chemotherapy for this patient, the β–HCG and AFP were decreasing more slowly than their usual $T^{1}/_{2}$ but adequate for chemotherapy killing of the malignancy (Fig. 112–7). He had CT documented masses in the chest (Figs. 112–2, 112–3) and in the abdomen (Fig. 112–5). There was at least a 40% chance these residual masses were teratomas, and there would be substantial benefit to him to remove the teratomas. There was a 20% chance of residual NSGCT, with a 50% possibility that further chemotherapy combined with surgical resection could cure him. Based on these probabilities, a retroperitoneal lymph node dissection was performed. The mass in the abdomen was found to be residual necrosis and fibrosis. Because the data are similar for residual chest masses, we explored the right thorax, the site of the largest mass (12). Again the pathologic findings were necrosis and fibrosis. When we approached the left chest nodule, there were several different considerations. Patient compliance was becoming an issue. The nodule in the left chest was readily seen on CT and chest radiograph and would be easy to watch. It had not changed in the 3 months since the

RPLND and right thoracotomy had been performed. His serum tumor markers had remained normal. For these reasons, the residual nodule in the left chest was not resected but instead only observed. He has subsequently remained disease free with normal markers for the last 3.5 years.

REFERENCES

1. Boring CC, Squires TS, Tong T. Cancer statistics, 1993. *CA Cancer J Clin* 1993;43:7–26.
2. Zbed MS. The probability of developing cancer. *Am J Epidemiol* 1977;106:6–16.
3. Richie JP. Detection and treatment of testicular cancer. *CA Cancer J Clin* 1993;43:151–75.
4. Li MC, Whitmore WF, Golbey R, Grabstald H. Effects of combined drug therapy on metastatic cancer of the testis. *JAMA* 1960;174: 1291–9.
5. Samuels ML, Johnson DE, Holoye PV. Continuous intravenous bleomycin (NSC-125066) therapy with vinblastine (NSC-49842) in stage III testicular neoplasia. *Cancer Chemother Rep* 1975;59: 563–70.
6. Higby DJ, Wallace HJ, Albert DJ, Holland JF. Diamminodichloroplatinum II: a phase I study showing response in testicular and other tumors. *Cancer* 1974;33:1219–25.
7. Bosl GJ. The treatment of germ cell tumors at Memorial Sloan-Kettering Cancer Center, 1960-1983. In: Garnick MB, ed. *Contemporary Issues in Urologic Cancer.* New York: Churchill Livingstone; 1985: 45–60.
8. Williams SD, Birch R, Einhorn LH, et al. Disseminated germ cell tumors: chemotherapy with cisplatin plus bleomycin plus either vinblastine or etoposide. A trial of the Southeastern Cancer Study Group. *N Engl J Med* 1987;316:1435–40.
9. Weiss RB, Stablein DEM, Muggia FM, et al. Toxicity comparisons between two chemotherapy regimens as adjuvant or salvage treatment in non seminomatous testicular cancer. *Cancer* 1988;62:18–23.
10. Vogelzang NJ, Lange PH, Goldman A, Vessela RH, et al. Acute changes of alpha-fetoprotein and human chorionic gonadotropin during induction chemotherapy of germ cell tumors. *Cancer Res* 1982; 42:4855–61.
11. Bajorin DF, Herr H, Motzer RJ, Bosl GJ. Current perspectives on the role of adjunctive surgery in combined modality treatment for patients with germ cell tumors. *Semin Oncol* 1992;19:148–58.
12. Einhorn LH, Williams SD, Mandelbaum I, et al. Surgical resection in disseminated testicular cancer following chemotherapeutic cytoreduction. *Cancer* 1981;48:904–8.

COMMENTARY by B.J. Kennedy

This patient presented to the physician with a classical example of stage III nonseminomatous testicular carcinoma with pulmonary and retroperitoneal metastases. The histology with yolk sac elements is a warning sign for high risk of persistent or resistant tumor. A standard four courses of cisplatin-based chemotherapy resulted in partial regression of tumor masses. Upon removal, these proved to be necrosis and fibrosis. Based on falling serum markers consistent with half-life decreases of 5 days, the authors describe a well person at 2 years, normal markers, yet with a persistent lung nodule.

Routine CT scans seem to be done regularly even when the chest roentgenogram clearly shows pulmonary nodules. The CT scan was done to "confirm" the chest nodules and for more details of the chest, which seems to be an unnecessary procedure.

The patient was given four courses of BEP chemotherapy. BEP was chosen on the basis of a slightly higher response rate and lower toxicity. No reference, however, is made to the potential of induced leukemia by etoposide (1).

Four courses of chemotherapy at 3-week intervals has become a national standard for stage III disease. Failures after such therapy are deemed resistant disease, and salvage therapies are recommended. The Australian Germ Cell Study Group does not believe that an arbitrary number of courses (four) is indicated (2). They emphasize that induction chemotherapy should continue in responding patients until the maximum response is achieved. The attainment of normal markers does not necessarily indicate abolition of all malignant tumor cells. Residual cells may be present that are not sufficient in quantity to produce measurable serum markers. Hence, others have recommended that after the serum markers become normal, then two additional courses of chemotherapy should be given (3). The initial chemotherapy program is the time that the highest rate of cure can be accomplished.

This patient had resection of residual tumor masses that revealed fibrosis and necrosis, implying that cure has been accomplished. Yet 2 years later, a residual pulmonary nodule remains, which might be a teratoma and a potential source of reactivation. It should be removed.

In view of a persistent pulmonary nodule and the initial yolk sac histology, the potential for recurrence of disease remains worrisome. Because recurrences beyond 5 years after chemotherapy have been noted (4), this patient will need to be carefully monitored because one cannot claim cure at this point.

REFERENCES

1. Boshoff CH, Begent RHJ, Oliver RTD, Newlands ES, et al. Secondary tumors following etoposide containing therapy for germ cell cancer. *Proc Am Soc Clin Oncol* 1994;13:245.
2. Levi JA, Thomson D, Sandeman T, Tattersall M, et al. A prospective study of cisplatin-based combination chemotherapy in advanced germ cell malignancy: role of maintenance and long-term follow-up. *J Clin Oncol* 1988;6:1154–60.
3. Kennedy BJ, Torkelson J, Fraley EE. Optimal number of chemotherapy courses in advanced nonseminomatous testicular carcinoma. *Am J Clin Oncol* 1995;18:463–468.
4. Nichols C, Baniel J, Foster R, Donohue JP, Einhorn LH. Late relapse of germ cell tumors. *Proc Am Soc Clin Oncol* 1994;13:234.

113

Young Man with a Stage I Nonseminomatous Germ Cell Tumor

Jerome Hoeksema

Surveillance versus nerve-sparing lymphadenectomy in stage I testis cancer

---

CASE PRESENTATION

B.H. is a 21-year-old white man who noticed a painless, nontender, 1-cm mass on his right testicle. Over the next month, he felt the mass double in size, and sought medical advice. He has no recent history of trauma or urinary complaints. There was no fever, weight change, cough, chest or abdominal pain, breast enlargement or tenderness.

He has no prior history of heart, renal, or liver disease; testicular or inguinal surgeries; and testicular trauma or mumps orchitis. There is a positive history for arthroscopic knee surgery.

There is no family history for cancer. Parents and grandparents are alive and in good health.

He is in his third year of college. The patient is not married. He is sexually active. He denies IV-drug or cigarette use. Alcohol consumption consists of approximately six beers per week.

On physical examination, the patient is a healthy-appearing man, 5'11" tall, weighing 78 kg; chest—clear to auscultation; abdomen—soft, nontender, without palpable masses or organomegaly; nodes—no supraclavicular, axillary, or inguinal nodes noted.

Both testicles are descended, with left being normal in size and consistency. The right is slightly larger with a hard nodule on the inferior medial aspect separate from a palpably normal epididymis and cord.

The laboratory results are as follows: Hgb and Hct—15.8 and 47%; WBC—6.8; BUN—16 mg/dl; creatinine—0.9 mg/dl; alkaline phosphatase —87 u/l; LDH—207 u/l; SGOT—32 u/l; SGPT—50 u/l; electrolytes and urinalysis—within normal limits; chest roentgenogram—normal.

CLINICAL COURSE

An ultrasound was performed at the time of his initial evaluation which confirmed a 2 × 2.5 cm mixed echogenic mass in the right testis. Serum for alpha-fetoprotein (AFP) and beta-human chorionic gonadotropin (HCG) were drawn, and the patient underwent a right orchiectomy through an inguinal incision.

The specimen consisted of a 30-g testis contained within a normal appearing fascia with an attached 11-cm spermatic cord. On opening the tunica vaginalis, the external surface of the testis appeared smooth and tan with a 1.7-cm firm bulging mass. On sectioning, the mass measured 2.8 × 2 cm, was well circumscribed, and did not appear to extend into the capsule. The tumor had a soft, friable, tan-pink appearance with focal areas of hemorrhage.

The tumor consisted of mixed germ cell tumor (embryonal carcinoma, yolk sac tumor, and teratoma) (Fig. 113–1). The tumor was well circumscribed and limited within the tunica albuginea. There was no extension of tumor into the rete, epididymis, or spermatic cord. Extensive sectioning failed to reveal areas of choriocarcinoma, vascular or lymphatic invasion. Preorchiectomy: AFP was 58.55 ng/mL; 6 days postorchiectomy: 24.3 ng/mL; 15 days postorchiectomy: 8.4 ng/mL. HCG was less than 3 MIU/mL, pre- and postorchiectomy.

During the CT scan of the abdomen, multiple contiguous images were obtained at 10-mm intervals. No abnormal intra-abdominal or pelvic adenopathy were identified.

Chest CT identified a single 2–3 mm peripheral nodule. Otherwise, no other pulmonary or mediastinal abnormalities were noted.

TUMOR BOARD COMMENTARY

Jerome Hoeksema: Testicular germ cell tumors have a peak incidence in men between the ages of 20 and 34, and in this age group, it is the most common solid malignancy. It is more prevalent in whites than nonwhites and is rare after the age of 50. For classification and treatment purposes, germ cell tumors (GCTs) are classified as either pure seminomas or nonseminomas. This patient falls into the latter category. Testicular tumors most commonly present as a painless hard mass. Patients often delay seeking medical attention due to a lack of symptoms. In addition, a small percentage (approximately 15%) present with pain which may be due to a rapidly growing tumor or associated hemorrhage, and further delays in diagnosis occur when it is confused with epididymo-orchitis. In this patient, the history and physical examination would lead to a rapid diagnosis, and a testicular ultrasound probably adds little. Ultrasound is, however, helpful in ruling out an underlying testicular cancer when the clinical presentation and findings suggest a benign condition, such as epididymitis, torsion, hydrocele/spermatocele, hernia, or in evaluating palpably normal testicles in young men presenting with distant disease.

A high inguinal approach to exploration and orchiectomy allows for early control of venous outflow during tumor manipulation, provides adequate local margins, and minimizes the risk of tumor spill or local recurrence. An altered pattern of lymphatic spread and risk of local recurrence complicate the management of patients when the scrotum has been violated through needle biopsy or scrotal incision.

Tumor markers, particularly HCG and AFP, are essential to the diagnosis, staging, and treatment decisions in patients with GCTs. The majority of pure seminomas, and as many as 20% of nonseminomatous germ cell tumors (NSGCT), do not produce elevated levels of markers. Therefore, the presence of markers usually does not influence the decision concerning orchiectomy. It is important, however, to obtain serum markers with the primary in place (or drawn immediately after removal). HCG is pro-

duced by syncytiotrophoblasts, and it is typically very high in choriocarcinoma. Since syncytiotrophoblasts may be found in pure seminomas, a modest elevation in HCG can be seen, but a markedly elevated HCG would indicate the presence of nonseminomatous elements. In addition, pure seminomas do not produce AFP, which is an embryonic protein produced mainly by the yolk sac elements of GCTs. With a markedly elevated HCG, or any elevation of AFP, even with histologic evidence of pure seminoma, patients are treated for NSGCT. The initial marker level along with subsequent change in levels following removal of the primary can help in differentiating Stage I patients from those with metastatic disease. Tumor markers failing to drop following the normal half-life degradation (approximately 5 days for AFP and 30 hours for HCG) would indicate the presence of metastatic disease even if radiologic evidence were absent. In the case presented, the elevated AFP is consistent with the pathologic diagnosis of NSGCT, and the subsequent drop follows the half-life of the marker.

Germ cell tumors spread via the lymphatic drainage following the testicular vasculature. Primary lymph node involvement is seen in the para-aortic and para-caval lymph nodes from the level of the renal hilum to the aortic bifurcation (Fig. 113–2). Supradiaphragmatic disease occurs via spread through the thoracic duct to the left supraclavicular region or via the retrocrural nodes to the posterior mediastinum. Blood-borne metastases usually lead to pulmonary lesions which occur with or without nodal involvement. Liver and bone metastases are rare and associated with extensive disseminated disease. Brain metastases also are rare but seen more commonly with choriocarcinoma. A preliminary metastatic work-up for patients with NSGCT would include an evaluation of the abdominal retroperitoneal nodes and the chest, along with serial evaluation of tumor markers. In this patient, the abdominal and chest CT were negative, and with markers that normalized following orchiectomy, the tumor is a clinical stage I NSGCT.

Suresh Patel: Computed tomography is the most commonly used imaging technique for assessing the abdominal retroperitoneum in patients with testicular cancer. It is accessible, noninvasive, and easily reproducible. The major limitation of CT is that size is the primary criterion used to evaluate lymph nodes. From 20% to 30% of patients with NSGCT and normal abdominal CTs are found to have positive lymph nodes when exposed to staging surgical lymphadenectomy.

Pedal lymphangiography opacifies the iliac and para-aortic chains. Unlike CT, filling defects can be identified in normal-size nodes, suggesting early metastatic disease. The limitations of pedal lymphangiography are that it is time consuming, operator dependent, invasive (skin incision on feet), and does not demonstrate all of the nodes in the primary lymphatic drainage of the testicles. It is questionable whether combining CT and lymphangiography

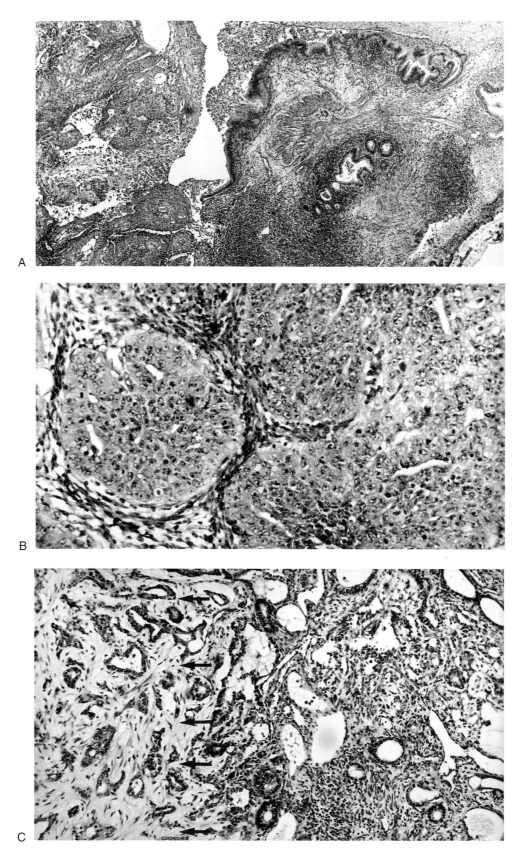

FIG. 113–1. Microscopic pathology. **A:** Low-power view of the tumor showing the multiple cell lines present. **B:** Sheets of poorly differentiated cells consistent with embryonal carcinoma. **C:** The yolk sac elements consisting of a tubuloalveolar pattern best seen on the left *(arrow).*

increases the accuracy of the retroperitoneal assessment. Some surgeons report an acute inflammatory reaction in the retroperitoneum following lymphangiography, making the surgical dissection more difficult. Therefore, when used, pedal lymphangiography is usually confined to patients who have a normal CT scan and are entering a surveillance program.

Chest CT has replaced conventional whole lung tomography. CT will be abnormal in up to 18% of patients with normal whole lung tomograms. In addition, CT gives a more-detailed assessment of the mediastinal lymph nodes. Small (2–4 mm) peripheral nodules, as seen in this patient (Fig. 113–4), can pose a problem in interpretation. If multiple, they probably represent metastatic disease. Solitary nodules are more likely benign granulomas, but they require follow-up.

Laurence A. Levine: This patient presents as a clinical stage I NSGCT. Because of the 20%–30% risk of occult disease in the retroperitoneum, surgical staging by retroperitoneal lymph node dissection (RPLND) has been, and continues to be, an integral part of the evaluation and management of these patients. In addition to giving prognostic information, RPLND is also therapeutic in patients with occult metastatic disease. Almost all patients who fail following RPLND for clinical stage I disease fail in sites other than the abdominal retroperitoneum. From 50% to 65% of patients with positive nodes at the time of RPLND have remained free of disease with no further treatment, and more than 90% of those patients failing can be salvaged with platinum-based chemotherapy. In experienced hands, the operation carries a near zero mortality and rela-

tively low morbidity. The standard lymph node dissection removes all lymphatic tissue from the renal hilum to below the aortic bifurcation and from ureter to ureter. Included in the dissection are the efferent sympathetic fibers, and essentially all patients are left anejaculatory. Clearly, fertility is an important issue in these patients, many of whom, as in the patient presented, have not had an opportunity to start their families. With our ability to salvage failures with effective chemotherapy reducing the morbidity of treatment, at the same time maintaining our better than 98% cure rate for patients with low-stage disease has become the focus of our efforts in recent years. By carefully mapping the location of positive nodes from past lymph node dissections, we can modify the template of dissection to preserve the contralateral sympathetic nerves. The nodes are evaluated by frozen section, and a more complete bilateral dissection is carried out if positive nodes are found. In addition, an anatomic nerve-sparing dissection of the ipsilateral sympathetic trunk has been developed by Donohue et al. (1). With these techniques the majority of patients maintain antegrade ejaculation. Those anejaculatory patients can often regain function with the administration of α–adrenergic drugs.

In addition to lymphadenectomy impacting on ejaculatory function, subsequent salvage chemotherapy can have a significant deleterious effect on fertility. Therefore, it is reasonable to consider and offer "sperm banking" prior to any therapeutic intervention. Unfortunately, as high as 50% of men can be found subfertile or infertile at the time of initial presentation. This may be secondary to hormonal effects of the primary tumor, underlying testicular

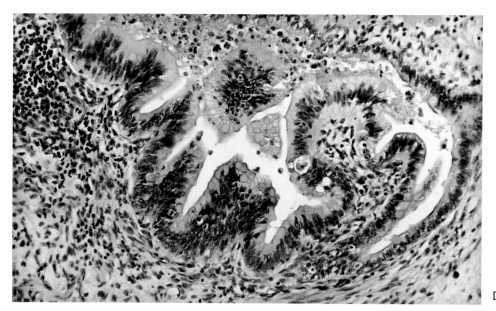

FIG. 113–1. Microscopic pathology. **D:** Benign mucinous glands surrounded by immature mesenchymal stroma, representing teratomatous elements.

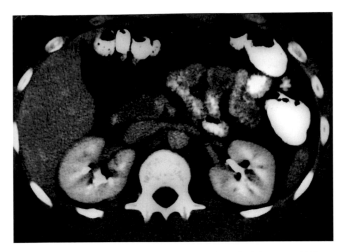

FIG. 113–2. CT of the abdomen at the level of the renal hilum with no demonstrable nodes.

dysplasia or the presence of CIS, autoimmune factors or other systemic effects from the stress of cancer diagnosis and orchiectomy on the germinal epithelium.

Melody Cobleigh: Seventy percent of clinical stage I patients who undergo appropriate surveillance will be cured. Those who relapse will do so with minimal metastatic disease. Current chemotherapy for minimal metastatic disease includes 11 weeks of treatment; three cycles of bleomycin, etoposide, and platinum. The short term toxicity of treatment is minimal. The new antiemetic regimens prevent nausea and vomiting in over 90% of patients. Hair loss is universal, but reversible. Azoospermia is universal, but substantial recovery of spermatogenesis occurs over time. In a report of 107 patients so treated, there was no mortality from the treatment. The survival rate was 97% (2). Stated another way, the cure rate from an observation strategy, including treatment of those who fail, is now 99%. Such a strategy spares 70 young men out of 100 any anticancer treatment beyond orchiectomy. Performing an RPLND on the entire cohort would expose everyone to a major surgical procedure, with its attendant morbidity, mortality, and expense, and still result in up to 10% of those men with negative nodes relapsing in the lung and requiring chemotherapy. In addition, approximately one third of patients with positive nodes will relapse following lymphadenectomy and require treatment.

Our ability to cure patients with disseminated GCT is dependent in part on extent of disease, and therefore the key to success with surveillance is rigid compliance to a strict and frequent follow-up routine. Monthly chest radiograph and serum markers with CT evaluation of the abdomen every 3 months is completed for the first year. Chest X-rays and markers are done every 2 months, with CT every 4 months for the second year. Although most patients on surveillance fail in the first 8 months, relapses

have been reported as late as 4 years, and therefore continued surveillance on a reduced schedule is required.

As the risk of relapse goes down, the advantages of surveillance are more pronounced. Many investigators have looked at how various factors affect the prognosis. One of the largest series looking at prognostic factors was compiled by the Medical Research Council (MRC), which evaluated more than two dozen histologic variables and their relationship to two-year disease-free rates (3,4). They identified four independent variables which had an adverse impact on relapse, namely venous invasion, lymphatic invasion, absence of yolk sac elements, and presence of undifferentiated elements (listed in order of importance). The 2-year relapse rates for patients with zero, one, or two of these risk factors present was 0%, 9%, and 25%, respectively. Patients with three, or all, risk factors present, had a near 70% chance of failing.

The patient presented fits into a low-risk category, with only one prognostic factor present—undifferentiated (embryonal) elements. In addition, the low tumor stage (T1) of the patient would make him a good candidate for surveillance. The patient should be further evaluated concerning his ability to comply with a surveillance program.

Status of the Patient

The options of RPLND and surveillance were presented to the patient, and surveillance was elected. The patient is now 2 years post orchiectomy and remains free of disease.

REFERENCES

1. Donohue J, Foster R, Rowland R, et al. Nerve-sparing retroperitoneal lymphadenectomy with preservation of ejaculation. *J Urol* 1990;144: 277.
2. Einhorn L, Williams S, Loehrer P, et al. Evaluation of optimal duration of chemotherapy in favorable prognosis disseminated germ cell tumors: a southwestern cancer study group protocol. *J Clin Oncol* 1989;7:387–91.
3. Freedman LS, Parkinson MC, Jones WG, et al. Histopathology in the prediction of relapse of patients with stage I testicular teratoma treated by orchiectomy alone. *Lancet* 1987;2:295–8.
4. Mead GM, Stemming SP, Parkinson MD, et al. The second medical research council study of prognostic factors in non-seminomatous germ cell tumors. *J Clin Oncol* 1972;10:85–94.

COMMENTARY by Jerome P. Ritchie

This case highlights the typical presentation of NSGCT—a painless mass discovered incidentally. The lack of pain leads to a delay in diagnosis, which is not uncommon in the age population in which this tumor occurs. This patient underwent expeditious, although not emergent, radical orchiectomy, and was evaluated in an appropriate fashion, including pre- and postoperative

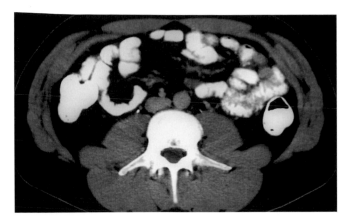

FIG. 113–3. CT of the abdomen at the level of L3 with two round structures anterior and one lateral to the vena cava. All are less than 6 mm in diameter.

tumor markers, CT scan of the abdomen (Fig. 113–3), and CT scan of the chest (Fig. 113–4). Imaging of the central nervous system is not necessary unless neurologic symptoms are present. Pedal lymphangiogram has been abandoned because of the lack of specificity and sensitivity as well as the invasive nature of the procedure.

Testicular cancer has become one of the most curable solid malignancies in the United States (1). This success story relates to numerous factors, including a cancer with well-defined metastatic pathways to the regional lymph nodes, presence of two tumor markers that can be measured by exquisitely sensitive assays, and the development of surgical and chemotherapeutic techniques which, in conjunction, have allowed for treatment of even advanced disease.

The availability of effective chemotherapy has allowed modifications of once fairly extensive or drastic treatment thought necessary to cure this disease process. The two major modifications have been modification of surgical technique to preserve sympathetic nerves, and thus, ejaculation and fertility, and the option of active surveillance protocols for patients with favorable disease processes.

Controversy exists concerning the preferred option for treatment. Surveillance protocols do spare unnecessary surgery, but do place the patient at increased risk for retroperitoneal recurrence and subsequent need for chemotherapy. The major problem with surveillance protocols is the relative inaccuracy of CT scan for staging of the retroperitoneum. Even though CT scanning represents the most accurate technique for depiction of retroperitoneal involvement, sensitivity and specificity are low, dependent upon size criteria alone for delineation of abnormal lymph nodes (2). The relative insensitivity of CT scanning mandates frequent CT scanning in patients who elect observation, in some protocols up to every 6 weeks for the first 6 months. Of additional concern is the need for reliability in patients who elect surveillance protocols. The doctor and patient must assume the burden of accurate follow-up and be certain that appointments are not missed. Surveillance must be carried out for a minimum of 5 years because of potential late relapse. Furthermore, in patients who relapse after surveillance, the mortality rate is higher than in patients who elect primary retroperitoneal lymph node dissection (3).

Modifications of surgical technique, including template procedures and nerve identifications procedures, have resulted in 95%–100% of patients retaining antegrade ejaculation (4,5). Nonetheless, retroperitoneal lymphadenectomy is a major procedure, with attendant risks, albeit well tolerated in young men.

In 1996, it would seem prudent to select patients for various protocols dependent upon risk factors. In patients with a low likelihood of failure, surveillance is an excellent option. Patients with vascular or lymphatic invasion, tumors greater than T2 with invasion of the epididymis, rete testis or cord, or patients with a high percentage of embryonal carcinoma, are at increased risk for failure. In such patients, modified retroperitoneal lymph node dissection may be a more rational approach than surveillance.

The availability of effective back-up therapy offers a luxury to the oncologist treating patients with testicular cancer that few other patients with solid tumor malignancies will enjoy. Nonetheless, one must continually weigh the risks of modifications against the incredible gains that have been made in the treatment of this once nearly uniformly fatal disease.

REFERENCES

1. Ritchie JP. Detection and treatment of testicular cancer. *CA* 1991;43: 151–75.

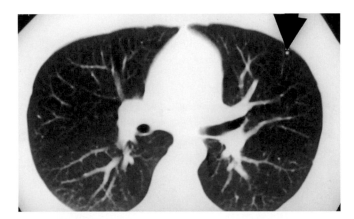

FIG. 113–4. CT of the chest with a solitary small peripheral nodule *(arrow).*

2. Stomper PC, Kalish LA, Garnick MB, et al. CT and pathologic predictive features of residual mass histologic findings after chemotherapy for non-seminomatous germ cell tumors: can residual malignancy or teratoma be excluded. *Radiology* 1991;180:711–14.

3. Raghavan D, Colls B, Levi J, et al. Surveillance for stage I non-seminomatous germ cell tumours of the testis: the optimal protocol has not yet been defined. *Br J Urol* 1988;61:522–6.

4. Ritchie JP: Clinical stage I testicular cancer: the role of modified retroperitoneal lymphadenectomy. *J Urol* 1990;144:1160–3.

5. Donohue JP, Foster RS, Rowland RG, et al. Nerve-sparing retroperitoneal lymphadenectomy with preservation of ejaculation. *J Urol* 1990;144:287–291.

114

Testicular Tumor with Metastases

James F. Glenn

The continuing saga of chemotherapy for stage III seminoma

CASE PRESENTATION

David P. Wood (Urology): P.T. is a 26-year-old white married man, who consulted his family physician 10 days ago because of weakness and weight loss of approximately 20 lbs over the past 3–4 months. Examination revealed a large, firm mass involving the left testicle. The patient stated that the enlargement had been progressive over the past year, but it was painless and he had sought no medical evaluation. With a diagnosis of probable testicular tumor, the patient was referred to the Markey Cancer Center for evaluation and treatment.

Examination revealed a pale and somewhat cachectic young white man. Vital signs were within normal limits, including blood pressure 122/78. Eyes, ears, nose, and throat were unremarkable. There were no palpable nodes in the neck or supraclavicular areas. The thyroid was not enlarged. Chest was clear to auscultation and heart sounds were normal. In the recumbent position, abdominal examination disclosed a firm mass, approximately 10 cm in diameter at the level of the umbilicus. The extremities were unremarkable. Genitalia were those of a normal adult circumcised male, except for an obvious mass in the left scrotal compartment. Palpation revealed this to be a hard, nodular mass, approximately 5 × 8 cm, irregular in contour, involving the left testicle and epididymis. The contralateral right testis was normal to palpation. Rectal examination was within normal limits.

Admission laboratory data included hemoglobin 11.2 g, hematocrit 32, white blood count 7,600. A complete panel of blood chemistries was within normal limits. Alpha-fetoprotein (AFP), β-subunit human chorionic gonadotropin (β-HCG), and lactic dehydrogenase (LDH)

studies were ordered. Radiologic evaluation of the chest and abdomen were requested, along with ultrasound evaluation of the left testicle.

Andrew M. Fried (Diagnostic Radiology): Coaxial tomography of the chest (Fig. 114–1) discloses a mixed density subcarinal nodal mass, which is indicated by the arrows and appears to measure approximately 2.5 × 4 cm. This is characteristic of mediastinal adenopathy, presumably secondary to the primary tumor. The abdomen, also examined by CT scans (Fig. 114–2), reveals significant retroperitoneal adenopathy anterior to vena cava near the lower pole of the right kidney. At a somewhat lower level (Fig. 114–2B), the scan demonstrates additional para-aor-

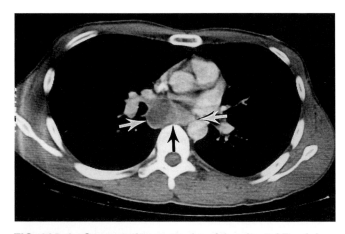

FIG. 114–1. Computed tomography of the chest. Mixed density subcarinal nodal mass *(arrows)* measuring 2.5 × 4 χm represents mediastinal adenopathy.

571

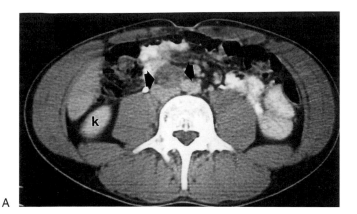

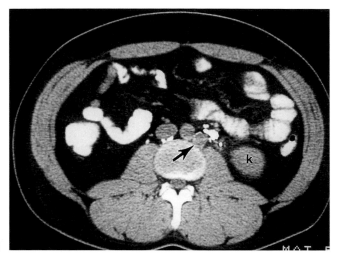

FIG. 114–2. Abdomen. **A:** Retroperitoneal adenopathy *(arrow)* is seen anterior to inferior vena cava at the level of lower pole of right kidney *(k)*. **B:** Scan taken at somewhat lower section demonstrates para-aortic adenopathy *(arrow)* medial to the lower pole of the left kidney *(k)*.

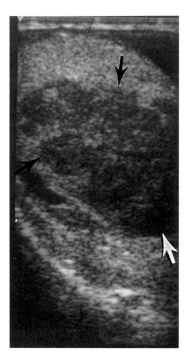

FIG. 114–3. Scrotum. Scan of the testicle demonstrates a large lobular hypoechoic mass *(arrows)* replacing the normal parenchyma.

tic adenopathy medial to the lower portion of the left kidney. Ultrasonic examination of the scrotal area reveals a large, lobular and hypoechoic mass replacing the normal parenchyma of the left testis (Fig. 114–3). All of these findings are compatible with a primary testicular malignancy with retroperitoneal and mediastinal metastatic disease. In accord with AJCC and UICC staging, this would be T2 N2 M1, stage III.

Dr. Wood: AFP, β-HCG, and LDH were all reported to be within normal limits. This information, coupled with the radiologic evidence of testicular tumor with retroperitoneal and mediastinal metastases led to the presumptive diagnosis of seminoma. For therapeutic and diagnostic reasons, left radical orchiectomy was undertaken. A high left inguinal incision was made, isolating the spermatic cord at the level of the internal inguinal ring. The cord was doubly cross-clamped and the entire contents of the left scrotal compartment were mobilized and externalized. Gross inspection confirmed obvious tumor. A frozen-section biopsy was not obtained. The spermatic cord was transected at its upper limit, ligated in the usual manner, and the entire specimen was submitted to Surgical Pathology for full evaluation.

Michael L. Cibull (Pathology): The specimen received in Surgical Pathology included an enlarged testis, epididymis, and attached cord structures. The testis contained a 5 × 7 cm firm, tan, circumscribed, but not encapsulated, mass that bulged above the cut surface. A thin rim of compressed testis was present at its periphery and the tunica was intact.

The histologic features of the tumor are typical of seminoma, with sheets and lobules of tumor cells surrounded by a delicate fibrovascular stroma that contains scattered small foci of lymphocytes. The tumor cells have enlarged vesicular nuclei containing one or two large nucleoli and abundant pale or cleared cytoplasm imparting a "fried egg" appearance to some cells. Infarctlike necrosis is seen in some areas but multinucleated tumor cells, unusually large numbers of mitoses, and a nonseminomatous component are absent (Fig. 114–4).

James F. Glenn (urology): This unfortunate young man ignored an enlarging mass in the left testicle for at least a year, possibly longer, and we are now presented with advanced metastatic disease, which is surgically incurable. On the basis of histologic findings, as well as negative tumor markers, this is pure seminoma. It is unlikely, but not impossible, that there are other malignant elements in the metastatic sites, such as teratocarcinoma, embryonal carcinoma or choriocarcinoma,

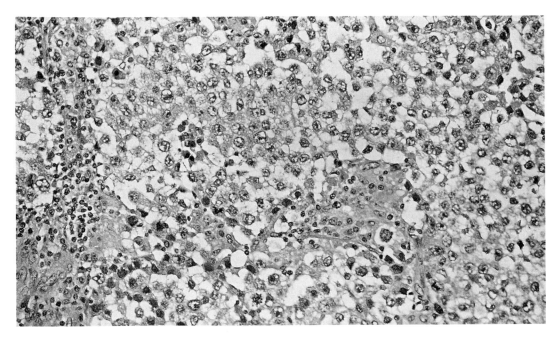

FIG. 114–4. Sheets of tumor cells with large vesicular nuclei, prominent nucleoli, and abundant clear cytoplasm. Note small clusters of lyphocytes and occasional mitotic figures (H&E stain, × 100).

because β-HCG, AFP or LDH are not elevated. As a seminoma, we have two effective modalities of treatment to consider: chemotherapy and radiation therapy. I would like to hear comments on the courses of treatment that might be pursued.

Rita K. Munn (Medical Oncology): Despite the marked radiosensitivity of seminoma, patients with stage III disease have only a 20–45% survival after radiotherapy. The development of cisplatin-based combination chemotherapy has dramatically improved treatment results, yielding 80-90% survival.

The development of chemotherapy for seminoma has paralleled that of chemotherapy for nonseminomatous germ cell tumors (NSGCT). The improved response rates seen with cisplatin, vinblastine, bleomycin (PVB) in NSGCT were reproduced in advanced stage seminoma.

Nineteen patients with advanced disease were treated with PVB with a 65% complete response. A multicenter collaborative study confirmed these single institution results.

The synergism of etoposide (VP-16) with cisplatinum noted in preclinical trials led to the first effective salvage regimen for any adult solid tumor. A randomized, phase III trial in previously untreated patients compared PVB to PVP$_{16}$B, revealing that PVP$_{16}$B has superior therapeutic effects and decreased toxicity.

Current clinical trials have focused on decreasing the toxicity associated with the PVP$_{16}$B regimen while maintaining its efficacy. The efficacy of bleomycin was less well documented in the treatment of seminoma as opposed to NSGCT in the pre-cisplatin era of chemother-

apy. The pulmonary toxicities associated with bleomycin have led investigators to evaluate two drug regimens. The Eastern Cooperative Oncology Group (ECOG) has demonstrated that three cycles of cisplatin, etoposide, and bleomycin are superior to cisplatin plus etoposide alone in patients with minimal to moderate disease. However, data from Memorial Sloan-Kettering Cancer Center indicate that when four cycles of therapy are given, etoposide and cisplatin alone is sufficient therapy for patients with good-risk GCT.

A multicenter study evaluating etoposide and cisplatin versus etoposide and carboplatinum has recently been completed. This randomized phase III study demonstrates that cisplatin remains the standard platinum analog in the treatment of patients with good-risk GCTs.

I recommend treatment with four cycles of cisplatin and etoposide. Treatment-related toxicities include alopecia, myelosuppression, and peripheral neuropathy. Renal insufficiency, high-frequency hearing loss, and neutropenic sepsis are rare complications.

Pushpa M. Patel (Radiation Medicine): Seminoma is the most common pure histologic subtype of testicular germ cell tumor. Treatment is influenced by the relatively indolent course and the extreme radiosensitivity and chemosensitivity of metastasis.

Optimum treatment of seminoma in early stages (A, B1, B2) has been, for the most part, clear and uncontroversial. High inguinal orchiectomy followed by moderate doses of 25 to 30 Gy to para-aortic and retroperitoneal lymphatics has resulted in high overall cure rates.

However, megavoltage irradiation as primary standard therapy for bulky abdominal metastases (>5–10 cm) and mediastinal disease (B3 or C) is not adequate; only 35% of these patients may be cured. Thus, cisplatin-based chemotherapy has become the conventional treatment for stage III and also for bulky abdominal disease. After chemotherapy for bulky disease, a residual mass may exist in as many as 75% of the patients. Surgical series have shown that only 10–12% of the residual masses have "viable" seminoma cells. Most have fibrosis only. Therefore, routine irradiation of residual masses is not indicated because 82–85% of the patients would receive irradiation unnecessarily.

It has been suggested by some authors that residual masses persisting after chemotherapy should merely be observed. On the other hand, the Memorial Sloan-Kettering Group has suggested that the likelihood of the persistent malignant disease correlates with the diameter of the residual mass. Residual masses less than 3 cm have about a one in three chance of containing persistent disease. This risk group has recommended surgical treatment for any individual who has a residual mass greater than 3 cm. However, this relationship was not confirmed in retrospective analysis at Indiana University. Both studies, however, are small, and the management of these patients remains controversial.

When radiation therapy is required for an enlarging mediastinal mass or abdominal mass after treatment with chemotherapy, the mass volume should be carefully defined by CT scan. The radiation fields should be tightly confined to the known site of residual disease, and the radiation dose should be limited to 25 Gy.

Dr. Wood: Because of the bulky retroperitoneal disease and very suspicious mediastinal adenopathy, we will elect to treat this patient with four cycles of cisplatin-based chemotherapy as recommended by Dr. Munn. The patient should tolerate chemotherapy well except for the expected nausea, vomiting, and alopecia. Dramatic reduction in the size of his retroperitoneal tumor after the first dose of chemotherapy will attest to the chemosensitivity of this seminoma. A CT scan of the chest and abdomen 2 weeks after the last dose of chemotherapy will indicate any evidence of disease in the mediastinum or abdomen. The patient will be having a physical examination, chest radiography, and B-HCG blood test every month for 1 year, then every 2 months the next year, then every 4 months the next year, then every 6 months the next year, then yearly for 3 years. A CT scan of the abdomen will be done every 6 months for 1 year, then yearly for 5 more years.

We will withhold radiation therapy because of the suspicious adenopathy in the mediastinum. In my opinion, this constitutes systemic disease, which is better treated with chemotherapy.

Dr. Glenn: What if the mediastinal disease appears to be eradicated and the abdominal disease improves, but a 3-cm mass remains as demonstrated by follow-up CT scans?

Dr. Wood: Because the tumor is a pure seminoma, this issue is controversial. There are two schools of thought: resect the residual mass, or follow the size of the mass with sequential CT scans. Unlike nonseminomatous germ cell tumors, the risk of small residual masses harboring viable tumor or teratoma is very low, less than 10%. However, for larger masses the risk increases significantly. A study by Motzer from Memorial Sloan-Kettering Cancer Center evaluated patients with advanced seminomatous tumors who received chemotherapy. Forty-two percent of patients with a residual retroperitoneal mass 3 cm or larger had viable residual tumor. None of the patients with less than a 3-cm mass had viable disease. However, resection of residual masses in patients with pure seminomas is difficult and can have a significant morbidity. Therefore, a "watch and wait" approach has been advocated by some groups. This entails frequent CT scans, and, unfortunately, many patients in this young age group are not compulsive enough to follow this regimen. If the disease grows substantially before being recognized, the patient will need additional chemotherapy and possibly surgery. Also, the cost of monthly CT scans rapidly becomes prohibitively expensive.

My opinion is that a residual mass of 3 cm or more should be resected if possible. During the operation, the surgeon should resect all visible disease. If the resection will jeopardize vital organs (i.e., the aorta or vena cava usually), then a subtotal resection is reasonable, combined with biopsies of the remaining tissue. If these biopsies are negative on frozen section, no further therapy is warranted. If viable tumor is identified, then further chemotherapy or radiation therapy is needed.

SELECTED READINGS

1. Thomas GM, Rider WD, Dembo AJ, et al. Seminoma of the testis: results of treatment and patterns of failure after radiation therapy. *Int J Radiat Oncol Biol Phys* 1982;8:165–74.
2. Horwich A, Dearnaley DP. Treatment of seminoma. *Semin Oncol* 1992;19(2):171–80.
3. Mendenhall WL, Williams SD, Einhorn LH, Donohue JP. Disseminated seminoma: re-evaluation of treatment protocols. *J Urol* 1981; 126:493–6.
4. Van Oosterom AT, Williams SD, Cordes Funes H, et al. The treatment of metastatic seminoma with combination chemotherapy. In: Jones WG, Ward AM, Anderson CK, eds. *Germ cell tumors II.* Oxford, England: Pergamon Press; 1986:229–33.
5. Williams SD, Birch R, Einhorn L, Irwin L, Greco FA, Loehrer L. Treatment of disseminated germ cell tumors with cisplatin, bleomycin, and either vinblastine or etoposide. *N Engl J Med* 1987;316: 1435–40.
6. Loehrer PJ, Elson P, Johnson DH, et al. A randomized trial of cisplatinum (P) plus etoposide (E) with or without bleomycin (B) in favorable prognosis disseminated germ cell tumors (GCT): an ECOG study. *Proc Am Cancer Soc* 1991;10:169(abstr 540).
7. Bosl GJ, Geller NL, Bajorin D, et al. A randomized trial of etoposide plus cisplatin versus vinblastine plus bleomycin plus cisplatin plus cyclophosphamide plus dactinomycin in patients with good-prognosis germ cell tumors. *J Clin Oncol* 1988;6:1231–8.
8. Bajorin D, Sarosdy M, Pfister D, Mazumdar M, et al. Randomized trial of etoposide andcisplatin versus etoposide and carboplatin in patients with good risk germ cell tumors: a multiinstitutional study. *J Clin Oncol* 1993;4:598–606.

9. Peckham MJ, Horwich A, Hendry WF. Advanced seminoma: treatment with cisplatin-based combination chemotherapy or carboplatin (JM-8). *Br J Cancer* 1985;52:7–13.
10. Motzer RJ, Bosl GJ, Heelan R, et al. Residual mass: an indication for further therapy in patients with advanced seminoma following systemic chemotherapy. *J Clin Oncol* 1987;5:1064–70.

COMMENTARY by Robert Dreicer

The case presented is that of a 26-year-old man with at least a 1-year history of a painless testicular mass, significant weight loss, and a palpable abdominal mass. He is taken to radical orchiectomy, and subsequent clinical staging demonstrates a stage III seminoma, marker negative with mediastinal and retroperitoneal metastases. He is anemic but has normal liver and renal function.

In any discussion of treatment outcome of testicular carcinoma, it is helpful to use one of the prognostically based staging systems. Using the Indiana staging criteria, this patient would be categorized as advanced disease, given his palpable abdominal mass and mediastinal adenopathy (1).

The pathology is read as a pure seminoma, and the normal value of AFP is at least consistent with this finding. Whether this tumor has additional nonseminomatous elements is initially moot, because the clinicians opt to treat this patient with systemic chemotherapy in lieu of radiotherapy.

The primary limitation of radiotherapy in this patient is not the quoted 20–45% survival, because many of those radiotherapy failures can be salvaged with chemotherapy. But as a consequence, these patients would require two treatment modalities, and despite the relatively low doses administered, the impact on bone marrow reserve would make subsequent salvage more difficult, therefore negatively impacting on survival (2).

The clinicians involved in this patient's care recommend four cycles of cisplatin and etoposide. The role of bleomycin as a component of cisplatin-based combination chemotherapy is somewhat controversial and two studies with different conclusions are cited. The study by the Eastern Cooperative Oncology Group (ECOG) compared three cycles of cisplatin and etoposide (PE) to three cycles of cisplatin, etoposide, and bleomycin (BEP) in good-risk patients. This study closed early after an unacceptably high incidence of failure was observed in the cisplatin-etoposide arm with the authors concluding that bleomycin was an essential component of this combination in good-risk patients treated with 3 cycles of therapy (3). In contrast, Bosl and colleagues found no differences in outcome when they compared their VAB-6 regimen to PE (4); however, no comparison between VAB-6 and BEP is available to clarify this issue. Two additional studies have recently evaluated the role of bleomycin. Levi and colleagues compared cisplatin and vinblastine (PV) with cisplatin, vinblastine, and bleomycin in 218 good-risk patients and found an unacceptably high death rate from progressive disease in the PV arm (5). Additionally, an update of the EORTC study that compared BEP with EP (four cycles compared with the ECOG study, which utilized three cycles) also demonstrates an inferior outcome with the EP regimen (4,6).

The management of residual masses in patients with seminoma following chemotherapy remains controversial with different approaches advocated by the Indiana and Memorial groups. While no definitive recommendation can be made, given the well-known difficulty in surgical removal of postchemotherapy (and radiotherapy) residual seminoma, this should only be attempted by a urologist with significant experience in performing RPLNDs in this population. Gallium scans (obtained pre- and post-chemotherapy) have been advocated by some as a method in which to discriminate viable residual seminoma post-chemotherapy (7). Patients with residual masses demonstrating disease progression after primary chemotherapy are best managed with salvage chemotherapy.

If this patient's postchemotherapy CT scans demonstrate resolution of all adenopathy, I would follow him up with physical exams, serum chemistry studies, chest roentgenography, and serum tumor markers monthly for 1 year and every 2 months the second year. The appropriate follow-up beyond 2 years is uncertain, with some questioning the need. I would not obtain subsequent CT scans of the abdomen in the absence of symptoms or other clinical indications of recurrence.

In summary, I would treat this patient with three cycles of BEP. If, after restaging, he had residual retroperitoneal or mediastinal adenopathy, I would discuss the pros and cons of adjunctive surgery with the patient, but I would opt for close observation.

REFERENCES

1. Birch R, Williams S, Cone A, et al. Prognostic factors for favorable outcome in disseminated germ cell tumors. *J Clin Oncol* 1986;4:400.
2. Loehrer PJ, Birch R, Williams SD, et al. Chemotherapy of metastatic seminoma: the Southeastern Cancer Study group experience. *J Clin Oncol* 1987;5:1212.
3. Loehrer PJ, Elson P, Johnson DH, et al. A randomized trial of cisplatin (P) plus etoposide (E) with or without bleomycin (B) in favorable prognosis disseminated germ cell tumors (GCT): an ECOG study. *Proc Am Soc Clin Oncol* 1991;10:169(abstr 540).
4. Bosl GJ, Geller NL, Bajorin D, et al. A randomized trial of etoposide + cisplatin versus vinblastine + bleomycin + cisplatin + cyclophosphamdie + dactinomycin in patients with good prognosis germ cell tumors. *J Clin Oncol* 1988;6:1231.
5. Levi JA, Raghavan D, Harvey V, et al. The importance of bleomycin in combination chemotherapy for good-prognosis germ cell carcinoma. *J Clin Oncol* 1993;11:1300.
6. Stoter G, Kaye S, Jones W, et al. Cisplatin and VP16 +/- bleomycin (BEP vs. EP) in good risk patients with disseminated nonseminomatous testicular cancer: a randomized EORTC GU Group study. *Proc Am Soc Clin Oncol* 1987;6:110.
7. Willan BD, Penney H, Castor WR, et al. The usefulness of gallium-67 citrate scanning in testicular seminoma. *Clin Nucl Med* 1987;10:813.

SECTION XXIV

Bladder

115

T3a NX M0, Grade 3 Bladder Tumor

John E. Garnett

Radical cystectomy or bladder conservation?

CASE PRESENTATION

Dr. Ofelein (Urology resident): Our patient is a 67-year-old white man, Italian national, who presented with a 3-month history of gross total hematuria. He has had incapacitating irritative voiding symptoms consisting of daytime frequency every 15 minutes and nocturia 15 times for which he had received antibiotic therapy in Italy. His past urologic history was significant for a bladder tumor (3 years ago), which was removed transurethrally. He has smoked one-half pack of cigarettes a day for the past 50 years. His general medical

health was excellent. He denied anorexia or recent weight loss. His physical exam was unremarkable, with an absence of abdominal masses and lymphadenopathy. His prostate was 2+ enlarged and was rubbery in consistency with normal landmarks. No pelvic masses were palpable. Urinalysis revealed red blood cells, too many to count. Chemistry profile showed normal renal and liver function, including an alkaline phosphatase of 45 mg/dl. Complete blood count revealed a mild anemia. A large sessile bladder tumor with papillary projections filling most of the bladder lumen was found during office cystoscopy. The tumor measured 15 × 10 × 10 cm arising from the left

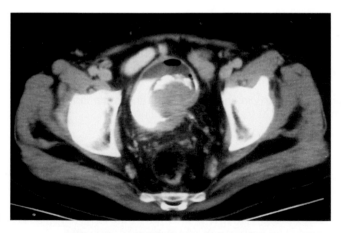 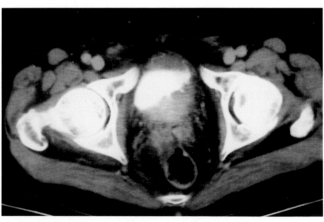

A   B

FIG. 115–1. A,B: Computed tomography scan of the pelvis showing a large intravesical tumor with associated bladder wall thickening. The left posterior lateral region demonstrates stranding in the perivesical fat suggesting extension of tumor through the bladder.

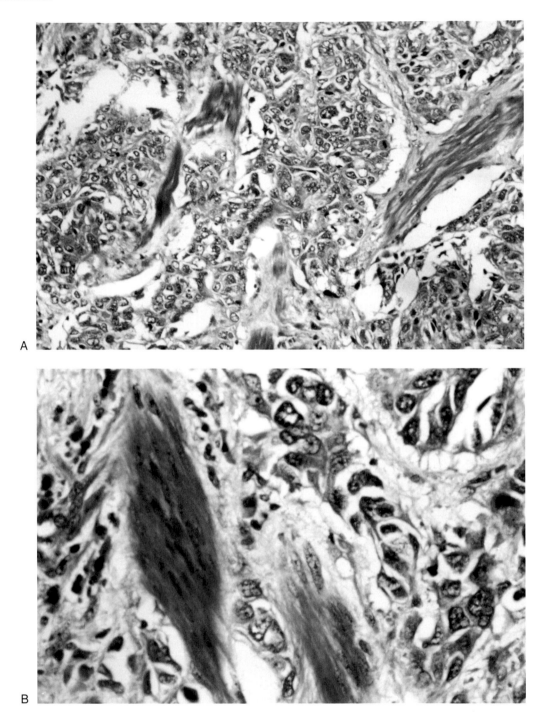

FIG. 115–2. Low- **(A)** and high-power **(B)** magnification of hematoxylin and eosin preparations demonstrating infiltrating high-grade transitional cell carcinoma obtained at transurethral resection.

lateral wall, extending to the anterior and posterior walls. A pelvic CT scan obtained prior to transurethral resection demonstrated the large, intravesical component of the tumor as well as adjacent bladder wall thickening and probable tumor extension into the perivesical fat (Fig. 115–1). Subsequent transurethral resection demonstrated a grade III transitional cell carcinoma weighing 41 g (Fig. 115–2) Extensive detrusor muscle invasion was found,

but the areas where the deep "bites" were taken showed no tumor. A complete metastatic work-up, including CT evaluation of the chest, abdomen, and pelvis, was negative. Flow cytometric evaluation of the resected specimen showed aneuploid cell populations.

Dr. Shetty: Dr. Ofelein, were random bladder biopsies obtained to assess the remaining urothelium? This information would be helpful for prognosis as well as assisting in selecting additional therapy, especially if a bladder-sparing approach is being considered.

Dr. Ofelein: Random bladder biopsies were not obtained for a number of reasons. First of all, this patient planned to return to his native Italy. He resides in a small village on a island in the Mediterranean which is remote from any large city. We anticipate that he would receive only the most basic medical care in the future. Certainly, a patient with an invasive bladder tumor in whom the bladder is spared will require very intensive follow-up because of the field change effect characteristic of transitional cell carcinoma. Second, although the deep biopsies did not demonstrate deeply invasive disease, the CT scan suggests that the tumor has extended into the perivesicular fat, indicating to us that an aggressive approach should be taken.

Dr. Shetty: It is my understanding in situations like this that the CT scan is no better than a flip of a coin, being about 50% accurate in determining true extravesical extension. If this patient were not from a remote part of Italy, I would think that he would be an excellent candidate for a bladder-sparing protocol. In fact, if the pathology is accurate, he may have been cured by the transurethral resection alone. A number of studies have shown 5-year disease-free survival similar to and superior to radical cystectomy in selected patients with superficially invasive bladder cancers. Certainly the loss of one's bladder is one of the more devastating things that can happen to someone, making these less drastic protocols attractive to patients.

Dr. Carter: Endoscopic staging of invasive bladder cancer has not proved to be very accurate. In protocols where delayed cystectomies have been performed, understaging has occurred in approximately 40% of cases where invasive bladder cancer was found in excised bladders thought to be tumor-free. This inaccuracy suggests that a "window of opportunity" for cure may be lost in some of these patients in whom aggressive therapy is delayed. On the other hand, in our practice we have had numerous patients who have not been candidates for major surgical undertakings, who, after removal of their primary invasive tumor, have been followed up with repeat transurethral biopsies and have done very well for extended periods of time.

Dr. Oyasu: A number of prognostic factors can be helpful in sorting out these patients. In addition to stage and grade of the tumor, the fact that this patient has had recurrent tumor puts him at higher risk for a poor outcome. Certainly, random bladder biopsies to determine if the tumor is multifocal would be helpful if a less-aggressive approach is being considered. DNA ploidy has not been particularly helpful in these tumors, with aneuploidy generally correlating with high-grade tumor, which holds true in this patient.

Dr. Garnett: Because this patient's tumor involves a large portion of the bladder and because of his place of res-

idence, he was not considered for segmental cystectomy. If circumstances were different, segmental cystectomy would have a number of advantages over radical cystectomy. Resnick and O'Connor and others have shown survival results similar to total cystectomy in selected patients with T3b disease. In these patients, normal bladder function is preserved as is sexual function, the latter being particularly important in younger patients. I do not believe segmental cystectomy has become a completely obsolete operation, despite the advent of continent urinary diversion and potency-sparing radical cystectomy, although with these two advances, we become even more selective to whom we recommend this operation. Only patients with small unifocal tumors, preferably located away from the trigone, and in whom incomplete endoscopic resection is suspected, should be considered if they otherwise would be candidates for a more-aggressive approach.

Dr. Shetty: Curative radiation therapy with bladder preservation has been used with only modest success in the past. Treatment results from Europe, where radiation therapy is standard, supports its avoidance with 5-year survival rates of approximately 20% for T3 tumors and 10% for T4 tumors. Currently, it is reserved for patients who either refuse surgery, are medically unable to undergo surgery, or who have inoperable disease. Preoperative radiation therapy with intent to improve survival by downstaging the disease has also been abandoned in most centers. Efforts have been made at bladder preservation by using combined TURBT, radiation therapy, and chemotherapy. George Prout reported in 1990 preliminary data indicating up to 70% local and distant tumor control at 2 years with functional bladder preservation in patients with invasive bladder cancer.

Dr. Shaw: We all recognize the advantage of bladder preservation as well as its risk of jeopardizing patients' lives if the treatment fails. Recently, protocols using adjuvant chemotherapy after transurethral removal of invasive bladder tumors are being completed with equivocal results. Chemotherapeutic regimens are toxic and have a complete response rate of only approximately 30%. Some of the early excitement with these protocols was probably due to patient selection. If the surgeon selects only minimally invasive tumors, he or she can expect up to 70% cure rates with TUR alone. Therefore, a high percentage of patients would receive a toxic therapy with no apparent benefit. On the other hand, patients with more deeply invasive tumors in whom TUR treatment alone is unlikely to succeed, and in whom an adjuvant therapy is therefore clearly indicated, fare less well if the bladder is to be preserved. In neoadjuvant protocols in which chemotherapy is given in an attempt to downstage deeply invasive T3b and T4 tumors, 50% of patients who are endoscopically thought to be tumor-free after chemotherapy are found to have persistent invasive tumor in their cystectomy specimens. In fact, downstaging to T0 disease occurs in less than 10% of these patients, and 40% are nonresponders, which suggests that a substantial number of patients will progress while chemotherapy is being delivered, thus delaying their definitive therapy. If our patient truly has T4 disease, as the CT scan suggests, then his prognosis with surgery alone is relatively poor, and some form of effective adjuvant therapy is needed. To date, a durable adjuvant therapy does not exist. Clearly, this patient should have a cystectomy. If the bladder were spared, this patient would have a substantial risk of subsequent tumors. He would have to be committed to a rigorous follow-up regimen, which because of distances involved, would be almost impossible.

Dr. Garnett: Dr. Ofelein, how was this patient treated and how has he done in follow-up?

Dr. Ofelein: Our patient underwent a radical cystectomy and ileal conduit urinary diversion. The surgical specimen showed no residual cancer, having been completely removed by transurethral resection. The patient recovered very well and returned to Italy 2 months after his surgery. It has been 3 years since his operation, and his relatives tell us that he continues to do quite well.

Dr. Garnett: In summary, our patient demonstrates the difficult choices encountered today in managing invasive bladder cancer. These choices are particularly acute because of the high stakes involved: loss of bladder function hopefully to avert a cancer death. The main confounding factor is the uncertainty of clinical staging, which necessitates that some patients will lose their bladders without demonstrable benefit, and others will die who could have survived had they been treated more aggressively. Hopefully, in the future, progress will be made in combating this disease, either through prevention, better treatment or if nothing else, through more effective staging so that current therapy can be applied more judiciously.

COMMENTARY by Anthony L. Zietman

From a purely clinical and pathologic point of view, this patient is an ideal candidate for combined modality bladder-conserving management. His tumor, though bulky, had had a visibly complete transurethral resection, a strong predictor of local control with a combined modality approach. Likewise, the strongest predictor of local failure, hydronephrosis, was absent. The only potential contraindication to a bladder-sparing approach is social. He may have little opportunity for close follow-up, and, in particular, check cystoscopy, on his return to Sicily. This will be a disadvantage only if the risk of bladder recurrence is very high. In series employing a modern, selective, organ-sparing approach with early cystectomy for nonresponders, recurrent invasive cancer is seen in less than 20%, a figure remarkably similar to the pelvic recurrence rates after cystectomy for T3–4 disease. This patient's major risk is therefore not local but metastatic, and this remains close to 50% regardless of the primary therapy.

Urologists have a deeply held concern that deferring cystectomy risks lives. Four studies reported over the last year have addressed this concern and greatly strengthened the argument for bladder conservation. These have been published by groups from the University of Erlangen in Germany (1), the University of Paris in France (2), the Massachusetts General Hospital (MGH) (3), and the Radiation Therapy Oncology Group (RTOG) (4). Three employed aggressive transurethral resection with radiation and cisplatinum-based chemotherapy (1–3), and three employed selection by initial tumor response (2–4). They all report overall survival rates of 45%–64% at 3 to 5 years. These figures are as good as any of the reported cystectomy series. This finding should not come as a surprise, as two previous randomized trials did not demonstrate any survival advantage when a bladder-conserving approach employing radiation alone was compared with immediate cystectomy (5,6). The surgeons argue that the cystectomy performed in these trials was not a modern radical operation and that current survival rates would be better. We argue that the bladder-sparing therapy used, radiation alone to only 60 Gy, was also less than radical therapy. Bearing in mind that most patients in the trials had T3 disease and no attempt at transurethral debulking was made, it is remarkable that as many patients had their primary disease controlled as did. This is great testimony to the relative radiosensitivity of transitional cell carcinoma.

Key to the success of the four bladder-conserving programs recently reported, and perhaps one of the reasons why their survival rates are better than the radiation arms of the two randomized trials, is their recognition that patients who are at high risk for local failure can be identified early and cystectomy promptly performed. Cystoscopies were carried out 4 to 8 weeks after completion of chemo-radiation, and any patient with persistent invasive tumor, referred for salvage cystectomy before local regrowth (and a second chance for metastasis) could occur. Those patients who had a complete response to therapy fared well with a 5-year survival of over 70%.

In those historic studies in which radiation alone was used for the management of T2-4 bladder cancer, pathologic complete response rates of about 40%, and durable local control rates of 30%, were usually reported (7). The Parisian program reported by Houssett et al. began life as induction therapy with concomitant cisplatin, 5-FU, and radiation prior to radical surgery (2). The first 18 complete responders underwent cystectomy as planned but there was no histologic evidence of residual tumor in any of the bladder specimens. Impressed by this striking evidence of tumor eradication, the program philosophy changed to one of bladder conservation. Seventy-four percent have had complete responses, and only 10% of these have subsequently failed within the preserved bladder. In the MGH, RTOG, and Erlangen studies, the complete response rates at cystoscopic re-biopsy were

58%–60%. Of those who had complete responses, 83%–89% remained free from invasive recurrence.

The urologists' fear that a conserved, irradiated bladder functions poorly is also answered by these studies. In the largest, that from Erlangen, only three cystectomies were necessary for bladder shrinkage among 192 preserved bladders (1.6%) (1). The Parisian group used less-conventional radiation fractionation, and still saw no late bladder problems (2). Furthermore, their urologists were still able to create continent diversions in the few patients who recurred locally, requiring salvage cystectomy. An excellent study by Lynch et al. reported in 1992 compared the bladder function of 69 patients rendered disease-free by 60 Gy in 30 fractions with an age and sex matched group of controls (8). No significant differences were observed.

Three of the studies emphasized the importance of an aggressive TURB, such as was received by the patient in this case study (1–3). Alone, a TURB may locally control a small proportion of T3 tumors. It cannot, however, usually be regarded as any more than a debulking procedure and does not obviate the need for irradiation, although it may allow a reduction in the dose required. A tailored approach to radiation dosing based on the completeness of the initial TURB should become a feature of all future protocols.

Over the last decade, multimodality organ-sparing treatment has become the standard of care for many of the common malignancies. Many radical and mutilating procedures, such as mastectomy and limb amputation, are no longer first-line management, and are reserved either for advanced cases or for the salvage of multimodality failures. Despite initial resistance, the weight of evidence has persuaded oncologic surgeons that survival, the bottom line, is not compromised, and that quality of life for most patients is enhanced. Bladder cancer should not be an exception.

REFERENCES

1. Dunst J, Sauer R, Schrott KM, Kuhn R, et al. Organ-sparing treatment of advanced bladder cancer: a 10-year experience. *Int J Radiat Oncol Biol Phys* 1994.
2. Houssett M, Maulard C, Chretien YC, Dufour B, et al. Combined radiation and chemotherapy for invasive transitional-cell carcinoma of the bladder: a prospective study. *J Clin Oncol* 1993;11:2150–7.
3. Kaufmann DS, Shipley WU, Griffin PP, Heney NM, et al. Selective preservation by combination treatment of invasive bladder cancer. *New Engl J Med* 1993;329:1377–82.
4. Tester W, Porter A, Asbell S, Coughlin C, et al. Combined modality program with possible organ preservation for invasive bladder carcinoma: results of RTOG protocol 85–12. *Int J Radiat Oncol Biol Phys* 1993;25:783–90.
5. Bloom HJG, Hendry WF, Wallace DM, et al. Treatment of T3 bladder cancer: controlled trial of pre-operative radiotherapy and radical cystectomy versus radical radiotherapy. *Br J Urol* 1982;54:136–51.
6. Sell A, Jakobsen A, Nerstrom B. Treatment of advanced bladder cancer category T2, T3, T4a. *Scand J Urol Nephrol* 1991;(Suppl)138:193–201.
7. Zietman AL, Shipley WU, Kaufman DK. Combined modality therapy in muscle-invading transitional cell carcinoma of the bladder. *Int J Radiat Oncol Biol Phys* 1993;27:161–70.
8. Lynch WJ, Jenkins BJ, Fowler CG. The quality of life after radical radiotherapy for bladder cancer. *Br J Urol* 1992;70:519–21.

116

Multiple Recurrent Noninvasive Papillary Carcinoma of the Bladder That Recurs Despite Multiple Transurethral Resections

William T. Sause

Multifocal low grade bladder cancer: surgery alone or with intravesical therapy?

CASE PRESENTATION

The patient is a 54-year-old woman who was initially seen in May, 1990. At that time she had experienced intermittent hematuria for 2 to 3 years. In the month before being seen she had experienced continued painless hematuria with every voiding. She was seen by her internist, who obtained an intravenous pyelogram. This revealed a large filling defect in the right side of the bladder measuring 5 × 5 cm (Fig. 116–1). With this history she was referred to a urologist.

Her past medical history is significant for a hysterectomy and bilateral salpingo-oophorectomy for "benign tumors" at age 43 and a rare episode of cystitis during her adult life. She took no medications at the time of her evaluation. She claimed to smoke one pack of cigarettes per day her entire adult life. Her physical exam was unremarkable for palpable pelvic masses or other abnormalities.

In May, 1990, she underwent cystoscopy and transurethral resection of a bladder tumor. At the time of cystoscopy a large tumor measuring approximately 4 to 6 cm in diameter occupied the right side of the bladder. It originated from the broad base superiorly and slightly laterally to the right ureteral orifice. It appeared papillary in nature. Small satellite papillary lesions were seen in several sites around the index lesion. Transurethral resection was accomplished with electrocauterization.

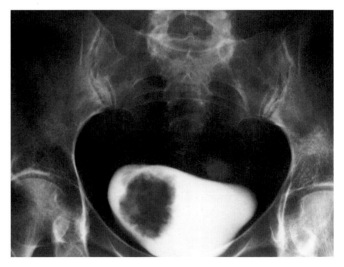

FIG. 116–1. A cystogram from the patient's intravenous pyelogram revealing mass in the bladder.

Postoperatively, the patient did well. The pathology report revealed a papillary transitional cell carcinoma of the bladder grade II without muscular invasion (Fig. 116–2).

In September, 1990, at the time of scheduled follow-up, two recurrent tumors were noted on the right side of the bladder at office cystoscopy. She was admitted to the hos-

584

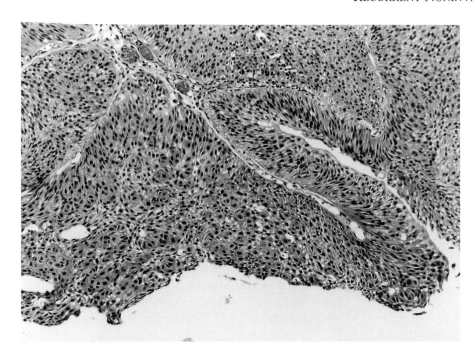

FIG. 116–2. Well-differentiated papillary transitional cell carcinoma. There is a papillary neoplasm with uniform multilayered transitional epithelium.

pital and subsequently underwent transurethral resection of these tumors. These tumors were small and were located on the right side of the bladder just lateral to the ureteral orifice. A resectoscope was used to completely resect these tumors. Pathology report revealed a grade I papillary tumor without muscle invasion.

In March, 1991, the patient underwent repeat scheduled cystoscopy. At that time she was noted to have three papillary tumors to the right of the trigone each measuring 0.5 to 1 cm in greatest diameter. The resection of the tumor was with a neodymium YAG laser.

In November, 1991, the patient again had scheduled cystoscopy. Two superficial tumors approximately 1 cm in diameter were noted to the right of the trigone. Because of technical reasons they were not easily treated with the Yag laser and the resectoscope was utilized to obtain complete resection of the tumors. The pathology report again revealed grade I papillary transitional cell carcinoma of the bladder without muscle invasion.

In July, 1992, at the time of surveillance cystoscopy, the patient was re-admitted to the hospital and two tumors were discovered in the bladder. One tumor was near the right ureteral orifice measuring 5 mm in diameter and at this time a 1-cm tumor was noted on the left anterior bladder wall. Cold-cut forceps were used to excise both lesions, and the resectoscope was used to cauterize the base. The pathology report revealed a transitional cell carcinoma of the bladder grade I (Fig. 116–3). No muscle invasion was noted.

Surveillance office cystoscopy was performed in March, 1993 and three tumors were noted: two on the left anterior wall measuring approximately 1 to 1.5 cm each; and one in the left posterior wall of the bladder measuring

approximately 1 cm. Repeated TURB was recommended to the patient.

Clinically, the patient has tolerated her multiple resections well. She has experienced no medical problems and an IVP performed on July 15, 1992, revealed a normal-appearing bladder.

COMMENTARY by Kenneth I. Wishnow

This woman presented initially with a large papillary grade II transitional cell carcinoma (TCC) of the bladder without muscle invasion. After "complete" transurethral resection of the tumor frequent recurrences of grade I or

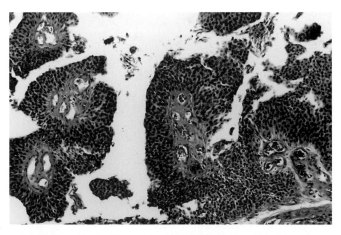

FIG. 116–3. Well-differentiated papillary transitional cell carcinoma. Note the papillary pattern with multilayered uniform transitional cells.

grade II papillary TCC were noted on multiple occasions at multiple sites within the bladder over a 3-year period. The recurrences were treated either by transurethral resection or Nd:Yag laser fulguration. Neither dysplasia nor carcinoma in situ were detected; and neither intravesicle chemotherapy nor immunotherapy were used to prevent recurrence.

The risk of progression of superficial bladder cancer to life-threatening muscle invasive disease was evaluated in a longitudinal multi-institutional prospective study by the National Bladder Cancer Group in 1983. The rate of progression to muscle invasion in 207 patients analyzed for a median of 39 months was 2% for grade I tumors, 11% for grade II, and 45% for grade III. Only 4% of intraepithelial tumors (stage Ta) progressed compared to 30% when the submucosa or lamina propria was invaded (stage I). Moderate to severe dysplasia elsewhere in the bladder was associated with progression in 33% compared with 8% when those changes were not present.

Although these data suggest that the risk of progression to muscle invasive disease in this patient was low, the risk of recurrence of superficial disease was significant. In the National Bladder Cancer Group study the recurrence rates at 1 year were 30% for grade I tumors, 38% for grade II, and 70% for grade III—whereas 50% of grade I tumors, 59% of grade II, and 80% of grade III recurred 3 years after "complete" transurethral resection. The recurrence rate for stage Ta tumors was 40% compared with 70% for stage I. Other findings likely to increase recurrence rates were (1) dysplasia elsewhere in the bladder; (2) positive urinary cytology; (3) multiple tumors; and (4) tumors larger than 5 cm in greatest diameter.

In this patient, the risk of progression was low but the risk of recurrence of superficial disease after transurethral resection alone or laser therapy was high. Accordingly, I believe treatment should have included intravesical chemotherapy or immunotherapy to reduce the rate of recurrence.

The four most commonly used intravesical agents are thiotepa mitomycin C doxorubicin and Bacillus-Camette-Guerin (BCG). These agents are instilled intravesically using varying dosages and treatment schedules. All have been documented to reduce recurrence compared with transurethral resection alone. BCG appears to be the most effective treatment when used as a prophylactic agent (after complete transurethral resection). BCG has demonstrated complete response rates from 63% to 100% at 1 year follow-up. Conversely, the recurrence rates at 1 year for mitomycin C is approximately 30%, doxorubicin 40%, and thiotepa 45%. In another study the net reduction in tumor recurrence was 42% for BCG, 12% for mitomycin C, 10% for doxorubicin, and 8% for thiotepa.

SELECTED READINGS

1. Heney NM. Natural history of superficial bladder cancer. *Urol Clin North Am* 1992;19:429.
2. Heney NM, Ahmed S, Flanagan MJ, et al. Superficial bladder cancer: progression and recurrence. *J Urol* 1986;135:265.
3. Brosman, SA. Bacillus Calmette-Guerin immunotherapy. *Urol Clin North Am* 1992;19:557.
4. Herr HW. Transurethral resection and intravesicle therapy of superficial bladder tumors. *Urol Clin North Am* 1991;18:525.

117

Squamous Cell Carcinoma of the Bladder with Vaginal Involvement and No Distant Metastases

John H. Texter, Jr.

Vague symptoms and advanced local disease at the time of diagnosis necessitated anterior exenteration

CASE PRESENTATION

S.R. is a 56-year-old black woman who was admitted to the Memorial Medical Center on October 1, 1992, because of a 40-lb weight loss, nausea, and hematuria. She is a known diabetic for the past 10 years and has been well controlled with diet and oral hypoglycemics. She was in her usual state of health until about 9 months before the admission when she began suffering episodes of nausea and occasional bouts of diarrhea. Her blood sugar remained stable, but she gradually began to lose weight despite continuing her regular dietary intake. On two occasions, one 6 months before admission and a second episode 2 months before admission, she experienced frequency and urgency of urination. During the last episode, the patient also noted dark urine with occasional passage of small blood clots. During both episodes the patient noted bilateral back pain with fever and chills. Both episodes responded promptly to oral antibiotics.

The patient is employed, and until the recent admission remained active, working full time. She is multigravid with the last menstrual period about 10 years ago. She has had several episodes of vaginal spotting since then but had undergone no evaluation or treatment. She has smoked about one-half pack of cigarettes per day for the past 25 years. She uses no alcohol. In addition to Diabeta, she takes Tagamet 200 mg twice daily and Restoril each evening. She is allergic to both penicillin and sulfa. There is a family history for hypertension and tuberculosis. An aunt recently died of cervical carcinoma.

On physical examination, the patient is a chronically ill appearing woman who is alert, cooperative, and oriented. There is an appearance of recent weight loss. Vital signs are normal except for a pulse of 106. There is a large lower abdominal mass measuring 10–12 cm just to the left of the midline, which feels firm and fixed. On pelvic examination, the mass feels fixed to the left perimetrium but not to the pelvic sidewall. No masses are felt on the rectal examination; however, the stool was hemocult positive.

The remainder of her exam was normal. She had a hemoglobin of 8.5 g, hematocrit of 28%, and white blood cell count of 14,100 with a slight shift to the left; blood sugar 178, BUN 12, and creatinine 1.0. The urine was grossly cloudy with 10–15 white cells and 40 red cells per high-powered field. Occasional rod bacteria were noted. Urine culture grew out a low colony counts of Enterobacter Cloacae and yeast.

A chest roentgenogram showed no infiltrates, masses, or cardiomegaly. A barium enema showed numerous diverticuli but no masses or bowel obstruction. A CT scan of the abdomen (Figs. 117–1 and 117–2) shows a lower abdominal solid mass with compression and deformity of the urinary bladder. The distal ureter is obstructed, producing left hydroureteronephrosis. Flexible colonoscopy identified only the multiple diverticuli. No other abnormalities were noted.

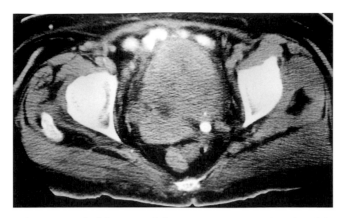

FIG. 117–1. A CT scan of the lower abdominal and pelvic area demonstrates the large solid mass with distortion of the anatomy and obstruction to the distal ureter. A small amount of contrast can be seen in the lumina of the small bowel as the mass distorts and compresses the bowel anteriorly.

A pelvic examination and cystoscopy was performed under anesthesia. On the anterior surface of the vagina there was obvious tumor, which was friable and bled easily. A dilation and curettage was performed. A biopsy specimen of the tumor was obtained. On cystoscopy, the bladder was filled with clots and a large necrotic tumor seemed to be arising from the left side of the bladder encompassing most of the trigone and the left bladder wall. The left ureteral orifice could not be identified. The right ureteral orifice was in normal position and did not appear to be involved with tumor. Multiple biopsies of the bladder and tumor were obtained. The biopsies were all reported as moderately well-differentiated squamous cell carcinoma of the urinary bladder with extension into the

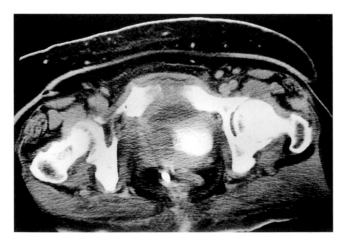

FIG. 117–2. This view obtained on the CT scan taken at the lower abdominal and pelvic area shows some partial filling with contrast in the urinary bladder; however, the lumen is greatly distorted and compressed by the bulk of the tumor mass. The limits of this tumor are difficult to define on these views.

anterior vaginal wall (Figs. 117–3 and 117–4). Tissue from the dilation and curettage was normal.

A joint consultation conference was obtained from Medical Oncology, Radiation Therapy, and Urologic Oncology. The medical oncologist acknowledged that while transitional cell carcinoma of the urinary bladder is responsive to the use of multiple chemotherapeutic agents such as MVAC, the squamous cell tumors are considerably less responsive. In view of the large volume of cancer, the anticipated response from multiagent neoadjunctive treatment would be minimal. Since there was already obstruction to the left ureter and possibly involvement of the right ureter on the trigone base, the possibility of renal failure from obstruction would be very likely in the future. In view of these findings, it was believed that debulking of the tumor and possibly urinary diversion would be appropriate, and then proceed with chemotherapy when the likelihood of ureteral obstruction and renal failure would be less. The planned postoperative chemotherapy would be the standard protocol developed at Memorial Sloan-Kettering Center using methotrexate, vinblastine, Adriamycin, and cisplatin (MVAC).

Radiation therapy would be an acceptable adjuvant; however, the response of squamous cell carcinoma of the urinary bladder is considerably less than that of transitional cell carcinoma. The effectiveness of radiation therapy with a large tumor mass would be less because of large central ischemia areas. It would be better to treat residual tumor with radiation therapy. Postoperative radiation therapy might be complicated by damage to the surrounding structure such as the bowel, because after operation, the bowel would be less mobile and receive the full effect of any radiation in the therapeutic fields. Nonetheless, it was believed that this complication would be of less concern than the problems encountered with a large bulky tumor.

The final recommendation was that the patient undergo surgery with the plan to perform an anterior exenteration with pelvic lymph node dissection. At that time, the bladder, anterior vagina, and uterus, along with the tubes and ovaries, would be removed. A conventional ileal conduit urinary diversion would be used for management of the urinary tract. This procedure was carried out on the 12th day following the hospital admission. At the time of surgery, a large bulky tumor was identified at the bladder base with extension into the vagina and also the anterior lower aspect of the uterus. There was no extension into the sidewalls, and the tumor was not identified in any lymph nodes. However, there were several small nodules in the mesentery of the small bowel overlying the bladder and uterus. It was recommended that during the postoperative period, the patient undergo combined chemotherapy using the MVAC routing. No radiation therapy was anticipated at this time but would be reserved for a later time if any metastatic lesions appeared.

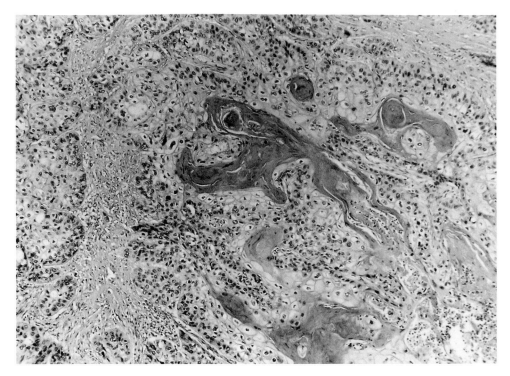

FIG. 117–3. Photomicrograph of the tumor obtained from a biopsy performed at the time of cystoscopy. The squamous cell carcinoma with abundant keratin formation is clearly identified on this low-power view.

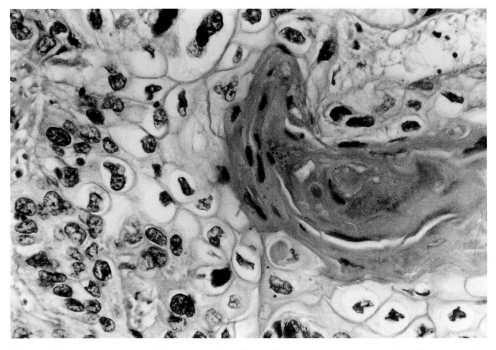

FIG. 117–4. High-power view of tissue obtained from the specimen removed at the time of the anterior exenteration shows the aggressive cellular pattern with large components of keratin and squamous cell carcinoma.

COMMENTARY by Carl A. Olsson

Squamous cell carcinoma of the bladder is a relatively uncommon vesical malignancy. In the Western world, it accounts for approximately 5% of all bladder cancers. In certain African and Near-Eastern countries the incidence of squamous cell cancer of the bladder is much higher, even exceeding the incidence of the more common transitional cell variety. The putative etiologic factor responsible for the increased incidence of squamous cancer in these geographic locales is the endemic prevalence of schistosomiasis (1–5). As compared with transitional cell cancer, in which a 3:1 male predominance is common, squamous cancers affect women at least with equal frequency as men (6).

A number of reports have indicated the relatively worse prognosis of squamous cell cancer of the bladder versus transitional cell variants (7,8). However, these reports may have been biased by the inclusion of the epidermoid variants of transitional cell carcinoma, generally regarded as grade IV lesions.

Furthermore, they may be biased by the observation (at least in some geographic locales) that squamous cell carcinoma of the bladder presents at a higher stage than its transitional cell counterpart. At least one compelling study has shown that, stage for stage, squamous cell carcinoma of the urinary bladder exerts no greater adverse prognosis than does transitional cell carcinoma (6).

As indicated in the case presentation, squamous cell cancer of the bladder is often overlooked until such time as a fairly large mass has arisen (7). In general, the symptomatic presentation of a squamous cell bladder cancer is dysuria alone, or microhematuria (6). This presentation is often misinterpreted as urinary tract infection and treated without further urologic investigation until such time as persistence of symptomatology prompts definitive urologic study.

With the presentation of a high stage malignancy, strategies incorporating adjunctive treatment are appropriate. In transitional cell cancers of the urinary bladder, preoperative chemotherapy is presently regarded as the appropriate adjunct (9). However, in pure squamous cell lesions, there is no patient who has unilateral renal obstruction. Even if this were a squamous variant of a transitional cell cancer, we would ordinarily carry out percutaneous nephrostomy drainage prior to the administration of MVAC, in order that maximal dosage regimens could be utilized.

Radiation therapy is generally regarded as an ineffective preoperative adjunct in transitional cell cancers of the bladder (10). Although a number of patients are downstaged, and such downstaged patients enjoy an excellent prognosis as compared with those individuals who do not experience downstaging, prospective randomized trials of surgery versus radiation therapy followed by surgery have shown no differences in overall survival.

In squamous cell cancers of the bladder, there has been only a single prospectively randomized study to analyze the influence of preoperative radiation therapy (11). Some studies suggest the favorable influence of preoperative radiation therapy; other studies have shown no influence whatever (11–13).

In the present, I would not disagree with a formal surgical approach to this patient with squamous cell cancer of the bladder. I would agree with the presenters that preoperative chemotherapy, consisting of methotrexate, phenblastine, Adriamycin, and cis-platinum should not be utilized. Prior studies with the MVAC regimen have shown no influence of this drug combination on pure squamous cell lesions (9). Although the combination may have some effect against transitional cell variants with epidermoid features (high-grade transitional cell carcinoma), there appears to be no effect on pure epidermoid cancers.

Whether or not preoperative radiation therapy might have played a role in this patient's management is unclear. Our usual prejudice is to agree with the presenters in a de novo surgical procedure.

Upon review of the pathology report in this case, it is clear that the patient has high-stage disease. The cancer has not only grown through the entire thickness of the bladder wall but has also invaded the adjacent vagina. An anterior exenteration as conducted in this patient is the appropriate management. Whether or not any postoperative adjunct should be used in this patient remains an enigma.

We have seen a patient with presumed pure squamous cell cancer of the bladder who, upon further histologic analysis of a final resected specimen, demonstrates that the squamous cancer is an epidermoid feature of a highly aggressive transitional cell lesion. In these circumstances, it is appropriate to consider postoperative administration of MVAC.

In contrast to the presenters' management, I would not consider postoperative MVAC because the lesion has been shown to be purely squamous in nature. Postoperative radiation therapy has not been documented to be a benefit. However, if any of the mesenteric nodules were left in situ, I would certainly consider the postoperative administration of radiation therapy, regardless of any potential adverse effects on bowel function.

REFERENCES

1. Sarma KP. Squamous cell carcinoma of the bladder. *Int Surg* 1970;53:313.
2. El Boulkany MN, Ghoneim MA, Mansour MA. Carcinoma of the bilharzial bladder in Egypt. *Br J Urol* 1972;44:561–4.
3. Khurana P, Morad N, Khan AR, Shetty S, Ibrahim A, Patil K. Impact of schistosomiasis on urinary bladder cancer in the southern province of Saudi Arabia: review of 60 cases. *J Trop Med Hyg* 1992;95:149–51.
4. Sharifi ARA, El Sir S, Beleil O. Squamous cell carcinoma of the urinary bladder. *Br J Urol* 1992;69:369–71.
5. Aghaji AE, Mbonu OO. Bladder tumors in Enugu, Nigeria. *Br J Urol* 1989;64:399–402.
6. Richie J, Waisman J, Skinner DG, Dretler SP. Squamous carcinoma of the bladder: treatment by radical cystectomy. *J Urol* 1976;115:670–2.

7. Miller A, Mitchell JP, Brown NJ. The bristol bladder tumor registry. *Br J Urol* 1969;41(suppl):24.
8. Besette PL, Abell MR, Herwig KR. A clinicopathologic study of squamous cell carcinoma of the bladder. *J Urol* 1974;112:66.
9. Sternberg CN, Yagoda A, Sher HI, Watson RC, Ahmed T, Weiselberg LR, Geller N, Hollander PS, Herr HW, Sogani PC, Morse MJ, Whitmore WF. Preliminary results of M-VAC for transitional cell carcinoma of the urothelium. *J Urol* 1985;133:403.
10. Radwin HM. Radiotherapy and bladder cancer: a critical review. *J Urol* 1980;124:43.
11. Ghoneim MA, Ashamallah AK, Awaad HK Whitmore WF, Jr. Randomized trial of cystectomy with or without preoperative radiotherapy for carcinoma of the bilharzial bladder. *J Urol* 1985;134: 266.
12. Swanson D, Liles A, Zagars G. Preoperative irradiation and radical cystectomy for stages T2 and T3 squamous cell carcinoma of the bladder. *J Urol* 1990;143:37–40.
13. Rundle JSH, Hart AJL, McGeorge A, et al. Squamous cell carcinoma of the bladder. A review of 114 patients. *Br J Urol* 1982;54:522.

SECTION XXV

Kidney

118 Carcinoma of the Kidney with Vena Cava Thrombus (T3b, N0, M0)

John Horton and Julio Pow-Sang

A tumor at high-risk for recurrence. Interleukin-2 and alpha-interferon may be beneficial

CASE PRESENTATION

T.C., a morbidly obese 38-year-old male aircraft construction worker, presented with exacerbation of a 2-week history of right flank pain. He had been evaluated in an emergency room elsewhere, where intravenous pyelography demonstrated multiple calcifications in, and poor excretion from, the right kidney. He had no gross hematuria. Cystoscopy was performed. Placement of a double J stent and analgesics were prescribed. The past history included hypertension for 4 years, and he had prior tonsillectomy, circumcision, and left elbow and shoulder surgery. He had smoked 60 cigarettes daily for 20 years, but drank no alcohol. The family history was unremarkable.

Examination showed a grossly obese man in mild distress from pain. His weight was 420 pounds, pulse 80/min and regular, blood pressure 150/90, temperature 98°F, performance status excellent. There was no evidence of cervical lymphadenopathy or a flank mass, but mild edema of the left ankle was present. Complete blood count, differential, platelet count, and chemical profile were all normal. Urinalysis showed red blood cells in the spun specimen. Electrocardiogram was normal. Chest radiography was normal, but computed tomography (CT) of the abdomen demonstrated a large right renal mass with a thrombus in the inferior vena cava (IVC) extending to the level of the superior mesenteric artery (Fig. 118–1). Arteriography was not possible because of the morbid obesity. Ultrasound showed no thrombus in the heart or superior vena cava. The preoperative diagnosis was right renal carcinoma with tumor extension to the inferior vena cava (Robson Stage C).

Anticoagulation with heparin was begun, and consultation with thoracic surgery obtained in case of need for cardiopulmonary bypass. He then underwent right radical nephrectomy with venacavotomy, resection of the vena cava tumor, and placement of a Greenfield filter.

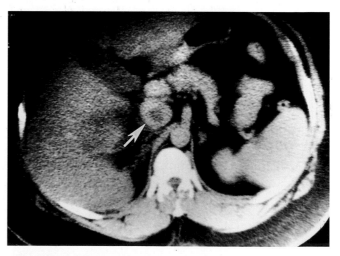

FIG. 118–1. Abdominal CT scan showing tumor thrombosis in the inferior vena cava. The technical quality of the study is not ideal because of morbid obesity.

595

The gross pathology showed the lateral and upper two thirds of the kidney to be replaced by tumor, with visible thrombus at the hilum extending into blood vessels. The microscopic diagnosis (Fig. 118–2) was renal carcinoma with vascular invasion at the hilum and in the perinephric fat. Removed aortocaval nodes were not involved by tumor.

The patient recovered after a stormy postoperative course with complications including deep vein thromboses in the legs, small bowel perforation, wound infection, and aspiration pneumonitis. No adjuvant cytotoxic, biologic, or radiation therapy was advised.

During follow-up, 6 months after operation, he was noted to have an isolated 5-cm mass in the left upper lung field (Fig. 118–3). This was excised and shown to be a metastasis. In vitro chemosensitivity testing suggested the tumor might respond to doxorubicin. He received this drug in a weekly schedule for 12 doses, but developed increasing pain due to new bone metastases. He died with disseminated metastases 1 year after his initial presentation.

COMMENTARY by Richard D. Williams

This case illustrates the not uncommon presentation of renal cancer (RCC) that has extended into the renal vein and vena cava below the hepatic veins (10%–12%). The patient presented with flank pain, microhematuria, and mild ankle edema. No other physical findings or paraneoplastic syndromes were present, with the possible exception of mild hypertension (liver function tests and serum calcium were not available). An IVP showed diffuse calcifications in the renal mass, which is commonly associated with renal cancer (more than 80% of such masses are RCC). CT of the abdomen showed no evidence of metastasis, and a chest radiograph showed no lesions. A full metastatic work-up to include chest CT and bone scan would have been optimal in this patient. To evaluate the renal mass, CT is usually adequate with no further information gained by arteriography unless the mass is equivocal on CT or a partial nephrectomy is contemplated. Evaluation of the thrombus is not optimal by CT alone

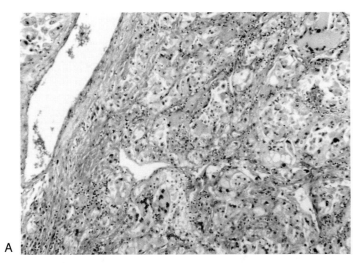

A

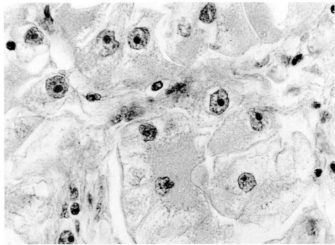

B

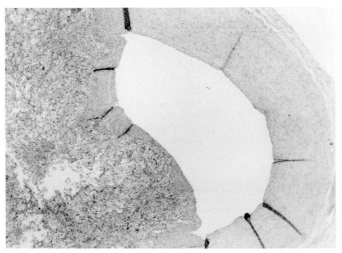

C

FIG. 118–2. Histopathology of the primary renal tumor. The large clear cells with rich vascularization, hemorrhage, and foci of necrosis are characteristic for adenocarcinoma of the kidney. **A:** Renal carcinoma, poorly differentiated clear cell. **B:** Renal carcinoma, high power. **C:** Renal carcinoma demonstrating involvement of the vena cava

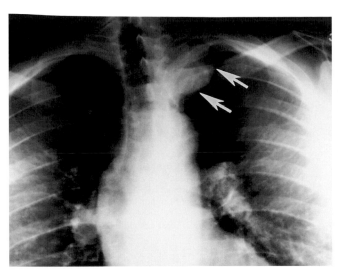

FIG. 118–3. Posteroanterior chest radiograph showing a 5-cm pleural-based nodule in the apex of the left lung (arrows).

and usually abdominal ultrasound, as was done in this case, or MRI can accurately depict the thrombus and its cephalic extent in the cava. Treatment of this patient with short caval extension by radical nephrectomy and caval tumor thrombectomy was routine without the need for cardiopulmonary bypass—the addition of anticoagulation and the Greenfield filter were prophylactic against pulmonary emboli in this obese man but not necessary in the usual caval thrombus patient.

Renal cancer can be cured surgically in nearly 70% of patients with stage T1 or T2 tumors. Patients with stage T3 tumors, as in this case, have a 15% to 24% 5-year survival after a radical nephrectomy. Recurrences are primarily in the lung (50%), long bones (10%–20%), or variable other sites. In this patient, metastasis at the time of presentation was likely, and an initial full metastatic work-up may have revealed the lesions discovered 6 months later. If a solitary metastasis was seen in the lung at the time of his initial presentation and no other lesions outside the primary were revealed, then a radical nephrectomy and simultaneous pulmonary resection would have been appropriate (20%–30% 5-year survival).

Consideration of adjuvant therapy would have been reasonable if there were appropriate agents of proven benefit. In general, cytotoxic chemotherapy has been of little value for metastatic RCC. Single agents, such as vinblastine, have shown a modest response rate, but few complete responses and fewer long-term survivors are reported. Combination chemotherapy has fared no better. *In vitro* chemosensitivity testing for RCC has shown no particular advantage in choosing therapeutic agents.

Adjuvant radiation therapy has not been shown to be of any benefit. Radiation to bone metastases to abate bone pain is the sole use of radiation therapy in RCC.

Immunotherapy has shown the most promise with regard to treatment of metastatic RCC. Alpha interferon

(IFN-A) can render responses in 15% to 20% of patients, few of which are complete, with only occasional long-term survivors. The toxicity is dose related, but tolerable in general. Vinblastine and IFN-A combined have not shown an improved response rate. Interleukin-II (IL-2) alone has shown a similar response rate (up to 20%) with a slightly increased complete response rate ±5%, which has resulted in FDA approval of IL-2 for the treatment of metastatic RCC. IL-2 is toxic in high doses, but low-dose outpatient regimens have recently shown similar results with less toxicity.

The addition of autologous lymphokine-activated killer cells (LAK) to IL-2 treatment has shown up to a 30% response rate at NCI but has not been duplicated in other venues. The addition of tumor-infiltrative lymphocytes (TIL) to IL-2 has been disappointing. The response rates are no better than IL-2 alone. Perhaps use of cytotoxic lymphocytes specific to autologous tumor cells will be more successful, but data are not yet available. Recently, autolymphocyte therapy has shown approximately the same efficacy as IFN-A alone, but data are incomplete. Current evidence suggests that the combination of IFN-A and IL-2 is the most efficacious regimen, giving up to a 35% response rate with an increased number of complete responses and perhaps long-term survivors. This combination, coupled with surgical removal of areas of incomplete response in selected patients, may improve survival, but again, long-term data are not available.

Based on these data, an inference could be drawn that adjuvant immunotherapy may be as efficacious using the same regimens as applied in patients with metastatic disease. The only data reported thus far from randomized adjuvant trials are the use of Provera versus placebo, and a recent trial of IFN-A versus placebo, neither of which has shown improved survival in the treated groups as compared with placebo groups.

In the patient presented, an initial full metastatic work-up might have shown disseminated disease, in which case IL-2 plus IFN-A could have been given before surgical intervention, and the kidney and any residual masses removed if a significant response was obtained. Surgical removal of the primary tumor (in a patient with metastases) without successful prior therapy or access to a promising adjuvant protocol would not be beneficial. In this patient, who had complete surgical removal of the primary tumor and thrombus with negative margins, adjuvant therapy would not have been chosen (presuming the complete preoperative metastatic work-up showed no evidence of tumor spread) because there is no evidence of survival benefit from any known adjuvant treatment. Despite this, if both the patient and the physician wished to initiate treatment, a combination of IFN-A and IL-2 would seem most promising at present.

In this young man, who was not treated by postoperative adjuvant therapy, another metastatic work-up should have been completed when he developed metastatic disease to the lung. If the lung lesion was solitary, excision was appropriate. If not solitary, the use of IFN-A and IL-2 or another promising protocol would be appropriate. If the lung lesion was completely removed, the same principles regarding adjuvant therapy mentioned above would be used.

SELECTED READINGS

1. Williams RD. Renal, perirenal and ureteral neoplasms. In *Adult and pediatric urology,* Gillenwater JY, Grayhack JT, Howards SS, Duckett JW, eds. New York: Year Book Medical Publishers; 1987;513–54; 2nd ed, 1991;571–614.

2. Figlin RA, Pierce WC, Belledegrun A. Combination biologic therapy with IL-2 and IFN-A in the outpatient treatment of metastatic renal cell carcinoma. *Semin Oncol* 1993;20:11–5.

3. deKernion JB, Ramming KP, Smith RB. The natural history of advanced renal cell carcinoma: a computer analysis. *J Urol* 1978;120: 148–52.

4. Montie JE, Stewart BH, Stratton RA, et al. The role of adjunctive nephrectomy in patients with metastatic renal cell carcinoma. *J Urol* 1977;117:272–5.

5. Krown SE. Interferon treatment of renal cell carcinoma: current status and future prospects. *Cancer* 1987;59:647–51.

6. Rosenberg SA, Lotze MT, Yang JC, et al. Experience with the use of high-dose Interleukin II in the treatment of 652 cancer patients. *Ann Surg* 1989;210:474–85.

7. Rosenberg SI, Spiess PJ, Lafrenier ER. A new approach to the adopted immunotherapy of cancer with tumor infiltrating lymphocytes. *Science* 1986;233:1318–21.

8. Yagoda A. Chemotherapy of renal cell carcinoma 1983–1989. *Semin Urol* 1989;7:199–206.

119

Stage IV Renal Cell Carcinoma with Resectable Primary Tumor

Robert Eyre, Charles Shapiro, and Richard Ober

What is the role of nephrectomy?

CASE PRESENTATION

A 53-year-old man presented to his physician with an episode of right-sided abdominal pain, two episodes of gross hematuria, and mild left shoulder pain. Physical examination was unremarkable. There were no palpable abdominal masses, extremity edema, or neurologic findings.

An IVP and subsequent abdominal CT scan revealed an 11 × 12 cm necrotic left renal mass with a soft tissue mass along the inferior vena cava at the level of the liver consistent with enlarged lymph nodes (Fig. 119-1). Chest CT revealed multiple nodules throughout both lung fields, the largest of which measured 7 cm in greatest diameter (Fig. 119-2). Several pleural-based nodules were also seen, as were small paratracheal lymph nodes. A bone scan showed increased uptake in the area of the left shoulder, and an MRI showed a 4 × 5 × 3 cm irregular mass involving the humerus and deltoid muscle origin (Fig. 119-3). A needle biopsy of a pleural-based chest nodule was felt to be consistent with renal cell carcinoma. He was referred to the Tumor Board for consideration of therapeutic options.

TUMOR BOARD DISCUSSION

This 53-year-old man presents with a potentially resectable large renal tumor metastatic to the parenchyma and pleura of the lung, and with a bone/soft tissue metastasis to the left shoulder. The question is raised whether there is a role for nephrectomy in this patient.

It is estimated that there will be 27,200 new cases of renal cell carcinoma (RCC) diagnosed in 1993, and 30%–40% of these will be stage IV at diagnosis (1). The disease remains refractory to conventional chemotherapeutic or radiotherapeutic options, and the prognosis for these patients is dismal, with 2-year to 5-year estimated survival rates of 20%, and less than 10%, respectively. Location of metastasis and tumor burden at diagnosis, reflected in tumor size, the number of metastatic sites (2), and weight loss of greater than 10% (3), appear to be the

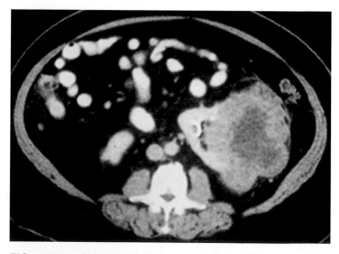

FIG. 119–1. Abdominal CT scan shows a large left renal mass. The inferior vena cava is of normal caliber.

599

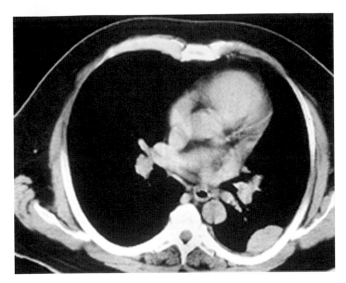

FIG. 119–2. Chest CT shows a large posterior pleural-based mass. Biopsy was consistent with metastatic renal cell cancer.

most important factors related to survival. The role of nephrectomy in stage IV disease must be critically evaluated with respect to three issues: symptom palliation; the possibility of spontaneous regression of metastasis; and the possibility of improved response rates to biologic therapy. Relatively firm indications for nephrectomy include the palliation of intractable pain or hematuria. Severe pain often indicates hemorrhage, or necrosis of the tumor, or malignant invasion of adjacent viscera or the abdominal wall. In the latter situation, surgical interven-

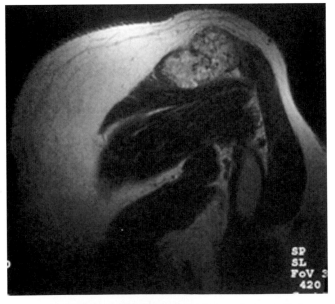

FIG. 119–3. MRI of left shoulder shows a large soft tissue mass. Biopsy was consistent with metastatic renal cell cancer.

tion may not relieve the pain and carries potentially high morbidity. It is rare that hematuria occurs to a degree that necessitates nephrectomy, and most patients can be managed with periodic transfusions to manage the symptoms associated with anemia. Since metastatic lesions may elaborate hormonal substances that produce paraneoplastic syndromes, cytoreductive nephrectomy for this indication is arguable. Thus, in the patient who currently has an ECOG performance status of 0, nephrectomy cannot be justified in order to provide palliation.

Several series have reported the incidence of spontaneous regression of metastasis following nephrectomy to be less than 1%. Such responses are usually of short duration and primarily occur in patients with low-volume, lung-only metastasis (4). Although deKernion reported significantly improved survival in a group of patients with stage IV disease who underwent nephrectomy, it was felt to represent selection bias, with patients in poor preoperative condition or with extensive disease not chosen for surgery (5).

With the advent of immunotherapy protocols for RCC has come the question of whether cytoreductive nephrectomy can provide improved response rates or confer survival advantage to patients treated with biologic therapies such as interleukin-2 or interferon-alpha (IFN-alpha). Before being considered for such programs, patients require a head CT, as CNS metastasis precludes the use of interleukin-2-based therapies. One also needs to assess cardiac, pulmonary, and renal function prior to therapy (6).

In a recent report from the National Cancer Institute, 40% of 93 patients undergoing nephrectomy failed to receive immunotherapy due to surgical complication or, more commonly, progression of disease postoperatively (7). The best predictor of failure to receive therapy was a preoperative ECOG performance status of 2. However, the study did demonstrate an improved response rate to IL-2-based therapy following nephrectomy. Recent reports have also indicated an improved response to IFN-alpha therapy following cytoredective nephrectomy (8,9). Again, selection bias may play a role in these studies.

Critics of cytoreductive nephrectomy argue that more patients might receive treatment if they did not incur the morbidity of surgery, and that response to immunotherapy should select that group of patients who are most likely to benefit from nephrectomy. Fleischmann and Kim (10) reported treatment of 10 patients with primary tumor in place. Of nine evaluable patients, three had complete regression of all sites of metastasis, and two were rendered tumor-free by nephrectomy after therapy. Clearly, the role for cytoreductive nephrectomy in patients who are candidates for immunotherapy awaits completion of prospective randomized trials comparing pretreatment nephrectomy to biologic therapy alone. Several recent studies have shown no therapeutic efficacy to lymphokine-activated killer cells plus IL-2 over IL-2 alone, equivalent responses with low-dose versus high-dose IL-2 (with significantly reduced morbidity), and increased response rates with combinations of IL-2, interferon, and conventional chemotherapeutic agents.

At the present time, I feel that nephrectomy for stage IV renal cell carcinoma should be reserved for patients without evidence of locally extensive disease who have low-volume metastatic disease to a single organ that is also potentially resectable (particularly lung), for those rare patients who are not palliated with more conservative measures as noted above, or for those patients whose ECOG performance status is 0-1 who will be enrolled in an immunotherapy protocol. For the patient presented here, I do not feel that nephrectomy is indicated unless he were to have a dramatic response to biologic therapy.

Follow-up

The patient was enrolled in a protocol to receive daily subcutaneous IL-2 injections. After three weeks of therapy he had noted mild fatigue and flu-like symptoms and a three-pound weight gain. He was restaged after three months of therapy. The renal tumor has slightly increased in size; the mediastinal and paratracheal lymph nodes had decreased slightly in size; the largest pleural-based metastasis had increased in size; and the left shoulder lesion had enlarged. No tumor was noted in the liver. He felt well.

REFERENCES

1. Thrasher JB, Paulson DF: Prognostic factors in renal cancer. *Urol Clin N Am* 1993;20(2):247–62.
2. Frank W, Stuhldreher D, Suffrin R, Shott S, Guinan S: Stage IV renal cell carcinoma. *J Urol* 1994;152:1990–9.
3. Neves RJ, Zincke H, Taylor WF: Metastatic renal cell cancer and radical nephrectomy: Identification of prognostic factors and patient survival. *J Urol* 1988;139:1173–6.
4. Flanigan RC: The failure of infarction and/or nephrectomy in stage IV renal cancer to influence survival or metastasis regression. *Urol Clin N Am* 1987;14:757.
5. deKernion JB, Ramming KP, Smith RB: The natural history of metastatic renal cell carcinoma: A computer analysis. *J Urol* 1978; 120:148.
6. Taneja SS, Pierce W, Figlin R, Belldegrun A: Management of disseminated kidney cancer. *Urol Clin North Am* 1994;21:625–37.
7. Walther MM, Alexander RB, Weiss GH, et al: Cytoreductive surgery prior to interleukin-2-based therapy in patients with metastatic renal cell carcinoma. *Urology* 1993;42:250.
8. Belldegrun AB, Koo AS, et al: Immunotherapy for advanced renal cell carcinoma: The role of radical nephrectomy. *Eur Urol* 1990;18:42.
9. Minasian LM, Motzer RJ, Gluck L, et al: Interferon alpha-2A in advanced renal cell carcinoma: Treatment results and survival in 159 patients with long-term follow-up. *J Clin Oncol* 1993;7:1368.
10. Fleischmann JD, Kim B: Interleukin-2 immunotherapy followed by resection of residual renal cell carcinoma. *J Urol* 1991;145:938.

COMMENTARY by Kenneth I. Wishnow

In general, patients with metastatic renal cell carcinoma have a dismal prognosis with five-year survival rates of 5%–10% and ten-year survival rates of 0%–7%. Accordingly, I believe that only palliative nephrectomy should be considered for patients with multiple metastatic lesions and concur with the authors that nephrectomy should not be performed in this patient with multiple pulmonary and bony metastases.

There is a small subset of patients with stage IV renal cell carcinoma, however, who may benefit from a complete resection. In 1967, Middleton reported a 35% five-year survival rate in fifty-nine patients with a solitary metastasis who were aggressively treated by nephrectomy and complete resection of the metastasis (1). In 1975, Tolia and Whitmore confirmed these results, again reporting a 35% five-year survival rate in nineteen patients who were treated by complete surgical resection (2). More recently, Dernevik et al (3) and Thrasher et al (4) reported increased survival in patients with multiple pulmonary metastases who were treated by nephrectomy and complete surgical resection of the pulmonary metastases.

It should be emphasized that patients with a solitary metastasis or even multiple pulmonary lesions which are easily amenable to complete surgical excision form a small subset of stage IV patients. However, nephrectomy and complete surgical resection may be beneficial and even curative in some of these highly selected patients.

REFERENCES

1. Middleton RG: Surgery for metastatic renal cell carcinoma. *J Urol* 1967;97:973.
2. Tolia BM, Whitmore WF Jr.: Solitary metastasis from renal cell carcinoma. *J Urol* 1975;114:836.
3. Dernevik L, Berggren H, Larsson S, et al: Surgical removal of pulmonary metastasis from renal cell carcinoma. *Scan J Urol Nephrol* 1985;19:133.
4. Thrasher JB, Clark JR, Cleland BP: Surgery for pulmonary metastases from renal cell carcinoma. Army experience form 1977–1987. *Urology* 1990;35:487.

120

Unresectable Carcinoma of the Urinary Bladder with Intractable Hematuria

Brian J. Moran

Successful palliation with local resection and radiotherapy

CASE PRESENTATION

W.S. is an 81-year-old white woman who was admitted to the Emergency Room with the complaint of having gross hematuria for approximately 1 month. Evaluation at this time revealed a hemoglobin of 7.0 g and hematocrit of 20.9%. The patient was evaluated with cystoscopy and IVP. A large tumor of the right bladder wall was noted. The tumor itself measured 4 × 4 cm in dimension, and extended inferiorly to involve the bladder neck. The patient was also found to have a concomitant urinary tract infection with large amounts of bacteria in the urine, and an elevated white blood count of 15.5. Past medical history is significant for coronary artery disease, myocardial infarction ×2, and coronary artery bypass grafts times four vessels. The patient also has significant chronic obstructive pulmonary disease. Medications included Lanoxin, Lasix, Ecotrin, Prinivil, Ventolin, and aspirin.

Radiographic Studies

The chest roentgenogram did not reveal any evidence of metastatic disease, however, there was some evidence of emphysema present. An intravenous pyelogram revealed a filling defect occupying the right lateral aspect of the urinary bladder, suggestive of malignant tumor (Fig. 120–1).

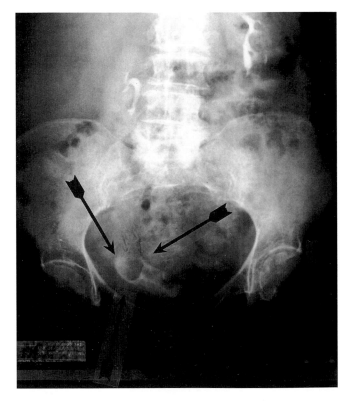

FIG. 120–1. An intravenous pyelogram revealing a filling defect occupying the right lateral aspect of the urinary bladder.

TUMOR BOARD DISCUSSION

Dr. Moran (Moderator): Dr. Flaster, in your opinion what would be the initial step in the management of this elderly woman with numerous other medical problems?

Dr. Flaster (Urologist): This is an elderly, frail woman with significant comorbid medical conditions. She did undergo cystoscopy, which confirmed the presence of this rather aggressive-appearing tumor. This was done, of course, after the patient was given whole blood so that she could tolerate such a procedure.

Dr. Moran (Moderator): Dr. Flaster, would this patient have been a candidate for cystectomy?

Dr. Flaster (Urologist): I do not think that this patient would be a good candidate for a cystectomy, given her medical condition at the time of diagnosis. Therefore, our approach was to maximally resect the tumor so as to control the problem at hand, which was her gross hematuria and resultant anemia.

Dr. Moran (Moderator): Can we now review the pathology report?

Dr. Bhatia (Pathologist): The pathologic finding is consistent with a necrotic grade III, poorly differentiated transitional cell carcinoma of the urinary bladder. There is extensive infiltration of the muscle wall with malignant tumor, and there is also extensive perineural invasion present (Fig. 120–2).

Dr. Moran (Moderator): Dr. Sowray, in your opinion is this patient a suitable candidate for systemic chemotherapy?

Dr. Sowray (Medical Oncologist): Systemic chemotherapy utilizing an MVAC protocol for the treatment of invasive transitional cell carcinoma is now becoming more popular. The therapy is given in an effort to downstage carcinomas of the bladder. Much of this work has been done in an effort to preserve the bladder while locally controlling the tumor. Certainly, there are variances of this protocol that have been proven to be effective against this disease. My concern, however, would be that this patient might not be able to tolerate the recommended doses of these drugs.

Dr. Moran (Moderator): It appears to me that, for this particular patient, aggressive therapy might not be indicated. I would now like to direct our discussion toward the role of palliative therapy and ask the radiation oncologist, Dr. Boyer, his opinion regarding local control of the tumor.

Dr. Boyer (Radiation Oncologist): I believe that this patient would respond at least temporarily to a palliative dose of radiation therapy directed to the urinary bladder. Our intent would be to treat the bladder with approximately 3,000 cGy. This would be done using conventional X-ray therapy produced from a linear accelerator. This dose could be given for approximately 2 to 3 weeks.

Dr. Moran (Moderator): Dr. Boyer, would you comment as to the side effects that this patient might experience?

Dr. Boyer (Radiation Oncologist): We all know that radiation therapy is a local treatment. Therefore, the side effects of the treatment would be confined to the field of radiation. I would anticipate some bladder irritation, but for the most part, I believe the treatment would be very well tolerated. The likelihood of controlling the hematuria, at least temporarily, is quite high. If then at a later date the patient develops recurrent hematuria, we could give an additional course of radiation. One could also pursue a course of more protracted radiation therapy; however, I believe that for this particular patient, palliative intent with a shorter course of therapy would be more suitable.

Follow-up of Patient

The patient did go on to receive localized radiation therapy to the urinary bladder, receiving a dose of 3,250 cGy given over 3 weeks. The treatment was well tolerated, and the patient's hematuria resolved for approximately 7 months. She then developed recurrent hematuria and underwent a repeat cystoscopy. Again, regrowth of tumor was noted at the primary tumor site along the right lateral wall of the bladder. This was maximally resected with the resectoscope by the attending urologist. The patient then received an additional course of external beam radiation to the urinary bladder. Again, this was effective in stopping the hematuria; the patient has now been 4 months without recurrent hematuria. It is important to note, however, that since the initial diagnosis, the patient's general medical condition has deteriorated as a result of her other medical problems. We therefore conclude that the appropriate management was recommended at the time of the initial multidisciplinary Tumor Board Conference.

COMMENTARY by Michael D. Blum

The case presentation summarizes the course of a frail, 81-year-old woman with invasive bladder cancer, managed with local therapy for recurrent significant hematuria and anemia. Treatment included aggressive local resection and palliative radiotherapy. At the time of the report, 11 months of survival has been achieved, with minimal apparent morbidity from therapy. I applaud the efforts of the treating physicians whose therapeutic decisions have been justified by the outcome.

The Tumor Board discussion reviews the options for treatment in these difficult situations. Attempts to cure the patient of her cancer were not entertained due to the

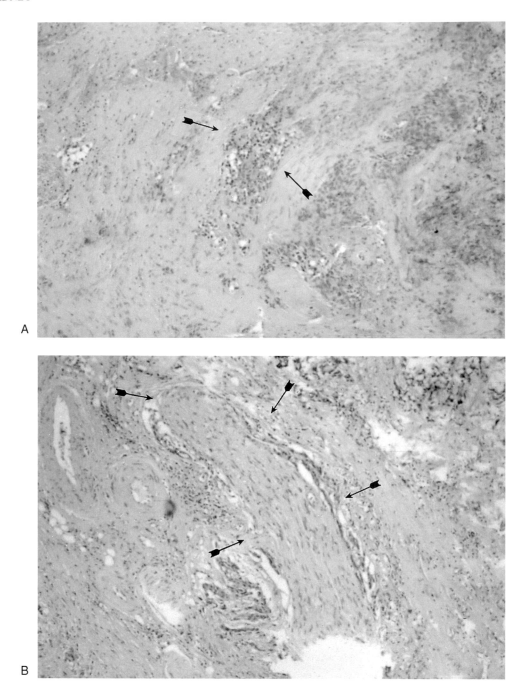

FIG. 120–2A–B. Pathologic specimen showing extensive infiltration of the muscle wall with malignant tumor; there is also extensive perineural invasion present.

patient's advanced age and medical condition. I assume that this decision was made at an early time in the evaluation of this patient, which explains the lack of further diagnostic staging studies, i.e., CT scanning of the abdomen and pelvis and perhaps bone scan. No comment was made regarding the presence of right hydronephrosis on the IVP, thus avoiding the difficult problem of management of the obstructed renal unit in invasive bladder cancer.

Though seldom curative, external beam radiation therapy can certainly accomplish palliation of advanced transitional cell carcinoma of the bladder. The radiotherapy, in concert with the urologist's surgical debulking, has achieved the desired goal of halting the hemorrhage for the duration of the patient's life without causing undue morbidity.

Chemotherapy has made significant advances in the treatment of unresectable transitional cell carcinoma of the bladder. However, the morbidity of the treatment is not inconsequential, and treatment with suboptimal dosage schedules to minimize morbidity will generally result in suboptimal results. Specifically, good cardiac reserve is necessary to tolerate full doses of MVAC therapy, and in this case, was likely lacking.

Surgical options include both endoscopic and open approaches. Endoscopy was successful in this case; and aggressive resection of the tumor mass with extensive efforts at electrocautery can achieve effective palliation. Often, however, the inability to completely resect an invasive tumor down to normal bladder wall can leave a friable, recurrently hemorrhaging tumor surface that remains difficult to manage. Endoscopic use of laser phototherapy using the Nd-Yag laser has been reported as effective in limited cases. Intravesical irrigations with a number of preparations, similar to the treatment of diffuse hemorrhagic cystitis from prior chemotherapy, radiation therapy, or coagulopathies are also effective. Examples of these treatments include silver nitrate, formalin, alum, hypothermic fluid, phenol, and prostaglandins have been reported (1). Systemic therapy with epsilon-amino caproic acid and conjugated estrogens may be effective. Finally, diversion of the urine from the bladder lumen can arrest the bleeding. In-dwelling externalized ureteral stents may eliminate the effect of urokinase-mediated clot lysis. Percutaneous nephrostomies achieve a similar goal and may provide a more long-term, though cumbersome, solution.

Open surgical procedures should not be abandoned, even in the critically ill patient. Open packing of the bladder with ureteral catheter urinary diversion may be a tolerable intervention. Formal urinary diversion with ileal conduit may be accomplished in less than 2 hours, and even total cystectomy with diversion may need to be considered, even with its attendant morbidity and mortality.

Angiographic embolization of the arterial supply of the bladder has been reported, similar to the therapeutic embolization of unresectable renal cell carcinomas with intractable bleeding. Selective embolization of the internal iliac vessels feeding the tumor with autologous clot, Gian-Turco coil, and gelatin foam have been used (2). Complications of bladder necrosis have been reported. Finally, hydrostatic tamponade with the Helmstein balloon has been used but largely abandoned due to complication of bladder rupture.

Intractable bleeding from unresectable urinary tract malignancies can be a vexing and recurrent problem, which was very well managed in this case. The Tumor Board participants are congratulated on their successful management in the case presented.

REFERENCES

1. Yang CC, Hurd DD, Case LD, Assimos DG. Hemorrhagic cystitis in bone marrow transplantation. *Urology* 1994;44:322–8.
2. Carmignai G, Belgrano E, Puppo P, Cichero A, Guiliani L. Transcatherter embolization of the hypogastric arteries in cases of bladder hemorrhage from advanced pelvic malignancies: follow-up in 9 cases. *J Urol* 1980;124:196–200.

121

Carcinoma of the Right Kidney Invading the Colon (T4 N0 M1)

Irving J. Weigensberg

Survival still depends on complete surgical resection. Clinical trials are needed to identify effective adjuvant therapies

CASE PRESENTATION

Dr. Irving Weigensberg: This 47-year-old divorced black woman had noted some mild aching pain in her right flank for several days prior to admission. On the day of admission, she noted abrupt increase of the right flank pain together with hematuria and presented to the Emergency Room. She denied any other urinary or abdominal symptoms. She had lost 22 lbs in weight but had been on a weight-reduction diet. The only positive finding in her past history was asymptomatic and uncomplicated hypertension. She had been normotensive for several months, and her medication had been discontinued. The review of her systems was negative. She denied any other serious illnesses or injuries, and had no prior surgery. Examination on admission revealed her blood pressure to be 157/82. She was markedly obese, weighing 231 pounds. There was minimal tenderness about the right flank. The abdomen was soft, and there were no palpable masses or enlarged abdominal organs. There were no other positive physical findings. Urinalysis confirmed the presence of hematuria. Her admission laboratory findings were otherwise unremarkable.

Acknowledgement:
The Tumor Board acknowledges the following participants: James DeBord, Alan DeBord, James Knost, Gerald Palagallo, John Taraska, and Irving J. Weigensberg

Dr. Gerald Palagallo: The first examination is an intravenous pyelogram. The pertinent finding is that the right kidney is essentially nonfunctioning. The exact etiology of this finding is not delineated on this examination.

On the following day, the patient had CT scan of the abdomen (Fig. 121–1). This demonstrated a large mass involving the right kidney. This is thought to be compatible with a primary neoplasm of the kidney. The interface between the liver and the kidney was poorly defined. There was poor definition of the fat surrounding Gerota's fascia indicating extension of the tumor beyond the capsule of the kidney. At the same time, the patient had a CT scan of the chest and two small indeterminate pulmonary nodules were identified at the lung base, raising the possibility of metastatic disease to the lung.

The patient then had a transfemoral aortogram and right renal arteriogram (Fig. 121–2) followed by an inferior venacavogram. The right renal arteriogram demonstrated a hypervascular right renal mass, the characteristics of which were consistent with a hypernephroma. The inferior venacavogram showed a small area of irregularity at the junction of the right renal vein and the inferior vena cava, indicating that the renal vein had been invaded, but no tumor was identified within the inferior vena cava.

Dr. James DeBord: The abdomen was approached through a large mid-line incision. Exploration revealed that the right colon was attached to, and possibly infil-

606

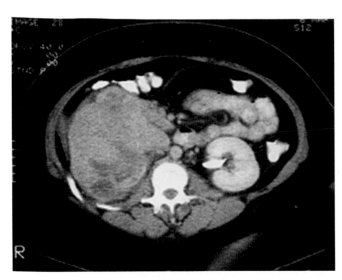

FIG. 121–1. Computed tomography section through the upper abdomen demonstrating the large tumor mass, with areas of necrosis, almost completely filling the right side of the abdomen.

trated by, the large right renal tumor mass. Therefore, the terminal ileum as well as the right and transverse colon were mobilized from their peritoneal attachments. Careful retroperitoneal dissection freed up the right kidney en bloc with the right colon. The retroperitoneal aorta and vena cava were then carefully dissected and the tumor separated by blunt dissection from the vena cava. Using a Satinsky clamp to partially occlude the vena cava, the right renal vein and a contiguous portion of the right lat-

eral wall of the inferior vena cava were excised. This contained within it a small bolus of intraluminal tumor extending from the renal vein and protruding minimally into the inferior vena cava. We were then able to repair the vena cava; the vascular clamp was removed and venous flow resumed. Although there was some deformity of the vena cava here, there remained adequate lumen for normal venous flow, in my opinion.

Dr. Alan DeBord: We dissected the retroperitoneal tissues with the right renal cell tumor. We thought that this would provide the best local resection with potentially curative intent for this large bulky tumor. Surgery with complete excision is still the only known cure for nephrocarcinoma. A primary ileo-transverse colon anastomosis was then performed and the wound closed in the usual manner.

Dr. John Taraska: In reviewing the slides (Fig. 121–3), the first thing we see is that the tumor is composed of large sheets and nests of cells, demonstrating a typical, clear cytoplasmic type of character. The only thing different from the usual renal cell carcinomas is there is more pleomorphism to the nuclei. We have some hyperchromatic nuclei with variation in size and shape and very prominent nucleoli. In many areas, the tumor has a spindloid appearance with the clear cells stretched out. Many other areas demonstrate a septum in between bundles of cells so they form small nodules. Examination of the peripheral portion of the tumor does demonstrate infiltration into the surrounding adipose tissue, and this was noted grossly to be adjacent to a portion of the intestinal tract. Again, what was demonstrated grossly is also demonstrated here microscopically, showing tumor plugs

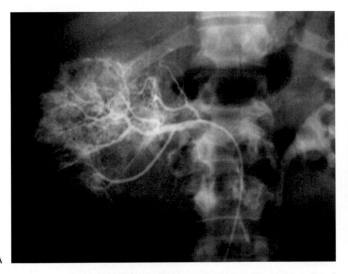

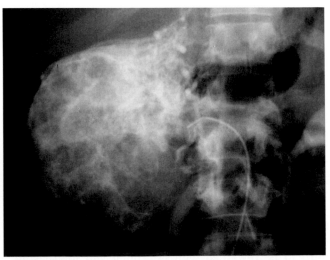

A   B

FIG. 121–2. A: Right renal arteriogram revealing hypervascularity with displacement of vessels around the renal tumor mass. **B:** Later phase in the arteriogram with abnormal vessels, "tumor staining," and collateral venous circulation.

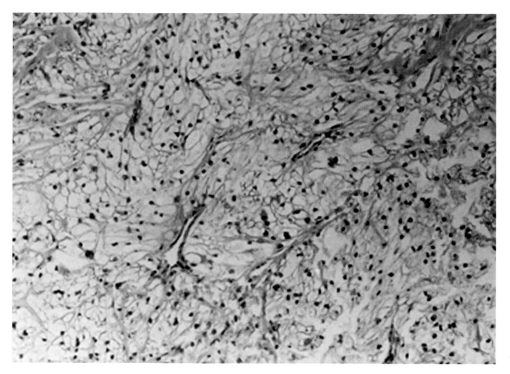

FIG. 121–3. Photomicrograph of the resected tumor.

in the renal vein even though the wall of the vein is not involved with attachment or invasion. Examination of the whole tumor demonstrates several large areas of necrosis and hemorrhage, indicating that these areas of tumor perhaps have outgrown their vascular supply.

Dr. James DeBord: In general, with renal cell carcinoma, an aggressive approach to surgical resection is indicated, including removal of directly involved contiguous organs. An aggressive approach also to intraluminal tumor thrombi in the inferior vena cava and renal vein is thought to be appropriate. Cases of large tumor thrombi into the inferior vena cava require special precautions and care to avoid intraoperative embolization of this tumor and fatal intraoperative massive pulmonary emboli. Occasionally, these patients are best managed by cardiopulmonary bypass in conjunction with a radical nephrectomy when extensive intracaval tumor thrombus is present. This emphasizes the importance of evaluation of the renal vein and vena cava in the initial work-up of patients with renal cell carcinoma where there is suspicion of possible tumor thrombus in the renal vein or inferior vena cava.

Dr. Irving Weigensberg: Radiation therapy has been utilized with advantage for symptomatic, localized lesions, particularly painful bone lesions. Such irradiation can be rewarded with gratifying and long-lasting palliation, but the response has not been consistent or predictable. Systemic forms of treatment for metastases include both hormones and chemotherapy. A small per-

centage of patients have been reported to respond to the administration of progestational agents. However, the frequency of response has been low and not of lasting duration. This is still used, particularly in the absence of other effective treatments and because of its low associated toxicity.

Dr. James Knost: Renal cell carcinoma, malignant melanoma, and nodular lymphoma are the adult solid tumors that are most likely to show spontaneous regressions. However, out of all patients with metastatic renal cell carcinoma, the 5-year survival rate is less than 3%.

In the early 1980s, genetically engineered interferons were used in renal cell carcinoma with roughly a 5%–15% response rate. Starting in the mid-1980s, Rosenberg and others began using IL-2 plus lymphokine-activated killer (LAK) cells in patients with metastatic malignant melanoma. This process, known as LAK/IL-2, has demonstrated quite conclusively that these LAK cells have the ability to kill in a nonspecific fashion. In the test tube, they will kill almost all tumor types. However, in vivo, they have certain "traffic" patterns that do not always bring them into the area of the tumor. This is one, if not the major reason, that LAK/IL-2 therapy is ineffective for certain subpopulations of patients with renal cell carcinoma. LAK cells kill by attaching themselves to the tumor and poking holes in the tumor. These holes are poked by using a molecule named Perforan. LAK cells can produce between 50 and 200 holes in each tumor cell.

An intergroup study showed that the response rate with LAK/IL-2 was roughly 10%-15%, and subsequent FDA information showed the response between LAK/IL-2 and IL-2 alone was essentially the same (1–4). Probably the most important fact to come out of the intergroup study and the work by Rosenberg is the following:

> If a patient with renal cell carcinoma has complete remission when treated with either IL-2 or IL-2 plus LAK, those have been durable, long-lived remissions and in some cases over 5 years.

The drawback to IL-2 is that it causes the "capillary leak syndrome." This leads to hypotension and fluid retention, which in many patients with renal cell carcinoma, makes the treatment prohibitive.

Rosenberg and others have also worked with what is referred to as TIL cells (tumor infiltrated lymphocytes). These are thought to be T-cells with the CD2, CD3, and CD8 cell-surface components that have a certain amount of memory in the T-cell receptor area, making them more specific for the individual's cancer rather than for cancer in general or for a specific subtype of cancer. Formerly, these were generated in polyolefin bags, which made the process cumbersome requiring four to eight incubators to house the developing TIL cells. That process has been streamlined and, today, by using dialysis cassette technology, they can be generated in a small space in a much more economical fashion. Dr. Rosenberg has labeled the TIL cells with the neomycin-resistant gene and has been able to demonstrate that these cells do localize to the tumor site.

The future for the treatment of metastatic renal cell carcinoma rests with the information that was generated in the 1980s, and hopefully, the marriage of T-cell immunology and macrophage immunology will allow for an effective cellular approach to renal cell carcinoma.

In the interim, we are left with using interleukins to treat this disease. There have been several studies from Europe and the United States using IL-2 subcutaneously once a day Monday through Friday for six weeks in a row with a rest period after the sixth week. It appears as if in some patients, this form of IL-2 is as effective as intravenous high-dose IL-2.

Early studies showed that bleomycin and Velban were effective agents in renal cell carcinoma. Subsequent large group studies have brought that into question. Recently, a study has been done with infusional FUDR (flourouracil desoxyriboside), which appears to be promising. The response rates in this study are somewhere between 35% and 40%. Our group is involved in using this form of therapy, either as first-line therapy or in patients who are IL2-resistant. The therapy consists of infusing FUDR for a period of 2 weeks, and then allowing the patient to rest for 2 weeks.

Dr. Irving Weigensberg: There are several interesting and unique aspects of renal carcinoma that merit mention

and further discussion (5,6). This tumor can often present with unsuspected, unique, and interesting manifestations. The primary tumor can be associated with a variety of systemic, paraneoplastic manifestations, such as fever, polycythemia, hypercalcemia, anemia, leukemoid reactions, amyloidosis, and hypertension. The natural history of this tumor can be varied, with a prolonged interval between manifestation of the primary tumor and metastases, a propensity to solitary metastasis, and the not unusual occurrence of metastases becoming clinically evident before the primary tumor in the kidney. These unique and interesting manifestations can be related to the anatomical relationships of the kidneys and their unique access to multiple and diverse routes of spread (Fig. 121–4). The well-known route of renal vein invasion (Fig. 121–4A) into the inferior vena cava and subsequently into the systemic circulation, is readily evident and well known. Tumor cells getting into the systemic circulation in this manner can travel through the right side of the heart into the lung. Although many of these cells will be trapped in pulmonary capillaries, a significant number will not be filtered out by the lung and will travel via the systemic circulation to such remote places as muscles and bones of the extremities, the brain, and so on (Fig. 121–4C). A second portal of access to the systemic circulation is via the regional lymph nodes and lymphatics into the thoracic duct, and thence into the left subclavian vein and superior vena cava (Fig. 121–4B). The tumor can invade small veins that connect with Batson's paravertebral plexus and thence emigrate the entire length of the axial skeleton, including the spine, calvarium, and pelvis

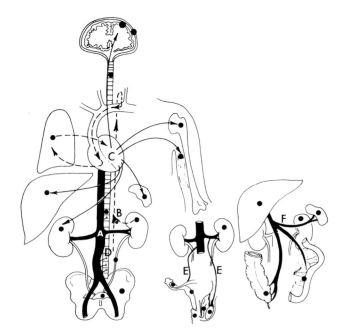

FIG. 121–4. Diagram of metastatic pathways of renal carcinoma (6).

(Fig. 121–4D). Invasion of the renal vein or inferior vena cava, mentioned previously, can also lead to retrograde extension into the spermatic or ovarian veins, and thence to the genitalia (Fig. 121–4E). This route results in metastases in the testes, vagina, vulva, uterus, and adnexae.

Finally, as in the case discussed here, the tumor can extend directly anteriorly into the bowel or mesentery (Fig. 121–4F). This invasion can lead to propagation into the portal venous bed and thence throughout the entire portal drainage bed, such as liver, spleen, and other sites in the bowel and mesentery.

Dr. Alan DeBord: Despite complete dissection with gross total removal in this patient, she developed a recurrence 1 year later. This was a large recurrence in the right renal fossa, which involved the bowel and diaphragm, requiring segmental small bowel resection. Her pulmonary metastases had also progressed, and postoperatively, she received chemotherapy. She expired 5 months later, 1½ years after her initial presentation.

REFERENCES

1. Rosenberg SA. The immunotherapy and gene therapy of cancer. *J Clin Oncol* 10:180–99.
2. Rosenberg SA, Lotze MT, Muul LM, Leitman S, et al. Observations on the systemic administration of autologous lymphokine-activated killer cells and recombinant interleukin-2 to patients with metastatic cancer. *N Engl J Med* 1985;313:1485–92.
3. Rosenberg SA, Lotze MT, Muul LM, et al. A progress report on the treatment of 157 patients with advanced cancer using lymphokine activated killer cells and interleukin-2 or high-dose interleukin-2 alone. *N Engl J Med* 1987;316:889–97.
4. Rosenberg SA, Lotze MT, Yang JC, Aebersold PM, Linehan WM, Seipp CA, White DE. Experience With the use of high-dose interleukin-2 in the treatment of 652 cancer patients. *Ann Surg* 1989;210:474–84.
5. Weigensberg IJ. The many faces of metastatic renal carcinoma. *Radiology* 1971;98:353–8.
6. Weigensberg IJ. Metastatic renal carcinoma: unusual and deceptive presenting features. *South Med J* 1972;65:611–16.

COMMENTARY by Donald G. Skinner

This case illustrates several points in the diagnosis and management of renal cell carcinoma. A nonfunctional kidney on IVP usually suggests the presence of venous involvement with tumor propagation into the renal vein and possibly the vena cava. A CT scan with contrast is the best study to establish the probable diagnosis of renal cell carcinoma and provides important information regarding the vena cava and possible presence of a tumor thrombus. Today, aortography, selective renal angiography, and venacavography are rarely indicated because the best study to determine presence of a vena caval thrombus and its cephalad extent is an MRI focused on the vena cava. Venacavography is usually reserved for those patients with a tumor thrombus extending up the vena cava close to, or possibly into, the right atrium. In these patients, we like to use a transbrachial approach to study the right atrium to determine whether the thrombus has extended into the atrium or can be controlled within the inferior vena cava at its junction with the right atrium.

In this case, a CT scan showed loss of interface between the liver and kidney, suggesting possible direct extension. Because the cancer in most primary renal tumors remains confined within Gerota's fascia, it is rare for renal cell carcinoma to invade directly contiguous structures, such as the liver, colon, pancreas, or spleen. If, however, the CT scan suggests direct extension, I would strongly recommend that the operation be done through a thoraco-abdominal approach. This surgical approach provides much better exposure to the retroperitoneum and is particularly suited to large tumors that may invade the liver, pancreas, spleen, or contiguous viscera. The authors are correct in their statement that the only proven treatment is surgical resection, and I believe the thoraco-abdominal approach provides a much better chance at successful outcome for large cancers than a mid-line approach.

It is unclear how the renal vessels were handled, but inasmuch as these tumors are extremely vascular, it is essential that the first step prior to any mobilization of the ascending colon or the primary tumor is ligation and division of the renal artery. This can be accomplished easily by tracing the inferior mesentery vein up to its junction with the splenic vein, identifying the origin of the superior mesenteric artery, and then identifying and mobilizing the left renal vein, which crosses over the aorta just distal to the origin of the superior mesenteric artery. This allows for early identification, ligation, and division of the right renal artery at its origin from the aorta. There is no mention made of a retroperitoneal lymph node dissection or whether there was any lymph node involvement by cancer. I believe that in large tumors such as this, particularly in a young patient or when the surgeon suspects extension through Gerota's fascia, that an en bloc retroperitoneal lymph node dissection should be part of the operation, as well as the en bloc removal of any involved adjacent organ. The presence or absence of lymph node involvement provides important prognostic information, and lymph node dissection may be curative in up to 25% of patients with positive nodes. The most important therapy is a properly performed radical nephrectomy, because local recurrence in the renal fossa or residual retroperitoneal nodes containing tumor usually results in the death of the patient. At the present time, there is no evidence that adjuvant therapy of any type, given either preoperatively or postoperatively, improves the survival of patients with renal cell carcinoma. Survival depends entirely on complete surgical resection, and prognosis is directly related to the nuclear grade of tumor and the pathologic stage of the primary neoplasm.

Based on Dr. Taraska's description, I suspect this was a grade III–IV tumor because there were prominent nucleoli, pleomorphism of the nuclei, and presence of spindle cells. We know this was at least a stage III tumor, based on the involvement of the renal vein, and possibly stage IV if there was actual tumor invasion of the ascending colon, liver, or if the small pulmonary nodules were in fact metastases. Given these facts, fewer than 30% of patients with stage III, grade IV renal cell carcinoma survive 5 years, and less than 5% of patients with stage IV, grades III or IV tumors survive 5 years.

The recent increase in knowledge of tumor immunology offers new hope for results of immunotherapy, and current clinical trials are well summarized by Dr. Knost. It should be emphasized, however, that to date, no clinical trial has yielded convincing long-term benefits in a significant number of patients with metastatic or advanced disease using any protocol of immunotherapy or chemotherapy. Survival depends entirely on complete surgical resection and, obviously, early diagnosis.

SELECTED READINGS

1. Skinner DG, Colvin RB, Vermillion CD, et al. Diagnosis and management of renal cell carcinoma: a clinical and pathologic study of 309 cases. *Cancer* 1971;20(28):1165–77.
2. Dickerson GR, Colvin RB. Pathology of renal tumors. In: Skinner DG, Lieskovsky G, eds. *Diagnosis and management of genitourinary cancer.* Philadelphia: W.B. Saunders; 1988:118–49.
3. Skinner DG, Lieskovsky G, Pritchett TR. Technique of radical nephrectomy. In: Skinner DG, Lieskovsky G, eds. *Diagnosis and management of genitourinary cancer.* Philadelphia: W.B. Saunders; 1988:684–93.

Spinal Cord

122 Sacrococcygeal Myxopapillary Ependymoma in a Young Man

Homer H. Russ

The importance of a precise pathologic diagnosis

CASE PRESENTATION

Samuel Idarraga (psychiatrist): The patient is a 38-year-old claims manager who works for a major insurance company. He complained of a burning, "grabbing" pain in the right side of the lower back, getting worse over the last 15 months. He had a past history of back pain and had a low lumbar laminectomy 12 years ago and said he felt 95% "normal" after recovering from that. Until his recent flare-up, he had been very active physically, playing golf and racquet ball. He had been taking ibuprofen, 800 mg, three or four times a day. and 25 to 50 mg of amitriptyline at night. A computed tomography (CT) scan and radiographs last year were said to show disc disease and scar tissue. He also complained that he sometimes goes 3 or 4 days without a bowel movement, and then has to take a laxative. This problem sometimes increases the back pain. He had an epidural and facet joint block hoping to relieve the pain, but it did not help much.

Physical examination was essentially normal except for the lower back. Straight leg raising caused pain in the lower back, especially on the right side. Muscle strength seemed normal, sensation was normal, but the right ankle jerk was hypoactive.

We decided to review the previous roentgenograms and CT scans, and to see him in a couple of weeks, at which time we would do electrodiagnostic studies.

When he returned he was much worse. He had a hard time walking, sitting, and laying down. Straight leg raising was intolerable. He claimed his right toes felt numb and that he had a constant pain in the right leg from the knee down on the lateral aspect. The electrodiagnostic studies supported a finding of right lumbosacral radiculopathy. A sedimentation rate was 1 mm per hour and a CBC and Chem. 19 panel was normal. We decided to put him on bedrest and schedule him for a myelogram, followed by a CT scan.

William Manor (diagnostic radiologist): The patient was seen in the Outpatient Radiology Department where we attempted a myelogram through a lumbar approach. Each time we got close to the dura during several attempts at different levels, we caused excruciating pain in the right leg. Finally, we abandoned the effort, thinking the patient probably had an arachnoiditis, and decided to admit him to the hospital and attempt to complete the study the next day, using a cervical approach with the help of Dr. Harris from Neurosurgery. The following day, a needle was inserted at the C1–2 area in the lateral neck and contrast slowly injected. The downward flow stopped at the first lumbar interspace, appearing to show a mass that caused a high-grade obstruction (Fig. 122–1). We thought this was most likely a neurofibroma, meningioma, or possibly an ependymoma. During this part of the exam, the patient again had excruciating back and right leg pain, requiring intravenous narcotics for relief. We scheduled a delayed CT scan.

The CT scan was arbitrarily done from the mid-body of T12 through the mid-body of L-2 and then the angle of the incident beam was changed to study the lower lumbar spine. The conus was found to be is normal, but the tip of conus was pushed from right to left. Starting at about the lower aspect of the L-1 body there was a low-density mass, virtually filling the thecal sac (Fig. 122–2). The mass seemed to extend lower, but no contrast material

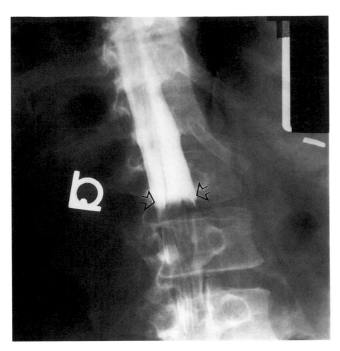

FIG. 122–1. Myelogram showing a block at the L1–2 interspace level. The contrast was injected at the upper cervical level.

was present below L-3. Soft tissue mass extended down to about L-5. In summary, the exam showed findings consistent with an intradural extramedullary mass, such as a meningioma, neurofibroma, or ependymoma.

The patient was then moved to the magnetic resonance imaging (MRI) suite and was examined using gadolinium for contrast. The axial postgadolinium study was quite informative, demonstrating a mass behind the bodies L-1, L-2 and L-3 (Fig. 122–3). We concluded that this mass was the cause of this man's symptoms. The exact tissue diagnosis would have to await surgical findings.

Frank S. Harris (neurosurgeon): I was impressed by this man's pain. He had been sleeping on the floor trying to get relief. Sometimes he would feel pretty good first thing in the morning, but by late afternoon the pain was bad. The pain was increased by walking or sitting, and at stool. Sometimes, at the end of the day, his right foot would be "flopping." Occasionally, he noted "numbness and tingling" involving the posterolateral aspect of his right thigh and calf. His sexual functions were normal and his bladder worked normally. His bowel problem seemed related to difficulty expelling stool, despite the fact that the stool was not hard and, in fact, was quite soft, because he took laxatives.

My neurologic examination was pretty much the same as has been described. I thought there was some decreased

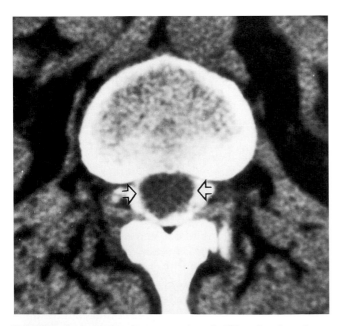

FIG. 122–2. Low density mass, virtually filling the thecal sac, seen on CT scan at L-1 level. Contrast injected for the myelogram surrounds the mass, which appears as a dark area surrounded by the white iodine-containing contrast used.

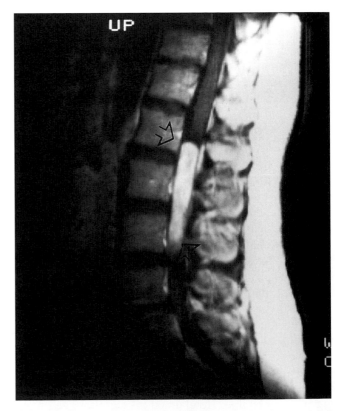

FIG. 122–3. The MRI, done with Gadolinium for contrast, demonstrates a mass behind the bodies of L-1, L-2, and L-3.

pin prick sensation on the lateral right foot and ankle area. The striking finding was severe pain elicited by straight leg raising, especially on the right side.

My impression was that this man had an intradural extramedullary tumor of the lumbar region, and that he would require surgery. I started him on high doses of dexamethasone. He was taken to the operating room the next day, where we did a four-level laminectomy (L-1, L-2, L-3, L-4) and gross removal of an intradural tumor. The tumor was in the region of the conus medullaris and, extending caudally from that point on, was intimately related to the proximal cauda equina. It was moderately vascular and made up of loosely cohesive tissue that could be removed with a 5F sucker. There was a very thin capsule to the tumor. Grossly, the tumor was removed, although certain portions of the capsule that were extremely thin seemed to envelope the pia surrounding the nerve roots; a clear line of demarcation was not always possible. The tumor extended from the upper part of the L-1 body to the lower aspect of the body of L-3.

Donald J. Schreiber (surgical pathologist): Frozen section favored the diagnosis of myxopapillary ependymoma. Permanent sections show a papillary tumor, portions of which are surrounded or invested by dural membrane. The tumor papillae are characterized by edematous, loosely textured fibrovascular cores surrounded by a layer of bland-appearing cuboidal or columnar cells, consistent with ependymal cells (Fig. 122–4). Our diagnosis is myxopapillary ependymoma.

Dr. Harris: Postoperatively, the patient was relieved of his severe pain. One week later he had soreness in both calves, but no swelling; Homan's sign was negative. The following day he experienced pleuritic right chest pain and dyspnea. Venograms showed multiple thrombi in the right lower leg and in the right lower lobe of lung. He was anticoagulated, accepting the risk of hemorrhage, and gradually improved. Postoperatively, we had him seen by Drs. Choucair and Greenlaw. He was discharged on Coumadin.

Robert H. Greenlaw (radiation oncologist): When the patient had recovered sufficiently, about 2 weeks after surgery, we embarked on a course of radiation treatment to the operative area, hoping to reduce the chance of recurrence of this tumor. The treatment ports went from the middle of the eleventh thoracic vertebra through the second sacral level. We gave 5,000 cGy of radiation in about 6 weeks, combining 24 MV photons and 6 MV photons. Giving about 165 cGy per treatment day, the patient experienced no particular difficulties with tolerance; in fact, he resumed part-time employment during the latter part of the treatment course.

Dr. Harris: We saw the patient in follow-up 5 weeks after surgery and he was doing exceedingly well. He was virtually asymptomatic. On examination, he continued to have slightly diminished reflexes at the right ankle and maybe some slight muscle weakness of his tibialis anterior and extensor hallucis longus on the right side. He was working part time, continuing on anticoagulants.

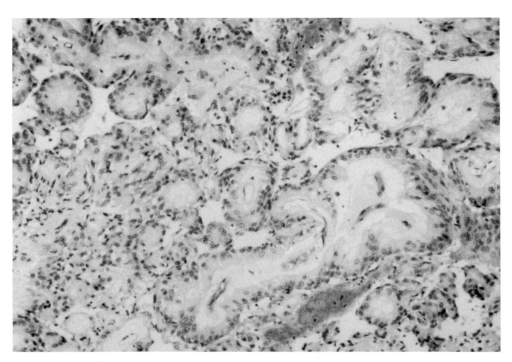

FIG. 122–4. Edematous, loosely textured fibrovascular cores surrounded by a layer of bland-appearing cuboidal or columnar cells, consistent with myxopapillary ependymoma.

Ali Choucair (neuro-oncologist): I have followed up this man at intervals of 6 months, and it is now 5 years after his diagnosis. We do an MRI study about every 6 months, and these have been consistently normal. His only residual neurologic deficit is a diminished right ankle jerk. There have been no complications from the surgery or radiation, and no further problems with pulmonary emboli. He maintains a full work schedule and is particularly active physically. We do recognize, however, that we will need to keep a close eye on him for a very long time. Tumors of this type may reappear after many years.

COMMENTARY by Nicholas A. Vick

The clinical presentation of this instance of myxopapillary ependymoma is characteristic. This tumor occurs in men nearly twice as often as in women. Most patients have low-back pain, often with sciatic radiculopathy, which on clinical grounds cannot be distinguished from benign lumbosacral conditions, such as protruded intravertebral discs (1). Magnetic resonance imaging is clearly the superior diagnostic test as compared with computed tomography or myelography. In fact, there is rarely a need to do either if an MRI scan is done first, since myxopapillary ependymomas have a very characteristic "sausagelike" appearance with striking gadolinium contrast enhancement.

It is important that myxopapillary ependymomas be separated from other ependymomas, especially those that are intra-axial and invade brain and spinal cord tissue as aggressively as astrocytomas (2). Myxopapillary ependymomas arise almost solely from the filum terminale and are often very well demarcated from the cauda equina that they compress. In some instances, they can be removed intact. Such patients have a very low recurrence rate, surely less than 10%. Patients who have gross total resections, with the tumor removed in a piecemeal manner by the neurosurgeon, still do well with a mean survival of 19 years in the largest reported series (1). Because this series included patients from the years 1924 to 1983, it is reasonable to believe that the results are even better now with the availability of MRI and the development of neurosurgical techniques. In fact, it is reasonable to withhold radiotherapy in those instances where postoperative MRI demonstrates gross total resection. This conservative approach has not, of course, been proven to be superior to the usual radiation treatment, as given in the case described. Nonetheless, it makes sense given the power of MRI for follow-up. Even the modest dose of 5,000 cGy, such as was delivered in the patient described, does not preclude radiation damage in long-term survivors. What is important in this decision is confidence that the tumor removed is, in fact, the *myxopapillary* variant of ependymoma. Definitive pathologic interpretation, combined with clinical knowledge of the benign nature of this tumor, as compared to most other ependymomas in adult spinal cords, is the central issue.

REFERENCES

1. Sonneland PRL, Scheithauer BW, Onofrio BM. Myxopapillary ependymoma: a clinicopathological and immunocytochemical study of 77 cases. *Cancer* 1985;56:883–93.
2. Russell DS, Rubinstein LJ. *Pathology of tumors of the nervous system.* 5th edition. Baltimore, MD: Williams and Wilkins; 1989:203–6.

123

Spinal Cord Meningioma

Kevin J. Murray

*Although "benign," this tumor must be diagnosed and
treated efficiently to avoid debility and recurrence*

CASE PRESENTATION

The patient is a 78-year-old woman who presented in May of 1990 with a 6-month history of progressive severe left hip and anterior thigh pain. During this time, she had no associated bowel or bladder dysfunction and noted no numbness, tingling, or other sensory changes. She finds that this pain has become very debilitating and feels that her life may not be worth living if she cannot achieve relief. The patient notes difficulty in sitting, walking, and has accentuation of the pain with laughing. An epidural steroid injection failed to provide relief, and the patient underwent a myelogram with CT scans. This revealed stenosis of the L4–5 segment from a combination of grade I spondylosis as well as facet hypertrophy and an intraspinal mass at the L-2 level.

The patient's past medical history is significant for hypertension and diabetes. She is currently taking Hydropres, Diabinese, Nalfon, and Tylenol. She is known to be allergic to penicillin.

Of significance, in February, 1990, she was diagnosed for a Bell's palsy, and was treated with steroid injections.

Physical examination reveals a very bright and alert 78-year-old woman of Polish descent. She ambulates with difficulty but is able to walk without assistance. She prefers to walk with her lumbar spine flexed approximately 20 degrees at the waist and declines to straighten her spine. She is able to walk on her heels and toes but complains of increased pain when attempting heel walking. Tandem gait is done with difficulty and the Romberg sign is negative. Limb coordination is excellent in the upper extremities and there is normal rapid alternating movement of all four limbs. Motor examination reveals

bilateral hamstring weakness, and sensory examination demonstrated decreased pinprick sensation of the dorsum of the left foot and a posterior aspect of the left thigh. Her joint position sense is normal in the great toes bilaterally. Deep tendon reflexes at the patella are +2/+4 in the right and 0–+1/+4 in the left. Ankle reflex is 0–+1/+4 on the right and absent on the left.

Laboratory evaluation at the time of her admission revealed her hemoglobin to be 14.6 and her hematocrit was 44. Her white blood cell count was 5,800 with a normal differential. Her urinalysis was unremarkable. Electrolytes were within normal limits. Her glucose was 117, creatinine was 0.9, and BUN was found to be 21.

Magnetic resonance images of the brain and the entire spinal cord were obtained. The images of the brain, and cervical and thoracic spinal cord were normal. In the lumbar spine region, at the level of L1–2 vertebral bodies, a 1.5 to 2.0 cm mass was identified. This mass is located intradurally, is well circumscribed, and shows homogenous enhancement (Figs. 123–1, 123–2, 123–3).

This patient's case was presented at the Tumor Board before her operative procedure. The involved neurosurgeon opened the discussion on spinal cord tumors by categorizing their location as being intradural or extradural. Of the intradural tumors, the majority (almost 85%) are extramedullary in location. Several histopathologic types are common with neurofibromas accounting for up to 30%, meningiomas 25%, and ependymomas 13%. Of the less common intradural intramedullary tumors, ependymomas make up a little over 50%, whereas astrocytomas are seen in 30%. For the extramedullary intradural tumors, tumors grow in relation to a nerve root, and chronic progressive radicular pain generally precedes all

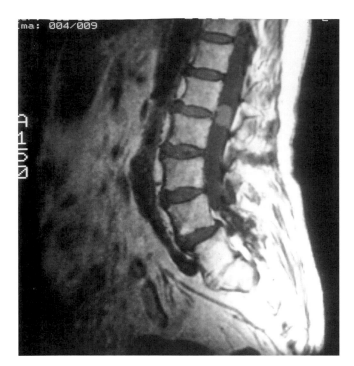

FIG. 123–1. Sagittal T1 MR image of the lumbar spine identifying a 2-cm mass at the L1–2 interspace.

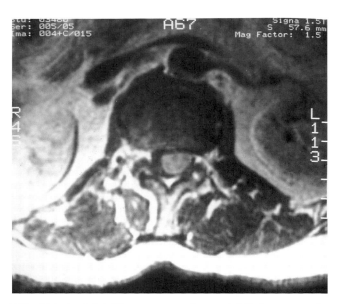

FIG. 123–3. Axial T1-contrast-enhanced MR image at the level of the L1–2 interspace demonstrating this enhancing lesion filling the left side of the spinal canal with deviation of the spinal cord and nerve roots to the right.

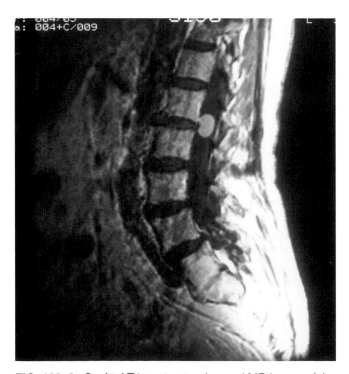

FIG. 123–2. Sagittal T1-contrast-enhanced MR image of the lumbar spine showing a homogeneously enhancing mass at the level of the L1–2 interspace.

symptoms. This agrees with what we have in the case under discussion. Because of the enhancing characteristics on the MR scan, this lesion was thought to be more compatible with a meningioma, although the neurosurgeon said he would not be surprised to see a neurofibroma. What is a bit unusual in this case is the location of this tumor. The majority of the meningiomas are found in the thoracic region, relatively few in the lumbar region.

The patient was admitted to the hospital on May 31 for a surgical decompression. On June 1, the patient underwent an L-1 through L-5 laminectomy with resection of the tumor mass. During the operative procedure, intraoperative ultrasound was utilized in the sagittal and axial plane to identify the intradural tumor. It was found to overlie the L1–2 intravertebral disk space. The dura was entered from the inferior aspect of the L-1 lamina, and this mass was found to attach to the dura at the left lateral aspect between the intervertebral foramina of L-1 and L-2. This did not appear to involve any nerve roots. Using a laser, this mass was resected from its dural attachment. The entire tumor was excised from its arachnoid attachments.

Postoperatively, the patient did quite well without any evidence of sensory or motor deficits. Her pain in the left leg resolved, although for a few days postoperatively, she had complaints of right anterior thigh pain, which were thought secondary to nerve root irritation. The patient was discharged on the eighth postoperative day without difficulty.

Pathologic examination reveals a 2.5 × 1.8 × 0.9 cm. mass that is pink-tan in nature and focally hemorrhagic. Frozen-section diagnosis was thought to be compatible with meningioma. Microscopic examination (Fig. 123–4) shows solid masses and bundles of spindle cells, which in other areas forms concentric whorls of cells. The cells have an oval- to elongated- to crescent-shaped nuclei and contain evenly dispersed chromatin and occasional indistinct nucleoli. Numerous psammoma bodies are identified. A few areas of necrosis are observed. Mitotic figures are rare; however, there is increased nuclear pleomorphism in the area near the necrosis. The final diagnosis was believed to be compatible with meningioma, although the presence of necrosis and cellular pleomorphism may indicate that this tumor is more aggressive than the usual meningioma.

A postoperative MR scan (Fig. 123–5) was done on September 17, which reveals that a laminectomy has been performed from L-1 through L-4. The intradural soft tissue mass previously identified has been removed. There is noted to be a very minimal increase of signal intensity at the posterior aspect of the thecal sac at L1–2, which most likely represents postsurgical change. Mild midline bulging of the L1–2 disk as well as at L3–4 and L4–5 is also identified. Slight spondylolisthesis of L4–5 persists. The L5–S1 disk space remains markedly narrowed. The final impression is no residual tumor is identified.

The patient has been seen in follow-up examination 6 months following her surgical procedure. She reports a

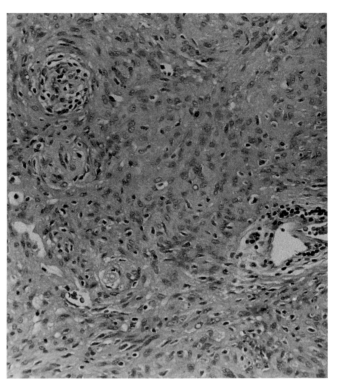

FIG. 123–4. The whorled arrangement of tumor cells is typical for meningioma. There is also a slight perivascular infiltrate of round cells.

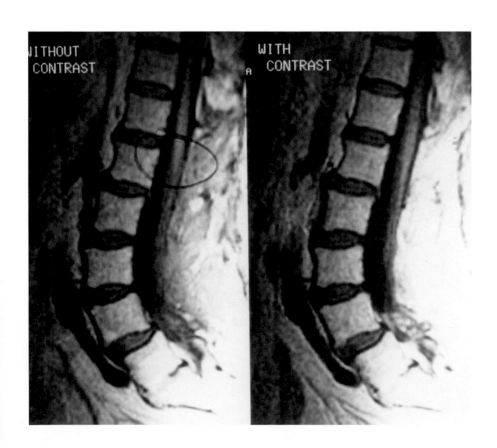

FIG. 123–5. Postoperative sagittal T1 MR images, with and without contrast, showing the complete disappearance of the tumor.

complete disappearance of her preoperative discomfort, and feels that she has returned to her normal baseline activity. Follow-up MR scans have been obtained, which show only postoperative changes. No suspicion for recurrence can be identified.

COMMENTARY by Edward R. Laws, Jr.

This case represents an excellent example of the diagnosis and surgical management of a benign meningioma affecting the spinal cord. Although the majority of meningiomas affect women in the fifth decade of life, it is not unusual for a much older woman, such as the one discussed here, to present with such a lesion. The clinical symptoms produced by this tumor were those of focal and progressive left hip and thigh pain. Of particular interest is the fact that her pain was accentuated with laughing, as this type of spinal cord tumor commonly causes partial obstruction of the spinal canal. The cardinal symptoms of such obstruction are accentuation of pain with cough, sneeze, strain, and laughing, and it is not at all uncommon for such patients to have accentuation of pain at night. The lack of response to conservative therapy prompted the diagnostic procedure of choice, namely an MR scan of the lumbar spine. The imaging characteristics were those of a homogeneously enhancing solid intradural extramedullary tumor, and the differential diagnosis was nicely covered in Dr. Murray's discussion.

Virtually all such meningiomas arise from the inner surface of the dura, and they can occur anywhere within the neuraxis in the spinal canal. A location in the lumbar spine is somewhat less common than more rostral locations.

The prognosis is uniformly good if the tumor can be removed without damaging the surrounding neural elements, and as long as the dural origin of the tumor is excised along with the lesion. In this situation, recurrence is rare, and adjunctive therapy is not necessary. One would follow such a patient with periodic follow-up MR scans and neurologic evaluation and anticipate an excellent prognosis.

124

Subtotal Resection of a High-Grade Glioblastoma

Raymond E. Sawaya

The roles of surgery, radiation therapy, and
neuropsychological testing for brain tumor patients

CASE PRESENTATION

Patient History, Physical Exam, and Neuropsychologic Assessment

The patient is a 57-year-old white man with a history of renal cell carcinoma, which was initially diagnosed in 1991. He presented in July, 1994, after experiencing incoherence while speaking during a funeral. While he was being evaluated in the emergency room for his episode of incoherence, he experienced a grand mal seizure, which began with arm stiffness. During the seizure, he was unable to speak and then passed out. When he awoke, he had some new onset of memory loss, especially with names. He has been seizure free since beginning Dilantin. He was referred to M.D. Anderson Cancer Center for evaluation of a metastatic tumor, the presumed diagnosis based on the imaging studies taken outside the institution. He had been given multiple treatment opinions, including treatment with radiation therapy without biopsy or a stereotactic biopsy followed by radiation therapy. He was specifically warned not to undergo a craniotomy because this was considered to be too risky.

Medical, Surgical History

His medical history includes asthma and the renal cell carcinoma noted above; and surgical history, a resection of a left scapular soft tissue mass in May of 1991 and removal of a soft tissue mass from his right thigh in November, 1993. Nephrectomies were performed on the same dates.

Medications

Dilantin 400 mg q hs; Proventil and Aero-Bid—he takes two puffs b.i.d. The patient has no known drug allergies.

Physical Examination

He was a well-developed, well-nourished man in no acute distress. Vital signs were stable. Head, eyes, ears, nose, and throat were normal. Cardiovascular status showed regular rate and rhythm, with no murmurs, gallops, or rubs. The lungs were clear to auscultation. The abdomen was soft and nontender, with normal bowel sounds and well-healed nephrectomy incisions. Neurologically, he was awake, alert, and fully oriented. His speech was clear and fluent, although he did relate that he had experienced some word-finding difficulties on occasions, especially upon arising in the morning. He remembered three out of three objects in five minutes, but he stated that he could not remember names. He did serial sevens without difficulty. The patient experienced some blurriness in his right visual fields, although the extraocular movements were normal and visual fields to confrontation were full. Bilateral cataracts were present, which had been reported to him by his ophthalmologist. The remainder of the neurologic examination was unremarkable.

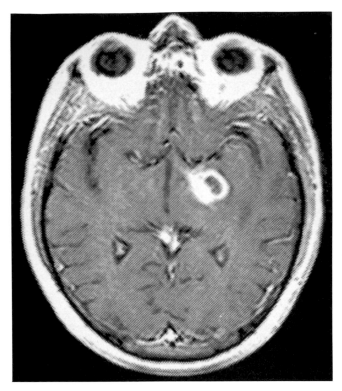

Fig. 124–1. MRI of the brain showing a ring-enhancing mass in the medial aspect of the left temporal lobe.

were obtained in our institution for the purpose of preoperative and intraoperative planning.

Surgical Planning

Several factors entered into the decision to recommend a craniotomy, and those were discussed extensively with the patient and his wife, both of whom are highly educated and were able to grasp the complexities of the decision making. It was the surgeon's opinion that the lesion most likely represented a primary brain tumor. The assessment, supported by a careful review with the neuroradiologist, was based on several factors, including the facts that the patient had been free of systemic disease and that, because of the lack of peritumoral edema and the amount of intratumoral necrosis seen on the MR scan, the characteristic of the lesion on the MR scan was not typical of a renal cell metastasis. In addition, the images obtained at our institution showed what appeared to be more extensive involvement of the left temporal lobe (Fig. 124–2), a finding that was not apparent on the MR scans performed outside. A craniotomy was recommended because it would provide a wider access to a larger portion of the

Neuropsychologic Evaluation

Test results revealed severe impairments of expressive speech, mostly word-finding and naming. In addition, he had visual motor scanning difficulties and fine motor coordination limitations on the right side. He was found to have significant right visual field neglect. Verbal memory, receptive language functions, visual-spatial analysis, and fine motor coordination on the left side were mildly to moderately impaired. This pattern of test results was considered to be consistent with a left-sided tumor that might be associated with diffuse effects of mass pressure or edema. These test results were in marked contrast to the routine neurologic evaluation and emphasize the need for more detailed assessment of patients with intracranial mass lesions.

Diagnostic Work-up

When first seen, the patient brought with him an MR scan performed in an outside institution. These images showed a ring-enhancing mass lesion involving the medial aspect of the left temporal lobe near the hippocampus and abutting the left hypothalamic region (Fig. 124–1). There was a slight degree of associated peritumoral edema. Although the images appeared to be of standard quality, they were not as clear or helpful as those that

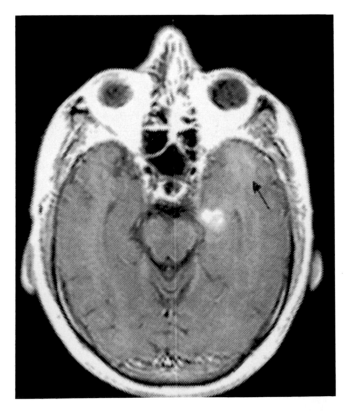

Fig. 124–2. MRI of the brain showing a tumor nodule in the medial aspect of the left temporal lobe. In addition, diffuse enhancement is seen in the anterior portion of the left temporal lobe (arrow).

temporal lobe and allow resection of a significant amount of tissue without producing increased neurologic deficits. In addition, it was considered that if the lesion were in fact a metastatic tumor, a resection would eventually lead to superior results as compared with those gained by performing a biopsy or administering radiation alone.

Surgical Procedure

The patient was taken to the operating room, where a left frontotemporal craniotomy was performed. A newly developed three-dimensional computer-guided technique was used to aid in accessing the lesion. The system, known as the viewing wand, is manufactured and developed by the ISG Company. Once the cortical surface of the temporal lobe was exposed, direct gross visual exploration of the surface of the brain indicated an area of discoloration highly indicative of an infiltrating glioma. A cortical incision was made at that level, and tissue was sent for frozen-section evaluation, the results of which confirmed the presence of a high-grade glioma. Because that area did not include necrosis, a diagnosis of glioblastoma could not be made and, therefore, the decision was made to proceed with a more extensive resection for better sampling of the tumor and for debulking of the mass. The deeper portion did include necrosis, and sampling of this portion was necessary for a more accurate diagnosis. The ISG viewing wand and ultrasound were used frequently to continually advance the vector toward the medial temporal lobe target (Fig. 124–3). An anterior and medial temporal lobectomy was accomplished, and the deeper portion was sufficiently sampled to reach the final diagnosis of a glioblastoma multiforme. Once the goals of the surgery were reached, hemostasis was achieved, and closure proceeded in the usual fashion. The patient recovered uneventfully from the operation, and was discharged from the hospital on the third postoperative day.

Pathology

The final pathology report indicated the presence of a diffuse glial tumor with malignant features and necrosis diagnostic of a glioblastoma (Figs. 124–4, 124–5). In addition, the immunohistochemistry, an antibody to BUDR used to measure the proliferation index of the tumor, showed a labelling index of 1.8% in selective portions of this glioblastoma multiforme (Fig. 124–6). This rate of proliferation is near the low range for glioblastoma and could represent a relatively more favorable prognosis.

TUMOR BOARD DISCUSSION

The patient's history, physical findings, and neuropsychologic assessments were all reviewed in detail at the

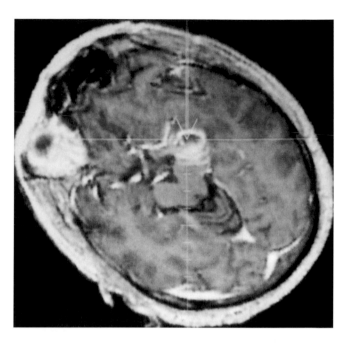

Fig. 124–3. Intraoperative MRI guidance using a frameless stereotactic system. The arrow points to the location of the tip of the probe during the operative exposure and indicates that the surgeon has already entered the ring-enhancing lesion.

Tumor Board, which was attended by a multidisciplinary team composed of neuro-oncologists, neurosurgeons, neuroradiologists, a neuropsychologist, and radiation oncologists with expertise in the management of brain tumors, in addition to nurse practitioners, trainees, and students.

Neuroradiologists: A careful review of the images demonstrated the necessity for high-quality MR images in the preoperative planning and emphasized the value of these images in differentiating between a primary brain tumor and a metastatic tumor. A most helpful aspect provided by the MR images we obtained was the ability to discern the presence of subtle abnormalities found diffusely in the temporal lobe.

Neuropathologist: The histologic slides and the immunohistochemistry slides were reviewed as described above and confirmed the presence of a glioblastoma.

Neurosurgeon: The planning of the surgery and the decision making were reviewed. In addition, the surgical findings and the fact that the resection was subtotal, were presented.

Radiation oncologist: Radiation therapy remains the most effective treatment against glioblastoma. External fractionated radiation therapy has become the standard, and the current tendency is strongly against whole brain radiation therapy and in favor of regionally focused radiation to the area of the abnormality, with a margin of approximately 2 to 3 cm around the tumor. Brachytherapy is another form of radiation that has been used in the treat-

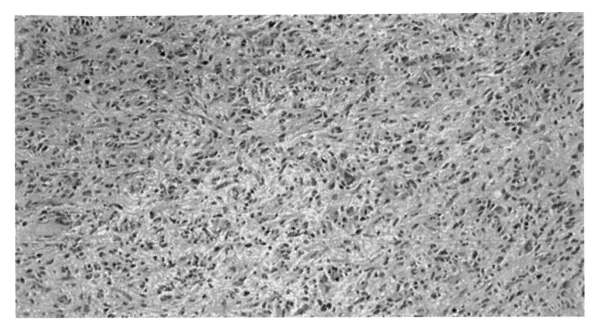

Fig. 124–4. Histologic demonstration of a hypercellular and pleomorphic malignant glioma.

ment of glioblastoma, but because the tumor in this case was located adjacent to the hypothalamus, this form of therapy was not advisable. Radiosurgery has also been used in some centers for treating malignant gliomas. It is, however, the opinion of this group, that in light of the diffuse nature of the tumor, stereotactic radiosurgery was not a viable option.

Neuro-Oncologist: Several chemotherapy protocols are under study at our institution. The use of chemotherapy in glioblastoma has shown some prolongation of survival, particularly in patients who are younger than 60 years of age. The benefit from chemotherapy for glioblastoma is not as prominent as that seen in the treatment of anaplastic astrocytoma. Chemotherapy in the form of

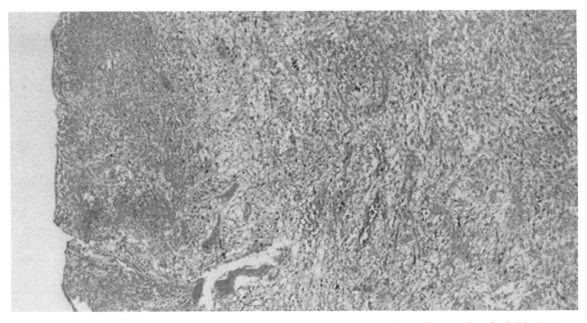

Fig. 124–5. Extensive zones of necrosis are found in the tumor and are diagnostic of glioblastoma multiforme.

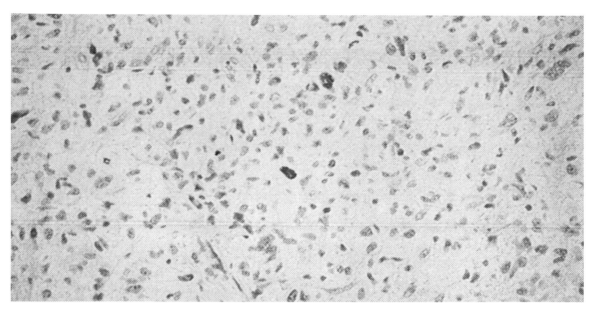

Fig. 124–6. A labelling index using an antibody against bromodeoxyuridine is reported to be 1.8%. Labelled cells are scarce and appear as dark brown cells.

hydroxyurea is used during radiation therapy as a radiosensitizer; it is also used in the postradiation phase in the form of multidrug therapy, namely as a combination of procarbazine, vincristine, and CCNU.

Consensus Opinion

Based on the discussion of the Tumor Board, the recommendation was that the patient undergo conventional radiation therapy to the focal area of the tumor in order to minimize the side effects of radiation on the temporal lobe and the memory and speech functions, which were already impaired in this patient. Chemotherapy was also recommended for this patient.

Status of Patient

As of the last follow-up, the patient was undergoing radiation therapy. His neurologic condition was described as stable.

Conclusion

The management of a patient with glioblastoma can be unrewarding because of the lack of cure for this disease. There are, however, multiple challenges along the course of management of these patients. These are highlighted in this case review. The first relates to the diagnosis, particularly in view of the past history of renal cell carcinoma and the fact that the patient was told he had a metastatic brain tumor. The second involves the surgical management of the tumor, and whether or not a debulking operation is superior to a biopsy. The open craniotomy provides additional information concerning the diffuse nature of the tumor and is likely to prevent any mass effect that could result from the radiation therapy and the peritumoral swelling. The third concerns several forms of radiation therapy that have been introduced, noting that, to date, the standard form of radiation remains the preferred one. In selected cases, however, brachytherapy and/or radiosurgery could provide additional benefits.

COMMENTARY by Kevin J. Murray

Primary malignant tumors of the CNS remains a puzzling and enigmatic process. While involvement of the brain due to either a metastatic or a primary tumor is relatively common (occurring in approximately 70,000 to 100,000 new cases per year), at most 25% represents a primary tumor process. While the current case raises many interesting issues, especially in the separation of a primary from a metastatic lesion, I would like to focus on two—the value of surgery and the usefulness of neuropsychologic evaluation.

In primary CNS tumors, the cornerstone of therapy remains surgery. The importance of surgical excision cannot be overstated. Resection is used both for the determination of histology as well as for the possibility of achieving a total or subtotal resection. As demonstrated in the current case, a more extensive surgical excision led to better sampling of the tumor and the determination of a more aggressive histology. This leads to an improved understanding of the probable natural history and an ability to describe the situation better to the patient.

In addition, the degree of surgical excision is an important determinant for long-term survival. Wood et al. (1), in describing a recent review from the Brain Tumor Cooperative Group, determined a direct relationship existed between the extent of postoperative tumor volume and long-term survival. This effect was noted to be independent of age, performance status, and histology. Simpson et al. (2) reviewed a total of 645 patients with a diagnosis of glioblastoma who were analyzed for survival with respect to known prognostic factors, such as age, Karnofsky performance status, extent of surgery, site, and size. Extent of surgery (biopsy only versus partial resection versus total resection) was determined to be a significant prognostic factor, with an improvement in median survival from 6.6 to 10.4 to 11.3 months, respectively. Besides surgery, age less than 40 years, a Karnofsky performance score of 80–100, and a frontal lobe location were also identified as significant determinants for long-term survival.

Psychologic evaluation and support of the cancer patient and family are important. It can include the assessment of patient and family to determine their psychologic frame of reference or to assist the patient and family in the development of coping skills for the many problems posed by the diagnosis and therapy. Success with rehabilitation can be improved with neuropsychologic or psychometric testing to identify deficits related to cancer and/or therapy.

With regard to the latter role, the current case demonstrates the value of an initial comprehensive assessment. Formal neuropsychologic evaluation showed multiple severe impairments, which were noted to be in marked contrast to the routine neurologic evaluation.

Following treatment, neuropsychologic evaluation also needs to be performed. While severe posttherapy (espe-cially radiation) effects can be seen on CT and MR scans, more subtle findings cannot be documented by these radiographic studies but can be found by neuropsychologic testing. The subject has been extensively explored in the pediatric population, where a large number of patients, either treated prophylactically to the whole brain (in cases of leukemia) or therapeutically for intracranial tumors, combined with an excellent long-term survival, has given rise to a large population of patients who are now more than 5 years from their initial therapy (3,4). The most commonly documented post-therapy effects have been on IQ scores, though other deficits, such as change in memory, cognitive flexibility, and problem-solving skills, do occur.

Psychologic outcome following treatment for brain tumors appears to be a multifactorial process. A high proportion of people treated for brain tumors may have chronic problems, although it is difficult to ascertain whether the problems are a direct casual effect of the tumor or treatment on the CNS. As we obtain more information regarding these late effects, more information will need to be made available to the patient and family and a more definite plan for intervening needs to be provided.

REFERENCES

1. Wood C, Green J, Shapiro W. The prognostic importance of tumor size in malignant gliomas: a computed tomographic scan study by the Brain Tumor Cooperative Group. *J Clin Oncol* 1988;6:338–43.
2. Simpson JR, Horton MD, Scott C, et al. Influence of location and extent of surgical resection on survival of patients with glioblastoma multiforme: results of three consecutive Radiation Therapy Oncology Group (RTOG) clinical trials. *Int J Radiat Biol Oncol Phys* 1993;26: 239–44.
3. Mulhern RK, Crisco JJ, Kun LE. Neuropsychologic sequelae of childhood brain tumors: a review. *J Clin Child Psychol* 1983;12:66–73.
4. Mulhern RK, Fairclough D, Ochs J. A prospective comparison of neuropsychologic performance of children surviving leukemia who received 18 Gy, 24 Gy or no cranial irradiation. *J Clin Oncol* 1989;9: 1348–56.

125

Giant and Invasive Prolactin-Secreting Pituitary Adenoma

Ivan Ciric

Early intervention is almost as important as cure

CASE PRESENTATION

History

M. M. is a 33-year-old laborer who presented with a 3-month history of progressive visual deterioration, especially in the left eye. Approximately 3 weeks prior to admission the patient also developed double vision and mild confusion. The confusion increased in severity to the point where he became lethargic some 5 days before admission. Finally, over a period of about a week the patient also became quite unsteady. The patient's past medical/endocrine history was unremarkable.

Examination

On examination the patient was lethargic although fully oriented. His attention span and power of concentration were clearly diminished. He had difficulty recalling recent events. The visual acuity was 20/80 on the right, 20/200 on the left. The patient had a weakness of the left lateral rectus and a partial ptosis on the left. His right arm drifted against gravity. He had diminished associated movements in the right arm when he walked and he dragged his right leg slightly. The deep tendon reflexes were more active on the right, and he had a right Babinski sign. He was also unsteady on his feet.

Laboratory Data

The serum prolactin level drawn on admission, but not obtained until the following morning, was greater than 4,000 ng/mL. The serum testosterone level was 150 ng/mL. The remainder of the admission laboratory studies were unremarkable.

Imaging Studies

The MRI showed a giant sellar/suprasellar tumor with asymmetric suprasellar extension more toward the left side with significant compression of the left hypothalamic/diencephalic regions. The tumor also compressed the medial aspect of the left temporal lobe. The suprasellar component of the tumor was associated with a cyst formation. Furthermore, the tumor was invasive into the cavernous sinuses with encasement of both carotid arteries (Fig. 125–1).

Clinical Impression

Giant invasive prolactin-secreting pituitary adenoma.

Treatment Plan

The patient was placed on dexamethasone 10 mg every 4 hours for about 2 weeks. He was also started on Parlodel

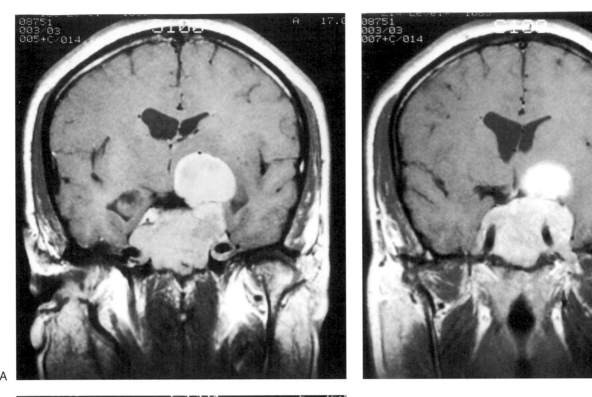

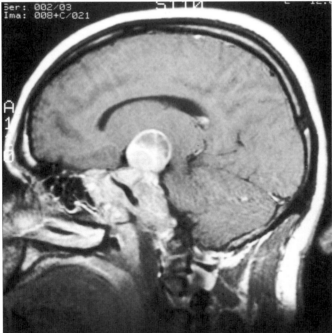

Fig. 125–1. Invasive prolactin-secreting adenoma. Preoperative coronal **(A,B)** and sagittal **(C)** MR images.

2.5 mg every 6 hours; this dosage was gradually increased to 20 mg a day for a period of about a month, when the dosage was gradually decreased to a maintenance dosage of 2.5 mg three times a day. The patient has remained on this dosage for the duration of the follow-up.

Course

The patient improved steadily, up to the point where he became fully alert with complete recovery of his premorbid cognitive functions. His visual acuity returned to normal and the ophthalmoplegia gradually recovered over a period of about 6 weeks. The hemiparesis improved over a period of 7 to 10 days.

Follow-up MRI studies showed steady improvement in appearance of the tumor to the point where it eventually was no longer identifiable.

At the present time, 4 years after initial admission, the patient is symptom-free and fully employed. His laboratory studies are unremarkable except for a mild residual prolactin elevation of about 75 ng/mL. The patient continues to take Parlodel 2.5 mg three times a day. He is also receiving testosterone replacement every 3 weeks. The last MRI obtained 4 years after initial admission shows no evidence of residual tumor tissue (Fig. 125–2).

TUMOR BOARD DISCUSSION

With the prolactin level as high as 4,000 ng/mL or more, this tumor is most assuredly a giant and invasive prolactin-secreting pituitary adenoma. These tumors are more often than not very fibrous and vascular. They invade dura and bone and are also intimately adherent to the neurovascular structures within the dural compartments such as the cavernous sinus. The treatment options include medical management with bromocriptine (Parlodel) or with other dopamine agonists, radiation therapy, and finally, surgical removal. The fundamental goals of any operative procedure are threefold: cure and thus prevention of recurrence; palliation and prevention of symptoms; and occasionally, diagnosis. It is our contention that giant and invasive prolactin-secreting pituitary adenomas

are not surgically curable. Any attempt at complete tumor removal in this patient would have likely resulted in unacceptable neurological sequelae, even in the most competent hands. Consequently, any claim that this tumor could have been removed completely with a cure would be not only unrealistic and unreasonable but also exceedingly dangerous. In fact, this tumor is probably incurable with any single means of therapy or succession of different therapeutic modalities.

The pivotal issue in this patient, therefore, is the need to obtain the best and fastest method of palliation for a tumor with a rapidly progressing clinical course. In addition, the goals of treatment should be to reduce the tumor size and delay or prevent re-growth, and thus a recurrence of the existing life-threatening clinical picture. Based on our experience with 21 giant and invasive prolactin-secreting pituitary adenomas, we believe that medical management with dopamine agonists is far superior in accomplishing these goals when compared with surgery. All of our patients were easily palliated with bromocryptine. Invariably, tumor size shrunk to either a very small residual tumor mass or became virtually nondemonstrable on follow-up imaging studies. In addition, medical management is also superior to surgical therapy in palliating the hyperprolactinemia. It is recognized, of course, that medical management only suppresses prolactin secretion, resulting in overall decrease in tumor size. Thus, lifelong therapy is indicated. Patients will respond in such a way that no other therapy is needed. We feel that an attempt at "decompressing" giant and invasive prolactin-secreting pituitary adenomas accomplishes very little, if anything,

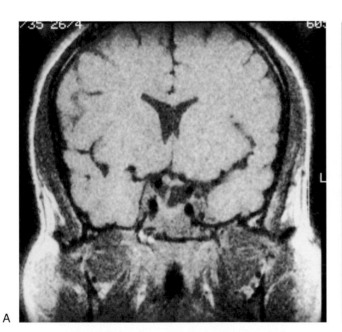
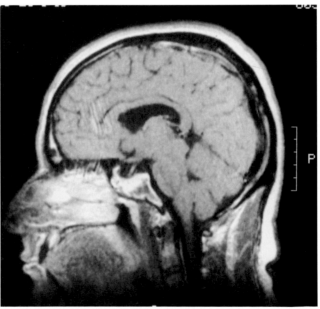

A   B

Fig. 125–2. Invasive prolactin-secreting macroadenoma, after 4 years of treatment with bromocryptine. Coronal **(A)** and sagittal **(B)** MR images.

in terms of an effective reduction in the tumor size, and may even be contraindicated because of hemorrhage and swelling in the residual tumor tissue with the possibility of a "stormy," if not catastrophic, postoperative course.

Surgical therapy, however, has a role in the treatment of enclosed, noninvasive prolactin-secreting pituitary macroadenomas. These tumors should also be pretreated medically with bromocriptine. If, after 6 to 12 weeks of medical management the tumor shrinks without disappearing completely, the residual tumor tissue can then be removed, preferably via the trans-sphenoidal approach. Consequently, some enclosed, noninvasive prolactin-secreting pituitary macroadenomas can be cured with surgical therapy.

In our experience, radiation therapy is ineffective not only in reducing the tumor size but also in achieving endocrine palliation. Occasionally, radiation therapy can be employed as a follow-up to either medical management or surgical removal of the tumor (or both). This would be true especially if there is a small residual prolactin-secreting tumor remaining in the confines of the cavernous sinus, where it is usually more resistant to shrinking with bromocryptine therapy. In such cases, focused radiation to the residual tumor is probably the treatment of choice.

COMMENTARY by Charles B. Wilson

This case, in my opinion, was very well managed, and the outcome is excellent. However, a result as good as this is not predictable, and problems with the use of Parlodel in this situation should be enumerated. Not all prolactin-secreting tumors are responsive to Parlodel, and most are not as responsive as the tumor in the present case. Although tumor volume and basal levels of prolactin decrease under the effect of bromocriptine, the basal level of prolactin is a far more predictable outcome than a change in volume. In fact, volume may change relatively little while the prolactin level falls into the normal range. A problem for many patients involves the patient's inability to tolerate the medication in any form. It seems that patients intolerant to one dopamine agonist are likely to be intolerant to other forms. Some patients cannot tolerate even the smallest bedtime dose, whereas others tolerate a daily dose up to a point, e.g., 7.5 mg, and yet at that level the prolactin has not fallen into the normal range. A final problem is medication-induced cerebrospinal rhinorrhea. If a prolactin-secreting tumor has destroyed the floor of the sella by plugging the opening with a "tongue" of tumor, shrinkage of the tumor under the influence of bromocryptine may allow CSF to drain into the sphenoid sinus through the unplugged opening in the sellar floor. In such a case, the development of cerebrospinal rhinorrhea presents an urgent situation because of the attendant risk of bacterial meningitis. My approach to such a situation is to carry out a limited objective trans-sphenoidal removal of accessible tumor and repair the sellar floor, followed by resumption of the previous regimen of bromocriptine.

Irradiation is highly effective in sterilizing prolactin-secreting adenomas, but because the tumor cells survive and remain metabolically active, continued production of prolactin maintains the elevated level of prolactin. Many years are required for attrition of the sterile cells, and with this a gradual decrease in prolactin level, often requiring many years to reach normal or near-normal levels. Irradiation may have a dramatic effect on the tumor volume, but in other tumors, perhaps those with a larger proportion of connective tissue, the tumor, while sterilized, does not show the diminution in bulk that one sees customarily in other neoplasms rendered incapable of replication following irradiation.

Finally, a tumor that has responded dramatically to bromocryptine may eventually escape its effect. This may occur while the tumor retains its phenotype as a prolactinoma, and in others the tumor that emerges is an endocrine-inactive or null-cell tumor. Consequently, the patients under long-term treatment with Parlodel should be followed at long intervals with scans.

Many prolactin-secreting adenomas can and should be treated surgically, and in general the younger the patient and the smaller the tumor, the more attractive a surgical option becomes. However, the safety and effectiveness of Parlodel provide excellent medical management of this neoplasm, and among all pituitary adenomas the prolactin-secreting tumor is the most benign because of its responsiveness to medication and irradiation and the frequency with which these tumors are recognized while still small and amenable to trans-sphenoidal removal.

126

T2 Adult Medulloblastoma

Christopher J. Schultz

Multimodality therapy has made a difference

CASE PRESENTATION

A 35-year-old white woman presented to her physician with a two-year history of occasional diplopia. Three to four weeks before her presentation, she also noted an increase in headaches, nausea without vomiting, and poor equilibrium. She denied fevers, chills, weight loss, or other systemic complaints. She, likewise, denied any other focal neurological complaints.

Her past medical history was remarkable for osteoarthritis of the spine and depression. Past surgical history included a right ovarian cystectomy three years before presentation, as well as a dilation and curettage that followed a miscarriage three years before presentation. The patient was on no medications, nor did she report any drug allergies. She denied tobacco use or recreational drug use. She reported occasional alcohol use. Her family history was noncontributory.

Physical examination revealed a well-developed and well-nourished woman appearing her stated age, in no acute distress. The patient was afebrile and vital signs were normal. Neurologic exam revealed intact cranial nerves. Sensory and motor function was symmetrically intact. Deep tendon reflexes were 2- and symmetric. Gait was slightly wide-based, though there was no gross ataxia. Mild dysmetria was present bilaterally, perhaps greater on the right than on the left.

A computed tomography (CT) scan of the head was obtained, which showed an enhancing cerebellar mass to the right of midline. Angiography demonstrated a right cerebellar hemispheric mass, without evidence of neovascularity. Anterior displacement of the basilar artery was suggestive of a diffuse mass effect. Cellular blood count and serum chemistries were unremarkable.

The patient underwent a suboccipital craniectomy, C1 laminectomy, and microsurgical exploration and excision of the right cerebral mass. A heterogeneous tumor was encountered with moderate vascularity and cystic formation extending from the pia to the vermis. The tumor was estimated to be 3 cm in diameter. Pathologic study demonstrated a medulloblastoma.(Fig. 126–1) Cytoplasmic GFAP staining was moderately positive. Staining for S100 and EMA were negative. Subsequent evaluation included a normal MRI evaluation of the spinal axis. Postoperative MRI of the head was consistent with tumor removal and postoperative changes. Cerebral spinal fluid obtained via lumbar puncture was without cytologic evidence of medulloblastoma. The patient's postoperative course was unremarkable.

The patient was evaluated by the Radiation Oncology Service for consideration of adjuvant therapy. Using the Chang/Harisiadis staging system, she was believed to have T2 M0 disease. Cranial spinal irradiation was recommended. The patient was also evaluated by the Medical Oncology Service who believed that there was no role for systemic chemotherapy for this stage of disease. The patient subsequently consented to proceed with adjuvant cranial spinal irradiation. Before initiating therapy, however, she was seen by the Gynecology Service for consideration of oophoropexy, displacing her ovaries out of the lower spine irradiation treatment portal to decrease the chance of radiation-associated ovarian failure. The patient agreed to the surgical procedure and underwent a right oophoropexy. Incidentally, a left ovarian benign serous cystadenoma was encountered, prompting a left ovarian cystectomy.

Approximately five weeks from her craniotomy and tumor removal, the patient began a course of cranial spinal

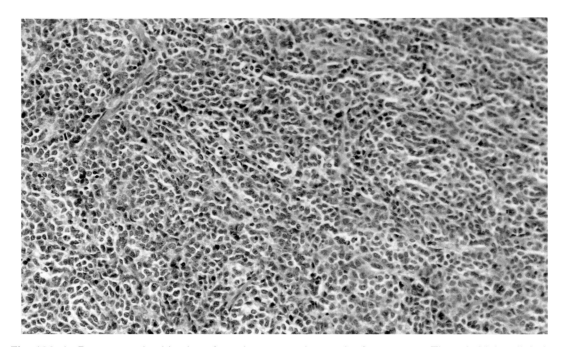

Fig. 126–1. Representative histology from the resected posterior fossa tumor. There is high cellularity, characterized by small cells with fairly uniform-sized nuclei with mild hyperchromatism to a moderately clumped chromatin pattern and scant cytoplasm. Rare mitotic figures are noted in other sections (not shown). Small back-to-back nests of cells showing a linear arrangement are noted. No rosette formation is identified within the tumor. The findings are consistent with medulloblastoma.

irradiation. A total dose of 36 Gy was delivered to the cranial vault, inclusive of the meninges. Following this, the field was reduced to include the posterior fossa. This volume was boosted to a total dose of 54 Gy. These fields were treated at 1.8 Gy per fraction. The remainder of the spinal axis was treated to a total dose of 30.3 Gy. Initially, this field was treated at 1.8 Gy per fraction; however, due to associated nausea and intermittent vomiting, the fractionation was reduced to 1.5 Gy. Therefore, a total dose of 30.3 Gy was delivered to the spinal axis, rather than 36 Gy as initially planned. 6 MV photons were used for the entirety of the treatment. Of note, in addition to the above change in fractionation, anti-emetic medications, including Compazine and Ativan, were used to treat her nausea and vomiting with a modest improvement in symptoms.

Follow-up imaging studies of the brain demonstrated complete tumor clearance. There was modest porencephaly and encephalomalacia noted in the cerebellar vermis at the site of the index lesion.(Fig. 126–2)

Her initial postradiation course was remarkable for persistent nausea and anorexia. She was evaluated by the Gastroenterology Service three months after completion of her irradiation. Their evaluation failed to disclose the cause for persistent nausea, which gradually improved with the use of dietary fiber. When last seen, these symptoms had resolved. Approximately three months after irradiation, the patient also noted cessation of her menstrual periods. Her menopausal status was confirmed with

elevation of luteinizing hormone and follicle stimulating hormone in the menopausal range. She has been maintained on Premarin and Provera regimen.

At seven months from completion of therapy, she is clinically and radiologically without evidence of recurrent disease. She has returned to work on a full-time basis.

COMMENTARY by Lawrence M. Cher, Lyndon J. Kim, Fred H. Hochberg

Medulloblastoma remains a rare adult tumor but is relatively common in pediatric neuro-oncologic practice and therefore most of the advances in management have been learned in that arena. These lessons are likely relevant to the adult patient. These tumors were first described by Bailey and Cushing (1), and were thought to arise from the putative embryonal medulloblast, a cell type that has still not been identified. However, the cell of origin does appear to be an early precursor as these tumors can differentiate along neural or glial lines. Classically, these tumors are midline cerebellar tumors, often briskly enhancing. In adults, they may be more laterally placed with less enhancement and may have cystic components. Pathologically, they consist of sheets of small blue cells, often indistinguishable from other tumors such as pineoblastomas. Some authors suggest that all such tumors should be considered together under the rubric of Primitive Neuroectodermal tumors (PNET). This is clinically a useful

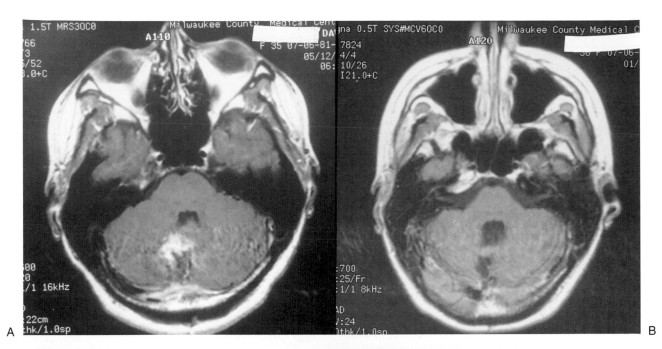

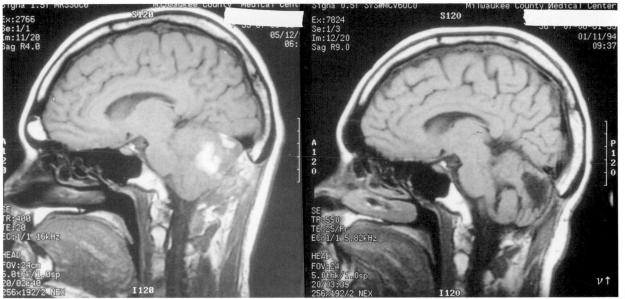

Fig. 126–2. Axial T1-weighted MRI scans with gadolinium demonstrate the surgical defect in the right cerebellar hemisphere to the right of the midline. These findings, 7 days postoperatively, are consistent with postoperative change **(A)**. Subsequent follow-up MR images 7 months from completion of therapy demonstrate complete tumor clearance with modest porencephaly and encephalomalacia in the right cerebellar vermis at the site of the index lesion **(B)**. Similar findings are noted in the sagittal views of these studies 7 days post-operatively **(C)** and 7 months postradiation therapy **(D)**.

concept as these tumors tend to behave in similar fashion (e.g. leptomeningeal spread) and are responsive to similar chemotherapeutic approaches. The validity of the concept remains still to be proven and remains controversial.

The case under discussion illustrates a number of points about the disease and its treatment. It tends to occur in younger adults with a median age of 25. Clinical signs may be subtle at presentation. Staging is important to assess disease spread. The standard therapy is craniospinal irradiation. Two of its complications here included significant nausea and vomiting from irradiation of the posterior fossa and amenorrhea (secondary to spinal irradiation despite the oophorexy) associated with elevated gonadotrophin level.

Medulloblastomas can be associated with a number of inherited conditions. (Table 126–1) Medulloblastoma

Table 112–1. *Genetic disorders associated with medulloblastoma*

Naevoid basal-cell carcinoma syndrome (Gorlin's syndrome)
Ataxia-telangiectasia
Li-Fraumeni syndrome
Turcot's syndrome
Blue rubber bleb nevus syndrome
Xeroderma pigmentosum

accounts for 7%–8% of all intracranial neuroepithelial tumors and 20% of all pediatric tumors. The presenting features are usually related to either progressive midline cerebellar dysfunction (ataxia, incoordination) or hydrocephalus secondary to fourth ventricular compression (headache, reduced level of arousal). A recent report from France (2) reviews more than 150 adults with the disease and provides a useful resource for understanding the disease in this group of patients. In that study, they found that the 5- and 10-year event-free survival rates, 61% and 48%, respectively, were comparable with pediatric series. The median time to recurrence was 30 months, but late relapses after 5 years remain frequent. The major prognostic factors, i.e., fourth ventricular floor involvement, histologic subtype, and radiation dose, were also identical with those observed in children. However, a new parameter—postoperative performance status—was identified. Postoperative craniospinal irradiation was the standard treatment, and no benefit of concomitant chemotherapy was demonstrated.

Radiologic Features

Neuroimaging usually shows a midline lesion that enhances briskly. Exceptions occur, particularly in adult patients. In this group approximately 50% percent of patients have laterally placed lesions. There may also be cystic components to the tumor, and occasionally, only minimal enhancement is seen.

Magnetic resonance imaging (MRI) is also useful for screening of the spinal access, although myelography and postmyelogram CT may be more sensitive.

Pathology

The tumor is a densely cellular "blue" tumor. The color is due to the small amount of cytoplasm and density of cell nuclei. This appearance is characteristic but other patterns may be seen. Occasionally, differentiation of the tumor may occur causing diagnostic confusion. Neuroblastic differentiation includes the presence of Homer–Wright rosettes and, rarely, widespread sheets of neuroblasts, even including mature ganglion cells. Spongioblastic differentiation is associated with rhythmic palisading,

whereas glial differentiation may show features of astrocytic, oligodendroglial, and ependymal differentiation.

Much has been written about the presence of desmoplasia (an intense fibrous reaction). In a number of studies this has been suggested to be a positive prognostic factor. This has been confirmed in adults. (2)

Staging

The investigation of patients with medulloblastoma includes examination of cerebrospinal fluid and radiologic staging of the spinal axis as discussed above. Metastases may occur at diagnosis. In the French study (2), 9% of patients had leptomeningeal spread, although not all were screened. A number of staging systems have been described based on factors thought to be of prognostic importance. The best known is the Chang/Harisiadis system (Table 126–2) (4). "Standard risk" has included those with T3a M0 or better, whereas more widespread disease was considered "high-risk." However, the prognostic importance of this system has been challenged. The POG group uses a system based on postoperative staging (5). (Table 126–3)

Treatment Options

The approach to treatment is dictated by the behavior of the tumor. In general, the surgeon should attempt as complete a resection of tumor as possible. This is generally relatively well tolerated. The aim is to debulk the maximum amount of tumor without neurologic compromise. Surgery alone is associated with a high-risk of both local and distant metastases. Focal radiation therapy is associated with a high-risk of distant recurrence. In children, the major advance has been in the use of craniospinal irradiation (CSRT) to control distant seeding. This has led to a major improvement in the five-year survival figures from all the large pediatric series. In Cushing's original series, the 3-year survival rate was 1.6%; and in series before 1970, the 5-year survival was approximately 20%. More recent series using CSRT show 5-year survival rates of

Table 126–2. *Chang staging system*

Stage	Description
T1	<3 cm
T2	>3 cm
T3a	>3 cm + Acq of Sylvius and For of Luschka
T3b	>3 cm + b/stem invasion
T4	>3 cm + past Acq of Sylvius or For magnum
M1	+ve CSF cytologies
M2	Intracranial nodular seeding
M3	Spinal subarach nodular seeding
M4	Extraneural metastases

Table 126–3. *POG postoperative staging system*

Stage	Description
I	Complete excision
II	Partial excision without posterior fossa extension
III	Extension outside posterior fossa
IV	Extraneural metastasis

60%-70%. More recently, chemotherapy has been used in children less than 3-years old to reduce the effects of RT on the developing nervous system by delaying radiation or in an effort to improve survival. However, in adults, its precise role remains unclear. There are not enough data to suggest the role of chemotherapy in regard to improved survival rate (3). High-risk patients appear to benefit from chemotherapy i.e., in the treatment of extraneural metas-tasis. Chemotherapy is also of benefit in those with recurrent disease following RT.

REFERENCES

1. Bailey P, Cushing H. Medulloblastoma cerebelli: a common type of mid-cerebellar glioma of childhood. *Arch Neurol Psychiatr* 1925;14: 192–224.
2. Carrie C, Lasset C, Alapetite C, et al. Multivariate analysis of prognostic factors in adult patients with medulloblastoma: retrospective study of 156 patients. *Cancer* 1994;74(8):2352–60.
3. Russell DS, Rubinstein LJ. Pathology of Tumors of the Nervous System. 5th ed. Baltimore: Williams and Wilkins, 1989:251–79.
4. Harisiadis L, Chang CH. Medulloblastoma in children: correlation between staging and results of treatment. *Int J Radiat Oncol Biol Phys* 1977;2:833–84.
5. Laurent JP, Chang CM, Cohen ME. A classification system for primitive neuroectodermal tumors (medulloblastoma of the posterior fossa). *Cancer* 1985;56:1807–9.
6. Cohen ME, Duffner PK. Medulloblastomas. In: Cohen ME, Duffner PK, ed. *Brain Tumors in Children: Principles of Diagnosis and Treatment.* 2nd ed. New York: Raven Press, 1994:177–201.

127 Solitary Brain Metastasis

Minesh P. Mehta and William R. Noyes

Treatment choices should be based on good data showing benefit and little or no toxicity

CASE PRESENTATION

L.W., a 65-year-old white man, underwent a work-up for a left flank mass in December 1985 that included an intravenous pyelogram, angiogram, chest roentgenogram, and abdomino-pelvic computed tomography (CT) scan, which demonstrated a hypervascular mass in the upper pole of the left kidney. The patient underwent a left nephrectomy in January 1986. Histopathologic findings demonstrated renal cell carcinoma with no lymph node metastasis. The patient was a pathologic stage III; T3a N0 M0. No further therapy was given. A routine chest roentgenography in August 1990 demonstrated a lung nodule, confirmed to be solitary by chest CT. Bone, abdomino-pelvic CT, and brain CT scans showed no other lesions. The patient underwent wedge resection with histopathologic results demonstrating metastatic renal cell carcinoma. He was treated with Acrivastine and vinblastine for three cycles, followed by interferon therapy, which was completed in September 1991. During his evaluation for an interleukin-II protocol, a head CT scan was performed, which revealed a small enhancing lesion in the right frontal cortex with associated vasogenic edema without mass effect or midline shift. The mass, adjacent to the falx cerebri in the right frontal cortex, measured 1 cm in diameter. He presently denies headaches, visual changes, muscle weakness, loss of memory, personality changes, nausea, vomiting, or lethargy. His past medical history is significant for hypertension, which is beign controlled with Dyazide. Review of systems as well as family history are noncontributory.

On physical examination, the patient is a pleasant elderly white man in no distress. Karnofsky performance score (KPS) is 100%. Pupils are equal, round and reactive to light and accommodation. Visual fields are full and intact. Funduscopic examination is normal. The facial musculature is symmetric. The tongue is midline with an intact gag reflex. There is no palpable adenopathy. His lungs are clear to auscultation in all fields. A thoracotomy scar is noted. His heart has a regular rate and rhythm without murmurs, clicks, or gallops. His abdomen is soft and without organomegaly, masses, or tenderness. A left nephrectomy scar is also noted. Muscular strength, deep tendon reflexes, mini-neuro status testing as well as finger-to-nose, heel-to-shin, gait, Romberg and pronator drift are normal.

TUMOR BOARD DISCUSSION

Neurosurgeon (Dr. NS): How certain are you of a diagnosis of metastasis to the brain from renal cell carcinoma?

Neuroradiologist (Dr. NR): The lesion is a 1-cm contrast-enhancing mass in the right frontal lobe at the junction of the gray-white matter and adjacent to, but definitely not arising from, the falx cerebri, thereby making the diagnosis of meningioma highly unlikely. A prior negative CT almost completely rules out meningioma. The mass has a small area of central necrosis and this, together with the associated vasogenic edema, is most consistent with either a metastasis or a high-grade glioma. The location of the mass at the gray-white junction, its relatively small size and almost spherical shape, and the patient's history of metastatic renal cell carcinoma to the lung diagnosed 7 months prior to the findings on the head CT scan, are most suggestive of metastasis rather than a primary CNS tumor.

Radiation Oncologist (Dr. RO): In a study reported by Patchell and colleagues (1), 6 of 54 patients (11%) with a history of a prior neoplasm, undergoing histopathologic confirmation at the time of radiographically suspected development of a single brain metastases, were found not to have metastatic brain tumors. Therefore, statistically, the patient has approximately an 11% risk of not having a brain metastasis. Another crucial factor to consider is the time to development of brain metastases. This patient developed lung metastases approximately 4 years after his diagnosis of renal cell carcinoma, and then developed a brain lesion within 7 months of his lung metastases with a prior negative head CT scan. The radiographic findings taken in context with this clinical presentation are highly suggestive of brain metastases.

Medical Oncologist (Dr. MO): Does this patient require whole brain radiation?

Dr. RO: In 1992, Coia reported the guidelines developed by a consensus workshop for the management of patients with brain metastases (2). The consensus workshop recommended that whole brain radiation is indicated in almost all patients with brain metastases, including those undergoing surgical resection because of the high-risk of relapse in the brain. The Mayo Clinic reported that adjuvant radiation therapy after surgical resection of a solitary brain metastasis decreased the brain relapse from 85% to 21%, and prolonged median survival from 11.5 months to 21 months (3). There are data from Stanford demonstrating that the addition of whole brain radiation decreases the incidence of regional intracranial recurrence as compared with radiosurgery alone (4). Therefore, in the United States, whole brain radiation would be regarded as the standard of care.

Dr. MO: What dose of radiation would you recommend for whole- brain irradiation?

Dr. RO: Presently, the standard of care is 30 Gy in 10 fractions, which has been proven to be as efficacious as the more prolonged regimens or schedules with higher doses (5–7). However, recent RTOG studies have demonstrated that accelerated hyperfractionation using 1.6 Gy b.i.d. to total doses ranging from 48 to 70.4 Gy result in a significant advantage in survival and neurologic improvement with higher doses (8). This most recent study implies that intracranial disease control is related to dose, and that prevention of neurologic deterioration will result in a survival advantage.

Dr. NS: There are data demonstrating the efficacy of surgical resection of a single brain metastases followed by postoperative radiation. Patchell and colleagues performed a prospective randomized study of patients with a single brain metastases (1). The patients underwent surgical removal of the brain tumor, followed by irradiation or a needle biopsy of the tumor, followed by radiation. The patients undergoing surgical resection had a local recurrence of only 20% versus 52% without surgery. In addition, the surgical group also experienced superior

survival with a median of 40 weeks compared with 15 weeks for the radiation group. Perhaps the most important finding was that patients treated with surgical resection remained functionally independent longer than patients treated with radiotherapy, a median of 38 weeks versus 8 weeks, respectively.

Dr. RO: An alternative to surgical resection for brain metastases would be stereotactic radiosurgery. There appears to be a dose-response relationship for local control of brain metastases, and improved local control translates into a survival benefit. Also, the majority of brain metastases are pseudospherical and located at the gray-white junction, thereby being ideal targets for radiosurgery and allowing the use of large fractions without excessive toxicity. Numerous institutions have reported local control rates of 80%–90% with radiosurgery (Table 127–1) (9). In a retrospective comparison of surgery versus radiosurgery, we have analyzed a patient population similar to Patchell's and reported a local failure rate of 13% for radiosurgery compared with 20% for patients undergoing surgical resection (15). The median survival was 40 weeks with surgery and 56 weeks with radiosurgery. The patients treated with radiosurgery maintained a KPS (Karnoffsky Performance Score) of 70% or greater for a median of 51 weeks versus 38 weeks as reported by Patchell (Table 127–2). Consideration should also be given to the histology of the primary tumor as well as the size of the metastases. Loeffler and colleagues have reported that tumors measuring 3.2 cm^3 or less had a local control rate of 93% as compared with 84% for tumors greater than 3.2 cm^3 (9). Interestingly, tumors believed to be "radioresistant," such as renal cell, actually had higher local control rates (Fig. 127–1)(9). We have also reported a relationship between size and response to radiosurgery. Tumors with a volume of 6 cm^3 or less had a radiographic response of 75%–78%, whereas tumors measuring greater than 6 cm^3 but less than 10 cm^3 had a response rate of 60%, and tumors greater than 10 cm^3 had a response rate of 50% (Table 127–3) (10).

Table 127–1. *Summary of brain metastates local control with radiosurgery*

Institution	Unit	No. of lesions	Dose (Gy)	% Control
Wisconsin	Linac	58	18.3	82
Cologne	Linac	66	18.0	83
Harvard	Linac	330	16.0	88
Heidelberg	Linac	102	17.2	95
Stanford	Linac	47	24.6	88
GK Users	Gamma	116	18.0	83
Karolinska	Gamma	300	29.0	94
Pittsburgh	Gamma	53	16.0	85
Sapporo	Gamma	132	27.0	95
Sendai	Gamma	77	26.0	99
Total		1281	16-29	82-99

Table 127–2. *Comparison of radiosurgery versus surgery*

Study	No. of patients	Median survival (wks)	Median KPS >70%	Local failure (%)	Neuro deaths(%)
Patchell	25	40	38	20	29
Auchter	122	56	51	13	25

Dr. NS: How does radiosurgery compare with interstitial brachytherapy?

Dr. RO: Presently, there are limited data supporting the use of interstitial brachytherapy for brain metastases (11,12). Due to the side effects of interstitial brachytherapy, it is best reserved for selected patients with malignant gliomas (13). In comparison, the acute complications of radiosurgery are very few. Loeffler has reported seizures in 6% of the patients treated within the first 24 hours, and transient motor weakness in 2% within 36 hours, all of whom had motor cortex lesions. Nausea was reported in 11% of patients within the first 24 hours of radiosurgery; all of these patients received more than 2.75 Gy to the area postrema. Loeffler has also reported symptomatic radiation necrosis in 8%, all of whom required resection, and cranial nerve palsies in two patients involving the trigeminal and vestibulocochlear nerves, respectively (14).

Dr. NS: Since the patient has known systemic metastases, would there be a role for chemotherapy or biologic therapy?

Dr. MO: Presently, there is no standard systemic therapy, but there are several experimental regimens that are being investigated.

Dr. MO: How then does one decide between surgical resection or radiosurgery?

Dr. RO: One must consider numerous factors before deciding which option is best for each patient, including location of the tumor, size, neurologic status, KPS, histology, and life expectancy. If all these factors are favorable so that a patient may undergo either surgical resection or radiosurgery, then the decision should be based upon the technique that has superior results. However, the data demonstrate that local control, overall survival and median duration of functional independence are equivalent for these two options. Therefore, in a time of health care reforms, one should recommend the most cost-effective treatment. We reviewed the costs incurred for patients undergoing surgical resection versus a similar patient population undergoing radiosurgery. The data were analyzed for a small subset of each patient population. The median length of hospitalization was 6 days for surgical resection versus 1 day for radiosurgery. The operating room charges were 12 times greater for surgical resection, and when all fees were combined, including both the professional and hospital charges, the total surgical resection invoice was 1.9 times larger than the radiosurgery invoice (Table 127–4). It appears that radiosurgery is the more cost-effective modality available for this patient. Three recent cost-effectiveness analysis studies have come to the same conclusion (16,17,18).

Addendum

The patient was treated on an in-house protocol, and received whole brain irradiation to 40 Gy in 20 fractions

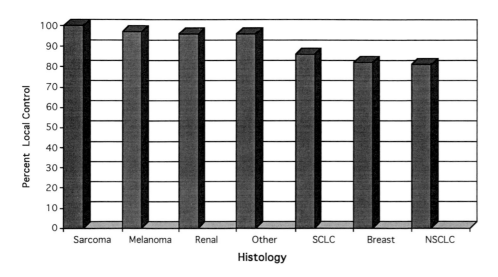

Local Control by Histology

FIG. 127–1. Histogram illustrates local control rate for brain metastases as a function of histologic origin. SCLC, small cell lung cancer; NSCLC, nonsmall cell lung cancer.

Table 127–3. *Tumor size versus response*

Volume (cm³)	No. of lesions	Mean volume (cm³)	Mean dose (Gy)	CR (%)	PR (%)	CR + PR (%)
<2	23	0.97	22.4	61	17	78
>2<6	16	3.27	17	43	32	75
>6<10	5	7.89	13.2	20	40	60
>10	10	19.9	13.2	10	40	50

CR, complete response; PR, partial response.

followed by stereotactic radiosurgery. The target volume of 0.4 cm³ was treated with a modified, linear-accelerator-based radiosurgery system with a 1.5-cm diameter collimator. The target volume received 27 Gy to the 80% isodose line, and 33.75 Gy maximum dose (Fig. 127–2). By 3 months, a partial response, as defined by more than 50% volume reduction, was achieved. At 24 months postradiosurgery, he had one episode of a grand mal seizure requiring phenytoin. The exact etiology of his seizure is unknown. He has also developed symptomatic thoracic spine metastases, necessitating thoracic spine irradiation. The patient has required no subsequent steroid therapy and has had no progression of his solitary brain metastasis or regional intracranial relapse at 31 months.

REFERENCES

1. Patchell RA, Tibbs PA, Walsh JW, Dempsey RJ, et al: A randomized trial of surgery in the treatment of single metastases to the brain. *N Engl J Med* 1990;322:494–500.
2. Coia LR, Aaronson N, Linggood R, Loeffler J, Priestman TJ. A report of the consensus workshop panel on the treatment of brain metastases. *Int J Radiat Oncol Biol Phys* 1992;23:223–7.
3. Smalley SR, Schray MF, Laws ER Jr., O'Fallon JR. Adjuvant radiation therapy after surgical resection of solitary brain metastases: association with pattern of failure and survival. *Int J Radiat Oncol Biol Phys* 1987;13:1611–6.
4. Fuller BG, Kaplan ID, Adler J, et al. Stereotactic radiosurgery for brain metastases: the importance of adjuvant whole brain irradiation. *Int J Radiat Oncol Biol Phys* 1992;23:413–8.
5. Borgelt B, Gelber R, Kramer S, Brady LW, et al. The palliation of brain metastases. Final results of the first two studies by the Radiation Therapy Oncology Group. *Int J Radiat Oncol Biol Phys* 1980;6:1–8.
6. Diener-West M, Dobbins TW, Phillips TL, Nelson DF. Identification of an optimal subgroup for treatment evaluation of patients with brain metastases using RTOG Study 7916. *Int J Radiat Oncol Biol Phys* 1989;16:669–73.
7. Swift PS, Phillips T, Martz K, Wara W, et al. CT characteristics of patients with brain metastases treated in RTOG study 7916. *Int J Radiat Oncol Biol Phys* 1993;25:209–14.
8. Epstein BE, Scott CB, Sause WT, Rotman M, et al. Improved survival duration in patients with unresected solitary brain metastases using accelerated hyperfractionated radiation therapy at total doses of 54.4 Gy and greater. Results of Radiation Therapy Oncology Group 85-28. *Cancer* 1993;71:1362–7.
9. Mehta MP. Radiosurgery for brain metastases. In: DeSalles AF, Goetsch SJ, eds. *Stereotactic surgery and radiosurgery.* Madison, Wis.: Medical Physics Publishing Corp.; 1993:353–68.
10. Mehta MP, Rozental JM, Levin AB, Mackie TR, et al. Defining the role of radiosurgery in the management of brain metastases. *Int J Radiat Oncol Biol Phys* 1992;24:619–25.
11. Lucas GL, Luxton G, Cohen D, Petrovich Z, et al. Treatment results of stereotactic interstitial brachytherapy for primary and metastatic brain tumors. *Int J Radiat Oncol Biol Phys* 1991;21:715–21.
12. Bernstein M, Laperriere N, Leung P, McKenzie S. Interstitial brachytherapy for malignant brain tumors: preliminary results. *Neurosurgery* 1990;26(3):371–9.
13. Prados MD, Gutin PH, Phillips TL, Wara WM, et al. Interstitial brachytherapy for newly diagnosed patients with malignant gliomas: the UCSF experience. *Int J Radiat Oncol Biol Phys* 1992;24(4):593–7.

Table 127–4. *Cost comparison: surgery vs. radiosurgery (relative ratios)*

	Charges				
	Hospital day Charges	OR Charges	Hospital Charges	Professional Charges	Total Charges
Radiosurgery	1	1	1	1.2	1
Surgery	6	12.1	2.98	1	1.86

OR, Operating room

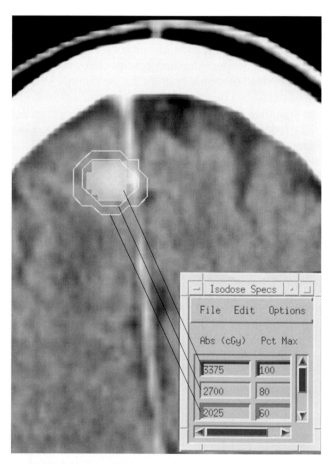

Fig. 127–2. Computer treatment plan for a solitary brain metastasis. Isodoses are shown for 100%, 80%, and 60%. Radiosurgery was performed to the 80% isodose.

14. Nedzi LA, Kooy H, Alexander E, Gelman RS, Loeffler JS. Variables associated with the development of complications from radiosurgery of intracranial tumors. *Int J Radiat Oncol Biol Phys* 1991;21:591–9.

15. Auchter R, Lamond J, Alexander E, et al. A multi-institutional outcome and prognostic factor analysis of radiosurgery (RS) for resectable single brain metastases. *Int J Radiat Oncol Biol Phys* 1996;35:27–35.

16. Rutigliano MH, Lunsford LD, Kondziolka, et al. A cost-effectiveness of stereotactic radiosurgery versus surgical resection in the treatment of solitary metastatic brain tumors. *Neurosurgery* 1995;37:445–53.

17. Sperduto PW, Hall WA. The cost-effectiveness for alternate treatment for single brain metastases. In: Kondziolka D, ed. *Radiosurgery 1995.* Basel, Switzerland: S. Karger Publishers, 1995:180–7.

18. Noyes WR, Auchter R, Craig B, et al. Lost analysis of radiosurgery versus resection for single brain metastases. In: Kondziolka D, ed. *Radiosurgery 1995.* Basel, Switzerland: S. Karger Publishers, 1995:188–92.

COMMENTARY by Roy A. Patchell

This case involves a 65-year-old man with renal cell cancer and a single brain metastasis. He had a history of a metastasis to his lung; however, at the time of presentation of the brain metastases, he had no other known cancer remaining in his body. He was also asymptomatic from his small right frontal brain lesion.

This report and the discussion presented in this chapter illustrate the difficulties with interpreting currently available information on the management of brain metastases. Considerable controversy exists about the role of the major treatment methods including radiation therapy, conventional surgery, and radiosurgery.

One of the longest-standing controversies involves the optimum dose of whole brain radiation therapy (WBRT) to be used for the treatment of brain metastases. So far, the best available evidence comes from several large randomized trials performed by the Radiation Therapy Oncology Group (RTOG) (1–4). These studies have shown that there is no relationship between dose and survival or prevention of neurologic recurrence once the total dose of WBRT is above 2,000 cGy. The RTOG study (5) quoted by the radiation oncologist showing an advantage in survival for accelerated hyperfractionated radiotherapy actually does not prove that a significant dose–response relationship exists. In that study, there was only a small (but statistically significant) difference between the highest dose used and all of the other arms in that study. Unfortunately, the authors were unable to demonstrate a significant difference in reduction of neurologic recurrence of disease, or of prevention of death due to neurologic causes. Therefore, it is impossible to conclude that the difference in survival was due to effect of treatment on the brain because the major endpoints that would be effected by treatment of the brain were not significantly different. The difference in overall survival was more likely due to chance or unidentified patient selection factors. There is evidence to show that higher doses per fraction may result in a higher percentage of CNS radiation damage in long-term survivors (6); however, the evidence for this is not conclusive. Currently, WBRT in total doses between 3,000 cGy and 5,500 cGy are given for brain metastases, whether single or multiple.

The role of surgery in the treatment of brain metastases has recently been clarified somewhat. There are now two randomized trials (7,8) that have shown a substantial benefit from surgery plus radiation when compared with radiation alone in the treatment of single brain metastases. In both studies, there was an increase in overall survival, a reduction in neurologic recurrence, and prevention of death due to neurologic causes in the patients treated with conventional surgery. Conventional surgery is now the treatment of choice for patients with single, surgically accessible lesions, who are candidates for surgical procedure. In both randomized trials, WBRT was given after surgery. However, it is unclear whether radiation therapy is actually needed in these patients—surgical resection is theoretically capable of totally removing the metastases, and there may not be a reason for giving it. There have been four retrospective studies (9–13) done to assess the need for postoperative WBRT following surgery. In only one of the trials (10,13) (a Mayo Clinic study) has any significant difference in survival or neurologic control been detected. In the other three trials, there was no difference in survival or neurologic control due to the addition of whole brain radiation therapy. In relatively radioresistant tumors, such as renal cell, it may be that postoperative WBRT is less effective and may not even be needed. Currently, a randomized trial is in process to assess the need for postoperative radiation therapy. Until that trial is completed, WBRT following surgery is the accepted standard of care.

The role of radiosurgery in the management of brain metastases is unclear at this writing (fall 1994). So far, there have been no controlled studies comparing radiosurgery with conventional surgery in the treatment of single brain metastases. What data do exist on radiosurgery consist exclusively of enthusiastic reports of uncontrolled series of highly selected (good prognosis) patients treated with radiosurgery. These studies, which were summarized earlier in the discussion, show a local control rate that is similar to that found with conventional surgery. However, many of these studies have very short follow-up times, and due to patient selection, the results are not directly comparable with the studies involving surgery. In addition, radiosurgery has long-term morbidity that needs to be considered when assessing its value. The rate of steroid dependence is substantially higher in patients treated with radiosurgery compared with that found after treatment with conventional surgery, and 10%–15% of patients treated with radiosurgery develop radiation necrosis of brain that is severe enough to require surgical debulking. The value of radiosurgery is unproven and should be considered experimental until conclusive evidence of its efficacy becomes available. Currently, the best available scientific evidence indicates that the good prognosis patients with single brain metastases should be treated with conventional surgery plus radiation therapy.

In summary, this case demonstrates the problems with interpretation of currently available data on treatment of brain metastases. This patient should probably have been treated with conventional surgical resection followed by WBRT. It is encouraging that the patient has done well following radiosurgery. However, at the current time, the treatment given to this patient has to be considered speculative.

REFERENCES

1. Hendrickson FR. The optimum schedule for palliative radiotherapy for metastatic brain cancer. *Int J Radiat Oncol Biol Phys* 1977;2:165–8.
2. Borgelt B, Gelber R, Kramer S, et al. The palliation of brain metastases: final results of the first two studies by the Radiation Therapy Oncology Group. *Int J Radiat Oncol Biol Phys* 1980;6:1.
3. Gelber RD, Larson M, Borgelt BB, Kramer S. Equivalence of radiation schedules for the palliative treatment of brain metastases in patients with favorable prognosis. *Cancer* 1981;48:1749–53.
4. Kurtz JM, Gelber R, Brady LW, Carella RJ, Cooper JS. The palliation of brain metastases in a favorable patient population: a randomized clinical trial by the Radiation Therapy Oncology Group. *Int J Radiat Oncol Biol Phys* 1981;7:891–5.
5. Epstein BE, Scott CB, Sause WT, et al. Improved survival duration in patients with unresected solitary brain metastasis using accelerated hyperfractionated radiation therapy at total doses of 54.4 gray and greater. Results of Radiation Oncology Group 85-28. *Cancer* 1993;71:1362–73.
6. DeAngelis LM, Delattre JY, Posner JB. Radiation-induced dementia in patients cured of brain metastases. *Neurology* 1989;39:789–96.
7. Patchell RA, Tibbs PA, Walsh JW, Dempsey RJ, Maruyama Y, Kryscio RJ, Markesbery WR, Macdonald JS, Young B. A randomized trial of surgery in the treatment of single metastases to the brain. *N Engl J Med* 1990;322:494–500.
8. Vecht CJ, Haaxma-Reiche H, Noordijk EM, Padberg GW, Voormolen JH, Hoekstra FH, Tans JT, Lambooij N, Metsaars JA, Wattendorff AR, et al. Treatment of single brain metastasis: radiotherapy alone or combined with neurosurgery? *Ann Neurol* 1993;33:583–590.
9. Dosoretz DE, Blitzer PH, Russell AH, et al. Management of solitary metastasis to the brain: the role of elective brain irradiation following complete surgical resection. *Int J Radiat Oncol Biol Phys* 1980;6:1727–30.
10. Smalley SR, Schray MF, Laws ER Jr, O'Fallon JR. Adjuvant radiation therapy after surgical resection of solitary brain metastasis: association with pattern of failure and survival. *Int J Radiat Oncol Biol Phys* 1987;13:1611–6.
11. Hagen N, Cirrincione C, DeAngelis, LM. The role of radiotherapy after resection of single brain metastases from melanoma. *Neurology* 1989;39(suppl 1):262.
12. DeAngelis LM, Mandell LR, Thaler HT, Kimmel DW, Galicich JH, Fuks Z, Posner JB. The role of postoperative radiotherapy after resection of single brain metastases. *Neurosurgery* 1989;24:798–805.
13. Smalley SR, Laws ER Jr, O'Fallon JR, Shaw EG, Schray MF. Resection for solitary brain metastasis. Role of adjuvant radiation and prognostic variables in 229 patients. *J Neurosurg* 1992;77:531–40.

SECTION XXVIII

Hodgkin's Disease

128

Stage IIIA Hodgkin's Disease in a Young Woman

Hugo V. Villar

Staging laparotomy: A relic of the past?

CASE PRESENTATION

Our case is a 30-year-old woman with a 4-month history of odynophagia and some neck swelling. She denies fever, chills, night sweats, or weight loss. When a new right-sided neck mass appeared 2 months later, she consulted the Arizona Cancer Center.

Her past medical history is relevant for a tonsillectomy and appendectomy. She is the second of three siblings. Review of her system was negative except for some coughing and some difficulties swallowing. Her menstrual periods were normal.

Physical examination reveals a young woman in no acute distress, with a height of 5'3" and a weight of 110 pounds. HEENT were normal. The neck shows multiple small "shotty" nodes on the posterior neck and anteriorly on the right side. There were supraclavicular nodes measuring about 5 cm on the right, and about 4 cm on the left, tender to the touch without any skin changes. The axillae were negative. Lungs were clear to auscultation and percussion. The heart had normal rhythms. The breasts were normal. The abdomen was nontender; neither the spleen nor the liver were palpable. There was no lymph adenopathy in the groin. Neurological examination was normal.

Laboratory assessment was as follows: CBC and differential were normal, chest roentgenogram showed a large anterior mediastinal mass (Fig. 128–1).

With a clinical diagnosis of probable Hodgkin's disease, clinical stage III A, the patient was referred to the surgical oncologist for a right supraclavicular lymph node biopsy.

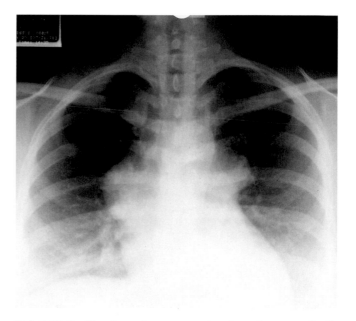

FIG. 128–1. Chest roentgenogram showing a large mediastinal mass.

Surgical oncologist: Under local anesthesia the patient underwent removal of a 2 × 3 cm right supraclavicular lymph node. The lymph nodes were matted against each other. The specimen was given fresh to the immunopathologist for touch preparations and immunophenopathology. The patient was discharged the same day. Her recovery was uneventful. On her first postoperative visit, the patient was told the diagnosis of nodular sclerosing Hodgkin's disease. Computed tomography of

649

her chest and abdominal and bone marrow biopsy were requested to complement her clinical staging.

Immunopathologist: The gross pathology examination reveals enlarged encapsulated lymphoid tissue, which on cross section has a fibrous and a nodular appearance. A cut section of the node is touched to glass for a touch imprint. Wright/Giemsa staining of this touch prep reveals small, regular, round lymphocytes, with admixed large polylobated lymphoid cells that have viral inclusion like nucleoli and chromatin clearing. The latter indicates the presence of Reed-Sternberg cells in a normal lymphoid reactive background as necessary for the diagnosis of Hodgkin's disease. The histologic sections with hematoxylin-eosin reveal small round regular lymphocytes, sclerosing bands of collagenosis, occasional large aberrant cells in tissue spaces known as *lacunar cells*, seen in the upper right quadrant, and finally, specific polylobated Reed-Sternberg cells as seen in the center of the figure. The classic Reed-Sternberg cell is characterized by viral inclusion-like nucleoli parachromatin clearing and multinucleation of the cell. Collectively, the findings are typical for a nodular sclerosis variant of Hodgkin's disease (Fig. 128–2).

Diagnostic radiologist: A posteroanterior view of the chest demonstrates bilateral loss of the clavicular companion shadows consistent with supraclavicular masses, larger on the right than the left. There is a bulky anterior mediastinal mass (Fig. 128–1). The heart is normal and the lungs are clear. No effusions are present. An axial section of the chest CT, approximately 3 cm below the carina, demonstrates the anterior mediastinal mass, which extends posteriorly to the pulmonary arteries. The right and left main stem bronchi are well visualized. They are not physically compromised by the bulky mass, and the airway is completely free of evidence of extrinsic compression throughout the other sections obtained on the CT scan. The lungs are normal (Fig. 128–3).

Cross section of the abdomen from the CT scan: A single axial section of the abdomen at the level of the inferior vena cava bifurcation demonstrates numerous lymph nodes (several about 2 cm in cross-sectional diameter) within the retroperitoneum. (Fig. 128–4).

An anteroposterior view of the abdomen after contrast injection into the retroperitoneum (lymphogram) demonstrates enlargement and a loss of normal internal architecture in several of the visualized nodes (Fig. 128–5).

Based on a summary evaluation of the imaging studies, including chest roentgenogram, chest and abdominal CT scans, and lymphogram, the diagnosis is likely Hodgkin's disease. The evidence suggests that this could be disease below the diaphragm but since reactive adenopathy can occur involving the infradiaphragmatic nodes, surgical confirmation to determine the stage is desirable.

Surgical oncologist: Preoperative assessment of the airway by our anesthesiologist places the risk of airway compression during induction as minimal; this complication has been observed with bulky mediastinal masses. Because concern about involvement of the periaortic lymph nodes, especially at the level of L-1 and L-2 as shown on the lymphogram, we agreed to perform a stag-

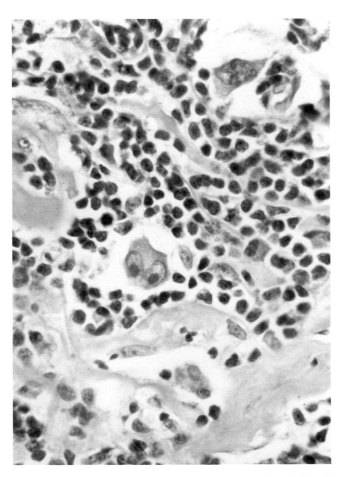

FIG. 128–2. Thin section of cervical lymph node. A Reed-Sternberg cell is clearly seen in the center.

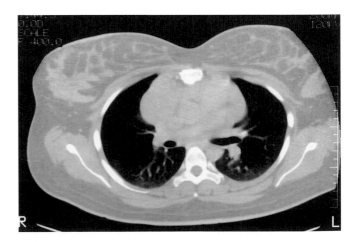

FIG. 128–3. Axial section of chest CT about 3 cm below the carina.

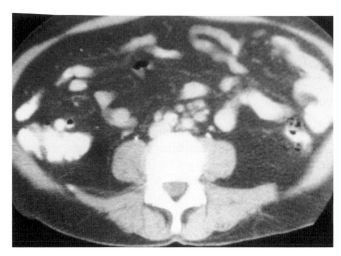

FIG. 128–4. Single axial section of the abdomen at the level of the IVC bifurcation showing numerous lymph nodes within the retroperitoneum.

ing laparotomy consisting of biopsy of both lobes of the liver, wedge and tru-cut, a splenectomy, and biopsy of the periaortic lymph nodes from the left renal vein to the bifurcation of the iliacs. The operation has a mortality of less than 0.5%. In our experience with 70 consecutive staging laparotomies, not one patient has died. Morbidity of a staging laparotomy includes bleeding, pancreatitis, and pneumonia. Small bowel obstruction may occur later,

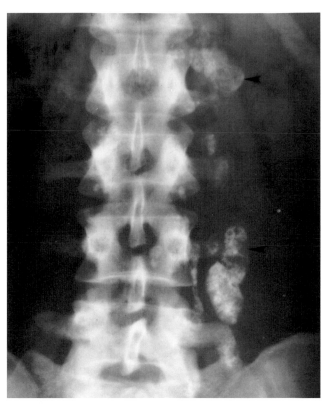

FIG. 128–5. AP view of the abdomen after contrast injection into the retroperitoneum showing enlargement and loss of normal internal architecture in several of the lymph nodes.

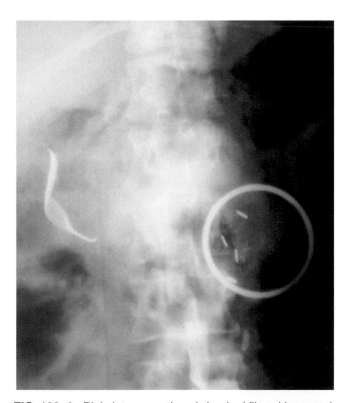

FIG. 128–6. Plain intraoperative abdominal film with a metallic ring to confirm removal of abnormal lymph nodes.

especially if the patient is subsequently radiated. In this particular patient, after standard removal of the periaortic lymph nodes, we placed a metallic ring at the level of L-2 and took a film of the abdomen to be sure we removed the lymph node in question (Fig. 128–6). In addition, we waited for a preliminary report from our pathologist to be sure that lymph node material was removed from the periaortic area rather than adipose tissue. We did not perform any plication of the ovaries behind the uterus because that procedure has been associated with dyspareunia. We were particularly careful during her splenectomy; and we divided all of the gastrocolic vessels and tied the splenic artery prior to mobilization of the spleen—this minimizes the risk of pancreatitis because the hilum of the spleen is divided under full view. The patient had an uneventful recovery. The final path report revealed involvement of the spleen with more than five nodules. Six of ten periaortic lymph nodes had Hodgkin's disease.

Medical oncologist: The treatment for young patients with pathologic-determined stage IIIA disease may include either total nodal irradiation or combination chemotherapy. In general, if the disease is extensive within the spleen, or extends below the bifurcation of the aorta, chemotherapy is indicated. Because the patient under discussion has more than five nodules within the spleen, the best choice for therapy would be a combination chemotherapy. Recent randomized trials have indicated that Adriamycin-containing regimens offer advantages over classical MOPP. Both ABVD (Adriamycin, bleomycin, vinblastine, DTIC) and the MOPP-ABV hybrid (nitrogen mustard, vincristine, procarbazine, and prednisone alternating with Adriamycin, bleomycin, and vinblastine) have been shown to be more active and less toxic than classic MOPP. These new regimens have a low incidence of sterility, especially among women, and a low incidence of acute leukemia. Furthermore, disease-free survival has been shown to be improved compared with MOPP. In general, treatment is delivered on monthly cycles for a minimum of 6 months. Many patients require 8 months of therapy; the duration of therapy is determined by the patient's response at the 4-month mark.

Of interest, this patient had nodular sclerosing Hodgkin's disease. In general, the histologic subtypes of Hodgkin's disease do not indicate different treatment options (the exception is lymphocyte-predominant Hodgkin's disease, which may be reclassified in the near future). Mixed cellularity Hodgkin's disease is frequently mistaken by pathologists. Consequently, many of the historical reports indicating a poor prognosis for mixed cellularity Hodgkin's disease are probably secondary to confusing some cases of non-Hodgkin's lymphomas with this disease.

Radiation oncologist: While total nodal irradiation has historically been an acceptable alternative to combination chemotherapy, the presence of relatively extensive subdiaphragmatic disease favor the use of combination chemotherapy, either as a primary treatment or in combination with radiation treatment.

However, when sites of relapse in patients with Hodgkin's disease treated with chemotherapy are examined, sites of initial bulk disease, particularly in the mediastinum, predominate. This suggests a role, at least in some patients, for consolidative radiation therapy following some number of cycles of chemotherapy. In addition, not all patients receiving primary chemotherapy obtain a complete response. In this group, radiation to both prior areas of bulk disease and residual incompletely responded sites of Hodgkin's disease has proved beneficial.

The presence of a large anterior mediastinal mass and apparently bulky neck nodes would make me favor the addition of irradiation to a mantel, or mini-mantel, field in this patient, following appropriate chemotherapy. This would be particularly true should response of the patient's Hodgkin's disease be inadequate or incomplete.

Most studies indicate that when radiation is given in conjunction with aggressive combination chemotherapy, the dose of irradiation can safely be lowered significantly; usually, in the 2,500 to 3,000 cGy range level and, in many instances, possibly lower. In patients who do not obtain an adequate response or whose tumor progresses despite chemotherapy, full-dose irradiation is appropri-

ate; numerous studies have demonstrated that radiation doses of 3,500 to 4,000+ cGy appear to more consistently produce long-term local control.

Follow-up

The patient underwent combination chemotherapy with ABVD. At the completion of her therapy, a mantle field of irradiation was given for a total dose of 3,500 centigrade.

Following completion of therapy, this patient would be followed by a clinical exam every 2 months for the first year, every 3 months for the second and third year, and every 6 months for the fourth and fifth year. Following the fifth year of follow-up the patient can be followed once each year. Follow-up would include an examination, a chest roentgenogram, peripheral blood counts, and routine chemistries. A CT scan may be obtained once a year or if the patient develops any signs or symptoms of concern.

COMMENTARY by Bruce A. Peterson

The major issue raised by this case of a young woman with Hodgkin's disease is the extent of her staging. Other than odynophagia and dysphagia, her presentation was not extraordinary for Hodgkin's disease. She had neck swelling and a right-sided neck mass, accompanied by a cough. There were no systemic symptoms. On physical examination, she had impressive bilateral supraclavicular lymph nodes and "shotty" nodes in the right anterior and posterior cervical regions. No other physical findings were apparent.

Both the location and size of this patient's lymph nodes are relevant to subsequent decisions in her management. Pangalis et al. have published their analysis of a systemic approach to the decision of whether to biopsy enlarged lymph nodes in 220 patients (1). An obvious acute infection or another identifiable illness may dictate the diagnostic approach to lymphadenopathy, but in the absence of these circumstances, among the factors indicating a need for biopsy are location and size of the lymph node(s). Sites in the neck, such as posterior/anterior cervical and suboccipital, are most often associated with benign conditions, but supraclavicular lymphadenopathy is associated with a specific cause in 95% of cases. The causes most commonly include Hodgkin's disease, non-Hodgkin's lymphoma, and metastatic carcinoma. Tuberculosis was the most frequent benign cause of enlarged supraclavicular nodes. In their study, size also became an important factor when the nodes surpassed 2.25 cm^2. Both criteria existed in this patient. She clearly required a biopsy, preferably an excisional biopsy, as was performed. This established her diagnosis and launched the process of staging to inform the selection of therapy.

The Ann Arbor staging system was developed and adopted for use in patients with Hodgkin's disease in 1971 (2) and modified slightly at a conference in the Cotswolds in 1989 (3). "Clinical" stage (CS) reflects the findings on physical, laboratory, and radiographic evaluation. A bone marrow biopsy that is negative is also reflected in the clinical stage, but a positive bone marrow biopsy or the findings of a staging laparotomy, positive or negative, determines the "pathologic" stage (PS). The current uses of staging are fourfold: (1) to provide guidance in selecting therapy for an individual patient; (2) to provide prognostic information related to that patient; (3) to identify pretherapeutic sites of disease so that these may be appropriately reassessed for response following therapy; and (4) to classify patients for the purposes of clinical investigation. Although thorough staging in the past has contributed enormously to understanding patterns of spread, the primary importance of staging today is to guide therapeutic decision making.

In addition to the history and physical examination, this patient's initial staging assessment included a limited series of laboratory tests, radiographic studies, and a bone marrow biopsy. She denied fever, night sweats, or weight loss—the three "symptoms" that require the designation "B" in the Ann Arbor system and indicate a worse prognosis. Laboratory testing routinely includes, in addition to CBC and differential, an erythrocyte sedimentation rate, serum tests of liver and renal function, as well as serum alkaline phosphatase and lactate dehydrogenase (4). The ESR, a very simple test, adds prognostic information, and an alkaline phosphatase can suggest bone involvement.

Radiographic evaluation usually includes PA and lateral chest roentgenograms, and chest and abdominal/pelvic CT scans. This patient's examinations disclosed a large anterior mediastinal mass and several 2-cm nodes at the level of the bifurcation of the inferior vena cava. Both findings are important. The accuracy of the abdominal CT findings in this case is sufficient for clinical staging (5). Lymphography in this patient was unnecessary. It is a cumbersome, uncomfortable test that now is used relatively infrequently. It requires special expertise that is often unavailable, and its routine use adds little of consequence to positive CT findings. Perhaps the most common indication for lymphography is in the patient with a negative abdominal/pelvic CT scan for whom irradiation alone is being contemplated as a therapeutic option. In that setting, especially if the results of the lymphogram will either influence treatment choice or a decision to proceed to staging laparotomy, it may be useful. In this patient, lymphography contributed little to her staging and subsequent management.

A bone marrow biopsy, a routine staging maneuver, was performed and was negative for involvement. Thus, this patient had Hodgkin's disease, nodular sclerosis, and based on the clinical evidence of nodal disease above and below the diaphragm and a negative bone marrow, the patient is CS IIIA. The next question is whether a staging laparotomy was necessary.

Staging laparotomy was originally a research tool introduced to document patterns of involvement in infradiaphragmatic sites and quickly became routinely employed to determine final stage (4). However, as noninvasive techniques for identifying subdiaphragmatic involvement improved and combination chemotherapy became increasingly and successfully used in earlier stages, its use and value have, like the lymphogram, been severely curtailed. The reason to do a staging laparotomy is to establish whether abdominal disease is present if knowing that information would directly determine whether irradiation alone is suitable. If treatment is to include chemotherapy, the value of any information obtained at staging laparotomy is minimal.

The clinical findings in this patient preclude the need for staging laparotomy. The involvement of multiple regions above the diaphragm, plus the large mediastinal mass, predict a high-risk of intra-abdominal disease (6–8). The additional findings on the abdominal CT scan are sufficient evidence of lower abdominal involvement to compel the use of chemotherapy, with or without irradiation, as her primary therapy. Finally, even if clinical evidence of intra-abdominal disease were absent, standard radiotherapy is not sufficient to cure a mediastinal mass of this size (9–11). Thus, since she requires chemotherapy as at least part of her treatment, she does not need a staging laparotomy and splenectomy, which expose her to both short-term and long-term risks, such as overwhelming postsplenectomy infections and a slightly increased risk of developing post-treatment acute leukemia.

REFERENCES

1. Pangalis GA, Vassilakopoulos TP, Boussiotis VA, et al. Clinical approach to lymphadenopathy. *Sem Oncol* 1993;20:570–82.
2. Carbone PP, Kaplan HS, Musshoff K, et al. Report of the committee on Hodgkin's disease staging classification. *Cancer Res* 1971;31:1860–1.
3. Lister TA, Crowther D, Sutcliffe SB, et al. Report of a committee convened to discuss the evaluation and staging of patients with Hodgkin's disease: Cotswolds Meeting. *J Clin Oncol* 1989;7:1630–6.
4. Weinshel EL, Peterson BA. Hodgkin's disease. *Cancer J Clin* 43:327-346, 1993.
5. Castellino RA, Hoppe RT, Blank N, et al. Computed tomography, lymphography, and staging laparotomy: correlations in initial staging of Hodgkin's disease. *Am J Roentgenol* 1984;143:37–41.
6. Mauch P, Larson D, Osteen R, et al. Prognostic factors for positive surgical staging in patients with Hodgkin's disease. *J Clin Oncol* 1990;8:257–65.
7. Leibenhaut MH, Hoppe RT, Efron B, et al. Prognostic indicators of laparotomy findings in clinical stage I-II supradiaphragmatic Hodgkin's disease. *J Clin Oncol* 1989;7:81–91.
8. Aragon de la Cruz G, Cardenes H, Otero J, et al. Individual risk of abdominal disease in patients with stages I and II supra-diaphragamatic Hodgkin's disease: a rule index based on 341 laparotomized patients. *Cancer* 1989;63:1799–1803.
9. Hoppe RT. The management of bulky mediastinal Hodgkin's disease. *Hematol Oncol Clin North Am* 1989;3:265–76.
10. Leopold KA, Canellos GP, Rosenthal D, et al. Stage IA–IIB Hodgkin's disease: staging and treatment of patients with large mediastinal adenopathy. *J Clin Oncol* 1989;7:1059–65.
11. Longo DL, Russa A, Duffey PL, et al. Treatment of advanced-stage massive mediastinal Hodgkin's disease: the case for combined modality treatment. *J Clin Oncol* 1991;9:227–35.

129

Long-Term Survival in Stage IV Hodgkin's Disease

B.J. Kennedy

Twenty-four plus years of good quality life can be a product of participation in clinical trials

CASE PRESENTATION

In October, 1970, this 38-year-old man complained of fever, chills, and hip pain of several months' duration. Examination revealed a left supraclavicular lymph node and a mediastinal mass on roentgenogram (Fig. 129–1). Biopsy of the node revealed nodular sclerosing Hodgkin's disease. The patient was referred to the University of Minnesota Hospitals where further evaluation revealed a bone marrow positive for Hodgkin's disease and a lymphangiogram revealing abdominal lymph nodes. The patient was judged to have stage IV-B Hodgkin's disease. The patient's occupation was that of a physicist in a nuclear power plant.

The patient was entered into a clinical research trial of chemotherapy with CVPP (cyclophosphamide, vinblastine, procarbazine, and prednisone) beginning in December, 1970. He tolerated this well, but because of myelosuppression 1 year later, testosterone enanthate was administered intramuscularly three times per week. By the end of the first year of chemotherapy, complete regression was recorded (Fig. 129–2). All tests were normal. He was continued on maintenance CVPP every 3 weeks for the next 2 years, during which time fluoxymesterone was substituted for the testosterone enanthate. Chemotherapy was discontinued in January, 1974 (a 3-year program).

The patient continued to do well. In February, 1977, the patient was re-evaluated for extent of disease. The lymphangiogram suggested slightly enlarged lymph nodes.

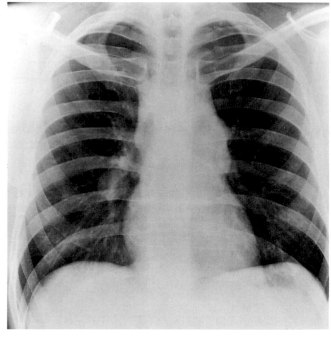

FIG. 129–1. Mediastinal lymphadenopathy at time of initial diagnosis of Hodgkin's disease.

Again, as part of a clinical research trial, a laparotomy was performed. A lymph node near the bile duct and a left periaortic node were positive for Hodgkin's disease, although other biopsies of mesenteric nodes and liver were normal. A splenectomy was performed.

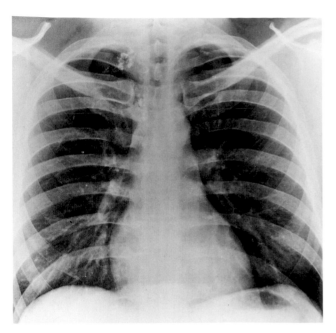

FIG. 129–2. Complete regression of mediastinal mass after CVPP chemotherapy.

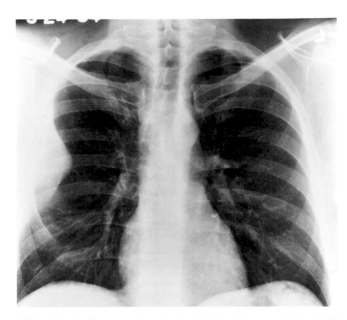

FIG. 129–3. Reactivation of Hodgkin's disease in the right thoracic wall.

The patient was entered into a third clinical trial consisting of chemotherapy with CCNU, doxorubicin, bleomycin, vincristine, and prednisone. After 26 months, a maintenance program was continued until December, 1978.

In September, 1979, as part of the clinical trial of vigorous search for recurrent disease, a laparotomy was performed. Biopsies of the lymph nodes and liver were negative. The patient did well. In October, 1981, the white blood count was 7,700. In September, 1982, it was 10,500; in September, 1983, 14,700. No evidence of recurrent tumor was noted.

In January, 1984, the white blood count had increased to 18,200, with a normal differential. Four months later, the patient complained of right chest pain. A chest roentgenogram was obtained (Fig. 129–3).On examination, there was a right posterior axillary mass. A CT of the chest revealed an intra- and extrathoracic mass along with an expanded rib. In the patient's occupation at the power plant, he had moderate exposure to asbestos. Biopsy again revealed recurrent Hodgkin's disease. Beginning in June, 1984, he was given seven cycles of CVPP resulting in a complete regression of the tumor mass (Fig. 129–4). Therapy was discontinued in January, 1985.

In October, 1988, a chest roentgenogram revealed a right pleural mass and enlarged mediastinal lymph nodes (Fig. 129–5). Biopsy of the pleural mass revealed Hodgkin's disease. The bone marrow biopsy was negative. A bone marrow transplant was carried out 1 month later.

On recovering from the bone marrow transplant, radiation therapy was delivered to the right pleural mass and

completed in March, 1989 (Fig. 129–6). He remains well more than 7 years after the bone marrow transplant.

COMMENTARY by Ilene Ceil Weitz and Cary A. Presant

This patient is a product of clinical research. Now, at age 62, over an expanse of 24 years, he has participated in four different clinical trials, two different chemotherapy

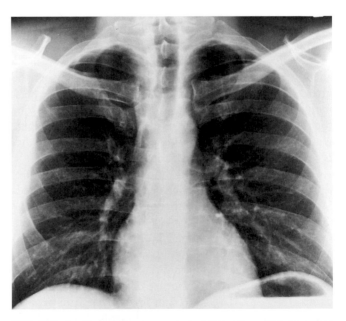

FIG. 129–4. Complete regression of thoracic wall mass after seven cycles of CVPP.

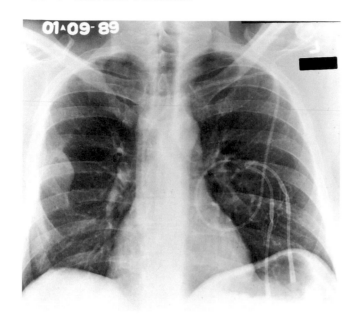

FIG. 129–5. Recurrent right pleural mass and enlarged mediastinal lymph nodes.

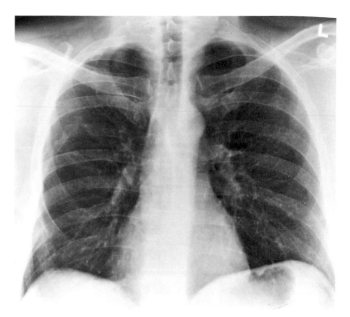

FIG. 129–6. Complete regression of right pleural mass after bone marrow transplantation and radiation therapy to chest wall.

regimens, surgical re-exploration of the abdomen and high-dose chemotherapy with bone marrow transplantation. The patient is convinced of the merits and advantages of clinical research programs.

The treatment of Hodgkin's disease is one of the true success stories in medical oncology. Prior to the 1960s, the disease was uniformly fatal. With contemporary therapy, 85%–95% of patients achieve remission, and approximately 70% of patients have long-term disease-free survival (1). This patient's 27-year odyssey with Hodgkin's disease highlights many of the advances made in treating this disease.

Hodgkin's disease affect people of all ages. However, in the United States and Europe, the peak incidence occurs in young adults aged 16–40 years, and in those aged 60 years and over. In less-developed countries, the greatest incidence occurs in childhood; in Japan, the peak incidence occurs over the age of 60. The specific reasons for this remain unclear. There is a male predominance, with the exception of the nodular-sclerosing subtype that is seen more often in young women (2).

The etiology of Hodgkin's disease remains obscure. Epstein-Barr virus DNA has been identified in Reed-Sternberg cells in 20% of patients with Hodgkin's disease (3). Ionizing radiation has also been implicated. Data from Hiroshima and Nagasaki indicated an increased incidence 10–15 years after exposure to atomic bomb radiation, and that the relative risk for developing a lymphoma, either Hodgkin's disease or non- Hodgkin's lymphoma (HD or NHL), was eight times greater for persons exposed to more than 100 Gy (4). It is interesting that this patient worked in a nuclear power plant, but we do not know the extent of his exposure to radiation.

This patient presented with stage IVB disease. Prior to the development of MOPP chemotherapy, less than 10% of patients treated with single-agent chemotherapy survived for 5 years. MOPP (and the related chemotherapy regimens) provided a major breakthrough in the treatment of Hodgkin's disease. The 20-year follow-up data on the MOPP regimen confirmed the very high complete remission (CR) rates (80%) and disease-free survivals (60% at 10 years) reported with the initial MOPP trial. Pathologic stage IV patients, like the patient in this case, have a 77% CR rate, with 65% remaining in remission at 5 years. Patients with bulky disease or B symptoms have a lower CR rate compared with those without symptoms, 78% versus 100%. However, even with B symptoms, 53% of patients treated with MOPP were alive in 10 years. In this report, the highest relapse rates were seen with the nodular sclerosing (NS) subtype, which this patient had. His course is fairly typical of patients with NSHD. These patients have chemosensitive disease (80% CR rate) but more frequent and earlier relapses compared to the other histologic subtypes (59% versus 70%–80% disease-free survival) (5).

For over 25 years, MOPP has been the primary chemotherapeutic regimen used to treat Hodgkin's disease. However, because of the toxicities associated with it, several other related regimens (CVPP, which this patient had, B-CVPP, CHL-VPP, etc.) have been used with comparable results (6,7). Most recently, a randomized trial comparing MOPP, MOPP-ABVD, and ABVD suggested that ABVD (Adriamycin, bleomycin, Velban, DTIC) has a superior CR rate to MOPP (82% versus 67%) as well as a superior 5-year survival rate (73% versus

66%). The ABVD regimen was also associated with less hematologic toxicity, and a lower rate of infertility and leukemia. Because of this, ABVD is considered by many to be the preferred therapy for stage IIIB and IV disease. Another important observation of this study was that MOPP appears to be a better salvage regimen for relapse following ABVD, as compared with ABVD following MOPP failures (61% CR versus 46%)(8). This patient, as part of the clinical trial, received maintenance therapy. The long-term MOPP data did not show any benefit for maintenance therapy (9).

Despite the high CR rates, there remain patients who fail to achieve a CR with conventional treatment. As mentioned, MOPP appears to be a better salvage regimen than ABVD. However, in patients who relapse more than 1 year after treatment, the same regimen may be used again to induce a remission.

When this patient first relapsed, he received a second type of chemotherapy regimen using CCNU, doxorubicin, bleomycin, vincristine, and prednisone, to which he responded. He was re-treated with CVPP at the time of his third relapse, 14 years later, and again responded.

After his fourth relapse, he underwent high-dose chemotherapy followed by bone marrow transplantation. Patients are usually treated with one or two cycles of standard-dose chemotherapy before high-dose chemotherapy in bone marrow transplantation, in order to reduce the tumor burden and to demonstrate chemosensitivity. The results with transplantation clearly indicate superior survival in patients with chemosensitive disease (50% alive at 3 years) versus median survival of 14 months in chemoresistant disease. Those patients undergoing bone marrow transplantation while in CR have a more favorable long-term outcome (10). In some patients who have received extensive chemotherapy in the past, the transplant conditioning regimen may be used as the induction regimen in an attempt to limit toxicity. It appears that this was the case with this patient. He was then consolidated with radiation therapy following the transplant. The results with allogeneic and autologous transplantation are comparable but there is significantly less morbidity associated with the autologous procedure (11). Data with peripheral blood stem cell transplantation appears to be comparable to that of autologous transplantation (12).

Radiation therapy was used to consolidate this patient's posttransplant remission. Clearly, radiation therapy has a curative role in early disease and may be used to treat initial sites of bulky disease to decrease local relapse. It may also be used to treat localized sites of relapse as well as for curative therapy in selected patients with relapsed disease (13–15).

This patient's case has been remarkable. However, one wonders what the future holds for him. He has had extensive exposure to alkylating chemotherapy as well as nitrosoureas, both which have been associated with the development of acute nonlymphocytic leukemia (ANLL),

particularly if patients have also received radiation therapy. In one study, the 12-year estimated risk of ANLL in patients receiving alkylating agents and radiation was 4.8%. In patients receiving MOPP and radiation therapy, the reported risk was 10.2%. The leukemic risk in patients receiving chemotherapy alone was 1.4 ± 2.3% (16). Myelodysplasia has been reported following autologous bone marrow transplantation for HD and NHL (17). Other second malignant tumors associated with treatment for Hodgkin's disease include Non-Hodgkin's lymphoma, basal cell carcinoma, skin carcinoma, and lung cancer. Most solid tumors occur in patients who have received radiation therapy (18).

Other long-term complications may include pulmonary fibrosis, related to either radiation or chemotherapy (such as bleomycin, BCNU, or melphalan) used as primary treatment or as part of the pretransplant conditioning regimen, cardiac dysfunction 2° to Adriamycin alone (and particularly if radiation has also been used), and pericarditis. Chemotherapy has also been associated with both male and female sterility (17).

This patient, along with thousands of others, participated in clinical therapeutic trials. The participation of these patients has greatly helped in the advances that have occurred with the treatment of Hodgkin's disease. We would encourage all physicians and patients to participate in clinical trials whenever possible so that we can answer the many critical issues concerning treatments and outcomes in many diseases.

REFERENCES

1. Bonadonna G. Systemic treatment of Hodgkin's disease. *Adv Oncol* 1987;3(3):7–15.
2. Liebman HA, Mauch P. Hodgkin's disease: a clinical perspective. *Semin Ultrasound CT MR* 1985;6(4):362–73.
3. Weiss LM, Movahed BS, Warnke RA, Sklar J. Detection of Epstein-Barr viral genome in Reed-Sternberg cells of Hodgkin's disease. *New Engl J Med* 1989;320:520–6.
4. The Committee for the Compilation of Materials on Damage Caused by the Atomic Bomb in Hiroshima and Nagasaki, Hiroshima and Nagasaki. Iwanami Shoten, Tokyo; 1979:273–5.
5. DeVita VT, Simon RT, Hubbard SM, Young RC, Berard CW, Moxley JH, Frei E, Carbone PP, Canellos GP. Curability of advanced Hodgkin's disease with chemotherapy. *Ann Int Med* 1980;92:587–95.
6. Liebman HA, Hum GL, Sheehan WW, Ryden VM, Bateman JR. Randomized study for the treatment of adult advanced Hodgkin's disease: mechlorethamine, vincristine, procarbazine and prednisone (MOPP) versus lomustine, vinblastine and prednisone. *Cancer Treat Rep* 1983;67(5):413–19.
7. DeVita VT, Hubbard SM. Hodgkin's disease. *New Engl J Med* 1993;328(8):560–5.
8. Canellos GP, Anderson JR, Propert KJ, Nissen N, Cooper NR, Henderson ES, Green MR, Gottlieb A, Peterson BA. Advanced Hodgkin's disease with MOPP, ABVD, or MOPP alternating with ABVD. *New Engl J Med* 1992;327:1478–84.
9. DeVita VT. The consequences of chemotherapy of Hodgkin's disease: the David A. Karnofsky Memorial Lecture. *Cancer* 1981;47(1):1–13.
10. Jones RT, et al. High-dose cytotoxic therapy and bone marrow transplantation for relapsed Hodgkin's disease. *J Clin Oncol* 1990;8(3):527–37.
11. Bierman P, Armitage JO. Role of autotransplantation in Hodgkin's diseases. *Hematol Oncol Clin North Am* 1993;6:591–611.

12. Bierman PJ, Vose J, Anderson J, Bishop M, Pierson J, Armitage JO, Kissinger A. Comparison of autologous bone marrow transplantation for patients with Hodgkin's disease. *Blood* 1993;82(suppl 10): 1763.
13. Mauch P, Tarbell N, Skarin A, Rosenthal D, Weinstein H. wide-field radiation therapy alone or with chemotherapy for Hodgkin's diseases in relapse from combination chemotherapy. *J Clin Oncol* 1987;5(4): 544–9.
14. Roach M, Kapp DS, Rosenberg SA, Hoppe RT. Radiotherapy with curative intent: an option in selected patients relapsing after chemotherapy for advanced Hodgkin's disease. *J Clin Oncol* 1987; 5(4):550–5.
15. Fox KA, Lippman SM, Cassaday JR, Heusinkveld RS, Miller TP. Radiation therapy salvage of Hodgkin's disease following chemotherapy failure. *J Clin Oncol* 1982;5(1):38–45.
16. Valagussa P, Santoro A, Fossati-Bellani F, Banfi A, Bonnadonna G. Second acute leukemia and other malignancies following treatment for Hodgkin's disease. *J Clin Oncol* 1986;4(6):830–7.
17. Traweek ST, Slovak MJ, Nademanee AP, Byrnes RK, Niland JC, Forman SJ. Myelodysplasia occurring after autologous bone marrow transplantation for Hodgkin's disease and non-Hodgkin's lymphoma. *Blood* 1993;82(10 suppl):1805.
18. Van Leeuwen FE, Somes R, Taal BQ, VanHeerde P, Coster B, Dozeman T, Heisman SJ, Hart AM. Increased risk of lung cancer, non-Hodgkin's lymphoma and leukemia following Hodgkin's diseases. *J Clin Oncol* 1989;7:1046–58.

130

Stage IIA Nodular Sclerosing Hodgkin's Disease with Bulky Mediastinal Disease

Reinhard W. von Roemeling and Michael J. Moffett

Treatment with intent to cure: It can be done

CASE PRESENTATION

History

E.P., a 23-year-old white woman, first noticed a painless swelling at the left side of her neck and a tight feeling in her neck and chest during the fall of 1990. She attributed this to stress. In February of 1991, she sought medical attention. No weight loss, fever, or night sweats were reported. The patient's previous medical and social history were unremarkable. She had no significant illnesses or allergies. There were no menstrual irregularities. She did not smoke or drink alcohol. She took multivitamins regularly but had no other medications. She was never exposed to hazardous materials. Her family history revealed lung cancer in her grandmother but had no other malignant tumors.

Physical Examination

The performance status was good (0 on the ECOG scale). She was 173-cm tall and weighed 63 kg. There was left neck adenopathy with a firm mass of approximately 5 cm diameter in the mid-neck region. There were no other suspicious nodes or other abnormalities.

Diagnostic Evaluation and Staging

Laboratory tests included complete blood count and differential count, PT, partial thromboplastin time, and chemical profile. Findings were within normal range including

alkaline phosphatase and lactate dehydrogenase. No eosinophilia was noted.

Radiographic studies included PA and lateral chest roentgenography, computed tomography of the chest, abdomen, and pelvis, and bipedal lymphangiography. These studies revealed a large upper, anterior mediastinal and left hilar mass of 11 cm in transverse diameter (greater than one third of chest diameter). Abdominal or pelvic lymph nodes did not exceed normal size limits and did not show characteristic filling defects on lymphangiographic films.

A cervical-node biopsy was performed. On microscopic examination, the regular lymph node structure was severely altered with thick dense bands of hyalinized connective tissue. Numerous lacunar cell and several classic Reed-Sternberg cells with many mononuclear Hodgkin cells were found. Numerous eosinophils, plasma cells, granulocytes, and lymphocytes were identified, leading to a diagnosis of Hodgkin's disease, nodular-sclerosing subtype (Fig. 130–1).

Bilateral iliac crest bone marrow biopsies revealed a normocytic marrow with slight reduction of iron stores, but no evidence of marrow involvement by Hodgkin's disease. It was concluded that she had nodular-sclerosing type Hodgkin's disease, stage IIA, with bulky mediastinal mass.

Treatment

Because of the large mediastinal mass, a multimodality treatment plan was adopted by medical and radiation

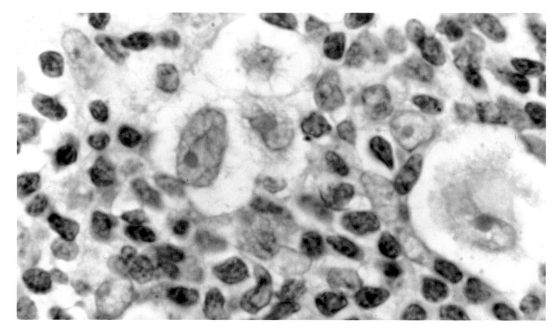

FIG. 130–1. Photomicrograph demonstrating classic lacunar cell variant of Reed-Sternberg cell with a background of mature lymphocytes.

oncologists, including primary chemotherapy with six cycles of standard MOPP (mechlorethamine, vincristine, procarbacine, and prednisone), followed by radiotherapy.

Chemotherapy

A ventral venous access was established (subcutaneous port). Standard MOPP doses were given for 6 courses. After 2 courses, the patient had mild peripheral polyneuropathy, which was thought to be secondary to vincristine. It was replaced by vinblastine for subsequent courses. Other side effects included moderate myelosuppression and mild nausea. Re-staging: After completion of chemotherapy in August, 1991, the patient underwent re-evaluation, including computed tomography of the chest and abdomen. There was residual adenopathy at the mediastinum measuring 3.5 × 2.5 cm, but no other abnormalities were found. On plain chest roentgenograms, this anterior mediastinal mass projected as 6 × 4 cm in size (Fig. 130–2). A gallium scan did not reveal pathological abnormality in the mediastinal mass. This evaluation indicated a complete clinical response with a residual mediastinal mass of unclear significance [CR(U)].

Radiation Therapy

Involved field radiation was given to the neck and mediastinum with total tumor doses of 4,000 cGy in 200 cGy fractions. (Involved field refers to treatment of involved lymph node chains only and is primarily used after systemic chemotherapy as consolidation therapy.) This treatment was completed in November 1991.

Follow-up

Examination in February, 1992, which included computed tomography of the chest, abdomen, and pelvis, revealed an unchanged mediastinal mass. In addition, interstitial densities in the lung parenchyma surrounding the mediastinal mass and several triangular-shaped patchy densities in the left mid-lung field were noted, reflecting radiation-therapy-induced scarring.

Subsequently, the patient continued with regular follow-up examinations in 4- to 6-month intervals. She has been free of symptoms and relapse for more than 3 years following her initial diagnosis. She has been in stable clinical complete remission of her disease, although a residual mediastinal mass is still detectable on plain chest films and CT scan [CR(U)].

TUMOR BOARD DISCUSSION

Epidemiology

In the Unites States, approximately 7,500 new cases of Hodgkin's disease are diagnosed annually, with a male:female predominance of 1.4:1. There is a bimodal incidence with peaks in young adulthood and in the later decades of life. Hodgkin's disease may represent a final common response to various pathologic processes,

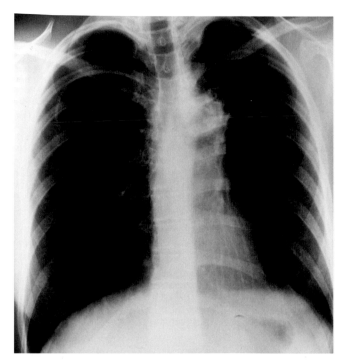

FIG. 130–2. Frontal chest radiograph demonstrating persistent left hilar AP window soft tissue density, which has remained unchanged since October, 1991.

including infections (e.g., EBV), environmental exposures, and genetic predispositions (1–3).

Pathology

Hodgkin's disease is a histologic diagnosis based on the recognition of mononuclear Hodgkin's cells and their multinucleated counterpart, Reed-Sternberg (RS) cells. RS cells are required for the diagnosis, but not pathognomonic, because they have been reported in benign conditions. They often account for only 1% of the cells present. The Rye classification identifies four subclasses (Table 130–1), based on the ratio of neoplastic to reactive cells, that have prognostic significance (1).

Humoral immunity is intact except in terminal stages, but several other immune defects may be present with Hodgkin's disease, whether being active or in remission, increasing the risk of opportunistic infection (4). This risk may be compounded by therapeutic interventions such as splenectomy, chemotherapy, and radiation.

Staging

The stage is based on the number of involved lymph nodes, whether nodes are involved on both sides of the diaphragm, whether there is visceral involvement, and whether B symptoms are present. Staging procedures are directed to guide therapy, which may be regional (radiation) or systemic (chemotherapy), and typically include radiologic procedures such as plain chest films and computed tomography of the chest, abdomen, and pelvis. A gallium scan at baseline is helpful in assessing mediastinal masses: a gallium-negative mass after treatment is likely to represent fibrosis, if it was positive prior to treatment; however, it would be indeterminate if the pretreatment gallium scan was negative. Bipedal lymphangiography (LAG) may complement CT scans of the pelvis and abdomen, as disease-specific filling defects may be detected in normal-size nodes. This procedure is infrequently performed and requires considerable experience. It is contraindicated in patients with large abdominal or mediastinal disease because of the risk of pneumonitis due to lipid microemboli. An exploratory laparotomy is only indicated if the findings are likely to significantly alter initial therapy. This may apply to clinical stages I–IIA (rarely IIIA), but the likelihood of upstaging (increased extent of disease) is low for women with stage II under 27 years of age (9%). The advantage of the most precise intra-abdominal staging must be balanced against procedure related mortality (1%) and morbidity. Bone marrow involvement is more frequent with unfavorable histology (lymphocyte-depleted subtype), splenic involvement, extensive disease, and B-symptoms, but rare in other cases.

Therapy is guided by stage of disease and factors that affect prognosis, including bulky disease, number of extranodal sites of the disease, the age of the patient, and the speed of response to chemotherapy in advanced stages (5). Radiation therapy alone is curative in more than 80% of cases presenting with localized disease. Chemotherapy cures more than 50% of patients with disseminated disease at presentation.

Early stage I–IIA disease is managed with megavoltage photon beam radiation with 10-year relapse-free survival of 75%–80% and survival of 90%. Most relapses occur within the first 3 years. However, bulky mediastinal disease carries a relapse risk of 50% when treated with radiation alone. Chest/mantle field irradiation is associated with

TABLE 130–1.

Subtype	Overall Frequency	Age/Gender	Prognosis
Lymphocyte-predominant	5–10%	Young, male	Favorable
Mixed cellularity	20–40%	Older patients	Intermediate
Lymphocyte-depleted	5–10%	Older, male	Unfavorable
Nodular sclerosing	30–60%	Younger, female	Good–intermediate

acute complications (anorexia, weight loss, fatigue, myelosuppression, pneumonitis, pericarditis) and late complications including hypothyroidism and fibrotic changes of normal tissues (e.g., lungs, heart). The cumulative risk of secondary solid tumors is increased with irradiation (9% at 10 years). For stage III$_1$A, radiation alone may be equally effective as combination chemotherapy; higher stages require initial chemotherapy. In the presence of B symptoms, chemotherapy is the treatment of choice, and staging laparotomy is unnecessary. A minimum of six treatment courses or continued chemotherapy for two additional cycles past clinical complete remission are standard. The combination of doxorubicin, bleomycin, vinblastine, and dacarbazine (ABVD) is now preferred by many oncologists over MOPP because of equal or better efficacy of full-dose treatment (90% vs. 80% complete response rate, respectively), with a reduced risk of late complications such as myelodysplasia, secondary leukemia, non-Hodgkin's lymphomas, and infertility (6). Late relapses from complete remissions (CR) that lasted at least 12 months have a high CR rate with any appropriate regimen, including the initial therapeutic regimen (5-year relapse free survival of 20%–50%). Early relapses (<12 mo.) must be treated with a non-cross-resistant regimen (e.g., ABVD after MOPP) and carry a worse prognosis (5-year relapse-free survival of <20%). Chemotherapy also is extremely effective for salvage after radiation therapy failures. Salvage chemotherapy combinations for second relapses after chemotherapy induce CRs in 20% of patients, but the duration of response is usually less than 1 year. Selected patients may benefit from high dose chemotherapy and bone marrow rescue (1). The combined use of chemotherapy and radiotherapy (involved field) has improved relapse rate and overall survival, especially in patients with advanced disease, but it is associated with an increased risk of second malignancies. Combined treatment is offered to patients with mediastinal masses greater than 10 cm.

Recent studies in patients with bulky mediastinal disease (>10 cm) have suggested that a reduced number of chemotherapy cycles may be equally effective as the standard six cycles when given with involved field radiotherapy; this may help reducing potential morbidity (7).

Specific Aspects of This Case

Nodular-sclerosing (N-S) Hodgkin's disease is more frequent than other subtypes, occurring in 30%–60% of all cases, but in nearly 90% of young women. Supradiaphragmatic lymph node involvement is most common (90%) and the cervical region is frequently involved (60%–80%). A mediastinal mass is less common, but it is more frequently seen with the N-S subtype than with others. Isolated subdiaphragmal disease is uncommon in young patients. A normal-size spleen does not rule out

disease involvement. However, the risk of abdominal involvement is low in clinical stage I and in younger women (<27 years) with stage II and two or three sites of involvement. Our patient's estimated chance of being upstaged by exploratory laparotomy was estimated at 5%–10%; this procedure would not have altered the treatment plan. Clinical staging procedures revealed stage IIA with bulky mediastinal mass. This carries an increased risk of hilar disease, contiguous parenchymal extension (E), and pericardial disease. These increase size of radiation therapy ports, necessitate a shrinking field technique, and are associated with marginal misses (50% chance of relapse). Similarly, bulky disease has a significant relapse rate when treated with chemotherapy alone, providing rationale for combined modality treatment (8,9). On a practical basis, chemotherapy is usually initiated first to decrease field size and volume of radiotherapy and to allow for full-dosage chemotherapy.

The patient's MOPP chemotherapy was given in six 28-day cycles: 6 mg/m^2 mechlorethamine IV on days 1+8; 1.4 mg/m^2 vincristine IV on days 1+8; 100 mg/m^2 procarbazine p.o. on days 1–14; 40 mg/m^2 prednisone on days 1–14. The maximal single vincristine dose is often attenuated to 2 mg as in this case. This practice has been challenged by DeVita (10), because reduced toxicity by dose attenuation may be more than counterbalanced by loss of antitumor activity and increased risk of relapse. Her chemotherapy was well tolerated; however, early intolerance of vincristine is uncommon. The replacement of vincristine with vinblastine (6 mg/m^2 IV on days 1+8) makes the MVPP combination equally effective to MOPP. The use of alkylating agents (mechlormethamine, procarbazine) carries a greater, cumulative dose-related risk of late complications (infertility, myelodysplasia, secondary leukemia, and non-Hodgkin's lymphoma after 2–10 years posttreatment; cumulative risk 10%–15%) than the ABVD combination. However, the latter is associated with a slightly increased risk of heart failure (doxorubicine) and pulmonary fibrosis (bleomycin); this risk may be increased if adjuvant radiotherapy to the chest is given.

The patient had a rapid tumor response to chemotherapy, resulting in a clinical complete response with residual mediastinal mass of unclear significance [CR$_{(U)}$]. The negative gallium scan did not rule out residual active disease, especially in the absence of a positive baseline. (MRI evaluation has not been performed.) However, after 3 years of relapse-free survival, her current risk of relapse is low (<25%). If relapse occurred now, the patient would have an excellent chance to respond to salvage chemotherapy. Radiographic studies still show a residual mass, which likely represents fibrosis; it may shrink further with time. Fibrotic changes in normal tissues within the radiation field are persistent, but they are functionally of no significance at the present time.

The patient now has a borderline elevated TSH level and is at risk for radiation-induced hypothyroidism, which occurs in 6%–25% of all cases. Lymphangiogram and its iodine load may predispose to thyroid dysfunction. Hypothyroidism may have a late onset (3–5 years post-treatment), necessitating prolonged surveillance (11). Other late complications include psychologic issues and increased risk of infection. Her risk of reactivating a latent herpes zoster/varicella infection is estimated at 50%. The patient's menstrual function is normal, and she may have the chance of a normal pregnancy. She is at risk for secondary malignancies from her treatment, such as leukemia (2%–3%); it would have been higher with more than six courses of chemotherapy and after splenectomy (1,12,13). Additional risks include development of non-Hodgkin's lymphoma, and solid tumors, especially lung and breast cancer.

REFERENCES

1. Takvorian T, Canellos G. Hodgkin's disease. In: Holland JF, Frei E, Bast RC, et al., eds. *Cancer medicine.* 3rd edition. Philadelphia: Lea & Febiger; 1993:1998–2027.
2. Sanford DB, Hagemeister FB. Hodgkin's disease. In: Pazdur R, ed. *Medical oncology: a comprehensive review.* Huntington, N.Y.: PRR; 1993:87–100.
3. Weinshel EL, Peterson BA. Hodgkin's disease. *CA Cancer J Clin* 1993; 43:327–46.
4. Slivnick DJ, Ellis TM, Nawrocki JF, et al. The impact of Hodgkin's disease on the immune system. *Semin Oncol* 1990;17:673–82.
5. Coleman M, Friedlander RJ. Semantics and the chemotherapy of Hodgkin's disease-resistance is not relapse: alternative chemotherapy lacks effectiveness for disease not totally responsive to initial MOPP treatment. *Cancer Invest* 1988;6:237–9.
6. Santoro A, Bonadonna G, Valagussa P, et al. Long-term results of combined chemotherapy-radiotherapy approach in Hodgkin's disease: superiority of ABVD plus radiotherapy versus MOPP plus radiotherapy. *J Clin Oncol* 1987;5:27–37.
7. Preti A, Hagemeister FB, McLaughlin P, et al. Hodgkin's disease with a mediastinal mass greater than 10 cm: results of four different treatment approaches. *Ann Oncol* 1994;5(Suppl 2):97–100.
8. Hoppe RT. The management of bulky mediastinal Hodgkin's disease. *Hematol Oncol Clin North Am* 1989;3:265–76.
9. Longo DL, Russo A, Duffey PL, et al. Treatment of advanced stage massive mediastinal Hodgkin's disease: the case for combined modality treatment. *J Clin Oncol* 1991;9:227–35.
10. DeVita VT Jr, Hubbard SM, Longo DL. Treatment of Hodgkin's disease. *J Natl Cancer Inst Mono* 1990;10:19.
11. Hancock SL, Cox RS, McDougall IR. Thyroid diseases after treatment of Hodgkin's disease. *N Engl J Med* 1991;325:599–605.
12. Kaldor JM, Day NE, Clarke EA, et al. Leukemia following Hodgkin's disease. *N Engl J Med* 1990;322:7–13.
13. van Leeuwen FE, Chorus AMJ, van den Belt-Dusebout AW, et al. Leukemia risk following Hodgkin's disease: relation to cumulative dose of alkylating agents, treatment with tenoposide combinations, number of episodes of chemotherapy, and bone marrow damage. *J Clin Oncol* 1994;12:1063–73.

EDITORIAL BOARD COMMENTARY

This case has been thoroughly discussed by the author and does not require a commentary. A bipedal lymphangiogram was performed, but the authors suggest that this is contraindicated in a patient with bulky mediastinal disease.

131

Hodgkin's Disease in Older Persons

David H. Garfield

*Don't compromise therapy in older persons–they do worse
than younger patients*

CASE PRESENTATION

An 81-year-old Caucasian woman was admitted to St. Joseph Hospital with a 2-month history of intermittent fevers to 103°F, night sweats, and chills. The symptoms would appear for several days and then disappear. There was also a 10-pound weight loss without anorexia. There was no pruritus or alcohol-associated pain.

Past history included the recent onset of non–insulin-dependent diabetes mellitus treated with Micronase, a previous myocardial infarct, and the use of quinidine and Lanoxin to control atrial fibrillation.

Physical examination was pertinent only in that right posterior cervical and supraclavicular nodes were enlarged. There was no other adenopathy or hepatosplenomegaly. There was slight evidence of weight loss with generalized muscle wasting; the patient appeared chronically ill.

Before admission, an aspiration biopsy of an enlarged right posterior cervical lymph node was performed but was nondiagnostic. Because of being ill, the patient was, therefore, admitted for surgery (excisional lymph node biopsy).

Laboratory studies included a hemoglobin of 9.0 and hematocrit of 28.5% (had been 33% 2 weeks prior); ESR was 66 and glucose was 196. All other labs, including LFTs, were normal. Chest radiograph was normal. The excised lymph node revealed Hodgkin's disease, nodular sclerosing.

Pathologist: Histologic sections of the lymph node show virtual effacement of normal nodal architecture. A vaguely nodular proliferation of cells is identified with focal areas of necrosis. On higher power, these areas are composed of large, atypical cells situated in an inflamma-tory background. The inflammatory background consists of small round lymphocytes, occasional cleaved lymphocytes, histiocytes, and occasional eosinophils. The large, atypical cells are somewhat variable morphologically and include classical binucleate Reed-Sternberg cells (Fig. 131–1), mononuclear Reed-Sternberg variants, and lacunar type Reed-Sternberg cells (Fig. 131–2). Immunohistochemical stains show positive staining with Leu-M1, BER-H2, and negative staining with common leukocyte antigen. Because of the vaguely nodular pattern of infiltration and the relatively frequent lacunar type Reed-Sternberg cells, a diagnosis of nodular sclerosing Hodgkin's disease was made. The Reed-Sternberg variants showed some clustering in the centers of tumor nodules, a feature felt to represent the "cellular phase" of nodular sclerosing Hodgkin's disease, classified as grade 1 of 2. However, some members of the department felt this could represent a peripheral T-cell lymphoma.

On occasion, the distinction between Hodgkin's disease and non-Hodgkin's lymphomas can be extremely difficult and requires specialized immunohistochemical studies and exhaustive morphologic review. In particular, peripheral T-cell lymphomas may pose diagnostic problems in that Reed-Sternberg–like cells may be present in peripheral T-cell lymphomas, and the distinction between peripheral T-cell lymphoma and Hodgkin's disease may rest solely on the morphologic analysis of the background inflammatory cell response. The inflammatory response in Hodgkin's disease should appear nonatypical and benign, whereas in pleomorphic T-cell lymphomas, dysplastic features of the background lymphocytes should be present. The distinction between T-cell lymphomas and Hodgkin's disease may be further blurred by recent evi-

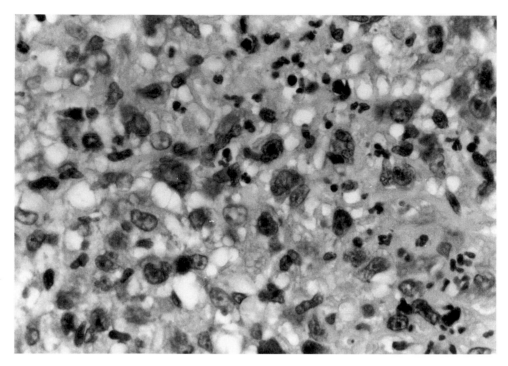

FIG. 131–1. High-power view showing Reed-Sternberg cell.

dence of T-cell receptor gene rearrangements in some cases of Hodgkin's disease.

DISCUSSION

Moderator: Why was a needle aspiration performed?

Surgeon: An aspiration biopsy is obviously easier than an incisional or excisional biopsy, but, in the case of lymphomas, this is often, although not always, nondiagnostic. It may be diagnostic in an adenocarcinoma or squamous cell carcinoma. However, in this case, lymphoma had to be at the top of the differential diagnosis.

Moderator: Why?

Surgeon: Because of the "B" symptoms of fever, weight loss, and night sweats.

Moderator: So, we now have a diagnosis. The referring physician refers the patient to a medical oncologist. Where do we go from here?

Medical oncologist: The patient must now be "staged." The stage will determine the type and extent of treatment as well as the prognosis. I would order an abdominal and pelvic CT scan as well as a bone marrow biopsy.

Moderator: Why not a chest CT?

Medical oncologist: Because with a normal chest radiograph the yield would be low at finding more pathology.

Moderator: CT scan showed retrocrural, celiac, splenic, peripancreatic, midcaval, periaortic, renal hila, and internal iliac nodes all to be slightly enlarged. The spleen was also slightly enlarged (Fig. 131–3). The liver was normal. The bone marrow was hypercellular with increased iron stores, but no lymphoma was found.

Moderator: If there had been clinically enlarged inguinal nodes, would you have ordered a CT scan?

Medical oncologist: No, because the stage would have been clinical IIIB. The CT scan would have revealed only liver involvement, unlikely with normal LFTs. There is little difference in treatment or prognosis between stages IIIB and IVB.

Moderator: How about a bone marrow?

Medical oncologist: Yes, because if there had been heavy involvement with Hodgkin's disease (HD), I may have modified the dose for the first course of chemotherapy, used a less myelosuppressive regimen, or used neupogen.

Moderator: Why is the patient anemic?

Medical oncologist: Either the "anemia of chronic disease" or because of multifocal, unrecognized involvement of HD in the bone marrow.

Moderator: Why not do bilateral bone marrow exams?

Medical oncologist: More pain and expense and, in this case, it does not much matter if the stage is IIIB or IVB. It is important to discover occult bone marrow involvement if it means that a patient will or will not have surgical staging, will or will not have only radiation therapy. She appears to have clinical stage (CS) IIIB.

Moderator: When is gallium scanning useful?

Radiologist: Not here. Mainly when there are equivocal chest findings on CT scan. The true positive value is 90%. False positives are unusual; false negatives frequent, usually in the abdomen. Six percent of the time occult disease may be found. Gallium is particularly useful to follow the response of disease that was initially positive, most often

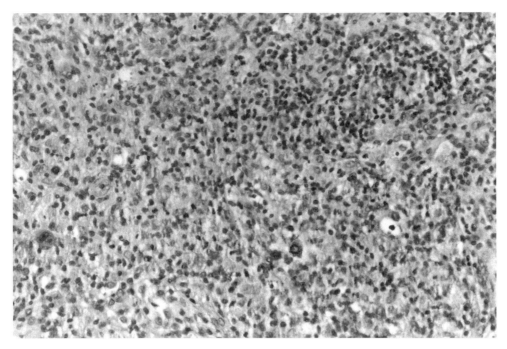

FIG. 131–2. Low-power view showing lacunar cell and Reed-Sternberg cells.

in the mediastinum. Otherwise, it is expensive, time consuming (3–4 days), and unpleasant for the patient.

Moderator: Is HD unusual in this age group?

Medical oncologist: Yes. Nonetheless, 10% to 15% of patients who have HD are older than 60 years at diagnosis. There are binodal peaks: an initial peak between 15 and 35 years and a second smaller peak at age older than 50 years. This is of interest because of the increasing proportion of older persons in Western countries. On the other hand, the incidence of HD appears to be declining in those over 50, primarily because of improved diagnostic accuracy.

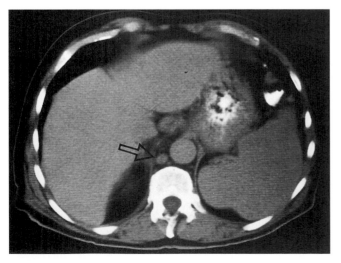

FIG. 131–3. Splenomegaly and enlarged periaortic lymph node (*arrow*).

Moderator: How else are the two groups different?

Radiation oncologist: In the young age group, HD may be caused by a biologic, granulomatous agent of low infectivity but be a true malignant neoplasm in the elderly.

Moderator: What about disease distribution?

Radiation oncologist: There is a high distribution of supraclavicular and mediastinal disease in the young and of inguinal nodes in the elderly. Initial infradiaphragmatic presentation is more frequent in the elderly, whereas bulky mediastinal disease is a distinctive feature of the young.

Moderator: What is the malignant cell in HD?

Pathologist: Although believed to be the malignant cell, the Reed-Sternberg (RS) cell has not been precisely characterized because no single phenotype can be readily assigned. Depending on histologic subtype, its morphology and antigen profile change.

Moderator: What is the etiology of HD?

Pathologist: The data suggest that oncogenes may be involved in HD pathogenesis. Also, the Epstein-Barr virus (EBV) is suspected of playing a role. Although not done as yet, a comparison of EBV expression in older and younger patients may be of interest in light of the suspicion that HD is distinctly different in the elderly. Assuming that ineffective elimination of EBV or another infectious agent contributes to the malignant transformation in HD, it may be noteworthy that in vitro lymphocyte-proliferative responses are lower in older than younger untreated patients.

Moderator: What is the etiology of "B" symptoms?

Medical oncologist: A variety of cytokines are overexpressed in primary and cultured RS cells. This may explain certain clinical features of HD such as eosinophilia and "B" symptoms. Because cytokine profiles change with normal aging, alterations in cytokine responses to the disease stimulus may explain some age-associated differences in clinical presentation.

Moderator: Is histology different in older patients?

Pathologist: Although success with current treatments has lessened its prognostic significance, histologic classification still remains an important clinical feature of HD. In the elderly there is a shift toward the less favorable histology of mixed cellularity (MC) and lymphocyte depletion (LD). LD proportion increases in those age 75 and older; LD is almost twice as frequent as the nodular sclerosis incidence. Tumor necrosis, background fibrosis, and lymphocyte depletion are more frequent as well in the older patient.

Moderator: Are there problems with diagnosis in older patients as compared with younger?

Pathologist: Yes. The reasons for this age-related finding are unclear but may be related to a confounding effect of an abnormal host response and/or immune deficit in older patients. This may change the histologic appearance of nodes in HD. Initial correct diagnoses may be seen in less than half of those with MC and less than a third of those with LD. Usually, the error is in mistaking non-Hodgkin's lymphoma (NHL) for HD. Problem areas include distinguishing (a) HD lymphocyte predominance (HDLP) from immune-reactive lymphadenitis and small-cell lymphocytic lymphoma, (b) HD nodular sclerosis (HDNS) and HDMC from peripheral T-cell lymphomas and Lennert lymphomas, as in this case, and (c) HDLD from the various large cell lymphoma variants.

Moderator: Is grading important?

Pathologist: Patients with grade I HDNS may do better than grade II, although this is not certain.

Moderator: What clinical features should alert the clinician to the possibility that the diagnosis is NHL rather than HD?

Medical oncologist: Involvement of extranodal sites such as lungs, bones, skin, ovaries, and thyroid gland; also, bulky abdominal disease, epitrochlear adenopathy, and hypercalcemia suggest NHL.

Moderator: Once the diagnosis is made and confirmed, what is the next step?

Medical oncologist: Clinical and, if possible, pathologic staging.

Moderator: Why?

Medical oncologist: To determine both treatment and prognosis.

Moderator: What are the problems in older patients?

Medical oncologist: Fortunately, more than 90% of patients with HD present with adenopathy so that the disease can usually be diagnosed without a laparotomy. However, older patients have a higher incidence of infradiaphragmatic disease, increasing the need to thoroughly evaluate the abdomen and sometimes necessitating an initial laparotomy just for diagnosis. This may, in part, be

related to the lower incidence of NS, which is usually above the diaphragm. Understandably, we are reluctant to do surgical staging in patients older than 60, but we may be doing them a disservice by understaging them. Laparotomy upstages about 25% of patients. The 5-year survival of older patients, stage II by pathologic staging (PS), is about 65% to 70%, those stage II by clinical staging (CS), 43%. However, it is generally felt that older patients with "B" symptoms should not be surgically staged because they probably do not have localized disease. In older patients the risk of postsplenectomy sepsis is relatively high. Even lymphangiogram carries a risk in older patients, being invasive, causing pulmonary emboli, although microscopic and transient, and leading to fluid overload. Also, especially in older patients, splenectomy, followed by multidrug chemotherapy using alkylating agents, leads to a higher incidence of secondary acute myelogenous leukemia.

Moderator: Once the stage has been determined, what should be the treatment?

Radiation therapist: Clearly, for localized disease, stages I and IIA, standard radiation therapy with curative intent, using the mantle technique, should be employed. If only involved field radiation therapy is used, more than one third will die of progressive disease. In patients with PS I and IIA, the cure rate may approach that of younger patients.

Medical oncologist: However, in older patients when HD recurs after curative radiation therapy, it becomes difficult to impossible to give them full-dose chemotherapy. On the other hand, the use of growth factors may help, somewhat. Multidrug chemotherapy should be given to all patients with stage III and IV, but it is clear that an older than 60-year age is an adverse prognostic feature.

In one large CALGB study of 73 patients older than 60 years with stage III or IV disease, the median survival was only 18 months; 28 similar patients in a SWOG study had a median survival of 16 months. Even in the subgroup that received full chemotherapy, the median survival was only 27 months. However, another study from Italy of 114 patients older than 60 years, stages III and IV, had a median survival of 50 months. In between these two extremes of reported results, a Stanford study of 18 patients older than 60 years with IIIB and IV given adequate therapy produced a median survival of 39 months. However, most of these patients still died of their disease.

In patients older than 70, the results of chemotherapy in some studies show the prognosis is no worse than for those aged 60 to 70 years. However, in another study, the median survival for those aged older than 70 in 25 patients was only 9 months.

Moderator: What are the causes of our inability to deliver full-dose chemotherapy to older patients?

Medical oncologist: Examples include (a) an increased risk of adriamycin-induced heart failure, and (b) progressive renal deterioration with age so that excretion of drugs like cyclophosphamide, BCNU, bleomycin, DTIC, and cis-

TABLE 131–1. *Ten-year survival (in percent) of patients with HD by age and pathologic stage. (From ref. 1.)*

| Pathologic stage | Age at diagnosis | | | | | Total[a] |
	<17	17–34	35–49	50–59	60+	
I	91.0 (124)[b]	90.0 (539)	80.6 (225)	72.6 (121)	64.9 (182)	83.0 (1191)
II	92.5 (163)	82.8 (719)	75.0 (185)	59.0 (92)	34.8 (141)	76.5 (1300)
III	77.6 (108)	73.0 (515)	62.0 (175)	41.9 (110)	22.0 (167)	61.0 (1057)
IV	72.1 (59)	56.9 (251)	43.0 (179)	32.2 (154)	21.3 (2155)	41.0 (898)
All[c]	86.0 (454)	79.0 (2024)	67.0 (746)	50.0 (477)	35.0 (745)	

[a] Adjusted for age
[b] Percent (number in parentheses)
[c] Adjusted for pathologic stage

platin is decreased. Also, the risk of developing acute non-lymphocytic leukemia is increased by using an alkylating agent, especially in older patients.

Moderator: What is the best regimen for older patients?

Medical oncologist: It may be that, in older patients, MOPP or ABVD or the MOPP/ABV hybrid are just too toxic. Perhaps the CHLVPP regimen (chlorambucil, vinblastine, procarbazine, and prednisone) is less toxic and just as effective.

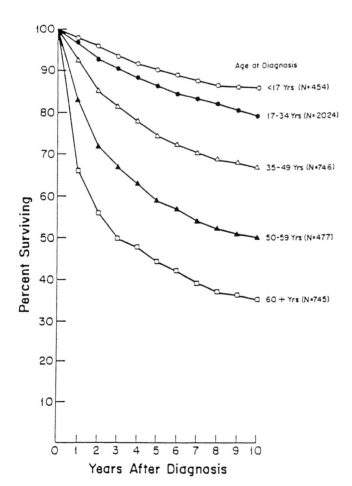

FIG. 131–4. HD-specific 10-year survival by age at diagnosis, adjusted for pathologic stage. (From ref. 1.)

Moderator: What is the outcome of older patients treated with curative intent?

Radiation therapist: At any stage they do worse than younger patients. The disease appears to have a different biologic behavior in the elderly (Fig. 131–4) (Table 131–1).

Medical oncologist: I would agree.

Moderator: For patients who cannot tolerate multidrug chemotherapy for whatever reason, what is the best single drug?

Medical oncologist: Vinblastine.

Moderator: What was the outcome of the patient presented in this case study?

Medical oncologist: She received the C-MOPP/ABV hybrid at 90% of full dosage in the first three cycles, but attained only a partial remission. After 4 months of chemotherapy, fevers returned and a CT scan showed splenomegaly and only partial decrease in abdominal nodes. Therapy was discontinued and she died 9 months after the diagnosis was made.

Moderator: What determines the curability of these patients?

Medical oncologist: Mainly the ability to obtain a complete remission which, in turn, is related to the ability to deliver full therapy, whether it be radiation therapy or chemotherapy.

REFERENCES

1. Kennedy BJ, et al. Survival in HD by stage and age. *Med Pediatr Oncol* 1992;20:100–4.
2. Bosi A, Poticelli P, Casini C, Messori A, Bellese G, et al. Clinical data and therapeutic approach in elderly patients with Hodgkin's disease. *Haematologica* 1989;74:463–73.

COMMENTARY by Bruce A. Peterson

The optimism that attends the diagnosis of HD in young adults is not warranted when it occurs in patients over 60 years of age. It has been known for many years that important characteristics of the disease vary greatly by age, and these characteristics include epidemiology, presenting symptoms and stage, histopathologic subtypes, response to therapy, and prognosis. The case presentation illustrates many of these points, and the discussion comprehensively addresses the major issues in HD of older people.

Although less than 25% of patients with HD present with fever, and a much smaller proportion have, as does this woman, cyclical bouts of high spiking temperatures separated by periods of days without fevers (Pel-Ebstein fevers), fever, night sweats, and weight loss are not uncommon in older individuals with HD. It is important to remember, however, that chronic inflammatory diseases and infections are even more commonly associated with these symptoms and must be excluded by diagnostic evaluation. Even after the histologic confirmation of HD in this patient, it still would be important to rule out an accompanying infection. Other malignancies must also be kept in mind with this presentation, because fever and weight loss are not restricted to HD. Weight loss is common in many advanced malignancies, and renal cell carcinomas, non-Hodgkin's lymphoma, and a variety of other cancers are sometimes heralded by fever.

Making the diagnosis of HD can be very difficult in older patients. In a recent study of 171 adults 60 years of age or older entered on national therapeutic trials for HD, a diagnosis of HD was confirmed on expert histopathologic review in only 67% of cases (1). The great majority of erroneously classified cases were actually diffuse non-Hodgkin's lymphomas, either mixed small cleaved and large cell or large-cell lymphomas. As in this case where there was some disagreement among pathologists, ancillary studies such as immunophenotyping can be essential. For these reasons, and because to classify correctly any lymphoma an excisional biopsy is almost always required, needle aspirations should be reserved for the clinical situation, where it is important first to rule out another malignancy (e.g., carcinoma).

Once the diagnosis is established, the next step is staging. The reasons for staging in this patient are simply to allow for the selection of the most appropriate treatment, to provide some prognostic information, and to allow for an assessment of the impact of the treatment. In the setting of a clinical trial, staging also ensures the relative uniformity or, at least, an accurate description of the population under study. As with the selection of treatment, the extent of staging undertaken must reflect an assessment of the needs of the individual and the goals of intervention. If the goal is to cure the patient, then staging is relatively extensive, although it must be emphasized that even in this setting a staging laparotomy is appropriate only if the results will affect the choice of treatment modality (i.e., irradiation alone vs. chemotherapy). In patients with B symptoms, staging laparotomy is almost never justified because contemporary treatment would include chemotherapy. If palliation is the goal, then the evaluation should be sufficient to permit the anticipation and prevention, if possible, of major morbidity (e.g., renal obstruction, liver function abnormalities, marrow involvement).

The staging of this patient is somewhere between the ends of the spectrum. There is nothing in the limited staging that would have prevented cure, but she was not evaluated to the extent that all reasonably known sites were identified before therapy so that they could be reassessed and demonstrated to have become negative before stopping therapy. A chest CT scan is an essential component in the evaluation of the thorax. It adds considerable information beyond that of a PA and lateral chest radiograph, whether the radiograph is normal or abnormal. Similarly, even in the face of enlarged inguinal lymph nodes, an abdominal-pelvic CT scan has a role in delineating unapparent sites of HD and assessing whether urinary obstruction is likely. A gallium scan would not be helpful in this case unless a chest radiograph and CT scan were inconclusive. However, in the different situation of a large mediastinal mass, gallium scans are also playing an increasing role in helping distinguish whether post-treatment residual masses reflect persistent HD (2,3). If a mass is known to be gallium-avid before treatment, the persistence of gallium uptake after treatment has substantially different implications (i.e., active HD) than one that has become negative (fibrotic mass). Finally, bilateral bone marrow biopsies are generally considered standard in the staging of HD. When HD involves the bone marrow, it is often focal, and the ability to detect it is directly related to the amount of tissue available for viewing. Again, the importance of establishing the sites of disease before treatment is so that the interval and post-treatment evaluations can be targeted appropriately and treatment not stopped prematurely.

The distribution of disease in this patient is fairly typical of the older patient with HD. A variety of studies have demonstrated that, when compared with younger patients, older individuals have more advanced stages of the disease (4) and lower rates of neck and mediastinal disease, but more inguinal, intra-abdominal, and splenic involvement (1,5,6,7).

Because more extensive disease is associated with advancing age, it is easy to comprehend why older patients do worse as an overall group. However, when matched stage for stage, older patients still do worse than younger patients, and in some instances much worse. In many trials the adverse impact of age becomes apparent in those 40 years of age and increases thereafter. The effect of age is undoubtedly due, in part, to an inability to tolerate full-dose chemotherapy, but even in analyses restricted to patients who received full-dose, the complete response rate, duration of response, and survival are markedly decreased compared with younger adults (8). A major study published recently again showed the major effect of age (9). Survival after chemotherapy for advanced HD at 5 years was 79% in those under 40 years, 63% in those 40 to 59 years, and 31% in those 60 years and older. The median survival in those over 60 years was still only 18 months. Clearly, all this suggests that there are biologic differences in HD for which age is simply a marker, and future progress may depend on understanding those differences.

REFERENCES

1. Mir R, Anderson J, Strauchen J, et al. Hodgkin's disease in patients 60 years of age or older. Histologic and clinical features of advanced-stage disease. *Cancer* 1993;71:1857–66.
2. Wylie BR, Southee AE, Joshua DE, et al. Gallium scanning in the management of mediastinal Hodgkin's disease. *Eur J Haematol* 1989; 42:344–7.
3. Hagemeister FB, Fesus SM, Lamki LM, et al. Role of the gallium scan in Hodgkin's disease. *Cancer* 1990;65:1090–6.
4. Newell G, Cole S, Miettinen O, MacMahon B. Age differences in the histology of Hodgkin's disease. *J Natl Cancer Inst* 1970;45:311–7.
5. Lokich JJ, Pinkus GS, Moloney WC. Hodgkin's disease in the elderly. *Oncology* 1974;29:484–500.
6. Rossi-Ferrine P, Bosi A, Casini C, et al. Hodgkin's disease in the elderly: a retrospective clinicopathologic study of 61 patients aged over 60 years. *Acta Haematol* 1987;78(suppl 1):163–70.
7. Specht L, Nissen NI. Hodgkin's disease and age. *Eur J Haematol* 1989;43:127–135.
8. Canellos GP, Anderson JR, Propert KJ, et al. Chemotherapy of advanced Hodgkin's disease with MOPP, ABVD, or MOPP alternating with ABVD. *N Engl J Med* 1992;327:1478–84.
9. Peterson BA, Pajak TF, Cooper MR, et al. Effect of age on therapeutic response and survival in advanced Hodgkin's disease. *Cancer Treat Rep* 1982;66:889–98.

SECTION XXIX

Non-Hodgkin's Lymphoma

132   Non-Hodgkin's Lymphoma

Janardan Khandekar and Lynne S. Kaminer

*A low-grade lymphoma may convert to a higher grade in the
course of the illness; to treat or not to treat early*

CASE PRESENTATION

M.M. was a 68-year-old man whose history dates to 1988 when he presented with watery, nonbloody diarrhea associated with mucous. A gastrointestinal evaluation included a barium enema and upper gastrointestinal series with small bowel follow-through (SBFT) that suggested inflammatory bowel disease (Fig. 132–1). He was treated with metronidazole and his symptoms were resolved.

The patient did well for 6 months, after which he noted a lump on the right side of his neck. He had noted a 15-lb weight loss and was having occasional night sweats. Physical examination revealed a 3 × 2 cm right upper cervical lymph node, 1.0-cm right supraclavicular, 1.0-cm posterior occipital node, and shoddy inguinal nodes bilaterally. An excisional biopsy of the node revealed a follicular mixed small cleaved and large-cell lymphoma. Further staging studies included a chest computed tomogram (CT), which was normal; abdominal and pelvic CT, which showed diffuse small adenopathy within the pelvis, a normal spleen, and an ill-defined right lower quadrant (RLQ) mass that had been seen previously on the SBFT and was presumed to be inflammatory. Bilateral bone marrow biopsies revealed one foci consistent with lymphoma. A colonoscopic evaluation of the terminal ileum showed findings more suggestive of Crohn's disease than lymphoma. Multiple biopsies of the ileum and ileocecal valve were consistent with Crohn's disease. The patient was staged as stage IV low-grade lymphoma. No specific therapy was initiated, and the patient was followed up and was examined every 2 months.

One year later, on repeat CT evaluation of the pelvis, shrinkage of the adenopathy and RLQ mass was noted

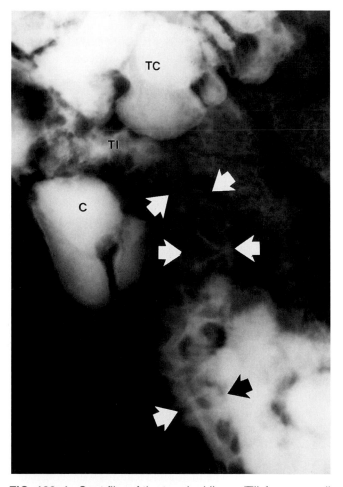

FIG. 132–1. Spot film of the terminal ileum (TI) from a small bowel follow-through series demonstrates a marked nodularity of the folds (*arrows*), creating a cobblestone appearance. *C,* cecum; *TC,* transverse colon.

673

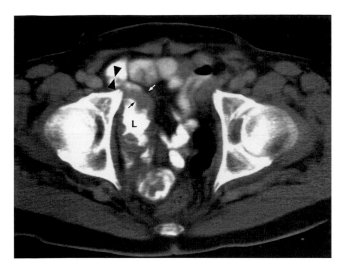

FIG. 132–2. CT scan of the pelvis at the level of the acetabulum shows marked mural thickening (*arrows*) of the distal ileum. Coarsened nodular folds indent the lumen (*L*). Normal thickness of the small bowel wall is indicated by the *arrowheads.*

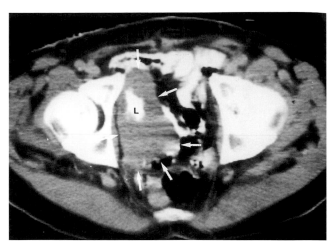

FIG. 132–3. With disease progression, the mural thickening has increased and there now is considerable mass effect (*arrows*) demonstrated on this scan obtained at the same level as Fig. 132–2.

(Fig. 132–2). In July 1990, his examination was notable for shoddy lymph nodes in the cervical, supraclavicular, and inguinal areas. Review of his peripheral blood smear showed "atypical lymphocytes," possibly consistent with lymphoma.

The patient continued to do well until November 1990, when he had recurrent gastrointestinal symptoms. Metronidazole was restarted. His examination was notable for increased adenopathy in his cervical area and a prominent mass in the pelvis on rectal examination. An abdominal and pelvic CT demonstrated extensive retroperitoneal adenopathy and a prominent RLQ soft tissue mass. Marked mural wall thickening was also noted (Fig. 132–3). UGI and SBFT now revealed changes more suggestive of lymphoma with a mass effect rather than Crohn's disease. A colonoscopic examination demonstrated a slightly ulcerated submucosal mass at the junction of the ascending colon. The patient was treated with chlorambucil, 16 mg/m^2 per day for 5 days, that is, for six cycles with excellent resolution of symptoms. Six months after his chemotherapy, his physical examination was normal. The CT scan evaluation exhibited a marked decrease in the size of the mesenteric and periaortic adenopathy. The RLQ mass and involvement of the terminal ileum had almost completely resolved (Fig. 132–4).

One year later, his gastrointestinal symptoms returned. The CT scans again demonstrated mesenteric and periaortic adenopathy. Chlorambucil was restarted and his symptoms resolved. A new left supraclavicular node was noted and was biopsied. The histologic features were consistent with a diffuse large-cell lymphoma. CT scans of the abdomen again showed diminution of the adenopathy in response to the previous chlorambucil. Chemotherapy

with CHOP (cyclophosphamide, doxorubicin, oncovin, and prednisone) was begun for the new large-cell histology. The left supraclavicular node shrank in size transiently but regrew within 2 weeks. The regimen was changed to ProMACE-CytaBOM (prednisone, methotrexate, leucovorin, adriamycin, cyclophosphamide, etoposide, cytarabine, bleomycin, and oncovin) with a slight improvement in response. Over the next several months, several palliative regimens were initiated because of persistent and rapidly enlarging supraclavicular adenopathy. The patient transiently responded to each intervention, including multiple courses of radiation therapy, but he expired in April 1994, 5 years after his initial diagnosis, from progressive disease.

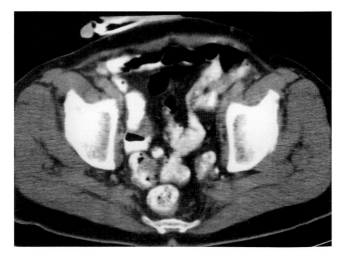

FIG. 132–4. After a successful course of chemotherapy, the involved distal ileum has almost returned to normal in appearance.

This case illustrates several important clinical features of lymphoma. The patient had a pre-existing diagnosis of Crohn's disease at the time he developed lymphoma. Inflammatory bowel disease is more often associated with an increased incidence of colon cancer, but an association with lymphoma has also been described. Ulcerative colitis specifically has been known to predispose to lymphoma of the colon. Patients with celiac sprue disease, another inflammatory condition of the bowel, have a 5% to 10% incidence of lymphoma. Similarly, nodular lymphoid hyperplasia of the gastrointestinal mucosa has been linked to the development of lymphoma.

Lymphoma can occur anywhere in the gastrointestinal tract and is the primary site in 5% of all newly diagnosed cases. The stomach is most frequently involved (40%–60%), followed by the small intestine (10%–30%), and more rarely in the colon (3%–15%). The various histologic appearances include the indolent MALT lymphoma (mucosa-associated lymphoid tissue), multiple lymphoid polyposis, enteropathy-associated T-cell lymphoma (more specifically associated with celiac sprue), as well as the more unusual lymphoma histologies. The presenting symptoms are usually nonspecific and include abdominal pain, symptoms mimicking peptic ulcer disease, nausea, vomiting, weight loss, and abdominal distention.

This patient was presented to the Tumor Board several times. At the time of his initial diagnosis from the supraclavicular node biopsy, his previous gastrointestinal films were carefully reviewed. The consensus opinion was that of an indolent lymphoma involving the mesenteric nodes, but of a different process than his known Crohn's disease. The decision was initially to observe him, and he was treated only with chemotherapy when there was marked progression of the abdominal adenopathy as well as the wall thickening. The patient went into complete remission after completion of his initial chemotherapy, and the marked improvement in his scans was noted. The patient never had significant problems with abdominal adenopathy again. Last, his histology transformed to a large-cell lymphoma. This underscores the necessity to rebiopsy lymph nodes after initial therapy. It has been demonstrated that transformation in histology occurs in many patients with indolent lymphoma. The discrepancy between the response of his abdominal disease, which never recurred, indicated the likelihood that the abdominal lymphoma was from an indolent clone, whereas his aggressive resistant supraclavicular disease probably originated from a different clone.

This 68-year-old gentleman presented with a low-grade lymphoma of the cecum and initially responded to treatment. The lymphoma then converted to a high-grade variety, became refractory to chemotherapy, and the patient ultimately succumbed to the disease. The discordance in the responsiveness of the abdominal lymphoma and that of the supraclavicular disease probably reflected dual clonality of the disease.

COMMENTARY by Carol Portlock

The case described is a typical patient with low-grade lymphoma presenting with generalized lymphadenopathy, an indolent clinical course, and the late development of histologic transformation to a more aggressive diffuse large-cell lymphoma (1).

The unusual twist in this case relates to the presence of Crohn's disease in the ileum and the decisions regarding simultaneous management of two diseases. As noted by the authors, benign gastrointestinal conditions may be associated with lymphomas at an increased frequency. The most recent association is that of *Helicobacter pylori* infection of the stomach and MALT (mucosa-associated lymphoid tumors) lymphoma (2).

The ileum is an unusual site for lymphomatous involvement, and when present, is more often associated with an intermediate- or high-grade lymphoma, such as Burkitt's lymphoma (3). For this reason, the authors proceeded with endoscopic evaluation because these more rapidly proliferating lymphomas may not be observed. Excluding lymphoma in the gastrointestinal tract permitted the authors to address management of the non-bulky, generalized lymphadenopathy of follicular mixed lymphoma.

This disease is a B-cell low-grade lymphoma with a unique surface immunoglobulin idiotype and the t(14;18) cytogenetic translocation of the Bcl-2 oncogene to the immunoglobulin heavy chain gene. These biologic characteristics make it possible to establish that the later emergence of a more aggressive lymphoma, as was seen in this case, is not due to a new lymphoma. Rather, there is the evolution of an aggressive subclone with the original lymphoma genetic fingerprint (unique idiotype and gene rearrangement) as well as the emergence of new genetic changes such as additional cytogenetic abnormalities or *p53* mutation. Histologic transformation is important to recognize, as it demands a change in treatment strategy and often connotes a poor prognosis. It is a biologic event that occurs with or without prior therapy and its likelihood increases over time from diagnosis, approaching at least 50% at 10 years.

The initial management strategy of this patient was observation (4). This remains a controversial approach, particularly in follicular mixed lymphoma, where the disease may progress quickly without therapy (usually requiring treatment in less than 1 year), and some report improved outcomes with combination chemotherapy. Nevertheless, in a 68-year-old patient with small bulk disease and a second complicating medical illness (Crohn's disease), it is an appropriate management strategy. Transient spontaneous regression, as seen in this case, has been reported in some patients.

Treatment was instituted with single alkylating agent therapy when progressive adenopathy and probable gastrointestinal tract disease was noted. No surgical intervention was undertaken to control the ileal involvement before chemotherapy. This has become an increasingly common approach in the management of gastrointestinal tract lymphoma. In gastric lymphomas, it is well recognized that the risks of bleeding/perforation are low enough to consider primary chemotherapy in the majority (5). However, in small or large bowel presentations these data are not available. Perhaps the Crohn's disease history influenced the surgical decision in this instance.

Recurrent lymphadenopathy after initial chemotherapy is best biopsied to evaluate a possible change in histology as documented in this case. The emergence of an intermediate-grade lymphoma (histologic transformation of the original low-grade clone) requires institution of combination chemotherapy and often connotes a poor prognosis.

Occasionally, the aggressive subclone may be eradicated by this systemic therapy and an indolent histology later recurs.

REFERENCES

1. Cheson BD. The biology and management of indolent B-cell lymphomas. *Semin Oncol* 1993;20:1–155.
2. Parsonnet J, Hansen S, Rodriquez L, et al. *Helicobacter pylori* infection and gastric lymphoma. *N Engl J Med* 1994;330:1267–71.
3. Haber DA, Mayer RJ. Primary gastrointestinal lymphoma. *Semin Oncol* 1988;15:154.
4. Armitage JO. Treatment of non-Hodgkin's lymphoma. *N Engl J Med* 1993;328:1023–30.
5. Maor MH, Velasquez WS, Fuller LM, Silvermintz KB. Stomach conservation in stage IE and IIE gastric non-Hodgkin's lymphoma. *J Clin Oncol* 1990;8:266–71.

133

A Young Patient with Mycosis Fungoides

Ann G. Martin and Mary K. Cullen

Itch, itch, itch: early diagnosis with biopsy

CASE PRESENTATION

L.P. is a 41-year-old Caucasian woman who presented in September 1988 with complaints of pruritus and xerosis. Past medical history was significant for lichen planus at age 13. Physical examination of the skin revealed mild eczema limited to the extremities and abdomen. She responded well to a regimen of medium potency topical steroids and emollients. In 1989, the patient was evaluated and believed to have keratosis pilaris of the extensor arms and anterior thighs. A topical lactic acid–containing preparation was added to the regimen.

The patient did well until January 1990, when she complained of a 2-month history of scalp alopecia and scaling accompanied by intense generalized pruritus. Physical exam revealed scaly, spiny, KOH-negative patches of alopecia present on the scalp. There were hypopigmented and erythematous spiny papules and plaques present on the extremities, trunk, and face (Fig. 133–1) covering approximately 40% of body surface area. No adenopathy or organomegaly were noted. Histologic examination of a scalp biopsy demonstrated follicular mucinosis with an atypical lymphohistiocytic infiltrate, suggestive of mycosis fungoides (MF) or cutaneous T-cell lymphoma (CTCL) (Fig. 133–2). Laboratory evaluations were significant only for an elevated white blood count of 14,000. The differential was normal and no Sezary cells were seen in the buffy coat smears. The patient was presented to Dermatology Grand Rounds, where the consensus was that follicular mucinosis is not necessarily a precursor of MF, and more biopsies of the skin were recommended.

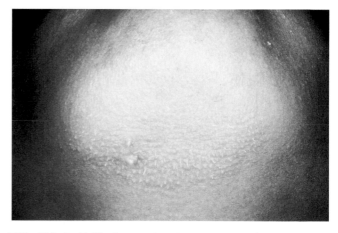

FIG. 133–1. Follicular mucinosis. A hypopigmented plaque composed of flesh-colored, follicular papules that are firm and rough to palpation.

Tissue examination of an erythematous, indurated plaque of the face and upper arm again demonstrated follicular mucinosis with an atypical lymphoid infiltrate suspicious of MF (Fig. 133–3). A 6-mm punch biopsy of the scalp was studied for gene rearrangement. Cell surface markers revealed a T-cell receptor β-chain rearrangement consistent with the presence of a clonal population of T cells. No immunoglobulin rearrangement was detected. The patient was presented to Dermatology Grand Rounds with the new data. The consensus recommendation was to initiate whole-body electron beam therapy for a diagnosis of cutaneous T-cell lymphoma, stage IB.

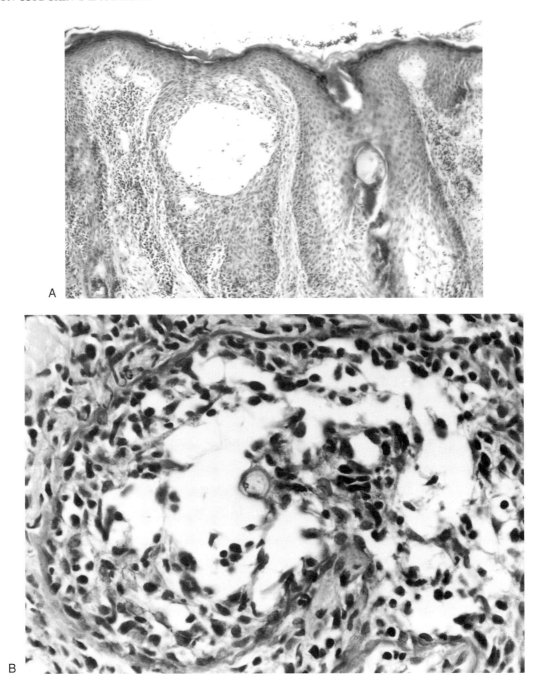

FIG. 133–2. A: Scalp ×10. Extensive perifollicular lymphohistiocytic infiltrate with mucin deposition of the hair follicle. **B:** Scalp ×40. Follicular structure with mucinous degeneration (alcian blue stain positive). There are atypical lymphohistiocytic cells with hyperchromatic convoluted nuclei.

The patient received total skin electron beam therapy as 3,200 cGy in 16 fractions over 8 weeks with a boost to the scalp. Side effects included further alopecia, loss of eyebrows and eyelashes, painful desquamation of the feet, hyperpigmentation, and xerosis. Two months after completing electron beam therapy, she presented with erythema and infiltration of the eyelids, an erythematous plaque with follicular papules on the right upper cheek, and erythematous papules on the arms and thighs. There was no palpable

adenopathy. Cheek biopsy demonstrated absence of adnexa, presence of deep dermal fibrosis, a dense superficial and mid-dermal lymphoid infiltrate with marked hyperchromasia, and irregularly shaped nuclei diagnosed as cutaneous T-cell lymphoma. Thigh biopsy revealed a deep neutrophilic infiltrate without evidence of cellular atypia. Topical corticosteroids were employed and the patient remained clear of lesions for the ensuing 9 months, at which time she developed recurrent lesions of the cheek

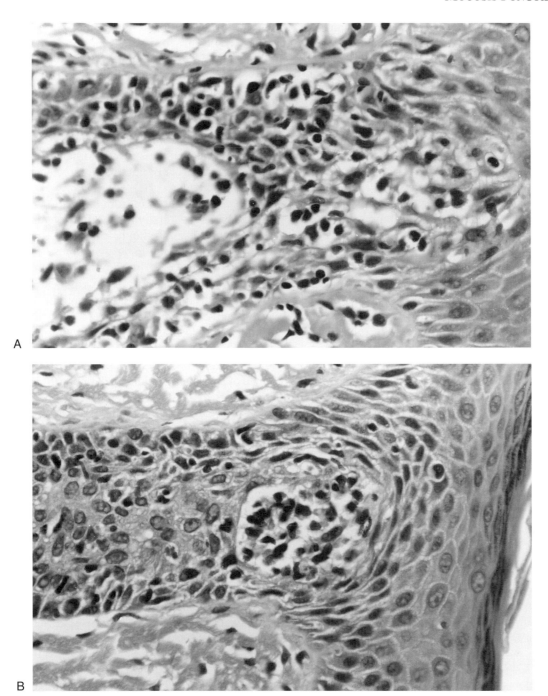

FIG. 133–3. A: Face ×40. Epidermotropism and mucinous degeneration with atypical mononuclear cells. **B:** Face ×40. Pautrier's microabscess formation.

and eyelids with new plaques present in the nasolabial folds, eyebrows, scalp, and thighs. A biopsy from the nasolabial fold demonstrated follicular mucinosis and findings of CTCL.

Psoralen plus ultraviolet A therapy (PUVA) was begun at 3 times per week. After a total cumulative dosage of 200 joules of UVA, a decrease in the induration of the facial plaques was noted. No further clinical changes were noted after a total cumulative dose of 327 joules. Isotretinoin (Accutane) 1 mg/kg orally was begun as adjunctive ther-

apy. At a total cumulative UVA dosage of 420 joules, all visible lesions had resolved with a small amount of eyebrow and eyelash regrowth.

In September 1991, after 625 joules UVA, the eyebrows and lashes had regrown, but new leg and face lesions were present. The PUVA therapy was intensified with resolution of the facial lesions. Serum chemistries and complete blood count remained normal, and no Sezary cells were seen on serum buffy coat exam. Blood for flow cytometry showed no evidence of malignant cells or monoclonal proliferation.

By June 1992, the patient had received 1,466 joules of UVA. The facial lesions had thickened with a pebbly appearance, and new lesions were present in a perioral and perinasal distribution with scattered plaques on the body. The patient was now complaining of intense pruritus and increasing alopecia.

The patient was presented to Dermatology Grand Rounds 2½ years after definitive diagnosis. The decision was made to add topical meclorethamine ointment 10% to the existing regimen and initiate photophoresis. Photophoresis was begun on a monthly basis with the patient receiving two consecutive 4-hour treatments in a 24-hour period. After 5 months of photophoresis, no clinical response was seen and the patient requested its discontinuation.

The patient continued to complain of marked pruritus, and supraclavicular and axillary adenopathy was present. Total body surface area involved with CTCL was estimated at 60%. Serum chemistries revealed an SGOT 59 (nl 11–47), LDH 298 (nl 90–200), and CK 178 (nl 20–170). She was anemic with a profound eosinophilia (28%) and elevated sedimentation rate of 37.

The patient was referred to an oncologist. In the interim, she developed herpes zoster in the right T6 dermatome successfully treated with acyclovir. Computed tomography (CT) scan of the chest and abdomen confirmed the axillary adenopathy. Bone marrow biopsies were normal. Her CTCL was staged as T3-T4, N2.

Three million units of interferon-alpha 2a administered subcutaneously three times a week was started in combination with Accutane 40 mg orally a day, and the patient discontinued PUVA. One month later, only the extremity lesions were present and a partial nodal response was documented. Accutane and topical meclorethamine ointment were continued, and the interferon dose was accelerated. One month later, the exam was unchanged, and PUVA therapy was restarted at two times per week. Ten days later, a continued nodal response and skin response were noted. Interferon dose was held at 9×10^6 units three times a week because of slight neutropenia. All serum chemistries had normalized and no eosinophils were seen on peripheral blood smear. After an additional month the physical exam was dramatically improved, showing only scaling of the lower extremities. Because of worsening neutropenia and anemia, the interferon dose was decreased to 3×10^6 units three times a week. Four months after starting interferon and Accutane, and 3 months after reinstating PUVA, dramatic improvement is noted with only one remaining palpable lymph node, and near clearing of all remaining skin lesions.

COMMENTARY by Cary A. Presant

The mean age of mycosis fungoides is between 50 and 55 years. The patient, who is 43 years old, is slightly young. The disease is equal in frequency in men and women. Because it is sometimes common to have a family history of other lymphoproliferative diseases, it would have been of interest to determine whether or not this patient had any family history of leukemia or lymphoma. This might be important to make recommendations for family surveillance of skin and nodal areas. Some patients with mycosis fungoides also have had occupational exposure to petrochemicals; it would have been of interest to determine whether or not this patient had such an employment history.

The average duration from onset of symptoms to diagnostic biopsy is usually long, often 3 years or longer. This patient was diagnosed quite promptly, 2 months after the onset of her dermatologic symptoms. This underscores the importance of early biopsy in patients with atypical dermatologic conditions, or patients with a poor response to clinical trials' dermatologic pharmaceuticals based on presumptive diagnosis without biopsy.

After the suspicion of mycosis fungoides, the patient had the sometimes crucial cell surface marker and gene rearrangement studies to confirm definitively the presence of a formal population of T cells (1,2). This made the diagnosis of mycosis fungoides unequivocal. The presence of Pautrier's microabscesses clearly indicated the high likelihood of the diagnosis of mycosis fungoides and would have been sufficient to have initiated therapy for mycosis fungoides.

The presenters have failed to emphasize the extreme importance of staging of patients. This patient presented with generalized plaques without evidence of lymph node enlargement. This patient was a stage IB at the time of presentation. The staging system helps to guide clinical therapy: stage IA is defined as limited plaques; stage IB is generalized plaques; stage IIA is any number of plaques plus lymphadenopathy; stage IIB is cutaneous tumors with or without lymphadenopathy; stage III is erythroderma; and stage IV is histologic evidence of lymphoproliferative disease in lymph nodes and or viscera.

The choices of therapy are many (3). Patients may be controlled at early stages (stage IA, stage IB, and stage IIA) with electron beam radiation therapy, as initiated in this patient, with PUVA therapy, and/or with topical nitrogen mustard (4). Indeed, all three treatments were used in this individual, with only brief periods of improvement.

Patients who have resistant stage I or stage II disease are often then treated with either systemic interferon or with systemic isotretinoin (5). This patient indeed received both such therapies with improvement in her condition, and a gradual near-complete remission. In addition, isotretinoin and/or interferon may be used at the initial diagnosis of stage III or stage IV disease, and/or Sezary syndrome.

Other treatments that have been useful for more advanced stages of disease (stage III, stage IV, or Sezary syndrome) include standard photon beam radiation therapy for extensive local symptoms, the administration of systemic chemotherapy with doxorubicin and/or cyclophosphamide combinations, and the more recent demonstrations that use of nucleoside chemotherapy with fludarabine, deoxycoformycin (pentostatin), or chlorode-oxyadenosine can be highly beneficial. Because of the greater side effects of these regimens (6), they are more appropriately reserved for treatment of stage I or II disease refractory to electron-beam radiation therapy, PUVA therapy, nitrogen mustard therapy, isotretinoin, and/or interferon; or in the initial treatment of aggressive stage III or stage IV disease, or Sezary syndrome.

This patient is now approximately 3 years after diagnosis. This result is consistent with the median survival in early-stage patients of greater than 5 years. Patients with stage II disease have a median survival of between 3 and 4 years, and patients with stage III or stage IV or Sezary syndrome have a more aggressive disease with a median survival of 1 to 2 years. The appropriate use of combinations of therapies mentioned above may extend the median survivals (5,7). Such studies, mostly in progress, show encouraging results that at present do not offer clear guidance as to which combinations are superior. Sequential use of these combination regimens is common practice.

New agents may offer additional therapeutic options. In early-stage patients, cutaneous chemotherapy may produce additional periods of control, as with topical pyridyl-methyl-deazaquanine BCX-34 (8). Novel biologic products may offer systemic therapy alternatives, alone or in combination, in patients with advanced stage disease, as for example thymopentin (an oligopeptide receptor site analogue) (9).

REFERENCES

1. Aisenberg AC, Kronteris TG, Mak TW, et al. Rearrangement of the gene for the beta chain of the T-cell receptor in T-cell chronic lymphocytic leukemia and related disorders. *N Engl J Med* 1985;313: 529–33.
2. Bakels V, VanOustreen JW, Gordijn RLJ, et al. Frequency and prognostic significance of clonal T-cell receptor beta gene rearrangements in the peripheral blood of patients with mycosis fungoides. *Arch Dermatol* 1992;128:1602–7.
3. Abel EA, et al. Mycosis fungoides: clinical and histologic features, staging, evaluation and approach to treatment. *CA Cancer J Clin* 1993;43:93–115.
4. Mostow EN, Neckel SL, Oberhelman L, et al. Complete remissions in psoralen and UV-A (PUVA)-refractory mycosis fungoides type cutaneous T-cell lymphoma with combined interferon alpha and PUVA. *Arch Dermatol* 1993;129:747–52.
5. Smith MA, Parkinson DR, Cheson BD, et al. Retinoids in cancer therapy. *J Clin Oncol* 1992;10:839–64.
6. Cohen RB, Abdallah JM, Gray JR, et al. Reversible neurologic toxicity in patients treated with standard dose fludarabine phosphate for mycosis fungoides and chronic lymphocytic leukemia. *Arch Internal Med* 1993;118:114–6.
7. Foss FM, Ihde DC, Breneman DL, et al. Phase II study of pentostatin and intermittent high dose recombinant interferon alpha 2a in advanced mycosis fungoides/Sezary syndrome. *J Clin Oncol* 1991;10: 1907–13.
8. Martin A, Blattel S, Fitzgibbon J, et al. Treatment of cutaneous T-cell lymphoma with BCX-34 dermal cream. *Proc Am Soc Clin Oncol* 1994;13:384 (abstr).
9. Foss F, Sznol M, Urba W, et al. Biological activity of thymopentin in cutaneous T-cell lymphoma. *Proc Am Assoc Cancer Res* 1994;35:237 (abstr).

134

Stage IIE Non-Hodgkin's Lymphoma of the Oropharynx

Elizabeth M. Gore and Stuart J. Wong

Radiotherapy versus chemotherapy versus both

CASE PRESENTATION

The patient is a 65-year-old Caucasian man with a diagnosis of diffuse histiocytic lymphoma of the right tonsil made in 1987. His first symptoms were that of mild throat pain for several weeks that did not resolve with antibiotics. On self-examination, he noted swelling and ulceration of the right tonsil. He was evaluated by an otolaryngologist in the community. He found no other abnormalities and obtained a biopsy of this lesion. Initially, this was thought to be a nonkeratinizing squamous cell carcinoma; but on more careful review and consultation with other pathologists, this was believed to be a small-cell cleaved lymphoma, histiocytic variant. The patient was evaluated by a medical oncologist in the community; however, because of the confusion regarding the pathologic diagnosis, he was referred to an outside cancer institute for a second opinion. In addition to the mass and ulceration of the right tonsil, a 1-cm soft, mobile, right submaxillary lymph node was identified. The original biopsy specimen was reviewed and thought to be most consistent with lymphoma of the right tonsil. A repeat biopsy was recommended, but the patient chose to return home and sought care at our institution, where the biopsy material had already been reviewed and was read as diffuse histiocytic lymphoma (Fig. 134–1).

The patient was referred to the Hematology Oncology Division. At the time of interview, 1 month after the biopsy, he denied mouth pain, dysphagia, odynophagia, or otalgia. He denied fever, chills, night sweats, or weight loss. The patient was an active smoker and drank alcohol only on occasion.

His past medical history was remarkable for hearing loss secondary to measles, cholecystectomy, and nasal polyposis.

Physical examination revealed a well developed, well nourished, Caucasian man in no acute distress. Vital signs were: weight 204 lbs, blood pressure 142/78, pulse 68 and regular, temperature 97.8°F. Skin exam was normal. Otolaryngologic examination revealed erythema of the right anterior tonsillar pillar. The right tonsil was absent. The left tonsillar fossa and pillars were normal. Indirect mirror examination revealed no abnormalities. A mobile, nontender 7- to 8-mm right lower anterior cervical lymph node was detected. No supraclavicular, axillary, epitrochlear, inguinal, or popliteal adenopathy was palpable. Lungs were clear to auscultation. Cardiovascular exam was normal. His abdomen was soft without masses or hepatosplenomegaly. Extremity and neurologic examinations were normal. A staging work-up was initiated.

Hematology profile, basic chemistry, and liver function tests were normal. ESR was 10 (nl 0–9). LDH was elevated at 200 (nl 90–160).

Radiographic staging work-up included chest radiograph, computed tomography (CT) scans of the neck, chest, abdomen, and pelvis, and a gallium scan. CT scan through the tonsillar region revealed no masses. A 1-cm homogeneous lymph node lateral to the right common carotid artery was seen. Several lymph nodes along the left jugular and right jugular chains measuring less than 1 cm were present. The remaining radiographic studies were normal. Bilateral bone marrow aspirates and biopsies were normal.

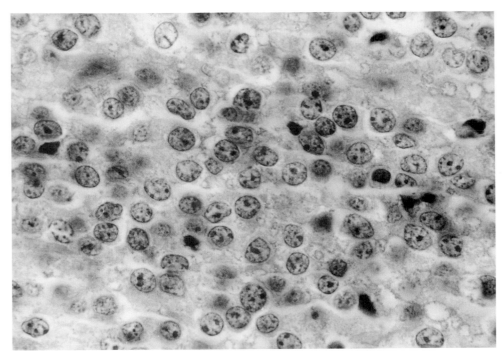

FIG. 134–1. Tonsil biopsy showing an infiltrative process composed of large lymphoid cells with round, vesicular nuclei containing one to three nucleoli, frequently subjacent to the nuclear membrane, and a moderate amount of pale cytoplasm. Scattered mitotic figures and occasional necrotic tumor cells are observed (original magnification ×240).

TUMOR BOARD DISCUSSION

Biopsy of the right submaxillary lymph node was considered to confirm the suspicion of regional nodal involvement. If negative, he would be staged as clinical IEA non-Hodgkin's lymphoma and his disease would be potentially curable with radiation alone or with radiation as the most important component of combined modality therapy. Alternatively, if the cervical lymph node were histologically confirmed, upstaging the patient to clinical stage IIEA, chemotherapy would be the primary treatment modality and radiation would be employed as adjuvant treatment. It was the joint opinion of Radiation Oncology and Medical Oncology that biopsy of the lymph node was unnecessary. The patient was felt to have clinical stage IIEA diffuse histiocytic lymphoma. He was treated with chemotherapy and consolidative irradiation.

Two cycles of chemotherapy were administered, followed by radiation therapy and an additional four cycles of chemotherapy. The chemotherapy regimen included cyclophosphamide 800 mg intravenously and doxorubicin 60 mg intravenously given on day 1 with prednisone 80 mg orally given on days 1 through 10. Cyclophosphamide 800 mg intravenously and vinblastine 6 mg intravenously were administered on day 8. Cycles were repeated every 4 weeks. The vinblastine was substituted for vincristine because of the patient's request to minimize the risk of neuropathy.

Radiation was initiated after the second cycle of chemotherapy. He was treated with 6 MV photons, with right and left lateral fields covering Waldeyer's ring and upper anterior cervical and posterior cervical lymph nodes. He received 1.8 Gy per fraction per day at midplane. The posterior neck was blocked after 39.6 Gy. The lateral fields were completed at 48.6 Gy. Left and right posterior neck nodes were treated with 10 MEV electrons at 2.0 Gy per fraction calculated at the 90% isodose line with an additional 10 Gy, for a total dose of 49.6 Gy. The lower cervical nodes were treated with an anterior supraclavicular field with 6 MV photons at 1.8 Gy per fraction at a 3-cm depth to 50.4 Gy.

The patient has been seen every 6 months since completion of therapy for complete physical examination and laboratory evaluation, including a hematologic profile, basic chemistry, liver function tests, LDH, and ESR, and yearly for chest x-rays. He has been without evidence of disease for 6 years and 5 months. He has had persistent xerostomia and no other clinically apparent side effects of therapy.

COMMENTARY by Eli Glatstein

Probably the first point to make on this case is that the confusion over the diagnosis is not that unusual; a comparatively anaplastic lymphoma can easily be confused with an anaplastic carcinoma. This is especially true if the carcinoma, presumably of a squamous cell origin, is thought to be nonkeratinizing. Once the biopsy has been made, the presence of a soft neck node in the vicinity of the biopsy is virtually impossible to interpret. Whether you wish to call it a positive node or not, the fact remains that the size of the node, less than 1 cm, is not especially obvious for cancer. In fact, it does not even meet most criteria that are arbitrary for diagnostic radiology. One of the points of staging is that when in doubt one is supposed to understage rather than upstage. One may wish to take this into account in one's recommendations for treatment, but on the basis of what is described, I would have called this stage I of the tonsil. The lymphoid tissue within Waldeyer's ring is considered part of the lymphatic system, and not a nonlymphatic lesion or an "E." Thus, as described, I would have staged this as a IA of the tonsil. If the node were unequivocally positive, then I would stage the patient as having stage IIA disease.

In terms of lymphomas, I consider them to be of two types: (a) indolent or (b) aggressive. The indolent lymphomas are predominantly of the follicular type, and I know of no evidence that multiagent chemotherapy can cure them at all. The aggressive types, on the other hand, represent one of the true success stories for chemotherapy, and I believe the treatment of choice for all stages of aggressive lymphoma is multiagent chemotherapy, to be followed by radiation if the target volume is small enough to be acceptable. Thus, whether it is a IA, IIA, IE, or IIE, I would have thought that multiagent chemotherapy was the basic treatment, with additional local control to be furnished by local field radiation for this aggressive histology (1). I do not have any trouble either recommending combined modality treatment for indolent lymphoma because the cure rate with radiation is relatively modest. Nonetheless, as noted above, the multiagent chemotherapy that is crucial for the management of aggressive histologies is, in my opinion, entirely lacking in evidence of curability for the indolent histopathologies. For indolent histology patients in whom curative treatment is a realistic goal (i.e., patients with stage I, II, IE, or IIE disease with good performance status), the major thrust of treatment at this time is radiation therapy, with or without adjuvant chemotherapy (2). Incidentally, for indolent histology disease, multiagent chemotherapy has never been shown to be superior to single agent chemotherapy in terms of outcome.

Given that the diagnosis here was one of the aggressive histologies with diffuse histiocytic lymphoma, I think the ideal treatment was multiagent chemotherapy to be followed by small volume radiation to the area of known disease. The likelihood of cure in that setting, with a questionable node for diffuse histiocytic lymphoma of IA type, should range from approximately 75% to 95%, depending on the kinds of patients who are treated (1). The value of the radiation on top of the chemotherapy for the aggressive histology lymphomas is not fully established. However, since the volume can be kept small after the chemotherapy, it makes sense because, in those patients who do relapse, the likely site of relapse is the area of initial involvement and its nearby vicinity. The additional local control achieved with radiation on top of the chemotherapy is probably worth approximately 10 percentage points in terms of long-term curability. Let there be no mistake, however, that the bulk of the curability comes from the chemotherapy. The xerostomia is a result of the radiation treatment but I believe is a reasonable price to pay for a successful outcome.

I must admit to being unhappy with the replacement of vinblastine for vincristine in the management of this patient. As a single agent, vinblastine is relatively ineffective against most aggressive histology lymphomas. It is true that vincristine is more likely to have peripheral neuropathy associated with it, but I do not believe that should serve as a reason for substitution. Our weapons for treatment represent a fairly limited arsenal, and I do not think we should casually substitute one drug for another to minimize side effects when our overall success rate is relatively poor. The fact that one was able to get away with it in this setting with a favorable early-stage lesion should not be construed as accepting this substitution. If the patient manifests a severe neuropathy to treatment, perhaps that substitution could then be rationalized, but the willingness to substitute in advance of the problem is, to my way of thinking, not a good decision. In this instance, it seems not to have mattered, but in the next patient one may not be so fortunate.

REFERENCES

1. Longo DL, Glatstein E, Duffy PL, et al. Treatment of localized aggressive lymphomas with combination chemotherapy followed by involved-field radiation therapy. *J Clin Oncol* 1979;7(9):1295–1302.
2. Paryani SB, Hoppe RT, Cox RS, et al. Analysis of non-Hodgkin's lymphomas with nodular and favorable histologies stages I and II. *Cancer* 1983;52:2300–7.

135

Stage IV Non-Hodgkin's Lymphoma (Favorable Histology) in a 70-Year-Old Man

Brian J. Moran and Frank Hussey

*An indolent disease that warrants serious consideration of
many treatment options*

CASE PRESENTATION

R.M. is a 70-year-old gentleman found to have a 3-cm mobile, nontender, right axillary mass. Excisional biopsy revealed non-Hodgkin's lymphoma of the follicular mixed type composed of both small-cleaved and large-cell type cells. The remainder of the physical examination was unremarkable and the patient was asymptomatic. A staging work-up was completed and there were found to be significantly enlarged lymph nodes in the retroperitoneal space and pelvis. The bone marrow biopsy was positive for malignancy. The patient was then considered to have stage IV favorable histology non-Hodgkin's lymphoma. Radiographic studies included a chest radiograph that was within normal limits; however, a computed tomography (CT) scan of the abdomen and pelvis did reveal significant lymphadenopathy.

The Tumor Board discussion is as follows.

Dr. Moran: Can we now review the radiographic finding on the CT scan?

Dr. Boyle (radiologist): There is marked periaortic and pericaval lymphadenopathy (Fig. 135–1). The CT scan of the pelvis reveals a large mass adjacent to the urinary bladder causing a filling defect (Fig. 135–2). There is also significant associated lymphadenopathy in the left side of the pelvis. When there is this degree of lymphadenopathy present, one is always concerned over

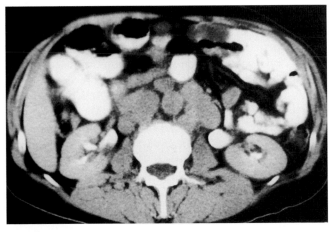

FIG. 135–1. Abdominal CT scan. A section through the level of the kidneys shows periaortic and pericaval lymphadenopathy.

the presence of hydronephrosis. There is no evidence of hydronephrosis at present.

Dr. Moran: Would a gallium scan offer any additional information?

Dr. Boyle: It may or may not, but it frequently will not with non-Hodgkin's lymphoma. Classically it is a better study for Hodgkin's disease.

Dr. Moran: We will now review the pathology.

Dr. Bernhardt (pathologist): In general, there are two features that one considers with non-Hodgkin's lym-

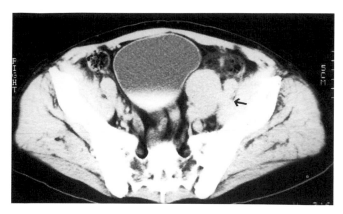

FIG. 135–2. CT scan of the pelvis. There is a large mass adjacent to the urinary bladder with displacement of the bladder wall. There is also adenopathy between the mass and the pelvic wall (*arrow*).

phoma. The first is architectural features, and that would be either a follicular pattern or a diffuse pattern of involvement. The other feature would be cytologic, meaning the size, shape, color, and other visible features of the individual cells. The small-cleaved cell has a relatively good prognosis when compared with the lymphoblast, which represents a much more aggressive variety (Fig. 135–3).

Dr. Moran: Would you comment please on the value of immunophenotyping?

Dr. Bernhardt: Immunophenotyping studies distinguish whether or not the B lymphocytic lesion is monoclonal or polyclonal. Monoclonal lesions represent malignancies whereas polyclonal lesions represent reactive nodes. Once the determination of a benign versus a malignant lesion is made, the subclassification is then done based primarily on hemotoxylin and eosin morphology. The aggressiveness of these non-Hodgkin's lymphomas can be predicted in more than 90% of cases with hemotoxylin and eosin morphology alone.

Dr. Moran: What is the role for surgical intervention in this case setting?

Dr. Sinha (surgeon): Traditionally, non-Hodgkin's lymphoma is not a disease that is treated surgically. Staging laparotomy, although useful for Hodgkin's disease, has minimal usefulness in the management of non-Hodgkin's lymphoma. Surgical intervention therefore is confined to the realm of biopsy and local problems if indicated. An example of this would be ureteral stents.

Dr. Moran: What is the role of radiation therapy in treatment of this patient?

Dr. Miller: External beam radiotherapy for stage IV non-Hodgkin's lymphoma is not the mainstay of treatment. Radiation therapy would be used, however, to treat local disease in an effort to decrease tumor bulk that may be causing local symptoms. An example of this would be hydronephrosis secondary to lymphadenopathy. In the past, before effective chemotherapy regimens, total nodal irradiation was used with some success, although it was not superior to the results obtained with chemotherapy. If one is to use radiation, a dose of 2,500 to 4,000 cGy usually is adequate for a complete response.

Dr. Moran: What is the role of chemotherapy?

Dr. Priest: Low-grade non-Hodgkin's lymphomas are controversial with regard to the best treatment. This particular class of lymphomas does respond well to chemotherapy, but there may be no survival benefit. This was demonstrated in the 1970s at Stanford, when a large group of patients with stage IV favorable histology non-Hodgkin's lymphoma was observed. These patients were asymptomatic and did as well as their cohorts with stage IV disease who did receive treatment. On the other hand, The National Cancer Institute and Memorial-Sloan Kettering have advocated a more aggressive approach. They recommend multiagent chemotherapy for these patients. They have postulated that there may be a subgroup of these patients that is potentially curable with aggressive chemotherapy. Needless to say, the controversy continues as to the best available therapy. The problem that can arise with observation alone is that untreated bulky disease can create problems. The possibility of hydronephrosis is always a concern in anyone with retroperitoneal or pelvic lymphadenopathy. One can therefore argue that there is a role for treatment to reduce disease bulk and prevent hydronephrosis. One could do this with a single-agent chemotherapy, which may not subject the patient to as much morbidity as if he were to receive multiagent chemotherapy.

Dr. Sowray: Essentially, there is no significant overall survival difference between patients treated with single-agent versus multiagent chemotherapy in this subgroup. There is a trade-off between treatment and observation for these patients. If they are treated they may have an excellent response, but it is not without risk for major complications. This could include second malignancies and acute cytotoxicity. These patients can experience significant granulocytopenia, risking infection.

Dr. Moran: Are there ways to minimize toxicity if you decide to treat that patient?

Dr. Sowray: Acutely, yes. Patient's on single-agent parambucil can be titrated so as to minimize the acute myelosuppression and resulting cytopenias.

Dr. Moran: With regard to the possibility of a second malignancy, I do not think this is an issue in this patient. The latency usually is 7 to 10 years and the incidence quite low.

Dr. Bank: Obviously, when you have different options including observation alone, it is of the utmost importance to educate your patient so as to involve him in the decision process. I believe that there are individuals with a pioneer spirit who would volunteer for a clinical trial. There are others, however, who are leery of potential toxicity and may prefer observation unless they became symptomatic.

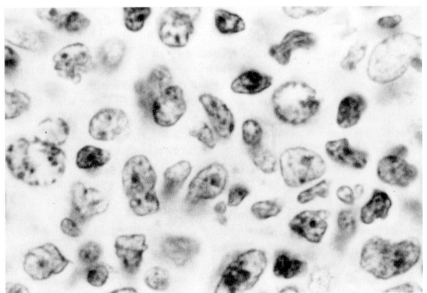

FIG. 135–3. Axillary lymph node manifesting follicular non-Hodgkin's lymphoma. **A:** H&E, ×40. Note irregular follicular configuration in the upper right and left quadrants. **B:** High-power field showing mixed-type follicular lymphoma composed of both small-cleaved and large-cell types.

It has been my experience that most patients are uncomfortable with the concept of sitting idly by with the knowledge that they do have a malignancy that is left untreated.

Dr. Moran: Would it be fair to say that at the present time we are able to increase the freedom from relapse for this type and stage of disease, and at the same time we cannot clearly demonstrate any improved survival with treatment?

Dr. Bank: Yes, I think that is a fair statement. There have been studies in Europe that have shown some improvement; however, there are others that have not. There are good data to suggest that we can generate complete responses for a significant period of time; however, we are not as fortunate with demonstrating improved overall survival.

Dr. Leibach: I think that the points mentioned demonstrate the extreme variability among patients presenting with these favorable histology lymphomas. It is for that reason that I recommend a very individualized approach to each case. I would also like to emphasize the importance of whether or not treatment is given. If the watch and wait approach is selected, then the patient will require regular follow-up. With this patient one would be concerned over the development of hydronephrosis. I would also like to mention that occasionally these favorable histology lymphomas can transform to a more aggressive unfavorable histology. Naturally, this would influence the treatment recommendations as we do not recommend observation alone for the more aggressive lymphomas.

Dr. Priest: The nomenclature that has been used can be misleading. It is ironic that the unfavorable histologies are the potentially curable lesions, whereas the favorable histologies have rather indolent courses but are incurable. In the future we will minimize the use of these terms and relate our discussions more to the exact histology of these lesions.

After thorough discussion with the patient regarding possible treatment options, he decided to receive chemotherapy. Cytoxan, vincristine, and prednisone were given for eight cycles and the patient did experience a 9-month complete remission. The disease recurred, however, and he received an additional eight cycles of CHOPP, resulting in a 4-month remission. The disease relapsed in the periaortic lymph node chain and was causing pain. A dose of 4,000 cGy was given to the retroperitoneal lymph nodes, and the patient experienced complete relief of his pain. Radiographically, the lymphadenopathy regressed considerably. He is doing well, his appetite is good, and his weight is stable. He is being monitored by serial physical examinations and CT scans of the abdomen as indicated.

COMMENTARY by Robert C. Young

This patient presents in a relatively typical manner for the follicular mixed non-Hodgkin's lymphomas (so-called indolent lymphomas.) Most patients present with asymptomatic nodal enlargement, and the diagnosis is made, as in this case, by biopsy and careful review by a skilled hematopathologist. Unlike other malignancies, it is often difficult to make a specific diagnosis from a frozen section. One cannot be confident of the diagnosis until final, permanent sections are available for review. Even under the best of circumstances, approximately 15% of non-Hodgkin's lymphomas are reclassified into another category when reviewed by another equally skilled hematopathologist (1). Fortunately, the subtle dif-

ferences in pathologic classification uncommonly convey a marked change in prognosis and, in general, the follicular small-cell and mixed-cell lymphomas are indolent and the diffuse large-cell lymphomas are more aggressive. Paradoxically, however, as Dr. Priest mentioned in his comments, the aggressive lymphomas are frequently now curable with combination chemotherapy or radiation therapy, and the so-called indolent lymphomas are treatable but generally incurable.

Although patients usually present with asymptomatic nodal enlargement, a more comprehensive staging (as in this case) generally reveals disseminated disease with nodal involvement above and below the diaphragm, and frequently with visceral involvement,

particularly the bone marrow and liver. Had this patient had a percutaneous liver biopsy performed, it is quite likely (40%) that this would have harbored non-Hodgkin's lymphoma (2). Despite the widespread dissemination of this disease, the finding of stage IV non-Hodgkin's lymphoma does not carry the ominous prognosis frequently associated with that stage in other malignancies. Indeed, long-term studies do not demonstrate a survival difference between stage III and IV patients.

At the present time, none of the existing therapies have convincingly demonstrated a survival difference between the conservative management approach either with no initial therapy or with minimal chemotherapy compared with a more aggressive combined modality approach at the outset (3). Nevertheless, the patient is 70 years of age and in most large survival studies the median survival is 9 years, regardless of initial therapy, so the prognosis in this instance is relatively good even though cure is not likely. The decision to initiate therapy should be based not on the survival impact, but on the need for therapy based on clinical findings or symptoms. In this instance, although the patient is asymptomatic, the large pelvic lymphadenopathy already displacing the bladder increases the risk for an asymptomatic ureteral obstruction with secondary hydronephrosis.

One could simply elect to follow this man with frequent pelvic CT scans and/or renal sonography to assess hydronephrosis, but the complexity and cost of this so-called no treatment approach would be substantial. It is frequently easier for the patient and cheaper in the long run to initiate therapy rather than use repeated and sometimes extensive disease reassessments while the patient is not receiving treatment.

Under the circumstances presented here, I would favor treatment and would select some form of chemotherapy, primarily because the patient's disease is widely disseminated and radiation therapy would not encompass all sites of disease. A wide range of chemotherapeutic regimens have been used and all are reasonably effective (3,4). In general, I prefer combination and intermittent chemotherapy rather than single-drug continuous alkylating agent therapy. Intermittent chemotherapy will allow immunologic recovery between treatments and appears to reduce the risk of second malignancies (5). It is of interest that the patients's histologic finding was follicular mixed lymphoma. In several studies, including those from the National Cancer Institute and from the St. Bartholomew's Hospital in London, this subset of follicular lymphoma has the longest disease-free survival after initial combination chemotherapy (6,7). It is also this histology that appears to include a subset of patients that may be cured with initial treatment (6).

Although no published regimen has yet demonstrated a difference in overall survival between patients treated with a watch and wait conservative approach compared with patients treated initially aggressively, the initial aggressive treatment by definition produces longer sustained disease-free intervals, and in many of these studies more than 30% of the patients are continuously disease-free after initial treatment for periods in excess of 7 or 8 years (8). The difficulty in interpreting these survival curves is that there continue to be relapses over time, and one cannot yet conclude that a subset of patients with indolent non-Hodgkin's lymphoma has been cured by aggressive initial intervention. It may require 15- or 20-year follow-up from these studies to resolve the question of whether a cured subset of patients has been produced.

Independent of whether or not cures have been achieved with existing therapies, it is important that a search for curative intervention continue to be undertaken. If we conclude that indolent lymphomas are incurable and the trial designs necessary to identify curative treatment are not initiated, we will have insured another self-fulfilling prophecy in medicine. Although it is true that these lymphomas are more indolent than others and the median survival of 9 years is substantial, many patients with this histology present in their 40s and survival into the next decade, for them, would not be considered a therapeutic triumph (9).

REFERENCES

1. NCI Non-Hodgkin's Classification Project Writing Committee. Classification of non-Hodgkin's lymphomas: reproducibility of major classification systems. *Cancer* 1985;55:91–5.
2. Chabner BA, Johnson RE, Young RC, et al. Sequential staging nonsurgical and surgical staging of non-Hodgkin's lymphoma. *Ann Intern Med* 1976;85:149–54.
3. Portlock CS. Management of the low-grade non-Hodgkin's lymphomas. *Semin Oncol* 1990;17:51–9.
4. Anderson T, Bender RA, Fisher RI, et al. Combination chemotherapy in non-Hodgkin's lymphoma: results of long term follow-up. *Cancer Treat Rep* 1977;61:1057–66.
5. Greene MH, Young RC, Merrill JM, et al. Evidence of a treatment-dose response in acute non-lymphocytic leukemias which occur after therapy of non-Hodgkin's lymphoma. *Cancer Res* 1983;43:1891–8.
6. Longo DL, Young RC, Hubbard SM, et al. Prolonged initial remission in patients with nodular mixed lymphoma. *Ann Intern Med* 1984;100:651–6.
7. Lister TA, Cullen MH, Beard MEJ, et al. Comparison of combined and single agent chemotherapy in non-Hodgkin's lymphoma of favorable histologic type. *Br Med J* 1978;1:533–7.
8. Young RC, Longo DL, Glatstein E, et al. The treatment of indolent lymphomas: watchful waiting vs. aggressive combined modality treatment. *Semin Hematol* 1988;25:11–6.
9. Longo DL, Young RC, DeVita VT. What is so good about the "good prognosis" lymphomas? In: *Recent advances in clinical oncology,* Williams CJ, ed. Edinburgh: Churchill-Livingstone; 1982:223–31.

136

High-Grade Stage IV Non-Hodgkin's Lymphoma

Letha E. Mills and Norman B. Levy

*A response to intensive chemotherapy with consideration of
the role of bone marrow transplant*

CASE PRESENTATION

The patient is a 35-year-old previously healthy woman, who presents with a six-month history of left-sided chest pain. She was jogging 3 miles a day before the time when she first noted the onset of sharp pleuritic pain. The pain was associated with numbness and tingling in her left arm. An EKG ordered by her local physician at that time was reported to her as normal. No further evaluation was done, and the pain resolved spontaneously allowing her to resume all normal activities, including vigorous exercise. Two weeks before admission, she again noted the onset of sharp debilitating left-sided chest pain radiating at times to her left arm. This time she started having nonproductive cough, dyspnea on exertion, and a low-grade fever. She was treated by her local physician with a ten-day course of erythromycin for presumed pneumonia. No chest radiography was done at that time. After antibiotic treatment was initiated, the sharp pain diminished but she was left with a persistent dull left-sided ache in her chest. Four days before admission, the sharp pain recurred and her dry cough worsened. She denied any weight loss or night sweats but did feel warm. Two days before admission, she had a syncopal episode while at work and was brought to her local hospital. A chest radiograph detected a large mediastinal mass. The patient was referred to a hematologist for further evaluation. The patient was admitted to the hospital because of concern that the mass might be impinging on ventricular outflow, leading to her episode of syncope. Her past medical history and family history were unremarkable. Her social history revealed that she was divorced and worked as a clerk at a greyhound race park. She denied any cigarette or alcohol use. On review of systems, she denied any other symptoms.

On physical exam in the emergency room, she was found to be in some distress due to the chest pain. Her temperature was 37.4°C, blood pressure 120/70 mm Hg, pulse 104, respiration 24. She had jugular venous distension, and her carotid upstroke was normal bilaterally. Cardiac exam revealed a normal S1 and S2, with a III/VI harsh systolic murmur heard best over the left sternal border and radiating to the axilla. No rubs or gallops were appreciated. Examination of her lungs revealed decreased breath sounds two-thirds of the way up her lung fields on the left side. She had no cervical adenopathy but had fullness in her supraclavicular area and shotty adenopathy in her left axilla. No inguinal adenopathy was noted. She had no hepatosplenomegaly, or palpable abdominal masses. She had no peripheral edema. Her neurologic exam was normal.

Pulse oximetry revealed an oxygen saturation of 98% on room air. Review of her chest radiograph confirmed the presence of a large mediastinal mass, a large left pleural effusion, and a small right pleural effusion (Fig. 136–1). The electrocardiogram showed a normal rhythm, with questionable Q waves leads II, III, and AVF. Laboratory studies showed a WBC of 10.1 × $10^3/\mu l$, with 68% neutrophils, 10 bands, 9 lymphocytes, 11 monocytes. She had a hemoglobin level of 12.9 gm %, a hematocrit reading of 38.2%, and a platelet count of

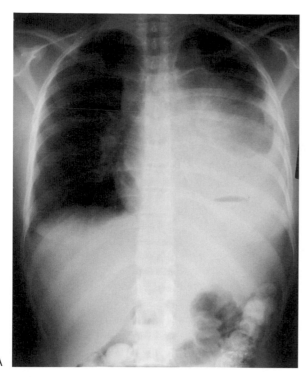

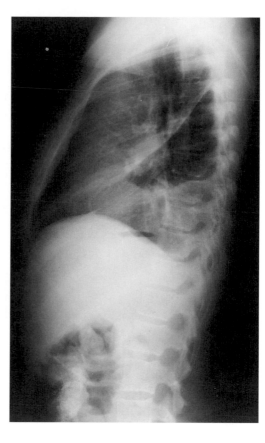

Fig. 136–1. Posteroanterior and lateral films of the chest demonstrating a large mediastinal mass with associated pleural effusions. **A:** The bulk of the fluid lies on the left; there is a small right-sided effusion. **B:** The lateral projection shows obliteration of the retrosternal space and mass in the region of the hilum.

$299,000 \times 10^3/\mu l$. Chemistries were normal except for a mildly elevated LDH at 723 U/L. Her sedimentation rate was elevated at 75.

An echocardiogram was done emergently, revealing normal function of the left and right ventricles with a left ventricular ejection fraction of 75%. A mass was seen anterior to the right ventricle compressing the right ventricular outflow tract and main pulmonary artery. A gradient of 25 mm Hg peak was found across the obstruction.

A computed tomography (CT) scan of the chest that evening revealed a large mediastinal mass with areas of decreased attenuation consistent with necrosis (Fig. 136–2). The mass extensively infiltrated the mediastinum, extending into the anteroposterior windows, precarinal area, right paratracheal region, subcarinal region and into the left hilum. The mass surrounded and encased the main pulmonary artery, the proximal left pulmonary artery, the aortic arch and proximal great vessels of the neck. All vessels were patent. There was moderate to severe narrowing of the left main stem bronchus and left upper lobe bronchus, with mild narrowing of the carina and lower trachea. The mass extended to the anterior and anterolateral chest wall. Inferiorly, the mass could not be separated from the pericardium, extending along the left heart border. A round opacity was seen in the left upper lobe consistent with pulmonary involve-

ment with tumor. Bilateral pleural effusions were present. The following day, a CT scan of the abdomen was performed, revealing normal liver, spleen, kidneys and bowel. Lymph nodes within upper limits of normal size were visualized in the region between the aorta and inferior vena cava were considered to be of unclear significance. There was no significant pelvic adenopathy. The differential diagnosis at this time included Hodgkin's or non-Hodgkin's lymphoma, thymoma, a mediastinal germ cell malignancy, soft tissue sarcoma or less likely, an epithelial malignancy such as an adenocarcinoma arising from the thyroid or parathyroid glands. She was placed on telemetry for cardiac monitoring, and treated with narcotics for pain control. Blood, urine, and sputum cultures were obtained to rule out an infection process contributing to her systemic symptoms. The following day, she underwent a biopsy by a cardiovascular surgeon via a mediastinotomy. The pathologic diagnosis was malignant lymphoma, diffuse large cell, with sclerosis (Fig. 136–3). Flow cytometry revealed the cells to be of B lymphocyte lineage. A bone marrow aspirate and bilateral biopsy specimens were obtained, demonstrating a mildly hypercellular marrow with no evidence of lymphoma. Iron stores were decreased.

The patient was presented to the lymphoma tumor board. Discussion at this time focused mainly on the issue

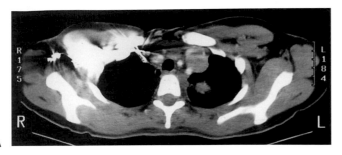

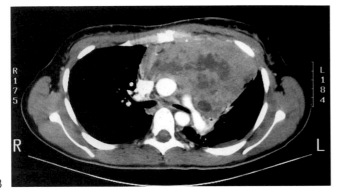

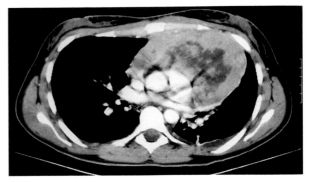

Fig. 136–2. Computed Tomography. **A:** Mediastinal adenopathy and parenchymal mass. **B:** Massive mediastinal involvement at the level of the carina with scattered areas of necrosis and involvement of the chest wall. **C:** Mass at the level of the hila with additional areas of necrosis and continued involvement of the chest wall.

of appropriate therapy for this patient with an aggressive lymphoma and a bulky mediastinal mass. The patient was believed to have probable stage IV disease on the basis of pulmonary parenchymal involvement that was not contiguous with the large mass. Treatment with systemic chemotherapy was believed to be the most appropriate, followed by consolidation with involved field radiation therapy (IFRT) to the mediastinal mass, because the size of this mass made local relapse a significant concern.

Chemotherapy regimens were discussed, recognizing the data from the Intergroup trial published by Fisher et al (1) demonstrating no substantial benefit to the use of the newer 7 or 8 drug combinations (m-BACOD, PRO-MACE-CytaBOM, MACOP-B) over the more standard four-drug chemotherapy of CHOP (cyclophosphamide, doxorubicin, vincristine, prednisone). However, this trial's results with CHOP were 15% better than most reported series, and the results of the more aggressive regimens were lower than previously reported.

Thus, the attending hematologist believed that the patient could tolerate more aggressive chemotherapy; and in view of the bulky disease in the mediastinum, his major concern was undertreating the patient. He chose to use PROMACE-CytaBOM (prednisone, doxorubicin, cyclophosphamide, etoposide, cytarabine, bleomycin, vincristine, and methotrexate), citing the published complete remission of 84% (2) and noting his favorable experience with this regimen in the treatment of prior patients with similar bulk disease. There was also discussion about supportive care measures to decrease the risks associated with this aggressive chemotherapy regimen. The use of G-CSF to shorten the period of neutropenia was dis-

cussed, as well as the use of trimethoprim-sulfamethoxazole prophylaxis three times per week to decrease the risk of *Pneumocystis carinii* pneumonia.

The patient improved dramatically with the therapy. Her chest pain significantly decreased, and there was a general improvement in her sense of well-being after only the first week of therapy. A baseline high-dose gallium scan done during this hospitalization did not show any sites of increased uptake. No tumor lysis syndrome was noted. She was discharged after 13 days in the hospital.

This patient was again presented to the lymphoma Tumor Board after 6 cycles of chemotherapy to consider whether she should be a candidate for high-dose chemotherapy and autologous bone marrow transplantation (ABMT). The patient's CT scan demonstrated a marked improvement in the mediastinal mass; however, there was still a residual mass present necessitating classification as a partial response (Fig. 136–4). Because gallium scanning was initially negative, it was unclear whether this residual mass represented active lymphoma or scarring. The possibility of re-biopsying or removing the residual mass was raised; however, this was thought to be a technically more difficult procedure with the prior surgery, and, unless the mass was completely excised, one could still not be sure there was not residual tumor. Options at this point therefore included: (1) 2 more cycles of chemotherapy; (2) involved field radiation; (3) 2 more cycles of chemotherapy followed by IFRT; (4) ABMT. It was noted that in the past, patients were very rarely considered for ABMT unless a relapse of their lymphoma was documented. However, the morbidity and mortality of ABMT has substantially improved since the use of G-CSF, and

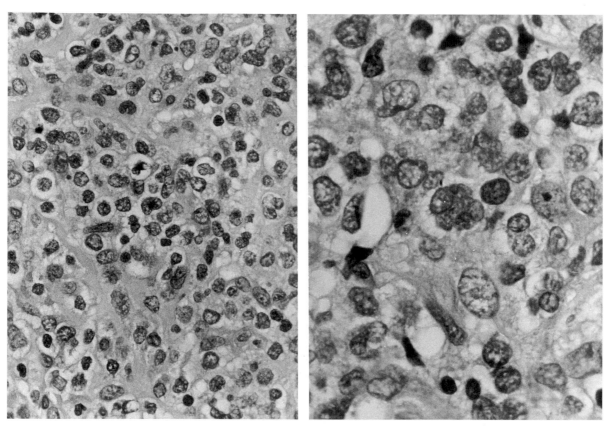

Fig. 136–3. Large cell malignant lymphoma with sclerosis.

the addition of G-CSF-primed peripheral blood progenitor cells as a source of stem cells has been given in conjunction with harvested bone marrow. The period of neutropenia has been shortened to the range of approximately 10 days, and the mortality has been decreased to less than 5%. The data in patients with relapsed lymphoma who are "chemosensitive" (responding to induction chemotherapy) has shown as good as a 50% long-term disease-free survival post-ABMT. However, if a patient is chemoresistant at this time, there are very few patients who achieve long-term disease-free survival.

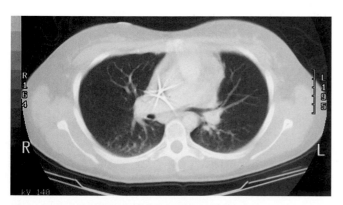

Fig. 136–4. Posttreatment computed tomography scan demonstrating residual mediastinal disease.

The patient chose to proceed with high-dose chemotherapy with ABMT, and presently, she remains in remission six months after ABMT.

REFERENCES

1. Fisher RI, Gaynor ER, Dahlberg S, et al. Comparison of a standard regimen (CHOP) with three intensive chemotherapy regimens for advanced non-Hodgkin's lymphoma. *N Engl J Med* 1993;328: 1002–6.
2. Longo DL, DeVita VT Jr., Duffey PL, et al. Superiority of ProMACE-CytaBOM over ProMACE-MOPP in the treatment of advanced diffuse aggressive lymphoma: results of a prospective randomized trial. *J Clin Oncol* 1991;9:25–38.

COMMENTARY by Bruce A. Peterson

This was obviously a very challenging case for the clinicians who took care of the patient, especially during her initial hospitalization. Lymphomas are the most common malignancy to present as a large mediastinal mass and, as was the case with this patient, when there is possible obstruction or interference with cardiac output or an airway, it is mandatory that a diagnosis be quickly established and rapidly followed by appropriate intervention. Because lymphomas are most often responsive to chemotherapy, it is usually not necessary to use irradiation once a lymphoma is diagnosed. However, the choice of a specific chemotherapy program will usually depend on the particular histologic subtype of lymphoma that is present.

This patient had a diffuse large cell lymphoma, one of the more common subtypes of non-Hodgkin's lymphoma in adults. Non-Hodgkin's lymphomas are currently classified by the International Working Formulation, a consensus classification used worldwide (1). It separates the non-Hodgkin's lymphomas into three grades: low, intermediate, and high with corresponding median survival times of approximately 10-12 years, 2-3 years, and 1-2 years, respectively. Patients with low-grade or indolent lymphomas tend to have widespread disease at diagnosis and, still, live for many years. Treatment can usually control these malignancies with relative ease, but almost all patients will experience relapses. Despite the shorter survival times seen in the intermediate- and high-grade malignancies, it is these patients, even with advanced stages of disease that may be predictably cured with current therapy. Patients with diffuse large cell lymphoma are included among the intermediate-grade lymphomas.

Based on a number of simple clinical features, it is possible to characterize the prognostic risk of an individual with large cell lymphoma. From an analysis of more than 3,000 cases collected from Europe and North America, a prognostic classification (the International Index) was devised that relies only on age, Ann Arbor stage, number of extranodal sites, performance status, and serum LDH (2). In patients under 60 years, the age-adjusted Index uses only stage, performance status, and serum LDH. Depending on the number of adverse factors present, individuals can be classified into one of four risk groups with five-year survival rates varying from 32% to 83%. This patient would most likely have been in the high-intermediate risk group and have an estimated five-year survival rate of approximately 45%.

One of the first questions faced by the clinician involved in the care of this patient was which of the several available treatment programs should be used. CHOP (cyclophosphamide, doxorubicin, vincristine and prednisone) was the first combination that resulted in a relatively high complete response rate and a reproducible fraction of cured patients. Subsequently, there were other regimens that were devised with various rationales. Some of these regimens, like the one chosen for this patient, appeared in phase II studies conducted at single institutions to be more promising than CHOP. There are now several mature phase III trials with CHOP in direct comparison to these newer regimens, and in every case, none was convincingly better than CHOP and they were all sometimes substantially more toxic (3–5). The use of CHOP will place about 50%-55% of patients into a complete remission and most of those will never relapse.

The next issue is the quality of response. It is only among those whose disease enters a complete remission that long-term survival can be expected. With the advent of modern imaging techniques, however, the small residual mass becomes problematic because we know that it does not always represent persistent tumor. Patients with a small defect on study may be considered to be only in partial response and, thus, we could underestimate the frequency of complete response and add unnecessary therapy. For clinical trials, the concept of "time to treatment failure" has been adopted and circumvents this problem. This approach measures the time from starting treatment until there is objective evidence of response failure and of progressive disease or death from any cause. In a sense, this is the sum of all positive and negative effects of intervention. It also allows investigators to be less concerned with complete or partial degrees of response because the factor of interest is only whether those patients ever progress. However, in an individual case this is not a useful concept. The clinician needs to come to a conclusion about whether a persistent abnormality represents malignancy.

This case presents a very real dilemma. She responded promptly to chemotherapy but was left with a small residual mass. In this patient, a persistent mass is not unexpected. She started with a very large tumor and it contained sclerosis, both characteristics associated with residual abnormalities that may not represent active tumor. Does this mass need additional therapy? Many oncologists would monitor such an incomplete response closely over two cycles of therapy. If after an initially good response there is no further regression, it is unlikely that the residuum is malignant or will have any effect on outcome (6). Others have used a change from positive uptake of gallium by the original tumor to no uptake on subsequent examination as ancillary evidence of a complete remission, an approach not possible in this patient because the original tumor did not take up the radionuclide.

High-dose chemotherapy plus autologous bone marrow transplantation (ABMT) was used in this patient to consolidate her response and attempt to prevent relapse. Clearly, ABMT can be effective in providing an extended disease-free interval for some patients with relapsed non-Hodgkin's lymphoma. However, to this date, studies of ABMT as part of the initial treatment strategy for patients with large cell lymphoma have largely failed to demonstrate an additional benefit conferred by ABMT beyond that supplied by standard chemotherapy (7–9). In one large study of 464 patients in complete remission (which included those with small residual masses) randomized to ABMT or modest consolidation therapy, there was no significant benefit attributed to transplantation even in the highest risk patients (8). However, for those patients who are in only a true partial response, ABMT may be beneficial (10). The risks and cost of ABMT are considerable. Until clear advantages are shown, its place in the initial management of patients with diffuse large cell lymphoma is solely limited to clinical investigation (11).

REFERENCES

1. The Non-Hodgkin's Lymphoma Pathologic Classification Project: National Cancer Institute sponsored study of classifications of non-Hodgkin's lymphomas. Summary and description of a working formulation for clinical usage. *Cancer* 1982;49:2112–35.
2. The International Non-Hodgkin's Lymphoma Prognostic Factors Project: a predictive model for aggressive non-Hodgkin's lymphoma. *N Engl J Med* 1993;329:987–94.
3. Cooper IA, Wolf MM, Tobertson T, et al. Randomized comparison of MACOP-B with CHOP in patients with intermediate-grade non-Hodgkin's lymphoma. *J Clin Oncol* 1994;12:769–78.
4. Fisher RI, Gaynor ER, Dahlberg S, et al. Comparison of a standard regimen (CHOP) with three intensive chemotherapy regimens for advanced non-Hodgkin's lymphoma. *N Engl J Med* 1993;328: 1002–6.
5. Gordon LI, Harrington D, Andersen J, et al. Comparison of a second-generation combination chemotherapeutic regimen (m-BACOD) with a standard regimen (CHOP) for advanced diffuse non-Hodgkin's lymphoma. *N Engl J Med* 1992;327:1342–9.
6. Coiffier B, Gissselbrecht C, Herbrecht R, et al. LNH-84 regimen: a multicenter study of intensive chemotherapy in 737 patients with aggressive malignant lymphoma. *J Clin Oncol* 1989;7:1018–26.
7. Hagenbeek A, Verdonck L, Sonneveld P, et al. CHOP chemotherapy versus autologous bone marrow transplantation in slowly responding patients with intermediate- and high-grade malignant non-Hodgkin's lymphoma. Results from a prospective randomized phase III clinical trial in 294 patients. *Blood* 1993;82(Suppl 1):332a (abstr).
8. Haioun C, Lepage E, Gisselbrecht C, et al. Comparison of autologous bone marrow transplantation with sequential chemotherapy for intermediate and high-grade non-Hodgkin's lymphoma in first complete remission. A study of 464 patients. *J Clin Oncol* 1994;12 (in press December).
9. Peterson BA. The role of transplantation in non-Hodgkin's lymphoma. *J Clin Oncol* 1994;12 (in press).
10. Mazza P, Tura S, Zinzani PL, et al. A multicenter randomized study on aggressive non-Hodgkin's lymphomas: an updated follow-up. *Proc Am Soc Clin Oncol* 1993;12:362 (abstr).
11. Coiffier B, Phillip T, Burnett AK, et al. Consensus conference on intensive chemotherapy plus hematopoietic stem-cell transplantation in malignancies: Lyon, France, June 4-6, 1993. *J Clin Oncol* 1994;83:226–31.

137

Non-Hodgkin's Lymphoma of the Central Nervous System in a 25-year-old HIV-Positive Man

Christopher J. Schultz and Michael Whittaker

CNS lymphoma is not curable

CASE PRESENTATION

A 25-year-old HIV-positive man presented with complaints of dysphasia and odynophagia. Evaluation, including EGD, revealed esophageal candidiasis. Blood cultures as part of his evaluation were remarkable for a *Mycobacterium avium intracellulare* and he was started on appropriate antifungal therapy. He was discharged and subsequently readmitted 1 week later with nausea, vomiting, and diarrhea. He was given intravenous hydration and was begun on antimicrobial therapy addressing an infectious diarrhea. On day 2 of admission, he developed a tonic clonic seizure. A computed tomography (CT) scan of the head with contrast was obtained and demonstrated a 4 × 6 cm ring-enhancing mass with mild surrounding edema in the right frontal lobe (Fig. 137–1). The radiologic interpretation favored abscess or toxoplasmosis. He was begun on empiric toxoplasmosis therapy and continued on his fungal and antimicrobial therapy. In addition, he was begun on Dilantin.

His past medical history was remarkable for positive HIV 3 months before admission on work-up for weight loss, adenopathy, and unexplained fevers. He had no prior operations. Medications at the time of admission included sulfadiazine, pyrimethamine, dideoxyinosine, nystantin, fluconazole, clotrimazole, leucovorian calcium, septra, folic acid, reglan, and pepsid. His family history was unremarkable. This patient was single and

did not use alcohol or tobacco, but he reported a past history of intravenous drug abuse.

On admission physical examination, the patient was a young, thin, well developed man. He was febrile at 104°F orally, pulse of 106, and respiration of 22. His blood pressure was 120/80. Otolaryngologic exam was unremarkable. His neck was supple with small adenopathy. Lungs were clear to auscultation and percussion. Abdomen was soft and nontender, without organomegaly. Cardiac exam revealed regular rhythm, although moderate tachycardia. There were normal heart sounds, with no murmurs, rubs, or gallop. Extremities disclosed no clubbing or edema. Small peripheral adenopathy was noted in the cervical, axillary, and inguinal areas. Neurologic exam revealed the patient to be alert and oriented ×3. Cranial nerves II–XII were intact. The strength in the upper and lower extremities was symmetrically intact. Sensory function was, likewise, intact. Reflexes were 2+ in the upper extremities and 3+ in the lower extremities. An upgoing toe was present on the left.

Approximately 1 week after admission following initiation of antibiotic, antifungal, and empiric toxoplasmosis therapy, the patient experienced two additional seizures, despite a therapeutic Dilantin level. A magnetic resonance image (MRI) was performed, which confirmed the presence of a right frontal mass. There was limited associated edema. The radiographic interpretation favored an inflammatory or infectious process,

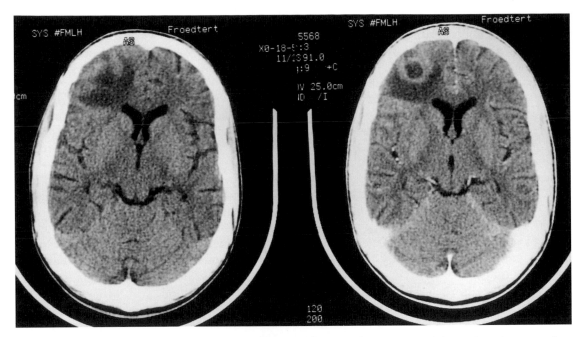

FIG. 137–1. Pre- (*left*) and post- (*right*) contrast axial CT scans demonstrate a ring-enhancing mass in the right frontal lobe with mild surrounding edema effacing the adjacent cortical sulci and causing minimal right-to-left shift of the anterior midline structures.

rather than a neoplasm, given the limited degree of edema and mass effect (Fig. 137–2).

The Radiation Oncology Service was consulted for consideration of empiric therapy for a possible central nervous system (CNS) lymphoma. The Radiation Oncol-

ogy Service recommended a biopsy to direct therapy, rather than proceed with empiric treatment. The patient was evaluated by the Neurological Service and was subsequently taken to surgery, where he underwent a stereotactic biopsy. Brain tissue demonstrated a malignant infil-

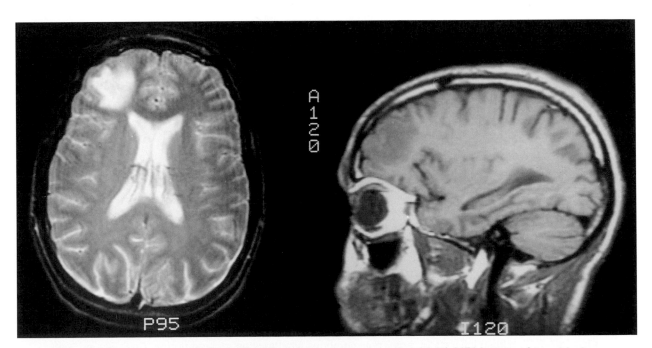

FIG. 137–2. Axial T2-weighted MRI (*left*) and T1-weighted sagittal (*right*) MRI images demonstrate a well defined process that is nearly spherical in shape in the right frontal lobe. The lower signal intensity center is faintly inhomogeneous as compared with the periphery.

trate consisting of cells with a high nuclear to cytoplasmic ratio and large pleomorphic nuclei. (Fig. 137–3) Immunoperoxidase stains for leukocyte common antigen were positive. Immunoperoxidase stains for cytokeratin, epithelial membrane antigen, S-100, and vimentin were negative. No organisms were identified on routine, acid-fast, or fungal stains. The morphologic diagnosis was malignant lymphoma, large cell, immunoblastic type. (Fig. 137–4)

Further evaluation, including CT scan of the chest, abdomen, and pelvis, failed to disclose any adenopathy suggestive of a systemic lymphoma. Bone marrow biopsy was negative. The patient was subsequently begun on Decadron, and his empiric toxoplasmosis therapy was discontinued. The patient received whole-brain irradiation delivered via right and left lateral treatment portals, inclusive of the meninges. A total dose of 30 Gy in 10 fractions was delivered over 12 days. The patient was discharged to a nursing home upon completion of his palliative brain irradiation. At the time of completion of this therapy, he had no focal neurologic complaints and had no further seizures.

The patient was seen in follow-up at 3 and 6 months and was without clinical evidence of progression of his CNS lymphoma. His physical examination was notable for partial alopecia corresponding to his radiation treatment portal, although was otherwise without demonstrable sequelae. He subsequently died from an opportunistic infection.

COMMENTARY by Eli Glatstein

Before the acquired immunodeficiency syndrome (AIDS) epidemic, primary CNS lymphoma was considered very rare, accounting for only 0.5% to 1.2% of intracranial neoplasms (1–3). After the recognition of AIDS, caused by infection of the human immunodeficiency virus (HIV-1), the complications of AIDS, including those affecting the nervous system, represent a direct consequence of the immune impairment.

There is a variety of neurologic complications of AIDS, but most are actually opportunistic infections. Involvement of the CNS by HIV-1 itself is still relatively unusual, but it is increasing in its frequency. Primary CNS lymphoma accounts for a little less than 2% of all the extranodal lymphomas that develop in the normal population (4). Fewer than 1% of HIV-1–infected patients will present with primary CNS lymphoma as their first manifestation of AIDS. However, throughout the entire course of the AIDS syndrome, between 2% and 13% of patients can be expected to develop a primary CNS lymphoma (5–9). This wide range of reported incidence of primary CNS lymphoma is really related to the method of data accumulation. Studies that include autopsy data consistently report a higher probability of primary CNS lymphoma in AIDS patients than studies confined to patients diagnosed in life. At least 50% of all cases of AIDS-related primary CNS lymphomas are

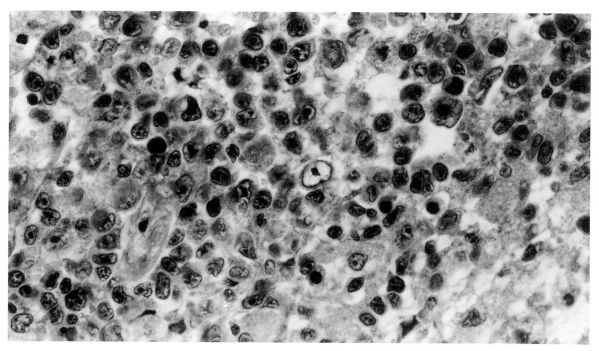

FIG. 137–3. A diffuse infiltrate of large, polymorphous lymphocytes replace normal CNS tissue. Scattered cells have large nucleoli in eccentrically placed nuclei, characteristic of immunoblastic differentiation. Individual necrotic cells are consistent with high cell turnover seen in high-grade tumors. (H&E, original magnification ×150.)

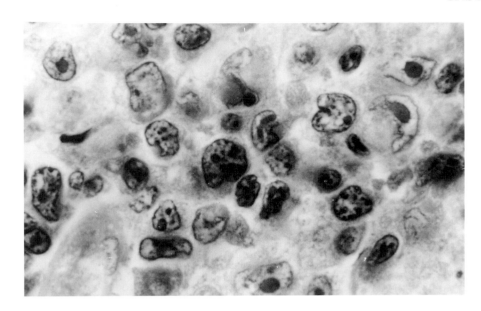

FIG. 137–4. Higher power evaluation illustrates immunoblasts, admixed with large cleaved and noncleaved malignant lymphocytes, typically seen in immunoblastic lymphoma. (H&E, original magnification ×250.)

diagnosed only at autopsy, and most of these were not suspected in life.

As can be expected, the large majority of patients with this tumor are adult men, typically with a homosexual background, but some who represent drug addiction as well. The clinical presentation can be very subtle. Fifty to sixty percent of patients will present with lethargy, confusion, and a personality change (10–13). Many patients will lack accompanying lateralizing neurologic signs; some will present with hemiparesis, seizure, or cranial nerve palsy.

Typically, a primary CNS lymphoma involves the deep periventricular region of the brain, which includes the basal ganglia and deep white matter. The frontal lobe is most frequently affected in the cerebrum; the posterior fossa is involved in fewer than 10% of patients.

AIDS-related primary CNS lymphoma is multifocal in 50% to 75% of patients on the basis of the CT or MRI scan at diagnosis (10,13). This is higher than the 22% to 44% frequency seen in nonimmunosuppressed patients who have primary CNS lymphoma, but it is still an underestimation of the problem because virtually all patients with AIDS who have CNS lymphoma prove to have multifocal disease at autopsy (10–15). The high frequency of multifocality and involvement of the frontal lobe account for confusion and lethargy, which are the most common symptoms at presentation. In this syndrome, the eye should be considered an extension of the CNS. About 20% of patients apparently immunocompetent who have primary CNS lymphoma will have ocular involvement at diagnosis (14,16,17). By contrast, 50% to 80% of patients with ocular lymphoma will develop primary CNS lymphoma, although the latency period may be years (17,18).

The CT or MRI images of the primary CNS lymphoma are usually distinctive and may suggest a diagnosis. In the non-AIDS patient, primary CNS lymphoma

lesions on CT scan are usually either hypointense or isointense before contrast administration. On the other hand, in the AIDS patients the lesions are virtually always hypointense (19–21). There is a prominent and diffuse enhancement that is seen after the administration of contrast and is usually the most notable radiographic feature of primary CNS lymphoma. Borders of the lesion are frequently indistinct, corresponding to the infiltrative margins that are seen microscopically. Unfortunately, opportunistic infections, especially toxoplasmosis, are more common in AIDS patients than primary CNS lymphoma. Such infections cannot always be distinguished radiologically from primary CNS lymphoma. Toxoplasmosis is virtually always ring enhancing, and AIDS-related primary CNS lymphoma can also enhance in this pattern (more frequently than in the non-AIDS patients). As a consequence, typically, such patients are treated with a 2-week trial of antitoxoplasmosis therapy and then the scan is repeated to determine if there has been radiologic improvement. Without improvement, patients are usually sent for brain biopsy; if malignancy is seen on biopsy, then radiation therapy is usually initiated, as was done in the reported patient. Antibody assays for toxoplasmosis in the serum are useful complements to the radiologic studies; the absence of such antibodies in the serum strongly suggests an alternative diagnosis. A positive cerebrospinal fluid (CSF) cytology has been reported in 25% of patients who have primary CNS lymphoma. Moreover, the early administration of corticosteroids can normalize the CSF (13,14, 22,23).

The typical primary CNS lymphoma has a diffuse, aggressive, non-Hodgkin's histology similar to systemic lymphomas of that subtype. Most are large-cell or immunoblastic subtypes (according to the working formulation). The vast majority of these tumors represent B-cell disease, but rare T-cell neoplasms have been reported (but not in the AIDS patients) (14,24,25).

There are data that implicate Epstein-Barr virus, especially in immunocompromised patients who develop this tumor (26). The initial acute infection with EBV is usually asymptomatic or very mild, often occurring in childhood. Infection later in life frequently causes infectious mononucleosis. The virus exists during acute infection apparently in a productive state and is capable of generating new virions that can cause cell lysis. After an acute infection with EBV, a small population of latently infected lymphocytes remains that may be immortalized for the life of the patient. The growth of this population of cells appears to be controlled by suppressor T cells, which have been specifically sensitized to EBV. EBV DNA has been detected in tumor tissue of AIDS patients with primary CNS lymphoma (7,27). It has been postulated that EBV may play a role in the genesis of primary CNS lymphoma, which is similar to the role that EBV presumably plays in the systemic lymphoid neoplasms that occur in these patients. Furthermore, the CNS is relatively isolated from what are presumed to be normal "immune surveillance" mechanisms.

As far as treatment is concerned, radiotherapy has been the most standard treatment modality used for the management of primary CNS lymphoma, both in AIDS and non-AIDS patients. A well defined dose response relationship has not been established, but most patients will receive whole-brain irradiation somewhere between 3,000 and 4,000 rad and then the recognized tumor volume is typically boosted to a total dose of 4,500 to 5,000 rad. As patients are detected later on in the course of their AIDS, one frequently uses smaller volumes and more rapidly applied doses, as was done in this patient. Personally, I try to avoid further complications by omitting corticosteroids unless either an overt seizure, hydrocephalus, or papilledema is present. On the other hand, if they have already been started before my evaluation, I do not deliberately discontinue such medications.

In the non-AIDS population, cranial irradiation appears to prolong survival, but the median is only 12 to 18 months (16,22,28). Although radiotherapy is effective in almost all patients in terms of alleviating symptoms, most patients experience significant clinical improvement along with a radiographic response. Unfortunately, the CNS tumor recurs in more than 90% of patients, leading typically to death within 2 years. Relapse frequently occurs in the brain, often in sites remote from the original tumor, and often in the meninges and in the eyes. Nodal relapses are seen less frequently. In the AIDS patients, cranial irradiation can be effective at producing clinical improvement and radiologic regression of neoplasm. However, the median survival is only 4 to 5 months (10,11,13,20). Untreated patients often die from progressive primary CNS lymphoma, but the autopsy findings on treated patients reveal that most die with systemic opportunistic infection or other neurologic process (18,11,20). In recent years, systemic chemotherapy has been added in many patients along with cranial irradiation therapy for the initial treatment of primary CNS lymphoma. It appears to delay the relapse substantially and prolong survival (14,16). In the non-AIDS patients, the best results reported have come from Neuwalt et al. at the University of Oregon, where chemotherapy has been used with and without radiation, but usually in the presence of blood–brain barrier disruption, using mannitol osmotic diuresis (29). The results in this small series suggest that about half the patients with primary CNS lymphoma in the non-HIV setting can be long-term survivors.

If the patient is in good performance status, leptomeningeal lymphoma should probably be considered in the treatment plan by means of intrathecal chemotherapy. This will usually mean the administration of methotrexate and cytosine arabinoside. An Ommaya reservoir improves the uniformity of drug delivery to the intrathecal space and is probably easier to administer than repeated lumbar punctures. Whenever ocular lymphoma is diagnosed, it is usually treated with bilateral ocular irradiation, usually 3,000 to 4,000 rad to the posterior globe (18), which causes tumor regression in the vast majority of such patients. Recurrent ocular disease can be treated with chemotherapy, especially high-dose methotrexate. However, the experience is moderate, and many drugs do not penetrate well into the vitreous humor.

REFERENCES

1. Jellinger K, Radaskiewicz TH, Slowik F. Primary malignant lymphomas of the central nervous system in man. *Acta Neuropathol* 1975;suppl VI:95–102.
2. Rubenstein LJ. *Tumors of the Central Nervous System. Atlas of Tumor Pathology,* Second Series, Fascicle 6, pp. 215–34, Armed Forces Institute of Pathology, Washington DC, 1972.
3. Zimmerman HM. Malignant lymphomas of the nervous system. *Acta Neuropathol (Berlin)* 1975;(suppl 16):69–74.
4. Freeman C, Berg JW, Cutler SJ. Occurrence and prognosis of extranodal lymphomas. *Cancer* 1972;29:252–60.
5. Levy RM, Bredesen DE, Rosenblum ML. Neurological manifestations of the acquired immunodeficiency syndrome (AIDS). *J Neurosurg* 1985;62:475–95.
6. Morgellos S, Petito CK, Mouradian JA. Central nervous system lymphoma in the acquired immunodeficiency syndrome. *Clin Neuropathol* 1990;9:205–15.
7. Rosenberg NL, Hochberg FH, Miller G, et al. Primary central nervous system lymphoma related to Epstein-Barr virus in a patient with acquired immuno-deficiency syndrome. *Ann Neurol* 1986;20:98–102.
8. Snider WD, Simpson DM, Nielsen S, et al. Neurolgic complications of acquired immune deficiency syndrome: analysis of 50 patients. *Ann Neurol* 1983;14:403–18.
9. Welch, Finkbeiner W, Alpers CE, et al. Autopsy findings in the acquired immune deficiency syndrome. *JAMA* 1984;252:1152–9.
10. Baumgartner JE, Rachlin JR, Beckstead JH, et al. Primary central nervous system lymphomas: natural history and response to radiation therapy in 55 patients with acquired immunodeficiency syndrome. *J Neurosurg* 1990;73:206–11.
11. Formente SC, Gill PS, Lean E, et al. Primary central nervous system lymphoma in AIDS. *Cancer* 1989;63:1101–7.
12. Rosenblum ML, Levy RM, Bredesen DE, et al. Primary central nervous system lymphomas in patients with AIDS. *Ann Neurol* 1988;23 (suppl):S13–6.

13. So YT, Beckstead JH, Davis RI, et al. Primary central nervous sytem lymphoma in acquired immune deficiency syndrome. *Ann Neurol* 1986;20:566–72.
14. Hochberg FH, Miller DC. Primary central nervous system lymphoma. *J Neurosurg* 1988;68:835–53.
15. Woodman R, Shin K, Pineo G. Primary non-Hodgkin's lymphoma of the brain. *Medicine* 1985;64:425–30.
16. DeAngelis LM, Yahalom J, Heinemann MH, et al. Primary CNS lymphoma: combined treatment with chemotherapy and radiotherapy. *Neurology* 1990;40:80–6.
17. Rockwood EJ, Zakov ZN, Bay JW. Combined malignant lymphoma of the eye and CNS (reticulum cell sarcoma). *J Neurosurg* 1984;61:369–74.
18. Char DH, Ljung BM, Miller T, et al. Primary intraocular lymphoma (ocular reticulum cell sarcoma) diagnosis and management. *Ophthalmology* 1988;95:625–30.
19. Cellerier P, Chicas J, Gray F, et al. Computed tomography in primary lymphoma of the brain. *Neuroradiology* 1984;26:485–92.
20. Gill PS, Levine AM, Meyer PR, et al. Primary central nervous system lymphoma in homosexual non-clinical immunologic and patholgic features. *Am J Med* 1985;78:742–8.
21. Lee YY, Brunner JM, Tassel PV, et al. Primary central nervous system lymphoma: CT and pathologic correlation. *Am J Radiol* 1986;147:747–52.
22. Murray K, Kun L, Cox J. Primary malignant lymphoma of the central nervous system. *J Neurosurg* 1986;65:600–7.
23. Schaumberg HH, Plank CR, Adams RD, et al. The reticulum cell sarcoma-microglioma group of brain tumors. *Brain* 1972;95:195–212.
24. Nakhle RE, Manivel JC, Hurd D, et al. Central nervous system lymphomas. Immunohistochemical and clinicopathologic study of 26 cases. *Arch Pathol Lab Med* 1989;113:1050–6.
25. Taylor CR, Russell R, Lukes RJ, et al. An immunohistological study of immunoglobin content of primary central nervous system lymphomas. *Cancer* 1978;41:2197–2205.
26. List AF, Greco FA, Yogler LB. Lymphoproliferative diseases in immuno-compromised hosts: the role of Epstein-Barr virus. *J Clin Oncol* 1987;5:1673–89.
27. Bashir RM, Harris NL, Hochberg FH, et al. Detection of Epstein-Barr virus in CNS lymphomas by in-situ hybridization. *Neurology* 1989;39:813–7.
28. Mendenhall NP, Thar TL, Agee OF, et al. Primary lymphoma of the central nervous system. Computerized tomography scan characteristics and treatment results for 12 cases. *Cancer* 1983;52:1993–2000.
29. Neuwalt EA, Goldman DL, Dahlberg SA, et al. Primary central nervous system lymphoma treated with osmotic blood–brain barrier disruption: prolonged survival and preservation of cognitive function. *J Clin Oncol* 1991;9:1580–90.

Cancers in the Immunosuppressed Host—HIV Positive

138

AIDS-Related Kaposi's Sarcoma with Mucosal Lesions

Jay S. Cooper

Therapy of this sarcoma is palliative

CASE PRESENTATION

The patient was a 25-year-old Caucasian, single, female, heterosexual school teacher who donated blood. Shortly thereafter she was contacted and told that her blood was infected with human immunodeficiency virus (HIV). As she had never used intravenous drugs, she contacted prior boyfriends and found that one of them had developed acquired immunodeficiency syndrome (AIDS). Over the next 4 years, although feeling well, she prophylactically took DDI, pentamidine, and nystatin. A violaceous lesion then appeared to arise from the gingiva just superior to her left upper incisor. It progressively grew and covered the tooth, became painful, began to bleed, and began to loosen the left upper incisor and left upper canine.

The patient was initially seen for consideration of radiotherapy approximately 3 months after first noticing the lesion. At that time it was $1^1/_2$ cm wide, 2 cm high, and approximately $^1/_4$ cm thick (Fig. 138–1). It appeared to arise from the gingiva just superior to the left upper incisor and extended over the left incisor. It was a uniformly violaceous color. The left incisor and canine teeth were both easily moved within their sockets upon light pressure. She had no other lesions suggestive of Kaposi's sarcoma either in her oral cavity or on her skin. She had shotty bilateral low cervical adenopathy (all nodes <1 cm in size). The rest of her physical examination was completely unremarkable. Biopsy of the lesion showed small, irregular, vascular-appearing channels and extravasated erythrocytes consistent with Kaposi's sarcoma.

TUMOR BOARD DISCUSSION

AIDS is a public health risk for the entire population. This young woman acquired the virus by having unprotected heterosexual intercourse. Although the risks of unprotected intercourse (and in particular homosexual intercourse) are now relatively well known in the medical community, transmission of HIV by heterosexual contact already accounts for more than 5% of new infections overall (1). For women, the importance is even greater because heterosexual contact currently represents the mode of transmission of the virus in approximately 40% of new cases.

To date, women account for only 10% of all cases of AIDS in the United States (1) and Kaposi's sarcoma arising in a woman who has AIDS is very unusual. Women account for only 1% of all patients who had Kaposi's sarcoma and AIDS who have been referred for consideration of radiation therapy at NYU. This frequency is even smaller than the 7% to 10% of patients who have non–AIDS–associated Kaposi's sarcoma who are women.

The lesion under consideration for treatment is the patient's first manifestation of AIDS (i.e., it was her AIDS-defining illness). At the beginning of the epidemic, Kaposi's sarcoma represented the AIDS-defining illness in 25% to 30% of patients; currently, because of changes in the epidemic and changes in the definition of AIDS, Kaposi's sarcoma accounts for the first manifestation of AIDS in approximately 15% of patients (2).

Oral lesions are fairly common in AIDS, occurring in approximately 50% of patients, although the incidence

705

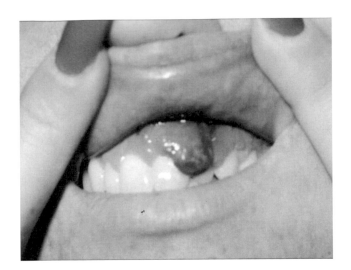

FIG. 138–1. Patient's appearance just prior to radiation therapy.

varies greatly among series (10,14). Gingival lesions comprise the second most common intraoral location of lesions, most lesions arising on the palate.

In terms of prognosis, the fact that our patient has no other evidence of AIDS than the clinically solitary lesion, which arose approximately 4 years after she was first known to be infected by HIV, is a relatively good sign. Rothenberg et al. (11) found that white homosexual men between the ages of 30 and 34 years who had Kaposi's sarcoma as their only manifestation of HIV infection had an approximately 80% likelihood of surviving for 1 year after diagnosis. Although women fared somewhat worse than men (40.2% vs. 49.7% 1 year survival overall), and patients who were between the ages of 30 and 34 years survived longer than those who were less than 30 years old (53.0% vs. 51.0% 1-year survival overall), she can be expected to survive for more than 1 year. We are not told the level of her CD4 lymphocytes, but that, too, could be used as a guide to indicate the likely subsequent course of her disease (15).

Our patient therefore needs a palliative therapy that is likely to be effective, relatively nontoxic, and relatively long-lived. Prolongation of life is not a consideration: localized treatments, virtually by definition, will not influence the course of a systemic illness and to date there has not been a convincing demonstration of life extension attributable to treatment of Kaposi's sarcoma by systemic therapy (9,16). Because the lesion is solitary, we can consider locoregional forms of therapy as sufficient for palliation but should also consider systemic forms of therapies for their locoregional effectiveness. For each possible form of therapy we would like to ask how effective that therapy is: (a) in improving the patient's cosmetic appearance, (b) in relieving pain, and (c) in improving function (strengthening her loose teeth), but the data reported in the literature simply are not sufficiently detailed for most

modalities to answer these questions definitively. We subsequently need to consider if any particular factors in this young woman's case influence the usual benefits, risks, and alternatives of each form of therapy.

Considerable evidence has now been amassed to demonstrate the palliative benefit of localized radiotherapy in the treatment of AIDS-related Kaposi's sarcoma. For cutaneous lesions, a relatively brief course of palliative radiotherapy will result in complete regression of a tumor mass in approximately two thirds of patients within 1 month of treatment. Because some residual purple pigmentation will be left behind in approximately 20% of instances, it is difficult to place a quantitative measure on the benefit of cosmetic improvement (3). In general, lesions that are flat can be covered by cosmetic make-up very effectively. Consequently, with proper case selection, the vast majority of patients have a very good to excellent cosmetic appearance after radiotherapy. Similarly, pain will be markedly diminished and functional improvement can be expected in most patients (3). However, it is important to consider other alternatives for this young woman. Schofer et al. (12) compared the results of different forms of palliative management for patients who had facial Kaposi's sarcoma. Liquid nitrogen, intralesional injections of vincristine, and local radiotherapy each induced 60% complete and 20% partial remissions of disease. The authors favored liquid nitrogen therapy for macular or only slightly nodular lesions that were less than 1 cm in size. More extensive lesions were better treated by either low-dose radiotherapy or intralesional vincristine. However, it is important to realize that the radiotherapy regimen they used—400 cGy every other day to a total dose of 1,600 cGy—is predicted by radiobiologic principles to yield an inferior cosmetic result to a more protracted fractionation scheme. De Wit et al. (5) reported palliation of cosmetic discomfort, pain, or edema in 90% of a variety of lesions treated with a single fraction of 800 cGy—a figure the authors comment is better than can be obtained with systemic therapy. However, the duration of response was relatively brief; for those patients who survived more than 4 months after treatment, approximately two thirds experienced recurrence of disease.

In this case, however, the choice of treatment is further complicated by the location of the lesion inside the oral cavity. Unlike cutaneous lesions, where radiotherapy can be expected to produce clinically important side effects in approximately 5% of patients, several authors have reported the frequent development of severe mucositis that precluded delivery of the planned course of radiotherapy in patients who had intraoral lesions (4,17). Although this finding has been subject to some dispute, particularly with low dose per fraction regimens and antifungal prophylaxis (8), it has been found in most reported series that examined this issue. On the other hand, the anterior placement of this lesion on the gingiva and the relatively small size of the lesion will permit the use of nonpenetrating radiation and intraoral shielding. This, at least in theory, would guard against undue toxicity.

Intralesional injections of Velban offer an alternative possibility for treatment. Epstein et al. (6) reported an approximately 50% decrease in the size of injected intra-oral lesions, but at the price of ulceration and pain that typically required oral analgesics. Photodynamic therapy also has been reported to provide local control of disease in the oral cavity (13). Systemic chemotherapy appears to be as effective for intraoral disease as it is for cutaneous disease (7) and likely will provide palliation of disease in one third to one half of patients that lasts for 3 to 4 months. Unfortunately, systemic chemotherapy (depending on the specific drugs used) also invokes the risk of peripheral neuropathy, leukopenia, and further immuno-suppression—risks that are not necessary in this patient at this point in her disease.

The patient was treated with 94 KV superficial radio-therapy. A custom-shaped lead cutout was made to bring her upper lip out of the field and to limit the volume of normal tissue irradiated. An intraoral shield was also fash-ioned and placed inside the oral cavity to prevent irradia-tion of normal mucosa deep in the oral cavity. A total dose of 3,000 cGy was delivered in 10 fractions over 2 weeks. After 1,500 cGy, the patient felt that she could detect that her teeth were slightly less loose than previously, although her objective physical examination was unchanged. By 2 weeks after completion of treatment, the lesion had markedly regressed and she was able to smile without embarrassment (Fig. 138–2). Her teeth were no longer loose and she was able to bite off a piece of a sand-wich without any difficulty or pain. She remained well for approximately 3 months, and her irradiated lesion contin-ued to regress (Fig. 138–3). Unfortunately, shortly there-after, the patient developed numerous diffusely placed,

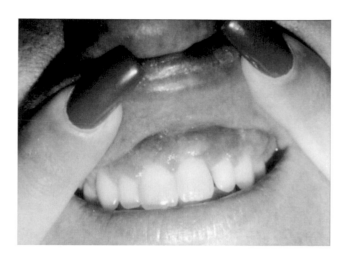

FIG. 138–3. Patient's appearance approximately three months following radiation therapy.

cutaneous lesions that required the institution of systemic therapy. She died approximately 1½ years later.

REFERENCES

1. Centers for Disease Control and Prevention, HIV/AIDS Surveillance Report. 1993;5(3):6–8.
2. Cho J, Chachoua A. Kaposi's sarcoma [published erratum appears in *Curr Opin Oncol* 1992 Oct;4(5):999]. *Curr Opin Oncol* 1992;4(4):667–73.
3. Greenspan JS. Initiatives in oral acquired immunodeficiency syndrome research. *Oral Surg Oral Med Oral Pathol* 1992;73:244–7.
4. Stafford ND, Herdman CD, Forster S, et al. Kaposi's sarcoma of the head and neck in patients with AIDS. *J Laryngol Otol* 1989;103:379–82.
5. Rothenberg R, Woelfel M, Stoneburner R, et al. Survival with AIDS. *N Engl J Med* 1987;317:1297–1302.
6. Taylor J, Afrasiabi R, Fahey J, et al. A prognostically significant clas-sification of immune changes in AIDS with Kaposi's sarcoma. *Blood* 1986;67:666–71.
7. Gelmann EP, Longo D, Lane HC, et al. Combination chemotherapy of disseminated Kaposi's sarcoma in patients with the acquired immune deficiency syndrome. *Am J Med* 1987;82(3):456–62.
8. Volberding PA, Kusick P, Feigal DW. Effect of chemotherapy for HIV associated Kaposi's sarcoma on longterm survival. *Proc ASCO* 1989;8:11.
9. Cooper JS, Fried PR. Defining the role of radiation therapy in the man-agement of epidemic Kaposi's sarcoma. *Int J Radiat Oncol Biol Phys* 1987;13(1):35–9.
10. Schofer H, Ochsendorf F, Hochscheid I, et al. Facial kaposi's sar-coma: evaluation of different palliative treatment modalities. *Int Conf Aids* 1991;7(1):2247.
11. de Wit R, Smit WG, Veenhof KH, et al. Palliative radiation therapy for AIDS-associated Kaposi's sarcoma by using a single fraction of 800 cGy. *Radiother Oncol* 1990;19(2):131–6.
12. Cooper JS, Fried PR. Toxicity of oral radiotherapy in patients having AIDS. *Arch Otolaryngol Head Neck Surg* 1987;113:327–8.
13. Watkins EB, Findlay P, Gelmann E, et al. Enhanced mucosal reactions in AIDS patients receiving oropharyngeal irradiation. *Int J Radiat Oncol Biol Phys* 1987;13:1403–8.
14. Geara F, Le Bourgeois JP, Lepechoux C, et al. Radiotherapy of mucosal and cutaneous epidemic kaposi's sarcoma (eks): a report on 285 patients (meeting abstract). *Proc Annu Meet Am Soc Clin Oncol* 1991;10:32.
15. Epstein JB, Lozada-Nur G, McLeo A, et al. Oral Kaposi's sarcoma in acquired immunodeficiency syndrome. *Cancer* 1989;64:2424–30.
16. Schweitzer VG, Visscher D. Photodynamic therapy for treatment of

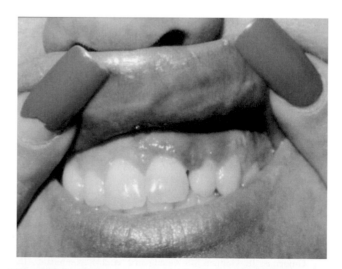

FIG. 138–2. Patient's appearance two weeks following radi-ation therapy.

AIDS-related oral Kaposi's sarcoma. *Otolaryngol Head Neck Surg* 1990;102:639–49.
17. Epstein JB, Silverman S Jr. Head and neck malignancies associated with HIV infection. *Oral Surg Oral Med Oral Pathol* 1992;73(2): 193–200.

COMMENTARY by Robert C. Young

AIDS-related Kaposi's sarcoma in a woman remains a relatively rare AIDS-defining complication. Heterosexual transmission accounts for only 6% of adult AIDS, and generally as in this case, occurs in individuals who have contact with partners in high-risk categories (bisexuals, intravenous drug users, or immigrants from endemic areas). Studies indicate that male-to-female transmission of AIDS is far more efficient than female-to-male transmission. Although many aspects of the disease appear to be similar in both sexes, there are some differences. Women with AIDS commonly manifest higher incidences of vaginal candidal infections and an increase in the incidence and severity of cervix cancer.

About a third of AIDS patients have Kaposi's sarcoma as a presenting manifestation of the disease. This is much more common in homosexuals and intravenous drug users than in patients who develop the disease from heterosexual contact, hemophilia, or other blood transfusions. There is evidence that the incidence of Kaposi's sarcoma in AIDS has decreased from 40% in 1981 to less than 20% in 1992. The dramatic difference in incidence associated with the different high-risk groups suggests that Kaposi's may be caused by an agent other than HIV, or a combination of agents including HIV. Laboratory evidence suggests that the HIV tat gene can produce skin lesions resembling Kaposi's sarcoma in transgenic mice, and it has been documented that retrovirus-infected CD4+ T cells produce growth factors that sustain the growth of Kaposi's sarcoma cells. Whether some unknown alteration in infectious exposure has altered the incidence of Kaposi's sarcoma is currently unknown.

A variety of therapies have been used in treating AIDS-related Kaposi's sarcoma and many have been moderately effective. Single-agent chemotherapy, combination chemotherapy, radiation therapy, and interferon all have a significant response rate. Generally, responses are substantial and palliative but rarely complete and generally are only of moderate duration. The 3-month duration seen in the present case is relatively typical. Radiation therapy for a localized singular lesion produces effective palliative benefit and is probably the treatment of choice in a situation as presented in this case. Appropriate shielding, as was used, can decrease the frequency of mucositis and avoid unnecessary complications and hospitalizations in patients with a limited anticipated survival. Single-agent chemotherapy with intravenous vinblastine, 4 to 8 mg/week intravenously, produces overall responses in approximately 50% of patients and is generally associated with minimal systemic toxicity. A randomized clinical trial in extensive mucocutaneous Kaposi's sarcoma compared low-dose adriamycin (20 mg/M²) alone with a combination of adriamycin, bleomycin, and vincristine. Although higher response rates (88%) were seen with the combination than with adriamycin alone (48%), both regimens had similar acceptable levels of toxicity. Median survival of both treated groups was 9 months. Recombinant interferon alpha has been associated with overall similar frequency of remissions but with occasional long-term durations. Interferon can be administered either subcutaneously or intramuscularly three times a week and can be given on an outpatient basis. Side effects include fevers, night sweats, chills, muscle pain, and fatigue.

The selection of dose and schedule of radiation therapy depend on the location of the lesion and the personal circumstances of the patient. One comparison of single-dose radiation therapy with conventional course radiation therapy yielded a better therapeutic result for the short-term high-dose approach. The University of California at San Francisco used various dose-fractionation regimens and achieved a 90% response to treatment regardless of fractionation schedule used. The median time to progression was 21 months and 69% of patients were free of any new or recurrent lesions at 6 months. Because a single fraction of 8 Gy was shown to be as effective as protracted courses of treatment with no increased morbidity, the single-course approach was preferred for quality of life benefits and cost effectiveness.

Although all these approaches can yield useful and palliative results in patients, as was apparent in the present case, the manifestation of Kaposi's sarcoma is usually an indication of falling CD4+ cells, cutaneous anergy, lymphocytopenia, decreased helper T cells, and hypergammuglobuminanemia and, therefore, a manifestation of progressive systemic disease. Survival, as seen in this instance, is generally compromised.

SELECTED READINGS

1. Centers for Disease Control. The Second 100,000 cases of acquired immunodeficiency syndrome—United States, June 1981–December 1991. *MMWR* 1992;41:28.
2. Padian NS, Shiboski SC, Jewell NP. Female-to-male transmission of human immunodeficiency virus. *JAMA* 1991;266:1664.
3. Spense MR, Reboli AC. Human immunodificiency virus infection in women. *Ann Intern Med* 1991;115:827.
4. Fauci AS, Masur H, Gelmann EP, et al. The acquired immunodeficiency syndrome: An update. *Ann Intern Med* 1985;l02:800.
5. Phillips TJ, Dover JS. Recent advances in dermatology. *N Engl J Med* 1991;326:167.
6. Gallo RC. Human retroviruses: a decade of discovery in link with human disease. *J Infect Dis* 1991;164:235.
7. Volberding PA, Abrams, DI, Conant M, et al. Vinblastine therapy for Kaposi's sarcoma in acquired immunodeficiency syndrome. *Ann Intern Med* 1985;103:335.
8. Gill PS, Ranick M, McCutchan JA, et al. Systemic treatment of AIDS-related Kaposi's sarcoma: results of a randomized trial. *Am J Med* 1991;90:427.
9. Groopman JE, Gottlieb MS, Goodman J, et al. Recombinant Alfa-2 interferon therapy for Kaposi's sarcoma associated with theacquired immunodeficiency syndrome. *Ann Intern Med* 1984;100:671.
10. Berson AM, Quivey JM, Harris JW, et al. Radiation therapy for AIDS-related Kaposi's sarcoma. *Int J Rad Oncol Biol Phys* 1990;19:569.

139

Non-Hodgkin's Lymphoma of the Cecum in a 55-Year-Old Woman with HIV Positivity After Multiple Blood Transfusions

Jules E. Harris and William T. Leslie

Immunocompromised patients (HIV positive) with lymphoma are a major therapeutic dilemma

CASE PRESENTATION

A 55-year-old woman was admitted with intermittent cramping, abdominal pain, and a 20-pound weight loss over 4 months. The pain would begin in the right lower quadrant and become more severe after eating. There was no change in the caliber of the stools, and no blood was seen. The patient noted occasional low-grade fevers up to 100.0°F, and her appetite was decreased.

Her past medical history included hypertension and insulin-dependent diabetes mellitus. The patient had a hysterectomy in 1984 for uterine fibroids. She had received several blood transfusions before surgery. She took Dyazide daily and Humulin 25 U scqd.

The patient smoked one pack of cigarettes a day for 35 years. She drank alcohol socially. She was divorced for 10 years and was not sexually active.

Her mother died of breast cancer, and her father, who had a history of diabetes mellitus, died of a myocardial infarction.

Physical examination revealed a temperature of 99.5°F, blood pressure 124/88, pulse 80 and regular, respiratory rate 20. Pupils were equal, round, and reactive to light. Extraocular movements were intact. The fundi were normal. The examination of the pharynx revealed mild oral candidiasis. The neck was supple without adenopathy.

The thyroid was normal to palpation. The chest was clear. No nodes were palpable in the axillae. Cardiac exam revealed a normal S1 and S2 without murmurs or S3. The breast exam showed no masses. The abdomen was soft and nontender, with no guarding. There was no palpable hepatosplenomegaly. No inguinal nodes were palpable. Pelvic exam was unremarkable. The stools were trace guaiac positive. The neurologic exam was normal. The skin was normal.

Laboratory data included Hgb 9.8, Hct 29.6, with an MCV of 74. White blood cell count was 5.8 with 72 polys, 4 bands, 20 lymphocytes, 2 monocytes, 1 eosinophil, and one basophil. The platelet count was 252,000, sodium 134, potassium 4.0, chloride 100, CO_2 26, blood urea nitrogen 10, creatinine 0.7. SMA 18 unremarkable except for a slight elevation in the LDH of 335 (nl 90–220). The chest radiograph was normal. No infiltrates or masses were seen. An electrocardiogram was normal.

After admission to the hospital, the patient had a plain film x-ray of the abdomen, which was unremarkable. Because of the guaiac-positive stools and microcytic anemia, the Gastroenterology Service was consulted. A lower gastrointestinal series had demonstrated a mass (Fig. 139–1). A colonoscopy showed a mass in the cecum. Biopsy of the mass revealed an immunoblastic lymphoma (Fig. 139–2). EBV DNA sequences were present in the

709

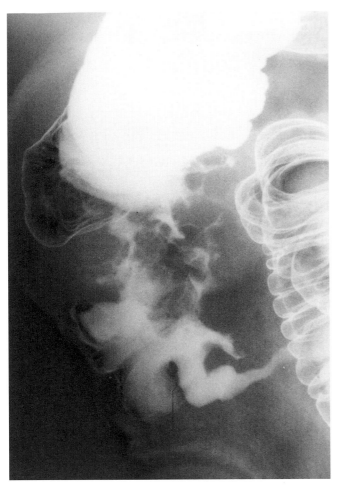

FIG. 139–1. Immunoblastic lymphoma of the cecum shown in lower gastrointestinal series.

tumor, and a cMYC rearrangement was found. A computed tomography (CT) scan of the chest, abdomen, and pelvis showed several enlarged retroperitoneal lymph nodes, but was otherwise negative. Bilateral bone marrow biopsies were performed, and an area of infiltration by immunoblastic lymphoma was found in the bone marrow biopsy from the left posterior iliac crest. A spinal tap was normal, and cytologic examination of the spinal fluid was negative for lymphoma. Because the patient had a history of multiple blood transfusions, she was tested for HIV. An ELISA was positive, and a positive Western blot confirmed the presence of HIV. The CD4 count was 40. The patient was eligible for the AIDS Clinical Trials Group protocol #142. In this study, the patients are randomized between standard doses of mBACOD chemotherapy with GM-CSF or a low-dose mBACOD chemotherapy regimen. Before beginning chemotherapy, the patient was started on allopurinol. She also had a MUGA scan, which showed a normal ejection fraction.

The patient was randomized to the low-dose mBACOD regimen, which included weekly prophylactic intrathecal cytosine arabinoside for 4 weeks. The patient

was seen by the Infectious Disease service. According to the protocol, patients cannot take zidovudine (AZT) while receiving chemotherapy. However, patients can receive dideoxyinosine (DDI) after the first week of chemotherapy. Because of the possibility of synergistic neurotoxicity with DDI and vincristine, it was decided to withhold all antiretroviral therapy during chemotherapy. After the first cycle of mBACOD, the patient had a marked decrease in her abdominal pain and gained 10 pounds. Her LDH decreased to normal. The chemotherapy was given every 3 weeks, and the patient tolerated the second and third cycles of chemotherapy well. However, when she returned for the fourth cycle, she complained of loss of appetite and a 5-pound weight loss. Liver enzymes were elevated. The alkaline phosphatase was 138 (nl 35–110), SGOT 42 (nl 5–35), SGPT 40 (nl 5–30), bilirubin 1.2. A CT scan of the abdomen and pelvis was repeated and showed several new lesions in the liver consistent with metastatic disease. The retroperitoneal adenopathy seen on the initial CT scan had increased significantly. It was felt that the patient was no longer responding to mBACOD chemotherapy and she was started on a salvage regimen of VP16, AraC, cisplatin, and solumedrol (ESAP). After the first cycle of salvage chemotherapy, the liver enzymes again returned to normal and the patient felt better. Two weeks later, the patient complained of blurred vision in the right eye. She was seen by an ophthalmologist who diagnosed CMV (cytomegalovirus) retinitis. A CT brain scan was normal. The patient was started on intravenous ganciclovir. Within a week the white blood cell count decreased to 1.1 and the next cycle of chemotherapy had to be held. The patient was started on Neupogen (GCSF) and the white blood count increased to 2.2. The patient was switched to Foscarnet, and the white count increased to a normal level but the serum creatinine increased to 2.6 and the patient developed hypokalemia. Foscarnet was stopped and the patient was restarted on ganciclovir and GCSF. During this time the patient was noted to have new inguinal lymph nodes, and the liver edge was palpable. The liver enzymes were mildly increased.

A week later the patient complained of dyspnea and cough and she also had temperatures to 100.8°F. An arterial blood gas showed mild hypoxia and a respiratory alkalosis. The chest radiograph did not show any new infiltrates. A bronchoscopy revealed invasive bronchial aspergillosis, and the patient was started on amphotericin, but her shortness of breath increased and she became more hypoxic. After discussion with the patient and her family, it was decided that she should not receive ventilatory support. Her pulmonary function continued to deteriorate and she died 2 weeks later. An autopsy showed immunoblastic lymphoma in the colon, liver, retroperitoneal nodes, and bone marrow as well as diffuse invasive bronchial aspergillosis.

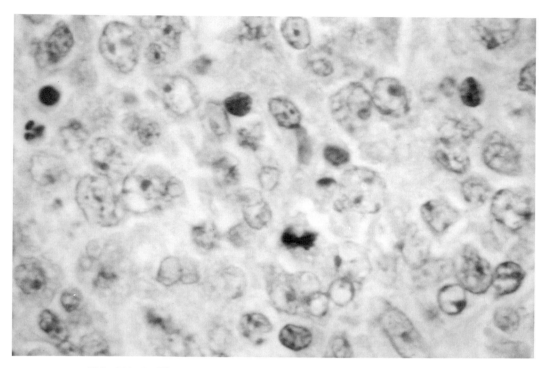

FIG. 139–2. Biopsy of cecal mass showing immunoblastic lymphoma.

COMMENTARY by George P. Canellos

This case represents the unusual occurrence of lymphoma of the cecum in a 55-year-old woman who was HIV positive. She subsequently showed an aggressive course and progression to the liver that was ultimately fatal.

All the features of this case are in concert with lymphoma in a severely immunodepressed population. This patient demonstrated a very low CD4 count, which is one of the poor risk factors for response to chemotherapy. Her tumor similarly was reflective of the usual histologic pattern seen with HIV-related lymphoma, namely, that a large percentage (usually about 60%–70%) of the tumors will be considered to be high grade by the Working Formulation. This includes immunoblastic (plasmocytic large cell lymphoma) and/or small cleaved with the feature of Burkitt's (1,2).

The protocol mentions that she has the oncogene *c-myc* rearranged, which is also a relatively common finding in some series of AIDS-related lymphoma. The rearrangement is because the patients have a translocation from chromosome 8, which is the normal residence of the *c-myc* oncogene. The genetic material is translocated to chromosome 14, 2, or 21. Unfortunately, there are no cytogenetics available on this patient. Rearrangement of chromosome of *c-myc* is usually associated with a very aggressive natural history (2).

This patient also showed evidence of Epstein-Barr virus (EBV) genomes in the DNA of material extracted from the tumor. A high order of detection of EBV infesta-

tion and incorporation into the DNA of the tumor is another cardinal feature of AIDS-related lymphoma (3,4). It is also known to occur in endemic Burkitt's lymphoma in Africa and represents in some ways a part of the pathogenesis of the disease, in contrast to the findings in the nonimmunosuppressed patient who presents with large cell lymphoma in the adult population. In the latter circumstance, most patients will have a large cleaved or noncleaved lymphoma, not usually of high-grade pathology. They will not have abnormalities of chromosome 8 or detectable EBV in their DNA. It is interesting that Burkitt's lymphoma has been reported primarily in HIV-related immunosuppression and not in other circumstances, such as immunosuppression related to transplantation. The large bowel, especially the cecum, is a rare extranodal site of lymphoma in the nonimmunosuppressed patient. The atypical extranodal presentations of lymphoma in HIV-positive patients reflect the abnormal biology in such immunosuppressed patients.

This patient's response to therapy again reflects the very poor prognostic features associated with severe immunodepression and low CD4 counts. Most series associate poor prognosis with CD4 counts below 100×10^{12}/mL and high-grade histology. The patient was offered chemotherapy with the mBACOD regimen, which is widely used for HIV lymphoma. It is to be noted, however, that in patients without poor prognostic features, durable complete remissions can be achieved with combination chemotherapy. The limiting factor has been death due to opportunistic infections. Recurrent lymphoma, which this patient showed, is known to occur between the cycles of chemotherapy. Various regimens have been tried with hematopoietic growth factors to improve the tolerance to cytotoxic agents, because bone marrow function is also compromised in HIV-positive patients. Thus, the effectiveness of chemotherapy is limited by the severe immunosuppression. The relative resistance of the tumor and its aggressive behavior, as well as the poor tolerance of the host to the side effects of chemotherapy, is the limiting problem. In AIDS as well as in other circumstances of immunodepression, central nervous system lymphoma is quite common with involvement of the cerebral cortex, meninges, and cranial nerves. Bone marrow, skin, and bowel represent the next most common sites, in addition to lung, liver, kidney, and pericardium (5).

A recent French report using a complicated regimen—known as LNH84—contains relatively high doses of chemotherapy of cyclophosphamide (1,200 mg/m^2), doxorubicin (75 mg/m^2), vindicine, and bleomycin for 2 days and prednisolone for 5 days (6). This treatment was followed by a consolidation phase with high-dose methotrexate and leucovorin factor rescue as well as asparaginase, ifosfamide, etoposide, and cytarabine. The regimen included AZT as part of maintenance after chemotherapy. Out of 144 patients, 60% had Burkitt's-like lymphoma, and most of them were in stage III–IV. Complete remissions were achieved in 89 patients, and 19 had a partial remission. A significant fraction of patients, however, died during the course of chemotherapy from complications, including those due to progressive disease. The median follow-up was 18 months, whereas the median survival and disease-free survival was 9 and 16 months, respectively. Almost 20% of the patients had opportunistic infections while in complete remission. Without negative factors such as CD4 counts and clinical AIDS, the probability of survival at 2 years is about 50%.

Clearly, this patient in question was in a poor prognostic category and succumbed early to her disease, as would be predicted by almost all series in the medical literature.

REFERENCES

1. Freter CE. Acquired immunodeficiency syndrome-associated lymphomas. *J Natl Cancer Inst Monogr* 1990;10:45–54.
2. Levine AM. Acquired immunodeficiency syndrome—related lymphoma. *Blood* 1992;80:8–20.
3. DeAngelis LM, Wong EL, Rosenblum M, Furneaux H. Epstein-Barr virus in acquired immunodeficiency syndrome (AIDS) and non-AIDS primary central nervous system lymphoma. *Cancer* 1992;70:1607–11.
4. Shibata D, Weiss LM, Hernandez AM, et al. Epstein-Barr virus-associated non-Hodgkin's lymphoma in patients infected with the human immunodeficiency virus. *Blood* 1993;81:2102–9.
5. Loureiro C, Gill PS, Meyer PR, et al. Autopsy findings in AIDS-related lymphoma. *Cancer* 1988;62:735–9.
6. Gisselbrecht C, Oksenhendler E, Tirelli U, et al. Human immunodeficiency virus-related lymphoma treatment with intensive combination chemotherapy. *Am J Med* 1993;95:188–96.

140

HIV-Associated Anal Cancer

Charles F. von Gunten, Jamie H. Von Roenn,
Mark S. Talamonti, and Bharat Mittal

Beware of rectal blood in an HIV-positive man

CASE PRESENTATION

C.W. is a 28-year-old white homosexual man with a history of acquired immunodeficiency syndrome (AIDS) and recent CD4 (T-helper cell) count of 96 cells/mL who presented to his primary physician complaining of low abdominal and rectal pain. These symptoms were accompanied by occasional bright red blood per rectum. The bleeding was not always associated with bowel movements. Physical examination was reported to show no distinct anorectal abnormality. Flexible sigmoidoscopy was nondiagnostic and random anorectal biopsies showed only inflammation. He was treated with antibiotics for a clinical impression of prostatitis without resolution of his symptoms. After 2 months of persistent symptoms, repeat rectal exam suggested an extrinsic mass. Pelvic computed tomography (CT) showed an irregular mass extending from the right side of the rectum into perirectal fat (Fig. 140–1). Rectal ultrasound-guided needle biopsy revealed only a few benign epithelial cells and granulocytes. CT-guided needle biopsy showed atypical squamous cells but was not diagnostic of squamous cell carcinoma. Repeat flexible sigmoidoscopy revealed a lesion at the anorectal junction. Brushings and needle biopsies showed squamous mucosa with severe dysplasia, ulceration, granulation tissue, and inflammatory exudate but no malignancy. Anorectal biopsy under general anesthesia was then performed, which showed infiltrating squamous cell carcinoma, grade II (Fig. 140–2). Six months elapsed between the initial complaint and definitive diagnosis.

The patient's past medical history was significant for one episode of *Pneumocystis carinii* pneumonia 18 months previously, chronic hepatitis B, and oral thrush. Medications included zidovudine 500 mg/day, trimethoprim/sulfamethoxazole 3 times per week, ciprofloxacin 500 mg b.i.d., metronidazole 500 mg t.i.d., acetaminophen with codeine, and hydromorphone p.r.n.

Physical examination showed a healthy-appearing man in moderate discomfort with a temperature of 102.4°F orally, pulse of 100, and blood pressure of 120/80. Physical examination was remarkable for no palpable inguinal adenopathy. Perirectal tenderness with a suggestion of focal fluctuance was noted. The prostate gland was not boggy or tender. Laboratory exam showed a hemoglobin of 10.1 mg/dL, and a white count of 4,800 cells/mL with platelets of 167,000/mL.

It has been known for some time that homosexual men with AIDS are at increased risk for developing anal cancer. This is probably related to infection with human papillomavirus (HPV). Women with AIDS are at increased risk of invasive cervical cancer in an analogous fashion. Although there was a prolonged period when the definitive tissue diagnosis could not be made in this patient, there was a strong clinical suspicion that he had anal cancer. Multiple needle biopsies did not show any evidence of malignant lymphoma, the principle alternative possibility. Because tissue diagnosis in epithelial derived anal cancer is not of prognostic significance and probably would not affect management, the medical oncologist and surgeon favored empiric treatment for anal cancer. However, the radiation oncologist was uncomfortable with this approach and preferred definitive diagnosis before therapy. Therefore, the patient was taken for open biopsy under general anesthesia.

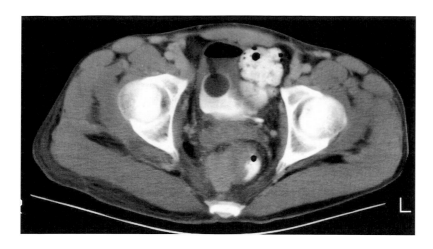

FIG. 140–1. Pelvic CT with intravenous and rectal contrast shows a right-sided perirectal mass displacing the rectum to the left.

Treatment of anal cancer outside the setting of human immunodeficiency virus (HIV) infection has changed over the past several decades. A primarily surgical approach with abdominal perineal (AP) resection was standard up until the 1970s. It is now generally accepted that radiation alone gives equivalent results in terms of long-term cure and local control while maintaining fecal continence in most patients. Some studies have suggested that chemotherapy combined with radiation (either con-

currently or sequentially) is superior to radiation alone, although this has not been conclusively demonstrated in a prospective controlled randomized trial. The standard approach in our institution is to give mitomycin C and 5-FU concurrently with radiation.

The question of metastatic spread to regional lymphatics was raised in this patient. Although his inguinal nodes were not palpable on examination, they looked to be of generous size on pelvic CT. This is a common dilemma in

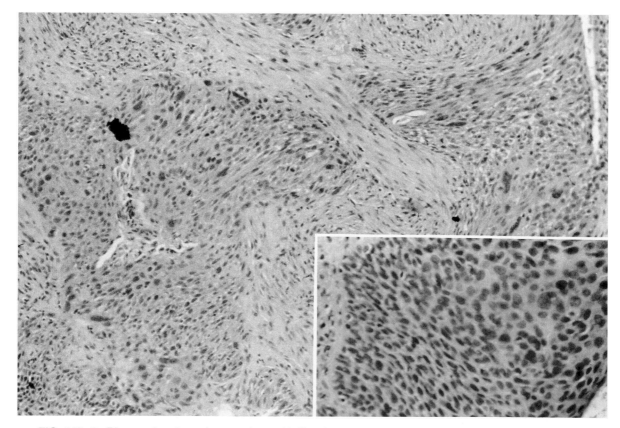

FIG. 140–2. Biopsy of perirectal mass showed infiltrating squamous cell carcinoma, grade II. The insert shows epithelial dysplasia and carcinoma in situ from the same specimen, which is thought to be the predisposing abnormality.

evaluating HIV-related malignancies. Although fine-needle aspiration could have been performed, it was the clinical consensus that this adenopathy reflected HIV adenopathy rather than metastatic disease because they were symmetrically and diffusely enlarged.

For this patient, who had an excellent performance status and a life expectancy of years before his rectal complaints, it was felt the diagnosis of AIDS should not affect the overall treatment approach. Therefore, the recommendation was to use mitomycin C and infusional 5-FU as radiosensitizers with concomitant radiation in a standard fashion.

He was treated with intravenous antibiotics for a presumed perirectal abscess. His temperature defervesced. His abscess drained spontaneously. A rectocutaneous fistula was also noted. After treatment for intercurrent staphylococcus bacteremia, the patient received combination chemotherapy/radiotherapy with one dose of mitomycin C 10 mg/m^2, then 5-FU 1,000 mg/m^2 as a continuous infusion for 5 days coincident with institution of radiation therapy. He received an additional 5-day course of 5-FU 1,000 mg/m^2 per day coincident with the final week of radiation, which was tolerated well. He received a total radiation dose of 4,500 cGy in daily fractions of 180 cGy. Treatment was complicated by the chronic draining rectal fistula and a mild perirectal cellulitis, which responded to oral antibiotics. Approximately 1 week after completion of therapy, he was admitted with profound diarrhea, increased fistula drainage, radiation dermatitis, and severe rectal pain. No infectious etiology for the diarrhea was identified. His symptoms were attributed to complications of the chemotherapy and radiation. A temporary diverting colostomy was performed to promote local healing.

Severe local toxicity requiring diverting colostomy due to either radiation therapy alone, or combination chemotherapy and radiation, has been reported in 10% to 15% of patients outside the setting of AIDS. There is a general clinical consensus that AIDS patients are more sensitive to the tissue effects of radiation and chemotherapy than patients without HIV infection. However, this has not been studied systematically.

COMMENTARY by Warren E. Enker

The case is that of a 28-year-old homosexual man known to have AIDS and a CD4 count of 96 cells/mL. With a normal CD4 count approaching 1,000 cells/mL, a CD4 count of 96 cells/mL suggests absolute immunoincompetence. Under the circumstances, atypical manifestations of disease should be regarded as the norm, and any cryptic complaints related to the anal region should be regarded as suspect for malignancy, unless otherwise proven.

The patient had a 6-month prodrome of symptoms until a diagnosis was established. The most unusual presenting feature is the absence of a palpable mass. Virtually every patient with anal epidermoid carcinoma has a discrete ulcerated mass crossing the dentate line. It is important here to distinguish between cancers of the anal margin, which are associated with excellent survival, and minimum treatment-related morbidity and cancers of the anal canal, which represent the model for multidisciplinary treatment. Although a 6-month delay was encountered until a histologic diagnosis was established, the clinical course is not unusual and the appropriate attempts at diagnosis were made. The diffuse infiltrative nature of the lesion prevented an accurate diagnosis until the lesion was no longer subtle.

Examination under anesthesia and anorectal biopsy represent an invaluable approach to the diagnosis of anal conditions, especially in the male patient. Male patients are generally muscular and for the most part not used to being examined routinely. Fear of pain and tense musculature prevent a thorough examination of a male patient under many circumstances. Examination under anesthesia, under a light general anesthetic (i.e., Versed and Propofol) provides an extremely favorable climate for anorectal examination or, in women, anorectal examination combined with pelvic examination in the presence of pain or anxiety. Biopsies can easily supplement such examinations. The infiltrative nature of this lesion confirms the importance of the incisional biopsy, even though it may have contributed to an abscess in this particular instance.

The patient presents with advanced disease. Although not mentioned in the description of physical findings, the CT scan suggests a large mass at the time of diagnosis, clearly one that measures more than 5 cm in diameter. Lesions larger than 5 cm are associated with poor response to combined chemotherapy and radiation at the normal clinical doses, and they are associated with significantly poorer survival than lesions smaller than 2 cm or smaller than tumors measuring 2 to 5 cm in diameter. Size and depth are both associated with poor outcome. The absence of palpable inguinal adenopathy is a favorable prognostic feature. The fact that symmetrical inguinal lymphadenopathy is observed on the CT scan is not totally reassuring, because rare patients will present with bilateral adenopathy. The absence of palpable inguinal adenopathy is more reassuring because metastases tend to be easily palpable, heterogeneous, and firm.

The patient went on to receive traditional doses of 5-FU, mitomycin C, and radiation therapy as primary definitive multidisciplinary treatment for his anal epidermoid carcinoma. The patient experienced spontaneous drainage of a perirectal abscess before the initiation of treatment. Whether any abscess that has drained spontaneously has resolved sufficiently for an immunoincompetent patient to undergo immunosuppressive treatment without risk of septicemia is unclear. Conceivably, the patient should have undergone a second examination under anesthesia and definitive drainage of the abscess before the initiation of treatment. Given the time course, little would have been lost by the delay of 7 to 10 days.

Typical for the HIV patient, this patient had a stormy course in response to the combined multidisciplinary treatment and ultimately underwent a diverting colostomy for what must have been considered the septic consequences of treatment to his primary tumor. It is the general impression of most people treating anal epidermoid carcinoma in conjunction with AIDS that such patients become profoundly ill under treatment. Whether or not the patient improved after fecal diversion is not clear.

In speaking of anal epidermoid carcinoma, one must distinguish between carcinomas of the anal canal and carcinomas of the anal margin. The latter represents skin cancers at the anal margin and are largely curable by excision alone. It is the rare margin cancer that extends upward to cross the dentate line.

Male homosexuality has been implicated in anal canal carcinoma. Case control studies suggest that anal-receptive intercourse is strongly associated with anal cancer. In patients under 35 years of age, anal carcinoma is more common in men. An exact etiology under these circumstances is not proven (1).

There is an association between human papilloma viruses and both precancerous and cancerous lesions of the anal canal. Human papilloma viruses (HPV) are associated with genital warts, as is the incidence of anal epidermoid carcinoma in young male homosexual patients. HPV has been identified in tumors of the anal canal both by in situ hybridization techniques and by immunohistochemistry. Most commonly, the DNA of

HPV type 16 is found in anal epidermoid carcinomas. In such studies, HPV DNA is not found in nonmalignant anal epithelium (2). Histologically, anal intraepithelial neoplasia (AIN) is a forerunner to anal epidermoid carcinoma in a significant number of patients infected with HPV (3). The incidence of AIN is significantly higher in homosexual men with HPV (7 of 28 patients) than in heterosexual men with HPV (1 of 28 patients). HPV RNA has been detected in 73% of epidermoid carcinomas with no HPV RNA detectable in anal or rectal adenocarcinomas (4). AIN was observed only in RNA+ tumors. A strong link connects homosexuality, HPV, and anal cancer, although causation is not proved by this association. Nevertheless, anal canal carcinoma seems to be related to immunosuppression and correlates highly with HPV and with condylomata acuminata. Other viral diseases and causes of immunosuppression in the male homosexual population may contribute to the etiology (5) (Fig. 140–3).

The AJCC/UICC staging system is most commonly employed in the staging of anal epidermoid cancer. With a decreasing number of surgical specimens, pathologic staging information is more limited. T stage is determined by size and by the invasion or adjacent organs. In this patient the lesion is both larger than 5 cm and deeply invasive of the levator muscles by virtue of CT scan findings. The N classification recognizes inguinal lymphadenopathy. Tumor size, depth of invasion, location across the dentate line, and presence of inguinal adenopathy are generally considered poor prognostic features. Histology, that is, basaloid or cloacogenic, is considered to be an inconsistent prognostic factor.

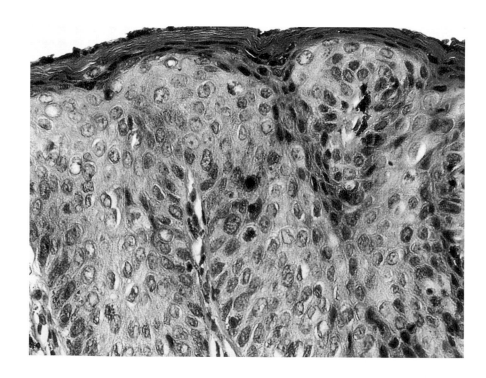

FIG. 140–3. Perianal intraepithelial neoplasia (AIN), also called Bowen's disease. Parakeratosis, pleiomorphic keratinocytes, and mitoses are present (H&E, ×400).

Before 1972, the treatment of anal epidermoid carcinoma, whether squamous, basaloid, or cloacogenic, was by radical surgery, that is, abdominoperineal resection of the rectum. Although varying from decade to decade, the overall 5-year survival for such lesions varied from 40% to 50%. Large lesions, that is, those over 5 cm in diameter, fared poorly, with survival averaging 40%. Since its introduction by Nigro, combined multidisciplinary therapy with 5-FU, mitomycin C, and radiation therapy has evolved to represent current definitive management. A common current treatment schedule would include 5-FU 1,000 mg/m^2 over 4 days, and mitomycin 10 to 15 mg/m^2 on day 1 of treatment with concurrent administration of 4,500 to 5,040 cGy to the whole pelvis. Five-year survival ranging from 65% to 90% is reported, with the vast majority of patients achieving sphincter preservation. Considerable controversy remains regarding the benefits of combined multidisciplinary therapy in patients with locally advanced lesions. For clinically T$_3$ lesions larger than 4 cm in diameter, initial responses to chemotherapy and radiation are common. Five-year survival and local control in such lesions nevertheless falls significantly short of the results quoted for survival as a whole or for lesions under 5 cm in diameter. Debate continues as to the appropriate course of action for patients with recurrent disease or persistent anal epidermoid carcinoma after definitive combined radiation and chemotherapy. Various authors advocate incremental increases in radiation therapy and platinum-based chemotherapy (6), whereas others suggest proceeding to salvage abdominoperineal resection of the rectum (7). Interstitial radiation has been advocated as well (8).

Recently, we have reviewed 38 patients in whom salvage abdominoperineal resection was performed for persistent/recurrent disease in the non-HIV+ setting. All patients had either failed definitive combined chemotherapy and radiation or had recurred after an interval of apparent response. In 22 female and 16 male patients, the actuarial 5-year survival was 44%. Recurrence after abdominal perineal resection was observed in the pelvis (isolated in 6, systemic in 12), liver (9), lung (6), and inguinal lymph nodes (5). Recurrence was related to inguinal lymphadenopathy, fixation to the pelvic sidewall, or involvement of the perirectal fat. These results suggested a moderate yield from aggressive surgery after failure of definitive chemotherapy and radiation. They also suggest the need for additional systemic treatment because of widespread systemic failure in those patients who succumb to the disease (9).

REFERENCES

1. Peters RK, Mack TM. Patterns of anal carcinoma by gender and marital status in Los Angeles County. *Br J Cancer* 1983;48:629–36.
2. Gal AA, Meyer PR, Taylor CR. Papillomavirus antigens in anorectal condyloma and carcinoma in homosexual men. *JAMA* 1987;257:337–40.
3. Scholefield JH, Sonnex C, Talbot IC, et al. Anal and cervical intraepithelial neoplasia: possible parallel. *Lancet* 1989;2:765–9.
4. Higgins GD, Uzelin DM, Phillips GE, et al. Differing characteristics of human papillomavirus RNA-positive and RNA-negative anal carcinomas. *Cancer* 1991;68:561–7.
5. Oriel JD. Human papillomaviruses and anal cancer. *Genitourin Med* [Editorial] 1989;65:213–5.
6. Magill GB, Quan S. Salvage chemotherapy of anal epidermoid carcinoma with cisplatin-based protocols. *Proc Am Soc Clin Oncol* 1989;8:117.
7. Sischy B. Doggett RLS, Krall JM, et al. Definitive irradiation and chemotherapy for radiosensitization in management of anal carcinoma: interim report on radiation therapy oncology group study No. 8314. *JNCI* 1989;81:850–6.
8. Papillon J. Montbarbon JG, Gerard JP, et al. Interstitial curietherapy in the conservative treatment of anal and rectal cancers *Int J Radiat Oncol Biol Phys* 1989;16:1161–9.
9. Ellenhorn, DI, Enker, WE and Quan SHQ. Salvage abdominoperineal resection for persistent or recurrent anal epidermal carcinoma after combined multi-disciplinary treatment. *Ann Surg Oncol* 1994;1:105–110.

Chronic Lymphocytic Leukemia

141

Chronic Lymphocytic Leukemia in an Asymptomatic 44-Year-Old Man

Richard F. Branda

A disease that a patient can live with

CASE PRESENTATION

The patient was first noted to have a lymphocytosis in 1972, during evaluation for a vasovagal syncopal episode. At the time, he was a 44-year-old U.S. Air Force pilot. Except for the syncopal episode, which cleared and did not recur, he had no other complaints. Past medical history, family history, and review of systems were negative. On physical examination, he was a well-developed, well-nourished Caucasian man in no distress. Examination was within normal limits; specifically, there was no adenopathy or hepatosplenomegaly. Laboratory tests showed a hemoglobin of 14.8 g%; hematocrit 43%; white count 24,000/mm^3 with 13% neutrophils, 80% lymphocytes, 2% eosinophils, 1% basophils, 4% monocytes; platelet count 286,000/mm^3. Examination of the blood film showed predominantly mature lymphocytes. A bone marrow examination showed diffuse infiltration with small lymphocytes. Erythroid, myeloid, and megakaryocytic elements were normal in number and morphology. The patient was diagnosed as having chronic lymphatic leukemia (CLL).

During the next 20 years the patient was seen by his physician once or twice per year for follow-up physical examinations and blood counts. From 1972 to 1985 he remained fully active. After leaving the military service he worked full time as a rural postman. He was a marathon distance runner and enjoyed long-distance bicycling. His physical examination remained within normal limits. His hematocrit was stable at about 42%, but his white count gradually rose and his platelet count

slowly dropped to the lower end of the normal range (Fig. 141–1).

In 1974, the patient's younger brother was diagnosed as having CLL, rather quickly became symptomatic, and expired in 1985 with overwhelming sepsis.

In early 1986 the patient noted an enlarged, tender lymph node in the right anterior cervical chain that measured 1.5 cm in diameter. There was no other adenopathy on examination. Later that year the lymph node was slightly more prominent, and enlarged cervical, axillary, and inguinal nodes were palpable for the first time. However, he remained physically active, jogging several times per week and logging more than 1,500 miles on his bicycle during the summer. His hematocrit had dropped to 39.5%, white count was 46,600/mm^3 with 86% lymphocytes, and platelet count of 127,000/mm^3.

Over the next 2 years, the right submandibular lymph node gradually increased in size, measuring 5 × 2.5 cm in 1988, and he continued to have generalized lymphadenopathy. Between 1988 and 1991 his lymph nodes remained stable in size, and he continued to work full time and exercise regularly, but his hematocrit and platelet count gradually declined (see Fig. 141–1).

In early 1991, he observed that the right submandibular lymph node had increased noticeably over a 1-month period and that he had decreased exercise tolerance. On examination, he had two hard movable masses in the right anterior cervical region, the larger measuring 3 × 4 cm. Laboratory evaluation showed a hematocrit of 38.6%; reticulocyte count 1.3%; Coombs' test negative; white count 50,800/mm^3 with 87% lymphocytes;

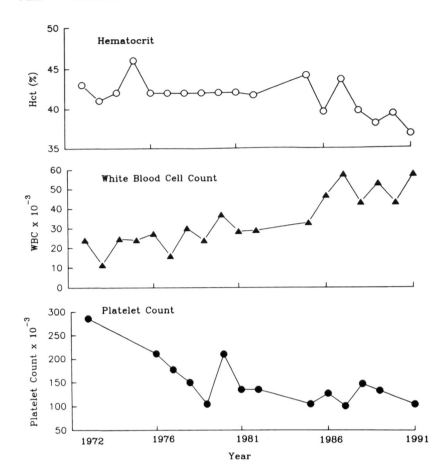

FIG. 141-1. Peripheral blood values of a patient diagnosed as having chronic lymphatic leukemia in 1972. White blood cell counts and platelet counts are per mm³ of blood.

platelet count 120,000/mm³; serum protein electrophoresis normal; quantitative immunoglobulins (IgG, IgA, and IgM) within the normal range; liver and renal function tests within normal limits.

The patient was seen at 3- to 4-month intervals during 1991. His adenopathy was relatively stable, but he had progressive anemia and thrombocytopenia. Chemotherapy was recommended but the patient was nervous and reluctant to proceed with therapy. By late summer his blood counts had dropped to a hematocrit of 35.9% and platelet count of 94,000/mm³. His white count was 53,500/mm³ with 84% lymphocytes. He agreed to begin chlorambucil in monthly cycles. After 2 months of treatment there was no discernible change, but a month later his lymph nodes had clearly decreased in size.

Nine monthly courses of chlorambucil were administered. By late 1992 only one 0.5-cm submandibular node was palpable and he had no other adenopathy. His white count gradually dropped to the range of 11,000 to 16,000/mm³, and his hematocrit increased to 37.9%, but his platelet count remained below the normal range.

Because of the discrepancy between his clinical improvement and persistent thrombocytopenia, a bone marrow examination was performed (Fig. 141–2). The bone marrow was diffusely infiltrated with small round

lymphocytes. Megakaryocytes were borderline adequate in number. There was no evidence of myelodysplasia. Smears showed 87% small lymphocytes (Fig. 141–3). Prednisone was added to his chemotherapy but his platelet count remained stable.

The patient was seen again in early 1993. He continued to work full time and was physically active. He had had no recent infections, bruising, or bleeding. On physical examination he continued to have a 0.5-cm right submandibular node but also had developed a new 1.5-cm right axillary node. There was no other palpable adenopathy, nor was there hepatosplenomegaly. His blood counts showed a hematocrit of 36.5%; white count 24,900/mm³ with 85% lymphocytes; platelet count 104,000/mm³.

QUESTIONS DISCUSSED AT TUMOR BOARD

1. *If this patient presented today to your clinic, what laboratory evaluation would be performed?*

There was consensus that a sustained lymphocytosis in an adult with no clinical evidence of infection or endocrine disorder is highly suggestive of CLL. It was noted that this patient was younger at presentation than the typical patient with CLL (90% are over 50). There-

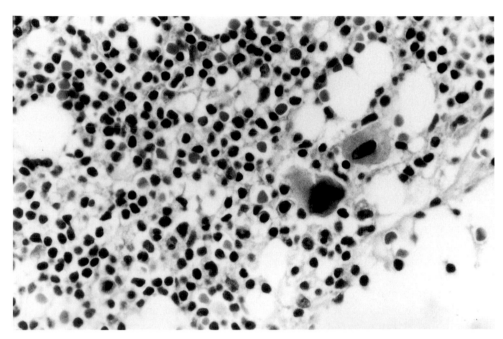

FIG. 141–2. Bone marrow examination of a patient with chronic lymphatic leukemia, performed in 1992. The bone marrow was hypercellular and diffusely infiltrated with small, well differentiated lymphocytes. Megakaryocyte morphology was normal. (Magnification ×400.)

fore, a careful clinical examination was warranted to consider other causes of lymphocytosis (such as lymphoma, thyrotoxicosis, chronic inflammatory conditions, and sarcoidosis). Examination of the peripheral smear was considered essential, and most participants felt that lymphocyte phenotype by flow cytometry was very important to establish that the patient had a clonal B-cell disorder. Evidence was cited indicating that the phenotype may provide prognostic information. A bone marrow examination, including biopsy, was not considered essential for diagnosis but might provide further prognostic information. Similarly, chromosome analysis was considered of

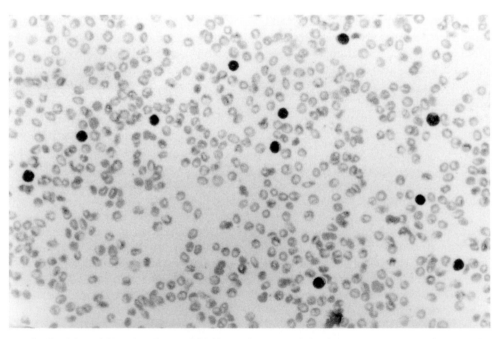

FIG. 141–3. Peripheral blood cell morphology at the time of the bone marrow examination. The predominant cell type was a small, well differentiated lymphocyte. (Magnification ×25.)

interest regarding prognosis. It was pointed out, however, that the current management of early stage CLL, even in a younger individual such as our patient, would not be changed by the pattern of bone marrow involvement or karyotypic abnormalities. Most participants would measure serum immunoglobulin levels. Low levels would identify patients at increased risk of infection who require additional education, more aggressive evaluation of fevers or other signs of infection, and prompt treatment. A serum protein electrophoresis to detect monoclonal gammopathies and a Coombs' test were also recommended at disease presentation.

2. *What stage was his disease at presentation?*

This patient was stage 0 by the Rai classification and stage A in the Binet system.

3. *What is the most appropriate follow-up (frequency, laboratory tests) for this patient?*

Most participants would perform a physical examination and measure blood counts once or twice per year. They would repeat the immunoglobulin level assays periodically, depending on the clinical progression of the patient.

4. *Should treatment have been initiated in 1972?*

The consensus was that early stage CLL should not be treated.

5. *At what point was treatment indicated?*

The indications for treatment are cytopenias, decreased performance status, and adenopathy or splenomegaly that causes functional disturbances.

6. *What is the current initial treatment of choice for CLL?*

Alkylating agent and prednisone.

7. *What are the possible causes of his anemia and thrombocytopenia after chemotherapy in 1992?*

Autoimmune phenomena, marrow infiltration, and splenic sequestration were discussed. An appropriate evaluation would include a physical examination, bone marrow aspirate and biopsy, Coombs' test, and antiplatelet antibody test.

8. *Which drug(s) should be used for retreatment?*

Most participants would treat again with alkylating agent and prednisone. If this treatment failed, most would chose fludarabine.

COMMENTARY by Kanti R. Rai

A 20-year-long clinical course of a patient with CLL provides an unusually attractive opportunity to review the natural history of this disease. The case history provides all the necessary and important data at the time of initial diagnosis and again at critical points during the long clinical course. In general, I am in complete agreement with the diagnostic and therapeutic decisions made on this case throughout this period. I also concur with the consensus opinions rendered by the Tumor Board that discussed this case. My specific comments relate to the questions concerning (a) the optimum work-up advisable to determine the extent of disease present at the time of initial diagnosis of CLL as well as at later points in its clinical course, and (b) the guiding principles to decide when to initiate therapeutic intervention in this disease.

1. *If this patient presented today to your clinic, what laboratory evaluation would be performed?*

Several diagnostic tests have now become available that were not a matter of routine in 1972. Lymphocyte immunophenotyping: Peripheral blood lymphocyte immunophenotyping is relatively easily accessible today. It is a good practice to establish that the blood lymphocytosis is produced by an increase in monoclonal B cells because in the rare event that these cells are found to be T lymphocytes, a somewhat different approach may be necessary. A T lymphocytosis would require us to look for H-TLV serology or for the presence of Sezary syndrome—diseases that are quite different from CLL. Even if the presence of monoclonal B-cell lymphocytosis is confirmed, low intensity of surface immunoglobulin and copositivity of B cells with CD5 are helpful to distinguish B-CLL from prolymphocytic leukemia or leukemic phase of non-Hodgkin's lymphoma. Once such a phenotype is established, it is not necessary to repeat the study because it does not offer any prognostic value and the phenotype does not change during the course of the disease. If, however, a patient is enrolled in a therapeutic research protocol and achieves a clinical complete remission (CR), a repeat phenotyping of blood lymphocytes may be advisable to determine if the normal B:T ratio has been established to prove that it is an immunologic CR as well.

I agree with the Tumor Board opinions concerning the value of bone marrow biopsy, chromosome analysis, and Coombs' test in CLL. The prognostic role of serial measurements of serum beta-2 microglobulin has not been established in CLL. Measurement of serum immunoglobulin levels at diagnosis, and yearly thereafter, is advisable to determine if significant hypogammaglobulinemia is present. In the actual case presented, we are informed that a younger sibling of the patient also developed CLL and died of overwhelming sepsis several years later but still at a relatively young age. The most frequent cause of death among patients with CLL is infection, and hypogammaglobulinemia (which is correctable with periodic intravenous immunoglobulin therapy) is a major basis for proneness to infections.

I do not routinely recommend computed tomography (CT) scans of the chest, abdomen, and pelvis on all patients newly diagnosed to have CLL. The extent of peripherally palpable adenopathy is usually a reliable indicator of presence or absence of mediastinal or retroperitoneal adenopathy.

2. *Is there anything special about CLL in younger age?*

With an increasing frequency of routine blood counts among ostensibly healthy people, larger numbers of patients are being diagnosed to have CLL while they are still in their late 30s or early 40s. I do not believe that the overall prevalence and epidemiology of the disease is changing; instead, it is just that we are diagnosing it at much earlier stages than before. Several studies (1–6) of CLL in younger ages have been published recently that indicate that the disease course and prognostic features are not different from the disease that typically affects a much older population. However, because a median life expectancy of 12 years for a person who is 44 years of age has a harsher connotation than a person who is in his 70s, suggestions are being made to take a more aggressive approach in therapy of younger patients. Although such suggestions have a laudable basis, there is no evidence that an aggressive approach would bestow younger patients a longer or a better quality of life.

The issue finally boils down to effective therapy of CLL. There has been no substantial increase in survival of patients with CLL over the past four decades. Whatever improvements have been observed are attributable to advances in supportive therapy. One of the time-honored prerequisites for prolongation of survival time in human malignancies has been that there is an effective therapy that results in a complete remission of the disease. In the past, complete remissions in CLL have been relatively rare. It is therefore interesting to note that in contrast to the "historical" less than 10% incidence, a 33% CR rate was reported with therapy with fludarabine in CLL patients who had received no treatment previously. These results, reported by Keating et al. (7,8), were from a single institution–based work, involved a relatively small number of patients, and the study did not include a control arm. A large multi-institutional, intergroup, controlled clinical trial is currently underway (conducted by Cancer and Leukemia Group B) in which previously untreated CLL patients who now need to be treated are randomized to one of the following three arms: (a) fludarabine, (b) chlorambucil (the "gold standard" in CLL), and (c) a combination of fludarabine and chlorambucil. The study is accruing patients at a rapid pace and it is likely that within the next few years will yield results to respond to the question whether a high rate of CR in CLL translates into a prolongation of survival and thus (for the first time in decades) improvement in the natural history of this disease. This, of course, will depend on confirmation of the premise that the study will reproduce Keating's results of 33% CR rate in previously untreated CLL. 2-Chlorodeoxyadenosine, a newly developed nucleoside analog with remarkable activity in hairy cell leukemia, is another candidate drug with promise and currently under clinical trials in previously untreated CLL (8,9).

REFERENCES

1. Dhodapkar M, Tefferi A, Su J, Phyliky RL. Prognostic features and survival in young adults with early/intermediate chronic lymphocytic leukemia (B-CLL): a single institution study. *Leukemia* 1993;7:1232.
2. Montserrat E, Gomis F, Vasespi T, et al. Presenting features and prognosis of chronic lymphocytic leukemia in younger adults. *Blood* 1991; 78:1545.
3. Pangalis GA, Reverter JC, Boussiotis VA, Montserrat E. Chronic lymphocytic leukemia in younger adults; preliminary results of a study based on 454 patients-IWCLL/Working group. *Leuk Lymphoma* 1991;5(suppl):175.
4. Lugassy G, Boussiotis VA, Ruchlemer R, Pangalis GA, Berrebi A, Pollack A. Chronic lymphocytic leukemia in young adults: report of six cases under the age of 30 years. *Leuk Lymphoma* 1991;5(suppl): 179.
5. De Rossi G, Mandelli F, Covelli A, et al. Chronic lymphocytic leukemia in younger adults: a restrspective study of 133 cases. *Hematol Oncol* 1989;7:127.
6. Bennett JM, Raphael B, Oken MA, Silbe R. The prognosis and therapy of chronic lymphocytic leukemia under age 50 years. *Nouv Rev Fr Hematol* 1988;30:411.
7. Keating MJ, Kantarjian H, O'Brien S, et al. Fludarabine: a new agent with marked cyto reductive activity in untreated chronic lymphocytic leukemia. *J Clin Oncol* 1991;9:44.
8. Keating MJ. Chemotherapy of chronic lymphocytic leukemia in chronic lymphocytic leukemia: scientific advances and clinical developments. In: Cheson B, ed. New York: Marcel Dekker; 1993;297–336.
9. Piro LD, Carrera CJ, Beutler E, Carson DA. 2-Chlorodeoxyadenosine: an effective new agent for the treatment of chronic lymphocytic leukemia. *Blood* 1988;72:1069.

Chronic Myelogenous Leukemia

142

Chronic Myeloid Leukemia

Steve Snyder and Linda Burns

A disease with continuing improvement in therapeutics

CASE PRESENTATION

B.M. is a 48-year-old Caucasian man who initially presented after minor trauma in December 1986 for arthroscopic surgery on his knee. During presurgical evaluation he was noted to have an elevated white blood count. When questioned, he had noted fatigue for 1 month and some night sweats. His family history was notable in that his maternal grandmother and maternal aunt each had succumbed to an unknown type of leukemia, and that he had two maternal half-siblings who died at age 3 years with some type of leukemia. His physical examination was unremarkable. Specifically, there was no adenopathy or organomegaly. Laboratory studies revealed a white blood count of 20.0×10^9/L with a left shift, hemoglobin of 14.7 g/dL, and platelet count of 261.0×10^9/L. LAP score was normal.

He was referred for evaluation to our institution in September 1987. During the preceding few months, he had noted increasing fatigue and continued night sweats. His physical examination now revealed an enlarged spleen. A complete blood count showed a white blood count of 115.0×10^9/L with 19.0×10^9/L metamyelocytes, 13.8×10^9/L myelocytes, 20.0×10^9/L bands, 45.0×10^9/L neutrophils, 9.2×10^9/L lymphocytes, and 6.9×10^9/L basophils; hemoglobin = 12.1 g/dL, and platelets = 219.0×10^9/L. A bone marrow aspirate and biopsy was obtained, which revealed a markedly hypercellular marrow, increased M:E ratio of 30:1, and basophilia. Thirty-three metaphase cells from the bone marrow were analyzed using G-banding. All the metaphases had a 46 XY male karyotype with a single Philadelphia chromosome arising from a complex translocation involving the short arm of one #4, and the long arms of one #12, one #21, and one #22 chromosome. The patient was diagnosed with chronic myelogenous leukemia (CML), chronic phase.

The patient did not have a matched sibling and therefore was not a candidate for allogenic bone marrow transplantation. In October 1987, he began a national cooperative group study using recombinant a2b interferon at a dose of 5×10^6 IU/m^2 SQ each day. He required some initial dose adjustment secondary to thrombocytopenia, and later because of a rise in liver transaminase levels. By April 1988, his splenomegaly had resolved and peripheral blood counts had normalized, with a white blood count of 3.5×10^9/L with 2.7×10^9/L neutrophils, 560×10^6/L lymphocytes, and no basophils; hemoglobin of 14 g/dL, and platelet count of 176.0×10^9/L. At that time, the bone marrow was mildly hypercellular with an M:E ratio of 2–3:1 and no basophilia. Cytogenetics revealed that 63% of the metaphases were normal. In August 1989, the bone marrow revealed morphologic remission, and cytogenetics revealed 100% normal metaphases. He currently is on 3.75×10^6 IU of a2bIFN each day and remains in a hematologic and cytogenetic remission. The bone marrow is negative for bcr-abl transcripts. He feels well except for mild fatigue.

TUMOR BOARD DISCUSSION

Chronic myeloid leukemia is characterized by a progressive course with most patients dying in the blast crisis stage of the disease. The median survival from the time of diagnosis is between 3 and 4 years. Neither standard chemotherapy (usually with hydroxyurea or Busulfan) nor aggressive regimens, such as those used in acute leukemia, have resulted in improved survival. These treatments are useful primarily for the control of peripheral blood counts. The only treatment to show a potential for prolonged survival is allogenic bone marrow transplantation. However, this form of treatment is available to only a small percentage of patients.

During the 1980s, several reports appeared from the M.D. Anderson Cancer Center suggesting a role for alpha-interferon in the treatment of CML (1). Patients in early chronic phase were treated daily with subcutaneous interferon alpha. Approximately 70% of the patients achieved hematologic remissions (defined as a normalization of peripheral blood counts and disappearance of splenomegaly). Moreover, complete suppression of the Philadelphia chromosome (cytogenetic remission) was observed in 20% of patients. With standard therapy, disappearance of the Philadelphia chromosome is rare.

Based on these encouraging findings, the Cancer and Leukemia Group B conducted a multicenter trial of 107 patients with newly diagnosed CML who were treated with recombinant alpha2b interferon (2). Hematologic remissions were achieved in 59% of patients (22% complete remissions). Cytogenetic remissions (complete suppression of the Philadelphia chromosome) occurred in 29% of patients. The median survival in this study (66 months) was similar to that observed in previous studies of alpha interferon. Side effects of treatment (principally fever, flulike illness, and thrombocytopenia) were largely reversible on discontinuation of therapy. However, major dose reductions (>50%) were required in 38% of the patients.

Despite the promising findings in these early studies, the effect of interferon treatment on survival of patients with CML was still unknown. In addition, it was also unclear whether attainment of a cytogenetic remission had any effect on patient survival. Several randomized clinical trials are currently underway to answer these questions.

The Italian Cooperative Study Group on CML recently published the findings of a randomized study comparing recombinant interferon alpha 2a with conventional treatment of chronic phase CML (3). Patients were eligible only if they had been diagnosed within the preceding 6 months and had received only minimal treatment. A total of 322 patients were randomized to either recombinant alpha interferon, given in an escalated dose schedule, or standard therapy with hydroxyurea or busulfan. The standard therapy dose and schedule were not specified, however. The median survival of the patients in the interferon group was reached at 6 years compared with a 29% survival in the conventional treatment group at 6 years. This difference was statistically significant. In addition, survival was significantly longer in patients who attained cytogenetic remissions. However, patients treated with interferon experienced significantly more side effects than the patients treated with conventional therapy. Nearly 50% of the patients treated with interferon discontinued therapy within 5 years compared with 30% of the patients treated with conventional therapy. The cost of interferon treatment is substantial (approximately 200 times the cost of hydroxyurea).

The cumulating evidence to date suggests that interferon should be considered as first-line therapy for patients with newly diagnosed CML who either do not wish or are not candidates for allogenic bone marrow transplantation. The results of other randomized trials are needed to confirm the Italian cooperative group's finding before general recommendations are made.

REFERENCES

1. Talpaz M, Kantarjian HM, McCredie KB, Kurzrock R, et al. Interferon-alpha produces sustained cytogenetic responses in chronic myelogenous leukemia. *Ann Intern Med* 1991;114:532–8.
2. Ozer H, George SL, Schiffer CA, et al. Prolonged subcutaneous administration of recombinant a2b interferon in patients with previously untreated Philadelphia chromosome-positive chronic phase chronic myelogenous leukemia: effect on remission duration and survival: Cancer and Leukemia Group B Study 8583. *Blood* 1993;82:2975–84.
3. The Italian Cooperative Group Study on Chronic Myeloid Leukemia. Interferon alpha-2a as compared with conventional chemotherapy for the treatment of chronic myeloid leukemia. *N Engl J Med* 1994;330:820–5.

COMMENTARY by John R. Durant

This patient represents many notable features important in the diagnosis and management of chronic myelogenous leukemia. Further, its management represents many of the advances made during the past 10 to 15 years.

First, the patient was discovered characteristically when a blood count done for another reason showed an increase in his total white blood cells with a left shift but LAP normal. Further work-up apparently was not considered seriously. He progressed rapidly, however, and over the next 9 months developed the characteristic findings of chronic myelogenous leukemia with the suggestion of fairly aggressive disease represented by night sweats and basophilia. The diagnosis was established firmly through cytogenetics with the presence of a Philadelphia chromosome, although the translocations were unusual for this particular abnormal chromosome.

The standard and variant forms of the Philadelphia chromosome carry a fusion gene from the bcr-abl loci. This gene produces a 210-kD protein with abnormal tyrosine kinase activity that is believed to be important in the pathogenesis of the disease. Identification of this protein by polymerase chain reaction (PCR) allows as few as one abnormal cell in $1 \times 10^{5,6}$ cells to be detected. The elimination of the chromosome is believed to be essential to the cure of the disease.

Because the data now indicate that allogenic transplantation is increasingly effective at eliminating the chromosome and producing cure, especially if done in the early phases of the disease, and because patients in the age group of this patient can now safely undergo transplantation, he was considered for this procedure; however, no match was found in his family. That approach was then abandoned. Some investigators have attempted to widen the use of transplantation by finding matched but unrelated donors through the use of large registries of potential donors that have been established. This approach, however, because of its greater hazards, is usually reserved for patients not responding to other alternatives, particularly interferon (see below). Another approach in the transplantation arena that has recently been pursued is the use of autologous bone marrow or stem cells. The long-term results from these alternatives are too preliminary to make recommendations, but they appear promising enough to continue to investigate.

It is clear, however, that if a patient is young, has some features suggesting poor prognosis, and has a matched sibling, early allogenic bone marrow transplantation is the best treatment. The trade-off, of course, is that if the patient dies as a result, he/she will have sacrificed several additional years of comfortable life for the hope of cure. Most would take this risk.

An important development, as illustrated by this case, is the use of recombinant alpha interferon which, when employed in the doses used in this patient and within the first year of diagnosis, has generally produced significant hematologic remission in most cases and has induced a cytogenetic remission in a modest percentage of these cases. There is controversy over the frequency with which the complete cytogenetic remission is truly complete, with studies using the PCR now being used to test its utility.

Finally, there are initial indications that interferon therapy, unlike the chemotherapy of the past (Myleran and Hydrea), does improve survival. What is not yet clear is whether the complete cytogenetic remissions are permanent, as those induced by allogenic bone marrow transplantation appear to be.

All these more recent treatments, that is, alpha interferon and the various types of transplantation, come at the expense of substantial toxicity, which is both biologic and financial, when compared with the conventional therapies of the past that improve the quality of life but do not lengthen survival. When cure is possible, particularly for the young, these are worth the cost.

Finally, in regard to this patient, the most intriguing question is what the mechanism of action of the interferons is that produces the reported results, and why early institution of therapy is so much more effective than delaying treatment into the second year or later of the chronic phase.

SELECTED READINGS

1. Deisseroth AB, Andreeff M, Champlin R, et al. *Cancer: principles and practice of oncology,* 4th ed. Philadelphia: JB Lippincott; 1993;55: 1970–9.
2. Tura S, Russo D, Zuffa E, Fiacchini M. A prospective comparison of human recombinant interferon (Roferon-A) and conventual chemotherapy in chronic myeloid leukemia (CML). Interim report of the Italian Study. *Blood* 1990;76(suppl 1):329A.
3. Lee MS, Chang KS, Freireich EJ, et al. Detection of minimal residual bcr/abl transcripts by a modified polymerase chain reaction. *Blood* 1988;72:893–7.
4. Beatty PG, Hansen JA, Longton GM, et al. Marrow transplantation from HLA-matched unrelated donors for treatment of hematologic malignancies. *Transplantation* 1991;51:443–7.

143

Acute Myelogenous Leukemia in a 40-year-old Man with Fatigue, Congestive Heart Failure, and a White Blood Cell Count of 1,000,000

Julie M. Vose

The complete remission rate of acute myelogenous leukemia is steadily improving

CASE PRESENTATION

The patient is a 40-year-old Caucasian man who had a 3-week history of fatigue, easy bruisability, and shortness of breath. He presented to his primary care physician, who performed a physical examination and found the patient to have evidence of congestive heart failure and tachycardia. A complete blood count was performed with a white blood count (WBC) of 1,000,000/mm³, hemoglobin 7.5 g%, and platelet count 23,000/mm³. A differential revealed 78% blasts, many containing Auer rods consistent with acute myelogenous leukemia (AML). A bone marrow aspirate was performed, which demonstrated a hypercellular bone marrow with 64% blasts (Fig. 143–1), which stained positively for myeloperoxidase, alpha-chloroacetate esterase, and Sudan black B, but negative for butyrate esterase. Cytogenetic examination revealed multiple abnormalities (Fig. 143–2).

The patient was admitted to the Hematology/Oncology Special Care Unit and started on intravenous fluids and allopurinol. Because of the extremely high blast count and evidence of leukostasis on chest radiograph and physical exam, leukopheresis was initiated. After two leukophereses, the patient was initiated on induction chemotherapy consisting of idarubicin 12 mg/M² per day for 3 days and cytarabine 100 mg/M² per day by continuous infusion for 7 days. The patient developed severe pancytopenia over the ensuing week after the initiation of therapy. The patient required platelet and packed red blood cell transfusion support as well as empiric antibiotics for neutropenia.

Fevers to 101°F developed in the second week after the induction chemotherapy was administered. Despite a change in the antibiotic regimen and addition of amphotericin, the high spiking fevers continued. A chest radiograph demonstrated a consolidation present in the upper lobe on the right. A chest computed tomograph (CT) demonstrated a well-circumscribed 2.5-cm abnormality with a "halo" effect. This was believed possibly to be consistent with a fungal infectious process. The patient was evaluated by the thoracic surgery team and subsequently underwent a right upper lobe resection without major complications. The histologic evaluation of the specimen revealed hyphae consistent with an *Aspergillus* infection. The patient was treated with amphotericin at 1 mg/kg intravenously daily for a total of 2 g of therapy. The patient

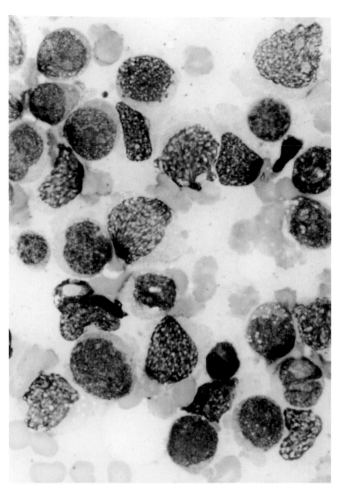

FIG. 143–1. Photomicrograph of the patient's bone marrow at presentation.

developed renal insufficiency with a creatinine up to 3.8 mg/dL; however, he was able to complete the intended amphotericin dosage.

A bone marrow biopsy was performed on day +14 after the initiation of therapy with idarubicin and cytarabine. The bone marrow was hypoplastic, with no evidence of acute leukemia at that time by morphology, and the cytogenetics did not demonstrate the previous cytogenetic abnormality. The patient was initiated on granulocyte-macrophage colony stimulating factor (GM-CSF) at 250 mcg/M^2 per day when a hypoplastic marrow was confirmed. Over the ensuing 10 days, the absolute neutrophil count recovered to 1,200/mm^3 and the patient became platelet transfusion independent. He was discharged from the hospital on day +27 after initiation of the induction chemotherapy.

The patient was readmitted 2 weeks later for intensification therapy with cytarabine 100 mg/M^2 per day by continuous infusion for 7 days and mitoxantrone 12 mg/M2 per day for 3 days. The patient tolerated the chemotherapy well with minimal toxicity. He was

placed on prophylactic amphotericin at 0.5 mg/kg per day when he became neutropenic to prevent any recurrence of the *Aspergillus* infection. His day +14 bone marrow was aplastic, with no evidence of AML. The patient became hypotensive and febrile on day +17, with a blood culture positive for *Pseudomonas aeruginosa*. The patient's antibiotics were changed, with ceftazidime and gentamicin added for double coverage of the gram-negative rod infection. His clinical condition improved on the antibiotics and as the neutrophil count recovered, he was discontinued from the antibiotics after a 14-day course.

Because of the high blast count and the poor prognosis cytogenetic abnormalities that he originally presented with, the patient was considered at high-risk for relapse, and consolidation with high-dose chemotherapy and a related allogeneic transplant were undertaken. Approximately 1 month after hospital discharge from the intensification therapy, the patient was readmitted for the allogeneic transplant. He received cyclophosphamide 60 mg/kg for 2 days, etoposide 1,800 mg/M^2 for one dose, and total body irradiation at 1,200 cGy as the preparatory regimen. The patient received his sister's 6-antigen HLA-matched bone marrow on day 0 without complications. Graft versus host disease (GVHD) prophylaxis consisted of cyclosporine and methotrexate as per standard protocol.

Complications that developed during the transplantation included the development of grade II/IV skin and liver GVHD. This complication was treated with intravenous solumedrol at 125 mg every 12 hours. The GVHD improved with the solumedrol therapy and the patient was discharged from the hospital on day +28 after transplant, when his hematopoietic engraftment was stable. A routine surveillance bronchoscopy was performed on day +35 with the cytomegalovirus (CMV) early antigen being positive. The patient was started on ganciclovir treatment, followed by maintenance therapy. Over the next few months the patient's steroids were able to be tapered, with no recurrence of the acute GVHD.

At day +100 after the allogenic bone marrow transplant, a bone marrow was performed that demonstrated no evidence of AML, normal cytogenetics, and all cells to be of donor origin. His cyclosporin and prednisone treatment was tapered over the next 3 months per protocol. At 9 months after transplantation, he developed sicca syndrome and evidence of chronic GVHD with skin and mouth involvement only. The patient was treated with an alternate-day cyclosporin and prednisone treatment regimen. The symptoms partially cleared after 1 month of therapy; however, the patient still remains on a low dose of alternate-day prednisone for adequate control of the chronic GVHD. At 1 year postallogenic transplant, the patient remains in complete remission from the AML, with only minimal evidence of chronic GVHD.

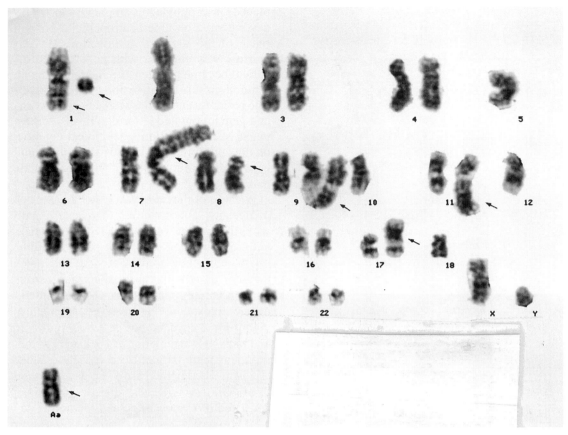

FIG. 143–2. Cytogenic examination revealing multiple abnormalities.

COMMENTARY by John R. Durant

The patient described in this report presented with a relatively short history and a very high blast count (780,000/m³). The most pressing immediate problem was leukostasis, demonstrated on chest radiograph and almost certainly responsible for the evidence of heart failure. He received two therapies for this acute emergency: leukopheresis and induction chemotherapy. Of the two, most evidence suggests that prompt institution of antileukemic therapy is the most important. Leukopheresis may only cause leukemic cells to enter the circulation from extravascular tissues because leukopheresis reduces the peripheral myeloblast count.

The patient was then treated with one of the several regimens most effective in induction remission, that is,. high-dose ara C and idarubicin. Combined results from two studies of 161 patients provided 72% complete remissions (CR). During induction, he had fever associated with a cavitary pulmonary lesion in the right upper lobe most compatible with a fungal infection. No amount of systemic antifungal therapy is likely to control this process rapidly enough to permit antileukemic therapy to proceed, so it was resected. That produced local control

and a specific diagnosis of the pulmonary lesion so that appropriate postoperative systemic antifungal therapy could be given. The patient responded nicely and went into CR.

He received intensification therapy, which is generally believed to prolong remission and improve survival. He had the common complication of *Pseudomonas* septicemia, was appropriately treated and recovered, still in CR.

The next issue was what to do next. Was he merely in clinical CR or was he cured? Did he need something more, that is, a transplant? About 20 years ago, I had a 17-year-old patient with this disease who failed induction therapy but developed a CR on an alternative regimen. He had numerous brothers and sisters, several of whom were a suitable genetic match. So, after achieving the remission, it was elected to refer him to the University of Washington for a transplant in remission. He went to Seattle, looked around, and decided to come home without undergoing transplantation. He did three things that I thought were foolish. He discontinued maintenance therapy, a decision we now know was reasonable; he got married; and he went to a faith healer. Today he is fine. This illustrates the dilemma. Patients in CR may be cured and need no more therapy. More therapy may be necessary, but not work. It may be necessary and work, but the patient may die from complications. Finally, it may be necessary and work. How are you to tell in advance? My patient clearly did not need any more therapy and might have died of therapy had it been given. No matter what, he would have been very sick for at least several months. Because of this dilemma, various prognostic factors have been used to select those patients with AML in first remission most likely to benefit from transplantation when there is a matched sibling, a possibility in only about 10% of all AML patients.

It was thought that the FAB classification of AML might be helpful in this regard. There are seven types with several subtypes. This classification is not highly reproducible and so provides uncertain prognostic guidance. This patient was M_2 based on differential staining and abundant Auer rods, which may be a favorable group. His blast count, however, was astronomical, a poor prognostic factor. His age of 40 was neutral. Younger age bears much the better prognosis. Cytogenetic abnormalities may also offer prognostic information. The best group are those with translocations between chromosomes 15 and 17 or an inversion of chromosome 16. Multiple abnormalities are usually considered a bad sign. The patient's physician considered the evidence and believed his poor prognostic fac-

tors far outweighed any others, and elected to do an allo-graft, which the patient survived. He had mild to moderate GVH, which in itself probably has a positive antileukemic effect. At 1 year, the patient is well except for mild chronic GVH and is likely cured. Was the transplant necessary? There is no conclusive evidence that it was, but most doctors would have chosen this option for this patient. Having survived the first year, it is likely that his chances of cure are better than if he had not had the transplant.

The years ahead will probably see a better definition of prognostic factors based on cytogenetic and clinical characteristics, and so remove some of the uncertainty surrounding the management of patients of this kind.

SELECTED READINGS

1. Berman E, Heller G, Santorsa J, et al. Results of randomized trial comparing idarubicin and cytosine arabinsoide with daunorubicin and cytosine arabinoside in adult patients with newly diagnosed acute myelogenous leukemia. *Blood* 1991;77:1666.
2. Wiernik PH, Banks PLC, Case DC Jr, et al. Cytarbine plus idarubicin or daunorubicin as induction and consolidation therapy for previously untreated adult patients with acute myeloid leukemia. *Blood* 199;79:313.
3. Butturini A, Gale RP. Chemotherapy versus transplantation in acute leukaemia. *Br J Haematol* 1989;72:1.
4. Keating MJ, Smith TL, Kantarjian H, et al. Cytogenetic pattern in acute myelogenous leukemia: A major reproducible determinant of outcome. *Leukemia* 1988;2:403.

SECTION XXXIII

Complex Cancer Management

144

The Excavating Pulmonary Lesion in a Patient with Prostate Cancer

Nael Martini

Second primary lung cancer, pulmonary metastasis, or
inflammatory lesion?

CASE PRESENTATION

A 66-year-old black man went for a physical examination to purchase insurance, and an enlarged prostate was found. He had a transrectal biopsy that was positive for adenocarcinoma, and on further investigation plain chest roentgenograms showed a pulmonary mass. This was confirmed on chest computed tomography (CT) scans. He had smoked for only 5 years and had stopped smoking altogether 6 years ago.

His physical examination was essentially normal. There was no palpable adenopathy. There were bilaterally clear breath sounds on chest auscultation. Heart sounds were normal with no murmurs or bruits. His abdomen was soft with no palpable organs or masses and the extremities were normal.

At the Tumor Board, discussion centered around how to handle the pulmonary mass and what to do with the prostatic tumor. A solitary pulmonary mass in a 66-year-old asymptomatic patient should be considered suspicious for a pulmonary neoplasm until proved otherwise. Cavitation does not preclude a cancer diagnosis; hence, the importance of establishing a firm histologic diagnosis. Recommendations were to pursue the investigation to rule out lung cancer and consult a urologist before considering definitive management.

A urologist was consulted. A transurethral biopsy and prostate scan were done to confirm the cancer diagnosis. The prostate specific antigen (PSA) was 49 ng/mL (nl 0–4). He was clinically staged to have a T3a tumor, and

periodic surveillance without treatment was recommended.

Review of the chest radiographs and CT scans showed a 4- to 5-cm cavitary mass in the right upper lobe without adenopathy in the hilum or mediastinum (Figs. 144–1, 144–2). The differential diagnoses of the pulmonary mass were inflammatory lung abscess, primary lung carcinoma, and metastatic prostatic cancer to the lung. Because of the peripheral position of the lesion, a diagnostic needle biopsy of the lung lesion under CT guidance was done and showed adenocarcinoma cells. Bronchoscopy was done to assess the status of the major bronchi and ascertain clear resection margins, and was found negative. Bone and brain scans were normal. No adrenal or hepatic metastases were suspected on CT scans. Pulmonary function evaluation showed a normal forced vital capacity and an FEV 1 of 71% (2,370 cc). The pulmonary diffusion capacity (DLCO) was 81% of predicted normal, and arterial blood gas analysis was also normal.

The lung lesion was considered to represent a separate primary lung cancer, and he was offered resection of the lung mass. He underwent a right posterolateral thoracotomy and a right upper lobectomy with a mediastinal lymph node dissection. Complete resection of the tumor was possible, and the resected margins were clear microscopically. His postsurgical stage was T2 N0 M0, stage I.

The histologic material from the resected lobe showed a predominantly squamous cell lung cancer with central cavitation and necrosis. The low- and high-power pho-

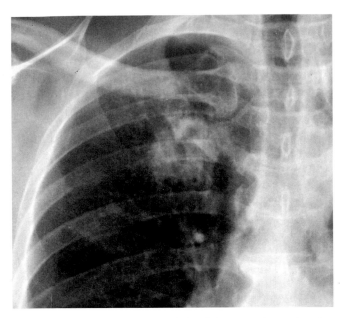

FIG. 144–1. A close-up view of the right upper lung showing a 4–5-cm mass with ill-defined borders and suspicion of central cavitation.

tomicrographs show a well demarcated tumor surrounded by normal lung (Figs. 144–3, 144–4).

The patient had an uneventful postoperative course. No further therapy was recommended. His expectation for a 5-year disease-free survival from his lung cancer was estimated to be 72%. Periodic follow-up exams by a chest surgeon and a urologist at 3- to 4-month intervals were recommended.

COMMENTARY by G. Alex Patterson

The case under discussion provides a number of interesting diagnostic and management dilemmas for the surgical oncologist. The patient presents with coexisting prostatic and lung lesions and the problem is how best to diagnose, stage, and manage both lesions. My comments will be restricted to the investigation and management of the lung lesion.

The patient has a limited smoking history and an absence of pulmonary symptoms. This does not exclude a diagnosis of bronchogenic carcinoma. Previous chest radiographs are always helpful but unavailable in this patient. The current chest radiograph demonstrates an apparently cavitated, ill-defined lesion having irregular borders. The lesion is seen to much better advantage on the CT image. The lesion is cavitated and has a thick outer margin with irregular borders. It is noncalcified. These are typical radiographic features of a bronchogenic squamous carcinoma. Although in the upper lobe, the cavity is not apical, a more typical location for benign cavitary lung disease. Of importance is the absence of enlarged

mediastinal nodes, which if present are suggestive of nodal metastatic disease.

A number of diagnostic options are available, including cytologic examination of sputum, bronchoscopic brushing or washings, as well as percutaneous fine-needle aspiration biopsy. Excisional biopsy of peripheral lesions suspected to be malignant is occasionally an option. However, the size and location of this lesion preclude wedge excision. A lobectomy would be required to achieve excisional biopsy. In the presence of another malignancy, preoperative diagnosis is the most prudent course. Percutaneous needle biopsy is an appropriate diagnostic maneuver in this patient and can be expected to have a high diagnostic yield (1). Having a malignant diagnosis preoperatively greatly simplifies the conduct of subsequent resection. The need for intraoperative diagnostic excisional biopsy is eliminated.

The cytologic diagnosis was adenocarcinoma. It is impossible to distinguish primary bronchogenic from metastatic prostatic cancer on the basis of a needle aspirate. Therefore, clinical judgment is required. An otherwise favorable prostatic cancer without local metastasis is unlikely to present with a solitary pulmonary metastasis without distant metastatic disease, especially to bone. Furthermore, the radiologic appearance is much more in keeping with a primary squamous bronchogenic carcinoma than that of a metastatic prostatic lesion. Finally, the cytologic diagnosis must be viewed with some suspicion, especially because the lesion has all the typical radiographic features of a bronchogenic squamous carcinoma. Mixed cellularly bronchogenic cancers can occur and may explain the adenocarcinoma obtained on needle aspirate.

It is important to exclude distant metastatic disease by imaging the most common sites of bronchogenic metasta-

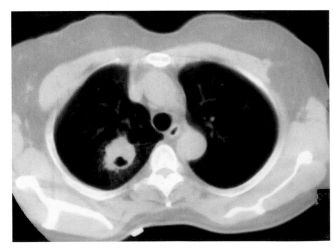

FIG. 144–2. CT scan of the upper chest showing a cavitated mass in the right upper lobe with a markedly irregular wall as well as multiple small stellate extensions from the main mass into surrounding lung parenchyma. This latter finding is more consistent with a primary lung neoplasm.

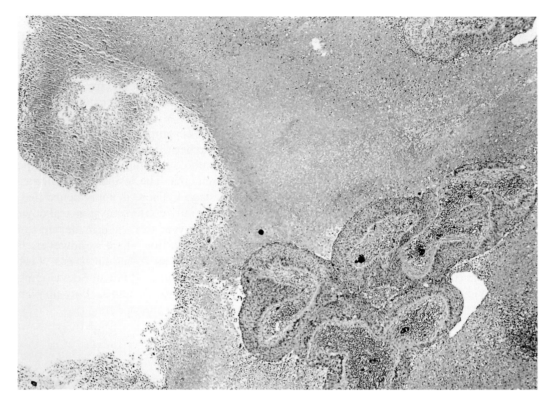

FIG. 144–3. Low-power appearance of the tumor showing central necrosis and cavitation with peripheral islands of viable carcinoma in the right lower quadrant of the photograph.

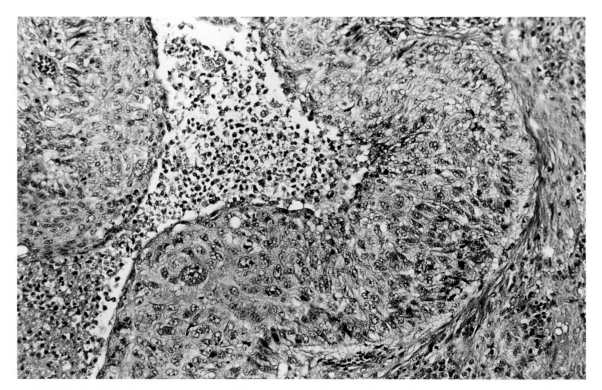

FIG. 144–4. High-power appearance of the tumor showing moderately differentiated squamous cell carcinoma.

sis (i.e., liver, adrenal, bone, and brain). A physiologic assessment of gas exchange and pulmonary function indicates that the patient will easily tolerate lobectomy, the most limited procedure likely to achieve complete resection. To summarize the preoperative investigation, it appears that the patient is relatively fit and has synchronous and favorable prostatic and non–small-cell lung cancers.

Survival in such a patient is determined by the presence of metastatic disease in regional nodes. Patients without metastatic disease have an excellent long-term survival after complete resection. Survival is reduced by 50% in patients having metastatic disease in bronchopulmonary or hilar lymph nodes (N1 disease). Ipsilateral mediastinal nodal metastasis (N2 disease) is associated with a marked reduction in long-term survival, with only 5% to 15% of patients surviving 5 years after resection. Contralateral mediastinal or supraclavicular nodal metastasis (N3 disease) indicates a lesion that cannot be completely resected and is therefore incurable.

Controversy exists regarding the importance of preresection surgical staging of the mediastinum by mediastinoscopy. We have previously reported the accuracy of mediastinoscopy to exceed CT scanning (2) and as a result use this strategy routinely. However, other authors as well as Dr. Martini have argued that the incidence of false-negative CT scans is low, particularly for squamous cancers. Therefore, although I would have performed a mediastinoscopy in this patient, a solid argument can be made for avoiding mediastinoscopy as long as a detailed node dissection at the time of resection was performed in this particular patient.

Without metastatic disease in the mediastinal nodes, the likelihood of a complete resection and cure is high. Therefore, neoadjuvant therapy is not required.

Complete excision by lobectomy is the standard operative procedure. A lesser resection by wedge or segmental resection is accompanied by an increased incidence of local recurrence (3) and decreased survival.

Final pathologic study reveals, as expected, a squamous carcinoma. The lesion is pathologically staged T2 N0 M0, stage I. There is no evidence that postoperative adjuvant therapy confers any survival advantage in these patients. Five-year survival is in the range of 70%, as indicated by Dr. Martini. There is, however, an incidence of distant as well as local metastasis. Furthermore, this patient is at an increased risk of developing a second primary. For these reasons, the follow-up plan posed for the patient is entirely appropriate.

REFERENCES

1. Todd TRJ, Weisbrod G, Tao LC, et al. Aspiration needle biopsy of thoracic lesions. *Ann Thorac Surg* 1981;32:154–61.
2. Patterson GA, Ginsberg RJ, Poon PY, et al. Prospective evaluation of magnetic resonance imaging, computed tomography, and mediastinoscopy in the preoperative assessment of mediastinal node status in bronchogenic carcinoma. *J Thorac Cardiovasc Surg* 1987;94:679–84.
3. Moores DWO, Miller SJ Jr, McKneally MF. *Current Problems in Surgery - Lung Cancer: A Surgeon's Approach*, volume XXIV, no. 11. Chicago: Year Book Medical Publishers; 1987.

145

Refractory Malignant Pleural Effusion

Willard A. Fry

*Limited parietal pleurectomy via video-assisted thoracic
surgery proved to be a good option*

CASE PRESENTATION

The patient is a 61-year-old woman who is a nursing educator. She developed cough and shortness of breath that caused her to consult her internist, who found her to be in good general condition but with findings of pleural effusion. A chest radiograph was obtained that demonstrated the effusion (Fig. 145–1). The patient's past history was unremarkable except for an extensive travel history. She had never used tobacco. She was nulliparous. She was active and had sustained no weight loss. Routine blood counts and chemistries were within normal limits. A diagnostic thoracocentesis was performed. The fluid was bloody and positive for adenocarcinoma with signet-ring features. Possible sites of origin mentioned were ovary, gastrointestinal tract, and breast. Evaluation of the gastrointestinal tract and pelvis was normal. A mammogram was normal.

The patient was seen by a thoracic surgeon, who believed that control of the pleural space was important for symptom control; and a tube thoracostomy was performed with complete re-expansion of the lung (Fig. 145–2). Doxycycline 500 mg was instilled into the pleural space the next day, and the tube was removed 2 days later, when the 24-hour pleural fluid drainage was less than 50 cc.

The patient was seen in consultation by a medical oncologist, who recommended chemotherapy with carboplatin and VP-16, to which the patient agreed. Initially, the chest radiographic picture was stable. However, 8

months after the chest tube therapy, she began to note increasing dyspnea and cough, and there was a change in the chest film, suggesting an increasing effusion (Fig. 145–3). Because of the previous attempt to obtain pleural symphysis, a computed tomogram (CT) of the chest was done to evaluate the amount of fluid and to evaluate the amount of loculation (Fig. 145–4). Because the patient's performance status was deteriorating because of her respiratory symptoms, her case was presented to the Tumor Board.

Several members of the board feel that the lung should also be considered as a possible primary source. Various options were listed, such as intermittent thoracocentesis, repeat tube thoracostomy with repeat instillation of a pleural irritant, insertion of a pleuroperitoneal shunt (Denver shunt), and parietal pleurectomy. There was a consensus that the anticipated life expectancy was not long enough to warrant parietal pleurectomy, as it probably would also require a major decortication based on the CT findings. Because fluid accumulation seemed loculated and focal, the possibility of doing a limited pleurectomy by thoracoscopy or video-assisted thoracic surgery (VATS) was entertained and so recommended to the patient, who accepted. It was felt that a Denver shunt could be held as a back-up or an "easy out" if the VATS would not allow for an easy and quick pleurectomy with re-expansion of the lung.

The VATS procedure went well, and it was possible to strip off the parietal pleura locally and gain lung re-expansion. The medical oncologist felt obligated to continue the

743

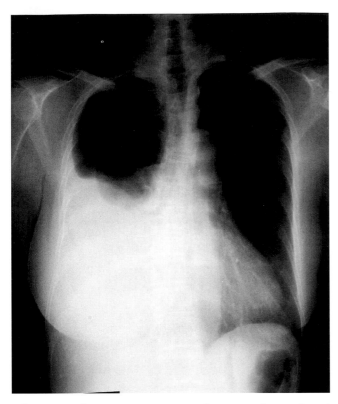

FIG. 145–1. Chest roentgenogram demonstrating a pleural effusion. Thoracocentesis procured bloody fluid positive for adenocarcinoma.

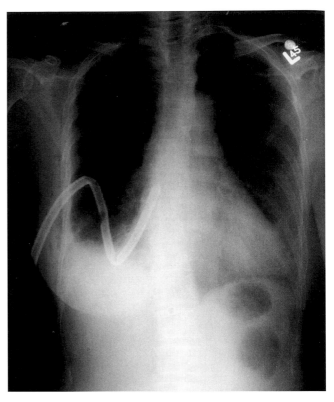

FIG. 145–2. Chest roentgenogram after tube thoracostomy. The lung is completely re-expanded. A rubber tube is used in preference to plastic because rubber is more irritating to the pleural surfaces and is felt to promote adhesions.

chemotherapy. Her respiratory symptoms were somewhat relieved by the VATS, but she continued to lose weight and strength and was planning to make a trip home to see her elderly mother. The time interval from the original presentation to now is 11 months. A chest film (Fig. 145–5) showed diffuse bilateral lung changes—presumed to be cancer. The medical oncologist is considering offering taxol therapy to the patient. A CT taken at this time again shows a focal accumulation of the malignant effusion. The thoracic surgeon thinks that the patient should be placed on a hospice program.

COMMENTARY by Michael Burt

This case report documents the morbidity associated with a malignant pleural effusion and the difficulty in management after tube thoracostomy with chemical pleurodesis fails. The percentage of pleural effusions that are determined to be secondary to malignancy has been reported to range from 10% to 50% in various series. The largest reported series found that of 5,888 pleural fluid specimens, 584 were malignant (10%)(1). The diagnosis of a malignant pleural effusion can usually be made by pleural fluid cytology and/or pleural biopsy. In the series of Salyer et al., the combination of

cytology and pleural biopsy established the diagnosis of malignancy in 90% of patients (2). For patients with suspected, but unproven, malignant pleural effusion, thoracoscopy plays an important role. In the series of Boutin, of 150 malignant pleural effusions not diagnosed by cytology or biopsy, thoracoscopy yielded a diagnosis of malignancy in 131 (87%) (3).

Malignant pleural effusions are a significant cause of morbidity, with very few, if any, patients totally asymptomatic. Since most patients (exceptions: lymphoma and germ cell carcinoma) with malignant pleural effusions are incurable, the objective is palliation of symptoms. Initially, therapeutic thoracentesis may be performed, but the effusion will usually accumulate quickly.

The treatment of patients with malignant pleural effusions ranges from observation, usually in patients with a life expectancy measured in weeks, to thoracotomy with pleurectomy. Most patients presenting with a new malignant pleural effusion requiring treatment are treated with tube thoracostomy, followed by instillation of sclerosing or antineoplastic agents. An excellent review of the literature by Austin and Flye (4) evaluated the results of treatment of malignant pleural effusions in 1,950 patients (89 articles). A summary of this report is listed in Table 145–1. All sclerosing and antineoplastic agents were instilled intrapleurally after tube thoracostomy; talc pon-

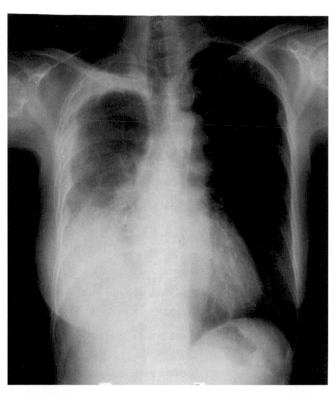

FIG. 145–3. Chest roentgenogram 8 months after the treatment shows re-accumulation of fluid.

drage and pleurectomy required general anesthesia. As is evident from the results listed in Table 145–1, the efficacy, defined as no recurrence of effusion in 1 month, ranged from 46% to 99%, with an overall efficacy of 63% in 1,950 patients. Although pleurectomy appears to be the gold standard by which other treatments are compared, less invasive methods are indicated before considering pleurectomy, with its associated 9% postoperative mortality (5).

Over the past 20 years, intrapleural tetracycline (after tube thoracostomy) emerged as the most common treatment of malignant pleural effusions for reasons that are not well documented in the literature but probably reflect less pain and fever compared with other agents (6). Bleomycin has also been used for treatment of malignant pleural effusions and some prefer it because there is little or no pain on intrapleural instillations. One randomized trial comparing intrapleural tetracycline with bleomycin suggested that bleomycin was more effective (7).

Currently, tetracycline is no longer available, and investigators have evaluated doxycycline or talc suspension as a substitute. One study evaluated 27 patients with malignant pleural effusions treated by tube thoracostomy and instillation of doxycycline and found it to be effective in 78% of patients (8). Another study evaluated a 5-g suspension of talc instilled intrapleurally by tube thoracos-

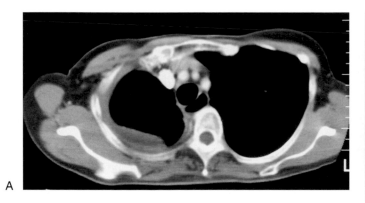

A

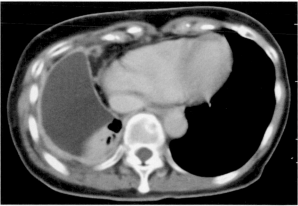

B

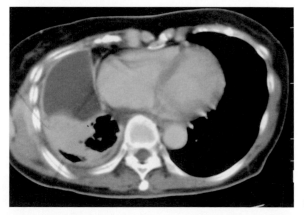

C

FIG. 145–4. A,B,C: CT confirms the recurrence of fluid and demonstrates focal loculation.

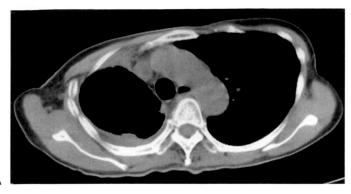
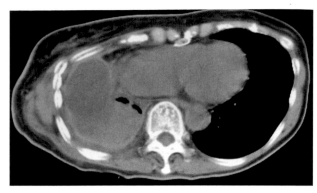

FIG. 145–5. A,B: CT obtained 11 months after initial diagnosis and 3 months after VATS. There is a persistent effusion.

tomy in 28 patients (9). The patients were followed for 1 to 21 months with no recurrence of pleural effusion. From these data and other studies, the treatment of a newly diagnosed malignant pleural effusion at our institution has been intrapleural instillation of talc suspension by tube thoracostomy.

Investigators have also evaluated pleuroperitoneal shunting in patients with malignant pleural effusions. Little et al. reported good to excellent results in 79% of 14 patients, with no documentation of peritoneal seeding, with a median survival of 4 months (10).

The patient described in this case report had satisfactory palliation of her malignant pleural effusion for 8 months by tube thoracostomy with instillation of doxycycline, but then recurred with a large loculated effusion. Tube thoracostomy could have been attempted, but the predicted success was very low. In this situation, decorti-

cation was contemplated because the chance of finding a trapped lung was high. The use of video thoracoscopy in place of thoracotomy was chosen and success achieved.

In summary, for patients with a newly diagnosed malignant pleural effusion, palliation of symptoms can be achieved in most patients by tube thoracostomy and intrapleural instillation of talc suspension, bleomycin, or doxycycline. Early recurrences are best treated by thoracoscopy and talc pondrage. Late recurrences should be considered for decortication/pleurectomy by open or VAT technique if the predicted survival is measured in months.

REFERENCES

1. Johnston WW. The malignant pleural effusion: a review of cytopathologic diagnoses of 584 specimens from 472 consecutive patients. *Cancer* 1985;56:905–9.
2. Salyer WR, Eggleston JC, Erozan YS. Efficacy of pleural needle biopsy and pleural fluid cytopathology in the diagnosis of malignant neoplasm involving the pleura. *Chest* 1975;67:536–45.
3. Boutin C, Viallat JR, Cargnino P, Farisse P. Thoracoscopy in malignant pleural effusions. *Am Rev Respir Dis* 1981;124:558–92.
4. Austin EH, Flye MW. The treatment of recurrent malignant pleural effusion. *Ann Thorac Surg* 1979;28:190–203.
5. Martini N, Bains MS, Beattie EJ Jr. Indications for pleurectomy in malignant effusion. *Cancer* 1975;35:734–8.
6. Bayly TC, Kisner DL, Sybert A, MacDonald JS, et al. Tetracycline and quinacrine in the control of malignant pleural effusions: a randomized trial. *Cancer* 1978;41:1188–92.
7. Ruckdeschel JC, Moores D, Lee JY, Einhorn LH, et al. Intrapleural therapy for malignant pleural effusions: a randomized comparison of bleomycin and tetracycline. *Chest* 1991;100:1528–35.
8. Heffner JE, Standerfer RJ, Torstveit J, Unruh L. Clinical efficacy of doxycycline for pleurodesis. *Chest* 1994;105:1743–7.
9. Webb WR, Ozmen V, Moulder PV, Shabahang B, Breaux J. Iodized talc pleurodesis for the treatment of pleural effusions. *J Thorac Cardiovasc Surg* 1992;103:881–6.
10. Little AG, Kadowaki MH, Ferguson MK, Staszek VM, Skinner DB. Pleuro-peritoneal shunting: alternative therapy for pleural effusions. *Ann Surg* 1988;208:443–51.

TABLE 145-1. *Efficacy of various treatments in patients with a malignant pleural effusion*[a]

Technique	N	Effective (%)
Thio-TEPA	39	46
Nitrogen mustard	338	52
Chest tube alone	69	55
Radioisotopes	980	55
5-Fluorouracil	35	66
Quinacrine	128	80
Tetracycline	31	87
Bleomycin	19	90
Talc suspension	59	90
Talc pondrage	105	92
Pleurectomy	147	99
Total	1,950	63

[a]Adapted from ref. 4.

146

Pathologic Fracture in Metastatic Breast Cancer

Frank J. Cummings

*Long-term survival and palliation were possible with
Tamoxifen, internal fixation, and radiation therapies*

CASE PRESENTATION

G.R. is a 77-year-old Caucasian woman who was admitted to the hospital with a chief complaint of acute severe pain in the right hip, suddenly noted while climbing stairs at home. She was unable to bear weight thereafter. Her past medical history was significant for a T2 N0 M0, stage IIA carcinoma of the breast treated with a modified radical mastectomy (Fig. 146-1). No adjuvant postoperative therapy was given. Estrogen receptors were highly positive at 165 fmols/mg cytosol protein. Progesterone receptors were negative.

The initial radiograph of the pelvis done in the emergency room showed a pathologic fracture of the right femoral neck in the area of a lytic lesion (Fig. 146-2). The orthopedic service was consulted. Internal fixation of the fracture was accomplished the day after admission, and the postoperative course was uneventful.

TUMOR BOARD DISCUSSION

Five years before sustaining the pathologic fracture, the patient had reported to her family physician that she noticed pain in the right thigh when walking. This was initially treated by rest and acetaminophen, but the pain progressed. Despite negative physical examinations, a bone scan was ordered, which revealed multiple areas of abnormal uptake.

The medical oncologist's initial assessment revealed no positive physical findings. A chest radiograph was ordered and was normal. Bone roentgenograms demonstrated lytic lesions of the skull, thoracic vertebrae, pelvis, and right femur. The CEA was elevated at 15 ng/mL. A complete blood count, liver function studies, and serum calcium were normal.

The patient was started on tamoxifen, 10 mg b.i.d., and tolerated it well for 3 weeks but then started to have increased pain that required narcotics for relief. The patient was re-evaluated and a repeat bone scan and serum calcium was done. The bone scan demonstrated progression and the serum calcium was 12.5 mg%. It was unclear at this point whether this represented rapidly progressive disease or a flare response to the initiation of hormonal therapy. The patient was managed with pain relief and the hypercalcemia treated with hydration and forced diuresis. When the patient became ambulatory, the calcium did not normalize, and biphosphonate was started. Over the course of the next 6 weeks there was gradual improvement. Her continued improvement suggested that the worsening of the osseous metastases and hypercalcemia represented a flare reaction.

The patient continued on tamoxifen after internal fixation and radiation therapy to the pathologic fracture. The patient experienced mild aching in the hips and back, aggravated by ambulation. A repeat bone scan showed multiple increased uptake in the spine, ribs, pelvis, and femur (Fig. 146–3).

The Tumor Board recommended that tamoxifen be discontinued and the patient observed for a withdrawal response. Given the long initial disease-free interval and

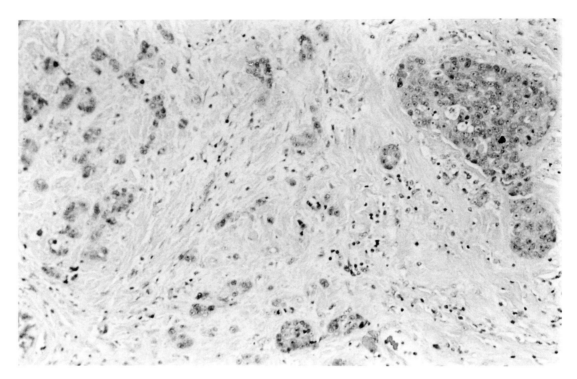

FIG. 146–1. Infiltrating and in situ ductal carcinoma of the breast.

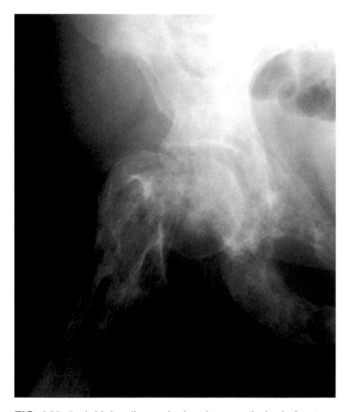

FIG. 146–2. Initial radiograph showing a pathologic fracture of the right femoral neck in the area of a lytic lesion.

subsequent response to tamoxifen after a flare reaction, there is a reasonable chance for obtaining another response from simply withdrawing the tamoxifen. Based on the patient's clinical course over the next 2 to 3 months, another decision will be made to continue the patient with no treatment until further progression, to start a different hormone, or to begin chemotherapy. Without visceral or life-threatening metastases, this approach appears to be justifiable. If the patient were to require chemotherapy, cytoxen, methotrexate, and 5-fluorouracil could be considered, or entry into a clinical trial evaluating the efficacy of newer agents in elderly women could be considered.

COMMENTARY by James D. Cox

The management of women with adenocarcinoma of the breast, especially in the setting of advancing age, allows many opportunities for reflection. The management of G.R., now 77 years old, 13 years after initial diagnosis of cancer of the breast, is a good example. Her care was thoughtful and quite effective.

At the age of 72, 8 years after her initial diagnosis, she began to have pain in the right thigh when walking. The roentgenograms of the bones revealed multiple lytic lesions including one or more in the right femur—the site of her pain. Treatment with tamoxifen was effective, although the early course of hormonal alteration was complicated by increased pain and hypercalcemia. From

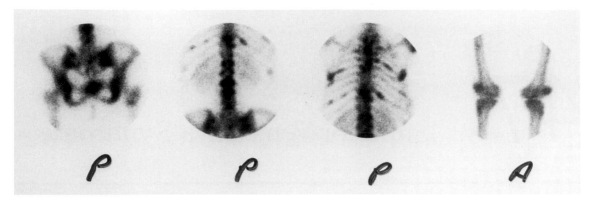

FIG. 146–3. Repeat bone scan showing areas of increased uptake in the spine, ribs, pelvis, and femur.

the time when a lytic process in the femur was first identified until the pathologic fracture of her right femoral neck 5 years later, one reasonably could have considered the use of radiation therapy to the proximal femur. In principle, it could have been particularly effective during the flare response to tamoxifen. Through the retrospectoscope, the most compelling time to have considered irradiation of the proximal right femur was the point in the recent past when she began to have increased discomfort and evidence of increased uptake on bone scan showing in multiple areas, including the femur. A course of irradiation lasting no more than 2 or 3 weeks might have retarded the lytic process in the right femur sufficiently to have avoided or delayed the pathologic fracture.

Irradiation of major weight-bearing bones in the absence of pain is one of the few legitimate undertakings in the dubious area of "prophylactic palliation." The role of irradiation in a patient with metastatic disease is confined to the relief of specific localized symptoms. When there are no symptoms, there is no justification for palliation. Irradiation of a weight-bearing bone is the one important exception to this rule. When the pain actually reappeared a month or so before the fracture, there was justification for consideration of irradiation to at least the proximal right femur. The current plan for irradiation after internal fixation is standard management.

Since the time of first recognition of distant metastasis in this lady, the management of her disseminated disease has appropriately been the primary focus. Some patients with this evolution of cancer of the breast can be treated effectively by repeated, brief courses of radiation therapy to areas of maximum discomfort. Because this elderly lady has now shown progression on tamoxifen, and the alternative is combination chemotherapy, which may be poorly tolerated by her bone marrow, reliance on such brief courses of treatment with radiation therapy could be a very important part of her care.

The addition of the bone-seeking radionucleid strontium-89 may improve the patient's quality of life by reduction of pain and also provide a reduction of costs.

SELECTED READINGS

1. Blitzer PH. Re-analysis of the RTOG study of the palliation of symptomatic osseous metastasis. *Cancer* 1985;55:1468–72.
2. Perez C, Bradield JS, Morgan HC. Management of pathologic fractures. *Cancer* 1972;29(3):684–93.
3. Porter AT, McEwan AJB. Strontium-89 as an adjuvant to external beam radiation improves pain relief and delays disease progression in advanced prostate cancer: results of a randomized controlled trial. *Semin Oncol* 1993;20(3)(suppl. 2):44–48.
4. Tong D, Gilick L, Hendrickson FR. The palliation of symptomatic osseous metastases. *Cancer* 1982;50(5):893–9.

147

Superior Vena Cava Syndrome

Ritsuko Komaki, Carmelita P. Escalante, and C.H. Carrasco

Is there a role for thrombolytic agents with a stent insertion?

CASE PRESENTATION

A 71-year-old man was admitted to the hospital with mediastinal, subcarinal, and paratracheal lymphadenopathy and right pleural effusion viewed on radiographs and computed tomography (CT) of the chest. He was well until 10 days earlier, when he noted difficulty in buttoning his shirt collar. He also noted facial erythema, edema, and a decrease in stamina and appetite. After admission, fine-needle aspiration of the mediastinal mass revealed poorly differentiated adenocarcinoma of the lung AJCC stage IIIB (T1 N3 M0). Radiation therapy was begun as initial treatment for superior vena cava syndrome (SVCS). He received 3 Gy in one fraction to the anterior mediastinum by Co^{60} external beam. Two days later he received 2 Gy daily for 5 consecutive days by using anteroposterior fields from the Co^{60}. He was then transferred to The University of Texas M.D. Anderson Cancer Center (MDACC) because of progression of facial and neck edema.

On arrival, he again noted the above symptoms, as well as dysphagia. His past medical history included hypertension and chronic atrial fibrillation first documented 15 years before admission, when he had an embolic stroke. His usual medications included warfarin sodium 5 mg daily, digoxin 0.25 mg daily, prazosin 2 mg twice daily, atenolol 50 mg daily, and ranitidine 150 mg twice daily. Furosemide 20 mg daily, dexamethasone 4 mg every 6 hours, and a potassium supplement were added to his medications before transfer.

Upon examination, his temperature was 37.9°C, blood pressure 152/90 mm Hg, pulse 90 per minute and irregular, and respiration 20 per minute. He was a tall, heavyset man with significant facial and neck edema and accompanying facial erythema. The supraclavicular fossae were full, and jugular venous distention to the mandible was noted. No adenopathy was appreciated. The lungs had decreased breath sounds in both bases, with dullness to percussion greater on the right. The heart had an irregularity. Abdominal examination was unremarkable; the liver and spleen were not palpated. His stools tested negative for occult blood, and he had an enlarged smooth prostate. The genitalia were normal. There was no peripheral edema, clubbing, or evidence of arthritis. Neurologic examination was unremarkable.

The hematocrit was 40.1%; the white cell count was 11,500 with 88% neutrophils, 6% lymphocytes, and 6% monocytes. The platelet count was 171,000. The prothrombin time was 11.4 s and partial thromboplastin time 24.4 s. Sodium was 132 mmol/L, potassium 4.1 mmol/L, chloride 97 mmol/L, and carbon dioxide 28 mmol/L. Lactic dehydrogenase was 226 IU, and blood urea nitrogen 32 mmol/L. The remainder of his biochemical survey was normal. A chest radiograph disclosed a right paratracheal azygos mass, a nodular density in the right upper lobe, and a right pleural effusion. Computed tomograms of the chest and abdomen revealed subcarinal and paratracheal adenopathy and a small peripheral lesion in the right upper lobe with bilateral pleural effusion, but no abnormalities in the abdomen.

An electrocardiogram revealed atrial fibrillation with a rate of 72 per minute. Echocardiogram revealed an ejection fraction of 78%; no pericardial effusion or thrombi within the atria or ventricles were noted. CTs of the brain showed a hypodensity in the left corona radiata compatible with a previous infarct; no metastatic disease was noted. A bone scan revealed an abnormal midthoracic spine and a focal area of abnormal tracer in the shaft of the right femur. Subsequent films of these areas revealed no abnormalities.

The cytology of the mediastinal mass was reviewed at MDACC and the patient was diagnosed with SVCS secondary to adenocarcinoma of the lung, and aggressive radiotherapy was instituted.

External radiotherapy was initiated using a "T"-shaped field to encompass bilateral supraclavicular and mediastinal nodes. Anteroposterior fields were used and the dose at the central axial midplane was 3.5 Gy from a linear accelerator 6 MV photon beam, which was given on days 1 and 2. He then received 2 Gy per fraction twice daily with 5 hours interfraction interval on days 3 and 4, followed by 2 Gy once daily on days 5 through 7 with improvement of his facial and neck edema. On the fifth hospital day, thoracentesis was performed and revealed fluid compatible with a transudate. Microscopic examination failed to reveal malignant cells. Before the thoracentesis, his daily warfarin sodium 5 mg was discontinued to prevent hemorrhage. Sixteen hours after the thoracentesis, on the sixth hospital day, he worsened acutely and complained of dysphagia. Examination revealed increasing facial and neck edema as well as upper extremity cyanosis (Fig. 147–1). The chest

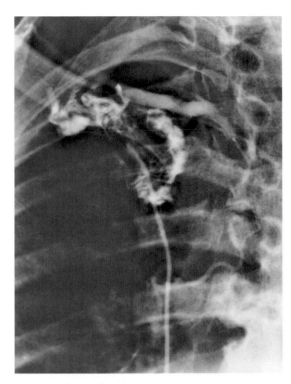

FIG. 147–2. Thrombosis located above the superior vena cava occlusion and extending to the subclavian vein.

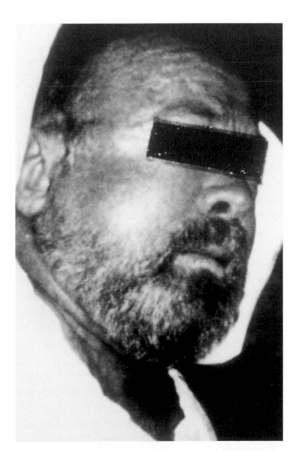

FIG. 147–1. Patient with increasing facial and neck edema and erythema.

radiograph showed no remarkable change. A venogram was performed with the intent of placing an expandable metallic stent in hopes of increasing the patency of the vena cava. However, thrombosis above the site of the superior vena cava occlusion was noted and extended bilaterally to the subclavian veins (Fig. 147–2). Ten mg of tissue plasminogen activator (t-PA) was administered intravenously via a right femoral catheter approach followed by 50 mg of t-PA over the next hour. Forty mg of t-PA was given over the subsequent 2 hours. A second venogram showed a reduced amount of residual clot but total thrombolysis had not been achieved. With the patient's informed consent, another 50 mg of t-PA was administered, with resolution of the thrombosis 4.5 hours after the initial injection of t-PA (Fig. 147–3). A "Z" double stent was inserted into the site of obstruction of the superior vena cava after thrombolysis with t-PA (Fig. 147–4). The stent did not open the stenotic segment, but the patient noted an immediate decrease in the pressure sensation in his head and neck. He was begun on an intravenous infusion of heparin to maintain his partial thromboplastin time at 60 seconds. On the third day after the procedure, his facial congestion was entirely resolved, and his wife felt that his face looked normal.

On the 13th hospital day, the patient developed visual blurriness and a CT of the brain revealed increased attenuation in the right occipital lobe compatible with a hemorrhagic infarct. A neurologic consultant felt that

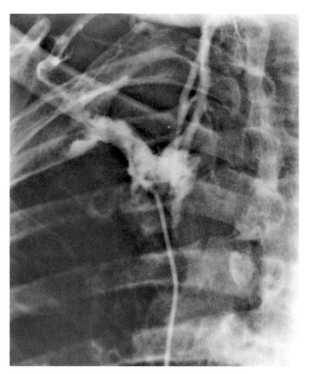

FIG. 147–3. Resolution of thrombosis 4.5 hours after the initial injection of t-PA.

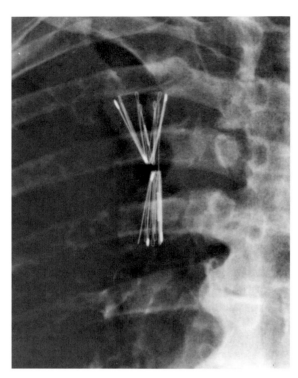

FIG. 147–4. An M.D. Anderson prototype "Z" double stent inserted into the site of obstruction of the superior vena cava next thrombolysis with t-PA.

this was unrelated to his prior thrombolytic therapy and most likely secondary to an embolic event. Anticoagulants were discontinued and his symptoms rapidly recurred. The patient expired the next day. His cause of death was attributed to superior vena cava obstruction secondary to adenocarcinoma of the lung.

TUMOR BOARD DISCUSSION

Patients who have SVCS may develop thrombosis superimposed on extrinsic compression. Thrombosis and thromboembolic events frequently complicate superior vena cava obstruction and a role for venography and anticoagulation therapy exists. Our case supports suggestions that randomized prospective trials be conducted. Tissue plasminogen activator may be useful as a thrombolytic agent in the treatment of superior vena cava syndrome complicated by thromboembolic events. Future clinical trials should help to define the role of thrombolytic, antiplatelet, and anticoagulation therapy in the evaluation and treatment of SVCS.

Patients with SVCS may develop thrombosis superimposed on extrinsic compression. Tissue plasminogen activator produced successful clot dissolution and may become a useful thrombolytic agent in treating SVCS that has associated thromboembolic events. Clinical trials should be conducted to help define the role of thrombolytic agents in the treatment of SVCS.

SELECTED READINGS

1. Marder VJ, Sherry S. Thrombolytic therapy: current status. *N Engl J Med* 1988;318:1512–20.
2. Adelstein DJ, Hines KD, Carter SG, Sacco C. Thromboembolic events in patients with malignant superior vena cava syndrome and the role of anticoagulation. *Cancer* 1988;62:2258–62.
3. Gaines P, Belli A, Anderson P, et al. Superior vena cava obstruction managed by the Gianturco Z stent. *Clin Radiol* 1994;49:202–6.

COMMENTARY by Lawrence R. Coia

Many of the difficult challenges in the evaluation and management of superior vena cava syndrome are apparent in the case presented by Komaki et al. Briefly summarizing, a 71-year-old man presented at an outside hospital with classic symptoms of SVCS, was found to have stage IIIB adenocarcinoma of the lung, and developed progressive symptoms despite thoracic irradiation, diuretics, and corticosteroid administration. (He was also taking warfarin for atrial fibrillation.) Upon transfer to M.D. Anderson Cancer Center, he received accelerated hyperfractionated radiation with some improvement. However, the patient's symptoms worsened after warfarin was discontinued in order to perform a thoracentesis. A venogram revealed thrombosis extending bilaterally to the subclavian veins. Tissue plasminogen activator was administered, a "Z" double stent was inserted, and intravenous heparin instituted with resolution of facial edema. Unfortunately, the patient developed a right occipital lobe hemorrhagic infarct and expired after thrombolytics were discontinued. In conclusion, Komaki et al. suggest that because thrombosis frequently complicates SVCS, trials to help define the role of thrombolytic agents in the treatment of SVCS should be conducted. In addition to the role of thrombolytics in SVCS, this commentary will briefly review some of the other challenges presented in SVCS management, such as the appropriate extent of evaluation, the use of radiation, and the value of stenting.

Although diagnosis of SVCS is usually apparent without extensive diagnostic testing, it is important to establish the etiology of SVCS to optimize the therapeutic approach. Common symptoms of SVCS and their appropriate incidence include dyspnea (>50%), facial swelling (43%), upper extremity and truncal swelling (40%), and chest pain, cough, and dyspnea (20% each) (1). On exam, most patients will have neck or thoracic vein distention or facial edema. About 20% to 25% will have a right pleural effusion. Less than 20% of patients presenting with SVCS have a nonmalignant primary pathologic diagnosis. The two major categories of malignancy causing SVCS are lung cancer (67%) and lymphoma (14%), with sarcomas, germ cell tumors, and metastatic carcinoma comprising a relatively small percentage of cases (1–4). Tumor tissue should be obtained from the most accessible site before initiation of therapy unless emergency treatment is required for life-threatening symptoms such as cerebral edema with impending herniation, or laryngeal edema with stridor (5). The chest radiograph may suffice to allow initiation of treatment; however, after pathologic diagnosis has been made, additional tests should be performed to adequately stage the patient's malignancy. An unresolved question is the need for venogram in a patient with malignancy causing SVCS. Because thrombosis is present in a third to one half of the cases, and venography is superior to most other imaging techniques in assessing the presence of thrombosis, this question is worthy of further examination (2,6). The risks of venography include bleeding at the puncture site, and this risk may be increased if the patient is taking anticoagulants, as was the circumstance in the case presented.

The primary management of SVCS due to malignancy is radiation for most solid tumors, particularly non–small-cell lung cancer, whereas chemotherapy is usually recommended as initial treatment for small-cell lung cancer and lymphoma (3,4,7). Radiation results in excellent symptomatic relief in approximately 70% to 90% of patients treated. One study indicated that initial high-dose radiation therapy (3–4 Gy daily for three fractions) yielded good symptomatic relief in less than 2 weeks in 70% of patients, whereas conventional dose radiation (2 Gy daily) yielded the same response in 56% of patients (p=0.09) (7). In another study, the use of large 8-Gy fractions twice or three times weekly to 24 Gy were compared, and the more rapid fractionation was felt to be superior (96% vs. 70% response) (8). Another means for delivery of a high radia-

tion dose in a relatively short period of time is to deliver multiple daily fractions, as was done for this patient during part of his treatment. Survival for patients with non–small-cell lung cancer treated with radiation alone is 15% to 20% at 1 year (7). Thus far, combinations of chemotherapy and radiation have not been shown to improve response rate or degree of symptomatic relief in patients with SVCS. Only 10% to 15% have no response to radiation or recurrence of symptoms. The most common side effect of radiation for SVCS is dysphagia due to radiation esophagitis.

The safety and efficacy of thrombolytic therapy for SVCS continues to be evaluated (9). More rapid clinical improvement has been suggested using fibrinolytic drugs in addition to radiation (10). Gray et al. found superior results with urokinase over streptokinase, with the use of a central venous catheter over no catheter, and when symptoms were of short, that is, less than a 5-day duration (9). The successful use of recombinant tissue type plasminogen activator (rt-PA) for the treatment of thrombosis due to malignant and nonmalignant causes has been reported (11,12). The risk of major hemorrhage from rt-PA increases with doses over 100 mg. Because thrombosis does not occur in most patients with SVC obstruction, and only 10% to 20% of irradiated patients fail to respond to radiation, routine administration of thrombolytic treatment for patients with SVC obstruction is not currently recommended. One possible clinical trial design to test the value of thrombolytics in SVC obstruction due to malignancy would be to randomize only those patients with thrombosis on venogram to radiation or chemotherapy versus radiation or chemotherapy plus rt-PA.

The use of stents to manage superior vena cava obstruction not responding to conventional antineoplastic treatment is gaining acceptance (13). Immediate relief of symptoms in a high percentage of patients has been reported with intraluminal self-expanding Gianturco Z stents (14). The Wallstent endovascular prosthesis was effective in 15 of 17 patients in relieving SVC obstruction, most of whom failed to respond to initial treatment with chemotherapy or radiation or recurred after chemotherapy or radiation (15). Intraluminal stenting is a useful adjunct in the management of patients with refractory SVC obstruction (16).

In summary, SVC obstruction due to malignancy is infrequently a true emergency and therefore calls for careful evaluation and individualized treatment. Radiation given relatively rapidly with attention to potential late effects is the mainstay of treatment. Although thrombolytics would likely benefit a significant number of patients, its routine use is not currently recommended. Finally, stent placement should be considered in refractory cases.

REFERENCES

1. Perez C, Present C, Amburg A. Management of superior vena cava syndrome. *Semin Oncol* 1978;5:123–4.
2. Lokich J, Goodman R. Superior vena cava syndrome. *JAMA* 1975; 231:58–61.

3. Baker G, Barnes H. Superior vena cava syndrome: etiology, diagnosis and treatment. *Am J Crit Care* 1992;1:54–64.

4. Chen J, Bongard F, Klein S. A contemporary perspective on superior vena cava syndrome. *Am J Surg* 1990;160:207–11.

5. Escalante C. Causes and management of superior vena cava syndrome. *Oncology* 1993;7:61–8.

6. Standorf W, Doty D. The role of venography and surgery in the management of patients with superior vena cava obstruction. *Ann Thorac Surg* 1986;41:158–63.

7. Armstrong B, Perez C, Simpson J, et al. Role of irradiation in the management of superior vena cava syndrome. *Int J Radiat Oncol Biol Phys* 1987;13:513–9.

8. Rodrigues C, Njo K, Karim A. Hyperfractionated radiation therapy in the treatment of superior vena cava syndrome. *Lung Cancer* 1993;10:221–8.

9. Gray B, Olin J, Groor R, et al. Safety and efficacy of thrombolytic therapy for superior vena cava syndrome. *Chest* 1991;99:54–9.

10. Salsali M, Clifton E. Superior vena cava obstruction with carcinoma of the lung. *Surg Gynecol Obstet* 1965;121:783–8.

11. Imberti R, Albertario F, Bellinzona G, et al. Fibrinolytic (rt-PA) therapy for superior vena cava thrombosis in a multiple trauma patient. *Acta Anesthes Belgic* 1991;42:233–6.

12. Greenberg S, Kosinski R, Daniels J. Treatment of superior vena cava thrombosis with recombinant tissue type plasminogen activator. *Chest* 1991;99:1298–1301.

13. Ouderk M, Heystraten F, Stoter G. Stenting in malignancy vena caval obstruction. *Cancer* 1993;71:142–6.

14. Gaines P, Belli A, Anderson P, et al. Superior vena cava obstruction managed by the Gianturco Z stent. *Clin Radiol* 1994;49:202–6.

15. Dyet J, Nicholson A, Cook A. The use of the Wallstent endovascular prosthesis in the treatment of malignant obstruction of the superior vena cava. *Clin Radiol* 1993;48:381–5.

16. Kumar P, Good R. Need for invasive procedures in the management of superior vena cava syndrome. *J Natl Med Assoc* 1989;81:41–7.

148 Hypercalcemic Crisis

Raymond P. Warrell, Jr.

Immobilization of a patient with bone metastases is a cause
of hypercalcemia and needs urgent management

CASE PRESENTATION

A 42-year-old woman was admitted from the emergency room. Two years previously, she had undergone a lumpectomy with axillary node dissection and postoperative radiation for invasive carcinoma of the breast. The primary tumor was 4 cm in diameter, and 9 of 20 axillary lymph nodes were involved. The tumor was positive for both estrogen and progesterone receptors. The bone and liver-spleen scans were normal. She received six cycles of adjuvant chemotherapy consisting of cyclophosphamide, doxorubicin, and 5-fluorouracil (CAF). Fifteen months later she developed low back pain. Two small nodules were observed on the anterior chest wall, and biopsy of one of the nodules revealed poorly differentiated carcinoma. Radiographs at that time showed a mixture of lytic and blastic areas in the lumbar spine, pelvis, and femurs. She was placed on tamoxifen.

On the day of admission, she slipped while getting out of a car and fell to the curb, immediately experiencing acute severe pain in the right leg and pelvis. She was brought to the emergency room unable to walk. Examination showed marked limitation of motion in the right lower extremity. A radiograph revealed a fracture of the intertrochanteric region of the right femur; she was admitted to the Orthopedic Service and was scheduled for open reduction and internal fixation.

On examination, she was fully alert and oriented, complaining only of pain. Otolaryngologic exam was normal. The lungs were clear; the cardiac rhythm was regular, and there were no extra heart sounds or murmurs. Neither the liver nor the spleen were palpable, and there were no other masses or lymphadenopathy. The right lower extremity

was inverted with a markedly decreased range of motion. The neurologic exam was grossly normal. The remaining skin nodule on the anterior chest was located and was not believed to have changed in size.

The hemoglobin was 11.0 g/dL, the hematocrit was 32.3%, the red blood cell indices were normal, the total leukocyte count was 4,200/mL with a normal differential, and the platelet count was 145,000/mL. Serum electrolytes, calcium, uric acid, bilirubin, SGOT, phosphorus, creatinine, and blood urea nitrogen (BUN) were within normal limits. The alkaline phosphatase was elevated to twice the upper limit of normal. The electrocardiogram showed a normal sinus rhythm. The chest radiograph was normal. A skeletal survey showed diffuse lytic involvement of the cervical, thoracic, and lumbar spine, and mixed lytic and blastic disease in the skull, pelvis, humeri, and both femurs.

The following morning the patient complained of persistent pain, moderate nausea, and constipation, which were attributed to her narcotic analgesics. The analgesic was switched to methadone, but the nausea persisted and she vomited in bed on two occasions. After she spontaneously voided in bed, a urinary catheter was inserted. She slept soundly that evening but was noted to be lethargic the following morning. Her speech was slurred and she complained of weakness. A neurologic exam showed no focal deficits; however, she was noted to be easily confused, her attention span was limited, and she was not oriented to the current date. A computed tomography (CT) scan with contrast was ordered to rule out intracranial metastases; when performed late in the afternoon, no abnormalities were observed. She was seen by the anesthesia service that evening and the confusional state was again noted. A routine electrocardiogram was obtained, which showed prolongation of the QT interval with shortening of the PR interval and nonspecific ST-T wave changes. The surgery for the following morning was canceled. A complete set of blood work was again ordered. At 10 p.m., results of these tests showed a hemoglobin of 12 g/dL, hematocrit of 36%, creatinine of 1.7 mg/dL (nl, 0.6–1.3 mg/dL), calcium of 13.7 mg/dL (nl, 9.0–10.5 mg/dL), and phosphorus of 4.1 mg/dL (nl, 2.5–4.2). Intravenous fluids were started (5% dextrose in 0.45% saline at 100 cc/hr).

The following day she had persistent lethargy, weakness, and nausea, but her mental status was somewhat improved. Repeat blood chemistries that afternoon showed a calcium of 14.9 mg/dL, creatinine of 1.7 mg/dL, and BUN of 29 (nl, 6–20 mg/dL); the intravenous fluids were increased to 150 cc/hr and serum chemistry examinations were ordered to be repeated the following morning. She remained nauseated and vomited several times during the night; she was again noted to be intermittently confused and somnolent. By midmorning she was markedly lethargic and disoriented; review of the serum chemistry exam results from 6 a.m. showed a calcium of 19.2 mg/dL, BUN of 40, creatinine of 2.3 mg/dL, and phosphorus of 4.0 mg/dL. The intravenous fluid rate was then increased to 200 cc/hr, and the serum chemistry exams were repeated on a stat basis. The ward was called back on an emergency basis from the laboratory with a report that the serum calcium was 32.4 mg/dL.

At that point, the running intravenous fluid line was opened wide. Because of the extreme abnormalities, another blood sample was sent to recheck the chemistry values. A central venous catheter was also quickly inserted, and 1,000 cc of normal saline was infused over the next 35 minutes. Intake and output were strictly monitored. Salmon calcitonin was injected (8 IU/kg intramuscularly) and was ordered to be repeated every 6 hours for 3 days. The laboratory exam confirmed the previous blood result. The patient received another 1,000 cc of normal saline over the next hour, and the saline infusion was then run at 500 cc/hr for the next 6 hours. In addition, an infusion of gallium nitrate was started (200 mg/m^2 running in over 24 hours). Five hours later, the urine output showed 800 cc of concentrated urine excreted over the previous 5 hours despite infusion of 4,000 cc of saline. The serum chemistries were rechecked and showed a serum sodium of 142 mEq/L, chloride of 102 mEq/L, CO_2 of 22 mEq/L, potassium of 3.4 mEq/L, calcium of 19.2 mg/dL, creatinine of 2.0 mg/dL, and BUN of 30 mg/dL. The intravenous rate was reduced to 400 cc/hr, the gallium nitrate infusion was ordered to be continued for 5 full days, and the serum chemistries were ordered repeated every 6 hours for the next 48 hours. Fluid retention and weight gain were recognized on the following day and furosemide was then administered. Over the next several days, her serum calcium gradually decreased into the normal range.

By the time the serum calcium level became extremely elevated, the patient was comatose and responsive only to deep pain. Despite normalization of the serum calcium, little improvement in her mental status was observed. Moreover, after the initial normalization, her serum calcium again increased on several occasions and the patient was retreated with gallium nitrate and mithramycin. After a prolonged hospital stay that eventually included internal fixation of the hip, the patient was discharged from the hospital. Her sole antitumor therapy at that time was oral medroxyprogesterone. When seen 4 months later, she had persistent bone pain but was ambulatory and normocalcemic.

TUMOR BOARD DISCUSSION

This patient's case presents a number of features. The first concerns the differential diagnosis of hypercalcemia. In this case, a patient with a known cancer diagnosis is admitted to the hospital with a normal serum calcium; but over the course of several days, she develops unusually severe hypercalcemia with a peak serum calcium of 32.4 mg/dL. A number of diseases are associated with hypercalcemia; however, in a patient who has a known cancer diagnosis (especially with an acute onset), the most likely cause is the underlying cancer itself rather than some other condition. Hyperparathyroidism can occasionally present as a hypercalcemic crisis, and several authors had previously reported an increased association between hyperparathyroidism and breast cancer. However, the former condition is now most commonly diagnosed in asymptomatic patients by routine screening tests, and the association of the two diseases is probably fortuitous. In addition, the normal level of serum phosphorus in this case (usually low in primary hyperparathyroidism) strongly suggests another diagnosis. Granulomatous diseases such as sarcoidosis and tuberculosis almost never present with such extreme calcium elevations, and there are usually other signs suggestive of these diseases such as mediastinal lymphadenopathy. Patients with cancer are recognized to be at increased risk for developing a second primary tumor, and this patient had also received an alkylating agent and irradiation. However, most secondary cancers related to anticancer therapy are hematologic in origin; with the exception of multiple myeloma, these disorders are rarely associated with hypercalcemia. Unlike the ambulatory setting in which hyperparathyroidism predominates, in hospitalized patients with hypercalcemia who ultimately prove to have cancer, the diagnosis is usually obvious on admission or apparent after limited testing.

The oncologist caring for this patient believed that the tumor was relatively well controlled with tamoxifen, and a normal serum calcium was documented at the time of admission. Therefore, a second feature of this case is establishing the factors that may have contributed to such an acute severe deterioration. One obvious reason would be tumor progression. Clearly, the skeletal survey had worsened since the initial appearance of bone metastasis, but a signal skin lesion was unchanged. However, there are two additional factors that appear critical. The first is the complete immobilization of a previously ambulatory patient with bone metastases due to a pathologic fracture. Even in patients with no underlying pathology, immobilization can lead to rapid loss of bone mass and hypercalcemia. The second factor is the decrease in oral intake. Nausea and constipation are frequently associated with hypercalcemia, although in this case an initiating factor may also have been the narcotic analgesics. In any event, the cessation of oral fluid intake (due to nausea and mental impairment) and polyuria (due to obligate fluid losses from hyercalciuria) set in motion a vicious cycle of rapid dehydration, hemoconcentration, decreased renal perfusion, and a rapid rise in serum calcium. Almost certainly, the combination of these secondary factors (immobilization, polyuria, decreased fluid intake, and dehydration) rather than tumor progression accounted for the acute decompensation.

The third feature of this case is the approach to management of a hypercalcemic patient with an immediately life-threatening problem. Because hypercalcemia is universally accompanied by some degree of dehydration, oral or parenteral fluids constitute first aid for any patient whether in the hospital or the outpatient setting. The rate and route of hydration obviously depends on the extent of dehydration and severity of hypercalcemia. In the evolution of this case, even though the hypercalcemia was recognized at a relatively moderate level, the potential risks of the condition were underappreciated and the fluid therapy was obviously inadequate. Fortunately, furosemide was not administered early; this agent should be used only to manage the fluid status and not to treat the hypercalcemia itself because early or repetitive use can actually worsen dehydration and cause additional metabolic abnormalities. Another important feature is the simultaneous use of multiple drugs to treat the condition rather than single agents sequentially. Intravenous fluid, with or without furosemide, rarely normalizes the serum calcium in hospitalized patients with hypercalcemia; in addition, such treatment is frequently associated with undesirable side effects such as fluid overload, pulmonary edema, and marked swelling of the lower extremities. Therefore, except in very mild cases, most patients should receive additional treatment. In this case, calcitonin and gallium nitrate were used. Calcitonin has the advantage of a very rapid onset of action (within hours); other than nausea, it does not commonly produce serious adverse effects. Its major disadvantage is low potency. On the other hand, gallium nitrate is probably the most potent drug currently available to treat this condition. Like the biphosphonates,

such as pamidronate and alendronate, gallium nitrate's onset of action occurs after 24 to 48 hours. Thus, the combination with calcitonin is desirable in acute emergencies. The rapid early decline from the peak serum calcium level was almost certainly due to the use of large quantities of fluids plus calcitonin; the later effect to restore the calcium completely to normal was an effect of gallium nitrate. The most common side effect of gallium nitrate is hypophosphatemia, which is usually asymptomatic; the drug should not be given to patients with a significant degree of renal impairment (i.e., serum creatinine >3.0 mg/dL).

Fourth, although the recovery of this patient's mental status was quite slow, this feature should not be surprising given the marked elevation in serum calcium to a level where most patients would have succumbed. The alteration in mental status commonly takes days to clear even after the serum calcium has been normalized; thus, persistent abnormalities need not prompt a search for other causes. Finally, the subsequent response to hormonal control as an outpatient illustrates that cancer-related hypercalcemia is not universally a terminal condition. Many patients can benefit greatly from rapid intervention with potent drugs.

SELECTED READING

1. Warrell RP Jr. Metabolic emergencies. In *Cancer: principles and practice of oncology,* 4th ed, DeVita Jr VT, Hellman S, Rosenberg SA, eds. New York: JB Lippincott; 1993:2128–40.

COMMENTARY by B.J. Kennedy

This young woman initially had a pathologic stage IIB or IIIA breast cancer that, despite adjuvant chemotherapy, would have a very high chance for recurrence, which did occur 15 months later. With skin nodules and osseous metastases she was given tamoxifen. She was 42 years old when given adjuvant chemotherapy. At the time of recurrence, if she still had menses, bilateral oophorectomy would have been an appropriate treatment. The tamoxifen seems to have produced a stable state of her disease, but 9 months later when she is admitted with a fracture of the femur the skin nodule is still present but unchanged.

On admission to the hospital, she was completely immobilized and over 48 hours gradually developed progressive nausea, vomiting, lethargy, and increasing confusion. The serum calcium level increased to 13.7 and, despite intravenous fluids at a very low volume (100 cc per hour), she had increasing symptoms with progressive rise of the serum calcium to 32.4 mg/dL.

Progressive hypercalcemia is characterized by progressive nausea, vomiting, polyuria, polydipsia, lethargy, and coma. Death can result from the acute increase in serum calcium. The syndrome should be recognized in any person with bone metastases acutely immobilized. The management of patients requires correction of dehydration, enhancement of renal excretion of calcium, inhibition of bone resorption, as well as treating the basic disorder (in this case immobilization and bone metastases from breast cancer). The depleted intravascular volume must be restored to normal with 2.5 to 4.0 L of isotonic saline daily, but hydration alone rarely leads to normalization of the serum calcium concentrations in severe hypercalcemia. In addition to hydration, specific therapy is required to inhibit osteoclast-mediated bone resorption. Several agents are available.

Calcitonin is a rapid but short-acting agent and only moderately effective. In the patient described it should be used only while considering the value of other agents.

Gallium nitrate is effective for hypercalcemia of malignancy, and it requires daily administration for several days.

Plicamycin (mithramycin) is a good choice for treating hypercalcemia because it produces a rapid decrease in the serum calcium. It can be used if there is no hepatic dysfunction, thrombocytopenia, or coagulopathy. Physicians tend to avoid this drug because its reported toxicities and underdosing is frequent. Twenty-five micrograms per kg repeated in 12 or 24 hours may be sufficient to normalize serum calcium concentration.

Biphosphonates, inhibitors of osteoclastic bone resorption, represent a new therapeutic approach to hypercalcemia. Three biphosphonates are available: etidronate, pamidronate, and clodronate. The latter is not available in the United States. Both etidronate and pamidronate require administration over time but appear to have few adverse effects.

In the patient presented, it was mandatory that rapid control of the hypercalcemia be accomplished. Saline rehydration and calcitonin followed by gallium nitrate were indicated. The patient's fracture was repaired and she was placed on a progestational agent. It is more likely that this woman will need intensive cytotoxic chemotherapy to control her disease.

SELECTED READINGS

1. Bilezikian JP. Management of acute hypercalcemia. *N Engl J Med* 1992;326:1196–1203.
2. Nussbaum SR, Younger J, VandePol CJ, Gagel RF, et al. Single-dose intravenous therapy with pamidronate for the treatment of hypercalcemia of malignancy: comparisons of 30-, 60-, and 90-mg dosages. *Am J Med* 1993;95:297–304.

149

Nonoperative Management of Biliary Tract Obstruction

Vincent P. Chuang and Sidney Wallace

To operate or not to operate

CASE PRESENTATION

A 76-year-old Caucasian woman developed malaise, anorexia, flushing, light-colored stool, dark urine, and pruritus in September 1992. She was treated with antibiotics for 1 week, but her jaundice progressed. She was then hospitalized for a detailed work-up. Abdominal ultrasonography and computed tomography (CT) revealed dilated intrahepatic ducts and a single gallstone. Her bilirubin was 15.4 mg%. An ERCP study disclosed stenosis of the left hepatic duct and a stent was placed between the left hepatic duct and the common bile duct (Fig. 149–1). Her past medical history included atrial fibrillation, hypertension, and mitral valve prolapse. She denied any history of gallstones, hepatitis, ethanol abuse, and any previous abdominal surgery.

One week following placement of the internal biliary stent, her bilirubin fell to 10 mg%, but alkaline phosphatase remained at 330 units/L, and she remained icteric clinically. Because of the persistent jaundice, she came to M.D. Anderson Cancer Center for further treatment. A CT scan of the abdomen revealed an infiltrating mass in the porta hepatis with possible extension to the pancreatic duct. A percutaneous transhepatic cholangiogram demonstrated involvement at the bifurcation of the common hepatic duct with severe stenosis of the right hepatic duct (Fig. 149–2). A 10F Cope-loop catheter was successfully placed into the duodenum for external-internal biliary drainage (Fig. 149–3). Five days later, her bilirubin level had decreased to 3.3 mg%. She underwent fine-needle aspiration biopsy of the tumor mass. Using the drainage catheter as a landmark, a 22 G needle was aimed at the

right hepatic duct near the bifurcation (Fig. 149–4) and the cytology revealed adenocarcinoma, compatible with cholangiocarcinoma.

Because of the extent of her tumor and other systemic diseases, she was not a candidate for surgery. She was placed on a systemic chemotherapy protocol consisting of PFLC, that is, cisplatin 12 mg in 250 cc 3% saline over 2 hours, followed by 5-fluorouracil (5-FU) 500 mg, and leucovorin 75 mg intravenous "piggyback" per day for 5 days. From November 1992 to March 1993, she received six courses of chemotherapy and had partial response clinically. Her biliary drainage catheter had to be exchanged once in February 1993. Her bilirubin level was maintained at 2% to 3 mg% since placement of the external-internal biliary stent. She was clinically stable with no limitation of activity. In November 1993 she had progressive disease and expired.

TUMOR BOARD DISCUSSION

Bile duct obstruction due to malignant tumor was traditionally treated with radical resection or bypass surgery. Because most of these patients have unresectable tumor, surgical procedures are usually a biliary-enteric anastomosis for palliative relief of the biliary obstruction. With continuous progress of the interventional and endoscopic technique and devices, these nonsurgical treatment modalities have been more widely used to treat biliary obstruction and to spare the patient a major surgical procedure.

Malignant neoplasm causing severe biliary obstruction can be from either primary tumors of the pancreas or bile

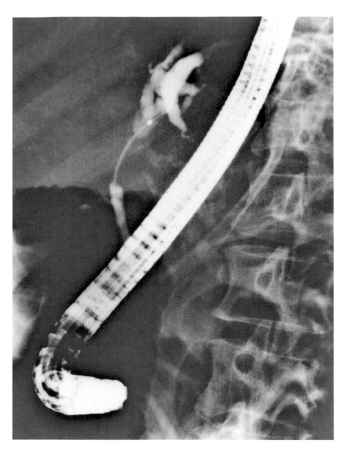

FIG. 149–1. Endoscopic retrograde cholangiogram reveals dilatation of left hepatic ducts and tumor encasement of common hepatic duct and proximal left hepatic duct.

duct, or metastatic tumor with porta hepatis adenopathy. Based on the location and extent of the disease, extrinsic biliary obstruction can be classified as (a) hilar, (b) mid-duct, and (c) distal duct obstruction (1). Although overall treatment options may slightly vary among various types of obstruction, the necessity to relieve the biliary obstruction as the first step of the treatment is the same.

Both endoscopic and percutaneous transhepatic approaches are important in the diagnosis and treatment of malignant biliary obstruction. The success rate in placing a biliary stent with a relatively low complication rate via either the endoscopic or percutaneous route depends largely on the expertise and experience of the performer. The endoscopic route has the advantage in that there is no hepatic parenchymal injury and less patient discomfort when compared with the percutaneous transhepatic route. Thus, the endoscopic route is performed first. The percutaneous transhepatic study is reserved for those who either fail the endoscopic approach totally or those in whom the endoscopically placed stent achieves only partial drainage, as in our illustrative case.

A malignant tumor at the bifurcation of the common hepatic duct frequently requires stents from both the right and the left hepatic ducts. In this case, the endoscopically

placed left hepatic duct stent was unsuccessful to totally relieve the patient's obstructive jaundice (see Fig. 149–1,2). Percutaneous transhepatic cholangiography revealed additional tumor encasement of the right hepatic duct, and an additional catheter for external-internal drainage (see Fig. 149–3,4) of the right hepatic ducts successfully relieved her jaundice and clinical symptoms.

Using the cholangiogram as a map, fine-needle aspiration of the tumor under fluoroscopy was performed for cytology to establish the diagnosis of the malignant tumor (see Fig. 149–4). This is the most economic and the least time-consuming approach to establish a diagnosis. Alternative nonsurgical approaches to establish a pathologic diagnosis include CT or ultrasound-guided fine-needle aspiration, and/or brush or forceps biopsy through the biliary catheter (2).

An endoprosthesis can also be used through this percutaneous route after establishment of external-internal drainage. Two types of stents are currently available: (a) in-dwelling catheter, 12 to 16F in size, e.g., Carey-Coons stent or Miller Mushroom stent, and (b) metallic stent, e.g., Gianturco expandable "Z" stent or Wallstent. The endoprosthesis has the physiologic and psychologic advantage of being catheter free. However, stenosis or occlusion of the internal stent is unavoidable either due to tumor, debris, or mucosal hyperplasia. The exchange of an in-dwelling internal stent is generally more difficult than that of an external-internal stent. A metallic stent cannot be exchanged.

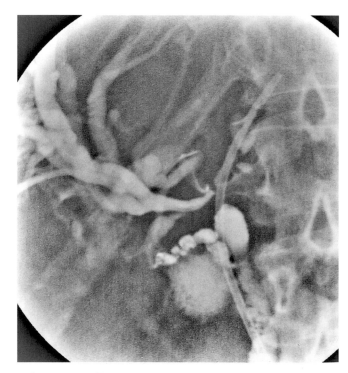

FIG. 149–2. Percutaneous transhepatic cholangiogram shows stenosis of the proximal right hepatic duct. The endoscopically placed left biliary stent is in place.

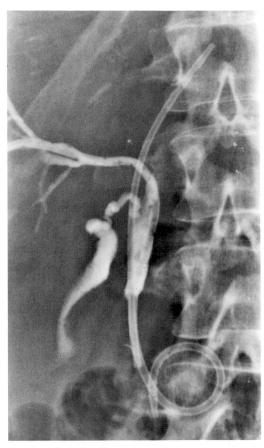

FIG. 149–3. A Cope-loop, multi–side holes catheter is placed across the stenotic right hepatic duct with the tip in the duodenum.

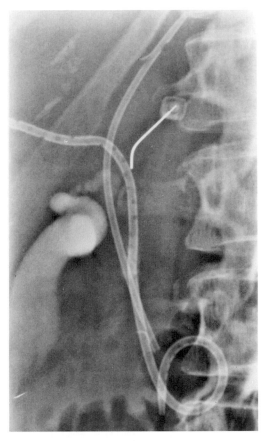

FIG. 149–4. Using biliary drainage catheter as a landmark, fluoroscopy-guided fine-needle aspiration reveals adenocarcinoma.

REFERENCES

1. Ring EJ. Radiologic approach to malignant biliary obstruction. *Cardiovasc Intervent Rad* 1990;13:217–22.
2. Coons H. Biliary intervention-technique and devices: a commentary. *Cardiovasc Intervent Rad* 1990;13:211–6.

COMMENTARY by David J. Fillmore and David G. Bragg

The management of malignant biliary obstruction is palliative by intent and designed to alleviate symptomatic pruritus, malabsorption, and progressive hepatocellular dysfunction that may accompany unrelieved malignant obstruction. There are three currently available principal approaches to achieve biliary tract decompression: surgical, radiologic, and endoscopic. The patient described underwent two of the three possible means of biliary tract decompression.

The ideal method for relief of malignant biliary obstruction should include minimal or no associated morbidity and mortality, long-term patency, and minimal cost. Such a technique is obviously not currently available; however, there are several randomized prospective trials that illustrate the relative advantages and disadvantages of each technique (1–5).

Three different prospective randomized trials of surgical bypass versus endoscopic stent placement have demonstrated no difference in survival by life table analysis (1–3). There is a higher acute mortality (18% vs. 7% 30-day mortality) associated with surgical treatment; however, the incidence of late duodenal obstruction is not surprisingly much higher (2% vs. 16%) for the endoscopically treated group. Despite rehospitalization for duodenal obstruction and biliary stent obstruction, patients treated endoscopically, as the illustrated patient was initially, spend less time in the hospital. It is important to consider local technical expertise in the choice of drainage technique but, in general, it appears that endoscopic stent placement should be the initial treatment modality of choice in the patient with neoplastic biliary obstruction. In the patient described here, because of the high nature of the obstruction, endoscopic or percutaneous drainage is obviously preferable.

Placement of biliary stents will require combined percutaneous and endoscopic techniques in up to 20% of patients. The single prospective randomized trial (4) comparing primary percutaneous radiologic versus endoscopic drainage suggests that, when possible, drainage via solely endoscopic techniques is associated with fewer complications, a lower 30-day mortality, and improved relief of jaundice. For these reasons, the endoscopic technique remains the initial procedure of choice.

When it is necessary to undertake percutaneous drainage for neoplastic biliary obstruction, the choice of endoprosthesis versus internal-external drainage catheters remains controversial. Recent prospective randomized endoscopic trial data (5) suggest that the use of a self-expanding metallic stent is associated with lower rates of reocclusion and is therefore more cost effective. This is true despite their markedly higher initial costs because of the substantially lower rate of stent occlusion from biliary sludge and tumor ingrowth. Despite this lower rate of reocclusion, survival is comparable regardless of the catheter type used. Retrospective analysis of outcome of plastic and metallic radiologic percutaneous stenting seems to demonstrate no difference in either outcome or length of hospitalization, probably because of the intrinsically short life expectancy of this patient group. The theoretical advantage of the larger lumen and presumed greater duration of patency from metallic stents has not been realized in practice. There has been no prospective randomized trial to date comparing internal versus external drainage catheters versus percutaneous placement of an internal stent.

It should be stressed that the evaluation of the patient's resectability, particularly when the tumor is a primary biliary tract cancer, should be completed before placement of metallic stents within the malignant biliary obstruction as metallic stents cannot be readily removed after the first week. The ideal technique for palliative drainage of malignant biliary obstruction remains to be developed.

REFERENCES

1. Shepard HA, Royle G, Ross APR, Diba A, Arthur M, Colin-Jones D. Endoscopic biliary endoprosthesis in the palliation of malignant obstruction of the distal common bile duct: a randomized trial. *Br F Surg* 1988;75:1166–8.
2. Anderson JR, Sorensen SM, Kruse A, Rokkjaer M, Matsen P. Randomized trial of endoscopic endoprosthesis versus operative bypass in malignant obstructive jaundice. *Gut* 1989;30:1132–5.
3. Smith AC, Dowsett JF, Hatfield ARW, et al. A prospective randomized trial of by-pass surgery versus endoscopic stenting in patients with malignant obstructive jaundice. *Gut* 1989;30:A1513.
4. Speer AG, Cotton PB, Russell RCG, et al. Randomized trial of endoscopic versus percutaneous stent insertion in malignant obstructive jaundice. *Lancet* 1987;ii:57–62.
5. Davids PHP, Groen AK, Rauws EAJ Tytgat GNJ, Huibregtse K. Randomized trial of self-expanding metal stents versus polyethylene stents for distal malignant biliary obstruction. *Lancet* 1992;340:1488–92.

EDITORIAL BOARD COMMENTARY

The authors describe that operation was not considered because of the extent of the tumor but to confirm extent would require Doppler ultrasound of the vessels or some modality that shows vascular invasion.

The authors treat the patient with systemic chemotherapy using Cisplatin, 5-FU, and leucovorin. The authors give no justification for the use of such a chemotherapeutic regimen in a 76-year-old woman. Many would favor radiation therapy as a primary modality or, indeed, consider biliary drainage alone.

The present description provides only one approach to the overall management of the malignancy. The authors appropriately emphasize the alternatives for biliary obstruction.

In the commentary, the authors focus on comparison between endoscopic stent placement versus surgical bypass. Most of the described studies, however, are done for distal biliary obstruction, which is not what the present patient presents with. The commentary also focuses on the presence of duodenal obstruction, which is unlikely to be seen in proximal biliary obstruction.

150

Thromboembolism in Cancer

Hau C. Kwaan, Illias Athanasiadis, and Jerry Hussong

A swollen leg may be the first sign of cancer

CASE PRESENTATION

W.W. is a 57-year-old man with no significant past medical history who presented with a painful swelling in his left lower extremity. Physical examination revealed tenderness of his left thigh and calf and a palpable mobile mass in the left upper quadrant of his abdomen. Laboratory findings including a complete blood picture and biochemical profile were normal. Urinalysis revealed persistent microscopic hematuria. Doppler studies confirmed the clinical diagnosis of a left iliofemoral deep vein thrombosis. He was given continuous intravenous heparin therapy for 5 days, followed by oral anticoagulation with coumadin, with the INR maintained between 2.0 and 3.0.

Shortly after recovering from the deep vein thrombosis, a computed tomogram (CT) of the abdomen and pelvis revealed a large left renal mass involving the mid- and lower pole of the left kidney. Magnetic resonance imaging (MRI) further showed that the mass did not involve the renal vein and that several small lymph nodes were demonstrated in the renal hilum. No other metastatic lesions were found in the rest of his staging evaluation. On laparotomy, the renal mass was found to be contained within Gerota's fascia. There was no vascular compression or involvement of the sigmoid colon. Pathologic examination revealed a tumor measuring 6 cm in diameter located in the lower pole of the left kidney. The renal pelvis, renal artery, and vein were not involved by tumor. Histologically, the tumor was found to be a clear cell carcinoma, nuclear grade II, with areas of necrosis (Fig. 150–1). No metastatic disease was found in the eight resected para-aortic lymph nodes. The final pathologic stage was T2 N0 M0, stage II. He had an uneventful postoperative course and was not given adjuvant treatment.

His subsequent follow-up has been negative for evidence of recurrent cancer or recurrent deep vein thrombosis.

TUMOR BOARD DISCUSSION

"Gentlemen: Those following my clinical work have surely noticed that there is a frequency of special diseases which attract attention due to the numerous circumstances in which they are observed. I want to talk about phlegmasia alba dolens. You do remember that we have studied together the white painful edema not only in women with recent parturition but more often in patients of both sexes affected with pulmonary phthisis or internal cancerous tumors. This is a rare example of generalized intravenous coagulation in the four limbs. What are the conditions where blood acquired this tendency of spontaneous coagulation? You know, gentlemen, in cachectic states in general, tuberculosis and cancer cachexia in particular, the blood is modified. . . "

Armand Trousseau (1801–1867)
Lecture at Hotel-Dieu, Paris 1865

Since the above, Trousseau's teachings (1) of the increased frequency of "phlegmasia alba dolens" in cancer patients, the association between "hypercoagulability" and cancer has been extensively studied. Today, it is generally recognized that thromboembolism is the second most common cause of death in cancer patients. Thromboembolism manifests as overt cases in 15% of cancer cases, but the true incidence may be much higher at autopsy. The existence of other risk factors would predispose an individual patient to thrombosis. These factors, commonly present in a cancer patient, include immobilization, dehydration, advanced age, smoking, diabetes, hypertension, and prior history of thromboembolism.

Not infrequently, thrombosis may be the first presentation of a cancer patient, as in the present case. This was

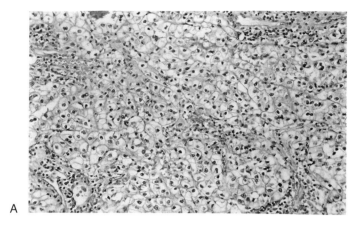

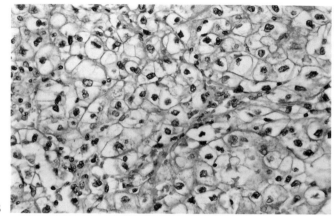

FIG. 150–1. Histologic appearance of patient's renal mass characteristic of a clear cell carcinoma. **A**, ×100; **B**, ×200.

first recognized by Gore et al. (2), who followed up 228 patients for 2 years after a work-up for pulmonary embolism by lung scan. Those who had a positive lung scan showed an incidence of cancer of 14.7%, whereas cancer occurred in none of those with negative lung scans. A similar study by Goldberg et al. (3) was carried out in 1,400 patients with impedance plethysmography (IPG) performed for evaluation of deep vein thrombosis. Over a 5-year period, those with positive tests showed an incidence of cancer of 6.3%, whereas those with negative tests had 2.4%. The difference was more remarkable among 490 of these patients who were over 50 years of age. The cancer incidence was 4.6% among those with positive IPG and only 0.3% in those with negative tests. A more recent study by Prandoni confirmed these observations (4). During a 2-year period after deep vein thrombosis, cancer was diagnosed in 16 of 153 patients (10.5%) with idiopathic deep vein thrombosis. In 5 of these 16 patients (31%), cancer was discovered at the time of the initial presentation, and in another 9 within the first year (56%). In contrast, only 2 of 107 patients (1.9%) with secondary deep vein thrombosis were found to have cancer during the 2-year follow-up period. They also observed that those with recurrences of their thrombosis have a

higher incidence of cancer (17%). This raises the issue that a diligent search for an "occult" malignant disease should be made when a patient, who has no obvious thromboembolic risk, first presents with deep vein thrombosis. This is especially true when the deep vein thrombosis is refractory to therapy and shows recurrence. Monreal et al. used more extensive diagnostic searches and observed an even higher incidence of 23% of cancer in those with idiopathic thrombosis (5). In our patient, the leg swelling leading to the diagnosis of deep vein thrombosis was the first manifestation of this illness. When examined by the physician initially, the renal tumor was palpated as a mass in the left upper quadrant of his abdomen. The awareness of the association between thrombosis and cancer in this case mandates a thorough work-up of the abdominal mass. The result was a discovery of his renal cell carcinoma at a relatively early stage of the disease.

Multiple etiologic factors for thrombosis have been recognized in the cancer patient, including those due to abnormalities of blood coagulation, defects in the fibrinolytic system, increased platelet count and aggregability, and local tumor destruction of the vascular integrity. Those of major significance are listed in Table 150–1. In renal cell carcinoma, certain features are notable. It has been recognized that the plasma fibrinogen is elevated, and this obviously will add to the tendency of the patient to thrombosis (6). Dysfibrinogenemia has also been reported (7). Whether the abnormal fibrinogen is more readily coagulable is not known. In addition, some patients have erythrocytosis due to the expression of erythropoietin by the tumor cells (8). This could produce hyperviscosity of the blood, contributing to an increased

TABLE 150–1. *Significant etiologic factors in thromboembolism in cancer patients*

Abnormalities of the content of blood
Activation of coagulation
    Tumor cell-derived tissue factor
    Tumor cell-derived cancer procoagulant
    Tumor cell-derived cytokines (IL-I, TNF)
    Tumor-associated leukocyte expression of procoagulants
Activation of platelets
Tumor cell-derived Le^a and Le^x glycolipid
    Thrombin activation
Presence of "thrombosis-induced activity"
Decreased natural anti-thrombotic factors
    Decreased antithrombin-III, prot C, free prot S
    Decreased fibrinolytic activity (increased inhibitors)
Lupus anticoagulant
Abnormal blood flow
Venous stasis from: immobilization
    tumor compression
Hyperviscosity from: paraproteins
    leukemic leukostasis
Abnormal blood vessel
Tumor invasion of blood vessel

risk of thrombosis. Our patient, however, has a normal hematocrit.

Thrombosis in cancer patients generally responds to anticoagulant therapy in a similar way to that in non-cancer patients. However, heparin resistance has been suggested in patients with malignancy (9). In our patient, we did not encounter any difficulty in obtaining the therapeutic range of activated partial thromboplastin time during his heparinization.

REFERENCES

1. Trousseau A. Phlegmasia alba dolens. In: *Lectures on clinical medicine.* Delivered at the Hotel-Dieu, Paris. London: New Sydenham Society; 1987:281–95.
2. Gore J, Applebaum JS, Greene HL, et al. Occult cancer in patients with acute pulmonary embolism. *Ann Intern Med* 1982;96:556–60.
3. Goldberg RJ, Seneff M, Gore JM, et al. Occult malignant neoplasm in patients with deep venous thrombosis. *Arch Intern Med* 1987;147:251–3.
4. Prandoni P, Lensing SWA, Buller HR, et al. Deep vein thrombosis and the incidence of subsequent symptomatic cancer. *N Engl J Med* 1992;327:1128–33.
5. Monreal M, Lafoz E, Cassals A, et al. Occult cancer in a patient with venous thrombosis: a systemic approach. *Cancer* 1990;67:541–5.
6. Sufrin G, Mink I, Moore FR. Coagulation factors in renal adenocarcinoma. *J Urol* 1978;119:727–30.
7. Dawson NA, Barr CF, Alving BM. Acquired dysfibrinogenemia. *Am J Med* 1985;78:682–6.
8. DaSilva JL, Lacombe C, Bruneval P, et al. Tumor cells are the site of erythropoietin synthesis in human renal cancers associated with polycythemia. *Blood* 1990;75:577–82.
9. Yudelman I, Greenberg J. Factors affecting fibrinopeptide-A levels in patients with venous thrombosis during anticoagulation therapy. *Blood* 1982;59:787–92.2

COMMENTARY by Joseph A. Caprini

The patient is a middle-aged man who presented with a swollen leg that proved to be an extensive deep vein thrombosis (DVT). An abdominal mass was also discovered, which represented a renal cell carcinoma that was eventually successfully removed. The tumor was confined inside Gerota's fascia, and the patient recovered without complications. His DVT resolved with anticoagulant therapy, and no apparent pulmonary emboli occurred. This presentation demonstrates beautifully the association between malignant tumors and thromboembolic disease first described by Trousseau, as pointed out by the authors. This clinical scenario raises a number of interesting management questions from both the medical and surgical perspectives.

We are told that the diagnosis of DVT was made by Doppler examination, but it is unclear about the exact method. We would assume that B-mode duplex ultrasonography was used, employing either a gray scale or color duplex scanner. Most feel that this is the method of choice for diagnosis of leg thrombosis in the symptomatic patient (1). Venography may be necessary in asymptomatic patients, those with indeterminate scans, or for accurate diagnosis of calf vein thrombi (2).

Is the diagnosis of iliofemoral thrombosis based on the clinical swelling or duplex visualization of the thrombosis? If the scanner were used, this would enable the extent of the thrombosis to be determined and would clarify two critical anatomic issues. The first is visualization of the top of the clot and whether it extends into the pelvis or vena cava. This is important because one management alternative in this patient would be the placement of a vena cava filter. If this option is selected, the extent of thrombosis would dictate the route of insertion of the filter. The presence of an acute iliofemoral thrombosis in a patient facing a major surgical procedure for cancer would be an indication to insert the filter to prevent extension of the thrombosis during and immediately after surgery, when only limited anticoagulant therapy can be used (3). Furthermore, some doctors feel that placement of a Greenfield filter as a primary therapy for venous thromboembolism is associated with fewer complications than conventional anticoagulant therapy in patients with cancer (4).

The second important anatomic issue is the degree of attachment of the proximal portion of the thrombus to the wall of the vein. The presence of a poorly attached clot may also be an indication to insert a vena cava filter to prevent the embolization of the clot. Berry and associates reported a 16% incidence of floating thrombi in a review of 400 cases of DVT with only 4 cases in which pulmonary emboli had occurred (5). This is a rare but potentially fatal event in the well anticoagulated patient, but the complicating factor of a surgical procedure in which anticoagulants may be limited or briefly discontinued increases the potential risk if an embolic event occurs. The decision to insert a vena cava filter in this setting may also revolve around the presence of existing pulmonary emboli. More than 25% of patients with acute DVT harbor asymptomatic pulmonary emboli (6), and the presence of these lesions may influence the decision to place a vena cava filter preoperatively, or if a poorly attached leg thrombus is present.

Another factor influencing the therapeutic approach is the urgency for surgical intervention. This is an early, relatively small tumor that should be removed within a reasonable period of time, but delaying the operation for 3 to 4 weeks to treat a thrombotic problem is most reasonable. This is apparently what was done, although we are not told the exact timing of the operative procedure relative to the diagnosis of DVT.

The issue of the leg swelling in these patients can be a serious, ongoing problem causing limitation of mobility and long-term disability if signs and symptoms of the postphlebitic syndrome appear. This syndrome was seen in 80% of patients with DVT followed for 5 to 10 years (7). We feel it is important to fit the patient with therapeutic compression stockings of at least 30 to 40 mm Hg to prevent clinical swelling and minimize the long-term sequelae from venous thrombosis. Frequently, antiembolism stockings are used in these patients; however, the 18-mm Hg pressures are insufficient to overcome swelling, and it may actually increase because ambulatory venous pressure in patients with venous obstruction sufficient to produce swelling may be 35 to 40 mm Hg.

Finally, we feel that management of patients with cancer and thrombosis can be difficult and requires an individual approach depending on multiple factors such as the extent of thrombosis, presence of pulmonary emboli, type of malignancy, and nature of the surgical treatment. The decision to use a vena cava filter must be carefully weighed, and therapeutic compression hose should be employed as part of the treatment plan.

REFERENCES

1. de Valois JC, van Schaik CC, Verzijlbergen F, et al. Contrast venography: From gold standard to "golden backup" in clinically suspected deep venous thrombosis. *Eur J Radiol* 1990;11:131–7.
2. Comerota AJ, Katz ML, Hashemi HA. Venous duplex imaging for the diagnosis ofä acute deep venous thrombosis. *Haemostasis* 1993; 23(suppl 1):61–71.
3. Cohen JR, Grella L, Citron M. Greenfield filter instead of heparin as primary treatment for deep vein thrombosis or pulmonary embolism in patients with cancer. *Cancer* 1992;70:1993–6.
4. Cohen JR, Tenenbaum N, Citron M. Greenfield filter as primary therapy for deep vein thrombosis or pulmonary embolism in patients with cancer. *Surgery* 1991;109:12–5.
5. Berry RE, George JE, Shaver WA. Free-floating venous thrombosis. *Ann Surg* 1990;211:719–23.
6. Monreal M, Ruiz J, Olazabal A, et al. Deep venous thrombosis and the risk of pulmonary embolism. *Chest* 1992;102:677–81.
7. Linder DJ, Edwards JM, Phinney ES, et al. Long-term hemodynamic and clinical sequelae of lower deep vein thrombosis. *J Vasc Surg* 1986;4:436–42.

151 Meningeal Carcinomatosis

Gershon Y. Locker

This grave disease site should be considered in a breast cancer patient with personality change, myelopathy, and radiculopathy

CASE PRESENTATION

J.H. was a 50-year-old premenopausal Caucasian woman in 1983 when she presented with a right breast lump. Biopsy was positive for infiltrating ductal carcinoma (Fig. 151–1). The patient underwent a right modified radical mastectomy and was found to have stage II disease: T2 (3 cm), N1 (2 of 21 nodes involved), M0, estrogen and progesterone receptor borderline positive (30 fmol/mg protein and 45 fmol/mg protein, respectively). The patient underwent 6 months of adjuvant cyclophosphamide/methotrexate/5-fluorouracil (5-FU) chemotherapy that was tolerated well but was associated with the onset of menopause.

She did well for 2½ years, then developed altered mentation and a seizure. Computed tomography (CT) scan of the brain with contrast revealed a single enhancing lesion of the right frontal lobe associated with edema. The patient had no other symptoms, but on general physical examination a right supraclavicular node and a chest wall papular rash were found. Biopsies of both were positive for adenocarcinoma of the breast; estrogen and progesterone receptors were borderline positive on both. Further restaging revealed minimal right pleural effusion blunting. There was no evidence of parenchymal lung, liver, or bone metastases on CT or bone scans. Because the brain lesion was single and possibly a second primary, the patient underwent a craniotomy and a total resection of the mass. Pathologically, it was an adenocarcinoma consistent with her original breast primary. She was treated with total brain irradiation to 3,000 Gy. The patient

received local radiation to the chest wall and supraclavicular fossa. She was started on tamoxifen, 10 mg, p.o., b.i.d. The adenopathy and rash resolved; her personality normalized.

Six months later as part of a routine evaluation, she was found to have an increase in her right pleural effusion on physical examination and chest radiograph. The patient had a thoracentesis, followed by a chest tube sclerosis of her effusion. Pathology revealed adenocarcinoma consistent with her breast primary. She was started on cyclophosphamide/methotrexate/5-FU chemotherapy, given on a day 1/day 8 basis monthly.

The patient did well, other than a deep vein thrombosis of her right leg, for 6 months, when she was noted again to have personality changes, new leg weakness, and difficulty urinating. General physical examination was within normal limits. There was no focal tenderness of the spine, hips, or legs; however, the patient was disoriented to place and time and she had asymmetric weakness of the legs with hyporeflexia and downgoing toes. Radiographs of her spine revealed no compression fracture or gross tumor. A bone scan was positive for uptake in the ribs and lumbar spine. CT of the head revealed no recurrence or new brain metastasis. A myelogram was performed, which revealed no evidence of extradural spinal cord or caudal compression; however, opening pressure was elevated at 220 mm of water, and the cerebrospinal fluid obtained at the time of the myelogram revealed a low glucose (30 mg%/120 mg% peripheral), elevated protein (200 mg%), and cytology positive for adenocarcinoma (Fig. 151–2). The patient was started on dexamethasone

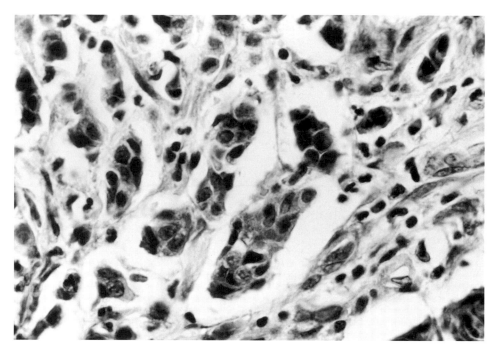

FIG. 151–1. Right breast biopsy revealing infiltrating ductal carcinoma.

and was re-evaluated again with CT scans of the chest and abdomen. There was no evidence of liver or lung metastasis or any other visceral spread, and no change in her pleural effusion/scar.

The patient's case was presented at Tumor Board. The consensus was that the patient had meningeal carcinomatosis causing her progressive neurologic symptoms but with relatively non–life-threatening systemic disease and no evidence of recurrence of her previous brain metastasis. Given the dire prognosis of her leptomeningeal cancer and the relatively limited effect of treatment

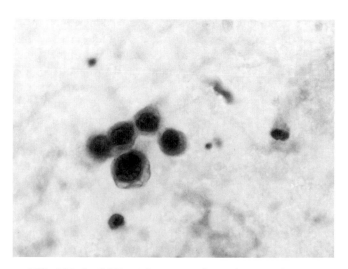

FIG. 151–2. CSF cytology revealing adenocarcinoma.

on this disease, there was some sentiment for palliative care using steroids +/- local radiation to the lumbar spine. The majority view was that given (a) the long duration of relatively non–life-threatening systemic disease, (b) her significant neurologic symptoms, (c) her young age and otherwise good health, and (d) the possibility of some response and palliation of symptoms with intrathecal treatment, that intrathecal treatment should be given in the hope of improving her neurologic status if not prolonging her life. There were concerns about the potential synergistic toxicity of intrathecal methotrexate and the previous brain irradiation on the central nervous system. Furthermore, the possibility of third spacing of intrathecal methotrexate in the effusion was discussed with recommendations that if treatment were given, peripheral methotrexate levels needed to be followed up.

At that time the patient had placement of an Ommaya reservoir and was started on intrathecal weekly methotrexate, 12 mg, with peripheral monitoring of her drug levels. Forty-eight hours after methotrexate treatment, there was no plasma drug measurable. Her systemic chemotherapy was switched to doxorubicin/thiotepa/vinblastine, intravenously, every 3 weeks, and was well tolerated. The decadron was tapered and then discontinued. The patient's confusion decreased and her leg strength improved to the point where she was able to ambulate with assistance; she continued to require a Foley catheter. Cerebrospinal spinal fluid cytology normalized after two weekly treatments, but her glucose and protein, although improving, did not normalize despite continued therapy.

The patient did well for 3 months, then was admitted to the hospital with gram-negative urosepsis and died. Postmortem examination was declined.

COMMENTARY by Dennis K. Burns

Leptomeningeal involvement by metastatic neoplasms other than leukemias and lymphomas is relatively uncommon, occurring in from 0.8% to 2.7% of patients with malignant solid tumors (1). The most common primary tumors in patients with meningeal carcinomatosis, in descending order of frequency, are carcinoma of the breast, carcinoma of the lung, and malignant melanoma. The clinical manifestations of meningeal carcinomatosis are variable but often include a global depression in mental status, as noted in the present case, accompanied by evidence of myelopathy, cranial nerve palsies, and spinal radiculopathies.

The presence of meningeal carcinomatosis is usually associated with the presence of concomitant nodular metastases in the brain parenchyma (2). On occasion, however, the leptomeninges may be the sole site of central nervous system metastases.

Leptomeningeal involvement is usually diffuse, although some cases are characterized by more discrete, multifocal lesions. Grossly, the meningeal carcinomatosis is characterized by variable opacification and thickening of the leptomeninges, particularly in the basal subarachnoid regions. Meningeal melanoma is usually pigmented and may produce a striking, diffuse pigmentation of the entire leptomeninges. The subjacent brain parenchyma is often edematous, with flattened gyral crests and narrowed sulci. Microscopically, the morphology of the metastatic leptomeningeal deposits recapitulates the appearance of the primary tumor. Neoplastic cells may be found anywhere within the subarachnoid space, including the perivascular Virchow-Robin spaces. On occasion, infiltration of the Virchow-Robin spaces represents the dominant pattern of involvement, a pattern sometimes referred to as the "encephalitic" form of meningeal carcinomatosis (3).

The route whereby neoplastic cells disseminate to the leptomeninges probably varies from case to case. In some cases, neoplastic cells may extend directly into the cerebrospinal fluid from localized parenchymal lesions. Less commonly, neoplastic cells may reach the subarachnoid cells via direct infiltration of cranial or spinal nerves (4), or from extension of hematogenous deposits within the choroid plexus (5,6). Although the role of other pathways in the development of leptomeningeal carcinomatosis remains to be established, the presence of leptomeningeal metastases in patients without concomitant disease in contiguous sites suggests that direct hematogenous seeding of the meninges may be an important additional route of dissemination.

The diagnosis of meningeal carcinomatosis is most often based on the cytologic examination of cerebrospinal fluid. Although CT scans may be of value in detecting the presence of concomitant brain parenchymal metastases, CT is generally of little value in defining the presence of leptomeningeal involvement. More recently, gadolinium-enhanced magnetic resonance imaging (MRI) has been shown to be a fairly sensitive technique in the detection of metastatic lesions in the leptomeninges (7). Definitive diagnosis of the presence of leptomeningeal carcinomatosis rests with the morphologic demonstration of malignant cells in biopsy or, more commonly, cytologic preparations. The cytologic demonstration of malignant cells may require examination of multiple CSF samples (8). Ancillary tests useful in the diagnosis of leptomeningeal metastases from carcinoma of the breast include assay of CSF β-glucuronidase levels, alone or in conjunction with b-2-microglobulin, carcinoembryonic antigen, and lactate dehydrogenase levels (9).

Treatment of the patient's initial central nervous system parenchymal lesion was reasonable. Although radiotherapy remains the standard treatment for brain parenchymal metastases, in the case of patients with a solitary brain parenchymal metastasis, surgical resection followed by radiotherapy has been associated with longer survival, lower recurrence rate, and a better quality of life than treatment with radiotherapy alone (10).

The treatment of the patient's leptomeningeal disease was somewhat conservative, although the prognosis of leptomeningeal carcinomatosis remains grim, regardless of the therapy used. Aggressive treatment of leptomeningeal disease may improve symptomatology and prolong survival in some patients, however (8). Treatment of leptomeningeal metastases usually involves the administration of radiation therapy to symptomatic sites of involvement, followed by the administration of chemotherapy. Because systemic chemotherapy penetrates quite poorly into the subarachnoid space, such agents are typically administered intrathecally, generally via an Ommaya reservoir. Current recommendations include intrathecal administration of methotrexate or cytosine arabinoside twice weekly during radiation therapy, followed by weekly or monthly doses after completion of radiation therapy (8,11,12). Additional chemotherapeutic agents suitable for intrathecal administration include thiotepa (12,13), an alkylating agent of proven efficacy in carcinoma of the breast, and 6-mercaptopurine (14). Intrathecal administration of an active metabolite of cyclophosphamide, 4-HC, is under current investigation for use in leptomeningeal carcinomatosis, as is the administration of intrathecal interferon (15). Other therapeutic maneuvers, including intrathecal immunotoxin (16) and intrathecal gene therapy (17), represent additional proposed, but incompletely evaluated, modalities in the treatment of meningeal carcinomatosis.

REFERENCES

1. Takakura K, Sano K, Hojo S, Hirano A. *Metastatic tumors of the central nervous system.* Tokyo-New York: Igaku-Shoin; 1982.
2. Chason JL, Walker FB, Landers JW: Metastatic carcinoma in the central nervous system and dorsal root ganglia: a prospective autopsy study. *Cancer* 1963;16:781–7.
3. Madow L, Alpers BJ. Encephalitic form of metastatic carcinoma. *Arch Neurol Psychiatry* 1951;65:161–73.
4. Griffin JW, Thompson RW, Mitchinson MJ, et al. Lymphomatous leptomeningitis. *Am J Med* 1971;51:200–8.
5. Grain GO, Karr JP. Diffuse leptomeningeal carcinomatosis. Clinical and pathologic characteristics. *Neurology* 1955;5:706–22.
6. Moberg A and Reis GV: Carcinosis meningum. *Acta Med Scand* 1961;170:747–55.
7. Watanabe M, Tanaka R, Takeda N. Correlation of MRI and clinical features in meningeal carcinomatosis. *Neuroradiology* 1993;35:512–5.
8. Wasserstrom WR, Glass JP, Posner JB. Diagnosis and treatment of leptomeningeal metastases from solid tumors: experience with 90 patients. *Cancer* 1982;49:759–72.
9. Twijnstra A, Van Zantan AP, Nooyen WJ, Ongerboer De Visser BW. Sensitivity and specificity of single and combined tumour markers in the diagnosis of leptomeningeal metastasis from breast cancer. *J Neurol Neurosurg Psychiatry* 1986;49:1246–50.
10. Patchell RA, Tibbs PA, Walsh JW, et al. A randomized trial of surgery in the treatment of single metastases to the brain. *N Engl J Med* 1990;322:494–500.
11. Holmes FA. University of Texas M.D. Anderson Cancer Center. Phase II chemotherapy with Ara-C in patients with leptomeningeal metastases from breast cancer, MDA-DM-8632, clinical trial, closed 01/29/82.
12. Stewart DJ, Maroun JA, Hugenholtz H, et al. Combined intraommaya methotrexate, cytosine arabinoside, hydrocortisone and thio-tepa for meningeal involvement by malignancies. *J Neuro-Oncol* 1987;5:315–22.
13. Gutin PH, Levi JA, Wiernik PH. Treatment of malignant meningeal disease with intrathecal thiotepa: a phase II study. *Cancer Treatment Rep* 1977;61:885–7.
14. Balis FM. Clinical Oncology Program, DCT, NCI, NIH. Phase I/II chemotherapy with intrathecal and/or intraventricular 6-MP in patients with refractory meningeal malignancies, NCI 86-C-78, clinical trial, active, 04/01/86.
15. Hankenson R, Hankenson A, Williams RM. Intrathecal interferon alpha 2B in meningeal carcinomatosis (Meeting abstract). *Proc Annu Meeting Am Soc Clin Oncol* 1993;12:P A513.
16. Mykelbust AT, Godal A, Fostad O. Targeted therapy with immunotoxins in a nude rat model for leptomeningeal growth of human small cell lung cancer. *Cancer Res* 1994;54:2146–50.
17. Ram Z, Walbridge S, Oshiro EM, et al. Intrathecal gene therapy for malignant leptomeningeal neoplasia. *Cancer Res* 1994;54:2141–5.

SECTION XXXIV

Adrenal Gland

152

Adrenal Cortical Carcinoma

David A. Goldfarb

Masculinizing adrenocortical carcinoma is usually fatal:
not this time

CASE PRESENTATION

This patient is a 23-year-old Caucasian woman. She had irregular menstrual periods for 5 years. Two years before presentation, she had a normal laparoscopy and was told that she had primary ovarian failure. Six to 10 months before presentation in our clinic, she was noted to have an increase in axillary, chest, abdominal, and facial hair. Her weight was labile and she lost 45 lbs, then subsequently gained 60 lbs. Her voice deepened. She also developed hypertension. Ultimately, she was referred for evaluation of a left upper quadrant abdominal mass. The referring physician provided a urogram suggesting the presence of a left adrenal mass.

On examination, her pulse was 88 and regular with a blood pressure of 154/100. She had a cushingoid appearance. She had facial plethora with frontal balding and facial acne. There was excessive facial hair. There was no adenopathy or thyromegaly. The breasts were normal. The chest and back demonstrated acne as well as an increased amount of hair. The lungs were clear. Cardiac examination was unremarkable. Abdominal exam was significant for the finding of a large left upper quadrant mass. Bowel sounds were present and there was no tenderness. Genitourinary examination was significant for an increase in the amount of pubic hair. There were no neurologic abnormalities.

Laboratory investigation revealed a normal complete blood count. The blood urea nitrogen (BUN) was 8 mg% and the creatinine was 0.6 mg%. Serum sodium was 142 mEq/L, and serum potassium was 4.7 mEq/L. An SMA12 panel was normal with the exception of a mildly elevated alkaline phosphatase at 105 mg% and a significantly ele-

vated lactate dehydrogenase (LDH) of 1,700 mg%. An 8:00 a.m. serum cortisol level was 23.1 µg%. After an overnight dexamethasone suppression test, the 8:00 a.m. cortisol remained at 25.0 µg%. Two days after receiving 0.5 mg of dexamethasone orally every 6 hours, serum cortisol did not suppress and remained at 22.3 µg%. Twenty four–hour urinary excretion of 17-ketosteroids (17-KS) were elevated at a level of 684 mg/24 hr. Twenty four–hour urinary excretion of 17-hydroxycorticosteroids (17-OHCS) were likewise elevated at a level of 51.6 mg/24 hr. The serum testosterone was elevated at 218 ng/dL.

A computed tomography (CT) scan of the abdomen demonstrated an extremely large mass in the left upper quadrant (Fig. 152–1). This appeared to be adrenal in origin. This was causing significant displacement of the kidney inferiorly and posteriorly. The mass was inhomogeneous, suggesting the presence of hemorrhage and necrosis. The liver was normal. An arteriogram was performed. This demonstrated a very large hypovascular abdominal mass that crossed the midline (Fig. 152–2). The mass was primarily supplied by the left inferior phrenic artery, the left middle adrenal artery, and the branches from the left renal artery. The remainder of the abdominal aorta appeared normal. Because of the finding of an elevated alkaline phosphatase, a bone scan was obtained. There was no evidence for any bony lesions. A chest radiograph demonstrated no evidence for pulmonary metastasis.

Given all clinical, biochemical, and radiographic data, it was felt that the patient had an adrenal cortical carcinoma with virilism and Cushing's syndrome. After a steroid preparation, the patient was brought to the operating room, where a left thoracoabdominal incision was employed. Exploration of the abdomen revealed an

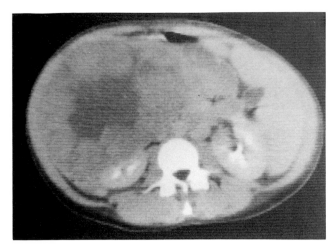

FIG. 152–1. Computed tomography scan of the abdomen demonstrating a large left adrenal mass with areas of hemorrhage and necrosis.

extremely large left upper quadrant mass. The liver was normal. A splenectomy was performed because of tumor adherence to the hilum of the spleen as well as to facilitate exposure to the mass. The left colon was reflected off the tumor. The mass was intimately associated with the tail of the pancreas and the tumor was dissected free from this structure. The tumor was excised en bloc with the left kidney. The entire specimen weighed 2,859 g. Careful hemostasis was achieved, a 32 F chest tube was left in the tenth intercostal space, and the abdomen and chest were closed.

The pathologic specimen measured 27.0 × 20.0 × 12.0 cm, and weighed 2,859 g. On cut section, the tumor had a variegated and nodular appearance with multiple foci of necrosis and hemorrhage. There were several tan, fleshy areas that appeared to be viable neoplasm. Microscopically, the tumor demonstrated pleomorphism, atypical mitoses, blood vessel invasion, and areas of necrosis (Fig. 152–3). Twelve lymph nodes were negative for metastatic tumor. A neoplastic nodule separate from the main mass was noted and it was uncertain whether this represented extension of the tumor or complete replacement of a single lymph node by tumor. The left kidney was normal. The spleen showed mild follicular hyperplasia.

Postoperatively, the patient did quite well. Oral intake resumed on the fourth postoperative day. The chest tube was removed on the fifth postoperative day. She was discharged home on the tenth postoperative day. She was maintained on intravenous steroids until she tolerated oral intake. She was begun on cortisone acetate 25 mg/q6h as well as florinef 0.1 mg/qam. Because the tumor was quite large with areas of vascular invasion and possible lymph node involvement, she was started on ortho-para' DDD (mitotane), 4 g/24 hr.

The patient returned in 4 months for a complete evaluation. The symptoms and signs of masculinization had improved. A chest radiograph and CT scan of the abdomen demonstrated no evidence for tumor recurrence. A serum testosterone was within the normal limit for an adult woman. Twenty-four-hour urinary values for 17-KS and 17-OHCS were within normal limits. She was tolerating mitotane 4.0 g/qd without any problems. At 1 year from the time of surgery, the patient continued to do well and was maintained on mitotane 4.0 mg/qd, cortisone acetate 37.5 mg/qd, and florinef 0.1 mg/qd. Again a CT scan of the abdomen as well as a chest radiograph showed no evidence for recurrent or metastatic disease. Plasma

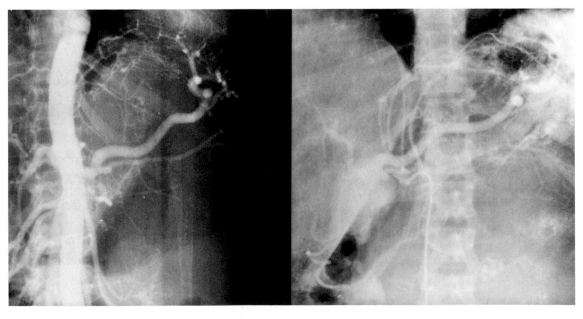

FIG. 152–2. Arteriogram demonstrating a large left-sided hypovascular mass.

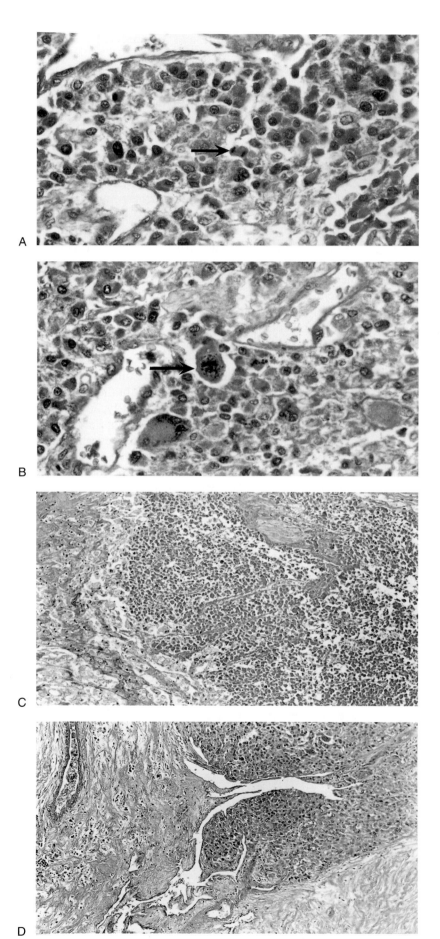

FIG. 152–3. Representative light microscopy of the pathologic specimen. **A:** Variably sized nuclei, occasional binucleate tumor cells, and a typical mitotic figure (*arrow*). **B:** Multinucleate tumor cells and an atypical mitotic figure (*arrow*). **C:** Large area of tumor cell necrosis. Tumor cells uniformly lack nuclei. **D:** Blood vessel invasion by adrenal cortical carcinoma cells.

testosterone remained within the normal limits for adult women, and 24-hour urinary studies for 17-KS and 17-OHCS were normal. An adrenocorticotropin-stimulating hormone (ACTH) simulation test at this time demonstrated no response indicating adrenal insufficiency.

Beginning 1½ years from the time of operation and continuing for 2 years, several recurrent problems developed. First, she was noted to have intermittent heavy menstrual bleeding. This at times required transfusion. Repeated Pap smears were normal. She underwent a dilatation and curettage of the uterus. The pathology showed benign endocervical glands, secretory phase endometrium with no atypia, dysplasia, or carcinoma. Episodes of heavy bleeding were treated initially with Provera and intermittently with oral contraceptives. A second problem developed consisting of a persistent hyperkalemia (K+=5–6 mEq/L) and hyponatremia (Na+=128–135 mEq/L). These laboratory abnormalities failed to respond to an increase in the dose of florinef to 0.3 mg/qd. A sodium sulfate infusion test demonstrated marked increase in urinary sodium excretion, fractional excretion of sodium, and a decrease in urinary potassium secretion and fractional excretion of potassium. These studies suggested the presence of a renal tubular defect as the cause of the chronic hyperkalemia and hyponatremia. The third development, which was most disturbing to the patient, was ataxia as well as a stuttering speech pattern. A CT scan of the head failed to show any evidence of a mass lesion and an electroencephalogram was normal. Examination of the cerebral spinal fluid demonstrated no abnormalities.

These three problems, vaginal bleeding, electrolyte abnormalities, and neurologic symptoms, all progressed and were of variable intensity between 1½ and 3½ years from initial excision of her tumor. During this time, there was never any clinical, biochemical, or radiographic evidence to suggest that she had recurrent disease. At 3 years and 8 months from the original surgery, mitotane was discontinued. Over the next year, her electrolytes gradually normalized. The neurologic symptoms gradually improved without any specific treatment. She was placed on oral contraceptives and had no further problems with severe vaginal bleeding.

She has subsequently been examined annually and has failed to demonstrate any evidence for tumor recurrence biochemically or radiographically. She has been maintained long-term on cortisone acetate 25.0 mg b.i.d. Florinef was maintained at 0.3 mg/24 hr for 5 years after discontinuation of mitotane, then gradually tapered to 0.1 mg/24 hr. She has continued to do well; and 10 years from her initial surgery, she was married. Subsequently, she has had two children. There were no problems with either pregnancy, and the children are healthy. At the present time, the patient is well and quite active. Her blood pressure remains normal.

COMMENTARY by Murray F. Brennan

This well-presented case demonstrates many of the features encountered in the diagnosis and management of adrenocortical carcinoma. Perhaps because the case was managed more than 10 years ago, there are some issues that might be approached a little differently at the present time.

In the clinical presentation, one would certainly have expected the patient to have demonstrated breast hair, a male escutcheon, and clitoral enlargement. The LDH and alkaline phosphatase elevations would be common, particularly in the patient who has central necrosis. No mention is made of fever, which commonly accompanies such a presentation. Weight loss and fever can be the major presenting symptoms in such patients. At the present time, we would not pursue dexamethasone suppression in a patient with such classical symptoms and signs. A CT remains the most commonly used localizing investigation, although MRI is increasingly used to demonstrate vascular and renal invasion. Arteriography would not be used at this time, as the tumor obtains its blood supply from the multiple small branches arising from all sites in the periphery. Clinically, one would expect this to be a highly malignant lesion. Few, if any, masculinizing tumors in an adult woman ever prove to be benign. This, combined with the large size, weight change, and central necrosis, all would predict a highly malignant tumor. The patient was appropriately prepared with perioperative steroids, as most such patients will have contralateral adrenal suppression. The surgical approach may be altered somewhat more recently, although basic premises remain the same. One might ask why the tumor, which was "intimately associated" with the tail of the pancreas, was resected without pancreatic resection when the left kidney was sacrificed. We learn progressively that we tend to sacrifice the organ of most ease of sacrifice rather than the necessarily limited adjacent organ of potential invasion. This is commonly encountered on the right-sided adrenal lesions where the right kidney is commonly sacrificed when the margin is the vena cava. Nevertheless, the procedure was well done and the subsequent outcome consistent with the described approach. The use of prophylactic ortho-para DDD is certainly highly controversial. Many would not use it, and the present case illustrates the potential toxic side effects. At doses greater than the 4 g described, virtually all patients have gastrointestinal upset and particularly in young patients depression is a major and problematic side effect. Not surprisingly, after a year of ortho-para DDD, an ACTH simulation did not show any function in the contralateral adrenal, consistent with the lifelong need for corticosteroid replacement.

Surgical resection remains the only potential curative approach to these difficult neoplasms. Unfortunately, many patients present with metastases and only a few patients with such a large and extensive tumor are as fortunate as the patient described. Management of metastatic disease is difficult; in selected patients surgical resection of metastasis, particularly in patients with functional tumors, can provide significant amelioration and palliation but rarely, if ever, prolonged survival. Current chemotherapeutic regimens have been extensively investigated, with some minimal response, but no one regimen has been found that promises significant or consistent response and results in any prolongation of survival.

SELECTED READINGS

1. Brennan MF. Adrenocortical carcinoma. *CA* 1987;3:348.365.
2. Pommier RF, Brennan MF. Management of adrenal neoplasms. In: Wells SA (ed): *Current Problems in Surgery*. Chicago: Year Book Medical Publishers, 1991, 659–739.
3. Pommier RF, Brennan MF. An eleven-year experience with adrenocortical carcinoma. *Surgery* 1992;112:963–971.

Subject Index

Subject Index

ISBN 0-397-51340-2